MN01493001

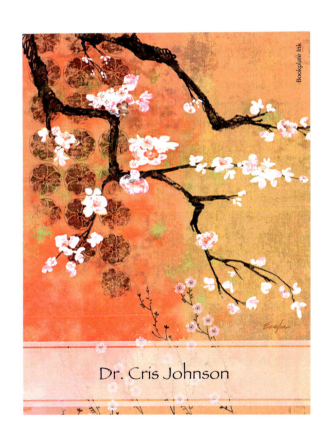

Bookplate Ink

Dr. Cris Johnson

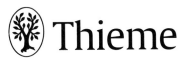

Neuro-Oncology
The Essentials

3rd Edition

Mark Bernstein, MD, BSc, MHSc, FRCSC
The Greg Wilkins-Barrick Chair in International Surgery
Professor
Department of Surgery, University of Toronto
Neurosurgeon, Toronto Western Hospital
Toronto, Ontario, Canada

Mitchel S. Berger, MD, FACS, FAANS
Berthold and Belle N. Guggenhime Professor
Chairman, Department of Neurological Surgery
Director, Brain Tumor Research Center
University of California San Francisco
San Francisco, California

With 377 figures

Thieme
New York • Stuttgart • Delhi • Rio

Thieme Medical Publishers, Inc.
333 Seventh Ave.
New York, NY 10001

Executive Editor: Kay Conerly
Managing Editor: Judith Tomat
Editorial Assistant: Haley Paskalides
Senior Vice President, Editorial and Electronic Product Development: Cornelia Schulze
Production Editor: Barbara A. Chernow
International Production Director: Andreas Schabert
International Marketing Director: Fiona Henderson
Director of Sales, North America: Mike Roseman
International Sales Director: Louisa Turrell
Vice President, Finance and Accounts: Sarah Vanderbilt
President: Brian D. Scanlan
Compositor: Carol Pierson, Chernow Editorial Services, Inc.
Printer: Sheridan Books

Library of Congress Cataloging-in-Publication Data

Neuro-oncology (Bernstein)
   Neuro-oncology : the essentials / [edited by] Mark Bernstein, Mitchel S. Berger. — Third edition.
     p. ; cm.
   Includes bibliographical references and index.
   ISBN 978-1-60406-883-2 (alk. paper) — ISBN 978-1-60406-884-9 (eBook)
   I. Bernstein, Mark, 1950 May 23– editor. II. Berger, Mitchel S., editor. III. Title.
   [DNLM: 1. Brain Neoplasms. WL 358]
   RC280.B7
   616.99′481—dc23
                                     2014015116

Printed in the United States of America
5 4 3 2 1
ISBN 978-1-60406-883-2

Also available as an eBook
eISBN 978-1-60406-884-9

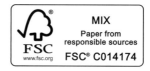

This book is dedicated to Lee, Lauren, Andrea, and Jody Bernstein,
and to Joan, Lindsay, and Alex Berger,
and to patients everywhere.

Contents

Preface

The first edition of this book, published in 2000, was unlike any other in neuro-oncology because of its relative brevity and because of the many special boxed features that highlighted selected important points in each chapter. This made the book readable and easily digestible, especially for residents, and for all practicing doctors for whom neuro-oncology is perhaps not their primary focus or area of specialty.

The second edition in 2008 was a great improvement on the first. We combined some chapters and dropped others that we felt were on somewhat outdated. In this new edition, we have again dropped some chapters (such as photodynamic therapy), but, as the field grows in complexity, we have added eight more chapters to keep the book contemporary and relevant. We have also included a number of new authors for this edition, all of whom are highly knowledgeable about their topics.

The main chapter changes include the creation of three chapters on surgical navigation, including stereotaxy, intraoperative magnetic resonance imaging, and other intraoperative aids. This reflects the huge role intraoperative navigation and guidance play in modern brain tumor surgery. We have also added chapters on endoscopy (because of the ever-expanding role of this important skill), intraventricular tumors (missing in the previous editions), pseudoprogression (because of its increasing importance in the assessment and management of patients after various treatments), seminal randomized controlled trials (because they are pivotal to guiding much of our care), and global neuro-oncology (as more effort and attention is being focused on patients and clinicians in less fortunate environments).

Another innovation for this edition is the addition of a brief editor's note at the end of each chapter. These notes summarize the topic, give a historical perspective, or highlight a point the editors feel requires emphasizing.

Many people feel that textbooks are outdated as soon as they are published, and that books on topics in medicine are becoming obsolete. But to have all the fundamental information on a topic that one can hold in one hand and carry around still has distinct scientific, educational, and aesthetic advantages. The treatment information in this book is as current as it can possibly be, and the essence of the book, the biological and pathological underpinnings of neuro-oncology, are to some degree timeless.

We believe this book has greatly improved on the first two editions and that it will become a useful resource for the many hard-working physicians engaged in the challenging job of managing patients with tumors involving the neurologic system, and for the neurosurgery, radiation oncology, and neuro-oncology residents and clinical fellows charged with learning about many topics in this field. We sincerely hope both the learning of neuro-oncology and its practice are facilitated by this book.

Mark Bernstein, MD, BSc, MHSc, FRCSC
Mitchel S. Berger, MD, FACS, FAANS

Acknowledgments

We would like to thank all of the authors for their excellent contributions and the staff at Thieme, especially Kay Conerly, Judith Tomat, and Haley Paskalides, who were gracious, expeditious, and helpful throughout the entire process. We also thank Lynn Nowen and Caroline Gunaratnam (Toronto) and Ilona Garner (San Francisco) for their invaluable assistance with this project. We also thank Barbara Chernow of Chernow Editorial Services, Inc.

Contributors

Kenneth D. Aldape, MD
Associate Professor
Department of Pathology
M.D. Anderson Cancer Center
University of Texas
Houston, Texas

Kaith K. Almefty, MD
Resident
Department of Neurosurgery
Barrow Neurological Institute
Phoenix, Arizona

Ossama Al-Mefty, MD
Director
Skull Base Program
Lecturer
Harvard Medical School
Brigham and Women's Hospital
Boston, Massachusetts

James Ayokunle Balogun, MD
Clinical Fellow
Surgical Neuro-Oncology
Division of Neurosurgery
Toronto Western Hospital
University Health Network
Toronto, Ontario, Canada

Fred G. Barker II, MD
Associate Professor
Department of Neurosurgery
Harvard Medical School
Attending Neurosurgeon
Director
Cranial Base Center
Brain Tumor Center/Neuro-Oncology
Massachusetts General Hospital
Boston, Massachusetts

Gene H. Barnett, MD, MBA
Director
Brain Tumor and Neuro-Oncology Center
Director
Cleveland Clinic Gamma Knife Center
Vice Chairman
Department of Neurosurgery
Cleveland Clinic
Cleveland, Ohio

Glenn S. Bauman, MD, FRCPC
Professor and Chair/Chief
Department of Oncology
London Regional Cancer Program
London, Ontario, Canada

Mitchel S. Berger, MD, FACS, FAANS
Berthold and Belle N. Guggenhime Professor
Chairman, Department of Neurological Surgery
Director, Brain Tumor Research Center
University of California San Francisco
San Francisco, Californiaa

Mark Bernstein, MD, BSc, MHSc, FRCSC
The Greg Wilkins-Barrick Chair in
    International Surgery
Professor
Department of Surgery
University of Toronto
Neurosurgeon
Toronto Western Hospital
Toronto, Ontario, Canada

Frederick A. Boop, MD
Professor and J.T. Robertson Chairman
Department of Neurosurgery
University of Tennessee Health Science Center, Memphis
St. Jude Children's Research Hospital
Semmes-Murphey Neurologic and Spine Institute
Chief
Pediatric Neurosurgery
LeBonheur Children's Hospital
Memphis, Tennessee

Henry Brem, MD
Professor
Department of Neurosurgery, Oncology, Ophthalmology,
    and Biomedical Engineering
Neurosurgeon-in-Chief
Johns Hopkins University School of Medicine
Department of Neurosurgery
Johns Hopkins Hospital
Baltimore, Maryland

Jeffrey N. Bruce, MD, FACS
Professor
Department of Neurological Surgery
Vice Chairman, Academic Affairs
Director
Bartoli Brain Tumor Research Laboratory
Co-Director, Brain Tumor Center
New York, New York

Soonmee Cha, MD
Professor
Departments of Radiology and Neurological Surgery
Program Director
Diagnostic Radiology Residency
Department of Radiology and Biomedical Imaging
University of California at San Francisco
San Francisco, California

Kaisorn L. Chaichana, MD
Neurosurgery Resident
Johns Hopkins Hospital
Baltimore, Maryland

Susan M. Chang, MD
Professor and Lai Wan Kai Chair
Neurological Surgery
Department of Neurological Surgery
University of California at San Francisco
San Francisco, California

Bryan D. Choi, MD
Duke Medical Scientist Training Program
Duke University
Durham, North Carolina

Elizabeth B. Claus, MD, PhD
Professor and Director of Medical Research
School of Public Health
Yale University
New Haven, Connecticut
Attending Neurosurgeon
Brigham and Women's Hospital
Boston, Massachusetts

William T. Couldwell, MD, PhD
Professor and Chairman
Department of Neurosurgery
University of Utah School of Medicine
Health Science Center
Salt Lake City, Utah

Ralph G. Dacey, Jr., MD, FACS, FAANS, FRCSI (Hon)
Henry G. and Edith R. Schwartz Professor
    and Chairman
Neurological Surgery
Neurosurgeon-In-Chief
Barnes-Jewish Hospital
Department of Neurological Surgery
Washington University School of Medicine
St. Louis, Missouri

Lisa M. DeAngelis, MD
Chair
Department of Neurology
Memorial Sloan-Kettering Cancer Center
New York, New York

Rebecca DeBoer, MD
Resident
Internal Medicine Residency Program
University of Chicago
Chicago, Illinois

Michael DeCuypere, MD, PhD
Department of Neurosurgery
University of Tennessee Health Science Center
Memphis, Tennessee

John F. de Groot, MD
Assistant Professor
Department of Neuro-Oncology
University of Texas M.D. Anderson Cancer Center
Houston, Texas

Peter B. Dirks, MD, PhD
Division of Neurosurgery
Program in Developmental and Stem Cell Biology
Hospital for Sick Children
Toronto, Ontario, Canada

Hugues Duffau, MD
Department of Neurosurgery
Gui de Chauliac Hospital
Montpellier University Medical Center
National Institute for Health and Medical Research
  (INSERM)
Institute for Neurosciences of Montpellier
Montpellier University Medical Center
Montpellier, France

Kadir Erkmen, MD
Assistant Professor
Department of Surgery and Neurology
Geisel School of Medicine
Lebanon, New Hampshire

Richard G. Everson, MD
Senior Resident
Department of Neurosurgery
University of California Los Angeles
Los Angeles, California

Peter E. Fecci, MD, PHD
Resident Physician
Department of Neurosurgery
Massachusetts General Hospital
Harvard Medical School
Boston, Massachusetts

Michael G. Fehlings, MD, PhD, FRCSC, FACS
Professor, Division of Neurosurgery
Halbert Chair in Neural Repair and Regeneration
Krembil Neuroscience Center
Head
Spine Program Toronto Western Hospital
University of Toronto
Toronto, Ontario, Canada

Marco Gallo, PhD
Research Fellow
Division of Neurosurgery
Program in Developmental and Stem Cell Biology
Hospital for Sick Children
University of Toronto
Toronto, Ontario, Canada

Sarah T. Garber, MD
Resident
Department of Neurosurgery
University of Utah School of Medicine
Salt Lake City, Utah

Roxanna M. Garcia, MD, MS
UCB School of Public Health
University of California Berkeley
Berkeley, California

Oren N. Gottfried, MD
Assistant Professor
Department of Surgery
Duke University School of Medicine
Durham, North Carolina

Jennifer Moliterno Gunel, MD
Neurosurgical Oncology Fellow
Memorial Sloan-Kettering Cancer Center
Memorial Hospital
New York, New York

Devon H. Haydon, MD
Resident
Department of Neurological Surgery
Washington University School of Medicine
St. Louis, Missouri

Wolf-Dieter Heiss, MD
Professor
Danube University Krems
Max Planck Institute for Neurological Research
Klaus-Joachim-Zuelch-Laboratories of the Max-Planck
  Society
University of Cologne
Cologne, Germany

Elizabeth J. Hovey, MBBS, FRACP, MSc
Conjoint Senior Lecturer
University of New South Wales
Honorary Associate
University of Sydney
Specialist, Medical Oncology
Prince of Wales Hospital
Sydney, Australia

B. Matthew Howe, MD
Department of Radiology
Mayo Clinic
Rochester, Minnesota

George M. Ibrahim, MD
Resident, Division of Neurosurgery
University of Toronto
Toronto, Ontario, Canada

John Kestle, MD, MSc, FRCSC, FACS
Pediatric Neurosurgery
Primary Children's Hospital
Salt Lake City, Utah

Osaama H. Khan, MD, MSc
Resident, Division of Neurosurgery
University of Toronto
Toronto, Ontario, Canada

Douglas Kondziolka, MD, MSc, FRCSC, FACS
Professor
Department of Neurosurgery and Department of Radiation
    Oncology
Vice-Chair
Clinical Research (Neurosurgery)
Director
Center for Advanced Radiosurgery
New York University Langone Medical Center
New York, New York

Lutz W. Kracht, MD
Senior Scientist
Max-Planck-Institute for Neurological Research
Klaus-Joachim-Zuelch-Laboratories of the Max-Planck
    Society
University of Cologne
Cologne, Germany

Khaled M. Krisht, MD
Chief Resident
Department of Neurosurgery
University of Utah School of Medicine
Salt Lake City, Utah

Walter Kucharczyk, MD
Radiologist and Scientist
Toronto Western Hospital, Toronto General
    Hospital
Institute of Medical Sciences
University of Toronto
Toronto, Ontario, Canada

Frederick Lang, MD, FACS, FAANS
Professor and Director
Clinical Research
Department of Neurosurgery
University of Texas
M.D. Anderson Cancer Center
Houston, Texas

Normand Laperriere, MD, FRCPC, FRANZCR (Hon)
Professor
University of Toronto
Department of Radiation Oncology
Princess Margaret Cancer Centre/University Health Network
Toronto, Ontario, Canada

Linda M. Liau, MD
Professor and Vice Chair
Department of Neurosurgery
University of California Los Angeles
Los Angeles, California

Daniel M. Mandell, MD, FRCPC
Staff Neuroradiologist
Toronto Western Hospital
Assistant Professor
Faculty of Medicine
University of Toronto
Toronto, Ontario, Canada

James M. Markert, MD
Division Director
Department of Neurosurgery
Professor
Departments of Neurosurgery, Physiology, and Pediatrics
University of Alabama
Birmingham, Alabama

Paul C. McCormick, MD, MPH, FAANS
Herbert and Linda Gallen Professor
Department of Neurological Surgery
Columbia University College of Physicians and Surgeons
New York Neurological Institute
New York, New York

Michael W. McDermott, MD
Professor in Residence
Department of Neurological Surgery
Halperin Endowed Chair
Neurosurgical Director
Gamma Knife® Radiosurgery Program
Vice Chairman
Department of Neurological Surgery
Robert & Ruth Halperin Chair
Meningioma Research
University of California San Francisco
San Francisco, California

Joseph H. Miller, MD
Resident
Division of Neurosurgery
University of Alabama at Birmingham
Birmingham, Alabama

Mustafa Nadi, MD
Postdoctoral Fellow
Arthur and Sonia Labatt Brain Tumour Research Center
Division of Neurosurgery
Hospital for Sick Children
Toronto, Ontario, Canada

Robert P. Naftel, MD
Assistant Professor
Department of Neurological Surgery
Vanderbilt University Medical Center
Nashville, Tennessee

Srikantan S. Nagarajan, MD
Professor
Department of Radiology and Biomedical Imaging
Director, Biomagnetic Imaging Laboratory
University of California at San Francisco
San Francisco, California

Anick Nater, MD
Resident, Division of Neurosurgery
University of Toronto
Toronto, Ontario, Canada

Kyle Richard Noll, PhD
Neuropsychology Fellow
Department of Physical Medicine and Rehabilitation
Baylor College of Medicine
Houston, Texas

Barbara J. O'Brien, MD
Fellow
Department of Neuro-Oncology
University of Texas M.D. Anderson Cancer Center
Houston, Texas

Alfred T. Ogden, MD
Director
Minimally Invasive Spine Surgery
Department of Neurological Surgery
Columbia University
New York, New York

Taemin Oh, BA
Pre-Doctoral Fellow
Department of Neurological Surgery
Northwestern Feinberg School of Medicine
Chicago, Illinois

Andrew T. Parsa, MD, PhD
Michael J. Marchese Professor and Chair
Department of Neurological Surgery
Northwestern University Feinberg School of Medicine
Chicago, Illinois

Akash J. Patel, MD
Resident Advisor
Department of Neurosurgery
University of Texas
M.D. Anderson Cancer Center
Houston, Texas

James Perry, MD, FRCPC
Associate Professor
Medicine
Crolla Family Chair of Brain Tumour Research
Division of Neurology, Department of Medicine
Sunnybrook Health Sciences Centre and Odette Cancer Centre
Toronto, Ontario, Canada

Michael J. Petr, MD, PhD
Minimally Invasive Cranial Surgery
Lyerly Neurosurgery
Jacksonville, Florida

Joseph M. Piepmeier, MD
Chief
Department of Surgical Neuro-Oncology
Yale University
New Haven, Connecticut

Ian F. Pollack, MD, FACS, FAAP, FAANS
Chief
Department of Pediatric Neurosurgery
Children's Hospital of Pittsburgh
Leland Albright Professor of Neurological Surgery
Vice Chairman for Academic Affairs
Department of Neurological Surgery
Co-Director, UPCI Brain Tumor Program
University of Pittsburgh School of Medicine
Pittsburgh, Pennsylvania

Michael D. Prados, MD
Charles B. Wilson Professor
Department of Neurosurgery
Professor
Department of Pediatrics (Neuro-Oncology)
Director
Division of Translational Research in Neuro-Oncology
Program Leader, Neurological Oncology Program
Comprehensive Cancer Center
University of California at San Francisco
Co-Project Leader
Adult Brain Tumor Consortium
Project Leader
Pacific Pediatric Neuro-Oncology Consortium
San Francisco, California

Aditya Raghunathan, MD, MPH
Senior Staff Pathologist
Departments of Pathology and Laboratory Medicine, and
  Neurosurgery
Henry Ford Health System
Detroit, Michigan

Vijay Ramaswamy, MD, FRCPC
Clinical Research Fellow
Hospital for Sick Children
Brain Tumour Research Centre
Toronto, Ontario, Canada

Marc Remke, MD
Division of Neurosurgery
Hospital for Sick Children
University of Toronto
Toronto, Ontario, Canada

David W. Roberts, MD
Section Chief
Department of Neurosurgery
Professor
Department of Surgery
Geisel School of Medicine
Dartmouth-Hitchcock Norris Cotton Cancer Center
Lebanon, New Hampshire

James T. Rutka, MD, PhD, FRCSC, FACS, FAAP
Professor and Chair
Department of Surgery
University of Toronto
Codirector and Principal Investigator
Arthur and Sonia Labatt Tumour Research Centre
Division of Neurosurgery
Hospital for Sick Children
Toronto, Ontario, Canada

Martin J. Rutkowski, MD
Resident
Department of Neurological Surgery
University of California at San Francisco
San Francisco, California

Arjun Sahgal, MD
Associate Professor
Department of Radiation Oncology
Sunnybrook Health Sciences Centre
University of Toronto
Toronto, Ontario, Canada

John H. Sampson, MD
Robert H. and Gloria Wilkins Distinguished Professor of
  Neurosurgery
Professor of Pathology, Immunology, and Radiation
  Oncology
Director
Duke Brain Tumor Immunotherapy Program
The Preston Robert Tisch Brain Tumor Center at Duke
Division of Neurosurgery, Department of Surgery
Duke University Medical Center
Durham, North Carolina

Nader Sanai, MD
Director
Neurosurgical Oncology and Barrow Brain Tumor Research
  Center
Barrow Neurological Institute
St. Joseph's Hospital and Medical Center
Phoenix, Arizona

Raymond Sawaya, MD
Professor and Chairman
Department of Neurosurgery
University of Texas
M.D. Anderson Cancer Center
Houston, Texas

Jason L. Schroeder, MD
Department of Neurosurgery
Harold F. Young Neurosurgical Center
Virginia Commonwealth University
Richmond, Virginia

Theodore H. Schwartz, MD
Associate Professor
Department of Neurosurgery
Codirector
Institute for Minimally Invasive Skull Base and Pituitary
  Surgery
Weill Cornell Medical College
New York Presbyterian Hospital
New York, New York

Cara Sedney, MD
Chief Resident
Division of Neurosurgery
Robert C. Byrd Health Sciences Center School of Medicine
West Virginia University
Morgantown, West Virginia

Ganesh M. Shankar, MD PhD
Neurosurgical Resident
Massachusetts General Hospital
Harvard Medical School
Boston, Massachusetts

Penny K. Sneed, MD, FACR
Professor in Residence
Department of Radiation Oncology
University of California at San Francisco
San Francisco, California

Adam M. Sonabend, MD
Resident
Department of Neurosurgery
Columbia University Medical Center
New York, New York

Mark M. Souweidane, MD
Neurological Surgeon
Weill Cornell Medical Center
New York Presbyterian Hospital
New York, New York

Robert J. Spinner, MD
Professor
Departments of Neurologic Surgery and
   Orthopedics
Mayo Clinic
Rochester, Minnesota

Michael D. Taylor, MD, PhD, FRSCC
Associate Professor
Division of Neurosurgery
Hospital for Sick Children
Toronto, Ontario, Canada

Elina Tsyvkin, MD
Fellow
Tufts Medical Center
Boston, Massachusetts

Pablo A. Valdes, PhD
MD/PhD Candidate
Dartmouth College
Geisel School of Medicine at Dartmouth and Thayer
   School of Engineering
Hanover, New Hampshire

Frederick Vincent, MD
Neurosurgeon
Providence Health and Services
Portland, Oregon

Kyle M. Walsh, PhD
Postdoctoral Scholar
Epidemiology and Biostatistics
University of California at San Francisco School of Medicine
San Francisco, California

Xin Wang
MD/PhD Program
Clinical Sciences
University of Toronto
Toronto, Ontario, Canada

Ronald E. Warnick, MD
Professor
Department of Neurosurgery
John M. Tew, Jr., M.D. Chair
Neurosurgical Oncology
Director
UC Brain Tumor Center
Cincinnati, Ohio

Jeffrey Scott Wefel, PhD, ABPP
Chief Ad Interim
Section of Neuropsychology
Associate Professor
Department of Neuro-Oncology
M.D. Anderson Cancer Center
Houston, Texas

Jon D. Weingart, MD
Professor
Department of Neurological Surgery and Oncology
Director
Neurosurgical Operating Room
Johns Hopkins Medicine
Baltimore, Maryland

Margaret R. Wrensch, MPH, PhD
Professor in Residence
Department of Neurological Surgery and Epidemiology and
   Biostatistics
Stanley D. Lewis and Virginia S. Lewis Endowed Chair
Brain Tumor Research
Codirector
Division of Neuroepidemiology
University of California at San Francisco
San Francisco, California

W. K. Alfred Yung, MD
Professor and Chairman
Department of Neuro-Oncology
University of Texas M.D. Anderson Cancer Center
Houston, Texas

Gelareh Zadeh, MD, PhD, FRCSC
Division of Neurosurgery
Toronto Western Hospital
University of Toronto
Toronto, Ontario, Canada

Corinna C. Zygourakis, MD
Resident
Department of Neurological Surgery
University of California at San Francisco
San Francisco, California

Biology

1

Epidemiology

Kyle M. Walsh, Elizabeth B. Claus, and Margaret R. Wrensch

In the United States, 70,000 new cases of primary malignant and benign brain and central nervous system (CNS) tumors are diagnosed each year, and 14,000 patients die; 31% of these tumors are gliomas and 37% are meningiomas.[1] There are two main types of epidemiological studies that contribute to our understanding of brain tumors: descriptive studies characterize the incidence of brain tumors and the mortality and survival rates associated with them in a given population by person, place, and time; analytic studies either compare the risk of brain tumors in people with and without certain characteristics (cohort studies) or, more commonly, because of the relative rarity of brain tumors, compare life histories of people with and without brain tumors (case-control studies). The main purposes of epidemiological studies are to characterize the distribution of brain tumors and understand their underlying causes. The distribution of these tumors may yield clues to their causes or point to high-risk populations requiring enhanced surveillance.

Descriptive Epidemiology

Descriptive epidemiological studies show variation in brain tumor incidence and mortality by time, geographic region, ethnicity, age, gender, histologic type, and intracranial site.

Although primary brain tumors are relatively rare compared with metastatic brain tumors or more common primary cancer sites such as lung, breast, prostate, and colorectal, they constitute an important source of morbidity and mortality. **Fig. 1.1** shows the percentages of brain tumors by major histological types.

Time Trends in Incidence and Mortality

Time trend studies report an increase in brain tumor incidence over the past three decades, with improved reporting, increased use of diagnostic imaging, and changing attitudes toward diagnosis in the elderly held responsible for much of the observed increase.[2] However, some researchers also suggest that the overall increase (especially among children) may be due to changes in etiologic factors.

Ethnic and Geographic Variation in Incidence and Mortality

Interpretations of ethnic and geographic variation in the occurrence of brain tumors are complicated by problems in as-

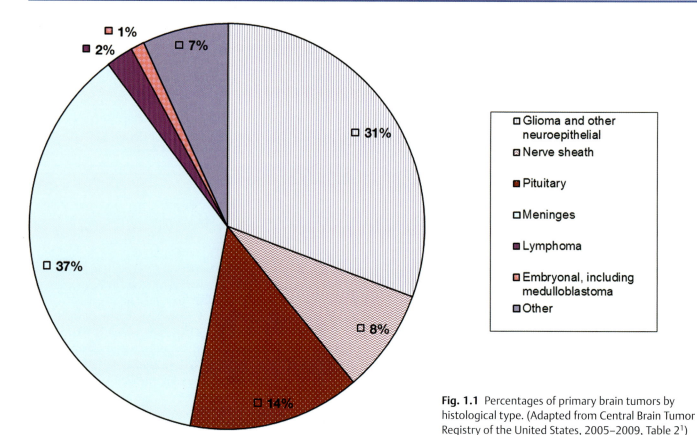

Legend:
- Glioma and other neuroepithelial
- Nerve sheath
- Pituitary
- Meninges
- Lymphoma
- Embryonal, including medulloblastoma
- Other

1%
2%
7%
31%
37%
8%
14%

Fig. 1.1 Percentages of primary brain tumors by histological type. (Adapted from Central Brain Tumor Registry of the United States, 2005–2009, Table 2[1])

certainment and reporting. Regions with the highest reported rates of primary malignant brain tumors (e.g., Northern Europe, the U.S. white population, and Israel; rates of 11 to 20 per 100,000 people) generally have more accessible and developed medical care than areas with the lowest rates (e.g., India and the Philippines; rates of 2 to 4 per 100,000 people).[3] However, some of the variation suggests ethnic differences in inherited susceptibility or cultural or geographic differences in risk factors.[4,5] For example, the rate of malignant brain tumors in Japan, an economically prosperous country, is less than half the rate in Northern Europe. In the United States, whites have higher rates of glioma than blacks but lower rates of meningioma; this would be difficult to attribute solely to differences in access to medical care or diagnostic practices in the two groups.[1]

The absolute variation in the occurrence of brain tumors between high-risk and low-risk areas is on the order of fourfold, compared with the 20-fold difference observed for lung cancer or the 150-fold difference observed for melanoma.[3] Thus, it seems unlikely that strong geographic risk factors for brain tumors exist in the same manner that they do for other neoplasms (e.g., cigarette smoking and asbestos exposures for lung cancer, sunlight intensity for melanoma).

Age and Gender Variation in Incidence and Mortality

Overall, the median age of onset for primary brain tumors is 59, and the median ages of onset for glioblastoma and meningioma are 64 and 65, respectively.[1] The age distributions of primary brain tumors vary by site and histological type (**Figs. 1.2, 1.3, 1.4**). As with other types of cancer, the increased incidence of most types of brain tumors with age could be due to length of exposure required for malignant transformation, the necessity of many genetic alterations prior to the onset of clinical disease, or diminished immune surveillance. Interestingly, there is a decline in the incidence of glioblastoma and astrocytoma among those 85 and older (**Fig. 1.2**), whereas the

Pearl

- Among the most consistent finding in the epidemiology of brain tumors is the difference in incidence rates between genders; glioma is more common in men and meningioma is more common in women.

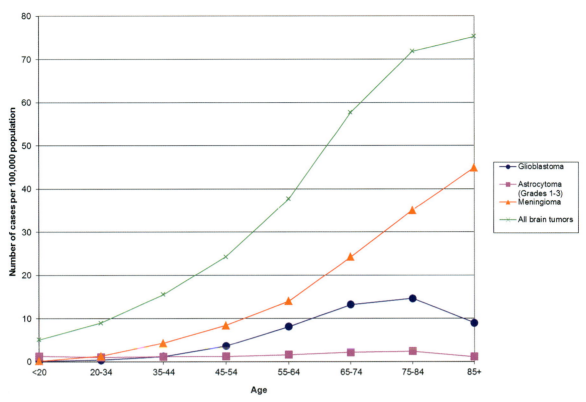

Fig. 1.2 Primary brain tumor incidence rates by age at diagnosis for all and most common histological types. (Adapted from Central Brain Tumor Registry of the United States, 2005–2009, Table 12[1])

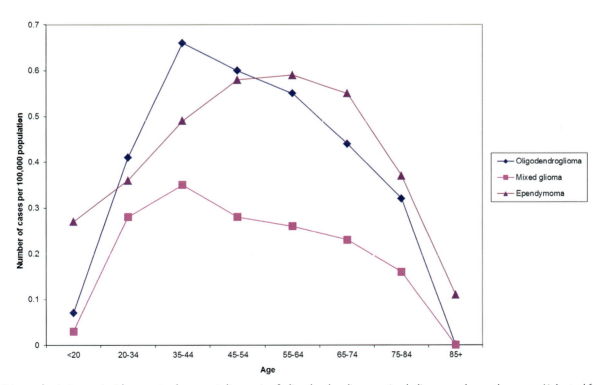

Fig. 1.3 Primary brain tumor incidence rates by age at diagnosis of oligodendroglioma, mixed glioma, and ependymoma. (Adapted from Central Brain Tumor Registry of the United States, 2005–2009, Table 12[1])

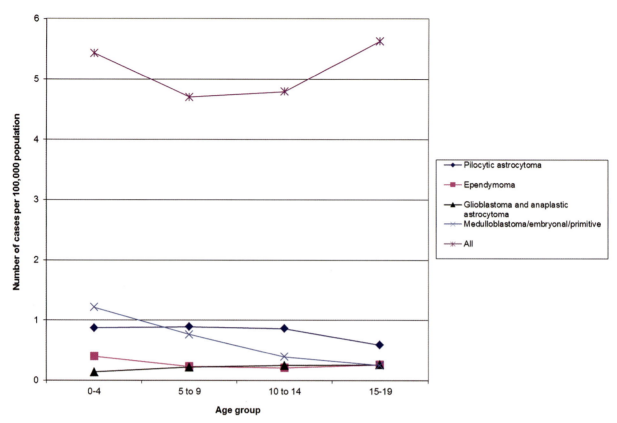

Fig. 1.4 Childhood primary brain tumor incidence rates by age and histologic type. (Adapted from Central Brain Tumor Registry of the United States, 2005–2009, Table 16[1])

incidence of oligodendroglioma and ependymoma peak in middle age (**Fig. 1.3**).

Glioma rates are higher in males and meningioma rates are higher in females (shown for U.S. data in **Fig. 1.5**). Because of the consistency of this finding across almost all ages and populations studied, a comprehensive theory of brain tumor etiology should account for this fact. However, this important epidemiological observation remains unexplained.

Survival and Prognostic Factors

For individuals with primary malignant brain tumors, histological type and age are strong prognostic factors (**Fig. 1.6**). In addition, grade of tumor, extent of lesion resection, tumor location, administration of radiotherapy (high-grade tumors only), and some chemotherapy protocols have been consistently linked with survival in both population registry and clinical trial data.[1,6] The Radiation Therapy Oncology Group and other clinical trial groups provide useful information on prognostic factors from patients whose pathological features have been reviewed and who are treated in clinical trials. However, many patients do not enter clinical trials, and thus these trial results may not be representative of the general population of patients with glioma.

One study examined changes in glioblastoma survival rates by age, race, and gender for the time period from 1993 to 2007.[7] A modest improvement in survival of 2 to 4 months was observed following widespread adoption of temozolomide treatment around 2005. No improvement in survival was observed for patients in the oldest age groups (80+). **Fig. 1.7** shows 1- to 10-year percent relative survival for glioblastoma and other common histologies.

Molecular Markers of Survival/Prognosis

The role of molecular markers in prognosis is a growing area of investigation that has led to some important findings. Combined losses of chromosomes 1p and 19q in oligodendroglial tumors are favorable prognostic indicators, as are mutations of the genes *IDH1* and *IDH2*.[8] A genetic signature often observed in oligodendrogliomas, consisting of mutations in *IDH1/2*, *CIC*, and *FUBP1*, correlates with improved overall survival. In astrocytic tumors, mutations in *IDH* and *ATRX* correlate with improved survival compared to astrocytic tumors without these mutations; however, these patients still experience poorer survival than patients with *IDH*-mutated oligodendroglioma.[9]

A large prospective trial of patients with newly diagnosed glioblastoma indicated that methylation of the *MGMT* pro-

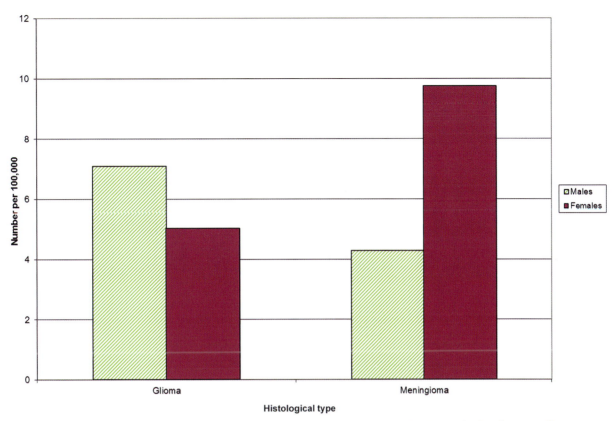

Fig.1.5 Primary brain tumor incidence rates age-adjusted to the 2000 U.S. standard population by gender for gliomas and meningiomas. (Adapted from Central Brain Tumor Registry of the United States, 2005–2009, Table 9[1])

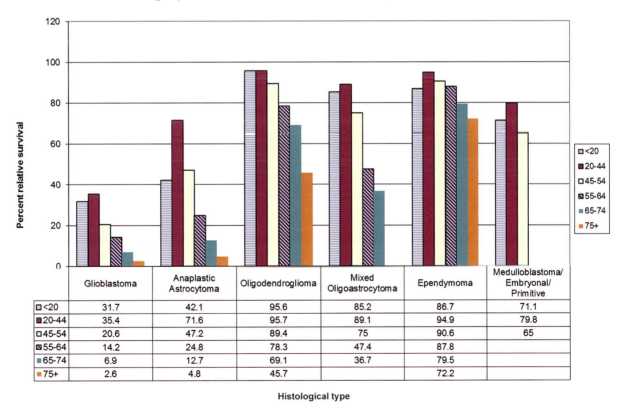

	Glioblastoma	Anaplastic Astrocytoma	Oligodendroglioma	Mixed Oligoastrocytoma	Ependymoma	Medulloblastoma/ Embryonal/ Primitive
<20	31.7	42.1	95.6	85.2	86.7	71.1
20-44	35.4	71.6	95.7	89.1	94.9	79.8
45-54	20.6	47.2	89.4	75	90.6	65
55-64	14.2	24.8	78.3	47.4	87.8	
65-74	6.9	12.7	69.1	36.7	79.5	
75+	2.6	4.8	45.7		72.2	

Histological type

Fig.1.6 Two-year relative survival rates for primary malignant brain tumors by age group. (Adapted from Central Brain Tumor Registry of the United States, 2005–2009, Table 22[1])

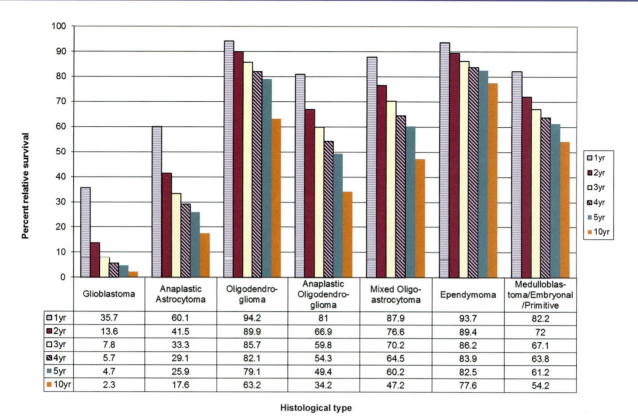

	Glioblastoma	Anaplastic Astrocytoma	Oligodendro-glioma	Anaplastic Oligodendro-glioma	Mixed Oligo-astrocytoma	Ependymoma	Medulloblas-toma/Embryonal /Primitive
1yr	35.7	60.1	94.2	81	87.9	93.7	82.2
2yr	13.6	41.5	89.9	66.9	76.6	89.4	72
3yr	7.8	33.3	85.7	59.8	70.2	86.2	67.1
4yr	5.7	29.1	82.1	54.3	64.5	83.9	63.8
5yr	4.7	25.9	79.1	49.4	60.2	82.5	61.2
10yr	2.3	17.6	63.2	34.2	47.2	77.6	54.2

Histological type

Fig. 1.7 One-, 2-, 3-, 4-, 5- and 10-year relative survival rates for primary brain tumors. (Adapted from Central Brain Tumor Registry of the United States, 2005–2009, Table 21[1])

moter is a marker of improved outcome.[6] Interestingly, *MGMT* methylation appeared to be more strongly associated with survival among patients who received temozolomide than among those who did not, raising the possibility that *MGMT* methylation may be a predictive marker of response to this alkylating agent. A genome-wide glioma-CpG island methylator phenotype (G-CIMP) has also been linked to improved survival in glioma patients. This hypermethylator phenotype is also associated with *IDH* mutations, indicating that there is overlap of glioma prognostic markers.[8]

A recent genome-wide association study of single nucleotide polymorphisms (SNPs) evaluated in similarly treated glioblastoma patients indicates that heritable variation in a gene called *SSBP2* may impact patient survival.[10] Another recent study indicated that somatic mutations in the *TERT* promoter are associated with poorer survival experiences among glioblastoma patients.[11] Both these findings await further validation.

Tumor Heterogeneity

Heterogeneity among tumors of varying histology and anatomic location has long been recognized. Cytogenetic and molecular studies show tumor heterogeneity exists within single histological categories. There are now several genetic and molecular changes thought to potentially cause primary CNS tumor formation.[9] Glioblastoma may arise by two pathways that can be defined in clinical terms: the first pathway results from tumor progression from lower grade astrocytoma, whereas a second pathway has no clinically evident precursor (i.e., de novo glioblastoma). *IDH* mutation, *TP53* mutation, and *EGFR* amplification appear to correlate with these clinical classifications (**Fig. 1.8**).

Primary glioblastoma is likely to harbor *EGFR* amplification, whereas secondary glioblastomas, arising from lower grade precursors, are more likely to harbor *TP53* and *IDH* mutations. The same appears true of somatic mutations in *TERT* and *ATRX*; the former is associated with primary glioblastoma, whereas the latter is found more commonly in lower grade astrocytomas and secondary glioblastomas.[11] Although this distinction is not absolute, it raises the possibility that distinct subtypes of glioblastoma, although similar histologically, may display substantial clinical differences.

Some important modifications that occur in 5 to 40% of glioblastoma and anaplastic astrocytoma include *EGFR* amplification and mutation, amplification of *CDK4* or *MDM2*, and deletion or mutation of *TP53*, *CDKN2A*, *RB1*, *PTEN*, *TERT*, or *ATRX*. In 30 to 40% of astrocytomas, *TP53* is deleted or mutated.[8] Chromosomes 1p and 19q are deleted in 40 to 90% of oligodendrogliomas. These tumors also frequently carry mutations in *FUBP1* (on chromosome 1p) and *CIC* (on 19q), as well as *IDH1* or *IDH2* mutation.[8] Chromosome 22 is deleted in

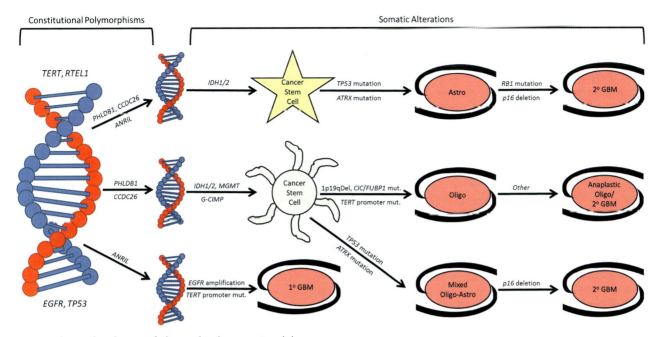

Fig.1.8 Hypothesized pathways of glioma development in adults.

25 to 50% of ependymomas. Varying proportions of medulloblastomas display amplification of *MYCN* and *CMYC*, deletion or mutation of *PTCH*, or deletion of chromosome 17p. About 20 to 30% of pilocytic astrocytomas have deletion of chromosome 17q. *NF2* is deleted or mutated in > 50% of meningioma or schwannoma, and *VHL* is deleted or mutated in about 15% of hemangioblastomas. Approximately 5 to 25% of non-*NF2* mutated meningiomas also carry mutations in *TRAF7*, *KLF4*, *AKT1*, or *SMO*.[12] This emphasizes the enormous heterogeneity of molecular modifications within and between histological types of primary brain tumors.

◼ Risk Factors

There are few established environmental risk factors for brain tumors, in part due to tumor heterogeneity and extended time since exposure. **Table 1.1** summarizes risk factors for adult and childhood gliomas, and **Table 1.2** does the same for meningiomas and other CNS tumors. Several excellent and comprehensive reviews of the epidemiological literature on primary brain tumors provide more detailed information about these factors.[2,13–16]

◼ Genetic and Familial Factors

Hereditary Cancer Syndromes

The heritability of brain tumors is suggested by reports of these tumors occurring more commonly in individuals with

hereditary syndromes. Many studies have attempted to identify rare genetic mutations conferring increased brain tumor risk within families.[17] Although such methods can identify genes contributing to brain tumor risk in families with rare mendelian diseases, these genes explain only a small proportion of brain tumor incidence at the population level. Common familial exposure to environmental carcinogens may also contribute to the induction of some brain tumors.[18] Although Li-Fraumeni syndrome (LFS) is the familial tumor syndrome most frequently associated with glioma, numerous other rare mendelian disorders also increase glioma risk. These syndromes are listed in **Table 1.1** (for glioma) and **Table 1.2** (for meningioma and other CNS tumors).

Familial Aggregation

Because only a small proportion of brain tumors are attributed purely to mendelian disorders, the remaining hereditary risk is likely associated with low-penetrance genetic variants and the effects of shared environment.[18] Several case-control studies suggest familial aggregation of primary brain tumors.[17,19] Segregation analyses of more than 600 adult glioma patients' families found a polygenic model best explained the pattern of brain tumor incidence.[20] Genome-wide association studies of common genetic variants, which contribute modest brain tumor risk, explains some of the missing heritability in brain tumor susceptibility.

Genome-Wide Association Studies

Genome-wide association studies (GWASes) have had far greater success in revealing the genetic etiology of primary

Table 1.1 Exposures Studied as Possible Risk Factors for Glioma

Established Risk Factors	Association (Magnitude and Direction)[a]	Subtype Specificity
High-dose radiation	+++	None
Male vs female gender	+	None
White vs African-American ethnicity	+	None
Increasing age	+++	Strongest for glioblastoma
Familial syndromes		
Neurofibromatosis type 1	+++	Astrocytoma
Neurofibromatosis type 2	+++	Ependymoma
Tuberous sclerosis	+++	Astrocytoma and ependymoma
Lynch syndrome	+++	Astrocytoma
Li-Fraumeni syndrome	+++	Strongest for glioblastoma
Melanoma-astrocytoma syndrome	+++	None
Ollier disease/Maffucci syndrome	+++	None
Inherited single nucleotide polymorphisms		
rs2736100-G (*TERT*)	+	None
rs2252586-T (*EGFR*)	+	None
rs11979158-A (*EGFR*)	+	None
rs55705857-G (*CCDC26*)	+++	Oligodendroglioma and *IDH*-mutated astrocytoma
rs1412829-C (*CDKN2B*)	+	Astrocytoma
rs498872-T (*PHLBD*)	+	*IDH*-mutated glioma
rs78378222-C (*TP53*)	++	None
rs6010620-G (*RTEL1*)	+	None
Probable Risk Factors		
Mutagen sensitivity	+	None
Allergies/asthma	–	None
Elevated immunoglobulin E	–	None
Chicken pox/anti–varicella-zoster virus VZV immunoglobulin G	–	None
Probably Not Risk Factors		
Diagnostic radiation	x	None
Head injury	x	None
Residential power lines/electromagnetic fields	x	None
Cigarette smoking	x	None
Alcohol consumption	x	None
Cell phone use	x	None

[a]+++, odds ratio ≥ 5.0; ++, 5.0 > odds ratio ≥ 2.0; +, 2.0 > odds ratio ≥ 1.0; x, odds ratio = 1.0; –, 1.00 > odds ratio ≥ 0.50.

brain tumors than previous candidate-gene studies.[16] In a GWAS, cases with the disease of interest and healthy controls are assayed at hundreds of thousands of SNP markers to identify genetic variants that are significantly more common in those with disease than in those without. This approach assumes that associated variants are linked to genes that influence disease susceptibility. Genomewide association studies of brain tumors have thus far investigated glioma and meningioma. For meningioma, a single GWAS identified a susceptibility locus in the *MLLT10* gene on chromosome 10, conferring a ~1.5-fold increased risk of meningioma.[21]

Five GWASs of glioma patients have been conducted to date, resulting in the identification of eight independently significant SNP associations located in seven genes.[22–25] Four of

these genes (*TERT, RTEL1, EGFR, TP53*) appear to contribute to development of all glioma grades and histologies, whereas the other three genes (*CDKN2B, PHLDB1, CCDC26*) contribute only to the development of certain grades/histologies/molecular subtypes (**Table 1.1**).[16] The SNPs near *CDKN2B* on chromosome 9 increase the risk of astrocytomas, regardless of grade, but do not seem to affect the risk of oligodendroglial tumors. The SNPs in *PHLDB1* increase risk of *IDH*-mutated gliomas, and therefore are most strongly associated with low-grade glioma risk.[26] In a similar but distinct manner, SNPs in *CCDC26* on chromosome 8 increase risk of *IDH*-mutated astrocytomas and also of oligodendroglial tumors regardless of *IDH* mutation status.[27] The *CCDC26* variant most strongly associated with glioma risk, rs55705857, confers a sixfold increased risk

Table 1.2 Exposures Studied as Possible Risk Factors for Brain Tumors Other Than Glioma

Established Risk Factors	Association (Magnitude and Direction)[a]	Subtype Specificity
High-dose radiation	+++	None
Female vs male gender	++	Meningioma
Increasing age	+++	Strongest for meningioma
Increased body mass index	+	Meningioma
Familial syndromes		
Neurofibromatosis type 2	+++	Meningioma, schwannoma
Von Hippel–Lindau disease	+++	Hemangioblastoma
Li-Fraumeni syndrome	+++	Medulloblastoma
Lynch syndrome	+++	Medulloblastoma
Familial adenomatous polyposis	+++	Medulloblastoma
Cowden syndrome	+++	Cerebellar gangliocytoma
Melanoma-astrocytoma syndrome	+++	Meningioma, medulloblastoma
Gorlin syndrome	+++	Medulloblastoma
Inherited single nucleotide polymorphism		
rs11012732-A (*MLLT10*)	+	Meningioma
Probable Risk Factors		
Allergies/asthma	–	Meningioma
Elevated immunoglobulin E	–	Meningioma
Family history of brain tumors	–	Meningioma
Dental X-rays	+	Meningioma, schwannoma
Cigarette smoking (in men)	+	Meningioma
Cigarette smoking (in women)	–	Meningioma
Probably Not Risk Factors		
Head injury	x	None
Residential power lines/electromagnetic fields	x	None
Reproductive factors	x	None
Cell phone use	x	None

[a]+++, odds ratio ≥ 5.0; ++, 5.0 > odds ratio ≥ 2.0; +, 2.0 > odds ratio ≥ 1.0; x, odds ratio = 1.0; –, 1.00 > odds ratio ≥ 0.50.

for this glioma subgroup. Because it confers such great risk, rs55705857 may be functionally related to gliomagenesis.

> **Pearl**
>
> • Heritable and acquired genetic variation in overlapping genes is revealing pathways involved in gliomagenesis. A GWAS identified risk SNPs in *TP53*, *CDKN2A/CDKN2B*, *EGFR*, and *TERT*, which also display somatic alterations in glioma tumor cells. Rare *TP53* and *CDKN2A* mutations also cause familial cancer predisposition syndromes associated with increased glioma risk.

Telomere Biology and Glioma

Telomeres act as a protective cap at the end of chromosomes, but are progressively shortened during mitotic divisions. Telomere depletion ultimately leads to replicative senescence, limiting the proliferative capacity of cells. With activation of telomerase, an enzyme that adds DNA sequence repeats to telomeres, dividing cells can replace lost telomeric DNA and continue proliferating. Of the tumors that do not maintain telomere length through activation of telomerase, a significant subset activates a secondary pathway referred to as alternative lengthening of telomeres (ALT).[28]

Inherited SNPs associated with glioma risk have been observed at the telomerase-related genes *RTEL1* and *TERT*. Additionally, sequencing has revealed recurrent somatic *TERT* promoter mutations in 75% of glioblastomas.[11] Glioblastomas that do not acquire *TERT* promoter mutations frequently have mutations of *ATRX*, a gene that participates in chromatin remodeling at telomeres. A strong correlation has been observed between inactivation of *ATRX* and activation of the ALT pathway.[29] As a result, a new model of gliomagenesis is being revealed in which cancer cell immortalization is enabled by telomere maintenance, either through *TERT* promoter mutation and telomerase-based telomere maintenance, or through *ATRX* mutation and telomerase-independent telomere maintenance (i.e., ALT). Whether the heritable variants in *TERT* and *RTEL1* interact with the somatic mutations in *TERT* and

ATRX remains to be determined, but it is noteworthy that the glioma risk SNPs in *TERT* and *RTEL1* have recently been associated with older ages at diagnosis in glioma patients.[30] Whether the increased risk associated with these variants in older age groups helps explain the glioblastoma incidence peak observed in individuals > 75 years of age merits further investigation.

Personal Medical History as a Risk Factor

Infections, Allergies, and Immunologic Risk Factors

Although infection with the Epstein-Barr virus in immuno-deficient patients is associated with increased risk of CNS lymphoma, it is unlikely that immunodeficiency plays a large role in the development of other primary malignant brain tumors.

Inverse associations between adult-onset glioma and history of allergies and chicken pox have been consistently reported in the literature. Additional studies report decreased glioma risk with increasing levels of immunoglobulin E and anti–varicella-zoster virus immunoglobulin G.[31]

Some investigators have studied the associations of glioma with genetic polymorphisms known to be associated with atopy.[32,33] The observed polymorphism–glioma associations were in the opposite direction of the polymorphism–atopy associations, and because germline polymorphisms were used as biomarkers of susceptibility to asthma/allergies, the results cannot be attributed to either recall bias or effects of glioblastoma on the immune system. Interestingly, it has been further demonstrated that a history of allergies is also inversely associated with meningioma, further supporting the hypothesis that brain tumor development has an immunologic component.[34]

Prior Cancers

Having a prior cancer may be associated with the development of intracranial tumors (e.g., breast cancer and meningioma), although the data are limited.[35] Shared environmental or genetic risk factors might also explain some of these associations. However, cancer patients treated with radiation to the head show a greatly increased risk for a number of brain tumors including glioma, acoustic neuroma, and meningioma.[36,37]

Ionizing Radiation

There is a strong increased risk of intracranial tumors following therapeutic ionizing radiation.[38] Even with the relatively low doses (averaging 1.5 Gy) used to treat tinea capitis in childhood, relative risks of 18, 10, and 3 have been observed

for nerve sheath tumors, meningiomas, and gliomas, respectively.[39] Atomic bomb survivors also show an increased risk of meningioma for high-dose levels of exposure.[38]

Studies have shown an increased risk of brain tumors in children after CNS radiation treatment for acute lymphoblastic leukemia (ALL).[38,39] One study showed that the incidence of brain tumors among irradiated children for ALL was 12.8%.

Evidence thus far does not support a role for diagnostic radiation in causing glioma, but the evidence is stronger for meningioma. A recent study reported that patients with meningioma were twice as likely as persons without meningioma to report receiving bite-wing dental X-rays on a yearly or more frequent basis.[40] Similar findings were recently noted for a hospital-based study of dental X-rays and risk of acoustic neuroma.[41] Because the radiation dosage has decreased dramatically since the time period during which patients in this study received X-rays, the public health impact of dental X-rays on brain tumor incidence is likely already on the decline.

A nonsignificant elevated risk for brain tumors has been reported in nuclear facility employees. Risks of the same magnitude have been reported for workers producing nuclear materials.[42] However, confounding or effect modification by chemical exposures makes interpretation of causality difficult.

Head Trauma

Serious head trauma has been a suspected cause of brain tumors but results are inconsistent.[43] Critics of causal association between head trauma and brain tumors suggest that the magnitude of the risk could be explained by preferential recall of head injuries by those with brain tumors or incidental identification of tumors following imaging at the time of trauma. To minimize these biases, a large cohort study of incident intracranial tumors after hospitalization for head injuries was conducted in Denmark.[44] There was no increased risk of glioma or meningioma during an average of 8 years of follow-up.

Seizures

History of seizures has been consistently associated with brain tumors in several cohort studies of epileptics and in case-control studies of adult glioma, although it is difficult to determine the temporal relationship of the two diagnoses.[45] The fact that some patients develop seizures many years prior to tumor diagnosis may suggest a true connection, but it is unclear if the seizures or the medications patients take to control them might increase tumor risk.

Exposure to Drugs and Medications

Few studies have looked at effects of medications and drugs on the risk of adult brain tumors. Nonsteroidal anti-inflammatory drug use was inversely associated with glioblastoma risk in at least two studies.[46] Studies of childhood brain tumors have considered prenatal exposures to some or all of the following drugs, with few significant or replicated findings: fertility drugs, oral contraceptives, sleeping pills or tranquilizers, pain medications, antihistamines, anesthetics, metronidazole, and diuretics.[47]

Hormones

Evidence of an association between hormones and meningioma risk includes the higher incidence in women versus men (most notably so before menopause); the presence of hormone receptors on some meningiomas; positive associations with uterine fibroids; endometriosis and possibly breast cancer; indications that meningioma size varies during the luteal phase of the menstrual cycle and pregnancy; a potential association with current oral contraceptive use; and a decreased risk for women who report ever smoking (which may impact hormone levels).[48]

Dietary Factors

Several mechanisms involving DNA damage through which N-nitroso compounds might operate to cause brain tumors are discussed in detail elsewhere.[49] The main points are that these compounds can initiate neuro-carcinogenesis both prenatally and postnatally, although fetal exposures result in more tumors in animals than postnatal exposures.

A meta-analysis of nine observational studies suggested a 48% increased risk of glioma development among adults ingesting high levels of cured meat.[50] However, the authors note that most studies failed to adjust for total energy intake, which may lead to spurious associations. Increased consumption of fruits and vegetables or vitamins that might block nitrosation or harmful effects of nitrosamines has been observed in some, but not all, studies.[49] In aggregate, results for adults suggest no increased risk for glioma with beer or wine consumption.[14]

Tobacco and Residential Chemicals

Because cigarette smoke is a major environmental source of carcinogens, many studies have examined its role in brain tumor pathogenesis. Results suggest no important effect of tobacco smoking on glioma risk, but a recent meta-analysis of meningioma, stratified by gender, did reveal significant associations; men who smoke were at an increased risk of meningioma, whereas women who smoke were at significantly reduced risk of meningioma.[51] Whether the observed gender differences are related to the hypothesized anti-estrogenic effects of smoking remains to be determined.

Studies of residential chemical exposures have focused on the role of pre- and postnatal pesticide exposures in childhood brain tumors. Although results are mixed, residential exposures during pregnancy or around delivery tend to be associated with higher risks of childhood brain tumors than exposures during childhood.[47] Further investigation of prenatal exposures may be justified.

Industry and Occupational Chemicals

The number of brain tumor cases reported in occupational cohort studies is often too small to conduct meaningful analyses. There has been no definitive link made between brain tumors and occupational exposures to specific chemicals, even known or strongly suspected carcinogens.[13] A meta-analysis of brain tumors and rubber workers concluded that occupational exposures in the rubber and tire industries do not increase brain tumor risk, despite synthetic rubber processing producing numerous potential carcinogenic by-products.[52]

Petrochemical production and oil refinery workers have long been studied with regard to brain tumor risk because of suspected clusters of brain tumors in several Texas petrochemical plants in the 1970s. However, a large meta-analysis found no overall increased brain cancer mortality in petroleum workers.[14] The inability to investigate the effects of specific agents has obstructed identification of causal exposures.

Scientists and biomedical professionals have also been examined for brain tumor risk. Although patients with glioma in the San Francisco Bay Area were more likely than controls to be physicians and surgeons, no specific medical specialty was singled out as being at increased risk for brain tumors, and the results were compatible with chance.[53] Negative findings have also been reported for employment in the aerospace industries, despite concerns that aircrews are exposed to low-level cosmic ionizing radiation.[54]

Parental Exposure to Carcinogens

Parental exposures could conceivably cause increased risks of cancer in their children. Significantly elevated risks of childhood brain tumors were reported for paternal work with paper and pulp, solvents, painting, printing, graphic arts, oil or chemical refining, farming, metallurgy, and the air and space industry.[14] Lack of specificity of exposures in the positive studies and inadequate numbers of exposed parents in the negative studies prevents meaningful conclusions.[47]

Cellular Telephones

Concern over possible health effects of using cellular telephones has prompted studies looking at the relationship between cellular phone usage and risk of brain tumors. Most case-control and cohort studies suggest that there is no association between cellular phone use or duration of cellular phone use and the incidence of most brain tumors.[55] After an 8-day review of the literature by 31 experts in 2012, the IARC classified mobile phone use and other radiofrequency electromagnetic fields as a possible carcinogen (group 2B). This means that there "could be some risk" of carcinogenicity and that "additional research into the long-term effects of mobile phone use is warranted."

The National Cancer Institute (NCI) states,

> Both IARC and NCI recommend continued monitoring of both brain cancer trends and new evidence from studies in humans and laboratory animals. In particular, it will be important to assess risk after long-term use, and for younger users. IARC further recommends specific actions to reduce exposure (e.g., hands-free use and texting) as further studies are undertaken. . . . However, we note that brain cancer incidence and mortality rates in the population have changed little in the past decade when cell phone use has increased markedly.

Electromagnetic Fields

Neither a large population-based study of adult glioma in the San Francisco Bay Area nor other epidemiological studies of adult brain tumors support the hypothesis that residential power frequency EMFs increase the risk of brain tumors.[14] A limitation with studies of EMF exposures and adult brain tumors is that the pertinent exposure period and the mechanisms through which EMF might contribute to brain tumor risk are unknown.

■ Conclusion

Gender differences, the most consistent feature in the descriptive epidemiology of primary brain tumors, provide a provocative etiologic clue that remains unexplained. Developing consensus in histopathological classification systems, increased use of molecular and genetic markers to form more etiologically homogeneous categories of tumors, and incorporation of potentially relevant inherited polymorphisms all may help to create a more complete picture of the natural history and pathogenesis of brain tumors. Current research suggests that gliomagenesis is influenced by common heritable variation in at least seven genes. Continued efforts to identify causal variants in the genes will help account for a more substantial proportion of glioma incidence. Many intriguing and promising possibilities remain to be pursued, and collaborative efforts will be required to further brain tumor research.

The Brain Tumor Epidemiology Consortium, Meningioma Consortium, and Gliogene Consortium have been formed to encourage innovative collaborations that will further the understanding of the etiology, prevention, and outcomes of brain tumors. Moreover, in the search for comprehensive explanations for this devastating disease, entirely new concepts about neuro-oncogenesis might emerge, making brain tumor epidemiology a particularly exciting area for continued epidemiologic research.

Editor's Note

Epidemiologists have taught clinicians as well as researchers a great deal about the overall trends in incidence and mortality for tumors that involve the CNS. The overall incidence throughout the years has remained steady, and, in general, any increased incidence rates have been largely linked to improved access to diagnostic imaging. There are subtle differences in the roles that geography, ethnicity, age, and gender play in incidence and mortality. Exceptions to this have to do with meningiomas, which are seen in much higher rates in females than males. We have learned a great deal from the molecular marker profile studies that have been done in patients with all types of tumors and, in particular, gliomas. These molecular markers have enabled us to better understand prognosis, and, through the GWASs of single nucleotide polymorphisms, to learn about the risk of developing a certain type of glioma based on the identification of certain high-risk chromosomal variations seen in patients.

With regard to environmental risk factors, there are very few established factors of this kind, which is largely due to the fact that these are very heterogeneous lesions. Tumors are sometimes seen in families, although this is not very common, as opposed to seeing an increased incidence of certain types of tumors associated with hereditary cancer syndromes. One of the more intriguing recent findings has been the inverse association between adult-onset glioma and a history of allergies. This certainly implicates the functioning of the immune system in the susceptibility to developing certain types of tumors such as gliomas. Another controversial area has been in the use of cell phones and whether or not exposure can be related to the formation of a brain tumor. Numerous case-control and cohort studies have been done in the past decade, a period of increased cell phones usage, yet overall the findings fail to implicate cell phones in any definitive way in the development of any type of brain tumor. The epidemiology community through its consortiums will continue to develop working collaborations to help all clinicians further understand the incidence as well as the risk of developing CNS tumors. This is a very important field for future research. (Berger)

Acknowledgments

This work was supported by the National Cancer Institute, grant numbers R01CA52689, CA109468, CA109461, CA109745, CA108473, CA151933, CA109475, P50CA097257, and R25CA112355, as well as by the Brain Science Foundation and the Meningioma Mommas.

References

1. Dolecek TA, Propp JM, Stroup NE, Kruchko C. CBTRUS statistical report: primary brain and central nervous system tumors diagnosed in the United States in 2005-2009. Neuro-oncol 2012;14(Suppl 5):v1–v49
2. Ohgaki H, Kleihues P. Epidemiology and etiology of gliomas. Acta Neuropathol 2005;109:93–108
3. Inskip PD, Linet MS, Heineman EF. Etiology of brain tumors in adults. Epidemiol Rev 1995;17:382–414
4. Dubrow R, Darefsky AS. Demographic variation in incidence of adult glioma by subtype, United States, 1992-2007. BMC Cancer 2011;11:325
5. Jacobs DI, Walsh KM, Wrensch M, et al. Leveraging ethnic group incidence variation to investigate genetic susceptibility to glioma: a novel candidate SNP approach. Front Genet 2012;3:203
6. Hegi ME, Diserens AC, Gorlia T, et al. MGMT gene silencing and benefit from temozolomide in glioblastoma. N Engl J Med 2005;352:997–1003
7. Darefsky AS, King JT Jr, Dubrow R. Adult glioblastoma multiforme survival in the temozolomide era: a population-based analysis of Surveillance, Epidemiology, and End Results registries. Cancer 2012;118:2163–2172
8. Goodenberger ML, Jenkins RB. Genetics of adult glioma. Cancer Genet 2012;205:613–621
9. Jiao Y, Killela PJ, Reitman ZJ, et al. Frequent ATRX, CIC, FUBP1 and IDH1 mutations refine the classification of malignant gliomas. Oncotarget 2012;3:709–722
10. Xiao Y, Decker PA, Rice T, et al. SSBP2 variants are associated with survival in glioblastoma patients. Clin Cancer Res 2012;18:3154–3162
11. Killela PJ, Reitman ZJ, Jiao Y, et al. TERT promoter mutations occur frequently in gliomas and a subset of tumors derived from cells with low rates of self-renewal. Proc Natl Acad Sci U S A 2013;110:6021–6026
12. Clark VE, Erson-Omay EZ, Serin A, et al. Genomic analysis of non-NF2 meningiomas reveals mutations in TRAF7, KLF4, AKT1, and SMO. Science 2013;339:1077–1080
13. Gomes J, Al Zayadi A, Guzman A. Occupational and environmental risk factors of adult primary brain cancers: a systematic review. Int J Occup Environ Med 2011;2:82–111
14. Wrensch M, Minn Y, Chew T, Bondy M, Berger MS. Epidemiology of primary brain tumors: current concepts and review of the literature. Neuro-oncol 2002;4:278–299
15. Wiemels J, Wrensch M, Claus EB. Epidemiology and etiology of meningioma. J Neurooncol 2010;99:307–314
16. Walsh KM, Anderson E, Hansen HM, et al. Analysis of 60 reported glioma risk SNPs replicates published GWAS findings but fails to replicate associations from published candidate-gene studies. Genet Epidemiol 2013;37:222–228
17. Hemminki K, Tretli S, Sundquist J, Johannesen TB, Granström C. Familial risks in nervous-system tumours: a histology-specific analysis from Sweden and Norway. Lancet Oncol 2009;10:481–488
18. Malmer B, Adatto P, Armstrong G, et al. GLIOGENE an International Consortium to Understand Familial Glioma. Cancer Epidemiol Biomarkers Prev 2007;16:1730–1734
19. Claus EB, Calvocoressi L, Bondy ML, Schildkraut JM, Wiemels JL, Wrensch M. Family and personal medical history and risk of meningioma. J Neurosurg 2011;115:1072–1077
20. de Andrade M, Barnholtz JS, Amos CI, Adatto P, Spencer C, Bondy ML. Segregation analysis of cancer in families of glioma patients. Genet Epidemiol 2001;20:258–270
21. Dobbins SE, Broderick P, Melin B, et al. Common variation at 10p12.31 near MLLT10 influences meningioma risk. Nat Genet 2011;43:825–827
22. Stacey SN, Sulem P, Jonasdottir A, et al; Swedish Low-risk Colorectal Cancer Study Group. A germline variant in the TP53 polyadenylation signal confers cancer susceptibility. Nat Genet 2011;43:1098–1103
23. Wrensch M, Jenkins RB, Chang JS, et al. Variants in the CDKN2B and RTEL1 regions are associated with high-grade glioma susceptibility. Nat Genet 2009;41:905–908
24. Sanson M, Hosking FJ, Shete S, et al. Chromosome 7p11.2 (EGFR) variation influences glioma risk. Hum Mol Genet 2011;20:2897–2904
25. Shete S, Hosking FJ, Robertson LB, et al. Genome-wide association study identifies five susceptibility loci for glioma. Nat Genet 2009;41:899–904
26. Rice T, Zheng S, Decker PA, et al. Inherited variant on chromosome 11q23 increases susceptibility to IDH-mutated but not IDH-normal gliomas regardless of grade or histology. Neuro-oncol 2013;15:535–541
27. Jenkins RB, Xiao Y, Sicotte H, et al. A low-frequency variant at 8q24.21 is strongly associated with risk of oligodendroglial tumors and astrocytomas with IDH1 or IDH2 mutation. Nat Genet 2012;44:1122–1125
28. Bryan TM, Englezou A, Dalla-Pozza L, Dunham MA, Reddel RR. Evidence for an alternative mechanism for maintaining telomere length in human tumors and tumor-derived cell lines. Nat Med 1997;3:1271–1274
29. Heaphy CM, de Wilde RF, Jiao Y, et al. Altered telomeres in tumors with ATRX and DAXX mutations. Science 2011;333:425
30. Walsh KM, Rice T, Decker PA, et al. Genetic variants in telomerase-elated genes are associated with an older age at diagnosis in glioma patients: evidence for distinct pathways of gliomagenesis. Neuro-oncol 2013,15.1041–1047
31. Wrensch M, Fisher JL, Schwartzbaum JA, Bondy M, Berger M, Aldape KD. The molecular epidemiology of gliomas in adults. Neurosurg Focus 2005;19:E5
32. Schwartzbaum J, Ahlbom A, Malmer B, et al. Polymorphisms associated with asthma are inversely related to glioblastoma multiforme. Cancer Res 2005;65:6459–6465
33. Wiemels JL, Wiencke JK, Kelsey KT, et al. Allergy-related polymorphisms influence glioma status and serum IgE levels. Cancer Epidemiol Biomarkers Prev 2007;16:1229–1235
34. Wiemels JL, Wrensch M, Sison JD, et al. Reduced allergy and immunoglobulin E among adults with intracranial meningioma compared to controls. Int J Cancer 2011;129:1932–1939
35. Custer BS, Koepsell TD, Mueller BA. The association between breast carcinoma and meningioma in women. Cancer 2002;94:1626–1635
36. Inskip PD. Multiple primary tumors involving cancer of the brain and central nervous system as the first or subsequent cancer. Cancer 2003;98:562–570
37. Hijiya N, Hudson MM, Lensing S, et al. Cumulative incidence of secondary neoplasms as a first event after childhood acute lymphoblastic leukemia. JAMA 2007;297:1207–1215
38. Claus EB, Bondy ML, Schildkraut JM, Wiemels JL, Wrensch M, Black PM. Epidemiology of intracranial meningioma. Neurosurgery 2005;57:1088–1095, discussion 1088–1095
39. Braganza MZ, Kitahara CM, Berrington de González A, Inskip PD, Johnson KJ, Rajaraman P. Ionizing radiation and the risk of brain and central nervous system tumors: a systematic review. Neuro-oncol 2012;14:1316–1324
40. Claus EB, Calvocoressi L, Bondy ML, Schildkraut JM, Wiemels JL, Wrensch M. Dental x-rays and risk of meningioma. Cancer 2012;118:4530–4537
41. Han YY, Berkowitz O, Talbott E, Kondziolka D, Donovan M, Lunsford LD. Are frequent dental x-ray examinations associated with increased risk of vestibular schwannoma? J Neurosurg 2012;117(Suppl):78–83

42. Rogel A, Joly K, Metz-Flamant C, et al. [Mortality in nuclear workers of the French electricity company: period 1968–2003]. Rev Epidemiol Sante Publique 2009;57:257–265

43. Preston-Martin S, Pogoda JM, Schlehofer B, et al. An international case-control study of adult glioma and meningioma: the role of head trauma. Int J Epidemiol 1998;27:579–586

44. Inskip PD, Mellemkjaer L, Gridley G, Olsen JH. Incidence of intracranial tumors following hospitalization for head injuries (Denmark). Cancer Causes Control 1998;9:109–116

45. Schwartzbaum J, Jonsson F, Ahlbom A, et al. Prior hospitalization for epilepsy, diabetes, and stroke and subsequent glioma and meningioma risk. Cancer Epidemiol Biomarkers Prev 2005;14:643–650

46. Scheurer ME, Amirian ES, Davlin SL, Rice T, Wrensch M, Bondy ML. Effects of antihistamine and anti-inflammatory medication use on risk of specific glioma histologies. Int J Cancer 2011;129:2290–2296

47. Baldwin RT, Preston-Martin S. Epidemiology of brain tumors in childhood—a review. Toxicol Appl Pharmacol 2004;199:118–131

48. Claus EB, Calvocoressi L, Bondy ML, Wrensch M, Wiemels JL, Schildkraut JM. Exogenous hormone use, reproductive factors, and risk of intracranial meningioma in females. J Neurosurg 2013;118:649–656

49. Berleur MP, Cordier S. The role of chemical, physical, or viral exposures and health factors in neurocarcinogenesis: implications for epidemiologic studies of brain tumors. Cancer Causes Control 1995;6:240–256

50. Huncharek M, Kupelnick B, Wheeler L. Dietary cured meat and the risk of adult glioma: a meta-analysis of nine observational studies. J Environ Pathol Toxicol Oncol 2003;22:129–137

51. Claus EB, Walsh KM, Calvocoressi L, et al. Cigarette smoking and risk of meningioma: the effect of gender. Cancer Epidemiol Biomarkers Prev 2012;21:943–950

52. Borak J, Slade MD, Russi M. Risks of brain tumors in rubber workers: a metaanalysis. J Occup Environ Med 2005;47:294–298

53. Krishnan G, Felini M, Carozza SE, Miike R, Chew T, Wrensch M. Occupation and adult gliomas in the San Francisco Bay Area. J Occup Environ Med 2003;45:639–647

54. Zeeb H, Hammer GP, Blettner M. Epidemiological investigations of aircrew: an occupational group with low-level cosmic radiation exposure. J Radiol Prot 2012;32:N15–N19

55. Repacholi MH, Lerchl A, Röösli M, et al. Systematic review of wireless phone use and brain cancer and other head tumors. Bioelectromagnetics 2012;33:187–206

2 Pathology and Molecular Classification

Kenneth D. Aldape and Aditya Raghunathan

Based on the principles established by Percival Bailey and Harvey Cushing almost a century ago, the classification of primary central nervous system (CNS) neoplasias is based on morphological similarities with preexisting normal cells from which these neoplasias are considered to originate. Brain tumors that are composed of cells that resemble astrocytes, oligodendrocytes, and ependymal cells are classified as astrocytomas, oligodendrogliomas, and ependymomas, respectively. Tumors composed of small round cells that resemble the neuronal precursor cells seen during normal neurodevelopment are classified as primitive neuroectodermal tumors (PNETs). When PNETs arise in the cerebellum, they are classified as medulloblastomas. To corroborate diagnoses that are based on microscopic analysis, tumors are further examined by immunohistochemistry to determine whether there is expression of specific proteins associated with specific types of normal CNS cells, alluding to the putative cell type of origin. For example, glial fibrillary acidic protein (GFAP) is expressed primarily in glial cells, and the presence of GFAP expression in a CNS neoplasm helps categorize it as a glioma.

In addition to the cell-of-origin relationship, CNS neoplasia are graded based on the identification of morphological features that have been associated with clinical behavior and patient outcomes, helping to guide the choice of therapy for that specific tumor type. Various grading schema have been proposed to classify CNS tumors based on their expected clinical behavior. Among these, the World Health Organization (WHO) Classification of Tumors of the Central Nervous System is the most widely accepted, and the most recent edition was published in 2007. Tumor classification includes an assessment of the extent of specimen anaplasia, which involves estimating tumor-cell to normal-cell similarity, combined with a determination of the presence or absence of microscopic features indicative of aggressive behavior, such as mitotic activity, tumor necrosis, and angiogenesis. Although the Bailey and Cushing system of classification has proven highly useful in neuro-oncology research and clinical practice, modern molecular profiling techniques are yielding a new layer of diagnostic and prognostic information, in addition to the conventional histopathological classification. However, it is important to recognize that comprehensive tumor molecular profiling is still at the relatively early stages of development and application, and the results of related studies are only just beginning to have a widespread impact on clinical practice. Nonetheless, as these approaches move toward consensus platforms and standardized methods, the prospect of their improving our ability to provide detailed and individualized information for appropriate therapy selection and improved patient outcomes looks very promising.

Methods for Tumor Molecular Profiling and Classification

During the 1980s and 1990s, the most commonly used molecular methods for examining cells and tissues enabled us to acquire results for single genes, transcripts, or proteins for each experiment conducted. Undoubtedly the Western or immunoblot for protein analysis, as well as Southern and Northern blots for DNA and RNA analysis, respectively, generated large and useful bodies of information that served to highlight the distinct features of normal versus malignant cells, but just as certainly these methods are labor intensive and relatively inefficient in yielding data. The rapid development and application of techniques for querying all, or at least large portions, of the genomes, transcriptomes, and proteomes for cells and tissues has led to giant strides in their application to the study of CNS neoplasia, and the most common representatives of these methods are discussed briefly in the following section.

Comparative Genomic Hybridization

The completion of the Human Genome Project brought with it the ability to organize cloned DNA sequences with respect to their linear and contiguous order on human chromosomes. A specific type of recombinant DNA, referred to as a bacterial artificial chromosome (BAC), proved highly useful for this purpose, and BAC clones containing human chromosomal DNA are now proving to be a critical resource for the genomic profiling of tumor DNAs. The BACs accommodate, on average, 100,000 base pairs of human chromosomal DNA (1.7×10^{-5} of the DNA in a normal human cell).

The DNA sequence contained in a BAC can be assigned to a specific chromosome location, and by arraying thousands of these BACs, it is possible to provide an orderly representation of all human chromosomes on very small surfaces. These arrayed BACs can be used for examining changes in tumor DNAs as follows. The DNA from a tumor and from a normal human DNA tissue/cell source are isolated, fragmented, and labeled through the incorporation of nucleotides that have been tagged with fluorescent dyes. Generally a red fluorescent dye

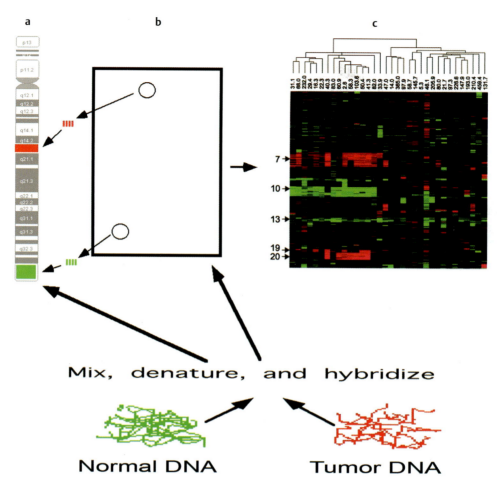

Fig. 2.1a–c Chromosomal and array comparative genomic hybridization. Diagram shows the mixing of labeled normal (*green*) and tumor (*red*) DNAs with subsequent hybridization to (**a**) metaphase chromosome or (**b**) arrayed bacterial artificial chromosome DNAs. Array comparative genomic hybridization (CGH) data output can be used to develop maps (*arrows pointing left*) showing regions of tumor chromosomal gain (*red*) or loss (*green*), or (**c**) the array CGH data can be analyzed for pattern associations with various patient clinical variables, such as survival (*arrow* pointing to the "heat map" at the right). (Reprinted with permission from the American Association for Cancer Research, Inc. Nigro JM, Misra A, Zhang L, et al. Integrated array-comparative genomic hybridization and expression array profiles identify clinically relevant molecular subtypes of glioblastoma. Cancer Res 2005;65:1678–1686.)

is used to label a tumor DNA, and a green fluorescent dye is used to label a normal DNA (**Fig. 2.1**). These DNAs are mixed and cohybridized to a slide or "chip," onto which BACs have been spotted or "arrayed." The fluorescent dye–labeled normal and tumor DNAs compete with each other for binding to the arrayed BACs, and for sequences in which there is overrepresentation in the tumor DNA, red fluorescence is preferentially emitted, whereas tumor DNA underrepresentation results in preferential green fluorescence emission. By reading the fluorescence emissions for all coordinates (spots) on the array (**Fig. 2.1b**), regions of tumor chromosomal gain or deletion can be deduced (**Fig. 2.1a**). This procedure is most commonly referred to as array comparative genomic hybridization (CGH). When applied to a series of tumors, the thousands of CGH data fields for each tumor can be compared against specific clinical behaviors, such as survival, in an attempt to identify array "fingerprints" that are consistently associated with the clinical feature of interest (**Fig. 2.1c**).

The lower-resolution precursor of array CGH involves the hybridization of labeled normal and tumor DNAs directly to metaphase chromosomes (**Fig. 2.1a**), followed by an analysis of the red-to-green fluorescence of the chromosomes to identify regions of gain or loss in the tumor genome. Array CGH technologies have rapidly supplanted direct chromosomal CGH and, as a result, much of the comparative genomic hybridization literature since 2000 involves this approach.

Fluorescence In-Situ Hybridization Analysis

Normally, there are two copies of each gene per cell. The same BAC clones already described can be used singularly to examine individual tumor cells for increased or decreased DNA con-

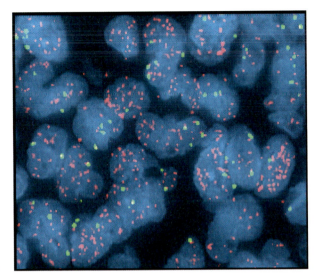

Fig. 2.2a,b Fluorescence in-situ hybridization (FISH) analysis for epidermal growth factor receptor (EGFR) amplification. **(a)** Tumor cells in which EGFR signals (*red*) far outnumber those of the control probe for chromosome 7 centromere (*green*), thereby indicating *EGFR* gene amplification in the corresponding tumor. **(b)** An *EGFR*/control signal ratio of approximately 1, thereby indicating a lack of *EGFR* amplification in the corresponding tumor.

tent of specific chromosome locations. This is accomplished by hybridizing a fluorescence-labeled BAC to sectioned tumor tissues, followed by fluorescence microscopy examination of the cells in the tissue to assess whether they show increased (> 2) or decreased (< 2) signals per cell, and that would indicate gain or loss, respectively, of the BAC sequence in tumor cells (there are normally 2 copies of each gene). A straightforward example of this fluorescence in-situ hybridization (FISH) analysis involves the hybridization of a BAC containing a gene that is amplified in a tumor, such as the epidermal growth factor receptor gene *(EGFR),* and that would produce many more than two signals in the cells of a tumor (**Fig. 2.2**), as compared with the two signals that we would see if the BAC were hybridized to a tumor in which the gene were not amplified. Though the results of FISH are often inferred from the results of array CGH, FISH is an essential corroboration of CGH information, especially in instances where a gene of interest encodes a potential therapeutic target.

Expression Profiling

Similar to the global as well as individual approaches for examining tumor DNA, there are comprehensive and individual approaches for examining expressed sequences (messenger RNAs [mRNAs]) in tumor tissues. The comprehensive analytic approach most commonly used is referred to as expression profiling. It shares some similarities with array CGH for DNA but has distinct features as well. Rather than the use of arrayed BAC clones containing very large genomic DNA inserts, short nucleotide sequences (oligonucleotides), complementary to all known expressed sequences, are fixed or synthesized on a solid support, with each oligonucleotide spotted at a defined coordinate. Tumor mRNA, rather than being directly labeled after isolation, is first converted to complementary DNA (cDNA) that is then used as a template for the synthesis of biotinylated complimentary RNA (cRNA), and which is then hybridized to the arrayed oligonucleotides. Subsequent to rinsing away unbound cRNA, the arrays are incubated with fluorescent dye–tagged streptavidin, which binds to the biotinylated cRNA. The array is then subjected to quantitative fluorescence analysis, and the relative expression levels of individual tumor transcripts are determined.

Real-Time Quantitative Polymerase Chain Reaction

Just as FISH analysis can be considered a validation for array CGH results, real-time quantitative polymerase chain reaction (PCR) is important to the validation of expression profile results. In brief, this approach involves the use of PCR and fluorescence detection to monitor the rate of amplification for a specific cDNA, the starting amount for which is determined by the tumor-associated expression of its corresponding transcript. A rapid amplification of a sequence of interest would be consistent with expression profile data indicating the same sequence as being overexpressed in the same tumor. Conversely, a tumor-specific reduced rate of sequence amplification would be consistent with expression profile data indicating a transcript's underrepresentation in a tumor. However, rather than simply reexamining tumors that have already been expression profiled, the approach that is used more often with quantitative PCR is to examine a set of genes, having been revealed as up- or downregulated in a few tumors by expression profiling, in an expanded series of tumors that have not been expression profiled. Alternatively, one can examine tumor tissues for corresponding protein expression. If appropriate antibodies are available for immunohistochemical (IHC) analysis, one can rapidly acquire data for a large number of tumor specimens using tissue microarrays (TMAs).

Matrix-Assisted Laser Desorption/Ionization Mass Spectrometry

In preparing to use this comprehensive protein detection method, a tissue section is deposited or mounted on a metal plate, coated with an ultraviolet (UV)-absorbing matrix, and subsequently exposed to a UV laser that ionizes the protein/peptide content coated by the matrix. The charged molecules in the matrix are accelerated down a flight tube, and each is detected based on its unique mass-to-charge ratio. The signals are separated according to this ratio, and the data output is a spectrum in which the peaks observed correspond to the peptides and proteins from the sample. In the case of direct tissue analysis, multiple regions of the tissue's surface are examined to account for cellular heterogeneity, and the data are collected as a series of mass spectra. Each spectrum contains signals from many hundreds of proteins and peptides specific to a corresponding tissue region.

As with the global/comprehensive approaches to DNA and RNA analysis, comprehensive protein analysis has corroborative approaches for validating individual biomarkers of interest (i.e., Western blot in instances where additional fresh tissue is available, and IHC analysis of formalin-fixed tissues). Comprehensive proteomic analysis has exciting potential but it is the least mature of the global approaches for investigating the molecular characteristics of a tumor tissue, although its use is gradually becoming more prevalent.

Next-Generation Sequencing for Brain Tumor Diagnosis

Recently, there has been a growing effort to better understand the genetic basis of various neoplasms, including gliomas, using highly refined high-throughput sequencing. The term *next-generation sequencing* (NGS) encompasses several different technologies to investigate the genome, epigenome, and transcriptome. Common to these methods is the concurrent analysis of multiple DNA templates (massively parallel sequencing) that extends far beyond the capabilities of prior standard methods, at a much lower overall cost. Next-generation sequencing refers to the technology only, and the exact template to be sequenced can range from the whole genome to a more targeted approach. For example, because the human exome (the portion of the genome that codes for known genes) makes up only 1% of the human genome, there is a gain in efficiency (not to mention lower sequencing costs) when targeted approaches, such as whole exome sequencing, are applied. In this method, there is initial enrichment of the exonic regions in the sample, followed by targeted sequencing.

Comparing the tumor exome to the nontumor exome from the same patient enables identification of tumor-specific variations (somatic mutations).

The efficiency of capturing the entire exome, or portions thereof, however, depends on the fidelity and efficiency of the enrichment methods utilized. Following the generation of raw data from the sequencer, various bioinformatics tools are required to analyze and interpret the results. These include aligning the sequences to the human genome, post-alignment processing to identify aberrations, and functional prediction. Interestingly, a major hurdle in the ability to apply NGS in the clinical setting is not the technology itself but rather the bioinformatics and data interpretation. A consensus regarding the standardized utilization of the available bioinformatics tools is only just beginning to form. Even with these challenges, NGS, by virtue of allowing simultaneous testing for multiple targets in a time frame appropriate for a clinical setting, holds great promise for clinical implementation of cancer diagnosis and management, including brain tumors.

Next-generation sequencing will most likely be utilized routinely in the near future as an adjunct to histopathology for tumor classification. Targeted drugs that show efficacy in a subset of patients will become personalized when known mutations or patterns of aberration (tumor signatures) are increasingly recognized. Acknowledging that histopathology offers only a first step toward biological classification, tumor subsets will be identified using clinically relevant mutations, DNA copy number alterations, and expression signatures, all of which can be determined by specific NGS applications, in the clinical setting.

■ Common Central Nervous System Tumors

Medulloblastoma

Medulloblastoma is a highly cellular, invasive, and malignant CNS tumor that occurs in the posterior fossa, with a peak incidence in childhood and occasional occurrences in adults of late middle age. Classic medulloblastomas consist of densely packed cells of round to oval shape, with hyperchromatic nuclei, minimal cytoplasm, and a "small round blue cell" tumor. They have high mitotic and apoptotic rates, and usually display neuroblastic rosettes (**Fig. 2.3**). Microvascular proliferation is relatively uncommon, and tumors may show evidence of neuronal, glial, or combined differentiation. Histological variants include desmoplastic/nodular medulloblastoma, which has nodular reticulin-free regions of neuronal maturation; anaplastic medulloblastoma, which has marked nuclear pleomorphism; and large cell medulloblastoma, which has larger nuclei with prominent nucleoli.

Medulloblastomas often invade the fourth ventricle, with occasional brainstem involvement. There is a high risk of seed-

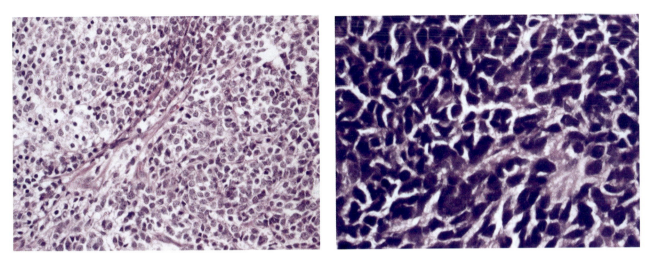

Fig. 2.3a,b Medulloblastoma histopathology. **(a)** Monotonous small, round, blue cells in a medulloblastoma. **(b)** Some medulloblastomas show prominent nuclear atypia.

ing through the subarachnoid space due to the tendency of the tumor to penetrate the ependymal surface. Many antigens have been identified as being focally expressed in medulloblastoma, including nestin, vimentin, neurofilament proteins, GFAP, retinal S-antigen, Trk-A, Trk-B, Trk-C, and neural cellular adhesion molecules (N-CAMs).

The study of genetic syndromes has contributed significantly to our understanding of the molecular biology of medulloblastoma. Gorlin's syndrome (hereditary nevoid basal cell carcinoma syndrome) and familial adenomatous polyposis (FAP) syndrome arise from mutations in the patched homolog 1, *PTCH1* (9q), and adenomatous polyposis coli, *APC* (5q) genes, respectively, and each confers predisposition to medulloblastoma formation. The products of these two genes take part in interconnected pathways that are of fundamental importance to neural development. Other genes being investigated for their significance in medulloblastoma development include *NMYC* and *MYCC,* which are amplified in ~10% of these tumors and are in fact associated with the large cell and anaplastic medulloblastoma variants, and have an especially aggressive clinical behavior.[1]

Among the common pediatric CNS tumors, substantial comprehensive genomic characterizations have been performed on medulloblastomas. The use of array CGH revealed chromosome 6q23 homozygous deletion in an extensively utilized medulloblastoma cell line, and novel medulloblastoma amplification targets PPM1D and CDK6. An alternative form of comprehensive genomic analysis, digital spectral karyotyping, also revealed the amplification of *OTX-2*, which encodes a transcriptional regulator of *CMYC*.[2–4]

With respect to transcriptome analysis, there has been substantial application of expression profiling to the study of medulloblastoma. The first such investigation,[5] which has proven to be highly influential as concerns the utility of global gene expression analysis in neuro-oncology research, demonstrated that transcriptome fingerprints can be used to distinguish histopathologically similar small round cell tumors of the CNS; specifically, medulloblastomas can be transcriptionally distinguished from other primitive neuroectodermal tumors and atypical teratoid/rhabdoid tumors, the latter of which has a consistently poor prognosis. The results of this same study additionally demonstrated that expression profiles can distinguish histopathological subtypes of medulloblastoma (i.e., desmoplastic from classical), and can reliably predict outcomes of medulloblastoma patients.

Recent genome-wide DNA copy number and mRNA expression profiles from a large cohort of primary medulloblastomas have been utilized to generate molecular classification schema that reliably predict patient prognosis. Current consensus classification based on these studies identifies four principal molecular subgroups of medulloblastomas, based on signalling pathway abnormalities, termed Wnt, Shh, Group 3, and Group 4.[6] These subgroups appear distinct in terms of patient demographics, histological features, DNA copy number aberrations, and clinical outcomes. Medulloblastomas in the Wnt subgroup frequently show somatic mutations of *CTNNB1* that encodes β-catenin, and deletions of one copy of chromosome 6. These tumors occur at all ages (but are relatively less common among infants), have an equal gender distribution, predominantly show classical medulloblastoma histology, and have relatively more favorable outcomes. Medulloblastomas in the Shh subgroup are driven by aberrations involving the sonic hedgehog signaling pathway, including mutations in the *PTCH, SMO,* and *SUFU* genes, and amplifications of *GLI 1/2*, almost exclusively show deletion of chromosome 9q that contains the *PTCH* gene, and frequently have *MYCN* amplification. These medulloblastomas have a bimodal age distribution, with infants and adults having these more frequently than children and appear to have an overall equal gender distribution. Desmoplastic/nodular medulloblastoma variants almost exclusively belong to this subgroup; however, it is important to note that a large proportion of medulloblastomas in the Shh subgroup are not desmoplastic/nodular. The Shh subgroup has an overall intermediate prognosis, and might have more favorable outcomes among infants. Group 3 and Group 4 medulloblastomas do not show aberrations in either of these two pathways. Medulloblastomas in these subgroups show classic, large cell and anaplastic histologies. Group 3 medulloblastomas have high-level expression of *MYC* but not *MYCN*. In contrast, Group 4 tumors have minimal expression of *MYC* and *MYCN*. Group 3 tumors have higher frequencies of gain of chromosome 1q and/or loss of chromosomes 5q and 10q as compared to Group 4 tumors. Loss of 17q is the most frequent cytogenetic change among Group 4 tumors, and is less frequently seen in Group 3 tumors. Group 3 tumors occur more commonly in males, are found in infants and children and are exceptionally rare in adults. Group 4 tumors also show a high male/female ratio, although a majority of these tumors that arise in females show loss of the X chromosome. Group 3 tumors have a high frequency of metastasis, whereas Group 4 cases have an intermediate prognosis, similar to Shh tumors. Epigenetic DNA methylation studies have also demonstrated four medulloblastoma subgroups that are highly related to these transcriptomic counterparts.[7]

Collectively, the results from studies of medulloblastoma genome and transcriptome characterizations suggest that these global approaches are generating information that, in conjunction with clinical and histological features, will be useful in tumor diagnosis and subsequent therapies targeted at specific aberrant pathways.

Gliomas

Gliomas are CNS tumors that are considered to arise from the normal glial cells in the CNS, namely astrocytes, oligodendroglial cells, and ependymal cells. In general, gliomas can be classified as circumscribed or diffusely infiltrating. Diffusely infiltrating gliomas are characterized by the presence of extensive infiltration of tumor cells into the adjacent brain parenchyma, and absence of a well-defined tumor–normal parenchyma interface. These gliomas include infiltrating astrocytomas and oligodendrogliomas. The most common examples of circumscribed gliomas are pilocytic astrocytomas and ependymomas.

Pearl

- The infiltrating gliomas (diffuse astrocytomas and oligodendrogliomas) must be distinguished from the circumscribed gliomas (e.g., pilocytic astrocytomas, ependymomas). The former are biologically aggressive (to varying degrees), whereas the latter are more amenable to surgical resection and have a more favorable clinical course.

Circumscribed Gliomas

Pilocytic Astrocytomas

Pilocytic astrocytomas are relatively circumscribed tumors that are most often present in the cerebellum of children, but can occur in the hypothalamic region as well as the optic nerve. These tumors show a wide spectrum of morphologies, though they generally present as biphasic tumors, with loose and dense areas, and are composed of cells with elongated nuclei and bipolar thin ("piloid," or hair-like) cytoplasmic processes. Rosenthal fibers and eosinophilic granular bodies are frequently seen in these tumors (**Fig. 2.4**).

Pearl

- Rosenthal fibers contain clumped GFAP filaments and might also be seen in the normal neuropil surrounding slowly expansile tumors. When present in a tumor, frequently accompanied by eosinophilic granular bodies, they suggest slow growth, such as in a pilocytic astrocytoma, pleomorphic xanthoastrocytoma, or ganglioglioma.

If present, the features typically associated with malignant biological behavior in diffuse adult astrocytomas, such as microvascular proliferation and mitoses, do not carry a negative prognostic implication. In fact, pilocytic astrocytomas are generally biologically nonaggressive and are remarkable among astrocytic tumors in maintaining their grade I status over many years. Consistent with this behavior is the favorable long-term prognosis for pilocytic astrocytoma patients where complete resection is often possible, especially for patients with cerebellar tumors.

With respect to comprehensive genome screens of these tumors, CGH (**Fig. 2.1a**) has demonstrated instances of 9q34.1-qter gain[8] and 19p loss,[9] suggesting the existence of specific gene targets whose alteration is associated with subsets of these tumors. The observation of gains of chromosome 7q34 in sporadic pilocytic astrocytomas[10] led to the subsequent identification of a novel *BRAF: KIAA1549* fusion/duplication product leading to activation of the BRAF-MEK-ERK signaling pathway.[8,11,12] Indeed, the activation of *BRAF* might be the initiating event that induces pilocytic astrocytoma.[13]

Anaplasia in pilocytic astrocytomas, a rare event associated with worse clinical outcomes, is histologically characterized by marked nuclear atypia, more frequent mitoses, and tumor necrosis. It has been associated with prior radiation therapy and neurofibromatosis type 1. Activation of the phosphatidylinositol 3′-kinase (PI3K)-Akt pathway has also been associated with clinically aggressive pilocytic astrocytomas.[14] The BRAF V600E mutation has also been described in a subset of pilocytic astrocytomas that occur in extracerebellar locations, and might be associated with a more aggressive clinical behavior.[14,15] However, this mutation is more frequently seen

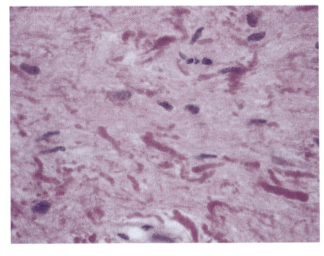

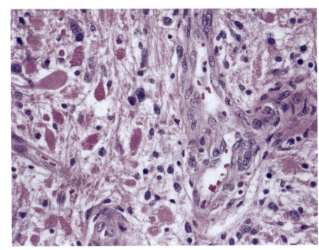

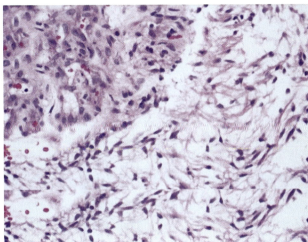

Fig. 2.4a–c Pilocytic astrocytoma histopathology. **(a)** Rosenthal fibers (dense red-pink elongated structures) in a pilocytic astrocytoma. **(b)** Eosinophilic granular bodies are seen in some pilocytic astrocytomas. **(c)** Microvascular proliferation (*upper left*) is often prominent in these tumors, but does not confer an ominous prognosis.

in pleomorphic xanthoastrocytoma and ganglioglioma, two other circumscribed glial/glioneuronal brain tumors.[15]

Pilomyxoid astrocytoma is a recently recognized variant of pilocytic astrocytoma. These tumors are histologically characterized by predominantly loose, myxoid stroma, and show pilocytic cells predominantly arranged around thin-walled blood vessels. These tumors show predilection for the hypothalamic region of young children, tend to undergo leptomeningeal dissemination, and are associated with worse prognosis, being categorized as malignancy grade II by the current WHO guidelines. Genome-wide copy number analysis of pilocytic and pilomyxoid astrocytomas suggest that while these two tumors are related, the frequency of copy number changes is different between the two, with a larger number of lost clones seen among pilomyxoid astrocytomas.[16]

Ependymoma

Ependymomas arise at or close to ependymal surfaces and may occur anywhere in the ventricular system as well as in the spinal cord, with the latter location common in adults. The most common location is in the fourth ventricle, followed by the spinal canal, lateral ventricles, and the third ventricle. Children have the highest incidence of ependymomas, but they can also occur into late middle age.

There are several ependymal tumor subtypes. The malignancy grade I variants consist of the subependymomas (intraventricular and are often without symptoms) and myxopapillary ependymomas (most commonly occurring in the cauda equina region). Grade II ependymomas show indication of an ependymal cell phenotype through formation of rosettes and canals that recapitulate the lining of the ventricular system (**Fig. 2.5**). Perivascular pseudorosettes are commonly identified, but are not specific to ependymomas.

Pearl

- Evidence of increased angiogenesis (microvascular proliferation) is not always associated with aggressive clinical behavior in glioma. Prominent arcades of glomeruloid vessels may be seen in pilocytic astrocytomas.

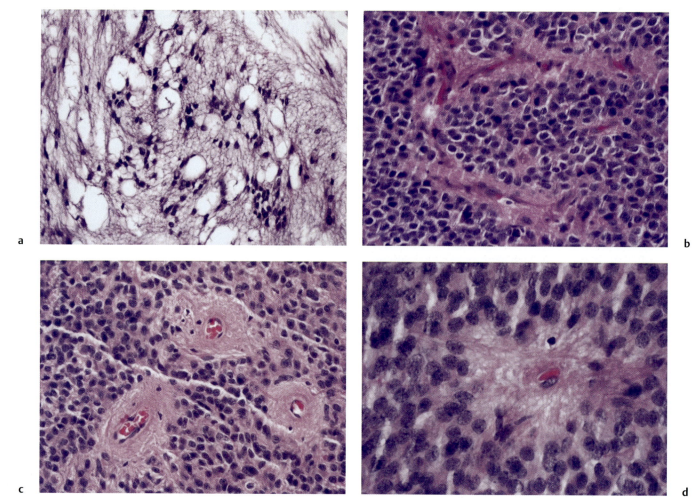

Fig. 2.5a–d Ependymoma histopathology. **(a)** Nuclear clusters in a fibrillary background with microcysts are typical of subependymoma. **(b)** Typical ependymoma. **(c)** Nuclear-free areas around three vessels (perivascular pseudorosettes) in an ependymoma. **(d)** High-power view of a perivascular pseudorosette.

The current WHO guidelines for grading ependymomas from all locations are based on the predominance of histological features that have been well established as markers of aggressive behavior, including tumor cellularity, cytological anaplasia, mitotic index, microvascular proliferation, and tumor necrosis. Grade III ependymomas have increased cellularity, marked nuclear anaplasia, and more frequent mitoses than grade II tumors. Areas of tumor necrosis as well as microvascular proliferation might be observed in grade III ependymomas. However, these do not have the same prognostic significance in this tumor type as in the adult astrocytic tumor.

With respect to immunohistochemical staining characteristics, most ependymomas show reactivity for GFAP and S-100 protein, consistent with their glial origin. The epithelial membrane antigen (EMA) might be reactive in the luminal aspects of ependymal rosettes, as well as intracytoplasmic "dot-like" staining, which reflects intracytoplasmic microlumina.

Special Consideration

- Gliovascular structuring, forming perivascular pseudorosette-like areas, can be present in some glioblastomas to the extent whereby ependymoma may be considered. In such a case, evidence for a diffusely infiltrating tumor (characteristic of astrocytic tumors but not ependymal tumors) should be sought.

The prognostic implications of clinical factors, including age at diagnosis, site of origin, and extent of tumor resection, have been well established. Chromosomally based CGH studies of ependymoma have demonstrated deletions of chromosome 22 in adult spinal tumors, and a significant proportion of these are known to have homozygous inactivation of the chromosome 22–localized *NF2* gene.[17] Comparative genomic hybridization has also demonstrated gain of 1q and homozygous deletion of cyclin-dependent kinase inhibitor 2A (*CDKN2A*) as independent indicators of unfavorable prognosis, whereas gains of chromosomes 9, 15q, and 18 and loss of chromosome 6 were associated with increased survival.[18] On gene expression profiling, ependymomas arising in the posterior fossa were clearly distinguished from ependymomas arising in the cerebral hemispheres,[19] a finding that might also be reflected in the differences in prognostically significant histological features in ependymomas arising in these two distinct compartments.[20]

Transcriptional profiling studies have described stereotypic genetic alterations that have helped identify two clinically distinct subgroups among posterior fossa ependymomas.[21] The first shows a largely balanced genomic profile, and was characterized by alterations involving numerous cancer-related networks, such as angiogenesis (Hypoxia-inducible factor-1a (HIF-1a) signaling, vascular endothelial growth factor (VEGF) signaling, cell migration), platelet-derived growth factor (PDGF) signaling, mitogen-activated protein kinase (MAPK) signaling, epidermal growth factor receptor (EGFR) signaling, transforming growth factor-β (TGF-β) signaling, integrin signaling, extracellular matrix assembly, tyrosine-receptor kinase signaling, and RAS/small guanosine triphosphatase (GTPase) signaling. These tumors tended to be more laterally located and were more likely to show invasive growth into the cerebellum, to occur in children, and to have a higher incidence of recurrence and mortality. In contrast, the tumors in the second group exhibited numerous cytogenetic abnormalities involving whole chromosomes or chromosomal arms, and were characterized by alterations in genes involved in microtubule assembly and oxidative metabolism. These tumors occurred predominantly in a more central location, in older patients, and were associated with better outcomes.

Diffusely Infiltrating Gliomas

Diffuse Astrocytomas

Diffuse astrocytic tumors are identified by the presence of abnormal, irregular, elongated nuclei. As per the current WHO guidelines, their grades of malignancy range from grade II to IV, with glioblastoma (GBM) being classified as a grade IV diffuse astrocytoma. The peak age incidence for these tumors parallels their malignancy progression, with the grade II tumors most commonly observed in individuals 25 to 50 years of age, and the glioblastomas showing peak incidence between 45 and 70 years. All are more common in males and most are located in the cerebral hemispheres. The relevance of the histologically based malignancy grading scheme is indicated by patient survival, with grade II astrocytoma patients having an average survival of approximately 7 years, grade III patients surviving about half as long, and GBM patients surviving approximately a year on average.

In general, increasing proliferative activity is associated with more aggressive behavior among diffuse astrocytomas.

Pearl

- Diffuse astrocytomas, WHO grade II, show a slight to moderate increase in cellularity as compared to the normal brain parenchyma. Mitotic figures are inconspicuous.
- Anaplastic astrocytomas, WHO grade III, show increasing cellularity, may show more nuclear atypia, and contain multiple identifiable mitoses (**Fig 2.6a,b**).
- Glioblastoma, WHO grade IV, is diagnosed by the presence of either tumor necrosis or microvascular proliferation. Tumor necrosis is not an absolute requirement for the diagnosis of GBM, and the presence of microvascular proliferation in a high-grade astrocytoma is sufficient. In practice, the majority of GBMs contain both tumor necrosis and microvascular proliferation.

Although clinically important, the histological distinction between grade II and grade III astrocytoma (**Fig. 2.6c,d**) is not well defined in the current WHO classification scheme and therefore is subject to some interobserver variability. Further, identification and scoring of mitoses can be subject to inaccuracies due to variation in tumor cellularity as well as technical artifacts.

Use of IHC markers of proliferation and mitotic activity might help in this regard.[14] Ki-67 is a labile, non-histone nuclear protein that is expressed in the G1 through M phases of the cell cycle. MIB-1 is a monoclonal antibody directed against the Ki-67 protein in formalin-fixed, paraffin-embedded tissues. Proliferating cells show strong nuclear staining for Ki-67/MIB-1, and widespread labeling among tumor cells is indicative of rapid proliferation.

During mitosis, histone H3, one of five histone proteins, is specifically phosphorylated at the serine 10 residue during chromatin condensation. The antibody to serine 10-phosphorylated histone H3 (pHH3) is a reliable and robust marker of mitoses and allows for the additional morphological validation of mitotic figures that are stained.[22] Among diffuse gliomas, the pHH3 staining has been shown to correlate well with the Ki-67/MIB-1 labeling index as well as other markers of proliferation.[23,24]

These markers have been shown to be significantly correlated with proliferative activity among grades II and III diffuse astrocytomas and to patient outcomes,[23–25] and uniform application of these markers may help to assess more accu-

Controversy

- It is agreed that the distinction of WHO grade II from WHO grade III (anaplastic) astrocytoma is based on mitotic activity. However, there is a lack of consensus as to the actual number of mitoses required to make the diagnosis of anaplastic astrocytoma.

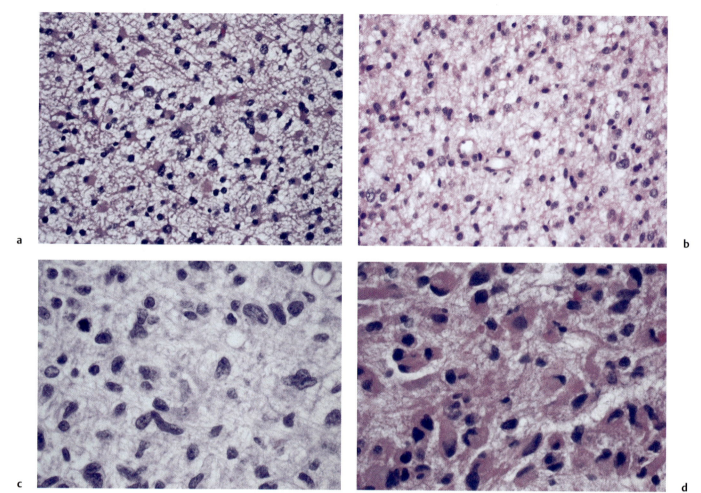

Fig. 2.6a–d Astrocytoma and anaplastic astrocytoma histopathology. **(a)** Irregular nuclei in a low-grade (grade II) infiltrating astrocytoma. **(b)** A random, patternless distribution of nuclei as seen in this astrocytoma (grade II) distinguishes it from reactive astrogliosis.

(c) Regularly elongate nuclei and mitotic activity (*upper left*) in an anaplastic (grade III) astrocytoma. **(d)** Gemistocytes (cells with prominent eosinophilic cytoplasm) in an anaplastic astrocytoma.

rately the proliferative activity and potential for biological aggressiveness among these tumors. However, other studies have failed to find a similar correlation on multivariate analysis, after taking into account clinical parameters known to be associated with patient survival.[26]

Further, variability in staining and counting techniques between laboratories renders establishing standardized cutoff values for the purpose of reproducible grading challenging.[27] Among these two markers, because pHH3 relies on both positive staining of morphologically identifiable mitosis, it has some theoretical advantage as compared to MIB-1 as a proliferation marker.

Proliferative activity, cellularity atypia, and pleomorphism are features all further accentuated in GBM, whose classification additionally requires tumor necrosis with pseudopalisading of tumor cells or endothelial cell proliferation (**Fig. 2.7**). Although the immunohistochemistry-based proliferation index may still be used in grade II to III astrocytomas, it has not shown clinical utility in GBM.

> **Key Concept**
>
> - Two clinically distinct types of GBM have long been identified, based on the initial presentation of the patient. "Secondary" (progressive) GBM arises from a previously diagnosed lower grade diffusely infiltrative astrocytoma. In contrast, "primary" or de novo GBM is fully evolved at the initial presentation, without the prior history of a lower grade astrocytoma.

Oligodendrogliomas and Oligoastrocytomas

Oligodendrogliomas occur mainly in the cerebral hemispheres of adults. They consist of moderately cellular, monomorphic tumors with round nuclei, often with artifactual perinuclear clear cytoplasm on formalin-fixed paraffin-embedded sections (**Fig. 2.8a,b**). Additional characteristic histological features of

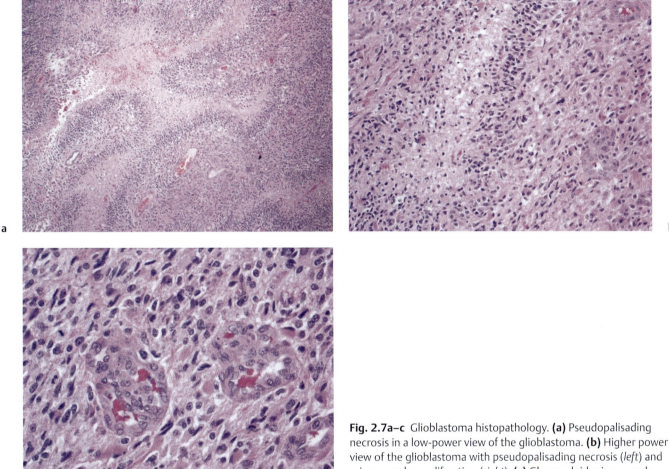

Fig. 2.7a–c Glioblastoma histopathology. **(a)** Pseudopalisading necrosis in a low-power view of the glioblastoma. **(b)** Higher power view of the glioblastoma with pseudopalisading necrosis (*left*) and microvascular proliferation (*right*). **(c)** Glomeruloid microvascular proliferation in a glioblastoma.

oligodendrogliomas include an intricate network of thin-walled blood vessels in a "chicken-wire" pattern, areas of microcystic change, and microcalcifications.

Although mitoses might be more readily found in oligodendroglioma than in diffuse astrocytoma, the presence of relatively few mitotic figures, the absence of microvascular proliferation, and the absence of necrosis correspond to WHO grade II. These WHO grade II oligodendrogliomas are relatively indolent, although they usually recur at the primary site and may display subependymal spread with cerebrospinal fluid (CSF) seeding. Increasing nuclear pleomorphism and hyperchromatism, and areas with pronounced hypercellularity, brisk mitotic activity, prominent microvascular proliferation, or tumor necrosis correspond to anaplastic oligodendroglioma (WHO grade III; **Fig. 2.8c**). Since 1990, when combination chemotherapy [procarbazine + chloroethyl-cyclohexyl-nitro-sourea (CCNU/lomustine) + vincristine (PCV)] was demonstrated to occasionally result in dramatic oligodendroglioma response, the identification of an oligodendroglial component in glial tumors has become extremely important for therapeutic decision making.

Oligoastrocytomas are composed of cells with astrocytic and oligodendroglial morphological features. Tumor cells with these morphologies can be diffusely admixed or exist in discrete areas of the tumor. The criteria suggested by the WHO guidelines to distinguish lower grade (grade II) oligoastrocytomas from anaplastic (grade III) oligoastrocytomas are similar to the criteria used to grade oligodendrogliomas. The use of the term *oligoastrocytoma* in diagnostic neuropathology is somewhat controversial because some neuropathologists regard it as a "wastebasket" diagnosis, rather than a distinct clinicopathological entity. But it is common to find this diag-

Pitfall

- Although perinuclear halos are characteristic of oligodendroglioma, they are not pathognomonic. The finding of irregular, pleomorphic nuclei in an infiltrating glioma nearly always suggests astrocytoma, even if perinuclear halos are present.

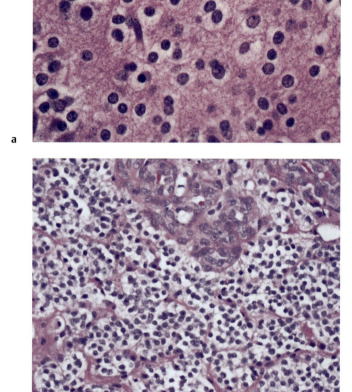

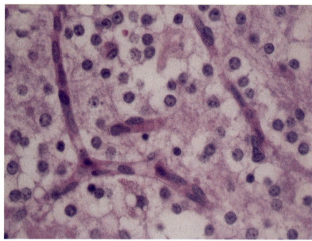

a

b

c

Fig. 2.8 Oligodendroglioma histopathology. **(a)** Round, uniform nuclei in an oligodendroglioma. **(b)** Delicate branching ("chicken wire") vasculature in a low-grade oligodendroglioma. **(c)** Microvascular proliferation in an anaplastic oligodendroglioma.

Controversy

- The diagnosis of oligoastrocytoma is the subject of much discussion among neuropathologists. Although some neuropathologists use this term frequently to describe low- to intermediate-grade infiltrating gliomas of indeterminate histology, others feel that this represents a "wastebasket" diagnosis and should be used rarely, if ever.

nostic term used for tumors with histological features that are intermediate between astrocytoma and oligodendroglioma.

Both grade II and grade III oligodendrogliomas show relatively specific genetic abnormalities that differ from those of other gliomas. Combined deletions of the short arm of chromosome 1 (1p) and the long arm of chromosome 19 (19q) have been found in a majority of oligodendroglioma.[28] The combined 1p/19q loss is strongly correlated with longer progression free survival and is an independent predictor of response to chemotherapy.[29,30] Although tightly correlated with

oligodendroglial histology, concurrent loss of the entire 1p and 19q may occasionally be identified among diffuse gliomas that lack characteristic features of oligodendroglioma.[31] In contrast, partial deletions of 1p or 19q may be identified in diffuse astrocytoma and GBM, but do not appear to be associated with improved overall survival.

The losses of chromosomal arms 1p and 19q have been associated with an unbalanced pericentromeric translocation that produces the derivative chromosome der (1; 19) (q10; p10).[32] The other derivative chromosome may not be formed or may be unstable, leading to a net concurrent loss of the 1p and 19q chromosomal arms. A recent deep sequencing study

---

Pearl

- Combined 1p/19q loss has been associated with classic histological features of an oligodendroglioma. Histologically diagnosed oligodendrogliomas without classic features are often intact for 1p/19q.

Special Consideration

- Combined 1p/19q loss in anaplastic oligodendroglioma is associated with improved outcome, and 1p/19q-intact anaplastic oligodendroglioma has a clinical behavior similar to that of anaplastic astrocytoma. This raises the possibility that this molecular marker may supersede morphological considerations for treatment decisions in the setting of anaplastic glioma in the future.

found inactivating mutations of the *FUBP1* gene (encoding far upstream element [FUSE] binding protein) on 1p and *CIC* gene (homolog of the *Drosophila* gene *capicua*) on 19q in a significant proportion of oligodendrogliomas.[33] In particular, *CIC* mutations appear to be correlated with classic oligodendroglioma morphology, 1p/19q co-deletion, and *IDH1* mutations, and are rare in tumors that lack the co-deletion.[34] Oligodendroglioma malignant progression is associated with additional genetic abnormalities similar to those described for the astrocytic tumors, especially those affecting Rb1 and p53 protein function.[35]

Oligoastrocytomas (low grade and anaplastic) tend to have aberrant genetic patterns similar either to the oligodendroglial tumors or to the diffuse astrocytomas[28]; as yet there are no specific abnormalities associated with these mixed glial tumors.

Common Molecular Alterations in Diffuse Gliomas

The molecular methods of choice in the 1980s and 1990s, although of low throughput and, in relation to current approaches, of low data yield, were nonetheless informative regarding the molecular genetics of malignant adult astrocytomas. For the grade II astrocytomas, these methods revealed loss of alleles on 17p, including the *TP53* locus. The p53 protein is a tumor suppressor that is involved in cell cycle arrest in G1 phase and initiation of apoptosis. Mutations of the *TP53* gene result in nonfunctional p53 protein, and have been identified in lower grade astrocytomas and in the secondary GBMs that evolve from these.[36–38] Although normally the p53 protein is labile, *TP53* mutations might result in more stable forms of the p53 protein, which might be detected by immunohistochemical staining.[39] On integrating genomic findings, the p53 pathway appears to be disrupted in a majority of GBMs,[40] either directly or through alterations in MDM2 (murine double minute 2) and INK4A-ARF (inhibitor of cyclin-dependent kinase 4a–alternative reading frame).[41–43]

Mutations of the *TP53* gene and the expression of the p53 protein have not been definitely correlated with prognosis or with response to therapy.[36] However, recent data suggest that p53 overexpression may be associated with improved progression-free survival among patients receiving prolonged therapy with adjuvant temozolomide.[44]

The nicotinamide adenine dinucleotide phosphate (NADP)-dependent isocitrate dehydrogenase-1, -2, and -3 enzymes (IDH1, IDH2 and IDH3) catalyze the oxidative decarboxylation of isocitrate to α-ketoglutarate in the citric acid cycle. The IDH1 enzyme is found in the cytoplasm and peroxisomes, and the *IDH1* gene is located at 2q33.3. The IDH2 enzyme is found in mitochondria, and the *IDH2* gene is located on 15q26.1. Mutations of these genes were initially observed among a small percentage of GBMs.[45] Subsequently, *IDH1/IDH2* mutations have been observed in a large proportion of WHO grade II and III diffuse gliomas and secondary GBMs in multiple data sets.[40,46–48] Mutations in *IDH3* have not been described.

In gliomas, these are almost exclusively point mutations, resulting in substitution of arginine at residue 132 of IDH1 (R132), or at residue 172 of IDH2 (R172).[47,49] The *IDH* mutations are associated with a younger age at presentation, with *IDH1* mutations being more common. Mutations involving *IDH2* are more frequently present in oligodendrogliomas than in diffuse astrocytomas, and the vast majority of diffuse gliomas with combined deletion of chromosomal arms 1p and 19q also show mutations in either IDH1 or IDH2.[47] In addition to aiding diagnosis of diffuse gliomas, *IDH* mutations have also been shown to be associated with clinical outcome. The effect of *IDH* mutation status on the response to chemotherapy has yet to be fully established.

The *IDH* mutation status of diffuse gliomas is conserved before the development of other aberrations during tumor progression from a lower to a higher grade, suggesting that this is an early event during glioma genesis.[50] The *IDH* mutations have been shown to repress lineage-specific cell differentiation by impairing histone demethylation, particularly of histone H3, via increased 2-hydroxyglutarate, supporting the role of these mutations as tumor-initiating events.[51,52] However, these mutations are rarely identified in pediatric gliomas, suggesting an alternative pathway may be involved in their evolution.

Whole exome sequencing of pediatric GBMs revealed recurrent mutations in genes coding for regulatory proteins that participate in chromatin remodeling: *H3F3A* (which encodes the replication-independent histone variant H3.3), *ATRX,* and *DAXX*.[53] Mutations in these genes and *IDH1* mutations appear to be mutually exclusive. These *H3F3A-ATRX-DAXX* mutations appear to be more prevalent in GBMs from pediatric, adolescent, and young-adult patients, and have not yet been identified in adult GBMs.

Key Concepts

- The *IDH* mutations are not seen in other types of common CNS tumors, and may help distinguish diffuse gliomas from other CNS tumors and nonneoplastic mimics.
- The *IDH* mutations are not seen in primary GBMs. The presence of an *IDH* mutation may practically be considered a key distinction between primary and secondary GBMs.

The most common *IDH* mutation involves *IDH1*, wherein adenine replaces guanine (G395A), resulting in histidine replacing arginine at position 132 (R132H). Immunohistochemistry (IHC) utilizing a mutation-specific mouse monoclonal antibody has been demonstrated to have high specificity and sensitivity for detecting the IDH1R132H mutant protein in histological sections from formalin-fixed paraffin-embedded tissue.[46,54,55]

Diffuse astrocytomas frequently show alterations in receptor tyrosine kinases and their downstream pathways. Amplification of the *EGFR*, located on chromosome 7p12, is the most prevalent such abnormality in GBMs.[40] A high level of EGFR amplification appears to be a late event during the tumorigenesis of GBMs.[56] Frequently, there is an associated mutant variant of EGFR, which is characterized by deletion of exons 2 to 7—the EGFR variant III (EGFR vIII).[57] This leads to ligand-independent constitutive activation of EGFR, resulting in persistent activation of the downstream PI3K signaling pathway. Activation of the EGFR-mediated signaling pathway has been observed in a small percentage of lower grade diffuse gliomas as well. Although EGFR overexpression and the presence of EGFR vIII have been reported as indicators of poor prognosis in anaplastic astrocytoma and GBM,[58,59] their association with patient outcomes remains to be further clarified.

The gene for the DNA-repair enzyme O-6-methylguanine-DNA methyltransferase (MGMT) is located on chromosome 10q26. Its promoter region contains 97 CG-dinucleotide (CpG)-rich sites, which are unmethylated in normal tissues. In tumors, however, the cytosine in these CpG-rich sites may become methylated, leading to binding of proteins to the DNA, altering the chromatin structure and preventing the binding of transcription factors, eventually causing silencing of *MGMT* expression. The effect of *MGMT* promoter methylation and silencing has been shown to be associated with response to alkylating chemotherapeutic agents that damage DNA by methylating the O-6 position of the guanine,[60] as well as radiation therapy.[61] It appears that *MGMT* silencing helps identify a subset of patients with high-grade gliomas and glioblastomas in whom adjuvant chemotherapy may significantly prolong overall survival at initial diagnosis[62] as well as at recurrence.[63]

The analysis of *MGMT*-promoter methylation appears to be a more reliable predictor of susceptibility and the prognosis of GBM than are MGMT protein and gene expression levels.[64] As a note of caution, different testing methodologies might not have reproducible results,[65,66] and the optimal technique to reliably identify the methylation status needs to be defined in order to reduce variability in the results from different laboratories.

Overall, *MGMT*-promoter methylation status appears to be, at least partially, a marker of better prognosis in high-grade astrocytoma and GBM,[62] and also might help identify patients who may benefit from radiation therapy and alkylating chemotherapy.[60-64] However, its imprecise correlation with the response to therapy suggests the presence of other prognostic and predictive genetic mechanisms in GBMs. The role of *MGMT* status in lower grade (grade II–III) astrocytomas is less clear.

The strength of the comprehensive molecular screening techniques is their generating thousands of data fields for each specimen analyzed, and from these data fields the ability to identify patterns or "fingerprints" associated with a clinical or biological property of interest (**Fig. 2.1**). This was exemplified by The Cancer Genome Atlas (TCGA) project recently identifying a distinct subset of gliomas that displays concerted hypermethylation at a large number of loci.[67] The presence of such a glioma-CpG island methylator phenotype (G-CIMP) was found to be significantly more prevalent among lower grade gliomas, particularly oligodendrogliomas, than among GBMs.[67,68] Patients with G-CIMP–positive tumors have been found to be younger at the time of diagnosis, and appear to have a significantly better survival on multivariate analysis, after adjusting for patient age, recurrence, and primary/secondary GBM status. The G-CIMP–positive status appears to be a better predictor of survival than *MGMT* methylation status alone,[69] and also appears to be correlated with improved patient outcome within each WHO grade. Whether positive or negative, the G-CIMP status appears to be retained at recurrence, suggesting the G-CIMP phenotype is stable over time and might be critical for tumor formation and maintenance.[67]

Among GBMs, *IDH* mutations appear to be strongly associated with a G-CIMP–positive status.[67,68,70] Indeed, the *IDH1* mutation might even be the molecular basis for gliomas acquiring a G-CIMP phenotype.[52] Further, a small proportion of G-CIMP–positive but *IDH1*–wild-type GBMs appear to have prolonged overall survival, suggesting that the G-CIMP–positive status may be an independent indicator of good prognosis.[67]

At present, there appear to be few genetic landmarks that are frequent among adult diffuse gliomas and that have

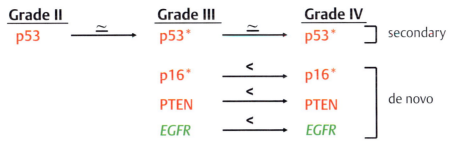

Fig. 2.9 Secondary and de novo glioblastoma. Diagram illustrates the genetic as well as the clinical distinction between the two classes of glioblastoma (GBM). Secondary GBMs are thought to arise from lower malignancy grade precursor gliomas and show similar frequency of p53 alterations as have been reported in grade II and grade III astrocytomas. De novo GBMs occur without known origin from a lower malignancy grade precursor, have infrequent mutation of p53, and have increased incidence of p16, Phosphatase and tensin homolog (PTEN), and *EGFR* alterations. Approximately 20% of grade III astrocytomas have gene alterations similar to those in GBMs, and these tumors generally display aggressive clinical behavior similar to that of GBMs. The asterisk is to alert the reader to the correct gene names for p53 and p16, which are *TP53* and *CDKN2A*, respectively. Alterations in red text involve tumor suppressor genes; green text indicates an oncogene alteration.

shown some utility in their classification (**Fig. 2.9**). These include the identification of *IDH* mutation in distinguishing primary GBM from secondary and lower grade diffuse gliomas, at the concurrent deletion of chromosomal arms 1p and 19q in distinguishing oligodendrogliomas from diffuse astrocytomas. Differences in the gene expression profiles between GBMs and lower grade diffuse gliomas have been well established, leading to various individual markers being associated with poor patient outcomes. Exploring global gene expression patterns to determine prognosis among diffuse gliomas has yielded two to four major subtypes in various studies, based on variations in patterns of DNA methylation, chromosomal copy numbers, DNA sequence alterations, and proteomic markers of signaling pathways.[71–75]

In 2006, three high-grade astrocytoma groups were defined based on the differential expression of prognostic markers, termed "proneural," "proliferative," and "mesenchymal," based on the predominant profiles of the molecular signatures identified within each group.[74] The proneural group was characterized by alterations in markers associated with neurogenesis, and was associated with the most favorable outcome. The proliferative group demonstrated alterations in markers of cellular proliferation and the mesenchymal group expressed markers found in tissues of mesenchymal origin. The GBMs in the proliferative group had elevated Ki-67/MIB-1 proliferation indices, and those in the mesenchymal group demonstrated increased angiogenesis. Both these groups were associated with worse outcomes than the proneural group.

Integrated genomic analysis of the TCGA data set demonstrated four GBM expression subtypes similar to those identified in the above-mentioned study. These were termed proneural, neural, mesenchymal, and classic.[75] Of these four, the most reproducibly identifiable subtypes are proneural and mesenchymal. The proneural subtype was strongly associated with *IDH1* mutations or PDGFRA amplification. The mesenchymal subtype was associated with loss or mutation of *NF1*, and the classic subtype was associated with *EGFR* amplifica-

> **Key Concept**
>
> - Proneural and mesenchymal phenotypes appear to show some consensus among a variety of investigators. The proneural signature is more frequently identified in lower grade gliomas and secondary GBMs. The mesenchymal signature is strongly associated with primary/de novo GBMs.

tion or mutations. The majority of G-CIMP tumors were also found to belong to the proneural subgroup on DNA methylation profiling.[67] Although the subgroups and the G-CIMP status were not perfectly concordant, among the proneural subgroup, G-CIMP–negative tumors were found to be similar to GBMs in the mesenchymal subgroup, whereas G-CIMP–positive tumors were distinct from this subgroup. Further, within the proneural subgroup, G-CIMP–positive patients had longer survival than G-CIMP–negative patients. The classical subtype demonstrated high rates of EGFR alterations and lack of TP53 mutations. The neural subtype was characterized by expression of genes that were typically expressed in neurons and were related to neuronal function, such as neuron projection and axon and synaptic transmission.

A meta-analysis compiling and comparing the results of these two studies found a strong agreement in the assignment of samples to the proneural and mesenchymal subgroups, indicating robust reproducibility in subcategorizing diffuse gliomas in this manner.[76]

As yet there is no consensus on the type and number of expression-based glioma subtypes, further complicated by the extent of overlap with the status of other prognostic molecular signatures, such as the status of *IDH* mutations, 1p/19q co-deletion, *MGMT* promoter methylation, and G-CIMP status. This may be a reflection of the multiple mechanisms that may be responsible for the heterogeneity in the clinical behavior of diffuse gliomas.

■ Conclusion

The goal of histopathologists is analyze the tissue received, so as to provide clinicians with as much useful information as possible, informing them of all the details of any pathological process present, forming the basis for accurate prognosis, and aiding the choice of the most appropriate treatment. Until recently this process was based mainly on morphological analysis that was occasionally accompanied with limited IHC information. However, as different forms of treatment become increasingly directed at specific molecular targets, the analysis of the specimens received must be extended to provide relevant data. This is, in fact, already occurring through the application of technologies for the comprehensive analysis of tumor genomes, transcriptomes, and proteomes. With the recent examples of molecularly defined subsets of various tumors responding to treatment with targeted therapies, there is good reason for optimism about the movement toward individualized therapies for improved outcomes for individuals afflicted with CNS cancer.

Editor's Note

For years we have relied on standard histology to make a diagnosis of a tumor, and one of the more striking aspects of this reliance is that there is a great deal of interobserver variability among neuropathologists. However, in the last several decades molecular techniques were used to uncover the specific aspects of these tumors that can be differentiated from one another. A lot of our current information was facilitated by the techniques used in the Human Genome Project that enabled researchers to perform genomic profiling on tumor DNA. Expression profiling also improved so that various messenger RNA sequences could be identified in tumor tissues. Recently there has been a great deal of success in developing high-throughput sequencing techniques such as in the form of next-generation sequencing. Overall these technologies have been fundamentally critical in allowing us to build expression profiles of different tumors and most importantly determine how these tumors are going to behave in the patient. The Cancer Genome Atlas study has proven highly useful in the field of neuro-oncology; for example, it has allowed clinicians to focus on the three most commonly aberrant pathways known in high-grade tumors namely p53, PI3K, and Rb. Now that we have a number of these pathways identified, we need to pick up the pace with regard to the development of therapeutic modalities that, it is hoped, can result in a more chronic and indolent clinical course for our patients. (Berger)

References

1. Stearns D, Chaudhry A, Abel TW, Burger PC, Dang CV, Eberhart CG. c-myc overexpression causes anaplasia in medulloblastoma. Cancer Res 2006;66:673–681

2. Bunt J, Hasselt NE, Zwijnenburg DA, et al. OTX2 directly activates cell cycle genes and inhibits differentiation in medulloblastoma cells. Int J Cancer 2012;131:E21–E32

3. Hui AB, Takano H, Lo KW, et al. Identification of a novel homozygous deletion region at 6q23.1 in medulloblastomas using high-resolution array comparative genomic hybridization analysis. Clin Cancer Res 2005;11:4707–4716

4. Mendrzyk F, Radlwimmer B, Joos S, et al. Genomic and protein expression profiling identifies CDK6 as novel independent prognostic marker in medulloblastoma. J Clin Oncol 2005;23:8853–8862

5. Pomeroy SL, Tamayo P, Gaasenbeek M, et al. Prediction of central nervous system embryonal tumour outcome based on gene expression. Nature 2002;415:436–442

6. Taylor MD, Northcott PA, Korshunov A, et al. Molecular subgroups of medulloblastoma: the current consensus. Acta Neuropathol 2012;123:465–472

7. Schwalbe EC, Williamson D, Lindsey JC, et al. DNA methylation profiling of medulloblastoma allows robust subclassification and improved outcome prediction using formalin-fixed biopsies. Acta Neuropathol 2013;125:359–371

8. Raabe EH, Lim KS, Kim JM, et al. BRAF activation induces transformation and then senescence in human neural stem cells: a pilocytic astrocytoma model. Clin Cancer Res 2011;17:3590–3599

9. Sanoudou D, Tingby O, Ferguson-Smith MA, Collins VP, Coleman N. Analysis of pilocytic astrocytoma by comparative genomic hybridization. Br J Cancer 2000;82:1218–1222

10. Bar EE, Lin A, Tihan T, Burger PC, Eberhart CG. Frequent gains at chromosome 7q34 involving BRAF in pilocytic astrocytoma. J Neuropathol Exp Neurol 2008;67:878–887

11. Cin H, Meyer C, Herr R, et al. Oncogenic FAM131B-BRAF fusion resulting from 7q34 deletion comprises an alternative mechanism of MAPK pathway activation in pilocytic astrocytoma. Acta Neuropathol 2011;121:763–774

12. Jones DT, Kocialkowski S, Liu L, Pearson DM, Ichimura K, Collins VP. Oncogenic RAF1 rearrangement and a novel BRAF mutation as alternatives to KIAA1549:BRAF fusion in activating the MAPK pathway in pilocytic astrocytoma. Oncogene 2009;28:2119–2123

13. Gronych J, Korshunov A, Bageritz J, et al. An activated mutant BRAF kinase domain is sufficient to induce pilocytic astrocytoma in mice. J Clin Invest 2011;121:1344–1348

14. Yeo YH, Byrne NP, Counelis GJ, Perry A. Adult with cerebellar anaplastic pilocytic astrocytoma associated with BRAF V600E mutation and p16 loss. Clin Neuropathol 2013;32:159–164

15. Schindler G, Capper D, Meyer J, et al. Analysis of BRAF V600E mutation in 1,320 nervous system tumors reveals high mutation frequencies in pleomorphic xanthoastrocytoma, ganglioglioma and extra-cerebellar pilocytic astrocytoma. Acta Neuropathol 2011;121:397–405

16. Jeon YK, Cheon JE, Kim SK, Wang KC, Cho BK, Park SH. Clinicopathological features and global genomic copy number alterations of pilomyxoid astrocytoma in the hypothalamus/optic pathway: comparative analysis with pilocytic astrocytoma using array-based comparative genomic hybridization. Mod Pathol 2008;21:1345–1356

17. Ward S, Harding B, Wilkins P, et al. Gain of 1q and loss of 22 are the most common changes detected by comparative genomic hybridisa-

tion in paediatric ependymoma. Genes Chromosomes Cancer 2001; 32:59–66

18. Korshunov A, Witt H, Hielscher T, et al. Molecular staging of intracranial ependymoma in children and adults. J Clin Oncol 2010;28:3182–3190

19. Johnson RA, Wright KD, Poppleton H, et al. Cross-species genomics matches driver mutations and cell compartments to model ependymoma. Nature 2010;466:632–636

20. Raghunathan A, Wani K, Armstrong TS, et al; Collaborative Ependymoma Research Network. Histological predictors of outcome in ependymoma are dependent on anatomic site within the central nervous system. Brain Pathol 2013;23:584–594

21. Witt H, Mack SC, Ryzhova M, et al. Delineation of two clinically and molecularly distinct subgroups of posterior fossa ependymoma. Cancer Cell 2011;20:143–157

22. Tapia C, Kutzner H, Mentzel T, Savic S, Baumhoer D, Glatz K. Two mitosis-specific antibodies, MPM-2 and phospho-histone H3 (Ser28), allow rapid and precise determination of mitotic activity. Am J Surg Pathol 2006;30:83–89

23. Colman H, Giannini C, Huang L, et al. Assessment and prognostic significance of mitotic index using the mitosis marker phospho-histone H3 in low and intermediate-grade infiltrating astrocytomas. Am J Surg Pathol 2006;30:657–664

24. Habberstad AH, Gulati S, Torp SH. Evaluation of the proliferation markers Ki-67/MIB-1, mitosin, survivin, pHH3, and DNA topoisomerase IIa in human anaplastic astrocytomas—an immunohistochemical study. Diagn Pathol 2011;6:43

25. Giannini C, Scheithauer BW, Burger PC, et al. Cellular proliferation in pilocytic and diffuse astrocytomas. J Neuropathol Exp Neurol 1999; 58:46–53

26. Rodríguez-Pereira C, Suárez-Peñaranda JM, Vázquez-Salvado M, et al. Value of MIB-1 labelling index (LI) in gliomas and its correlation with other prognostic factors. A clinicopathologic study. J Neurosurg Sci 2000;44:203–209, discussion 209–210

27. Hsu CY, Ho DM, Yang CF, Chiang H. Interobserver reproducibility of MIB-1 labeling index in astrocytic tumors using different counting methods. Mod Pathol 2003;16:951–957

28. Reifenberger J, Reifenberger G, Liu L, James CD, Wechsler W, Collins VP. Molecular genetic analysis of oligodendroglial tumors shows preferential allelic deletions on 19q and 1p. Am J Pathol 1994;145:1175–1190

29. Mikkelsen T, Doyle T, Anderson J, et al. Temozolomide single-agent chemotherapy for newly diagnosed anaplastic oligodendroglioma. J Neurooncol 2009;92:57–63

30. Thiessen B, Maguire JA, McNeil K, Huntsman D, Martin MA, Horsman D. Loss of heterozygosity for loci on chromosome arms 1p and 10q in oligodendroglial tumors: relationship to outcome and chemosensitivity. J Neurooncol 2003;64:271–278

31. Vogazianou AP, Chan R, Bäcklund LM, et al. Distinct patterns of 1p and 19q alterations identify subtypes of human gliomas that have different prognoses. Neuro-oncol 2010;12:664–678

32. Jenkins RB, Blair H, Ballman KV, et al. A t(1;19)(q10;p10) mediates the combined deletions of 1p and 19q and predicts a better prognosis of patients with oligodendroglioma. Cancer Res 2006;66:9852–9861

33. Bettegowda C, Agrawal N, Jiao Y, et al. Mutations in CIC and FUBP1 contribute to human oligodendroglioma. Science 2011;333:1453–1455

34. Yip S, Butterfield YS, Morozova O, et al. Concurrent CIC mutations, IDH mutations, and 1p/19q loss distinguish oligodendrogliomas from other cancers. J Pathol 2012;226:7–16

35. Watanabe T, Yokoo H, Yokoo M, Yonekawa Y, Kleihues P, Ohgaki H. Concurrent inactivation of RB1 and TP53 pathways in anaplastic oligodendrogliomas. J Neuropathol Exp Neurol 2001;60:1181–1189

36. Kraus JA, Wenghoefer M, Glesmann N, et al. TP53 gene mutations, nuclear p53 accumulation, expression of Waf/p21, Bcl-2, and CD95

(APO-1/Fas) proteins are not prognostic factors in de novo glioblastoma multiforme. J Neurooncol 2001;52:263–272

37. Louis DN, von Deimling A, Chung RY, et al. Comparative study of p53 gene and protein alterations in human astrocytic tumors. J Neuropathol Exp Neurol 1993;52:31–38

38. von Deimling A, Eibl RH, Ohgaki H, et al. p53 mutations are associated with 17p allelic loss in grade II and grade III astrocytoma. Cancer Res 1992;52:2987–2990

39. Lotfi M, Afsharnezhad S, Raziee HR, et al. Immunohistochemical assessment of MGMT expression and p53 mutation in glioblastoma multiforme. Tumori 2011;97:104–108

40. Comprehensive Genomic Characterization Defines Human Glioblastoma Genes and Core Pathways. Nature 2008;455:1061–1068

41. Hede SM, Nazarenko I, Nistér M, Lindström MS. Novel perspectives on p53 function in neural stem cells and brain tumors. J Oncol 2011; 2011:852970

42. Kumar M, Lu Z, Takwi AA, et al. Negative regulation of the tumor suppressor p53 gene by microRNAs. Oncogene 2011;30:843–853

43. Sato A, Sunayama J, Matsuda K, et al. MEK-ERK signaling dictates DNA-repair gene MGMT expression and temozolomide resistance of stem-like glioblastoma cells via the MDM2-p53 axis. Stem Cells 2011; 29:1942–1951

44. Malkoun N, Chargari C, Forest F, et al. Prolonged temozolomide for treatment of glioblastoma: preliminary clinical results and prognostic value of p53 overexpression. J Neurooncol 2012;106:127–133

45. Parsons DW, Jones S, Zhang X, et al. An integrated genomic analysis of human glioblastoma multiforme. Science 2008;321:1807–1812

46. Capper D, Reuss D, Schittenhelm J, et al. Mutation-specific IDH1 antibody differentiates oligodendrogliomas and oligoastrocytomas from other brain tumors with oligodendroglioma-like morphology. Acta Neuropathol 2011;121:241–252

47. Hartmann C, Meyer J, Balss J, et al. Type and frequency of IDH1 and IDH2 mutations are related to astrocytic and oligodendroglial differentiation and age: a study of 1,010 diffuse gliomas. Acta Neuropathol 2009;118:469–474

48. Ichimura K, Pearson DM, Kocialkowski S, et al. IDH1 mutations are present in the majority of common adult gliomas but rare in primary glioblastomas. Neuro-oncol 2009;11:341–347

49. Yan H, Parsons DW, Jin G, et al. IDH1 and IDH2 mutations in gliomas. N Engl J Med 2009;360:765–773

50. Watanabe T, Nobusawa S, Kleihues P, Ohgaki H. IDH1 mutations are early events in the development of astrocytomas and oligodendrogliomas. Am J Pathol 2009;174:1149–1153

51. Lu C, Ward PS, KApoor GS et al. IDH mutation impairs histone demethylation and results in a block to cell differentiation. Nature. 2012; 483(7390):474–478.

52. Turcan S, Rohle D, Goenka A et al. IDH1 mutation is sufficient to establish the glima hypermethylator phenotype. Nature. 2012; 483(7390): 479–483.

53. Schwartzentruber J, Korshunov A, Liu XY, et al. Driver mutations in histone H3.3 and chromatin remodelling genes in paediatric glioblastoma. Nature 2012;482:226–231

54. Capper D, Zentgraf H, Balss J, Hartmann C, von Deimling A. Monoclonal antibody specific for IDH1 R132H mutation. Acta Neuropathol 2009; 118:599–601

55. Preusser M, Wöhrer A, Stary S, Höftberger R, Streubel B, Hainfellner JA. Value and limitations of immunohistochemistry and gene sequencing for detection of the IDH1-R132H mutation in diffuse glioma biopsy specimens. J Neuropathol Exp Neurol 2011;70:715–723

56. Attolini CS, Cheng YK, Beroukhim R, et al. A mathematical framework to determine the temporal sequence of somatic genetic events in cancer. Proc Natl Acad Sci U S A 2010;107:17604–17609

57. Sugawa N, Ekstrand AJ, James CD, Collins VP. Identical splicing of aberrant epidermal growth factor receptor transcripts from amplified rearranged genes in human glioblastomas. Proc Natl Acad Sci U S A 1990;87:8602–8606

58. Quaranta M, Divella R, Daniele A, et al. Epidermal growth factor receptor serum levels and prognostic value in malignant gliomas. Tumori 2007;93:275–280

59. Heimberger AB, Hlatky R, Suki D, et al. Prognostic effect of epidermal growth factor receptor and EGFRvIII in glioblastoma multiforme patients. Clin Cancer Res 2005;11:1462–1466

60. Hegi ME, Diserens AC, Gorlia T, et al. MGMT gene silencing and benefit from temozolomide in glioblastoma. N Engl J Med 2005;352:997–1003

61. Rivera AL, Pelloski CE, Gilbert MR, et al. MGMT promoter methylation is predictive of response to radiotherapy and prognostic in the absence of adjuvant alkylating chemotherapy for glioblastoma. Neuro-oncol 2010;12:116–121

62. Olson RA, Brastianos PK, Palma DA. Prognostic and predictive value of epigenetic silencing of MGMT in patients with high grade gliomas: a systematic review and meta-analysis. J Neurooncol 2011;105:325–335

63. Sadones J, Michotte A, Veld P, et al. MGMT promoter hypermethylation correlates with a survival benefit from temozolomide in patients with recurrent anaplastic astrocytoma but not glioblastoma. Eur J Cancer 2009;45:146–153

64. Uno M, Oba-Shinjo SM, Camargo AA, et al. Correlation of MGMT promoter methylation status with gene and protein expression levels in glioblastoma. Clinics (Sao Paulo) 2011;66:1747–1755

65. Kreth S, Thon N, Eigenbrod S, et al. O-methylguanine-DNA methyltransferase (MGMT) mRNA expression predicts outcome in malignant glioma independent of MGMT promoter methylation. PLoS ONE 2011;6:e17156

66. Preusser M, Elezi L, Hainfellner JA. Reliability and reproducibility of PCR-based testing of O6-methylguanine-DNA methyltransferase gene (MGMT) promoter methylation status in formalin-fixed and paraffin-embedded neurosurgical biopsy specimens. Clin Neuropathol 2008;27:388–390

67. Noushmehr H, Weisenberger DJ, Diefes K, et al; Cancer Genome Atlas Research Network. Identification of a CpG island methylator phenotype that defines a distinct subgroup of glioma. Cancer Cell 2010;17:510–522

68. Laffaire J, Everhard S, Idbaih A, et al. Methylation profiling identifies 2 groups of gliomas according to their tumorigenesis. Neuro-oncol 2011;13:84–98

69. van den Bent MJ, Gravendeel LA, Gorlia T, et al. A hypermethylated phenotype is a better predictor of survival than MGMT methylation in anaplastic oligodendroglial brain tumors: a report from EORTC study 26951. Clin Cancer Res 2011;17:7148–7155

70. Christensen BC, Smith AA, Zheng S, et al. DNA methylation, isocitrate dehydrogenase mutation, and survival in glioma. J Natl Cancer Inst 2011;103:143–153

71. Brennan C, Momota H, Hambardzumyan D, et al. Glioblastoma subclasses can be defined by activity among signal transduction pathways and associated genomic alterations. PLoS ONE 2009;4:e7752

72. Maher EA, Brennan C, Wen PY, et al. Marked genomic differences characterize primary and secondary glioblastoma subtypes and identify two distinct molecular and clinical secondary glioblastoma entities. Cancer Res 2006;66:11502–11513

73. Nigro JM, Misra A, Zhang L, et al. Integrated array-comparative genomic hybridization and expression array profiles identify clinically relevant molecular subtypes of glioblastoma. Cancer Res 2005;65:1678–1686

74. Phillips HS, Kharbanda S, Chen R, et al. Molecular subclasses of high-grade glioma predict prognosis, delineate a pattern of disease progression, and resemble stages in neurogenesis. Cancer Cell 2006;9:157–173

75. Verhaak RG, Hoadley KA, Purdom E, et al; Cancer Genome Atlas Research Network. Integrated genomic analysis identifies clinically relevant subtypes of glioblastoma characterized by abnormalities in PDGFRA, IDH1, EGFR, and NF1. Cancer Cell 2010;17:98–110

76. Huse JT, Phillips HS, Brennan CW. Molecular subclassification of diffuse gliomas: seeing order in the chaos. Glia 2011;59:1190–1199

3 Molecular Markers and Pathways in Brain Tumorigenesis

Mustafa Nadi and James T. Rutka

Neoplastic transformation is a multistep process precipitated by the loss of cellular mechanisms controlling cell proliferation and cell–cell interaction. This tumorigenic process involves the interplay between at least two gene classes: oncogenes and tumor suppressor genes (TSGs). Activated oncogenes result in exaggerated cellular signaling that promotes expansion of the aberrant cell population. The TSGs are normal genes that act to inhibit cell proliferation and growth, and inactivation of these genes results in tumor formation or progression. The most common scenario for TSG inactivation results when there is mutation of one allelic copy, followed by loss of all or part of the chromosome bearing the second allele. Consequently, the identification of regions of recurrent chromosomal loss in specific tumor types suggests that a TSG resides in that chromosomal region. These basic themes of oncogene activation and TSG inactivation, coupled with chromosomal loss of heterozygosity, underlie the current molecular understanding of human tumor formation. This chapter reviews the emerging knowledge on the molecular basis of brain tumorigenesis, and discusses primary tumors of the brain as well as other common primary intracranial neoplasms.

Signaling Pathways Regulating Gliomagenesis

Gliomas are the most common primary neoplasm of the brain, accounting for 40% of all central nervous system (CNS) tumors. The two main types of tumors in the World Health Organization (WHO) classification, astrocytomas and oligodendrogliomas, are named according to their presumed cell of origin and graded according to their histopathological appearance. The system is based primarily on subjective observations of morphological characteristics such as nuclear atypia, mitotic figures, microvascular proliferation, and focal pseudopalisading necrosis. Although tumor grade is currently the most accurate prognostic indicator for clinical outcome, it has been less helpful in determining optimal therapies.

Molecular genetic data gathered since the early 1990s suggest that histologically defined subtypes are even more diverse at a biological level. For instance, the majority of glioblastoma multiforme (GBM) tumors (WHO grade IV) manifest after a short clinical history, thus appearing to arise de novo without clinical or histological evidence of a less malignant precursor lesion. These primary GBMs share mutations affect-

Special Consideration

- It remains to be shown whether primary and secondary GBMs differ significantly with respect to prognosis, but it appears likely that they will respond differently to specific novel therapies. Ongoing clinical trials and future classification schemes will require incorporation of molecular subtyping.

ing two common mechanisms of gliomagenesis: overactive growth factor (mitogen) signaling and disruption of cell cycle control (reviewed below). In contrast, secondary GBMs develop slowly by malignant progression from lower grade gliomas, and the accumulation of genetic alterations over time is a hallmark of these tumors. An unambiguous histopathological distinction of these subtypes has remained elusive, but they clearly evolve through different genetic pathways[1,2] (**Fig. 3.1**).

Growth Factor-Regulated Pathways

Overactive signaling from several mitogens and their cognate membrane receptors have been implicated in gliomagenesis. Epidermal growth factor (EGF) and its receptor (EGFR), platelet-derived growth factor (PDGF)-A and –B and their respective receptors (PDGF-α, -β), transforming growth factor-α (TGF-α) acting through EGFR, and insulin-like growth factor-I (IGF-I) and its receptor (IGFR) are often involved in stimulating tumor cell proliferation.[3,4] Frequently, components of these mitogenic pathways are overexpressed in gliomas, or their upstream receptors harbor constitutively active mutations.[5]

Epidermal growth factor receptor amplifications and mutations have long been recognized as common (40%) gain of function alterations in GBMs.[3,6] Polymorphism in the 5′-untranslated region of EGF has also been implicated in gliomagenesis.[7] Patients with the –GA/–GG genotypes had higher levels of EGF within tumor tissue, irrespective of EGFR status, and had significantly shorter overall progression-free survival, compared to the common –AA genotype.

Three key signaling pathways downstream of aberrant growth factor/receptors involve Ras-Raf-MAPK (mitogen activated protein kinase), PI3K/Akt-PKB (phosphoinositide 3′kinase/ Akt-protein kinase B), and PLC-γ/PKC (phospholipase C-γ/protein kinase C) (**Fig. 3.2**). These signaling pathways regulate

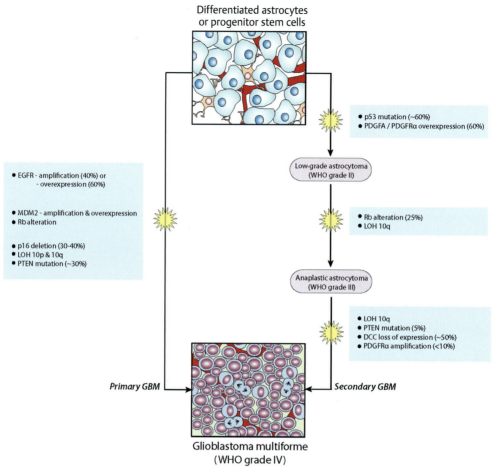

Differentiated astrocytes
or progenitor stem cells

- p53 mutation (~60%)
- PDGFA / PDGFRα overexpression (60%)

- EGFR - amplification (40%) or
   - overexpression (60%)

- MDM2 - amplification & overexpression
- Rb alteration

- p16 deletion (30-40%)
- LOH 10p & 10q
- PTEN mutation (~30%)

Low-grade astrocytoma
(WHO grade II)

- Rb alteration (25%)
- LOH 10q

Anaplastic astrocytoma
(WHO grade III)

- LOH 10q
- PTEN mutation (5%)
- DCC loss of expression (~50%)
- PDGFRα amplification (<10%)

Primary GBM   *Secondary GBM*

Glioblastoma multiforme
(WHO grade IV)

Fig. 3.1 Two distinct genetic pathways have been proposed for primary versus secondary glioblastoma multiforme (GBM). Primary GBMs are characterized by epidermal growth factor receptor (EGFR) amplification (~40% of cases) and/or overexpression (60%), tyrosine phosphatase/tensin (PTEN) mutations (30%), p16 deletion (30–40%), murine double minute 2 (MDM2) amplification (< 10%) or overexpression (50%), and, in 50 to 80% of cases, loss of heterozygosity (LOH) on the entire chromosome 10. In contrast, secondary GBMs contain TP53 mutations (~60% of cases), platelet-derived growth factor (PDGF)-A/PDGFRα overexpression (~60%), and Rb alteration (~25%). The pathway to secondary GBMs is further characterized by allelic loss of chromosomes 19q and 10q.

cellular processes including proliferation, differentiation, and apoptosis, and have traditionally been thought to influence nuclear factors to alter cellular transcription and hence potential transformation.[8] However, both the Ras and PI3K pathways primarily alter existing growth-promoting messenger RNA (mRNA) to become associated with polysomes and hence actively transcribed.[9] The PI3K/Akt-PKB pathway, in particular, has received much attention given its negative regulation by the tyrosine phosphatase/tensin (PTEN) homolog protein,[10] the most common loss of functional genetic alteration in GBMs. Additionally, the PI3K/Akt-PKB pathway modulates, through intermediate signal transducers, EGFR-regulated activation of the transcription nuclear factor (NF)-κB involved in inflammatory and transformation pathways.[11,12]

The Ras-Raf-MAPK signaling pathway is known to transduce mitogenic signals in a variety of cells, including astrocytomas. Ras is a small (21 kd) intracellular protein that exists bound to a guanine nucleotide (such as guanosine diphosphate, GDP) in its inactive state. Upon delivery of an appropriate stimulus, its intrinsic guanosine triphosphatase (GTPase) activity is upregulated through a series of intermediary adapter molecules. Accumulation of Ras–guanosine triphosphate (GTP) ultimately leads to increased expression or repression of specific target genes.

Special Consideration

- Study findings justify targeting the EGF/EGFR-regulated pathways and suggest that a single nucleotide polymorphism in EGF may be a useful marker for identifying patients with poor prognosis and who may benefit from anti-EGF/EGFR targeted biological therapies.

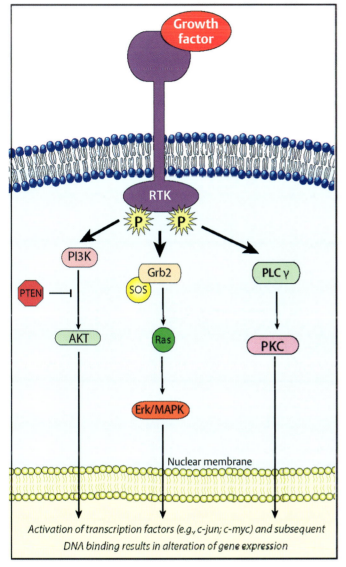

Fig. 3.2 Binding of a growth factor, such as epidermal growth factor (EGF), platelet-derived growth factor (PDGF), or fibroblast growth factor (FGF), to receptor tyrosine kinases (RTK) leads to activation of several signaling cascades through phosphorylation: the PI3K/Akt-PKB, Ras-Raf-MAPK, and PLC-γ/PKC pathways. These signaling pathways activate biological responses (through transcription factor–DNA binding) including cell proliferation and differentiation, antiapoptosis, migration, and metabolism. Tyrosine phosphatase/tensin (PTEN) functions as a tumor suppressor by inhibiting the PI3K/Akt-activated signaling cascade. P, phosphate group in the process of phosphorylation; SOS, son of sevenless.

Ras activation is implicated in other key processes such as cell adhesion through activation of integrin-mediated focal adhesion kinase (FAK) in astrocytomas.[13] The GBMs are known to overexpress FAK, which, if exogenously expressed in GBM cells, activates Ras, presumably by interaction of FAK with adapter molecules such as Shc. Mutations of other small-GTPase members of the Ras superfamily, including Rac1, have

also been linked to cytoskeletal alterations and invasion of glioma cells.[14] Rho, a related GTPase family member, has also been implicated in cell shape and motility, with recent evidence that inhibition of Rho leads to radiosensitization.[15] Significantly, expression of p190Rho-GAP, the endogenous inactivator of Rho, inhibits PDGF-mediated oligodendroglioma development.[16]

Cell Cycle–Regulated Pathways

A variety of signaling pathways converge at various checkpoints to tightly regulate progression through the cell cycle. Alterations in the retinoblastoma (Rb)- and p53- dependent pathways are implicated in glial transformation through control of progression at the G1 and G2 checkpoints.[17,18] These pathways are regulated by the tumor suppressor proteins p16INK4a and p14ARF, respectively, which are encoded by the INK4a-ARF (inhibitor of cyclin-dependent kinase 4a–alternative reading frame) locus.[19]

The retinoblastoma (Rb) gene was initially identified as a tumor suppressor and, within the CNS, Rb null mice demonstrate aberrant cell division and apoptosis, revealing a role in cell proliferation and survival.[20] Rb mutations have been found in about 20% of WHO grade III gliomas, thus supporting a role in their formation.[21,22] Low-level phosphorylation of Rb by cyclin-dependent kinase 4/6 (CDK4/6)-cyclin D1 complexes disrupts interactions between Rb and E2F, which relieves Rb-mediated repression of E2F-target genes required for cell cycle progression.[22] Loss of the tumor suppressor p16INK4a results in deregulated Rb phosphorylation and, consequently, in unchecked G1-S progression (**Fig. 3.3**).

The p53 transcription factor activates target genes that promote cell cycle arrest or apoptosis in response to cellular stresses such as oncogene activation.[23] The activity of p53 is regulated by the interplay between MDM2 (murine double minute 2)-mediated degradation and p14ARF-mediated inhibition of MDM2[24] (**Fig. 3.3**). Over two thirds of GBMs and anaplastic astrocytomas exhibit deregulated G1-S transition associated with inactivation of the p53 pathway, with either mutation of p53, amplification of MDM2, or homozygous deletion/mutation of p14ARF.[25]

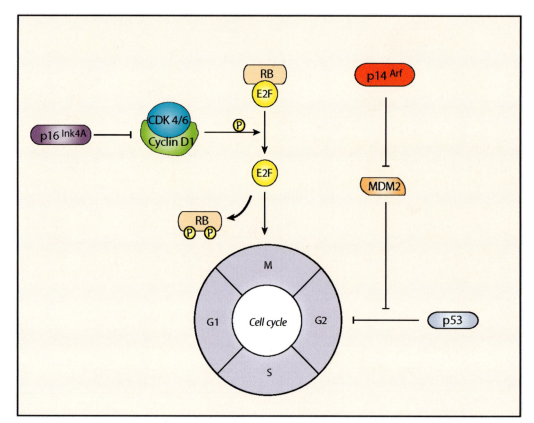

Fig. 3.3 The retinoblastoma protein (Rb) normally maintains G1 arrest by sequestering E2F transcription factors whereas mitogenic signals promote G1-S progression through a variety of mechanisms. Cyclin D1 and CDK4/6 form an active kinase complex and promote low-level phosphorylation of Rb family proteins. Interaction between Rb and E2F proteins is disrupted, thus relieving Rb-mediated repression of E2F-target genes required for cell-cycle progression and growth. The tumor suppressor p16^INK4A binds to and disrupts cyclin D1-CDK4/6 complexes, thereby inhibiting Rb phosphorylation and blocking G1-S progression. p53 maintains G1 or G2 arrest and directs apoptosis of cells with severe DNA damage. p53 activity is counteracted by the E3 ubiquitin ligase MDM2. MDM2 activity is also counteracted by the tumor suppressor p14^ARF. Therefore, binding of p14^ARF to MDM2 inhibits MDM2-mediated p53 transcriptional silencing and degradation, leading to cell-cycle arrest or apoptosis.

■ Medulloblastomas

Deregulated Developmental Signaling in Medulloblastomas

Medulloblastoma (MB), the most common malignant brain tumor of childhood, is a primitive neuroectodermal tumor arising from the granule cell progenitors of the cerebellum.[26] It accounts for up to 40% of all posterior fossa neoplasms.[26] Medulloblastoma is currently diagnosed on histopathological examination of tumor tissue; however, recent integrated genomic approaches have demonstrated that MB is composed of multiple clinically and molecularly distinct subgroups.[27,28] Emerging evidence indicates that the different precursor cell populations that form the cerebellum and the cell signaling pathways that regulate its development likely represent distinct compartments from which the subtypes of MB arise.

The main limitation in current therapies for MB is the lack of specificity of drugs used. Advances in understanding the molecular mechanisms have provided clues on the pathogenesis of MBs and could substantially improve the management of these neoplasms by employing targeted treatments. At least four subgroups of MB have now been described—Wnt, Shh, Group 3, and Group 4—and there may be other subtypes within these subgroups.[29]

Sonic-Hedgehog-Patched Signaling

The Sonic Hedgehog (Shh)-Patched (Ptch) signaling pathway is a major mitogenic regulator of cerebellar granule cell progenitors (CGCPs).[30,31] During cerebellar development, the glycoprotein Shh is primarily synthesized and secreted by pyramidal neurons and upon binding to the receptor Ptch, is mainly expressed on granule precursor cells, which activates the pathway by relieving Smoothened (Smoh)-mediated

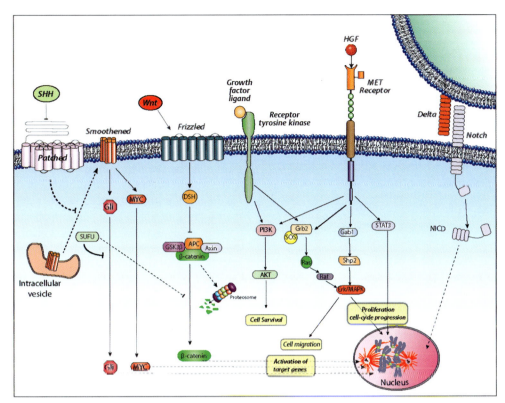

Fig. 3.4 The Shh-Ptch and Wnt-Frz-β-catenin signaling networks control the proliferation of cerebellar granule progenitor cells. The Ptch receptor normally inhibits the Smoh receptor in the absence of Shh signaling. SUFU binds to Gli and promotes its degradation and transport out of the nucleus. By bonding the membrane-bound Ptch receptor, Shh removes the inhibition of Smo and prevents SUFU binding of Gli, thus allowing Gli entry into the nucleus to promote target gene transcription. In the absence of Wnt signaling, the GSK3β/APC/Axin complex phosphorylates β-catenin, leading to its degradation. The Wnt ligand binds to Frizzled (Ftz) receptor, inducing activation of Dishevelled (Dsh), which inhibits the multimeric complex so that β-catenin accumulates in the cytoplasm. β-catenin can translocate into the nucleus and bind to LEF/TCF and activate target gene transcription. The Notch signaling pathway regulates cell proliferation; the receptors for this pathway are single-pass trans-membrane proteins. The Notch intracellular domain (NICD) is released from the membrane and translocates to the nucleus and forms a complex with the DNA-binding protein CBF1, activating the transcription of effector genes. The HGF/cMET pathway overpromotes cancer through increased cell proliferation and cell-cycle dysregulation and leads to metastatic behavior. This pathway starts by phosphorylation and activation of the growth factor receptor–bound protein 2 (Grb2), Grb2-associated adaptor protein (Gab1), son of sevenless (SOS), SRC homology protein tyrosine phosphatase 3 (Shp2), phosphatidylinositol 3-kinase (PI3K), and signal transducer and activator of transcription 3 (STAT3). This leads to the activation of downstream signaling pathways that include the mitogen-activated protein kinase (MAPK), PI3K/AKT, and STAT pathways, which mediate Met-dependent cell proliferation, migration, and invasion.

inhibition (**Fig. 3.4**). Disruption of Ptch activity causes aberrant Smoh activation of downstream target genes, such as the Gli family of transcription factors, to induce oncogenesis. Overexpression of Shh or Gli leads to oncogenic transformation.[32,33]

The crucial role of this pathway in progenitor proliferation has been linked to cell-cycle control at the G1 checkpoint, wherein Shh induces Cyclin D1 and Cyclin D2 expression, Rb hyperphosphorylation, and E2F activation.[34]

A subset of MB patients was shown to express mutated SUFU (suppressor of fused),[35] a protein originally isolated as a downstream repressor of Shh signaling that functions by exporting Gli proteins from the nucleus for degradation. SUFU mutants that fail to export Gli proteins from the nucleus result in aberrant Shh signaling. Therefore, MB can arise from deregulation of Shh-Ptch signaling in granule cell precursors via mutations of various pathway components. Mutations

Pearl

- The role of *PTCH1* mutations in the genesis of MB is supported by murine models, where approximately 14% of mice with a heterozygous deletion of Ptc (Ptc+/2) develop MB by 10 months of age, with peak tumor incidence occurring between 16 and 24 weeks of age.

affecting *PTCH1* and other components of the Shh signaling complex, namely *SUFU, PTCH2,* and *SMO,* have been identified in up to 25% of sporadic cases of MB.[35,36]

Wnt Signaling

The Wnt signaling pathway has been well studied in multiple developmental systems and has been implicated in tumorigenesis of many tissues.[37] The binding of Wnt to its cell surface receptor, Frizzled (Frz), activates a cascade of downstream events, resulting in the destabilization of an otherwise stable multiprotein complex containing APC, the product of the adenomatous polyposis coli gene that functions as a tumor suppressor by modulating the levels of cytoplasmic β-catenin, GSK3β (glycogen synthetase kinase), axin, and β-catenin (**Fig. 3.4**). The disruption of the multiprotein complex, either by Wnt signaling or as a result of mutations in one of its components, leads to the nuclear accumulation of β-catenin, which transactivates *TCF/LEF* (T-cell factor/lymphoid enhancer factor) resulting in activation of cell proliferation genes including *Cyclin D1* and *c-Myc*[38] (**Fig. 3.4**).

The constitutive activation of Wnt signaling, either by expression of the active form of β-catenin or by the inactivation of APC, inhibit neural differentiation and promote cell-cycle reentry and tumorigenesis. Approximately 15% of sporadic

MBs bear mutations affecting Wnt signal transduction, with the detection of elevated nuclear β-catenin levels.[39] These data suggest a role for abnormal Wnt signaling in contributing to a subset of sporadic MBs.[40]

Notch Signaling Pathway

The Notch signaling pathway regulates cell proliferation, cell-fate determination, and cell survival during development. It promotes the proliferation of granule neuron precursor cells (GNPCs) and prevents their differentiation.[30] Four receptors have been identified (Notch1–4) that are single-pass transmembrane proteins. Binding of the Notch receptor by its ligand triggers proteolytic cleavage and activation of the receptor. The Notch intracellular domain (NICD) is released from the membrane and translocates to the nucleus.[41] In the nucleus, the NICD forms a complex with the DNA-binding protein CBF1, activating the transcription of effector genes including *Hes1, Hes5, p21,* and *cyclin D1.*

Growth Factor Mutations

Receptor activation through ligand binding leads to EGF dimerization, autophosphorylation, and activation of downstream PI3K and MAPK signaling cascades (**Fig. 3.4**). This process is essential for normal CNS development. Aberrant activation of this pathway results in upregulation of downstream signaling elements, leading to increased cell proliferation and altered cell migration through the activation of transcription factor target proteins. In line with this, upregulation of RAS–MAP kinase downstream components (such as MAP2K1, MAP2K2, and MAPK1/3) and overexpression of the EGFR family member ERBB2 have been correlated with metastatic behavior of MBs.[42]

The hepatocyte growth factor (HGF)/cMET signaling pathway is also implicated in MB formation (**Fig. 3.4**); HGF signaling through the cMET receptor plays a critical role in cerebellar GNPCs proliferation and survival. Overactivation of this pathway can thus promote cancer through increased cell proliferation and cell-cycle dysregulation and lead to metastatic behavior by abnormal cell migration and invasion. In MB, *MET* gene copy number gains have been detected in 38.5% of primary tumor.[43]

The amplification of *MYC* and *MYCN* proto-oncogenes has been detected in 5 to 15% of primary MBs.[44] *MYCN* activation by Shh promotes the expression of the cell-cycle proteins Cyclin D1 and Cyclin D2, leading to GNPCs proliferation. A high

Table 3.1 Key Pathway and Gene Aberrations in Medulloblastoma

Pathway	Gene	Aberration
Shh	PTCH	Loss of function
	SUFU	Loss of function
	SMO	Activation
	MYC	Amplification and overexpression
Wnt	APC	Loss of function
	β-catenin	Activation
	AXI1	Loss of function
	GSK3-β	Decreased expression
Notch	NOTCH2	Gain
	HES1	Overexpression
EGF	ERBB2	Overexpression
	MAP2K1	Activation
	MAP2K2	Activation
	MAP2K3	Activation
HGF/cMET	CMET	Gain

expression level of MYC has been linked to poor clinical outcome. **Table 3.1** summarizes these genes and pathways.

Ependymoma

Ependymoma is a CNS tumor that occurs in both children and adults and is incurable in nearly 45% of patients.[45] It can arise almost anywhere along the neuraxis including the supratentorial region, comprising the cerebral hemispheres, the posterior fossa, the cerebellum and brainstem, and the spinal cord.[46] To date, surgery and adjuvant radiotherapy are the mainstays of ependymoma treatment. Transcriptional profiling studies have shown that, despite histological similarity, ependymomas from different regions of the CNS exhibit distinct gene expression signatures, and harbor numerous distinct subgroups.[47,48] Genomic characterization of these subgroups has led to the identification of molecular drivers of ependymoma such as EPHB2 amplification and INK4A deletion in supratentorial ependymoma.[49] Copy number alterations have also been beneficial in the prognostic stratification of ependymoma, such as the risk classification scheme proposed in 2010,[45] and in the further validation of gain of 1q25 as an indicator of poor clinical outcome.[50] However, despite extensive characterization of ependymoma at a copy number level, and in contrast to other CNS neoplasms, few oncogenes and TSGs have been identified in the form of recurrent focal genomic amplifications or deletions.[29] In the case of posterior fossa ependymoma, the most common location of occurrence in children, up to 50% of cases exhibit a balanced genomic profile.[49]

Aberrant promoter methylation of CpG islands is a well-recognized feature seen in numerous cancers.[51] RASSF1A has been shown to be the most frequently hypermethylated TSG, reported in up to 100% of ependymomas and occurring in all clinical and pathological subtypes.[52] HIC1 has also been reported to be commonly methylated in up to 83% of ependymomas, with a higher incidence in intracranial tumors.[53] Furthermore, the CDKN2A/INK4a locus, which is focally and recurrently deleted in supratentorial ependymoma,[45] has been shown to be hypermethylated in 21% of cases, followed by CDKN2B and p14ARF in 32% and 33% of tumors, respectively.[54] To a lesser extent, putative TSGs found to be hypermethylated in ependymoma include BLU, GSTP1, DAPK, FHIT, MGMT, MCJ, RARB, TIMP3, THBS1, TP73, and the TRAIL gene family CASP8, TFRSF10C, and TFRSF10D.[55] Despite the frequency of methylation of these potential TSGs in ependymoma, their role and significance in tumor formation remains unclear, requiring validation in independent cohorts and functional investigation in appropriate ependymoma models.

Intracranial Germ Cell Tumors

Primary intracranial germ cell tumors are rare and usually localized in the pineal and the suprasellar regions. They are divided into the following histological types: germinoma, teratoma (mature, immature, malignant), choriocarcinoma, embryonal carcinoma, endodermal sinus tumor (yolk sac tumor), and mixed tumors. Clinically, they manifest with ocular signs or signs of obstructive hydrocephalus.[56] If the tumors secrete β-human chorionic gonadotrophin (β-hCG) or α-fetoprotein (AFP), these tumor markers can be used to accurately monitor response to treatment. Prognosis is best for germinomas and mature teratomas and worst for choriocarcinomas and embryonal carcinomas.[56]

Molecular studies with fluorescence in-situ hybridization (FISH) have demonstrated X chromosomal gains in nearly all intracranial germ cell tumors, regardless of histological subtype.[57] FISH demonstrating amplification on chromosome 12p, particularly 12p13, is helpful diagnostically because it occurs in all germ cell tumors.[58] In a case of a malignant mixed teratoma–embryonal carcinoma, chromosomal analysis demonstrated a near-triploid complex karyotype (62 chromosomes), including two copies of an isochromosome 12p, suggesting that isochromosome 12p formation may be associated with the development of this tumor.[59] HOP/NECC1 is a gene located on human chromosome 4q11–q12, and it comprises an open reading frame of 219 base pairs (bp) encoding 73 amino acids. HOP/NECC1 has been shown to be a suppressor of choriocarcinogenesis, and loss of its expression is involved in malignant conversion of placental trophoblasts.[60] Germ cell tumors may demonstrate overexpression of the proto-oncogene c-kit. In 18 surgical germinoma specimens, c-kit was diffusely expressed on the cell surface of the germinoma cells, but not on lymphocytes or interstitial cells. In seven of eight immature teratomas, only some mature components such as cartilage and glands were immunoreactive for *c-kit*. Syncytiotrophoblastic giant cells also demonstrated negative findings, suggesting that only germinoma cells express *c-kit*. In addition, cerebrospinal fluid (CSF) examination of patients with germ cell tumors showed significantly higher levels of s-kit (a soluble isoform of *c-kit*) in germinomas than in patients with teratomas or non–germ cell brain tumors, or in CSF collected from controls. These results indicated that the concentration of s-kit in CSF may be a useful clinical marker for germinomas, especially for detecting recurrence or subarachnoid dissemination of these lesions. Other genetic abnormalities include expression of p53 protein in 94% of intracranial germ cell tumors and expression of p21(*WAF1/Cip1*) in 20%, associated with decreased sensitivity to radiotherapy, chemotherapy, and poor prognosis.[56]

Tumor Markers for Intracranial Germ Cell Tumors

Serological evaluation is an important part of the evaluation of marker-producing germ cell tumors. Histologically verified germ cell tumors of the pineal and suprasellar regions have been studied immunohistochemically using antiserum to human β- hCG, AFP, carcinoembryonic antigen (CEA), human placental lactogen (HPL), pregnancy-specific β-1 glycoprotein (SP-1), glial fibrillary acidic protein (GFAP), S-100, and neuron-specific enolase (NSE). In germinomas, the presence of β-hCG has been occasionally demonstrated in cells presenting as syncytiotrophoblastic giant cells, and GFAP and S-100 positive cells were found in the surrounding gliotic lesions. Teratomas were positive for CEA in their epithelial components. Endodermal sinus tumors were positive for AFP, choriocarcinomas for β-hCG and SP-1, and embryonal carcinomas for AFP, β-hCG, and SP-1.[61]

■ Oligodendrogliomas

Oligodendrogliomas are identified by tumor cells that mimic oligodendroglial differentiation. It is unclear, though, whether this histological appearance is truly reflective of a derivation from oligodendroglial cells. According to the WHO classification, oligodendrogliomas are diffusely infiltrating tumors and are divided into grade II and anaplastic grade III tumors.

Their incidence is about 4% of primary brain tumors and 10 to 15% of the gliomas. Most occur in adults of ages 50 to 60 years and are found in men more often than in women. Oligodendroglial tumors are different from the diffuse astrocytic gliomas, as these tumors respond favorably to chemotherapy and are associated with longer survival. These differences in response to therapy and in prognosis have been associated with the following distinct genetic aberrations: (1) loss of

alleles on chromosome arms 1p and 19q in oligodendroglial tumors, (2) homozygous deletion of the *CDKN2A* gene at 9p21, (3) mutation of the *PTEN* gene at 10q23, and (4) amplification of the *EGFR* gene at 7p12.[62]

In oligodendroglioma, loss of heterozygosity on chromosomes 1p and 19q *(LOH 1p/19q)* is associated with chemosensitivity; these patients benefit from intensive chemotherapy early in the disease course. Two large randomized trials in Europe and North America have investigated this notion in patients with anaplastic tumors.[63,64]

Of importance, in the subgroup of patients presumed to have particularly chemotherapy-sensitive pure oligodendroglioma with *LOH 1p/19q*, no improvement in survival was achieved with early chemotherapy. However, this subgroup of patients had a more protracted disease course irrespective of treatment modality; median survival of patients without *LOH 1p/19q* was 3 to 3.5 years, compared with more than 6 years for patients with *LOH 1p/19q*.[65]

■ Atypical Teratoid/Rhabdoid Tumors

Atypical teratoid/rhabdoid tumors (AT/RTs) of the brain are clinically aggressive malignancies that have overlapping clinical, histological, and imaging features with MB/primitive neuroectodermal tumor (PNET).[66] An AT/RT of the brain is almost exclusively a tumor of infants, with the majority of patients being diagnosed in the first 2 years of life. In the past, the majority of AT/RTs had been misclassified as MB/PNETs because two thirds of AT/RTs contain fields of primitive neuroepithelial cells characteristic of MB/PNET.[66] Cytogenetic and molecular studies are a useful adjunct in the differential diagnosis of children with these tumors. Isochromosome 17q is present in approximately 30 to 40% of MBs and has not, to date, been observed in AT/RT.[67] Identification of *hSNF5/INI1* as a TSG on chromosome 22 for malignant rhabdoid tumors has been reported.[68] The *hSNF5/INI1* gene is a component of the mammalian switch/sucrose nonfermenting complex, which functions in an adenosine triphosphate (ATP)-dependent manner to remodel chromatin, thus allowing transcription factor binding to DNA.[69]

Pearl

- Merlin is defined as a putative TSG, as its inactivation or loss of expression is found in all NF2 tumors as well as 60% and 80% of sporadic meningiomas and schwannomas, respectively.

Molecular Pathogenesis of Meningiomas

Meningiomas are common, slow-growing, benign (WHO grade I) tumors that arise from the meningeal coverings of the CNS. Rarely, grade II and III variants show aggressive local behavior and are associated with a less favorable prognosis. Genetic analysis of neurofibromatosis type 2 (NF2) has identified a causal mechanism underlying the formation of meningiomas. The *NF2* gene (chromosome 22q) encodes a 595-amino-acid protein named merlin that is closely linked to the ERM (ezrin, radixin, moesin) family of proteins involved in linking the actin cytoskeleton to cell surface molecules.[70,71]

Studies on mice bearing *NF2* germline mutations have identified merlin inactivation as a critical step in tumor formation and metastasis. Conditional inactivation of NF2 in meningeal or myelin precursor cells promotes meningioma and schwannoma formation.[72] NF2+/– mice are prone to developing a variety of nonmeningeal tumors and NF2–/– mouse embryonic fibroblasts grow unchecked in vitro despite achieving confluence or when deprived of growth factors. This phenotype is reversed by reintroduction of merlin expression.[73]

Merlin is associated with adherens junction components including N-cadherin, as well as α- and β-catenin.[73] Loss of merlin inhibits normal actin cytoskeleton and stable cadherin-mediated cell–cell junction formation. These findings highlight the critical role of merlin and the cytoskeleton in suppressing metastases.

Several candidate merlin-interacting proteins have been identified, including CD44, actin, βII-spectrin, β1-integrin, paxillin, syntenin, and hepatocyte growth factor–regulated tyrosine kinase substrate (HRS). In particular, HRS is a tyrosine phosphorylated protein involved in growth factor receptor endocytosis and has been linked to the EGFR and TGF-β signaling pathways.[74] As with merlin, HRS overexpression in rat schwannoma cells induces growth arrest, thus suggesting potentially overlapping functional pathways.[75]

Merlin-induced growth suppression is transduced through its interaction with the transmembrane hyaluronic acid receptor CD44.[76] In this model, growth arrest occurs when merlin is bound alone in a tight intramolecular configuration to the cytoplasmic tail of CD44. However, this process is attenuated when merlin is bound in a complex with ERM proteins, resulting in cellular proliferation and motility.

Another merlin-related protein, termed DAL-1/4.1B, has been found to act as a tumor suppressor in meningiomas.[77]

DAL-1/4.1B reexpression in lung tumor and meningioma cells results in growth suppression, and overexpression impairs cell motility and disrupts the cytoskeleton. DAL-1/4.1B also interacts with a subset of proteins that also bind merlin, such as CD44 and the ERM proteins, further suggesting a shared mechanism of growth suppression. Of note, DAL-1/4.1B also specifically interacts with 14-3-3 proteins, which have been linked to mitogen signal transduction, cell-cycle control, and apoptosis.[78]

Future Prospects

Our current histological grading system has proved useful for predicting the overall survival for groups of brain tumor patients. However, it provides limited insight into the underlying molecular perturbations. Furthermore, clinically relevant subsets that might significantly differ in their clinical course and response to therapy cannot be identified by the current classification system.

Recent advances in cancer genetics and the development of animal models have shown that chronic activation of key intracellular pathways that are critical for normal development might be crucial for the formation and progression of CNS tumors. In turn, the same pathways that promote tumorigenesis may sensitize tumor cells to targeted pathway inhibitors. Therefore, new classification systems for CNS cancer need to be developed that incorporate information on associated molecular pathway alterations. For instance, molecular criteria are currently employed to distinguish among different types of oligodendrogliomas; a more favorable chemotherapeutic response is predicted for tumors carrying loss of heterozygosity of chromosomes 1p and 19q as compared with tumors bearing p53 mutations.[79]

The high frequency of signaling pathway alterations in brain tumors, such as chronic PI3K pathway activation in malignant gliomas and Shh signaling in MBs, enables identification of potential therapeutic targets for small-molecule inhibitors. The recent development of high-throughput methods of gene expression and tissue analysis via microarrays will speed the discovery of novel molecular markers and potentially result in faithful predictions of clinical progress and outcome. Such predictive molecular diagnostics may lead to individualized tumor diagnosis with knowledge of patient-specific tumor susceptibilities allowing for precisely targeted molecular therapies.

Editor's Note

The current histological grading system provides guidance on the best treatment, and is useful for predicting the overall survival for groups of brain tumor patients. But it provides little insight into the molecular abnormalities causing these tumors or at least associated with them. Furthermore, subsets of patients who might significantly differ in their response to therapy and clinical course cannot be identified by the current classification system. Molecular markers will help better identify certain subsets of brain tumors or even individual brain tumors, and help better predict prognosis and responsiveness to treatment. The next challenge is to translate this knowledge into therapeutic interventions, specifically targeted molecular therapies designed to alter the growth of these tumors, and individualized to a specific tumor's molecular identity. At present, this is arguably one of the single greatest potential areas of hope to substantially alter the outcome of patients with brain tumors. (Bernstein)

Acknowledgment
The authors would like to thank Christian Smith, PhD, from the Arthur and Sonia Labatt Brain Tumor Research Centre, the Hospital for Sick Children, Toronto, Canada, for his assistance with the figures for this chapter.

References

1. von Deimling A, von Ammon K, Schoenfeld D, Wiestler OD, Seizinger BR, Louis DN. Subsets of glioblastoma multiforme defined by molecular genetic analysis. Brain Pathol 1993;3:19–26
2. Lang FF, Miller DC, Koslow M, Newcomb EW. Pathways leading to glioblastoma multiforme: a molecular analysis of genetic alterations in 65 astrocytic tumors. J Neurosurg 1994;81:427–436
3. Ekstrand AJ, James CD, Cavenee WK, Seliger B, Pettersson RF, Collins VP. Genes for epidermal growth factor receptor, transforming growth factor alpha, and epidermal growth factor and their expression in human gliomas in vivo. Cancer Res 1991;51:2164–2172
4. Guha A, Dashner K, Black PM, Wagner JA, Stiles CD. Expression of PDGF and PDGF receptors in human astrocytoma operation specimens supports the existence of an autocrine loop. Int J Cancer 1995;60:168–173
5. Ekstrand AJ, Longo N, Hamid ML, et al. Functional characterization of an EGF receptor with a truncated extracellular domain expressed in glioblastomas with EGFR gene amplification. Oncogene 1994;9:2313–2320
6. Frederick L, Wang XY, Eley G, James CD. Diversity and frequency of epidermal growth factor receptor mutations in human glioblastomas. Cancer Res 2000;60:1383–1387
7. Bhowmick DA, Zhuang Z, Wait SD, Weil RJ. A functional polymorphism in the EGF gene is found with increased frequency in glioblastoma multiforme patients and is associated with more aggressive disease. Cancer Res 2004;64:1220–1223
8. Schlessinger J. Cell signaling by receptor tyrosine kinases. Cell 2000; 103:211–225
9. Rajasekhar VK, Viale A, Socci ND, Wiedmann M, Hu X, Holland EC. Oncogenic Ras and Akt signaling contribute to glioblastoma formation by differential recruitment of existing mRNAs to polysomes. Mol Cell 2003;12:889–901
10. Cantley LC, Neel BG. New insights into tumor suppression: PTEN suppresses tumor formation by restraining the phosphoinositide 3-kinase/AKT pathway. Proc Natl Acad Sci U S A 1999;96:4240–4245
11. Kapoor GS, Zhan Y, Johnson GR, O'Rourke DM. Distinct domains in the SHP-2 phosphatase differentially regulate epidermal growth factor receptor/NF-kappaB activation through Gab1 in glioblastoma cells. Mol Cell Biol 2004;24:823–836
12. Stambolic V, Suzuki A, de la Pompa JL, et al. Negative regulation of PKB/Akt-dependent cell survival by the tumor suppressor PTEN. Cell 1998; 95:29–39
13. Hecker TP, Ding Q, Rege TA, Hanks SK, Gladson CL. Overexpression of FAK promotes Ras activity through the formation of a FAK/p120RasGAP complex in malignant astrocytoma cells. Oncogene 2004;23:3962–3971
14. Murai T, Miyazaki Y, Nishinakamura H, et al. Engagement of CD44 promotes Rac activation and CD44 cleavage during tumor cell migration. J Biol Chem 2004;279:4541–4550
15. Ader I, Delmas C, Bonnet J, et al. Inhibition of Rho pathways induces radiosensitization and oxygenation in human glioblastoma xenografts. Oncogene 2003;22:8861–8869
16. Wolf RM, Draghi N, Liang X, et al. p190RhoGAP can act to inhibit PDGF-induced gliomas in mice: a putative tumor suppressor encoded on human chromosome 19q13.3. Genes Dev 2003;17:476–487
17. Taylor WR, Stark GR. Regulation of the G2/M transition by p53. Oncogene 2001;20:1803–1815
18. Serrano M, Lee H, Chin L, Cordon-Cardo C, Beach D, DePinho RA. Role of the INK4a locus in tumor suppression and cell mortality. Cell 1996;85:27–37
19. Ueki K, Ono Y, Henson JW, Efird JT, von Deimling A, Louis DN. CDKN2/p16 or RB alterations occur in the majority of glioblastomas and are inversely correlated. Cancer Res 1996;56:150–153
20. Lee EY, Hu N, Yuan SS, et al. Dual roles of the retinoblastoma protein in cell cycle regulation and neuron differentiation. Genes Dev 1994;8:2008–2021
21. Ichimura K, Schmidt EE, Goike HM, Collins VP. Human glioblastomas with no alterations of the CDKN2A (p16INK4A, MTS1) and CDK4 genes have frequent mutations of the retinoblastoma gene. Oncogene 1996;13:1065–1072
22. Lipinski MM, Jacks T. The retinoblastoma gene family in differentiation and development. Oncogene 1999;18:7873–7882
23. Sharpless NE, DePinho RA. p53: good cop/bad cop. Cell 2002;110:9–12
24. Zhang Y, Xiong Y, Yarbrough WG. ARF promotes MDM2 degradation and stabilizes p53: ARF-INK4a locus deletion impairs both the Rb and p53 tumor suppression pathways. Cell 1998;92:725–734
25. Ichimura K, Bolin MB, Goike HM, Schmidt EE, Moshref A, Collins VP. Deregulation of the p14ARF/MDM2/p53 pathway is a prerequisite for human astrocytic gliomas with G1-S transition control gene abnormalities. Cancer Res 2000;60:417–424

26. Sardi I, Cavalieri D, Massimino M. Emerging treatments and gene expression profiling in high-risk medulloblastoma. Paediatr Drugs 2007; 9:81–96

27. Thompson MC, Fuller C, Hogg TL, et al. Genomics identifies medulloblastoma subgroups that are enriched for specific genetic alterations. J Clin Oncol 2006;24:1924–1931

28. Kool M, Koster J, Bunt J, et al. Integrated genomics identifies five medulloblastoma subtypes with distinct genetic profiles, pathway signatures and clinicopathological features. PLoS ONE 2008;3:e3088

29. Northcott PA, Shih DJ, Peacock J, et al. Subgroup-specific structural variation across 1,000 medulloblastoma genomes. Nature 2012;488: 49–56

30. Behesti H, Marino S. Cerebellar granule cells: insights into proliferation, differentiation, and role in medulloblastoma pathogenesis. Int J Biochem Cell Biol 2009;41:435–445

31. Wetmore C. Sonic hedgehog in normal and neoplastic proliferation: insight gained from human tumors and animal models. Curr Opin Genet Dev 2003;13:34–42

32. Pasca di Magliano M, Hebrok M. Hedgehog signalling in cancer formation and maintenance. Nat Rev Cancer 2003;3:903–911

33. Wetmore C, Eberhart DE, Curran T. The normal patched allele is expressed in medulloblastomas from mice with heterozygous germ-line mutation of patched. Cancer Res 2000;60:2239–2246

34. Kenney AM, Rowitch DH. Sonic hedgehog promotes G(1) cyclin expression and sustained cell cycle progression in mammalian neuronal precursors. Mol Cell Biol 2000;20:9055–9067

35. Taylor MD, Liu L, Raffel C, et al. Mutations in SUFU predispose to medulloblastoma. Nat Genet 2002;31:306–310

36. Raffel C, Jenkins RB, Frederick L, et al. Sporadic medulloblastomas contain PTCH mutations. Cancer Res 1997;57:842–845

37. Peifer M, Polakis P. Wnt signaling in oncogenesis and embryogenesis—a look outside the nucleus. Science 2000;287:1606–1609

38. Marino S. Medulloblastoma: developmental mechanisms out of control. Trends Mol Med 2005;11:17–22

39. Koch A, Waha A, Tonn JC, et al. Somatic mutations of WNT/wingless signaling pathway components in primitive neuroectodermal tumors. Int J Cancer 2001;93:445–449

40. Taylor MD, Zhang X, Liu L, et al. Failure of a medulloblastoma-derived mutant of SUFU to suppress WNT signaling. Oncogene 2004;23:4577–4583

41. Carlotti CG Jr, Smith C, Rutka JT. The molecular genetics of medulloblastoma: an assessment of new therapeutic targets. Neurosurg Rev 2008;31:359–368, discussion 368–369

42. Gilbertson RJ, Clifford SC. PDGFRB is overexpressed in metastatic medulloblastoma. Nat Genet 2003;35:197–198

43. Li Y, Lal B, Kwon S, et al. The scatter factor/hepatocyte growth factor: c-met pathway in human embryonal central nervous system tumor malignancy. Cancer Res 2005;65:9355–9362

44. Aldosari N, Bigner SH, Burger PC, et al. MYCC and MYCN oncogene amplification in medulloblastoma. A fluorescence in situ hybridization study on paraffin sections from the Children's Oncology Group. Arch Pathol Lab Med 2002;126:540–544

45. Korshunov A, Witt H, Hielscher T, et al. Molecular staging of intracranial ependymoma in children and adults. J Clin Oncol 2010;28:3182–3190

46. Louis DN, Ohgaki H, Wiestler OD, et al. The 2007 WHO classification of tumours of the central nervous system. Acta Neuropathol 2007;114: 97–109

47. Jones DT, Jäger N, Kool M, et al. Dissecting the genomic complexity underlying medulloblastoma. Nature 2012;488:100–105

48. Witt H, Mack SC, Ryzhova M, et al. Delineation of two clinically and molecularly distinct subgroups of posterior fossa ependymoma. Cancer Cell 2011;20:143–157

49. Johnson RA, Wright KD, Poppleton H, et al. Cross-species genomics matches driver mutations and cell compartments to model ependymoma. Nature 2010;466:632–636

50. Kilday JP, Mitra B, Domerg C, et al. Copy number gain of 1q25 predicts poor progression-free survival for pediatric intracranial ependymomas and enables patient risk stratification: a prospective European clinical trial cohort analysis on behalf of the Children's Cancer Leukaemia Group (CCLG), Societe Francaise d'Oncologie Pediatrique (SFOP), and International Society for Pediatric Oncology (SIOP). Clin Cancer Res 2012;18:2001–2011

51. Hanahan D, Weinberg RA. Hallmarks of cancer: the next generation. Cell 2011;144:646–674

52. Rogers HA, Kilday JP, Mayne C, et al. Supratentorial and spinal pediatric ependymomas display a hypermethylated phenotype which includes the loss of tumor suppressor genes involved in the control of cell growth and death. Acta Neuropathol 2012;123:711–725

53. Waha A, Koch A, Hartmann W, et al. Analysis of HIC-1 methylation and transcription in human ependymomas. Int J Cancer 2004;110:542–549

54. Rousseau E, Ruchoux MM, Scaravilli F, et al. CDKN2A, CDKN2B and p14ARF are frequently and differentially methylated in ependymal tumours. Neuropathol Appl Neurobiol 2003;29:574–583

55. Koos B, Bender S, Witt H, et al. The transcription factor evi-1 is overexpressed, promotes proliferation, and is prognostically unfavorable in infratentorial ependymomas. Clin Cancer Res 2011;17:3631–3637

56. Kyritsis AP. Management of primary intracranial germ cell tumors. J Neurooncol 2010;96:143–149

57. Okada Y, Nishikawa R, Matsutani M, Louis DN. Hypomethylated X chromosome gain and rare isochromosome 12p in diverse intracranial germ cell tumors. J Neuropathol Exp Neurol 2002;61:531–538

58. Juric D, Sale S, Hromas RA, et al. Gene expression profiling differentiates germ cell tumors from other cancers and defines subtype-specific signatures. Proc Natl Acad Sci U S A 2005;102:17763–17768

59. Losi L, Polito P, Hagemeijer A, Buonamici L, Van den Berghe H, Dal Cin P. Intracranial germ cell tumour (embryonal carcinoma with teratoma) with complex karyotype including isochromosome 12p. Virchows Arch 1998;433:571–574

60. Asanoma K, Matsuda T, Kondo H, et al. NECC1, a candidate choriocarcinoma suppressor gene that encodes a homeodomain consensus motif. Genomics 2003;81:15–25

61. Yamagami T, Handa H, Yamashita J, et al. An immunohistochemical study of intracranial germ cell tumours. Acta Neurochir (Wien) 1987; 86:33–41

62. Reifenberger G, Louis DN. Oligodendroglioma: toward molecular definitions in diagnostic neuro-oncology. J Neuropathol Exp Neurol 2003; 62:111–126

63. van den Bent MJ, Carpentier AF, Brandes AA, et al. Adjuvant procarbazine, lomustine, and vincristine improves progression-free survival but not overall survival in newly diagnosed anaplastic oligodendrogliomas and oligoastrocytomas: a randomized European Organisation for Research and Treatment of Cancer phase III trial. J Clin Oncol 2006;24:2715–2722

64. Cairncross G, Berkey B, Shaw E, et al; Intergroup Radiation Therapy Oncology Group Trial 9402. Phase III trial of chemotherapy plus radiotherapy compared with radiotherapy alone for pure and mixed anaplastic oligodendroglioma: Intergroup Radiation Therapy Oncology Group Trial 9402. J Clin Oncol 2006;24:2707–2714

65. Stupp R, Hegi ME. Neuro-oncology: oligodendroglioma and molecular markers. Lancet Neurol 2007;6:10–12

66. Rorke LB, Packer RJ, Biegel JA. Central nervous system atypical teratoid/rhabdoid tumors of infancy and childhood: definition of an entity. J Neurosurg 1996;85:56–65

67. Biegel JA, Zhou JY, Rorke LB, Stenstrom C, Wainwright LM, Fogelgren B. Germ-line and acquired mutations of INI1 in atypical teratoid and rhabdoid tumors. Cancer Res 1999;59:74–79

68. Versteege I, Sévenet N, Lange J, et al. Truncating mutations of hSNF5/INI1 in aggressive paediatric cancer. Nature 1998;394:203–206

69. Muchardt C, Yaniv M. The mammalian SWI/SNF complex and the control of cell growth. Semin Cell Dev Biol 1999;10:189–195

70. Twist EC, Ruttledge MH, Rousseau M, et al. The neurofibromatosis type 2 gene is inactivated in schwannomas. Hum Mol Genet 1994;3:147–151

71. Ruttledge MH, Sarrazin J, Rangaratnam S, et al. Evidence for the complete inactivation of the NF2 gene in the majority of sporadic meningiomas. Nat Genet 1994;6:180–184

72. Kalamarides M, Niwa-Kawakita M, Leblois H, et al. Nf2 gene inactivation in arachnoidal cells is rate-limiting for meningioma development in the mouse. Genes Dev 2002;16:1060–1065

73. Lallemand D, Curto M, Saotome I, Giovannini M, McClatchey AI. NF2 deficiency promotes tumorigenesis and metastasis by destabilizing adherens junctions. Genes Dev 2003;17:1090–1100

74. Miura S, Takeshita T, Asao H, et al. Hgs (Hrs), a FYVE domain protein, is involved in Smad signaling through cooperation with SARA. Mol Cell Biol 2000;20:9346–9355

75. Gutmann DH, Haipek CA, Burke SP, Sun CX, Scoles DR, Pulst SM. The NF2 interactor, hepatocyte growth factor-regulated tyrosine kinase substrate (HRS), associates with merlin in the "open" conformation and suppresses cell growth and motility. Hum Mol Genet 2001;10:825–834

76. Sun CX, Robb VA, Gutmann DH. Protein 4.1 tumor suppressors: getting a FERM grip on growth regulation. J Cell Sci 2002;115(Pt 21):3991–4000

77. Gutmann DH, Donahoe J, Perry A, et al. Loss of DAL-1, a protein 4.1-related tumor suppressor, is an important early event in the pathogenesis of meningiomas. Hum Mol Genet 2000;9:1495–1500

78. Hermeking H. The 14-3-3 cancer connection. Nat Rev Cancer 2003;3:931–943

79. van den Bent MJ. Advances in the biology and treatment of oligodendrogliomas. Curr Opin Neurol 2004;17:675–680

4   Brain Tumor Stem Cells

Marco Gallo and Peter B. Dirks

The Cancer Stem Cell Hypothesis

Cancer tissues are recognized to be heterogeneous, composed of cells with different morphologies and expressing different markers. Evidence accumulated in the last 50 years suggests that intratumoral morphological heterogeneity is accompanied by functional heterogeneity; that is, not every cancer cell carries the same tumor-propagating potential.

Functional differences between cancer cells are not immediately evident on the pathology examination of specimens, but they become apparent under specific experimental settings. Experiments performed in the 1950s and 1960s, and not ethically performable today, showed that cancer cells could be transplanted subcutaneously in human subjects to generate nodules, although high numbers of cells were required for successful engraftment.[1,2] These studies suggested, but did not prove, that cancers might be hierarchically organized, with only a small fraction of cells in a tumor being required for tumor growth and maintenance, hence the high number of cells required for transplantation. It was not until 1997 that a functional hierarchy was definitively and experimentally proven to exist in leukemia.[3]

The discovery in leukemia was rapidly followed by similar findings in breast cancer[4] and in brain tumors.[5–9] The key findings of these studies consisted in the identification of a small population of cells characterized by defined cell surface markers in human tumors that can be experimentally transplanted orthotopically in immunocompromised mouse recipients to initiate tumor formation. Histological evaluation of the resulting tumor xenografts showed that the transplants recapitulated the main characteristics of the patients' tumors from which they were isolated. In other words, transplantation of a small number of phenotypically defined cells into recipients was enough to generate a tumor that reproduced the entirety of the cellular heterogeneity found in the initial human specimen. These results support a "cancer stem cell" (CSC) hypothesis to explain tumor growth, by showing that tumors are organized hierarchically; not all cells in a tumor can transplant the diseases in recipients, but the ones that do produce all the cell types observed in a tumor (**Fig. 4.1**).

This hierarchical organization of tumor cells is reminiscent of the hierarchical structure of normal tissues. In most adult tissues, somatic stem cells maintain homeostasis by replenishing damaged or aged cells with new ones. This process requires stem cells to have the following properties: (1) self-renewal, because they need to be able to generate more stem cells to guarantee lifelong tissue homeostasis; (2) generation of progenitor cells with extensive proliferative potential; and (3) multi-lineage differentiation, in order to provide a supply of all cell types present in a given tissue that are required for tissue functional integrity.

The term *cancer stem cell* derives from the biological similarity between tumors and normal tissues, in that both require a small number of cells that can self-renew and generate all the cell types observed in situ. The definition of a cancer stem cell does not require that it be derived from a normal somatic cell, although this is the case in leukemia and probably in other tumors. As the use of the term *cancer stem cell* has generated some confusion because it is seen as suggestive of a cell of origin for tumors, the alternative term *tumor-initiating cell* (TIC) has been used to provide a less phylogenetically biased and more functionally accurate definition of the cellular population residing at the top of the tumor hierarchy.

It is important to point out that the CSC hypothesis is not the only model for the organization of tumors. Another theory, the stochastic model, postulates that any cell in a tumor can acquire tumor-initiating functions, without the need for a stable functional hierarchy within the tumor.[10] In light of these competing models, experimental evidence suggests that some malignancies might be organized hierarchically according to a CSC model, whereas others seem to be more in line with a stochastic model. For example, primary malignant brain tumors[6,7] and acute myeloid leukemia[3] appear to follow the CSC model. In contrast, B-cell lymphoblastic leukemia[11] and melanoma[12] appear to follow a stochastic model. Execution of in vivo transplantation experiments of primary tumor cells will be fundamental in determining the functional organization of different cancers. The key challenge to the concept of a hierarchical cellular organization in human brain tumors is that it sheds light on therapeutic failure and then leads to the development of more durable and even curative treatments (**Fig. 4.2**).

Evidence for Cancer Stem Cells in Brain Tumors

Glioblastoma

Cells in brain tumors are morphologically heterogeneous, and they are known to express different markers. In the case of

CSC hierarchy

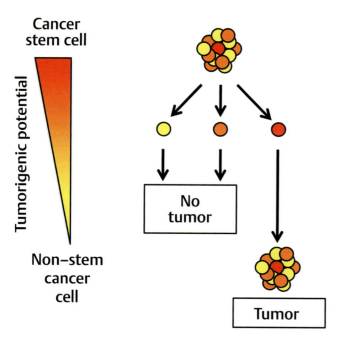

Fig. 4.1 Cancer stem cell (CSC) hierarchy. According to the CSC hypothesis, tumors are organized hierarchically, with CSCs residing at the top of the hierarchy and being necessary and sufficient to give rise to all cell types found in the malignancy. A gradient of tumor-initiation abilities exists in tumors, with CSCs (*red*) having strong tumor-initiation potential, and bulk tumor cells (*yellow*) having little or no tumor-initiation potential.

> **Controversy**
>
> • GBM CSCs may contribute to tumor vasculature by transdifferentiation.

evidence suggests that GBM is functionally organized as a hierarchy.

Research in the early 2000s showed that cells isolated from GBM specimens based on expression of the cell surface marker CD133 (CD133+ cells) are enriched for tumorigenic potential.[5–7] Notably, researchers showed that orthotopic injections of as few as 100 patient-derived CD133+ cells in immunocompromised mice resulted in the formation of GBMs that could be serially transplanted in recipients. Serial transplantation is a functional assay for long-term self-renewal potential. In contrast, transplantation of over 100,000 CD133– cells did not generate any tumors in mouse recipients.[6]

More recently, another group identified integrin α6 as a putative cancer stem cell marker in GBM.[13] Integrin α6 is the receptor for the extracellular matrix protein laminin, and therefore it serves to illustrate a potentially important interaction between the cancer stem cells and their cellular milieu or niche. In normal development and tissue homeostasis, the stem cell niche, or microenvironment, plays an important role in regulating the self-renewal and differentiation properties of stem cells. Analogously, it is possible that the brain tumor niche affects the tumor-initiating properties of GBM stem cells. It is important to point out that the markers mentioned above represent tools to *enrich* for CSCs, but by no means do they capture the full heterogeneity of CSCs. Ultimately, CSCs are identified by determining their in vivo tumorigenic potential.

Another interesting function of GBM CSCs is their putative role in contributing to tumor vasculature. It was known for some time that GBMs are hypervascularized, probably in re-

glioblastoma multiforme (GBM; World Health Organization [WHO] grade IV), the most aggressive and lethal adult brain tumor, the level of phenotypic heterogeneity is so noticeable that it is highlighted in the name of the disease itself. Recent

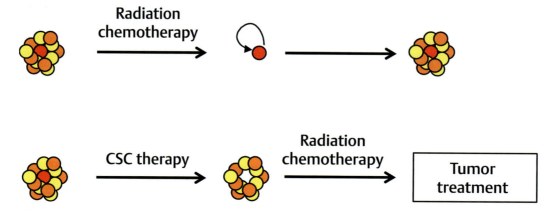

Fig. 4.2 The need for a CSC therapy. Experimental evidence suggests that CSCs are largely resistant to radiation and chemotherapy. Whereas these treatments may be effective at removing fast-proliferating bulk tumor cells, CSCs are spared. The CSCs then go on to self-renew and generate a new tumor. The goal of current research is to identify compounds that specifically target the CSC compartment, thereby removing self-renewing cells and the potential for tumor regeneration.

Special Consideration

- CSCs might be responsible for GBM recurrence after treatment.

sponse to the high metabolic needs of a growing tumor. Furthermore, GBM CSCs may induce angiogenesis by secreting high levels of vascular endothelial growth factor (VEGF).[14] Recent and controversial work provocatively suggested that GBM CSCs contribute to the tumor vasculature by transdifferentiation. Work from two different laboratories indicated that GBM CSCs can give rise to the endothelium upon transplantation in mouse recipients.[15,16] A third group obtained similar results in a mouse model of glioma.[17] The most compelling evidence that GBM CSCs transdifferentiated into CD31+ endothelial cells was the identification of GBM-specific mutations—namely amplification of the gene *EGFR* and of chromosome 7—in endothelial cells. These findings have now been rendered more controversial by the recent publication of data suggesting transdifferentiation of GBM CSCs into pericytes—specialized support cells of the vasculature—but not into endothelial cells.[18] Elucidation of the transdifferentiation potential of GBM CSCs is an interesting topic that needs to be examined further because of its possible implications for treatment.

Finally, recent work in an experimental model of glioblastoma in mice showed that CSCs might be responsible for GBM recurrence after treatment,[19] thereby highlighting the clinical significance of targeting CSCs to achieve lasting treatments. The authors induced glioma formation in mice carrying mutations in *Nf1*, *p53* and *Pten*, three important tumor suppressors. They then treated mice with temozolomide to reduce tumor size. Their key finding was that a cell population expressing the neural stem cell and CSC marker *Nestin* contributed to repopulating the tumors after treatment. These results strongly implicate the existence of a CSC population in maintaining tumor growth in this mouse model.

Medulloblastoma

There is evidence that medulloblastoma, the most common pediatric malignancy of the brain, is also hierarchically organized. Transplantation of medulloblastoma cells positive for the marker CD133 into immunocompromised mice results in tumor formation.[6] More recently, two separate groups showed that the marker CD15 enriches for a CSC population in a mouse model of the Sonic Hedgehog (Shh) subtype of medulloblastoma.[8,9] The authors isolated CD15+ and CD15– cells from medulloblastomas originated in the Shh mouse model, and showed that the CD15+ fraction had a much higher efficiency in transplanting the disease in allogeneic recipients. As GBM, medulloblastoma seems therefore to be organized hierarchically. Evidence has been provided that Shh medulloblastomas arise from both stem cells and committed granule

neuron precursors, the latter being progenitor cells with more limited self renewal and differentiation potential than stem cells.[20] This group found that tumor development is faster if Shh mutations are induced in stem cells, compared to the mutation arising in granule neuron precursors. Similar to leukemia, medulloblastoma might therefore represent an instance of a tumor characterized by a CSC hierarchy and initiated by mutations in the normal stem cell compartment.

◼ Application of Stem Cell Biology Concepts to Cancer

The advent of the CSC hypothesis has enabled the application of stem cell concepts to the study of cancer. Notwithstanding the current debate on the cell of origin for brain tumors, it can easily be appreciated how some biological properties, like self-renewal, are shared by normal and cancer stem cells and are inherent in the ability of cells to transplant the disease in serial recipients. Therefore, the application of stem cell concepts to cancer may result in a novel focus on developing therapies that target self-renewal abilities. Importantly, self-renewal can be decoupled from cell proliferation, as the former entails maintenance of specific stem-like or tumor-initiation properties, whereas the latter is concerned with the rate of cell division. Current therapies that target proliferating cells in brain tumors have not been especially successful, in particular for GBM, for which average patient survival is still 11 to 15 months.[21]

From the biological point of view, GBM CSCs express genes and pathways that are characteristic of normal stem cells. One instance is the high expression of the pluripotency transcription factor SOX2. SOX2 is expressed in a wide array of progenitor cells, including neural stem cells. It was recently shown that turning off the *SOX2* gene in GBM CSCs resulted in arrested proliferation and loss of tumorigenic potential upon transplantation in mouse recipients.[22] Another example of a developmental pathway that plays a role in normal and cancer stem cells is the Wnt pathway. Wnt signaling is required for the self-renewal potential of hematopoietic stem cells[23] and other stem cells. A recent study found that Wnt signaling was fundamental for the self-renewal properties of GBM CSCs.[24] Silencing of β-catenin, a downstream effector of Wnt signaling, reduced tumorigenic potential by 80 to 90%, depending on patient sample. It is interesting to note that the markers traditionally used to enrich for brain tumor stem cells, for example, CD133 and CD15, are also expressed on neural stem cells.

Special Consideration

- Developing therapies that target self-renewal abilities may be essential in the fight against malignant brain tumors.

Brain Tumor Stem Cells as Necessary Therapeutic Targets

Standard therapies to treat high-grade tumors have not produced the desired improvement in patient outcome. Although chemotherapy to treat medulloblastoma has been successful in decreasing mortality rates, especially for the Wnt molecular subgroup, treatment toxicity to the central nervous system results in long-term learning and behavioral deficits in survivors. Regarding GBM, the use of temozolomide as the standard of care produced the biggest increase in median patient survival in the last century, but it still represented a mere 4-month increase in life span.[21] It is therefore apparent that targeting indiscriminately proliferating cells in brain tumors will not lead to lasting cures for these diseases and more targeted approaches are required. This is especially true based on evidence that leukemia[25,26] and GBM[27] possess populations of tumor-initiating cells that are quiescent or more slowly cycling.

The CSC hypothesis postulates that pharmacological targeting of the cells at the top of the hierarchy—the tumor-initiating cells—will be fundamental to curing patients. Gaining a better understanding of the stem-like properties of CSCs, including self-renewal and tumorigenic potential, will be fundamental to achieving new benchmark standards of care. Furthermore, there are now multiple lines of evidence suggesting that CSCs are responsible for tumor recurrence, especially in the case of GBM. As mentioned above, it appears that CSCs are responsible for repopulating temozolomide-treated gliomas in a mouse model.[19] These data corroborate previous studies that showed GBM tumor-initiating cells to be radio- and chemoresistant.[28,29] Radioresistance seems to be determined by efficient upregulation of the DNA damage response, whereas chemoresistance arises from increased expression of prosurvival genes like *BCL-xL* and *BCL-2* and the downregulation of proapoptotic genes like *BAX*.

Based on the putative ability of GBM CSCs to contribute to tumor vasculature, it has been speculated that targeting angiogenesis might be a viable strategy to treat this tumor.[14–17]

Indeed, treating mice transplanted with GBM CSCs with bevacizumab, a VEGF-neutralizing antibody, has resulted in a marked decrease in tumor growth.[14] However, results from a recent clinical trial showed only a limited effect of bevacizumab on progression-free survival, with no effects on overall patient survival.[30] These results could be explained by the direct transdifferentiation of GBM CSCs into the vasculature. In any event, they also emphasize the need to identify novel therapies that directly target the CSC population.

Conclusion

The CSC hypothesis introduced a new way of thinking about cancer and the relationship between cells in a tumor. Moreover, by showing that we can apply stem cell concepts to the study of malignancies, the CSC hypothesis made an important conceptual contribution to oncology. In particular, a number of groups applying the conceptual and methodological framework of normal neural stem cell biology to the study of brain tumors has revealed a real "stemness" feature, and is leading to new insights into mechanisms of tumor growth and resistance. All the accumulated evidence implicating a CSC in generating the entirety of the heterogeneous populations of cells in a tumor stresses the importance of identifying therapies that selectively target the CSC, which, it is hoped, will provide more long-lasting cures for primary malignant brain tumor.

References

1. Moore AE, Rhoads CP, Southam CM. Homotransplantation of human cell lines. Science 1957;125:158–160
2. Brunschwig A, Southam CM, Levin AG. Host resistance to cancer. Clinical experiments by homotransplants, autotransplants and admixture of autologous leucocytes. Ann Surg 1965;162:416–425
3. Bonnet D, Dick JE. Human acute myeloid leukemia is organized as a hierarchy that originates from a primitive hematopoietic cell. Nat Med 1997;3:730–737
4. Al-Hajj M, Wicha MS, Benito-Hernandez A, Morrison SJ, Clarke MF. Prospective identification of tumorigenic breast cancer cells. Proc Natl Acad Sci U S A 2003;100:3983–3988
5. Singh SK, Clarke ID, Terasaki M, et al. Identification of a cancer stem cell in human brain tumors. Cancer Res 2003;63:5821–5828
6. Singh SK, Hawkins C, Clarke ID, et al. Identification of human brain tumour initiating cells. Nature 2004;432:396–401
7. Galli R, Binda E, Orfanelli U, et al. Isolation and characterization of tumorigenic, stem-like neural precursors from human glioblastoma. Cancer Res 2004;64:7011–7021
8. Ward RJ, Lee L, Graham K, et al. Multipotent CD15+ cancer stem cells in patched-1-deficient mouse medulloblastoma. Cancer Res 2009;69: 4682–4690
9. Read TA, Fogarty MP, Markant SL, et al. Identification of CD15 as a marker for tumor-propagating cells in a mouse model of medulloblastoma. Cancer Cell 2009;15:135–147
10. Shackleton M, Quintana E, Fearon ER, Morrison SJ. Heterogeneity in cancer: cancer stem cells versus clonal evolution. Cell 2009;138:822–829
11. Williams RT, den Besten W, Sherr CJ. Cytokine-dependent imatinib resistance in mouse BCR-ABL+, Arf-null lymphoblastic leukemia. Genes Dev 2007;21:2283–2287
12. Quintana E, Shackleton M, Foster HR, et al. Phenotypic heterogeneity among tumorigenic melanoma cells from patients that is reversible and not hierarchically organized. Cancer Cell 2010;18:510–523
13. Lathia JD, Gallagher J, Heddleston JM, et al. Integrin alpha 6 regulates glioblastoma stem cells. Cell Stem Cell 2010;6:421–432
14. Bao S, Wu Q, Sathornsumetee S, et al. Stem cell-like glioma cells promote tumor angiogenesis through vascular endothelial growth factor. Cancer Res 2006;66:7843–7848
15. Wang R, Chadalavada K, Wilshire J, et al. Glioblastoma stem-like cells give rise to tumour endothelium. Nature 2010;468:829–833
16. Ricci-Vitiani L, Pallini R, Biffoni M, et al. Tumour vascularization via endothelial differentiation of glioblastoma stem-like cells. Nature 2010; 468:824–828
17. Soda Y, Marumoto T, Friedmann-Morvinski D, et al. Transdifferentiation of glioblastoma cells into vascular endothelial cells. Proc Natl Acad Sci U S A 2011;108:4274–4280
18. Cheng L, Huang Z, Zhou W, et al. Glioblastoma stem cells generate vascular pericytes to support vessel function and tumor growth. Cell 2013;153:139–152
19. Chen J, Li Y, Yu TS, et al. A restricted cell population propagates glioblastoma growth after chemotherapy. Nature 2012;488:522–526
20. Yang ZJ, Ellis T, Markant SL, et al. Medulloblastoma can be initiated by deletion of Patched in lineage-restricted progenitors or stem cells. Cancer Cell 2008;14:135–145
21. Stupp R, Mason WP, van den Bent MJ, et al; European Organisation for Research and Treatment of Cancer Brain Tumor and Radiotherapy Groups; National Cancer Institute of Canada Clinical Trials Group. Radiotherapy plus concomitant and adjuvant temozolomide for glioblastoma. N Engl J Med 2005;352:987–996
22. Gangemi RM, Griffero F, Marubbi D, et al. SOX2 silencing in glioblastoma tumor-initiating cells causes stop of proliferation and loss of tumorigenicity. Stem Cells 2009;27:40–48
23. Reya T, Duncan AW, Ailles L, et al. A role for Wnt signalling in self-renewal of haematopoietic stem cells. Nature 2003;423:409–414
24. Zhang N, Wei P, Gong A, et al. FoxM1 promotes β-catenin nuclear localization and controls Wnt target-gene expression and glioma tumorigenesis. Cancer Cell 2011;20:427–442
25. Graham SM, Jørgensen HG, Allan E, et al. Primitive, quiescent, Philadelphia-positive stem cells from patients with chronic myeloid leukemia are insensitive to STI571 in vitro. Blood 2002;99:319–325
26. Holyoake T, Jiang X, Eaves C, Eaves A. Isolation of a highly quiescent subpopulation of primitive leukemic cells in chronic myeloid leukemia. Blood 1999;94:2056–2064
27. Deleyrolle LP, Harding A, Cato K, et al. Evidence for label-retaining tumour-initiating cells in human glioblastoma. Brain 2011;134(Pt 5): 1331–1343
28. Bao S, Wu Q, McLendon RE, et al. Glioma stem cells promote radioresistance by preferential activation of the DNA damage response. Nature 2006;444:756–760
29. Liu G, Yuan X, Zeng Z, et al. Analysis of gene expression and chemoresistance of CD133+ cancer stem cells in glioblastoma. Mol Cancer 2006;5:67
30. Lai A, Tran A, Nghiemphu PL, et al. Phase II study of bevacizumab plus temozolomide during and after radiation therapy for patients with newly diagnosed glioblastoma multiforme. J Clin Oncol 2011;29: 142–148

Evaluation

5 Anatomic Imaging

Daniel M. Mandell and Walter Kucharczyk

Imaging is essential for the care of patients with cranial and spinal tumors. Imaging is used to detect and characterize lesions, establish a differential diagnosis, guide invasive diagnostic tests and therapy, and monitor change over time. This chapter provides an introduction to imaging the neuro-oncology patient, and discusses a general imaging approach, technique, tumor characterization, mass effect, and follow-up imaging.

◼ Imaging Approach

Computed tomography (CT) and magnetic resonance imaging (MRI) are the main imaging modalities for cranial and spinal neoplastic disease. When a patient presents with acute neurologic symptoms and a suspected or known cranial tumor, it is best to begin with a CT scan of the brain, as this is the quickest way to exclude conditions such as intracranial hemorrhage, brain herniation, and acute hydrocephalus, which may require urgent neurosurgical treatment. Computed tomography is widely available, and current multidetector scanners cover the whole head in about 30 seconds. Whether the CT is normal or abnormal, if a brain tumor is suspected, contrast-enhanced MRI is usually warranted for further evaluation. If symptom progression is subacute (over weeks to months) and MRI is available within a few days, it is reasonable to begin with MRI.

When a patient presents with symptoms of acute spinal cord or cauda equina compression (in the absence of trauma), imaging should begin with MRI, which provides excellent contrast among the spinal cord, cerebrospinal fluid (CSF), and other tissues in the spinal canal. If MRI is not possible, then the study of choice is CT myelography. This technique involves lumbar, or rarely C1-C2 cisternal, puncture and injection of iodinated contrast medium into the thecal sac under fluoroscopic guidance, followed by CT scanning through the spinal levels of interest. The contrast medium distributes in the CSF and delineates the subarachnoid space.

Pitfall

- Not all iodinated contrast agents are safe for intrathecal use; the agent must be chosen carefully.

◼ Technique

Computed tomography images are obtained by transmitting precisely collimated beams of X-rays through the body at multiple angles. Some X-rays are absorbed or scattered, and the remainder are transmitted through the patient to a detector opposite the X-ray source. From these data on X-ray transmission along each path, a computer algorithm derives the X-ray attenuation attributable to each location within the region imaged. These attenuation values, measured in Hounsfield units, are then displayed as two-dimensional images. Advantages of CT compared with MRI are lower cost, wider availability, better access to critically ill patients during the examination, and greater tolerance of patient motion. Disadvantages include exposure to ionizing radiation and less contrast between soft tissues.

Whereas CT relies on X-ray transmission to create contrast between tissues, MRI uses electromagnetic waves in the radiofrequency range, and relies on a more complex interaction between this incident energy and tissue to generate images. The MRI scanner has a very strong and constant main magnetic field and additional milder time-varying magnetic fields. The latter magnetic fields are used to transmit electromagnetic waves into the body and then spatially localize the electromagnetic signals that are returned from the body. Advantages of MRI compared with CT are superior contrast between tissues[1]; availability of many different kinds of contrast between tissues; flexibility of adding a variety of advanced imaging techniques, such as spectroscopy, perfusion, diffusion tensor, and functional mapping of the cortex in the same examination as routine imaging; and lack of ionizing radiation.

Magnetic Resonance Imaging: Pulse Sequences

After a radiofrequency wave emitted by the scanner "excites" nuclei in the body, the body returns a signal to the MRI receiver. The characteristics of this returned signal depend on the local physical, chemical, and biological environment of the nuclei from which the signal arises; thus, the MRI signal reflects tissue characteristics. In particular, the waveform of the signal returned to the MRI receiver depends on how quickly the excited nuclei "relax" back to their initial state after radiofrequency excitation. There are two main types of relaxation: longitudinal and transverse. The time it takes for longitudinal magnetization to return to 63% of its equilibrium value after excitation is called "T1." The time it takes for transverse magnetization to return 63% of the way to its equilibrium value (of zero) after excitation is called "T2."

Different patterns ("pulse sequences") of incident radiofrequency waves yield images with different types of contrast between tissues. A pulse sequence that generates images with tissue contrast reflecting mainly differences in T1 is called "T1-weighted," and a sequence reflecting mainly differences in T2 is called "T2-weighted." T2-weighted pulse sequences correct for inhomogeneities in the magnetic field. If this correction is removed, the resulting images are called "T2*-weighted" (pronounced "T2 star") and are particularly sensitive to blood and calcification. Unfortunately, T2*-weighted images are also very sensitive to the magnetic inhomogeneities at interfaces between tissue and air, so the images are often distorted near the air-containing paranasal sinuses and temporal bones. T2*-weighted images are generated using a "gradient echo" type of pulse sequence. So-called susceptibility-weighted imaging is a newer variant of this sequence.

T2-weighted fluid-attenuated inversion recovery (FLAIR) is a type of T2-weighted pulse sequence that suppresses (i.e., turns black) signal from CSF. This sequence is helpful for detection of lesions near the margins of the ventricular system and at the surface of the brain. It is technically challenging to obtain complete suppression of CSF signal, especially in the posterior fossa, resulting in artifacts on FLAIR images. A diffusion-weighted pulse sequence yields images that reflect the degree of thermal or brownian motion of water molecules in tissue. Highly cellular tumors demonstrate restricted diffusion, as do some tumor mimics such as abscess. A diffusion-weighted sequence generates diffusion-weighted images, which have a combination of T2 weighting and diffusion weighting, and an "apparent diffusion coefficient" (ADC) map that is only diffusion weighted. It is important to review both kinds of information to determine whether restricted diffusion is truly present. Steady-state pulse sequences are a group of sequences often used to obtain high spatial resolution images with very strong T2 weighting. They are ideal for examining cranial nerve lesions such as vestibular schwannomas, but offer poor tissue contrast within soft tissues such as the brain.

Each sequence has specific uses as well as advantages and disadvantages relative to the others. The MRI vendors have created unique names for their proprietary versions of these sequences, resulting in a confusing plethora of sequence names. A routine MRI protocol for brain tumor imaging includes a T1-weighted sequence before intravenous injection of contrast medium, an axial T2-weighted or T2-weighted FLAIR sequence, an axial diffusion-weighted sequence, an axial T2*-weighted sequence, and contrast-enhanced T1-weighted sequences.

Vascular Imaging

Vascular abnormalities are often apparent on images obtained using routine pulse sequences, and such findings can be important (**Fig. 5.1**). There are several methods for obtaining dedicated images of the arteries and veins. One option is the gadolinium-bolus magnetic resonance (MR) angiogram, but there are also options that do not require gadolinium such as time-of-flight MR angiography and phase-contrast MR angiography. The time-of-flight technique is based on nuclei from elsewhere in the body flowing into the slice that is being imaged, resulting in increased signal in vessels in that image.

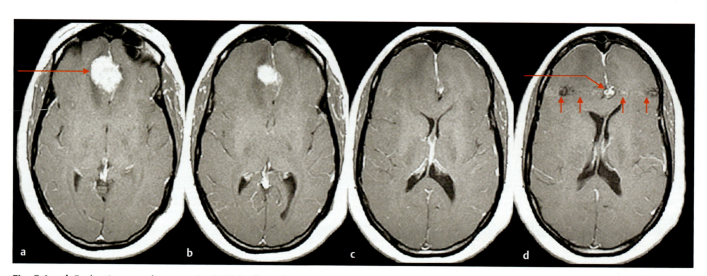

Fig. 5.1a–d Evaluating vessels on routine MRI. (**a-d**) Axial contrast-enhanced T1-weighted images were obtained prior to resection of a presumed meningioma. Images demonstrate an extra-axial mass along the falx cerebri consistent with a meningioma (**a**, *long arrow*), but also a lesion along the course of the anterior cerebral arteries (**d**, *long arrow*) adjacent to the meningioma. The second lesion has "phase ghosting" artifact (**d**, *small arrows*) indicating that it is a vascular structure, and subsequent CT angiography confirmed a 9-mm aneurysm.

Computed tomography angiography is another technique for evaluating the arteries of the head and neck. It provides higher spatial resolution than MR angiography, but poorer contrast between arteries and background tissues. Catheter angiography is now rarely performed for diagnostic purposes in patients with tumors apart from occasional preoperative embolization of a highly vascular tumor. For preoperative planning, it is important to view not only postprocessed images, which provide a three-dimensional depiction of the blood vessels in isolation, but also the "source" images, which show the blood vessels in relation to the tumor.

Tumor Appearance

Tumors generally have the appearance of a mass lesion; that is, they occupy space and displace normal structures. However, the mass effect of a small tumor may be difficult to appreciate, and primary brain tumors often infiltrate rather than grossly displace parenchyma, yielding less mass effect for their size than metastases or extra-axial tumors. Apart from lesion size and mass effect, the other main determinate of detectability is the CT attenuation or MR signal intensity contrast between a lesion and background tissue.[2] Once a lesion is detected, the next step is characterization.

Tumor Characterization

Location

The first step is to determine whether a tumor arises from within the brain parenchyma (intra-axial) or from outside the

brain (extra-axial). This initial distinction is a major determinant of the differential diagnosis, and to a degree, also portends prognosis. Several imaging findings suggest that a lesion is extra-axial: abnormality in the adjacent bone such as hyperostosis associated with a meningioma, a broad base of the lesion along the inner table of the calvaria or dura, associated dural enhancement, displacement of the brain away from the calvaria, dura between an epidural mass and the brain, widening of the subarachnoid space around the mass, a cleft of CSF or pial vessels coursing between the mass and the brain, and cortex between the mass and the white matter (**Fig. 5.2**).

Once a tumor is categorized as intra-axial or extra-axial, more precise localization will help narrow the differential diagnosis, as many tumors tend to occur in specific locations. For example, oligodendroglioma typically arises at the junction between the cortex and subcortical white matter, whereas primary central nervous system (CNS) lymphoma typically arises in the periventricular region. Extra-axial lesions arise from specific structures such as the calvaria, dura, leptomeninges, vessels, and cranial nerves. For spinal lesions, it is helpful to categorize location as intramedullary, that is, arising from within the spinal cord, extramedullary intradural, or extradural (**Fig. 5.3**).

Multiplicity of tumors is a hallmark of metastatic disease, but metastatic disease can present as a single lesion, and many other neoplastic and nonneoplastic diseases can yield

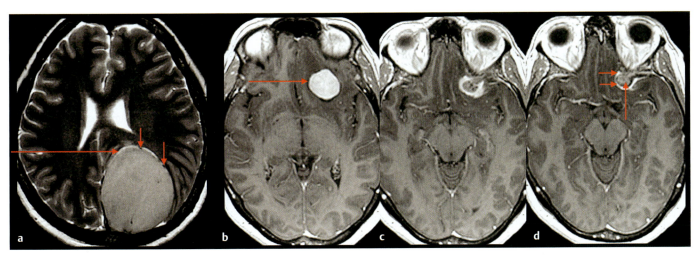

Fig. 5.2a–d Features that indicate that a mass is extra-axial. **(a)** Axial T2-weighted image demonstrates a large mass in the left parietal region. There is a cleft of cerebrospinal fluid (*long arrows*) and there are vessels (*short arrows*) between the mass and the brain.

(b–d) Contrast-enhanced axial T1-weighted images in a different patient shows an enhancing mass (*long arrow in* **b**) with adjacent dural enhancement (*short arrows*) and hyperostosis (*long arrow in* **d**) of the underlying bone of the anterior clinoid process.

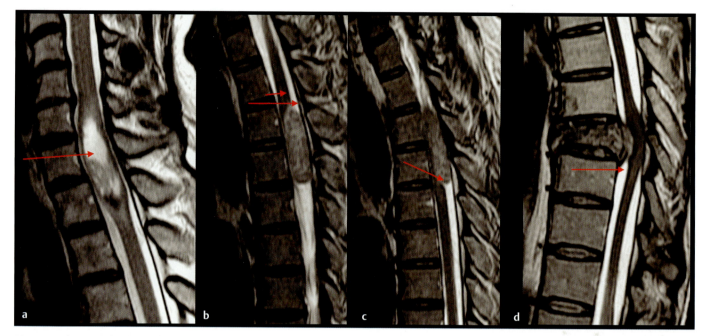

Fig. 5.3a–d Tumor localization in the spinal canal. **(a)** Sagittal T2-weighted image demonstrates an intramedullary tumor expanding the spinal cord. **(b,c)** Sagittal T2-weighted images in a different patient demonstrate a tubular mass between the spinal cord (**b**, *short arrow*) and dura (**b**, *long arrow*). The meniscus of CSF at the margin of the lesion (**c**, *arrow*) confirms that the lesion expands the subarachnoid space, indicating that it is in the extramedullary intradural compartment. This was a schwannoma. **(d)** Sagittal T2-weighted image in a third patient shows a mass arising from a partially collapsed vertebral body extending into the spinal canal and compressing the spinal cord. The mass narrows (*arrow*) the CSF space rather than expands it, indicating that the mass is extradural. This was a rectal carcinoma metastasis.

> **Special Consideration**
>
> • The presence of multiple lesions is not specific for metastatic disease. Primary tumors can be multifocal and many tumor mimics are multifocal.

multiple lesions. For example, high-grade primary tumors such as glioblastoma can present with multiple sites of involvement, and patients with genetic disorders such as neurofibromatosis type 1 (gliomas and neurofibromas), neurofibromatosis type 2 (meningiomas, ependymomas, schwannomas), and von Hippel–Lindau syndrome (hemangioblastomas and endolymphatic sac tumors) commonly have multiple tumors.

Composition

Tumors typically have greater water content than does brain parenchyma and are therefore hypoattenuating on CT, hypointense on T1-weighted images, and hyperintense on T2-weighted images relative to parenchyma. However, this pattern is commonly altered due to the presence of hemorrhage, necrosis, fat, proteinaceous fluid, calcification, or very high tumor cellularity.

Tumors, such as metastases from melanoma and from thyroid and renal cell carcinoma, are highly vascular and have a tendency to hemorrhage. On CT images, hematoma is hyperattenuating in the acute phase, subsequently isoattenuating to parenchyma, and, after a few weeks, hypoattenuating and similar in density to CSF. On MRI, the appearance of hemorrhage is more complex, as the hemoglobin molecule's magnetic properties change as it is metabolized within red blood cells from oxyhemoglobin to deoxyhemoglobin to methemoglobin, and then red blood cells lyse yielding extracellular methemoglobin, and then hemosiderin. In general, intraparenchymal hematoma evolves through corresponding stages: isointense on T1- and hyperintense on T2-weighted images in the first few hours, isointense to hypointense on T1- and hypointense on T2-weighted images after hours to days, hyperintense on T1- and hypointense on T2-weighted images after a few days, hyperintense on both T1- and T2-weighted images after a week, and hypointense on both T1- and T2-weighted images after several weeks. However, intratumoral hematoma is often heterogeneous and may not evolve as rapidly as other hematomas due intratumoral hypoxia[3] and repeated episodes of hemorrhage.[4]

The presence of blood product can help with differential diagnosis, but hemorrhage can also obscure visualization of a tumor. When a patient presents with an intraparenchymal hematoma and tumor is a possibility, follow-up imaging is needed to provide time for the hematoma to resolve and unmask any underlying lesion (**Fig. 5.4**). The timing of this

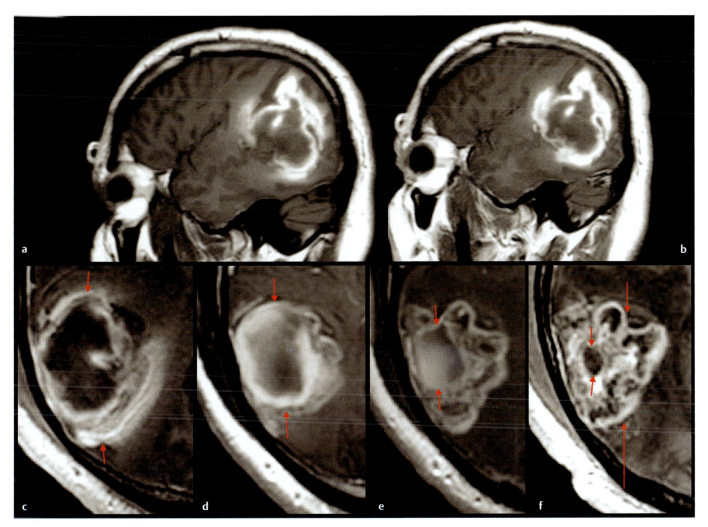

Fig. 5.4a–f Hematoma with underlying tumor. Sagittal T1-weighted images before **(a)** and after **(b)** intravenous contrast injection demonstrate a peripherally hyperintense mass in the parietotemporal region, with a similar appearance on the nonenhanced and enhanced images, suggesting that the hyperintensity is due to blood product rather than tumor. On axial contrast-enhanced T1-weighted images at the same time **(c)**, 1 month **(d)**, 2 months **(e)**, and 3 months **(f)** later, an underlying tumor (*long arrows*) becomes apparent as the hematoma (*short arrows*) resolves.

follow-up depends on the size of the hematoma, but a moderate to large hematoma will usually require at least 2 to 3 months to resolve. Other clues that there may be a tumor underlying an acute hematoma include edema or mass effect greater than expected for the hematoma size, or lack of a complete hemosiderin rim at the periphery of the hematoma.

Certain tumors have a tendency to calcify. Among these are intra-axial tumors such as oligodendroglioma and gangliocytoma, intraventricular tumors such as ependymoma, and extra-axial tumors such as craniopharyngioma and meningioma. On CT images, calcification is hyperattenuating, usually greater than 100 Hounsfield units. On MRI, calcification is typically hypointense on both T1- and T2-weighted images, but the signal intensity depends on the crystalline structure of the calcification, and calcification is sometimes hyperintense on T1-weighted images.

High-grade enhancing tumors commonly have a central necrotic region that is nonenhancing. The thickness and irregularity of the enhancing rim helps differentiate these tumors from other ring-enhancing masses such as abscesses. Other tumors, such as pilocytic astrocytoma, have a nonenhancing component that is sharply marginated and represents a cyst rather than necrosis. Whether a cyst contains simple fluid with similar CT and MRI appearance to CSF or it has protein-

---

Pitfall

- Fat will not be appreciated unless the window and level settings of a CT image are adjusted to accentuate the difference in density between fat and CSF.

aceous or hemorrhagic content can be helpful for differential diagnosis. For example, an extra-axial cyst with the appearance of CSF is usually an arachnoid cyst, a similar cyst with proteinaceous content in certain locations is likely a neurenteric cyst, and a similar cyst with internal restricted diffusion is usually an epidermoid cyst.

Intralesional fat is not a common finding, but when present, it narrows the differential. On CT images, fat is hypoattenuating—approximately 100 Hounsfield units. On MRI, fat is demonstrated in several ways: hyperintensity on T1-weighted images, a chemical shift artifact at lipid–water interfaces, manifest as high and low signal at the boundaries of the lesion, and reduced signal on fat-suppressed pulse sequences.

Tumor cellularity is another feature that is sometimes apparent on CT and MRI. Tumors, such as lymphoma and medulloblastoma, have tightly packed cells and high nucleus-to-cytoplasm ratio, with reduced free water. Computed tomography demonstrates hyperattenuation, and there is typically hypointensity on T2-weighted images and restricted diffusion. Nontumoral lesions such as a colloid cyst also demonstrate hyperattenuation CT and reduced signal on T2-weighted images due to protein content.

Contrast Enhancement

The blood–brain barrier is a functional barrier to cerebral capillary permeability. It is the result of several features of cerebral capillaries: continuous basement membranes; narrow intercellular gaps; a paucity of pinocytosis; and, perhaps most importantly, fused membranes between the endothelial cells, known as tight junctions. The macromolecules that make up the commonly used MRI and CT contrast agents are too large to pass through this barrier, but can leak into the brain parenchyma when the barrier is disrupted. This leakage is apparent on images as contrast enhancement. The commonly used MRI contrast agents are based on gadolinium, which exerts a paramagnetic effect that alters local tissue T1 and T2. Gadolinium is a rare earth element and, like lead, it is toxic in its elemental form, so it must be chelated with a protein to ensure that it is excreted from the body. It is important to be aware of the disorder nephrogenic systemic fibrosis, which is a rare but severe complication of gadolinium contrast use in patients with renal failure. Computed tomography images are based on spatial variations in tissue electron density, so iodinated substances that have very high electron density are used as CT

> **Pitfall**
>
> - The degree of enhancement alone does not indicate the grade of a tumor.

contrast media. In general, MRI is more sensitive than CT for detection of tumor enhancement.

The brain does not normally enhance, with a few exceptions, where the blood–brain barrier is absent, for example, in the pituitary gland and pineal gland. Contrast enhancement on MRI is usually evaluated using T1-weighted sequences, but contrast-enhanced T2-weighted FLAIR images are also useful, particularly to search for enhancement in the CSF spaces. Lesion conspicuity on contrast-enhanced images varies with the time between injection of contrast medium and imaging. A greater number of small brain metastases are visible 20 minutes after injection than at 10 minutes or immediately after injection.[5] Apparent lesion volume of an enhancing lesion may also depend on the time between contrast injection and imaging.[6] T2-weighted, T2*-weighted, and diffusion-weighted sequences can be performed after contrast injection to provide an adequate delay between the injection and the contrast-enhanced T1-weighted sequences.

Low-grade intra-axial tumors often have no or minimal enhancement, whereas high-grade intra-axial tumors enhance, likely reflecting the underlying maturity of the capillaries in low-grade tumors compared with the immature leaky capillaries in high-grade tumors. However, presence or absence of enhancement is not an absolute indicator of tumor grade; some low-grade tumors such as pilocytic astrocytoma commonly enhance and some high-grade tumors do not. Contrast enhancement is still extremely useful for lesion detection and characterization. For example, tiny metastases are often apparent only on contrast-enhanced sequences. Extra-axial tumors generally lack a blood–brain barrier so they tend to enhance. Spatial patterns of enhancement differ among tumors. For example, primary CNS lymphoma typically demonstrates homogeneous enhancement, hemangioblastoma has an enhancing nodule along the wall of a cyst, oligodendroglioma has patchy enhancement, and glioblastoma has thick irregular rim enhancement. Subacute infarcts, infections, granulomatous disease, acute demyelination, radiation necrosis, and many other nonneoplastic lesions also enhance.

> **Pitfall**
>
> - Checking for the brightness of the vascular structures is not a reliable way to determine if a sequence was performed with intravenous contrast material because vessels can appear bright simply due to the MRI "inflow phenomenon."

> **Special Consideration**
>
> - Contrast-enhanced T1-weighted images cannot be used to search for vertebral metastases. Vertebral marrow is intrinsically hyperintense on T1-weighted images, so there is commonly very little tissue contrast between tumor and normal marrow on these images.

Tumor Margin

Glial tumors, and most intra-axial tumors in general, lack a capsule, so tumor cells can migrate away from the discrete mass. The margins of contrast enhancement around an infiltrating intra-axial tumor do not accurately indicate the margins of most brain tumors; rather, the entire region of abnormal signal on T2-weighted images should be viewed as possible tumor extension.[7] For radiation therapy planning, gross tumor volume is commonly defined as the macroscopic tumor visible on contrast-enhanced T1-weighted images, but the clinical target volume includes the region of hyperintensity on T2-weighted images to provide a safety margin for microscopic spread. Certain tumors such as glioblastoma, primary CNS lymphoma, and ependymoma may also seed the subarachnoid space, and contrast-enhanced MRI of the spine is a consideration to screen for drop metastases.

> **Pitfall**
>
> - Whereas the vasogenic edema surrounding an extra-axial tumor or a noninfiltrating intra-axial tumor such as a metastasis is truly edema, the nonenhancing signal alteration around a high-grade brain tumor does not differentiate between brain edema and infiltrating tumor.

Leptomeningeal Metastases

Cerebrospinal fluid cytology is the traditional gold standard method for detection of subarachnoid space seeding of metastatic disease, but its sensitivity is limited. Contrast-enhanced MRI is complementary to cytology and may demonstrate leptomeningeal metastases as curvilinear or nodular enhancement along the pial surface of the brain, spinal cord, and nerve roots. In a cohort of patients who had CSF or MRI positive for leptomeningeal disease, both tests were positive in 54% of patients, only CSF was positive in 25%, and only MRI was positive in 21%.[8] Of note, some of these patients did not have the entire brain and spine covered during the MRI exam. The study found that MRI was more sensitive for detection of leptomeningeal metastases from solid primaries, whereas cytology was more sensitive for disease from hematopoietic primaries.

■ Tumor Mimics

Many nonneoplastic conditions mimic the appearance of a neoplasm on imaging (**Fig. 5.5**). These mimics span the full spectrum of pathology. A bacterial or fungal abscess can mimic a high-grade brain tumor. Herpes simplex encephalitis can mimic a low-grade glioma. Subacute infarction, tumefactive demyelination, sarcoidosis, and radiation necrosis are a few of the many other mimics.

■ Mass Effect

A unique feature of intracranial and spinal tumors is that they reside within relatively noncompliant osseous compartments. Consequently, the mass effect of tumors can be devastating. Brain herniation is the displacement of brain parenchyma through the openings in the rigid falx cerebri or tentorium cerebellum or through the foramen magnum (**Fig. 5.6**). Subfalcine herniation is displacement of the cingulate gyrus under the free margin of the falx. This is quantified on axial CT images as the degree of rightward or leftward displacement of the septum pellucidum. Descending central herniation is downward displacement of brain parenchyma through the tentorial incisura. Uncal herniation, a subtype of descending herniation, involves displacement of the temporal lobe uncus inferomedially between the free edge of the tentorium and the brainstem. Axial images show the displaced uncus, indentation and displacement of the brainstem, and effacement of the contralateral perimesencephalic cistern. Ascending central herniation is displacement of the cerebellum upward through the tentorial incisura with compression of the brainstem. Axial images show effacement of the superior cerebellar and quadrigeminal plate cisterns. Tonsillar herniation is displacement of the cerebellar tonsils through the foramen magnum. Axial images show parenchyma rather than CSF surrounding the medulla at the foramen magnum. Tumors may also exert mass effect on the ventricular system, resulting in obstructive hydrocephalus.

■ Follow-Up Imaging

Magnetic resonance imaging performed soon after resection can help identify residual tumor.[9] Enhancing granulation tissue begins to develop 3 days after surgery, persists for weeks to months, and mimics tumor, so early postoperative imaging should be performed within 48 hours of surgery.[10] It is important to obtain contrast-enhanced T1-weighted images but also nonenhanced T1-weighted images, as postoperative blood product has a similar appearance to enhancement on the contrast-enhanced images.[11] Diffusion-weighted imaging is also useful, as regions of restricted diffusion at the resection margin on the early postoperative MRI will often demonstrate enhancement on subsequent follow-up MRI, mimicking tumor. However, the presence of restricted diffusion on the initial MRI indicates that these regions represent tissue injury, which will enhance but then evolve into gliosis or encephalomalacia. For longer term follow-up, high-grade tumors are commonly imaged every 6 to 12 weeks and low-grade tumors are imaged yearly or biyearly.

"Pseudo-progression"[12-14] refers to a usually self-limited type of treatment-related tissue injury that is common in the first 3 to 6 months after temozolomide and radiation therapy, and mimics tumor progression, but then stabilizes or decreases

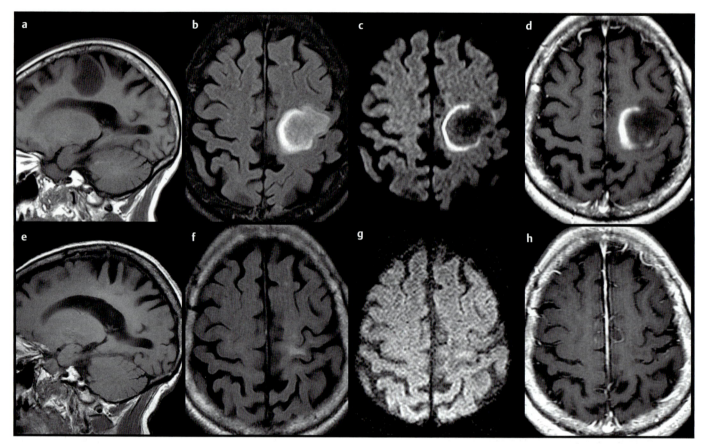

Fig. 5.5a–h Tumefactive demyelination. **(a)** Sagittal T1-weighted, **(b)** axial T2-weighted FLAIR, **(c)** axial diffusion-weighted, and **(d)** axial contrast enhanced T1-weighted images show a mass lesion in the left frontal lobe. The mass is nonenhancing apart from a rim of intense enhancement and corresponding restricted diffusion and hyper- intensity on FLAIR along its deep margin. The patient received no treatment for this lesion. **(e–h)** Follow-up imaging 1 year later with the same sequences demonstrates near-complete resolution of the lesion.

Pitfall

- When comparing studies, the size and shape of a tumor can appear substantially different due to differences in the angle of the imaging, slice thickness, and gaps between slices.

(**Fig. 5.7**). This phenomenon is distinguished from classic radiation necrosis, the latter also mimicking tumor progression, but typically more severe and more delayed in onset. Contrast enhancement beyond the radiation field is suspicious for tumor, but routine imaging has limited utility for differentiating between tumor progression and pseudo-progression within the radiation field.[15] It is not that studies have failed to find features for differentiation, but rather that inconsistent results among such studies preclude routine clinical use of such features. The largest such study of this kind found that the only indicative sign was subependymal spread of enhancement, which was not sensitive for tumor progression, but, when present, suggested true tumor progression rather than pseudo-progression.[16] Pseudo-progression is also seen with radiosurgery treatment of brain metastases. A large study found that one third of gamma knife–treated metastases increased in size typically 3 to 6 months after treatment, but increase in lesion size was associated with better prognosis, and was usually due to inflammation and necrosis rather than tumor.[17]

"Pseudo-response"[13] is a phenomenon that has emerged with the use of angiogenesis inhibitors such as Bevacizumab (Avastin). These drugs can cause a decrease in contrast enhancement due to a change in blood–brain barrier permeability rather than true reduction in tumor volume (**Fig. 5.8**). However, there is also evidence that pseudo-response is an indicator of subsequent favorable tumor response. For patients on an angiogenesis inhibitor, an increase in lesion extent and new restricted diffusion are clues to progression. These phenomena have led to updated response assessment criteria for high-grade gliomas.[18] There are many other treatment-related effects seen on imaging such as chemotherapy toxicities, radiation-induced leukoencephalopathy, and radiation-induced vascular malformations.

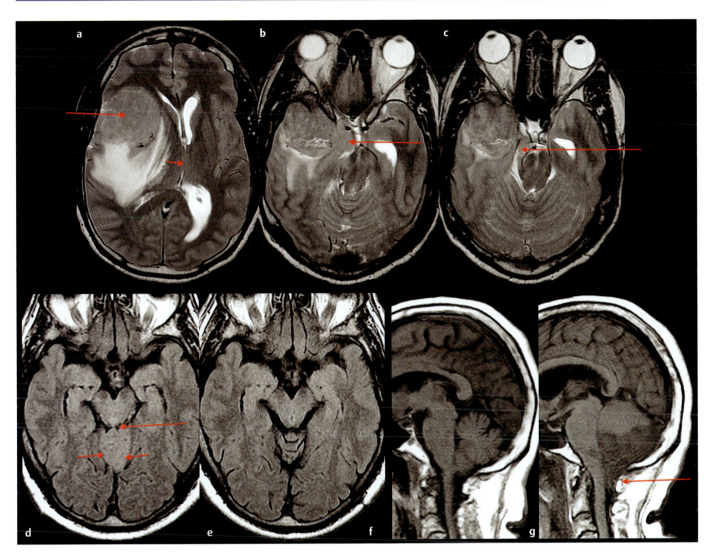

Fig. 5.6a–g Brain herniation. **(a–c)** Axial T2-weighted images demonstrates an extra-axial tumor in the right middle cranial fossa (*arrow*) with leftward subfalcine herniation (**a,** *short arrow*), right uncal herniation (**b,c,** *long arrows*), and obstructive hydrocephalus with enlargement of the left lateral ventricle. **(d)** Axial T2-weighted FLAIR image in a different patient demonstrates partial effacement of the supracerebellar cistern (*short arrows*) and quadrigeminal plate cistern (*long arrow*), indicating ascending transtentorial herniation. **(e)** A follow-up image in the same patient demonstrates resolution of these findings. **(f)** Sagittal T1-weighted image in a third patient is unremarkable. **(g)** A subsequent image in the same patient demonstrates infarction of the inferior half of the cerebellum with herniation of the cerebellar tonsils through the foramen magnum (*arrow*).

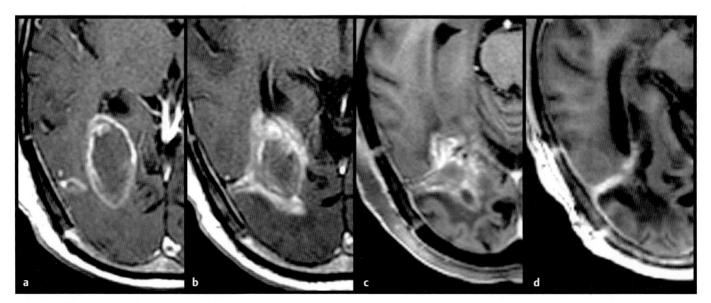

Fig. 5.7a–d Pseudoprogression. This patient with a right occipital glioblastoma was treated with surgical resection, temozolomide chemotherapy, and radiation therapy. All images are axial T1-weighted contrast-enhanced MRI. **(a)** Three weeks after completing radiation therapy, there is a rim enhancing lesion with a small enhancing nodule anteriorly. **(b)** Six months later, there is increased thickness of the enhancing rim and increase in size of the nodule. **(c,d)** MRI obtained at 12 months and at 30 months demonstrates progressive decrease in size of the lesion, indicating that the increased enhancement on the 6 month scan was pseudoprogression.

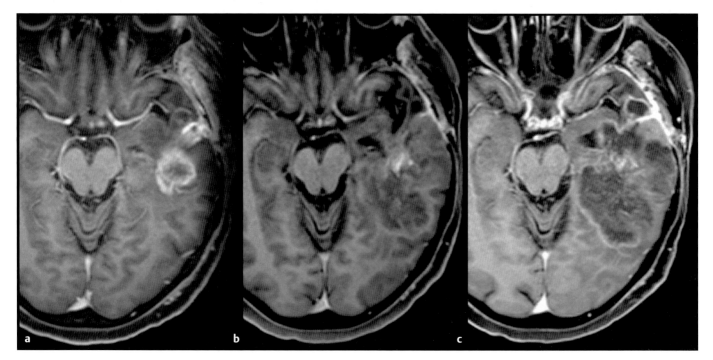

Fig. 5.8a–c Pseudoresponse. This patient with a left temporal glioblastoma was treated with surgical resection, chemotherapy (temozolamide), and radiation therapy. The tumor progressed despite treatment and the patient was started on the angiogenesis inhibitor Bevacizumab (Avastin). All images are axial T1-weighted contrast-enhanced MRI. **(a)** MRI before starting Avastin demonstrates a peripherally enhancing lesion in the left temporal lobe. **(b)** MRI 3 months after starting the drug demonstrates reduction in size of the enhancing lesion, but marked enlargement of the overall size of the lesion, which is now predominantly nonenhancing. This paradoxical response is consistent with tumor progression in a patient treated with Avastin. **(c)** MRI at 5 months demonstrates further enlargement of the lesion with new peripheral enhancement.

Editor's Note

Older neurosurgeons, radiation oncologists, neuro-oncologists, and neuroradiologists have witnessed a remarkable evolution in anatomic imaging of the lesions we diagnose and treat in the brain and spine. In the old days, indirect imaging with displacements of recognizable structures like nerves, arteries, veins, and CSF spaces (as in myelography, angiography, and pneumoencephalography) allowed us to deduce roughly where tumors were, and positive imaging then evolved from radionuclide scan to CT to MRI to pinpoint the geography of lesions and their effects on the brain such as cerebral edema. For younger physicians, life without MRI would be unthinkable. The real beneficiaries are patients who now receive precise imaging to diagnose, treat, and follow their tumor but with much less time, discomfort, and risk. The innovations in anatomic imaging are arguably one of the most important developments in the practice of neuro-oncology, and it is hard to imagine further imaging improvements beyond MRI, but it will be surprising to none of us if they develop. (Bernstein)

Acknowledgment

This chapter is based in part on the Anatomical Imaging chapter by Kei Yamada and A. Gregory Sorenson in the second edition of this book. We acknowledge their contributions.

References

1. Schellinger PD, Meinck HM, Thron A. Diagnostic accuracy of MRI compared to CCT in patients with brain metastases. J Neurooncol 1999;44:275–281
2. Healy ME, Hesselink JR, Press GA, Middleton MS. Increased detection of intracranial metastases with intravenous Gd-DTPA. Radiology 1987; 165:619–624
3. Gatenby RA, Coia LR, Richter MP, et al. Oxygen tension in human tumors: in vivo mapping using CT-guided probes. Radiology 1985;156: 211–214
4. Atlas SW, Grossman RI, Gomori JM, et al. Hemorrhagic intracranial malignant neoplasms: spin-echo MR imaging. Radiology 1987;164:71–77
5. Yuh WT, Tali ET, Nguyen HD, Simonson TM, Mayr NA, Fisher DJ. The effect of contrast dose, imaging time, and lesion size in the MR detection of intracerebral metastasis. AJNR Am J Neuroradiol 1995;16: 373–380
6. Engelhorn T, Schwarz MA, Eyupoglu IY, Kloska SP, Struffert T, Doerfler A. Dynamic contrast enhancement of experimental glioma an intra-individual comparative study to assess the optimal time delay. Acad Radiol 2010;17:188–193
7. Earnest F IV, Kelly PJ, Scheithauer BW, et al. Cerebral astrocytomas: histopathologic correlation of MR and CT contrast enhancement with stereotactic biopsy. Radiology 1988;166:823–827
8. Clarke JL, Perez HR, Jacks LM, Panageas KS, Deangelis LM. Leptomeningeal metastases in the MRI era. Neurology 2010;74:1449–1454
9. Albert FK, Forsting M, Sartor K, Adams HP, Kunze S. Early postoperative magnetic resonance imaging after resection of malignant glioma: objective evaluation of residual tumor and its influence on regrowth and prognosis. Neurosurgery 1994;34:45–60, discussion 60–61
10. Forsting M, Albert FK, Kunze S, Adams HP, Zenner D, Sartor K. Extirpation of glioblastomas: MR and CT follow-up of residual tumor and regrowth patterns. AJNR Am J Neuroradiol 1993;14:77–87
11. Meyding-Lamadé U, Forsting M, Albert F, Kunze S, Sartor K. Accelerated methaemoglobin formation: potential pitfall in early postoperative MRI. Neuroradiology 1993;35:178–180
12. Hygino da Cruz LC Jr, Rodriguez I, Domingues RC, Gasparetto EL, Sorensen AG. Pseudoprogression and pseudoresponse: imaging challenges in the assessment of posttreatment glioma. AJNR Am J Neuroradiol 2011;32:1978–1985
13. Clarke JL, Chang S. Pseudoprogression and pseudoresponse: challenges in brain tumor imaging. Curr Neurol Neurosci Rep 2009;9:241–246
14. Brandsma D, Stalpers L, Taal W, Sminia P, van den Bent MJ. Clinical features, mechanisms, and management of pseudoprogression in malignant gliomas. Lancet Oncol 2008;9:453–461
15. Mullins ME, Barest GD, Schaefer PW, Hochberg FH, Gonzalez RG, Lev MH. Radiation necrosis versus glioma recurrence: conventional MR imaging clues to diagnosis. AJNR Am J Neuroradiol 2005;26:1967–1972
16. Young RJ, Gupta A, Shah AD, et al. Potential utility of conventional MRI signs in diagnosing pseudoprogression in glioblastoma. Neurology 2011;76:1918–1924
17. Patel TR, McHugh BJ, Bi WL, Minja FJ, Knisely JP, Chiang VL. A comprehensive review of MR imaging changes following radiosurgery to 500 brain metastases. AJNR Am J Neuroradiol 2011;32:1885–1892
18. Wen PY, Macdonald DR, Reardon DA, et al. Updated response assessment criteria for high-grade gliomas: response assessment in neuro-oncology working group. J Clin Oncol 2010;28:1963–1972

6 Metabolic Imaging

Lutz W. Kracht and Wolf-Dieter Heiss

■ Positron Emission Tomography

Positron emission tomography (PET) provides metabolic in vivo measurement of local tracer activity at a very high sensitivity. This is a unique property unmatched by other imaging modalities. As major structural lesions, brain tumors are diagnosed and clinically managed primarily with computed tomography (CT) and magnetic resonance imaging (MRI). However, it is possible to improve clinical management by using PET to provide physiological and biochemical information related to tumor metabolism, proliferation rate, and invasiveness as well as relation to functionally important tissue.[1]

In this context, image registration is extremely important for accurately correlating abnormalities on the MRI with findings on the PET scan. Different modalities, such as *methyl*-[11C]-L-methionine ([11C]-MET) and 2-[18F]fluoro-2-deoxy-D-glucose ([18F]-FDG), can be co-registered to magnetic resonance images in glioma patients.

If the images are not registered, the location of a small abnormality on MRI cannot be accurately identified on PET. The registration with MRI permits the accurate characterization of even small MRI lesions. The image registration permits the interpreting physician to be more accurate and confident in the diagnosis.

Imaging Glucose Metabolism

Glucose is the main substrate for energy supply of the brain by oxidation. It is transported into the brain by the insulin-dependent carrier GLUT 1, which is expressed in brain capillary endothelial cells. Transport rates depend on the plasma glucose levels in accordance with Michaelis-Menten kinetics for facilitated transport. The standard PET tracer for measuring cerebral metabolic rate of glucose (CMRGlc) is [18F]-FDG. [18F]-FDG is transported into the tissue and phosphorylated to [18F]-FDG-phosphate but does not undergo significant further metabolism. It accumulates in brain in proportion to local CMRGlc. Methods for quantification are based on physiological monitoring. Because [18F]-FDG is an analogue tracer and has different physiological properties than glucose, conversion factors like the "lumped constant" are necessary to calculate CMRClc.[2]

Glucose consumption measured by [18F]-FDG-PET is increased in most malignant gliomas.[3] Although uptake correlates with degree of malignancy, there are concerns about the use of the [18F]-FDG model to calculate the CMRClc in brain tumors. The lumped constant used in the model to estimate glucose consumption from [18F]-FDG uptake seems to be higher in tumors and therefore overestimates the glucose consumption if the value for the normal brain is used. Changes in the lumped constant in tumors compared to normal brain may be due to increased expression of hexokinase II in tumors. Hexokinase II has a higher affinity to [18F]-FDG compared to hexokinase I, which is expressed in the normal brain.[4] Increased transport may also play a role together with increased glycolysis compared to oxidative metabolism of glucose.

In clinical routine, [18F]-FDG images are analyzed visually or the relative [18F]-FDG uptake compared to normal brain structures that are not affected by the tumor is calculated. Preferably, uptake in the cerebral cortex or the deep white matter is used to calculate relative uptake ratios by using average uptake in regions of interest.

Imaging for Primary Diagnosis

At the point of first diagnosis, patients with brain tumors most often have either new-onset generalized or focal seizures or demonstrate progressive focal neurologic symptoms. They are referred for CT or MRI, and in most cases the diagnosis of a primary brain tumor can be made from MRI alone. But it is not uncommon that other differential diagnoses, such as acute inflammatory lesions or ischemic or hemorrhagic stroke, cannot be excluded by MRI findings. Differentiating tumors from nontumorous lesions with [18F]-FDG is difficult because of the high [18F]-FDG-uptake in normal cortex (**Figs. 6.1** and **6.2**). Low [18F]-FDG uptake is frequently seen in brain tumors; low-grade gliomas especially show [18F]-FDG levels comparable to those of white matter and cannot be distinguished from nontumorous lesions like inflammation or acute stroke. On

> **Pitfall**
>
> - For the interpretation of FDG brain scans, the similarity of FDG uptake of tumor and cortex is a limiting factor, which is especially critical for small lesions. Due to the limited spatial resolution of PET and partial volume averaging, FDG uptake can be underestimated in small lesions. The best assessment of FDG uptake in brain tumors is obtained if co-registration with MRI permits reliable localization of PET data.

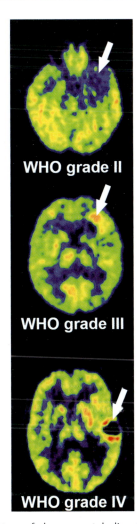

Fig. 6.1 Typical pattern of glucose metabolism in astrocytic brain tumors of different World Health Organization (WHO) grade. Low-grade astrocytoma (WHO grade II) is demonstrated with decreased [18F]-FDG uptake when compared to gray matter, and these tumors cannot be distinguished clearly from nontumor lesions. Malignant astrocytoma (WHO grade III and IV) show [18F]-FDG uptake in the range of or slightly above cerebral gray matter. Arrows point to tumor.

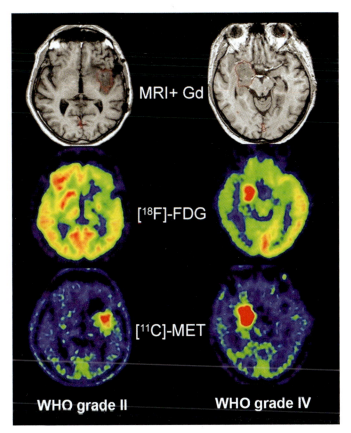

Fig. 6.2 MRI, [18F]-FDG-PET, and [11C]-MET-PET in low- and high-grade gliomas. [18F]-FDG clearly distinguishes between the low-grade and the high-grade tumor in contrast to MRI. [11C]-MET shows higher uptake in the malignant tumor but a clear differentiation is not possible in these examples. (From Jacobs AH. PET in gliomas. In: Schlegel U, Weller M, Westphal M, eds. Neuroonkologie. Berlin: Thieme-Verlag, 2003:72–76. Copyright 2003, Thieme-Verlag. All rights reserved. Reproduced with permission.)

the other hand, high [18F]-FDG uptake is not specific for brain tumors, but may also be seen in inflammatory lesions (e.g., sarcoidosis, acute demyelinating encephalomyelitis), focal epilepsy, and recent ischemic infarcts with nonoxidative glycolysis. On [18F]-FDG-PET imaging tumors often demonstrate a wide rim of reduced [18F]-FDG uptake, which might be also due to functional inactivation by the infiltrating tumor growth or edema formation (**Figs. 6.1** and **6.2**).

The sensitivity to detect lesions is further decreased by the high variance of [18F]-FDG uptake and its heterogeneity within a single tumor that has areas of low uptake and areas of high uptake near each other. Therefore, [18F]-FDG grading of newly discovered gliomas must be applied with caution, and the high variability must be taken into consideration. Delayed imaging (3 to 8 hours after injection) can improve the dis-

tinction between tumor and normal gray matter,[5] because excretion of the tracer is faster in normal brain than in tumor tissue.[6]

The amount of accumulation of FDG in a primary brain tumor correlates to histological tumor grade,[7] to cell density,[8] and to survival.[9]

Low-grade tumors have [18F]-FDG uptake similar to or less than that of normal white matter, whereas high-grade tumors have [18F]-FDG uptake equal to or exceeding that of normal gray matter (**Figs. 6.1, 6.2**). In a study of 58 patients tumor-to-white matter (T/WM) and tumor-to-gray matter (T/GM) ratios were able to distinguish benign (grades I and II) from malignant tumors (grades III and IV).[10] T/WM ratios greater than 1.5 and T/GM ratios greater than 0.6 showed a sensitivity of 94% and a specificity of 77% for the detection of malignant tumors.[10] Glucose consumption in normal brain tissue is reduced in most patients with malignant brain tumors.[11] The impairment of tissue metabolism is related to prognosis.[12] The most malignant gliomas (grade IV, glioblastoma) show high uptake, which is often heterogeneous due to necroses typical for this tumor type. Relatively benign tumors with high FDG uptake include pilocytic astrocytoma, which is characterized by metabolically active fenestrated endothelial cells, and ganglioglioma. In meningiomas FDG uptake is variable and may be related to aggressiveness and probability of recurrence.[13] Other malignant tumors in the brain—primitive neuroectodermal tumors, medulloblastomas, malignant lymphomas, and brain metastases from systemic cancers—often show high FDG uptake (review in[14]).

Differentiation Between Recurrent Tumor and Necrosis

After tumor resection, normal postsurgical changes do not show increased FDG uptake. Therefore, hypermetabolic activity after surgery is highly indicative of residual tumor, and [18F]-FDG-PET can be performed within a few days after surgery.[15]

One of the most important applications of PET tracers is in the post–radiation therapy setting, where it can be used to differentiate between radiation-induced changes like necrosis or recurrent or residual tumor.[3] Generally, the question "tumor or necrosis" is an oversimplification, as in most cases both tumor and necrotic tissue can be found next to each other in individual patients.

Several weeks after treatment, the therapeutic effects of radiotherapy can be visualized. [18F]-FDG shows a transient increase of uptake in the initial phase caused by infiltrating macrophages consuming [18F]-FDG.[16,17] A newly detected hypermetabolism weeks after therapy indicates a recurrent tumor and progression from low-grade to high-grade glioma.[15] One study showed that the sensitivity of [18F]-FDG-PET for the detection of recurrent tumor versus radiation necrosis was 75% and the specificity was 81%.[18] Another study showed that there is a certain overlap in [18F]-FDG uptake in recurrent tumor and radiation necrosis.[19] Disadvantages of [18F]-FDG-PET include accumulation of [18F]-FDG in macrophages that may infiltrate the sites having received radiation therapy. Therefore, radiation necrosis may be indistinguishable from recurrent tumor.

Patients with brain tumors have decreased glucose metabolism in the contralateral cortex and the degree of decrease correlates with tumor size.[20] This phenomenon might also be caused by corticosteroids, but a functional inactivation of the contralateral hemisphere by deafferentation of the input from the ipsilateral hemisphere cannot be excluded.[20]

Biopsy Planning

Gliomas are characteristically heterogeneous and may present with areas of different histological grade when they progress to a more malignant subtype. This smaller part of the tumor that already has progressed to a more malignant grade might not show contrast enhancement on MRI or CT. Therefore, MRI- or CT-guided biopsies may be associated with signifi-

cant sampling error and potentially incorrect staging. Trajectory planning in stereotactic biopsy based on [18F]-FDG-PET improves the detection of tumor tissue when compared to anatomic imaging alone.[21]

Therapy Response Assessment

It is very important to detect responders and nonresponders as early as possible during chemotherapy regimens, and it is crucial not to forfeit bone marrow reserve and quality of life to an ineffective treatment.

One study of patients with recurrent high-grade gliomas undergoing treatment with temozolomide (TMZ) looked at early evaluation of tumor metabolic response using [18F]-FDG–PET.[16] The metabolic rate of glucose was quantified in nine patients prior to and 14 days after TMZ treatment and was compared with objective response after 8 weeks. Pretreatment metabolic rate of glucose was higher in responders than nonresponders. The responding patient group had a greater than 25% reduction in CMRGlc in regions of high focal tumor uptake after 8 weeks.[16] FDG-PET imaging has been shown to predict tumor metabolic response to TMZ versus TMZ plus radiotherapy in recurrent high-grade glioma.[22] Therefore, monitoring of therapeutic response by PET imaging is now done to provide an early assessment of therapy efficacy and aid oncologists in optimizing therapeutic management of brain tumors.

Another study evaluated the ability of FDG-PET to detect response to a mammalian target of rapamycin (mTOR) inhibitor used to treat glioblastoma multiforme.[23] mTOR functions within the phosphatidylinositol 3-kinase (PI3K)/Akt signaling pathway as a critical modulator of cell survival. On the basis of promising preclinical data, the safety and tolerability of therapy with the mTOR inhibitor everolimus in combination with radiation therapy and TMZ was evaluated in a phase I study. The study concluded that changes in tumor metabolism could be detected by FDG-PET in a subset of patients within days of initiating everolimus therapy.[23]

Special Consideration

- Positron emission tomography imaging is now used in the clinical setting to assess early response to certain therapies and help guide further therapeutic strategies

---

■ Imaging Amino Acid Metabolism

Several studies using different amino acid tracers demonstrate that increased amino acid uptake in gliomas is not a direct measure of protein synthesis but rather seems to be due to increased transport mediated by type L amino acid carriers.[24,25] In a rat tumor model, facilitated transport of amino acids was upregulated, which suggested that tumors can influence transporter expression in their vasculature.[25] At the normal blood–brain barrier the sodium-independent L-transporter system in the luminal membrane of endothelial cells is the main mechanism of methionine and tyrosine transport into brain tissue.[26,27] Movement of an amino acid across sodium-independent transporter systems is driven by its extra- to intracellular concentration gradient, but it is frequently associated with countertransport of a second amino acid. The gradient of this second amino acid can be established by one of the sodium-dependent carriers like the A-system, which is located in the abluminal endothelial cell membrane at the blood–brain barrier and transports amino acids with short, polar side chains.[26,27] Transport system A is overexpressed in neoplastic cells and seems to be positively correlated with tumor cell growth rate.[28] This increased growth rate requires an efficient and increased supply of nutrients for protein synthesis, energy metabolism, and proliferation. Therefore, elevated transport of amino acids is not only a result of increased protein synthesis but also reflects the increased demand for the different metabolic activities in the tumor cell. It is well known that tumors can influence growth of their vasculature and therefore can regulate their nutrient supply, including amino acids.

Amino acid uptake in the normal cortex is higher than in white matter, but relatively low when compared to the high background activity of the normal cortex in [18F]-FDG-PET (**Fig. 6.2**).

Tracers

The most frequently used radiolabeled amino acid is *methyl-*[11C]-L-methionine ([11C]-MET).[29] Various amino acids have been labeled for tumor imaging especially with PET. As [11C]-labeled tracers can only be used in centers with an onsite cyclotron, there were several attempts to label amino acids with [18F]-fluorine to facilitate a wider use of amino acid tracers. Clinically relevant findings have been obtained mainly with two of them: (1) O-(2-[18F]fluoroethyl)-L-tyrosine (18FET), which showed similar results when compared to [11C]-MET; and (2) [18F]fluoro-Dopa (18F-Dopa), which is a very interesting amino acid tracer that has been successfully used in movement disorders for several years and that also showed comparable results to [11C]-MET.[29]

18FET and 18F-Dopa are transported into the brain and tumor, but no further metabolism takes place; thus they reflect transport only. [11C]-MET, in contrast, is used in different metabolic pathways. It is incorporated into proteins, used for methylation, and is needed for DNA translation.

[11C]-MET uptake ratios compared with background activity in tumors is in the range of 1.2 to 6.0 for gliomas. Uptake correlates to cell proliferation in cell culture, Ki-67 expression, proliferating cell nuclear antigen expression, and microvessel density,[30] indicating its role as a marker for active tumor pro-

liferation and angiogenesis. Of all the gliomas, the highest uptake is observed in anaplastic oligodendrogliomas World Health Organization (WHO) grade III.

Imaging for Primary Diagnosis

In a study of 89 patients, [11C]-MET demonstrated a sensitivity of 76% and a specificity of 87% for distinguishing brain tumors from nontumoral brain lesions.[31] Low-grade tumors are especially better detected by amino acid tracers because of the low background activity of normal brain (**Fig. 6.3**) and increased uptake in the absence of blood–brain barrier damage. On the other hand, a small portion of low-grade astrocytomas demonstrates only low tracer uptake, and again acute inflammation or ischemic stroke might present with increased amino acid uptake. Brain lesions that show hypo- or isometabolism on [18F]-FDG-PET can be detected and differentiated with high sensitivity and good contrast using [11C]-MET. [11C]-MET can provide additional information when used in combination with [18F]-FDG-PET in the evaluation of these patients.

Although there is a good correlation between amino acid uptake and histological tumor grade, there are overlaps in tracer uptake in the different histological tumor types and grades, and amino acid tracers might be not suitable for noninvasive grading[31] (**Fig. 6.3**). Other studies found good differentiation properties between high- and low-grade tumors.[32] Generally, from our experience it is very difficult to determine the histological grade from [11C]-MET-PET without knowing the histological subtype or with additional information from MRI or computed tomography (CT) (**Fig. 6.3**). This might be different when an increased [11C]-MET-PET uptake is detected in the follow-up of the same patient.[33] There is also a relationship between angiogenesis and amino acid uptake.[30]

In many instances the extent of increased MET uptake is larger than that of contrast enhancement,[34] and it indicates tumor infiltration and tumor margins. Especially in low-grade gliomas, amino acid uptake is related to prognosis and survival.[35] MET-PET is therefore most useful in low-grade gliomas for differentiation from nontumorous lesions, for detection of recurrences, for indicating changes in grade of progressing disease,[33] and for potentially allowing a better prediction of prognosis. MET-PET is related to prognosis in gliomas and is better than FDG-PET and MRI in predicting survival in low-grade gliomas.[36] MET-PET was useful in differentiating tumorous from nontumorous lesions in children and young adults when the decision about further therapy was difficult or impossible to make from routine structural imaging alone.[37] MET uptake differs with tumor type; in oligodendrogliomas, uptake tends to be higher than in astrocytomas of the same histological grade, although they are less aggressive.[38] In oligodendrogliomas, [11C]-choline PET may be useful in evaluating the potential malignancy, but MET-PET is superior in detecting "hot lesions."[39] MET uptake is increased in other malignant intracranial tumors, but also in benign neoplasias, such as meningiomas.[14]

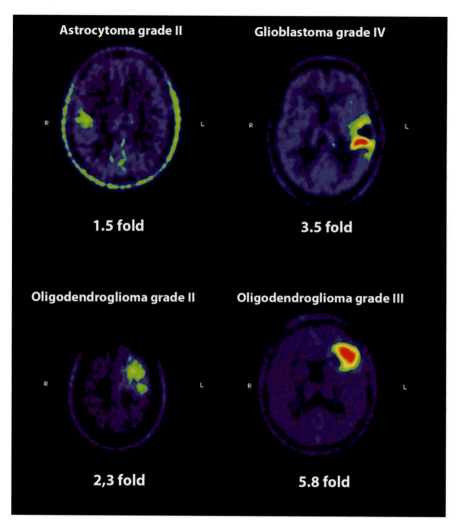

Fig. 6.3 Images and corresponding [^{11}C]-MET uptake ratios compared to corresponding contralateral region in patients with different histological subtypes and different grades of gliomas. There are overlaps of uptake ratio especially in astrocytoma (WHO grade III) and oligodendroglioma (WHO grade II). The highest uptake ratios can be observed in anaplastic oligodendrogliomas (WHO grade III).

Pearl

- Using MET-PET to monitor amino acid uptake is especially useful in low-grade gliomas to differentiate from nontumorous lesions, detect recurrence, detect changes in grade of progressing disease, and predict prognosis

Because of the short half-life of [^{11}C] (20 minutes), [^{18}F]-labeled aromatic amino acid analogues have been developed for tumor imaging. Tumor uptake of [^{18}F]-fluoroethyl-L-tyrosine (FET) and dihydroxy-[^{18}F]-fluoro-L-phenylalanine (FDOPA) is similar to that of MET.[29] In a large study, FDOPA demonstrated excellent visualization of high- and low-grade tumors and was more sensitive and specific than FDG, but no significant relation to tumor grade or to contrast-enhancement was observed.[40] Especially in newly diagnosed tumors, uptake was related to proliferation, whereas this correlation was not observed in recurrent gliomas.[41] High FET uptake indicative of tumor cell infiltration was associated with markers of neuronal cell loss seen on magnetic resonance spectroscopy.[42]

Differentiation between Recurrent Tumor and Necrosis

Amino acid tracers seem to be more useful in the differentiation between postradiation changes and recurrent tumor. Necrosis and glioses after therapy show a reduction of amino acid uptake in contrast to recurrent or residual tumor growth. Therefore, [^{11}C]-MET-PET successfully differentiates between recurrent tumor and radiation necrosis with the detection of recurrent tumor at high sensitivity and high specificity (**Figs. 6.4** and **6.5**) Again, MET-PET is more sensitive than FDG-PET for differentiation between recurrent tumor and radiation necrosis[43] despite its limitations in tumor grading,[44] and is especially effective in combination with MRI.[45] Even in brain lesions that did not show increased uptake in FDG-PET a sensitivity between 89% (tumors) and 92% (gliomas) with a specificity of 100% was obtained (detailed elsewhere[46]).

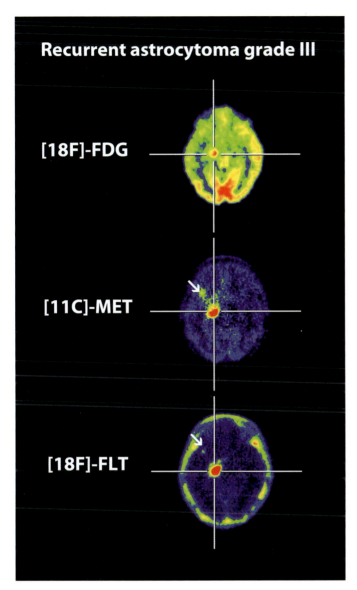

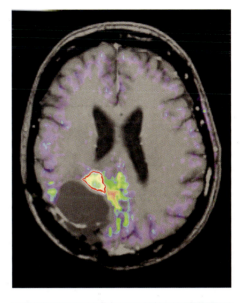

a

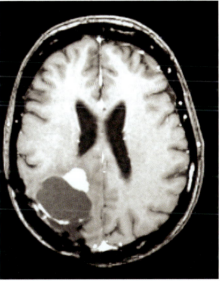

b

Fig. 6.4 [18F]-FDG, [11C]-MET-PET, and [18F]-FLT-PET in a patient suffering from a recurrent astrocytoma (WHO grade III). The high background activity of normal brain is seen in the [18F]-FDG-image. In contrast there is a very low background activity in the [18F]-FLT image, resulting in a high tumor-to-background ratio. There is an additional area at the right temporal pole with increased uptake in [11C]-MET-PET and [18F]-FLT-PET (*white arrows*) but not in the [18F]-FDG image.

Fig. 6.5a,b Differentiation between recurrent tumor and radiation necrosis in 11C-MET-PET **(a)** and MRI **(b)**. Biopsy of this clinically worsening tumor, taken from the region with positive magnetic resonance contrast enhancement, evidenced only necrosis. However, a second biopsy from the area of increased amino acid uptake revealed the findings of recurrent tumor. (From Thiel A, Pietrzyk U, et al. Enhanced accuracy in differential diagnosis of radiation necrosis by positron emission tomography-magnetic resonance imaging coregistration: technical case report. *Neurosurgery* 2000;46:232–234. Copyright © 2000, Lippincott Williams & Wilkins. All rights reserved. Reproduced with permission.)

A recent systemic review and meta-analysis demonstrated that FET-PET has good sensitivity (82%) and average specificity (76%) for diagnosis of brain tumors; it distinguishes between infection and tumoral lesions and between tumor recurrence and radionecrosis.[47] In another recent large multicenter retrospective study, sensitivity and specificity for detection of brain tumors were 87% and 68%, respectively, but significant differences were seen for high– and low-grade tumors as well as among inflammatory and other brain lesions.[48] The speci-

ficity of FET-PET as a single modality was low and limited by passive tracer influx through a disrupted blood–brain barrier and tracer uptake in nonneoplastic lesions, for example, inflammatory lesions, acute and subacute ischemic infarctions, and intracranial hemorrhage. The diagnostic accuracy can be improved by combination with MRI[49] and MR spectroscopy.[50]

Kinetic analysis of FET uptake significantly improved sensitivity for detection of high-grade gliomas even for lesions with low or diffuse tracer uptake[51]; the uptake kinetic of FET was an independent predictor of overall and, to a lesser extent, progression-free survival.[52]

Tumor Delineation

Many studies have shown that the margins of tumors in [11C]-MET are frequently wider when compared to MRI or CT.[53] This phenomenon is even more pronounced in low-grade tumors and in diffuse gliomatoses because of the often missing contrast enhancement in MRI.[54] [11C]-MET-PET is superior to [18F]-FDG-PET in the assessment of tumor extent[55] (**Figs. 6.2** and **6.4**).

In one study, a patient was described with an anaplastic astrocytoma who was examined with CT and PET using [68Ga]–ethylenediaminetetraacetic acid (EDTA), [11C]-glucose, and [11C]-MET.[55] The patient died 15 days after the [11C]-MET-PET, and histological evaluation at autopsy showed excellent agreement between tumor extent and [11C]-MET uptake. More than 50% of the tumor would not have been detected without the [11C]-MET-PET. Studies integrating [11C]-MET-PET images in radiation therapy planning procedures confirm these discrepancies among MRI, CT, and [11C]-MET-PET.[56]

> **Pearl**
>
> - [11C]-MET-PET is superior to [18F]-FDG-PET for defining tumor extent and is an excellent method for further therapy planning.

[11C]-MET-PET detects solid parts of brain tumors as well as an infiltration zone with high sensitivity and specificity.[57]

Monitoring Therapy Response

Because of the high cortical background activity, FDG is limited in the detection of residual tumor after therapy.[58] The effects of radiation and chemotherapy can only be shown after a few weeks of treatment[16] and recurrent tumor or malignant transformation is marked by newly occurring hypermetabolism.[16] Hypermetabolism after radiotherapy, however, can also be mimicked by infiltration of macrophages. With these limitations, FDG-PET is not the preferred method for the assessment of therapeutic effects.[59] For this application amino acid and nucleoid tracers are better suited.[60,61] Several studies suggested that outcomes are better for patients in whom MET- or FET-PET co-registered to MRI is applied for treatment planning and follow-up than for patients diagnosed by MRI alone.[60]

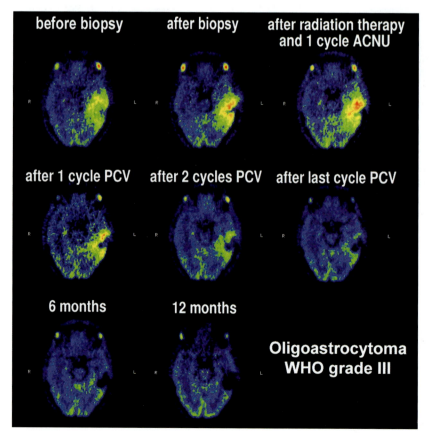

Fig. 6.6 Chemotherapy monitoring. Follow-up of a patient with oligoastrocytoma WHO grade III in the left temporal lobe. After the radiation therapy and first cycle of ACNU chemotherapy, tumor showed a clear progress in [11C]-MET-PET. Chemotherapy regimen was changed to PCV and [11C]-MET-uptake decreased which was clearly detectable even after the first cycle of chemotherapy. Patient reached a complete remission and no significant [11C]-MET-uptake was detectable after 8 cycles of chemotherapy and in one year of follow-up.

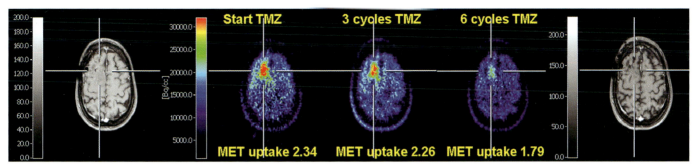

Fig. 6.7 Chemotherapy monitoring. Follow-up of a patient with a recurrent glioblastoma. From the first to the sixth cycle of temozolomide (TMZ) chemotherapy, a clear decrease of [¹¹C]-MET uptake can

be observed compared with no changes in signal abnormalities in contrast-enhanced MRI.

For the management of patients with brain tumors, differentiating between recurrent tumor as a sign of treatment failure and necrosis as an indicator of success is essential. For that application, MET-PET co-registered to MRI has high sensitivity and specificity (~75%).[43,62] Malignant progression in nontreated as well as treated patients was detected with high sensitivity and specificity by MET-PET (**Figs. 6.6** and **6.7**). The increase in MET uptake during malignant progression was also reflected by an increase in angiogenesis-promoting markers as vascular endothelial growth factor.[63] The volume of metabolically active tumor in recurrent glioblastoma multiforme was underestimated by gadolinium–diethylenetriamine penta-acetic acid (Gd-DTPA)-enhanced MRI.[64] The additional information supplied by MET-PET changed management in half of the cases.[65] Responses after chemotherapy can be detected by amino acid PET early in the course,[66] suggesting that deactivation of amino acid transport is an early sign of response to chemotherapy. FET-PET co-registered to MRI was more sensitive in detecting the effects of a multimodal treatment than was conventional MRI alone and reached a sensitivity of more than 80% and a specificity of close to 100%.[67]

The currently available data suggest that a reduction of amino acid uptake by a glioma is a sign of a response to treatment. Recently, a prospective study evaluated the prognostic value of early changes of ¹⁸F-FET uptake after postoperative radiochemotherapy in glioblastomas.[68] It could be demonstrated that PET responders with a decrease of the tumor/brain ratio of > 10% had a significantly longer disease-free survival and overall survival than patients with stable or increasing tracer uptake after radiochemotherapy in glioblastomas. Multimodal imaging including various PET and MRI modalities will be of great impact on the development of new therapeutic strategies, such as targeting proliferating cells or applying gene therapy vectors and to angiogenesis.

Imaging Tumor Proliferation

Labeled nucleosides are indicators of cellular proliferation and should provide information on histological grading. The thymidine analogue 3-deoxy-3-[¹⁸F]-fluorothymidine (FLT) was developed as a noninvasive tracer of tumor cell proliferation. The uptake of FLT correlates with thymidine kinase-1 activity, an enzyme expressed during the DNA synthesis phase of cell cycle, which is high in proliferating and low in quiescent cells. With this tracer an excellent delineation of grade III and IV tumors with high tumor-to–normal brain ratio was obtained[69] (**Fig. 6.4**), whereas grade II gliomas and stable lesions did not show considerable tracer uptake; additionally, a high correlation of FLT uptake was seen with Ki-67 expression as a surrogate marker for tumor proliferation.[70] Despite that, absolute tumor uptake of FLT was lower than that of MET, tumor-to–normal brain uptake ratios were higher than for MET due to the low FLT concentration in normal brain (**Fig. 6.4**).

Gadolinium-enhanced MRI yields complementary information on tumor extent, because FLT uptake occurs also in regions with disrupted blood–brain barrier, and sensitivity for detection of low-grade gliomas is lower than with MET.[71] A kinetic analysis of FLT tracer uptake permits assessment of tumor proliferation rates in high-grade gliomas, whereas uptake ratios of MET and FLT fails to correlate with the in vitro determined proliferation index by Ki-67 immunostaining.[69] In another study FLT-PET was superior to MET-PET in tumor grading and assessment of proliferation in different gliomas, and the combination with MET-PET added significant information.[72] In a direct comparison of FDG, [¹⁸F]-Dopa and [¹⁸F]-FLT in primary and recurrent low-grade gliomas FLT uptake was low (Standardized uptake value [SUV] = 1.8) in comparison to F-Dopa (SUV = 5.75) and FDG (SUV = 8.5), and tumor-to–normal brain ratios were 2.3 ± 0.5 for F-Dopa, 1.8 ± 0.9 for FLT, and 1.0 ± 0.6 for FDG. The authors concluded that F-Dopa is superior to the other tracers for evaluation of low-grade gliomas.[73]

In another study only the FLT influx rate, but not SUV, could separate recurrence from radionecrosis.[74] In high-grade gliomas FLT-PET–derived proliferative volume predicted overall survival of patients.[75] FLT uptake investigated at different time points in the course of treatment was able to differentiate between responders and nonresponders by an SUV decrease of more or less 25%, and the responders survived 3 times as long as nonresponders.[76] As shown by several groups, the kinetics of FLT uptake are closely related to prognosis, to early efficacy of treatment, and to outcome.[77] These therapeutic effects may be related to normalization of neovascularization, for example, by bevacizumab and/or permeability changes by chemotherapy,[77] and can serve as early surrogate markers of long-term survival.

■ Future Perspectives

Combining the unsurpassed soft tissue contrast of MRI with the sensitivity of PET will be the goal for multimodality imaging in brain tumors. Integrating the indirect measure of cell density with apparent diffusion coefficient (ADC) maps and an indirect measure of cell amino acid transport with dynamic FET-PET enables assessing different and complementary tumor characteristics reflecting tumoral aggressiveness potential. If used for better selecting patients who can benefit from aggressive first-line therapy, sensitivity can be improved to 86% and specificity to 100%.[47] This combination of imaging modalities may best be achieved by hybrid MRI-PET, which additionally can be used to perform simultaneously magnetic resonance spectroscopy in selected regions. Such integrated MRI-PET assessing simultaneously morphological, dynamic, and various molecular parameters might be the gold standard for diagnosis of gliomas in the future.[78]

Editor's Note

Positron emission tomography imaging has been the gold standard for the in vivo detection of metabolic activity within a tumor or in the adjacent brain. There have been different types of imaging substrates used in this field with the main player thus far being [18F]-FDG. This measures glucose consumption, which is typically elevated in high-grade gliomas. The problem has always been that [18F]-FDG uptake is not specific for brain tumors and can be seen in inflammatory situations that may be related to treatment effect or response to tumor immunotherapy protocols. Also, FDG is not the ideal isotope to use for low-grade tumors because these lesions have similar metabolism to normal white matter. That said, PET imaging can be accurately used to add to the armamentarium of the treating physician in making a diagnosis of a glioma and to help differentiate tumor recurrence from treatment effect such as radiation necrosis. Where we think this technique becomes less robust is in actually defining the true extent of the tumor away from the obvious margin of the lesion. That said, PET scanning will continue to be a very useful modality for monitoring response to therapy, and newer isotopes such as fluorothymidine will be able to more specifically demonstrate certain components of the cell cycle that is a surrogate marker of proliferation, which could be very helpful in terms of actually grading the tumor and determining the response to therapy, such as in the case of vascular normalization following bevacizumab. (Berger)

References

1. la Fougère C, Suchorska B, Bartenstein P, Kreth FW, Tonn JC. Molecular imaging of gliomas with PET: opportunities and limitations. Neuro-oncol 2011;13:806–819

2. Reivich M, Kuhl D, Wolf A, et al. The [18F]fluorodeoxyglucose method for the measurement of local cerebral glucose utilization in man. Circ Res 1979;44:127–137

3. Patronas NJ, Di Chiro G, Brooks RA, et al. Work in progress: [18F] fluorodeoxyglucose and positron emission tomography in the evaluation of radiation necrosis of the brain. Radiology 1982;144:885–889

4. Tyler JL, Diksic M, Villemure JG, et al. Metabolic and hemodynamic evaluation of gliomas using positron emission tomography. J Nucl Med 1987;28:1123–1133

5. Spence AM, Muzi M, Mankoff DA, et al. 18F-FDG PET of gliomas at delayed intervals: improved distinction between tumor and normal gray matter. J Nucl Med 2004;45:1653–1659

6. Prieto E, Martí-Climent JM, Domínguez-Prado I, et al. Voxel-based analysis of dual-time-point 18F-FDG PET images for brain tumor identification and delineation. J Nucl Med 2011;52:865–872

7. Alavi JB, Alavi A, Chawluk J, et al. Positron emission tomography in patients with glioma. A predictor of prognosis. Cancer 1988;62:1074–1078

8. Herholz K, Pietrzyk U, Voges J, et al. Correlation of glucose consumption and tumor cell density in astrocytomas. A stereotactic PET study. J Neurosurg 1993;79:853–858

9. Barker FG II, Chang SM, Valk PE, Pounds TR, Prados MD. 18-Fluorodeoxyglucose uptake and survival of patients with suspected recurrent malignant glioma. Cancer 1997;79:115–126

10. Delbeke D, Meyerowitz C, Lapidus RL, et al. Optimal cutoff levels of F-18 fluorodeoxyglucose uptake in the differentiation of low-grade from high-grade brain tumors with PET. Radiology 1995;195:47–52

11. DeLaPaz RL, Patronas NJ, Brooks RA, et al. Positron emission tomographic study of suppression of gray-matter glucose utilization by brain tumors. AJNR Am J Neuroradiol 1983;4:826–829

12. Hölzer T, Herholz K, Jeske J, Heiss WD. FDG-PET as a prognostic indicator in radiochemotherapy of glioblastoma. J Comput Assist Tomogr 1993;17:681–687

13. Di Chiro G, Hatazawa J, Katz DA, Rizzoli HV, De Michele DJ. Glucose utilization by intracranial meningiomas as an index of tumor aggressivity and probability of recurrence: a PET study. Radiology 1987;164:521–526

14. Herholz K, Herscovitch P, Heiss WD. NeuroPET—Positron Emission Tomography in Neuroscience and Clinical Neurology. Berlin: Springer, 2004

15. Glantz MJ, Hoffman JM, Coleman RE, et al. Identification of early recurrence of primary central nervous system tumors by [18F]fluorodeoxyglucose positron emission tomography. Ann Neurol 1991;29:347–355

16. Brock CS, Young H, O'Reilly SM, et al. Early evaluation of tumour metabolic response using [18F]fluorodeoxyglucose and positron emission tomography: a pilot study following the phase II chemotherapy schedule for temozolomide in recurrent high-grade gliomas. Br J Cancer 2000;82:608–615

17. Reinhardt MJ, Kubota K, Yamada S, Iwata R, Yaegashi H. Assessment of cancer recurrence in residual tumors after fractionated radiotherapy: a comparison of fluorodeoxyglucose, L-methionine and thymidine. J Nucl Med 1997;38:280–287

18. Chao ST, Suh JH, Raja S, Lee SY, Barnett G. The sensitivity and specificity of FDG PET in distinguishing recurrent brain tumor from radionecrosis in patients treated with stereotactic radiosurgery. Int J Cancer 2001;96:191–197

19. Levivier M, Becerra A, De Witte O, Brotchi J, Goldman S. Radiation necrosis or recurrence. J Neurosurg 1996;84:148–149

20. Roelcke U, Blasberg RG, von Ammon K, et al. Dexamethasone treatment and plasma glucose levels: relevance for fluorine-18-fluorodeoxyglucose uptake measurements in gliomas. J Nucl Med 1998;39:879–884

21. Levivier M, Goldman S, Pirotte B, et al. Diagnostic yield of stereotactic brain biopsy guided by positron emission tomography with [18F]fluorodeoxyglucose. J Neurosurg 1995;82:445–452

22. Charnley N, West CM, Barnett CM, et al. Early change in glucose metabolic rate measured using FDG-PET in patients with high-grade glioma predicts response to temozolomide but not temozolomide plus radiotherapy. Int J Radiat Oncol Biol Phys 2006;66:331–338

23. Sarkaria JN, Galanis E, Wu W, et al. North Central Cancer Treatment Group Phase I trial N057K of everolimus (RAD001) and temozolomide in combination with radiation therapy in patients with newly diagnosed glioblastoma multiforme. Int J Radiat Oncol Biol Phys 2011;81:468–475

24. Bergström M, Lundqvist H, Ericson K, et al. Comparison of the accumulation kinetics of L-(methyl-11C)-methionine and D-(methyl-11C)-methionine in brain tumors studied with positron emission tomography. Acta Radiol 1987;28:225–229

25. Miyagawa T, Oku T, Uehara H, et al. "Facilitated" amino acid transport is upregulated in brain tumors. J Cereb Blood Flow Metab 1998;18:500–509

26. Knudsen GM, Pettigrew KD, Patlak CS, Hertz MM, Paulson OB. Asymmetrical transport of amino acids across the blood-brain barrier in humans. J Cereb Blood Flow Metab 1990;10:698–706

27. Sánchez del Pino MM, Peterson DR, Hawkins RA. Neutral amino acid transport characterization of isolated luminal and abluminal membranes of the blood-brain barrier. J Biol Chem 1995;270:14913–14918

28. Bading JR, Kan-Mitchell J, Conti PS. System A amino acid transport in cultured human tumor cells: implications for tumor imaging with PET. Nucl Med Biol 1996;23:779–786

29. Becherer A, Karanikas G, Szabó M, et al. Brain tumour imaging with PET: a comparison between [18F]fluorodopa and [11C]methionine. Eur J Nucl Med Mol Imaging 2003;30:1561–1567

30. Kracht LW, Friese M, Herholz K, et al. Methyl-[11C]-l-methionine uptake as measured by positron emission tomography correlates to microvessel density in patients with glioma. Eur J Nucl Med Mol Imaging 2003;30:868–873

31. Herholz K, Hölzer T, Bauer B, et al. 11C-methionine PET for differential diagnosis of low-grade gliomas. Neurology 1998;50:1316–1322

32. Kuwert T, Morgenroth C, Woesler B, et al. Uptake of iodine-123-alpha-methyl tyrosine by gliomas and non-neoplastic brain lesions. Eur J Nucl Med 1996;23:1345–1353

33. Ullrich RT, Kracht L, Brunn A, et al. Methyl-L-11C-methionine PET as a diagnostic marker for malignant progression in patients with glioma. J Nucl Med 2009;50:1962–1968

34. Ericson K, Lilja A, Bergström M, et al. Positron emission tomography with ([11C]methyl)-L-methionine, [11C]D-glucose, and [68Ga]EDTA in supratentorial tumors. J Comput Assist Tomogr 1985;9:683–689

35. Ribom D, Eriksson A, Hartman M, et al. Positron emission tomography (11)C-methionine and survival in patients with low-grade gliomas. Cancer 2001;92:1541–1549

36. Singhal T, Narayanan TK, Jacobs MP, Bal C, Mantil JC. 11C-methionine PET for grading and prognostication in gliomas: a comparison study with 18F-FDG PET and contrast enhancement on MRI. J Nucl Med 2012;53:1709–1715

37. Galldiks N, Kracht LW, Berthold F, et al. [11C]-L-methionine positron emission tomography in the management of children and young adults with brain tumors. J Neurooncol 2010;96:231–239

38. Derlon JM, Petit-Taboué MC, Chapon F, et al. The in vivo metabolic pattern of low-grade brain gliomas: a positron emission tomographic study using 18F-fluorodeoxyglucose and 11C-L-methylmethionine. Neurosurgery 1997;40:276–287, discussion 287–288

39. Kato T, Shinoda J, Oka N, et al. Analysis of 11C-methionine uptake in low-grade gliomas and correlation with proliferative activity. AJNR Am J Neuroradiol 2008;29:1867–1871

40. Chen W, Silverman DH, Delaloye S, et al. 18F-FDOPA PET imaging of brain tumors: comparison study with 18F-FDG PET and evaluation of diagnostic accuracy. J Nucl Med 2006;47:904–911

41. Fueger BJ, Czernin J, Cloughesy T, et al. Correlation of 6-18F-fluoro-L-dopa PET uptake with proliferation and tumor grade in newly diagnosed and recurrent gliomas. J Nucl Med 2010;51:1532–1538

42. Stadlbauer A, Prante O, Nimsky C, et al. Metabolic imaging of cerebral gliomas: spatial correlation of changes in O-(2-18F-fluoroethyl)-L-tyrosine PET and proton magnetic resonance spectroscopic imaging. J Nucl Med 2008;49:721–729

43. Van Laere K, Ceyssens S, Van Calenbergh F, et al. Direct comparison of 18F-FDG and 11C-methionine PET in suspected recurrence of glioma: sensitivity, inter-observer variability and prognostic value. Eur J Nucl Med Mol Imaging 2005;32:39–51

44. Ceyssens S, Van Laere K, de Groot T, Goffin J, Bormans G, Mortelmans L. [11C]methionine PET, histopathology, and survival in primary brain tumors and recurrence. AJNR Am J Neuroradiol 2006;27:1432–1437

45. Pöpperl G, Gotz C, Rachinger W, Gildehaus FJ, Tonn JC, Tatsch K. Value of O-(2-[18F]fluoroethyl)-L-tyrosine PET for the diagnosis of recurrent glioma. Eur J Nucl Med Mol Imaging 2004;31:1464–1470

46. Chen W. Clinical applications of PET in brain tumors. J Nucl Med 2007;48:1468–1481

47. Dunet V, Rossier C, Buck A, Stupp R, Prior JO. Performance of 18F-fluoro-ethyl-tyrosine (18F-FET) PET for the differential diagnosis of primary brain tumor: a systematic review and Metaanalysis. J Nucl Med 2012;53:207–214

48. Hutterer M, Nowosielski M, Putzer D, et al. [18F]-fluoro-ethyl-L-tyrosine PET: a valuable diagnostic tool in neuro-oncology, but not all that glitters is glioma. Neuro-oncol 2013;15:341–351

49. Pauleit D, Floeth F, Hamacher K, et al. O-(2-[18F]fluoroethyl)-L-tyrosine PET combined with MRI improves the diagnostic assessment of cerebral gliomas. Brain 2005;128(Pt 3):678–687

50. Floeth FW, Pauleit D, Wittsack HJ, et al. Multimodal metabolic imaging of cerebral gliomas: positron emission tomography with [18F]fluoro-ethyl-L-tyrosine and magnetic resonance spectroscopy. J Neurosurg 2005;102:318–327

51. Jansen NL, Graute V, Armbruster L, et al. MRI-suspected low-grade glioma: is there a need to perform dynamic FET PET? Eur J Nucl Med Mol Imaging 2012;39:1021–1029

52. Niyazi M, Jansen N, Ganswindt U, et al. Re-irradiation in recurrent malignant glioma: prognostic value of [18F]FET-PET. J Neurooncol 2012; 110:389–395

53. Jacobs AH, Winkler A, Dittmar C, et al. Molecular and functional imaging technology for the development of efficient treatment strategies for gliomas. Technol Cancer Res Treat 2002;1:187–204

54. Mineura K, Sasajima T, Kowada M, Uesaka Y, Shishido F. Innovative approach in the diagnosis of gliomatosis cerebri using carbon-11-L-methionine positron emission tomography. J Nucl Med 1991;32:726–728

55. Bergström M, Collins VP, Ehrin E, et al. Discrepancies in brain tumor extent as shown by computed tomography and positron emission tomography using [68Ga]EDTA, [11C]glucose, and [11C]methionine. J Comput Assist Tomogr 1983;7:1062–1066

56. Nuutinen J, Sonninen P, Lehikoinen P, et al. Radiotherapy treatment planning and long-term follow-up with [(11)C]methionine PET in patients with low-grade astrocytoma. Int J Radiat Oncol Biol Phys 2000; 48:43–52

57. Kracht LW, Miletic H, Busch S, et al. Delineation of brain tumor extent with [11C]L-methionine positron emission tomography: local comparison with stereotactic histopathology. Clin Cancer Res 2004;10: 7163–7170

58. Würker M, Herholz K, Voges J, et al. Glucose consumption and methionine uptake in low-grade gliomas after iodine-125 brachytherapy. Eur J Nucl Med 1996;23:583–586

59. Ricci PE, Karis JP, Heiserman JE, Fram EK, Bice AN, Drayer BP. Differentiating recurrent tumor from radiation necrosis: time for re-evaluation of positron emission tomography? AJNR Am J Neuroradiol 1998;19: 407–413

60. Vees H, Senthamizhchelvan S, Miralbell R, Weber DC, Ratib O, Zaidi H. Assessment of various strategies for 18F-FET PET-guided delineation of target volumes in high-grade glioma patients. Eur J Nucl Med Mol Imaging 2009;36:182–193

61. Nariai T, Tanaka Y, Wakimoto H, et al. Usefulness of L-[methyl-11C] methionine-positron emission tomography as a biological monitoring tool in the treatment of glioma. J Neurosurg 2005;103:498–507

62. Terakawa Y, Tsuyuguchi N, Iwai Y, et al. Diagnostic accuracy of 11C-methionine PET for differentiation of recurrent brain tumors from radiation necrosis after radiotherapy. J Nucl Med 2008;49:694–699

63. Ullrich RT, Kracht L, Brunn A, et al. Methyl-L-11C-methionine PET as a diagnostic marker for malignant progression in patients with glioma. J Nucl Med 2009;50:1962–1968

64. Galldiks N, Ullrich R, Schroeter M, Fink GR, Jacobs AH, Kracht LW. Volumetry of [(11)C]-methionine PET uptake and MRI contrast enhancement in patients with recurrent glioblastoma multiforme. Eur J Nucl Med Mol Imaging 2010;37:84–92

65. Yamane T, Sakamoto S, Senda M. Clinical impact of (11)C-methionine PET on expected management of patients with brain neoplasm. Eur J Nucl Med Mol Imaging 2010;37:685–690

66. Galldiks N, Kracht LW, Burghaus L, et al. Patient-tailored, imaging-guided, long-term temozolomide chemotherapy in patients with glioblastoma. Mol Imaging 2010;9:40–46

67. Mehrkens JH, Pöpperl G, Rachinger W, et al. The positive predictive value of O-(2-[18F]fluoroethyl)-L-tyrosine (FET) PET in the diagnosis of a glioma recurrence after multimodal treatment. J Neurooncol 2008;88:27–35

68. Piroth MD, Pinkawa M, Holy R, et al. Prognostic value of early [18F] fluoroethyltyrosine positron emission tomography after radiochemotherapy in glioblastoma multiforme. Int J Radiat Oncol Biol Phys 2011; 80:176–184

69. Ullrich R, Backes H, Li H, et al. Glioma proliferation as assessed by 3′-fluoro-3′deoxy-L-thymidine positron emission tomography in patients with newly diagnosed high-grade glioma. Clin Cancer Res 2008; 14:2049–2055

70. Yamamoto Y, Ono Y, Aga F, Kawai N, Kudomi N, Nishiyama Y. Correlation of 18F-FLT uptake with tumor grade and Ki-67 immunohistochemistry in patients with newly diagnosed and recurrent gliomas. J Nucl Med 2012;53:1911–1915

71. Jacobs AH, Thomas A, Kracht LW, et al. 18F-fluoro-L-thymidine and 11C-methylmethionine as markers of increased transport and proliferation in brain tumors. J Nucl Med 2005;46:1948–1958

72. Hatakeyama T, Kawai N, Nishiyama Y, et al. 11C-methionine (MET) and 18F-fluorothymidine (FLT) PET in patients with newly diagnosed glioma. Eur J Nucl Med Mol Imaging 2008;35:2009–2017

73. Tripathi M, Sharma R, D'Souza M, et al. Comparative evaluation of F-18 FDOPA, F-18 FDG, and F-18 FLT-PET/CT for metabolic imaging of low grade gliomas. Clin Nucl Med 2009;34:878–883

74. Spence AM, Muzi M, Link JM, et al. NCI-sponsored trial for the evaluation of safety and preliminary efficacy of 3′-deoxy-3′-[18F]fluorothymidine (FLT) as a marker of proliferation in patients with recurrent gliomas: preliminary efficacy studies. Mol Imaging Biol 2009;11:343–355

75. Idema AJ, Hoffmann AL, Boogaarts HD, et al. 3′-Deoxy-3′18F-fluorothymidine PET-derived proliferative volume predicts overall survival in high-grade glioma patients. J Nucl Med 2012;53:1904–1910

76. Chen W, Delaloye S, Silverman DH, et al. Predicting treatment response of malignant gliomas to bevacizumab and irinotecan by imaging proliferation with [18F] fluorothymidine positron emission tomography: a pilot study. J Clin Oncol 2007;25:4714–4721

77. Wardak M, Schiepers C, Dahlbom M, et al. Discriminant analysis of 18F-fluorothymidine kinetic parameters to predict survival in patients with recurrent high-grade glioma. Clin Cancer Res 2011;17:6553–6562

78. Catana C, Drzezga A, Heiss WD, Rosen BR. PET/MRI for neurologic applications. J Nucl Med 2012;53:1916–1925

7 Physiological Imaging

Soonmee Cha

The past three decades have seen the implementation and widespread clinical use of noninvasive anatomic and physiological magnetic resonance imaging (MRI) methods in the field of neuroimaging of brain tumors. Along with advances in neuroimaging, tremendous progress has been made in other fields of neuro-oncology such as stereotactic and navigational neurosurgical techniques, intraoperative cortical and subcortical stimulation mapping methods, immunohistochemical methodologies, and a variety of conformal radiation therapies such as gamma knife radiosurgery and cyberknife radiation therapy. More recently, the unraveling of molecular biology, of the origin of neural stem cells, and of the cancer genetics of brain tumors has led to an entirely new era of exploring the pathogenesis and therapeutic targeting of brain tumors.

Neuroimaging plays a critical role in the diagnosis and preoperative planning of brain tumor cases and also serves as a means for evaluation during or after therapy. Recent advances in technology have fostered the development and clinical application of several new physiology-based MRI methods that provide information not readily available from traditional anatomic imaging. Combined anatomic and physiological MRI promises more comprehensive characterization of tumor and a better understanding of tumor biology. Recent developments and clinical trials of highly selective chemotherapeutic agents, such as those that target specific cancer signaling pathways, tumor-produced growth factors, or angiogenic tumor vessels, promise much hope and reinforce the conviction of every practitioner in the field of neuro-oncology that growth control, albeit not cure, of malignant brain tumors is potentially within reach in the next decade.

Controversy

- Despite their potentially powerful role in advancing knowledge of brain tumor biology, physiology-based MRI methods still await much-needed validation and correlation with clinical outcomes data.

■ Brain Tumor Imaging

Computed tomography (CT) of the brain is very sensitive in detecting acute hemorrhage, hydrocephalus, and herniation, and can be helpful in detecting areas of blood–brain barrier and defining the contrast–enhancing tumor border. However, CT is primarily reserved as an initial screening method to exclude a potentially life–threatening intracranial process, and it suffers from several important limitations. First, CT is not optimally suited for detecting subtle changes in brain parenchyma, such as nonenhancing tumor or infiltrative changes, due to its intrinsically low soft tissue contrast.[1] Computed tomography findings can be rather subtle in cases of infiltrating tumor and easily overlooked. Second, CT does not provide flexible multiplanar acquisition, thus limiting the three–dimensional depiction of tumor. Third, CT involves ionizing radiation, and its iodinated contrast agent can cause serious allergic reaction. Finally, CT is largely confined to providing anatomic information. Even with the addition of intravenous contrast agent, CT is still inferior to MRI in terms of soft tissue resolution, multiplanar capability, and physiology–based applications.

Contrast–enhanced MRI provides exquisite anatomic detail, has multiplanar capability, and does not require ionizing radiation; therefore, it is the current imaging standard for brain tumor diagnosis and therapy monitoring. In clinical practice, the most widely accepted standard imaging protocol includes at least the following two sequences: contrast–enhanced T1–weighted imaging and fluid–attenuated inversion recovery (FLAIR) imaging.

Unfortunately, anatomic MRI is largely limited to depicting morphological abnormality and suffers from nonspecificity. Different disease processes can appear similar or a single disease entity may have varied imaging findings. The underlying metabolic or functional integrity of the brain cannot be adequately evaluated based on anatomic MRI alone. To that end, several physiology–based MRI methods have been developed and have become part of an armamentarium of imaging paradigm to improve tumor characterization. It should be noted that most of these advanced MRI methods are still considered investigational and require further clinical validation and outcomes data to determine their role in clinical management of patients.

Physiology–Based Magnetic Resonance Imaging

Diffusion–Weighted Magnetic Resonance Imaging

Diffusion of water in biological systems, particularly within the brain, is affected not only by the complex interaction between the intra– and extracellular compartments but also by the cytoarchitecture of the microstructures and permeability barriers. Diffusion of water molecules through the magnetic field gradient produces intravoxel dephasing and a loss of signal intensity. Because this microscopic diffusional motion is so small, a large gradient strength or duration is needed to produce observable signal loss from diffusion. By utilizing bipolar pulsed gradient methods, microscopic diffusional motion is detected by a change in the magnitude of moving spins due to phase dispersion. To detect this highly sensitive motion, an ultrafast imaging method, such as the echo planar technique, is needed to acquire a sufficient number of images in the range of milliseconds to produce meaningful information.

Apparent diffusion coefficient (ADC) characterizes the rate of diffusional motion (given in millimeters squared per second). The ADC takes into consideration the heterogeneous environment of brain cytoarchitecture and factors other than diffusion, such as temperature, perfusion, and metabolic rates, that can affect the measurement of microscopic thermal motion. High ADC implies relatively unrestricted water motion. Low ADC indicates restricted diffusional motion, as seen in acute cerebral ischemia. The diffusion sensitivity parameter, b value, is related to duration, strength, and time interval between the diffusion–sensitizing gradients. A typical b value used in clinical imaging is in the range of 900 to 1,000 seconds/mm[2]. The higher the b value, the more sensitive the diffusion imaging is in obtaining greater contrast and detecting areas of restricted water motion.

Anisotropic diffusion is defined as having different diffusional motion in different directions, as is the case in normal myelinated white matter tracts in the brain. Diffusion of water molecules is far less restricted along the parallel plane of the axonal fibers than in perpendicular direction. White matter anisotropy can be demonstrated by comparing diffusion–weighted images with bipolar gradients placed in three orthogonal directions in which hyperintensity in the white matter

---

Pitfall

- Physiological imaging methods based on the echo planar imaging technique are prone to susceptibility artifact and geometric distortion. The susceptibility artifact is most pronounced at the brain–bone–air interface such as the anterior and middle cranial fossa or cerebellar hemisphere near the petrous apex.

---

is visible when the diffusion encoding is perpendicular to the fiber orientation. By combining the information from the three orthogonal data, an orientation–independent image is created without the artifact from normal white matter anisotropy.

Echo planar imaging (EPI) is currently the most widely used MRI technique for clinical application of diffusion–weighted imaging for the diagnosis of acute stroke and other brain disorders such as abscess, epidermoid cyst, traumatic shearing injury, or necrotic encephalitis. It is the fastest available MRI method, which allows the entire set of echoes needed to form an image to be collected within a single acquisition period of 25 to 100 ms.[2] The data are obtained by forming a train of gradient echoes by repeated reversal of a large gradient capable of very rapid polarity inversion to complete k–space filling after a single radiofrequency (RF) pulse. Each gradient echo is phase encoded separately by a very brief blipped gradient or a weak constant phase–encoding gradient. Although the long echo train renders the images sensitive to chemical shift and magnetic susceptibility artifacts, EPI virtually eliminates motion artifact. The chemical shift artifact is overcome by routine use of lipid suppression, whereas the magnetic susceptibility artifact is manifested prominently at air–bone–tissue interfaces such as those at the skull base, paranasal sinuses, orbits, and petrous temporal bone.[3–5]

Clinical Application of Diffusion–Weighted Magnetic Resonance Imaging

Diffusion–weighted MRI is now considered the standard imaging method to diagnosis early cerebral ischemia. With the onset of ischemia, there is breakdown of the cell membrane. There is failure of Na^{2+}–K^+–adenosine triphosphatase (ATPase) pumps, resulting in an influx of Na^{2+} into the cell and subsequent cell swelling. At this time the cells are still viable; however, the extracellular space is compressed and restricted in mobility secondary to expansion of the intracellular compartment. This impaired diffusion within the areas of ischemia is due to cytotoxic edema and microstructural changes within the damaged cells. Localized hyperintensities appear on diffusion–weighted EPI images within minutes of the onset of cerebral ischemia well before conventional MRI shows any changes. These rapidly appearing diffusion abnormalities and the decrease in ADC represent the failure of the energy–driven membrane pumps and the subsequent changes in membrane permeability and regional cytoarchitecture restricting water motion. Changes seen on conventional MRI, including the FLAIR sequence, are delayed until there is a breakdown of the blood–brain barrier, which occurs after the membrane pump failure. Ischemia–induced diffusion abnormality may persist up to 14 days following the acute event, and it precedes later-occurring, permanent structural alterations signifying complete infarction. The abnormality on diffusion–weighted MRI and ADC maps returns to baseline approximately 7 to 14 days following the acute event. The sensitivity and specificity of diffusion imaging in the diagnosis of acute infarct exceeds 95% and is far superior to conventional MRI and CT examinations.

In addition to early diagnosis of cerebral ischemia, diffusion–weighted MRI is extremely sensitive in detecting other intracranial disease processes, including cerebral abscess, epidermoid cyst, traumatic shearing injury, toxic or infectious encephalitis, and immediate postoperative brain injury. The exact mechanism of diffusion restriction in each of these disease entities remains not entirely certain, but diffusion–weighted MRI can be extremely helpful in making the diagnosis. Cerebral abscess, for example, can appear indistinct from a cystic brain tumor, and preoperative diagnosis is critical for proper surgical and medical management. Diffusion–weighted MRI demonstrates profound restricted–diffusion abnormality in cerebral abscess (**Fig. 7.1**), most likely attributable to the increased viscosity of the pus fluid. Similarly, an epidermoid cyst contains highly viscous material, which can explain the characteristic restricted diffusion associated with this entity as shown in (**Fig. 7.2**). Diffuse axonal injury following trauma represents areas of permanent brain injury due to the rotational shearing force that results in destruction of cytoarchitecture of the affected brain. In toxic or infectious encephalitis, herpes being the prototype, there is widespread necrotizing tissue destruction due to direct injury to the neurons and oligodendrocytes. Again, the end result is altered membrane integrity and shift of water into the intracellular compartment and corresponding restriction of extracellular space and water motion.

Diffusion–weighted MRI can be extremely valuable in accurate interpretation of new abnormal contrast enhancement that develops soon after tumor resection. **Fig. 7.3** depicts an area of reduced diffusion on the immediate postoperative MRI

> **Pearl**
>
> • Diffusion–weighted MRI can be extremely valuable in accurate interpretation of new abnormal contrast enhancement that develops soon after tumor resection.

following resection of a glioma. On 1-month follow–up MRI, there is a clear focus of abnormal contrast enhancement along the resection margin corresponding to the area of the reduced diffusion on the postoperative MRI. This new enhancement, which can be easily misinterpreted as recurrent tumor, represents an area of brain injury with subsequent blood–brain barrier disruption rather than recurrent tumor. A study shows that this enhancement within the area of diffusion abnormality invariably evolves into a gliotic cavity, as one would expect in any permanently injured brain, and does not represent tumor recurrence.[6] Therefore, it is imperative to evaluate any new enhancement within the first few months after surgery in the context of diffusion abnormality on the immediate postoperative MRI following tumor resection.

Diffusion tensor imaging is the latest application of diffusion–weighted MRI, where white matter integrity can be depicted on a three–dimensional map.[7] Although still in their clinical infancy, diffusion tensor imaging and tractography are promising, noninvasive tools to study the white matter tracts and are likely to become an important and integral part of preoperative planning of brain tumors in the future.

One of the major pitfalls of diffusion–weighted imaging is related to the technique's intrinsic sensitivity to lesions containing high magnetic susceptibility, such as blood products,

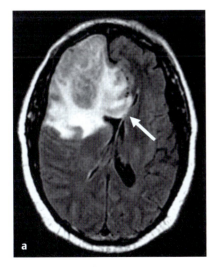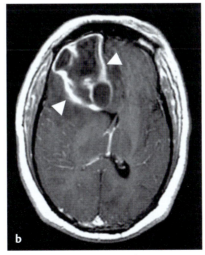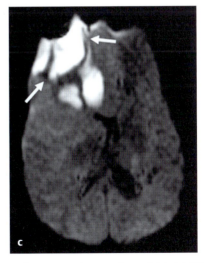

Fig. 7.1a–c A 41–year–old man with right frontal pyogenic cerebral abscess. (**a**) Axial fluid–attenuated inversion recovery image demonstrates a large mass into the corpus callosum (*arrow*). (**b**) Axial postcontrast T1–weighted magnetic resonance image shows a large rim–enhancing, centrally necrotic mass (*arrowheads*) within the right frontal lobe, suggestive of an aggressive neoplasm. (**c**) Axial diffusion–weighted image clearly demonstrates marked reduced diffusion (*arrows*) within the mass consistent with a pyogenic abscess, which was confirmed in surgery.

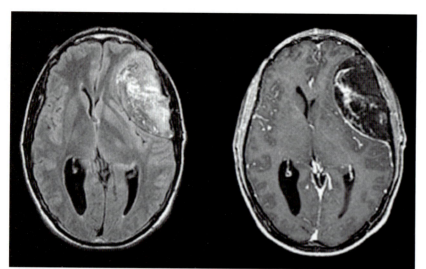

a

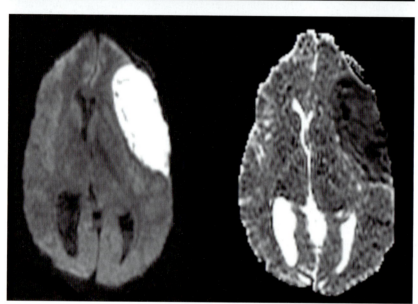

b

Fig. 7.2a,b A 31–year–old man with left frontal epidermoid cyst. (**a**) Axial fluid–attenuated inversion recovery (*left*) and postcontrast T1–weighted images (*right*) show a well–circumscribed left frontal extra–axial mass with heterogeneous internal architecture. (**b**) Axial diffusion–weighted image (*left*) and apparent diffusion coefficient map (*right*) demonstrate marked reduced diffusion associated with this extra–axial mass, pathognomonic for an intracranial epidermoid tumor. At surgery, an epidermoid cyst containing thick mucinous, viscous material was found.

calcium or metal, and bone or air. The susceptibility artifact caused by the paramagnetic or ferromagnetic material can cause spurious signal changes on an MRI that simulate pathological processes such as infarct or abscess, and hence the interpretation of diffusion–weighted images must be done by concomitant review of anatomic MRI. This is particularly true in the immediate postoperative state, in which there is usually a combination of blood products and surgical material within the surgical bed that can cause prominent susceptibil-

ity artifacts on diffusion–weighted imaging. As demonstrated in **Fig. 7.4**, an intracranial parenchymal hematoma can show apparent reduced diffusion on diffusion–weighted imaging due to susceptibility effect caused by subacute and chronic blood products, methemoglobin, and hemosiderin.

Dynamic Contrast–Enhanced Perfusion Magnetic Resonance Imaging

Dynamic contrast–enhanced perfusion MRI of the brain provides hemodynamic information that complements the anatomic information attainable with conventional MRI. Contrast–enhanced perfusion MRI methods exploit signal changes that accompany the passage of a paramagnetic contrast agent through the cerebrovascular system and can be used to derive information on blood volume and flow.[8–10] Dynamic perfusion MRI data analyzed using the radiotracer

---

Pitfall

- Para– or ferromagnetic materials such as blood products or calcium within the brain can simulate pathology on diffusion–weighted and perfusion MRI.

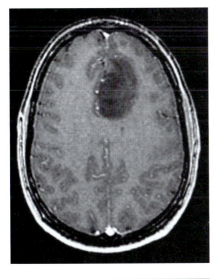
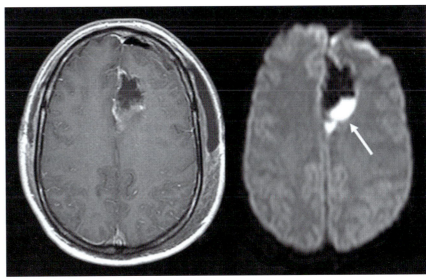
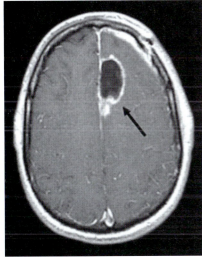

Fig. 7.3a–c A 35–year–old man with left medial frontal low–grade astrocytoma. (**a**) Axial postcontrast T1–weighted image shows a nonenhancing left medial frontal lobe mass. (**b**) Axial postcontrast T1–weighted image immediately following surgery demonstrates gross total resection of the mass. Axial diffusion–weighted image shows a nodular area of reduced diffusion (*arrow*) posterior to the resection cavity. (**c**) Axial postcontrast T1–weighted image 4 months after the surgery shows a nodular area of abnormal enhancement along the posterior margin of the resection cavity suspicious for recurrent tumor (*arrow*). However, this enhancing region, which corresponds to the area of reduced diffusion on the immediate postoperative image, most likely represents an area of cytotoxic injury related to surgical trauma rather than recurrent tumor. On 1–month follow–up, the enhancement completely resolved and was replaced with a gliotic cavity.

kinetic theory yield quantitative estimates of cerebral blood volume that reflect the underlying microvasculature and angiogenesis. Hence, this quick and robust technique is increasingly used as a research tool to evaluate and understand intracranial disease processes and as a clinical tool for diagnosis, management, and understanding of intracranial mass lesions, especially brain tumors. The vascularity of intracranial lesions, such as gliomas,[11–13] cerebral lymphomas,[14] and tumor–mimicking demyelinating lesions,[15] has been assessed with perfusion MRI.

Clinical Application of Perfusion Magnetic Resonance Imaging

Vascular morphology and the degree of angiogenesis are important elements in evaluating different tumor types and determining the biological aggressiveness of intracranial neoplasms, especially gliomas.[16,17] Tumor angiogenesis can be indirectly assessed using perfusion MRI–derived in vivo maps

of cerebral blood volume that depict the overall tumor vascularity. Perfusion MRI measurements of relative cerebral blood volume have been shown to correlate with both conventional angiographic assessments of tumor vascular density and histological measurements of tumor neovascularization. Increased tumor vascularity, however, is not synonymous with malignancy. Several intracranial neoplasms, especially those that are extra–axial, such as meningiomas or choroid plexus papillomas, can be highly vascular but rather benign in biological behavior.

In patients receiving antiangiogenesis cancer therapies that directly attack tumor vessels, perfusion MRI is a noninvasive method to assess changes in the relative cerebral blood volume of the tumor during treatment and thus can be used to monitor the efficacy of therapy. Conventional MRI is limited by its nonspecificity and inability to differentiate between tumor recurrence and therapy–related necrosis. Findings of perfusion MRI have been shown to correlate better with clinical responses of patients undergoing antiangiogenic therapy.

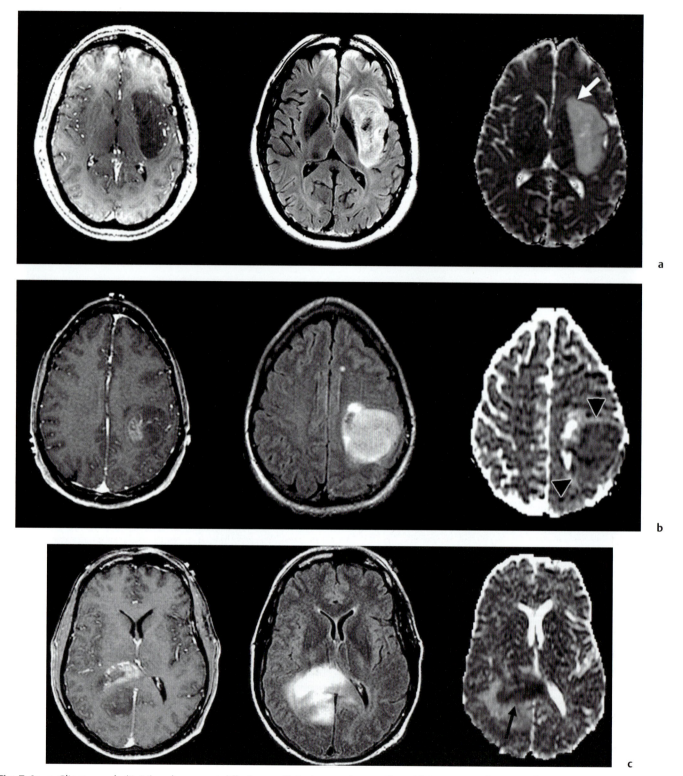

Fig. 7.4a–c Glioma grade (II–IV) and apparent diffusion coefficient (ADC) map. (**a**) Low–grade astrocytoma. (**b**) Anaplastic astrocytoma. (**c**) Glioblastoma multiforme. Axial postcontrast T1–weighted (*left*) and axial fluid–attenuated inversion recovery (*middle*) images demonstrate increase in tumoral enhancement and degree of T2 abnormality with increasing glioma grade. Axial ADC maps (*right*) show increased diffusion in low–grade astrocytoma (*white arrow*), mildly reduced diffusion (*arrowheads*) in anaplastic astrocytoma, and moderately reduced diffusion (*black arrow*) in glioblastoma multiforme.

Gliomas

Several studies have found a statistically significant correlation between the relative cerebral blood volume in a tumor and glioma grading. Studies have also shown statistically significant correlation between relative cerebral blood volume in a tumor and tumor vascularities determined using conventional catheter angiography.[13] Because MRI can be used to quantitatively assess tumor vascularity, contrast–enhanced perfusion MRI can be used to measure cerebral blood volume of the tumor, which reflects underlying tumor vascularity. Therefore, perfusion MRI–derived relative cerebral blood volume measurements can serve as noninvasive surrogate markers of tumor angiogenesis and malignancy. The implications of these findings are important because in primary high–grade gliomas, vascular morphology is a critical parameter in determining the potential for malignancy and for survival.

Low–grade astrocytomas have significantly lower mean relative cerebral blood volume than anaplastic astrocytomas or glioblastomas.[11,12] Low–grade astrocytomas show little or no elevation in the cerebral blood volume in the tumor compared with the contralateral uninvolved brain. Anaplastic astrocytomas tend to have a higher relative cerebral blood volume than low–grade astrocytomas but lower relative cerebral blood volume than glioblastomas. The progressive increase in relative cerebral blood volume from low grade to high–grade tumors is consistent with studies showing that microvascular density in low–grade astrocytomas is significantly lower than in anaplastic astrocytomas or glioblastomas, with glioblastomas being the most vascularized type of tumor. However, not only do the measurements of relative cerebral blood volume in different glioma grades overlap, but also relative cerebral blood volume measurements can and do vary considerably because of the inherent extreme histological heterogeneity of gliomas. Therefore, maps of relative cerebral blood volume of gliomas should not be interpreted without a concomitant evaluation of conventional MRI, which can provide other valuable information, such as the integrity of the blood–brain barrier or the degree and characteristics of T2 abnormality.

Biopsy remains the definitive method of determining tumor type and grade. The sampling error rate in biopsies of high–grade gliomas, however, is well known and is caused in part by the extreme geographic heterogeneity within a single tumor. Ideally, the grading of gliomas should be based on histological evaluation of tissue from the most malignant area in the tumor. Identifying this region can be quite difficult, however. In most biopsies, the imaging modality used for guidance is contrast–enhanced T1–weighted MRI or CT,[18] which depict areas of blood–brain barrier breakdown that may not correspond with the most malignant or most vascular portion of the tumor. Selecting a biopsy target on the basis of contrast–enhanced T1–weighted MRI alone may be quite challenging. Maps of cerebral blood volume can depict regions of increased vascularity that can serve as additional targets for stereotactic

biopsy. At my institution, maps of relative cerebral blood volume are routinely used to select biopsy sites for both enhancing and nonenhancing tumors and to help reduce sampling error and nondiagnostic biopsies. The relative cerebral blood volume map is particularly useful in patients with nonenhancing tumors because the map can be used to locate the "hot" area, or the presumed site of increased tumor vascularity.

Radiation Necrosis and Recurrent Tumor

Differentiation between radiation necrosis and recurrent tumor carries obvious therapeutic implications. Patients with recurrent tumors may benefit from undergoing a second operation and receiving adjuvant chemotherapy or targeted high–dose radiotherapy, whereas patients with radiation necrosis may be treated conservatively with steroids. Currently, the only definitive means of differentiating between radiation necrosis and recurrent tumor is histological evaluation of tissue from biopsy or resection. However, surgical manipulation of areas of radiation necrosis can cause further damage to the adjacent brain parenchyma. Delayed radiation necrosis is usually indistinguishable from recurrent tumor, both clinically and radiologically. Clinically, patients with either entity can present with progressive focal neurologic deficits and signs of increased intracranial pressure. On imaging, both entities can appear as a mass lesion with surrounding edema.[19,20] Conventional contrast–enhanced CT or MRI cannot be used to reliably distinguish radiation necrosis from recurrent tumor (**Fig. 7.5**). Both processes can cause extensive edema and varying degrees of disruption in the blood–brain barrier that result in mass effect and abnormal contrast enhancement, respectively. Pathologically, however, radiation necrosis and recurrent tumor are markedly dissimilar. Although the exact pathogenesis of delayed radiation necrosis remains obscure, a consistent pathological feature is extensive endothelial injury and ultimate fibrinoid necrosis; in contrast, recurrent tumor is characterized by vascular proliferation.[21,22] The MRI–derived cerebral blood volume maps can show the pathological differences in vascularity between therapy–induced necrosis and recurrent tumor and may help differentiate the two.

Metastases

Metastatic tumors, which make up almost 50% of all brain tumors, enter the central nervous system either hematogenously or by direct extension. Metastatic tumors induce neovascularization as they grow and expand. The newly formed capillaries resemble those of the primary systemic tumor with

---

Pearl

- Perfusion MRI may be useful for differentiating a solitary metastasis from a primary glioma.

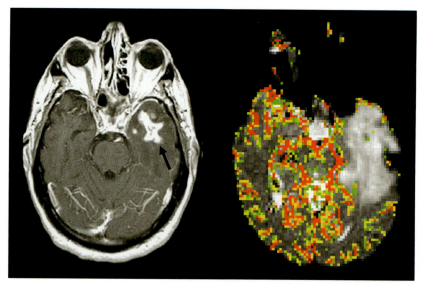

a   b

Fig. 7.5a,b A 55–year–old man with left temporal radiation necrosis, status post–external beam irradiation for clival chordoma 5 years prior. (**a**) Axial postcontrast T1–weighted image shows an irregularly enhancing left temporal lobe mass (*arrow*). (**b**) Axial relative cerebral blood volume map shows absent vascularity within the lesion suggestive of a nonneoplastic process. At surgery, radiation necrosis without evidence of tumor was found.

fenestrated membranes and open endothelial junctions, all of which differ from normal brain capillaries that possess a well–developed blood–brain barrier with tight junctions, a continuous basement membrane, and astrocytic foot processes.[23] Intracranial metastases tend to be multiple lesions that enhance avidly on enhanced T1–weighted images with varying degrees of associated edema, and they are characteristically located near the junction of the gray and white matters. Hence, differentiating a metastatic brain lesion from a primary glioma usually presents no diagnostic dilemma. However, when a metastatic brain tumor presents as a solitary lesion, it can have an appearance similar to that of a glioma both on enhanced T1–weighted MRI and on relative cerebral blood volume maps.

Perfusion MRI may be useful in differentiating a solitary metastasis from a primary glioma on the basis of the difference in the measurements of peritumoral relative cerebral blood volume.[19] This difference in the blood volume can be explained, in part, by the difference in the pathophysiology of metastatic tumors. The peritumoral edema (defined as the area of hyperintensity on T2–weighted images in immediate contact with the enhancing tumor margin) is purely vasogenic edema that is caused by the increased interstitial water from leaky capillaries.[24] In other words, in metastatic tumors, there is no histological evidence of tumor beyond the outer contrast–enhancing margin of the tumor, and the peritumoral region represents the reaction of the surrounding intrinsically normal but edematous brain parenchyma. In high–grade gliomas, on the other hand, the peritumoral region represents a variable combination of vasogenic edema and tumor cells infiltrating along the perivascular spaces. It has been shown that neoplastic cells can be found in some high–grade gliomas not only outside the contrast–enhancing margin but also well beyond the outer edge of the peritumoral zone visualized on T2–weighted MRI.[18] As shown in **Fig. 7.6**, by exploiting the pathophysiological differences in the peritumoral region, perfusion MRI–derived blood volume measurements may help differentiate tumor–infiltrated edema (in cases of high–grade gliomas) from purely vasogenic edema (in cases of metastasis).

Meningiomas

Meningiomas are highly vascular, extra–axial tumors that derive blood supply mostly from meningeal arteries with tumor capillaries that completely lack a blood–brain barrier. Angiographically, meningiomas appear as hypervascular extra–axial masses that exhibit diffuse, homogeneous, and prolonged staining. Similarly, meningiomas are hypervascular on perfusion MRI. Because of the lack of a blood–brain barrier within the tumor, the capillaries of meningioma are highly leaky and permeable. This phenomenon is apparent during the first–pass

Pitfall

- Perfusion MRI for meningioma is especially challenging. Because these tumors can be highly vascular, relative cerebral blood volume measurements may not correlate with malignancy. Perfusion MRI for meningiomas is also hampered by their location in the brain, which produces artifact due to echo planar and T2* effect of the technique.

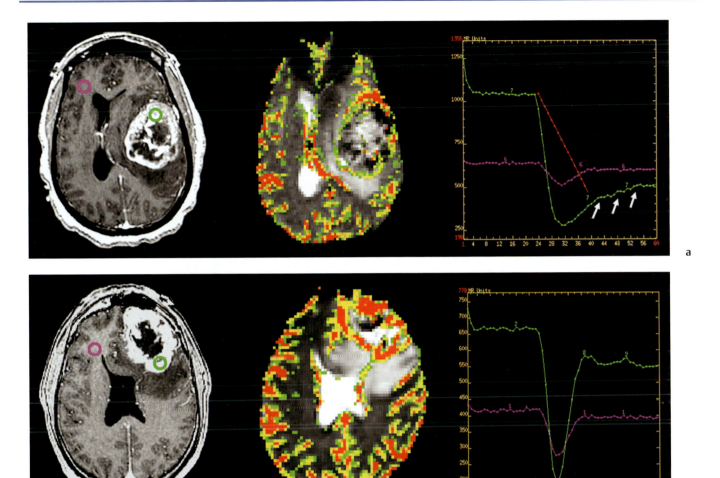

Fig. 7.6a,b Perfusion magnetic resonance imaging of metastatic brain tumor and glioblastoma multiforme. (**a**) A 37–year–old woman with pulmonary adenocarcinoma metastasis to the brain. Axial postcontrast T1–weighted image shows a large necrotic mass in the left frontal lobe. A relative cerebral blood volume (rCBV) map of the mass reveals increased blood volume, mostly around the periphery of the tumor. Regions of interest for perfusion analysis were placed over the tumor (*green circle*) and the contralateral normal white matter (*pink circle*). Dynamic T2* signal intensity time curve shows marked leakage of contrast material immediately after the bolus phase within the region of interest (ROI) placed over the tumor, suggesting highly leaky vasculature (*green curve with white arrows*) when compared with the normal white matter (*pink curve*). (**b**) A 52–year–old man with left frontal glioblastoma multiforme. Axial postcontrast T1–weighted image and rCBV map demonstrate an irregularly enhancing mass with central necrosis in the left frontal lobe. The ROI placed over the tumor (*green circle*) and the normal white matter (*pink circle*) for perfusion analysis show only mild leakage of contrast material within the tumor (*green curve*).

contrast agent bolus when there is immediate contrast agent leakage without any substantial recovery of T2* signal loss back to the baseline. Therefore, the perfusion MRI–derived relative cerebral blood volume measurements of meningiomas may be grossly over– or underestimated because of first–pass leakage, which essentially renders the intravascular compartmentalization of contrast agent impossible.

Similar to diffusion–weighted imaging, perfusion MRI is highly sensitive to susceptibility artifact due to echo planar and T2* effect of the technique. Therefore, any paramagnetic or ferromagnetic material can cause severe artifact, particularly near the brain–bone–air interface near the middle cranial fossa or posterior fossa. Perfusion MRI of tumors in these locations is therefore intrinsically limited and challenging. In the immediate postoperative setting, perfusion MRI is often hampered by susceptibility artifact caused by blood products and surgical material.

Proton Magnetic Resonance Spectroscopy

Basic Physics

Magnetic resonance spectroscopy (MRS) is a noninvasive MRI technique that produces metabolic spectra instead of generating anatomic images. There are several nuclei (e.g., proton, phosphorus, carbon, sodium, fluorine) that can be used to produce MRS, but proton is the most commonly used due to its abundance and high nuclear magnetic sensitivity. Proton MRS captures the biochemical signature of normal and diseased brain in vivo. Despite a large number of metabolites present in the brain, only freely mobile metabolites are detectable by MRS. Because water protons far outnumber the protons of other metabolites, it is critical to suppress water signal adequately to detect the minuscule amount of important metabolites that are normally obscured by water proton signal.

The acquisition of MRS involves first defining the three-dimensional volume of interest (VOI) to be studied. Localization of VOI can be done by either single voxel or chemical shift technique. In single voxel spectroscopy, a small region (usual minimum of 1 cm^3) of brain is interrogated to obtain metabolic information. It is a fast and easy technique but is limited by tissue coverage. Chemical shift imaging, on the other hand, offers larger coverage and improved signal detection. For brain tumors, chemical shift imaging is preferable due to its ability to provide metabolic information on a larger target area. This method does, however, require longer imaging time and complex data processing. Two essential steps involved in MRS acquisition involve sufficient water suppression and shimming the magnetic field to ensure homogeneity.

The major brain metabolites detected by proton MRS are *N*-acetyl aspartate (NAA), choline, creatine, myoinositol, lipid, lactate, glutamine, and glutamate. Each metabolite has corresponding proposed biochemical correlates: NAA, a marker of neuronal integrity; choline, a membrane turnover; creatine, an energetic; myoinositol, an astrocytic marker; lipid, a tissue destruction/necrosis marker; lactate, a hypoxia marker; glutamine and glutamate, excitatory markers. Each metabolite is characterized by its specific resonance frequency with peak height, width, and area. Height or area under the peak can be calculated to yield a relative measure of the concentrations of protons. Because actively dividing cells require membrane turnover, choline peaks tend to be high in brain tumors, whereas NAA peaks tend to be low due to destruction of neurons.

Clinical Application of Proton Magnetic Resonance Spectroscopy

Several potential clinical applications of proton MRS have been proposed, including guiding surgical brain biopsy and tumor grading. Although proton MRS has shown much promise as a helpful diagnostic tool to further characterize intracranial mass lesions, its contribution to altering outcome remains unknown.

Image-Guided Surgical Brain Biopsy

Proton MRS has been used in guiding surgical biopsy to the area of high cellularity.[25] Three-dimensional proton MRS using

---

> **Pitfall**
>
> - There is limited coverage of the brain in perfusion MRI and proton MRS; hence, not all of the brain tumor in question may be included in the imaging plane. This limited coverage is particularly true in large brain tumors or brain tumors located near the cortex and skull.

chemical shift imaging can capture metabolic information from a large portion of tumor (**Fig. 7.7**). This may locate the most active or aggressive portion of tumor that can serve as a site for biopsy. Areas of high choline metabolites have been shown to correlate with high tumor proliferative index. It is important to recognize, however, that the minimum voxel size for MRS is 1 cm^3, whereas a biopsy tissue specimen may be smaller than 1 mm^3. This discrepancy in size must be considered when choosing a biopsy site based on MRS and interpretation of biopsy result.

Glioma Grading

Similar to perfusion MRI, MRS is a promising noninvasive tool to assess tumor grade preoperatively (**Fig. 7.7**). The presence of lipid on MRS is highly suggestive of higher grade gliomas because lipid is a marker of tissue necrosis more often found in malignant gliomas.[26] However, there are several important limitations associated with clinical application of proton MRS for brain tumor imaging. First, due to limitations in MRS voxel size, the entire tumor volume may not be interrogated. Thus important areas of tumor may be missed. Second, there is no one signature MRS characteristic that correlates with tumor malignancy, and nonspecific spectral findings are not uncommon. Third, MRS data processing remains cumbersome, especially in cases of multidimensional data sets, and requires an offline workstation and sophisticated software program.

Functional Magnetic Resonance Imaging

Functional magnetic resonance imaging (fMRI) is used for mapping changes in cerebral hemodynamics of neuronal and motor events related to brain activation based on changes in tissue blood oxygen level dependence (BOLD).[27] As a method to depict and quantify brain activation, fMRI has several advantages: it is noninvasive, has excellent spatial and good temporal resolution, is easy to implement. Over the past decade fMRI has provided new insight to the investigation of language, formation of memory, pain, learning, emotion, and other brain functions to name but a few areas of active research. Functional MRI is also being more widely used in clinical settings to map out major motor, sensory, and visual pathways.

With an increasing prevalence in the last several years, fMRI data are being incorporated into neuronavigational systems in the operating room to guide brain tumor surgery. The

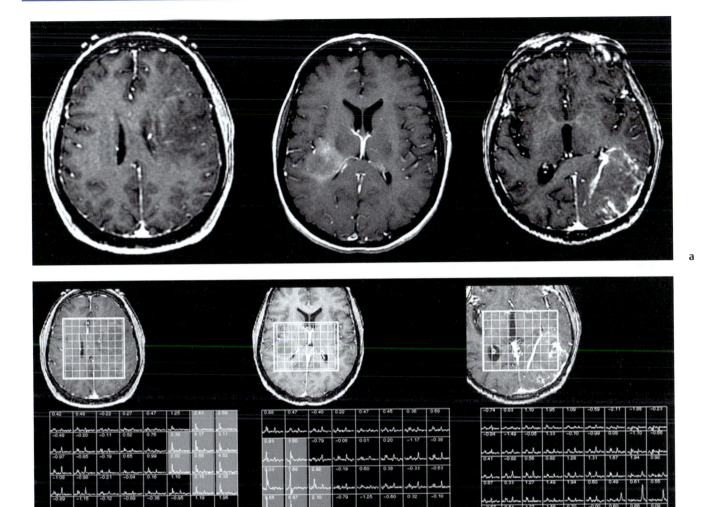

Fig. 7.7a,b Glioma grade and proton magnetic resonance spectroscopy (MRS). (**a**) Axial postcontrast T1–weighted images of grade II astrocytoma (*left*), grade III astrocytoma (*middle*), and grade IV astrocytoma (*right*) show definite abnormal contrast enhancement associated with the grade IV tumor. (**b**) Corresponding proton MRS spectra through the same axial plane as in part **a** show high choline metabolite within both grade II and grade III astrocytomas (*shaded area*). In grade IV astrocytoma, the most abnormal metabolite is lipid (*lower half of the right three columns*).

fMRI data have been widely used and validated for precise and accurate localization of the motor cortex.[28–30] A preoperative fMRI with a bilateral finger-tapping paradigm can show the spatial relationship between the tumor and motor activation (**Fig. 7.8**), contralateral hemispheric motor activation, and supplemental motor activation. Localizing the motor cortex and co-registering the results to a surgical MRI scan prior to a neurosurgical intervention can help guide the direct cortical stimulation during an awake craniotomy and possibly shorten operation time. In some cases, using fMRI to confirm the expected location of the motor cortex may avoid awake neurosurgery altogether.

Imaging for Pediatric Patients with Brain Tumors

Brain tumors in childhood differ significantly from adult lesions in their sites of origin, histological features, clinical presentations, and likelihood to disseminate throughout the nervous system early in the course of disease. As one study

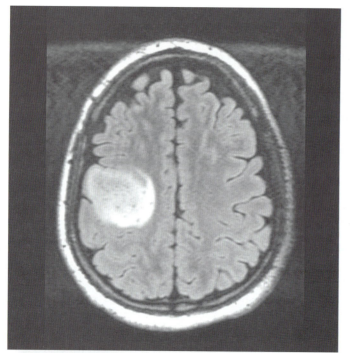

a

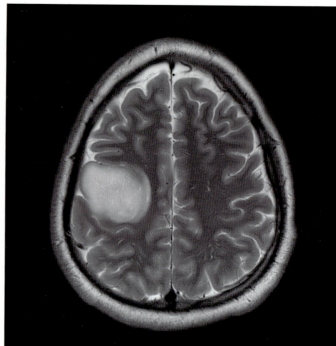

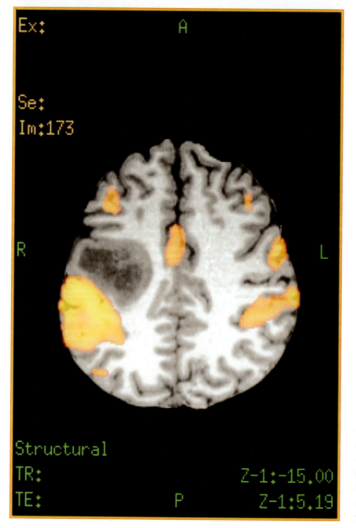

c

Fig. 7.8a–c Functional magnetic resonance imaging (MRI) of low-grade glioma (grade II astrocytoma) near motor cortex in a 22-year-old man. (**a**) Axial fluid attenuated inversion recovery (FLAIR) and (**b**) axial fast spin echo T2-wieighted image show a hyperintense expansile mass in the right frontal lobe. (**c**) Functional MRI map obtained with left finger tapping paradigm shows activation of right motor strip (*large yellow area* just posterior to the right frontal tumor).

Special Consideration

- Pediatric brain tumors are prone to occur in the posterior fossa where they can be obscured or distorted by the susceptibility artifact associated with the echo planar imaging technique. However, susceptibility artifact can be greatly reduced with a thinner slice technique.

summarized,[20] there are vast differences in epidemiology, topography, histology, and prognosis of brain cancer between adults and children. Whereas the great majority of adult tumors arise in the cerebral cortex, about half of childhood brain cancers originate infratentorially—in the cerebellum, brainstem, or fourth ventricular region. Brain metastases from systemic cancer are rare in children and mainly represent leptomeningeal dissemination from a primary brain lesion such as medulloblastoma, pineoblastoma, or germinoma. Hence, it is important to image the entire neuraxis in these patients (i.e., brain and entire spine). Headache, posterior fossa symptoms (such as nausea and vomiting), ataxia, and cranial nerve symptoms predominate in children because about half of pediatric brain cancer occurs infratentorially.[31–33]

The predilection for pediatric brain tumors in the posterior fossa creates a unique challenge in performing physiological MRI. As mentioned in the previous section, brain tumors in the posterior fossa can be obscured or distorted by the echo planar imaging technique due to susceptibility artifact and geometric distortion. However, by using a thinner slice technique, the degree of susceptibility artifact can be substantially reduced, allowing a diagnostic imaging study. For perfusion MRI, the dose of contrast agent, gadolinium complexed with diethylenetriamine pentaacetic acid (Gd–DTPA), remains the same for pediatric patients (0.1 mmol/kg of body weight), but the injection rate should not be higher than 4 mL/s because the size of intravenous catheters tends to be smaller. The minimum size of the intravenous catheter should be 23 gauge to allow the minimum injection rate of 2 mL/s, ensuring bolus delivery of contrast agent to the brain.

Editor's Note

It is imperative for all physicians dealing with patients who have central nervous system tumors to consider various advanced techniques involving physiological imaging. This is largely in the form of magnetic resonance spectroscopy, diffusion weighted imaging, perfusion imaging, and functional scans. Prior to operating on anyone it becomes essential to gain as much physiological imaging as possible to understand the areas that are most active with regard to the tumor based on the degree of cellularity (diffusion weighted imaging), vascularity (perfusion), and metabolic function (spectroscopy). In addition, surgeons must learn to rely on functional imaging as it relates to motor and sensory localization in addition to cerebral dominance and language. It is critical to understand that functional imaging cannot detect specific areas for such functions as comprehension and reading, for example, and that the only way to map these functions is with intraoperative stimulation mapping. One form of diffusion weighted imaging, namely diffusion tensor imaging, enables surgeons to define subcortical pathways of function that can be verified with stimulation mapping during surgery. We are beginning to unravel the mysteries of pseudo-progression with perfusion imaging, and with newer high-resolution spectroscopy paradigms we soon will be able to sort out the difference between gliosis and infiltrative tumor cells. Thus, it is essential for all of us managing patients with central nervous system tumors to make physiological imaging part of the evaluation and follow-up process in addition to standard, yet advanced, anatomic imaging. (Berger)

References

1. Ricci PE. Imaging of adult brain tumors. Neuroimaging Clin N Am 1999;9:651–669
2. Edelman RR, Wielopolski P, Schmitt F. Echo-planar MR imaging. Radiology 1994;192:600–612
3. Castillo M, Mukherji SK. Diffusion-weighted imaging in the evaluation of intracranial lesions. Semin Ultrasound CT MR 2000;21:405–416
4. Schaefer PW, Grant PE, Gonzalez RG. Diffusion-weighted MR imaging of the brain. Radiology 2000;217:331–345
5. Holodny AI, Ollenschlager M. Diffusion imaging in brain tumors. Neuroimaging Clin N Am 2002;12:107–124, x x
6. Smith JS, Cha S, Mayo MC, et al. Serial diffusion-weighted magnetic resonance imaging in cases of glioma: distinguishing tumor recurrence from postresection injury. J Neurosurg 2005;103:428–438
7. Ito R, Mori S, Melhem ER. Diffusion tensor brain imaging and tractography. Neuroimaging Clin N Am 2002;12:1–19
8. Rosen BR, Belliveau JW, Vevea JM, Brady TJ. Perfusion imaging with NMR contrast agents. Magn Reson Med 1990;14:249–265
9. Weisskoff R, Belliveau J, Kwong K, Rosen B. Functional MR imaging of capillary hemodynamics. In: Potchen E, ed. Magnetic Resonance Angiography: Concepts and Applications. St. Louis: Mosby, 1993:473–484
10. Weisskoff RM, Rosen BR. Noninvasive determination of regional cerebral blood flow in rats using dynamic imaging with Gd(DTPA). Magn Reson Med 1992;25:211–212
11. Aronen HJ, Gazit IE, Louis DN, et al. Cerebral blood volume maps of gliomas: comparison with tumor grade and histologic findings. Radiology 1994;191:41–51
12. Knopp EA, Cha S, Johnson G, et al. Glial neoplasms: dynamic contrast-enhanced T2*-weighted MR imaging. Radiology 1999;211:791–798
13. Sugahara T, Korogi Y, Kochi M, et al. Correlation of MR imaging-determined cerebral blood volume maps with histologic and angiographic

determination of vascularity of gliomas. AJR Am J Roentgenol 1998; 171:1479–1486

14. Sugahara T, Korogi Y, Shigematsu Y, et al. Perfusion-sensitive MRI of cerebral lymphomas: a preliminary report. J Comput Assist Tomogr 1999;23:232–237

15. Cha S, Pierce S, Knopp EA, et al. Dynamic contrast-enhanced T2*-weighted MR imaging of tumefactive demyelinating lesions. AJNR Am J Neuroradiol 2001;22:1109–1116

16. Burger PC, Vollmer RT. Histologic factors of prognostic significance in the glioblastoma multiforme. Cancer 1980;46:1179–1186

17. Burger PC, Vogel FS, Green SB, Strike TA. Glioblastoma multiforme and anaplastic astrocytoma. Pathologic criteria and prognostic implications. Cancer 1985;56:1106–1111

18. Kelly PJ, Daumas-Duport C, Scheithauer BW, Kall BA, Kispert DB. Stereotactic histologic correlations of computed tomography- and magnetic resonance imaging-defined abnormalities in patients with glial neoplasms. Mayo Clin Proc 1987;62:450–459

19. Law M, Cha S, Knopp EA, Johnson G, Arnett J, Litt AW. High-grade gliomas and solitary metastases: differentiation by using perfusion and proton spectroscopic MR imaging. Radiology 2002;222:715–721

20. Hutter A, Schwetye KE, Bierhals AJ, McKinstry RC. Brain neoplasms: epidemiology, diagnosis, and prospects for cost-effective imaging. Neuroimaging Clin N Am 2003;13:237–250, x–xi

21. Valk PE, Dillon WP. Radiation injury of the brain. AJNR Am J Neuroradiol 1991;12:45–62

22. Ricci PE, Karis JP, Heiserman JE, Fram EK, Bice AN, Drayer BP. Differentiating recurrent tumor from radiation necrosis: time for re-evaluation of positron emission tomography? [see comments] AJNR Am J Neuroradiol 1998;19:407–413

23. Vajkoczy P, Menger MD. Vascular microenvironment in gliomas. J Neurooncol 2000;50:99–108

24. Machein MR, Plate KH. VEGF in brain tumors. J Neurooncol 2000; 50:109–120

25. Burtscher IM, Skagerberg G, Geijer B, Englund E, Ståhlberg F, Holtås S. Proton MR spectroscopy and preoperative diagnostic accuracy: an evaluation of intracranial mass lesions characterized by stereotactic biopsy findings. AJNR Am J Neuroradiol 2000;21:84–93

26. Li X, Lu Y, Pirzkall A, McKnight T, Nelson SJ. Analysis of the spatial characteristics of metabolic abnormalities in newly diagnosed glioma patients. J Magn Reson Imaging 2002;16:229–237

27. Ogawa S, Menon RS, Tank DW, et al. Functional brain mapping by blood oxygenation level-dependent contrast magnetic resonance imaging. A comparison of signal characteristics with a biophysical model. Biophys J 1993;64:803–812

28. Fandino J, Kollias SS, Wieser HG, Valavanis A, Yonekawa Y. Intraoperative validation of functional magnetic resonance imaging and cortical reorganization patterns in patients with brain tumors involving the primary motor cortex. J Neurosurg 1999;91:238–250

29. Yetkin FZ, Mueller WM, Morris GL, et al. Functional MR activation correlated with intraoperative cortical mapping. AJNR Am J Neuroradiol 1997;18:1311–1315

30. Lehéricy S, Duffau H, Cornu P, et al. Correspondence between functional magnetic resonance imaging somatotopy and individual brain anatomy of the central region: comparison with intraoperative stimulation in patients with brain tumors. J Neurosurg 2000;92:589–598

31. Becker LE. Pathology of pediatric brain tumors. Neuroimaging Clin N Am 1999;9:671–690

32. Miltenburg D, Louw DF, Sutherland GR. Epidemiology of childhood brain tumors. Can J Neurol Sci 1996;23:118–122

33. Pollack IF. Pediatric brain tumors. Semin Surg Oncol 1999;16:73–90

8 Functional Imaging

Srikantan S. Nagarajan and Mitchel S. Berger

The surgical management of brain tumors requires detailed functional mapping of cortical regions around a tumor. Traditional intraoperative methods are electrical cortical stimulation (ECS) or electrocorticography (ECoG). Although these methods are considered gold standards, they are not helpful for presurgical planning. Preoperative localization of functionally intact brain tissue helps guide neurosurgical planning and limits the region of resection, allowing for improved long-term patient morbidity and neurologic function. Various techniques are available to preoperatively and noninvasively map functional brain organization, such as positron emission tomography (PET), functional magnetic resonance imaging (fMRI), and magnetoencephalographic imaging (MEGI). This chapter reviews each of these methods for noninvasive functional brain imaging.

Surgery is often used in the management of patients with brain tumors or pharmacologically resistant epileptic foci. However, there is a trade-off between the margin of excision used to ensure complete removal and the potential loss of function that may arise as a consequence of removing normal surrounding brain tissue. There are several invasive approaches used in neurosurgery to define eloquent areas of the cortex prior to surgical excision. One approach is to perform electrophysiological mapping of the cortex in the awake patient at the time of the operation. A second approach routinely used prior to surgery is the Wada test, in which the predominant side of the brain used for language and memory is identified by the invasive sequential injection of sodium amytal (which transiently stops the brain from working) into each of the two main blood vessels supplying different sides of the brain, during standard neuropsychological testing.

Preoperative mapping techniques can result in a precise estimation of the location of functional areas in relation to a tumor or epileptic focus, therefore reducing surgical risk. Although traditional brain imaging methods such as magnetic resonance imaging (MRI) and computed tomography (CT) provide detailed knowledge of the *structure* of the brain, these methods do not tell us about brain *function*. Several

> **Pearl**
>
> • Preoperative functional imaging can result in a precise estimation of the location of functional areas in relation to a tumor, therefore reducing surgical risk.

> **Pearl**
>
> • Positron emission tomography (PET), functional magnetic resonance imaging (fMRI), and magnetoencephalographic imaging (MEGI) are the most popular preoperative functional brain imaging methods.

studies have shown that considerable variability exists in anatomic identification of functional brain areas, even by experts.[1] This variability can be significantly reduced by functional brain mapping methods.

Functional brain imaging allows us to look inside the brain of humans in "real time" and appreciate the neural mechanisms underlying behavior, rather than just observing the consequences of these effects in lesion studies. Functional brain imaging has revealed the neural basis for several behaviors, such as how we are able to make sense of and integrate large amounts of dynamic information in our environment, understand language, learn new skills, and remember important facts. Preoperative functional brain imaging techniques can be integrated with neuro-navigational systems to provide intraoperative guidance to the surgical team.[2-8] Preoperative functional brain imaging can provide significant information for determining the surgical approach, screening of patients for awake craniotomy, planning for intraoperative mapping, and the limits of resection.

The earliest studies of preoperative mapping in brain tumors were PET studies of sensorimotor, language, and visual areas. Since its advent in 1990, fMRI has quickly become widely available and has also been extensively used before surgery. More recently, MEGI has become more widely available for planning and guiding tumor surgery and can also measure tumor infiltration.

■ Positron Emission Tomography

Positron emission tomography is a nuclear medicine technique requiring a tracer compound of physiological interest that is introduced into the body. This tracer is labeled with radioactive isotopes of atoms (such as oxygen, carbon, or nitrogen) that emit positrons. Once a positron is emitted from the nucleus of the atom, it will speed in an unpredictable direction, and before it traverses a distance of less than a millimeter, it will collide with one of the electrons in its environment. As a result of this collision, the positron and electron will be annihilated and converted to high-frequency photons in the gamma frequency range that will fly with equal speed in diametrically opposite directions. The energy of these photons is sufficient to propel them without distortion clear through the brain tissues and the skull to the surface of the head. Scintillation detectors arranged outside the head consist of a crystal coupled to a photomultiplier tubes or avalanche photodiodes.

When a photon hits a crystal, visible light is emitted. The light interacts with the cathode plate inside the photomultiplier tube, causing emission of electrons, which in turn interact with a series of dynodes that successively multiply their number such that each photon results in a sufficiently amplified electrical pulse to be handled by large-scale timers and counters. The precise timing and counting of pulses generated by a series of such detectors is the basis for determining where each positron emission originates. Specifically, it is the simultaneous or coincident detection of the pair of photons moving in approximately opposite direction that is the basis of PET reconstruction. Photons that do not arrive in temporal pairs, that is, within a timing-window of a few nanoseconds, are ignored.

Reconstruction algorithms enable tomographic reconstruction images of the distribution of positron-emitting radioactivity in the body. Using statistics collected from tens of thousands of coincidence events, a set of simultaneous equations for the total activity of each parcel of tissue can be solved by a number of techniques, and, thus, a map of radioactivity as a function of location for parcels or bits of tissue (also called voxels) may be constructed and plotted. The PET scans are often read alongside CT or MRI scans, giving co-registered anatomic and metabolic information. Modern PET scanners are now available with integrated CT, or more recently MRI scanners. Because these multimodality scans can be performed in immediate sequence during the same session, with the patient not changing position between the two types of scans, the two sets of images are more precisely registered; that is, they are in alignment, so that areas of abnormality on the PET imaging can be more perfectly correlated with anatomy on the CT or MR images.

Positron emission tomography can be used to trace the biological pathway of any compound in living humans provided it is radiolabeled with a PET isotope. Radioisotopes or radionuclides used in PET scans are typically isotopes with short half-lives such as carbon-11 (~20 minutes), nitrogen-13 (~10 minutes), oxygen-15 (~2 minutes), fluorine-18 (~110 minutes), or rubidium-82 (~1.27 minutes). These radionuclides are incorporated either into compounds normally used by the body, such as glucose (or glucose analogues), water, or ammonia, or into molecules that bind to receptors or other sites of drug action. Such labeled compounds are known as radiotracers. Using radiotracers, the specific processes that can be probed with PET are virtually limitless, and radiotracers

for new target molecules and processes are continuing to be synthesized. There are already dozens of compounds in clinical use and hundreds used in research. By far the most commonly used radiotracer in clinical PET scanning is fluorodeoxyglucose (FDG; also called fludeoxyglucose), an analogue of glucose that is labeled with fluorine-18.

Functional brain imaging with PET is based on an assumption that areas of high radioactivity are associated with brain activity. What is actually measured indirectly is the flow of blood to different parts of the brain, which is, in general, believed to be correlated, and has been measured using the tracer oxygen-15. However, because of its 2-minute half-life, O-15 must be piped directly from a medical cyclotron for such uses, which restricted PET scans to a few centers. More recently, however, the development of ligands such as [^{11}C] raclopride and [^{18}F] fallypride for dopamine D2/D3 receptors, [^{11}C]McN 5652 and [^{11}C] DASB for serotonin transporters, or enzyme substrates (e.g., 6-fluoro-Dopa [F-Dopa] for the AADC enzyme) permit the visualization of neuroreceptor pools in the context of a plurality of neuropsychiatric and neurologic illnesses.

Thus, highly accurate measurements of blood flow, volume, glucose, oxygen and protein metabolism, neuroreceptor and transmission system function, and blood–brain barrier permeability can be achieved with PET. However, regional cerebral blood flow (rCBF) is the favored functional brain imaging technique because it can be measured quickly using oxygen-15–labeled water with a half-life of 123 seconds, which allows for repeat measurements in the same patient.

A typical PET functional image is obtained by subtraction of a scan obtained during a baseline condition from a scan obtained during an active condition. Studies with PET have brought to light the fact that metabolic changes accompanying brain activation do not appear to follow the time-honored notion of a close coupling between blood flow and oxidative metabolism of glucose. Changes in blood flow appear to be accompanied by changes in glucose utilization that exceed the increase in oxygen consumption, suggesting that oxidative metabolism of glucose may not supply all of the energy demands encountered transiently during brain activation. Rather, glycolysis alone may provide the energy needed for transient changes. The above issues confound inferences about neuronal activity from PET. Nevertheless, successful functional localization accomplished by activation studies in which PET scanning has been used has been shown to correlate well with the results of intraoperative cortical stimulation mapping.[9-12]

Functional Magnetic Resonance Imaging

Functional magnetic resonance imaging (fMRI) in general may refer to any MRI technique to measure physiological function. However, the term typically refers to techniques developed in the early 1990s that exploit a phenomenon called blood oxygen level dependence (BOLD) response. The BOLD response is based on the fact that properties of water molecules in the brain change slightly between areas that are near blood, with its oxygen exhausted relative to those near freshly oxygenated blood. Local increase in energy requirements arising as a consequence of neuronal firing is largely met through an increase in oxygen-based metabolism, with the increased demand for oxygen being delivered seconds later by an increase in the local blood flow. Changes in the oxygenation level of the blood, therefore, occur as a consequence of neuronal activity, and the magnitude of change in signal intensity can be used as an indirect measure of excitatory input to neurons. The MRI signal can be made sensitive to the amount of oxygen in hemoglobin, and changes in blood oxygen content at sites of brain activation can be detected. Thus, increased neuronal activity causes a BOLD signal and is reflected as a small increase in signal intensity on the MRI scan. Activation patterns in working human brain can be mapped with high temporal and spatial resolution using fMRI based on the BOLD effect.[13]

Although BOLD activations have been demonstrated with many different MRI schemes, most fMRI work is done with single-shot echo planar imaging (EPI), in which a single slice of the brain can be acquired in 30 to 100 ms. The key advantage of single-shot EPI is that the speed of data collection renders the images insensitive to physiological motions that would create artifacts in standard images (e.g., pulsatile flow). Similar to PET, fMRI activation maps are obtained by statistical methods that are equivalent to subtraction of images obtained during baseline conditions from images obtained during active conditions. A standard mapping protocol in fMRI is a block design experiment, where blocks of the stimulus or task are presented typically for 20 to 30 seconds, alternating with periods of rest, or a control condition. The control task is chosen carefully such that it activates all of the neural processes common to the stimulus task, with the exception of the cognitive process of interest. By subtracting the brain regions recruited during the performance of the control task from the brain regions recruited during the test condition, the areas of the brain having activity associated specifically with the cognitive process of interest can be identified.

An alternative experimental approach is to present stimuli as isolated brief events separated in time so that the individual response to single events can be identified. The principal advantage of this event-related approach is that it avoids the potential confounding factors of habituation or fatigue, which may arise in a block design as a consequence of the presentation of repeated identical stimuli. Although this approach can

preserve much of the temporal information in the hemodynamic response, it is not often used in functional brain mapping studies. Typically, changes in signal intensity are on the order of a few percent; hence the need for effective statistical methods to extract meaningful signals.

The hemodynamic response (occurring over seconds) is much slower than the neuronal response (occurring over tens to hundreds of milliseconds). Although there is typically a delay of 4 to 6 seconds between the onset of the task and the peak latency of the hemodynamic response, the temporal resolution of fMRI as a technique would not be compromised if the shape of the hemodynamic response function was fixed and was simply convolved with the time course of the task-induced neural activity. However, there is some evidence that characteristics of the hemodynamic response may vary between different individuals, between different brain regions, with the nature of the task, or in the presence of disease. The unknown potential variability in the latency of the hemodynamic response limits precise interpretations of the magnitude and the temporal resolution of the signal. The latter problem, however, does not generally limit uses of fMRI as a "mapping" technique. For such experiments, the time course of the response is itself not the most critical issue.[14]

Several studies have reported the effectiveness of fMRI in correctly identifying the localization of the main motor strip or language area preoperatively in patients with lesions near these eloquent regions and for preoperative evaluation of patients with intracranial tumors, and have correlated sensorimotor and language activation with ECS.[15–20] Patients with tumors close to eloquent sensorimotor or language areas have been assessed with motor, sensory, and language paradigms. Motor and sensory paradigms are more effective than language paradigms. Many activation maps often yield high or adequate quality and are useful in the decision to operate, as well as in the decision of surgical approach and extent of resection.[21–24]

Functional MRI is more prone to artifacts caused by visualization of the draining veins, which may explain the more cranial and lateral activation, whereas PET depicts capillary perfusion changes and therefore shows activation closer to the parenchyma. Although a variety of studies have discussed its potential, there is still some doubt about the localization accuracy, which might be impaired, at least in part, by the low signal-to-noise ratio (SNR), susceptibility artifacts, and draining veins. Fluorodeoxyglucose-PET and fMRI have good correspondence. Advantages of fMRI over PET are higher spatial temporal resolution, shorter examination time, wider

Pearl

- Advantages of fMRI over PET are higher spatial and temporal resolution, shorter examination times, wider availability, and no exposure to radioactivity.

availability, and lack of exposure to radioactivity. When evaluating fMRI, however, caution is needed because of multiple sources of artifacts. Correction of distortions and motion-related artifacts is important. Positron emission tomography has a higher SNR and lesser susceptibility to artifacts, and is amenable to patients with MRI contraindications. Pathophysiological factors might cause neurovascular uncoupling and facilitate artifactual findings with fMRI in patients with direct tumor infiltration, neovascularity, cerebrovascular inflammation, and arteriovenous malformation (AVM)-induced hemodynamic effects. Lesion-induced neurovascular uncoupling causing reduced fMRI signal in perilesional eloquent cortex, in conjunction with normal or increased activity in homologous brain regions, may simulate hemispheric dominance and lesion-induced homotopic cortical reorganization.

Magnetoencephalographic Imaging

Magnetoencephalographic imaging (MEGI) refers to the reconstruction of the spatiotemporal activation of brain sources from noninvasive magnetoencephalography (MEG) measurements. Magnetoencephalographic imaging is increasingly being used for preoperative functional brain imaging. When combined with MRI data, preoperative functional localization with MEGI can be integrated with neuronavigational systems to provide intraoperative guidance to the surgical team. By mapping relevant somatosensory, auditory, and occasionally motor cortices preoperatively, retained areas of function can be delineated, reducing the time needed for intraoperative mapping. Such preoperative mapping of somatosensory cortex has been validated by comparison with intraoperative mapping.[3,4,6,7,25,26] In contrast to other functional brain techniques that measure indirect hemodynamic and metabolic changes due to neuronal activity, MEG measurements measure direct neural activity in the millisecond time scale with high temporal resolution. Magnetoencephalography measures tiny magnetic fields generated by the human brain and is enabled by superconducting quantum interference devices (SQUIDs), used in conjunction with flux-couplers and flux-locked loop circuitry, which have adequate sensitivity on the order of tens of femtotesla (seven orders of magnitude smaller than the earth's magnetic field). Modern MEG systems are capable of whole-head coverage with simultaneous measurements of about 300 channels. Magnetoencephalography is the magnetic analogue of electroencephalography (EEG), which measures electric potentials on the scalp surface due to neural currents, and the two are complementary modalities of underlying neuronal currents.

Magnetoencephalography imaging is unique among functional imaging techniques for its ability to provide spatiotemporal brain activation profiles that reflect not only where activity occurs in the brain but also when this activity occurs in relation to the presentation of the external stimulus and

the activity in other brain regions. Advanced reconstruction algorithms enable detailed spatiotemporal reconstructions of brain activity from MEG data, thereby making it an imaging method. Typically, MEGI algorithms involve two major components—a forward model and an inverse model. The forward model consists of three subcomponents: a source model, volume conductor, and measurement model. Typical source models assume that the MEG measurements outside the head are generated primarily by electric current dipoles located in the brain. This model is consistent with available measurements of coherent synaptic and intracellular currents in cortical columns that are thought to be major contributors to MEG signals. Volume conductor models refer to the equations that govern the relation between the source model and the sensor measurements (i.e., the electric potentials or the magnetic fields). These surface integral equations, obtained by solving Maxwell's equations under quasi-static conditions, can be solved analytically for special geometries of the volume conductor, such as spheres and ellipsoids.

Measurement models refer to the specific measurement systems used in MEG. For instance, different MEG systems measure axial versus planar gradients of the magnetic fields with respect to different locations of reference sensors. The measurement model incorporates information about the type of measurement and the geometry of the reference sensors. The source, volume conductor, and measurement models are typically combined in the forward field, which describes a linear relationship between the sources and the measurements. Usually, we assume that the forward-field matrix is known. We can easily calculate the forward field for electric current dipoles in a spherical volume conductor model for a whole-head axial gradiometer MEG system. In this model, MEG is sensitive only to the tangential component of the primary current dipoles. In contrast, EEG signals are sensitive to all components but sensitive to uncertainties in the head model. Simultaneous MEG and EEG can be acquired in most modern MEG systems and require some modification to the forward-field matrix for combined MEG and EEG measurements, especially for more realistic source, volume conductor, and measurement models.

Inverse modeling refers to the algorithm or procedure that is used to reconstruct sources based on a forward model and MEG measurements. Inverse algorithms are used to solve the bioelectromagnetic inverse problem (i.e., estimating neural source model parameters from MEG and EEG measurements obtained outside the human head). Because the source distributions are inherently four-dimensional (three in space and one in time) and only a few measurements are made outside the head, estimation is generally ill posed. To reduce this problem and to improve the spatial resolution of MEGI, various estimation procedures that incorporate prior knowledge and constraints about source characteristics, such as possible source locations, the source spatial extent, the total number of sources, and the source frequency/time frequency characteristics, have been developed.

Magnetoencephalographic imaging has been successfully used for functional mapping in patients with gliomas.[27-29] It has been used for localization of the sensorimotor cortex along the central sulcus[30-33] as well as mapping the primary auditory[34,35] and visual cortices.[36] Identifying the hand region[30,31,37-39] and the mouth region[37,40] of the primary sensorimotor cortex has been useful for presurgical evaluation, and also confirmed with intracranial direct cortical stimulation mapping. **Fig. 8.1** shows an example of parametric dipole localization in the context of a somatosensory evoked response, and shows that responses to vibrotactile stimuli can often be localized to activity arising from primary somatosensory cortex in the contralateral hemisphere. **Fig. 8.2** shows integration

of MEG source reconstructions with diffusion magnetic resonance (MR) findings.

Motor evoked fields can also be recorded by time-locking the MEG signal corresponding to movement,[41] and single equivalent current dipole (ECD) fitting of the corresponding evoked field generated from the average sensor data.[31,37,38,40,42] **Fig. 8.3** shows how MEG signals from motor cortex can be reconstructed. When magnetic source imaging (MSI) was compared to intraoperative mapping in tumor patients receiving painless tactile somatosensory stimulation to the lip, hand, and foot, it was found that both approaches had a favorable degree of quantitative correlation.[37] Similarly, a favorable degree of quantitative correlation was also seen from utilizing dipole fitting with MEG versus fMRI.[42] Confirmed with ECOG, dipole fitting of evoked magnetic fields to median nerve stimulation proved to be superior to fMRI for 15 patients in identifying the sensorimotor cortex.[31] Following dipole fitting of the mouth motor cortex, ECS sites were usually anterior and lateral to MEG localization of the lip somatosensory cortex.[40]

The use of MEG spatial filtering holds promise for a more robust method for mapping the motor cortex in presurgical

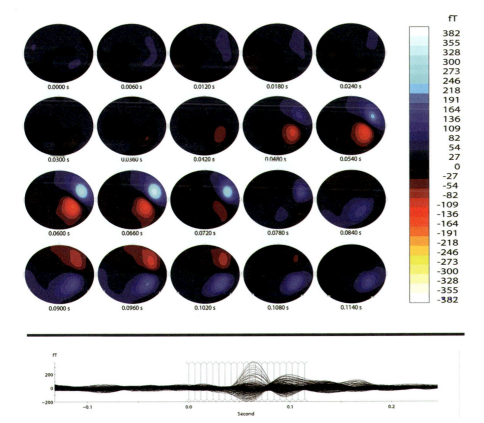
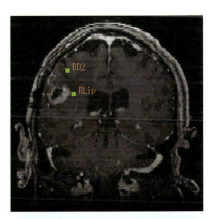
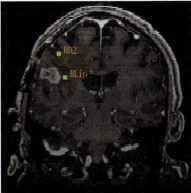

Fig. 8.1 Example case of parametric dipole localization of somatosensory stimuli to the right lip (RLip) and right index finger (RD2). Multiple stimulus trials are performed for each site and cortical magnetic fields are recorded. The trials are averaged and a single dipole is reconstructed for each site using the least-square fit method. The resulting dipoles are then displayed on a co-registered, T1-weighted, post-gadolinium coronal magnetic resonance (MR) slice.

patients.[30,39,43] The use of a spatial filter beam former while subjects performed a self-paced index finger movement can generate high-resolution imaging of the spatiotemporal patterns of premotor and motor cortex activity.[43] Peaks of the tomographic distribution of beta-band event-related desynchronization sources reliably localized the hand motor cortex in a group of 66 patients, which was confirmed with ECS.[39]

Magnetoencephalographic imaging also offers a noninvasive and potentially a more accurate alternative for deter-

mining hemispheric dominance of language. Using MEGI, language laterality can be measured by determining the asymmetry of equivalent dipole sources between both hemispheres.[44] Using this approach, MEGI and Wada tests were concordant in determining dominant hemisphere in 86% of a group of 35 patients with high sensitivity and specificity.[45] Dipole sources of the late auditory evoked field components in both hemispheres can also be determined while subjects undergo a recognition task for spoken words or listening to

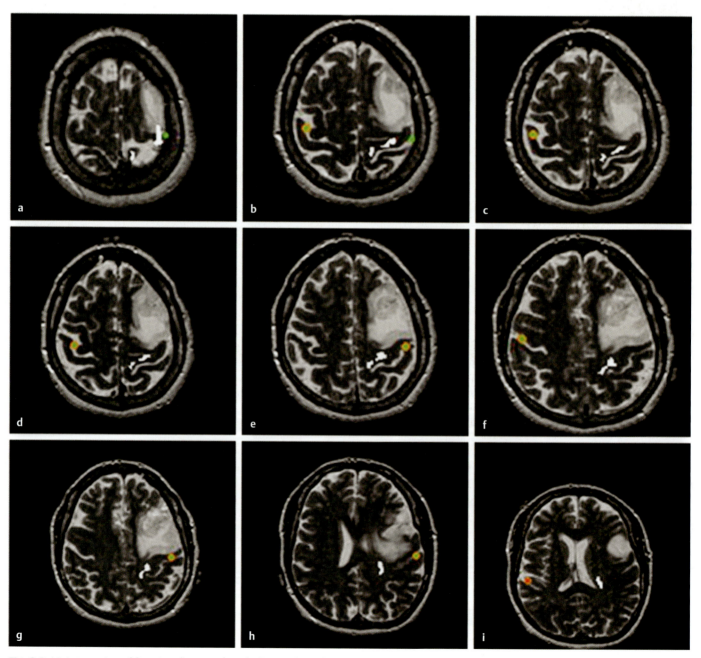

Fig. 8.2a–i Integration of functional mapping with electromagnetic source imaging (ESI) and white-matter tractography. Axial slices are shown in color, with functional locations overlaid that were obtained from ESI dipole modeling procedures. The functional areas mapped and shown in relation to a tumor are (**a**) hand–motor cortex, (**b**) left and right digit 5 (i.e., pinky), (**c**) left thumb, (**d**) left index finger, (**e**) right index finger, (**f**) left lip, (**g**) right index, (**h**) right thumb, and (**i**) auditory cortex.

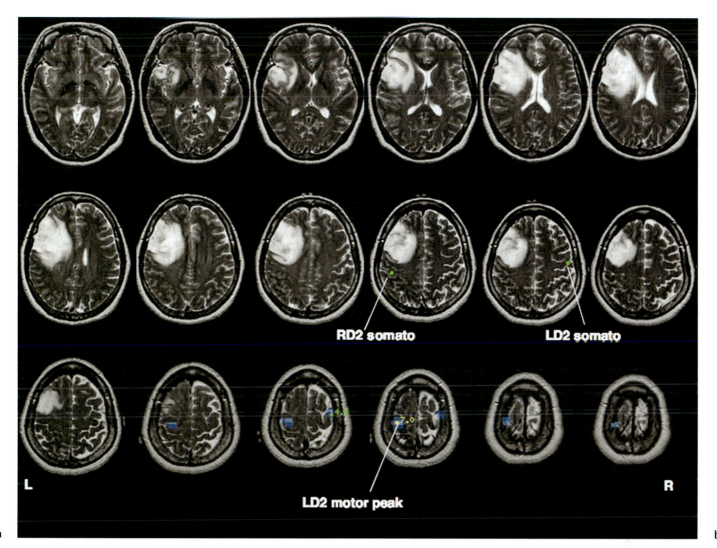

Fig. 8.3a,b **(a)** Localization of β-band desynchronization preceding right index finger flexion for a subject with a frontal tumor. The location of hand motor cortex relative to a single dipole localization of hand somatosensory cortex is also shown. **(b)** Localization of β-band desynchronization due to left index finger flexion in the same subject, showing contralateral hand motor cortical activation in the right hemisphere.

synthesized vowel sounds.[44,46] The laterality of increased suppression of MEG activity in the 8- to 50-Hz range in the inferior frontal gyrus regions corresponded to the dominant hemisphere and was consistent with the Wada test among 95% of the patients.[47]

Location of the language cortex (i.e., Broca's area and Wernicke's area) also holds clinical value, as mass lesions can distort the anatomy, and also because of interindividual anatomic variation among patients. One study compared MEG to fMRI

in locating Wernicke's area and Broca's area in 172 patients.[48] These language areas were localized in all patients; however, 4% of cases differed in MEG and fMRI and in 19% one modality showed activation whereas the other did not. Similarly, a group of investigators using spatially filtered MEG located Wernicke's area in the posterior part of the left superior temporal gyrus and motor speech area in the left inferior frontal gyrus.[49]

A prospective study using MEGI to determine language lateralization found high concordance with Wada testing and intraoperative cortical stimulation results.[50] An extension of this approach has been used to characterize dynamics of language dominance using MEG. One study was able to detect decreases in power in the beta-frequency band during the process of verb generation. With these data, a laterality index (LI) could be calculated, which quantified the "leftness" or "rightness" of the subject's language function (**Fig. 8.4**). These

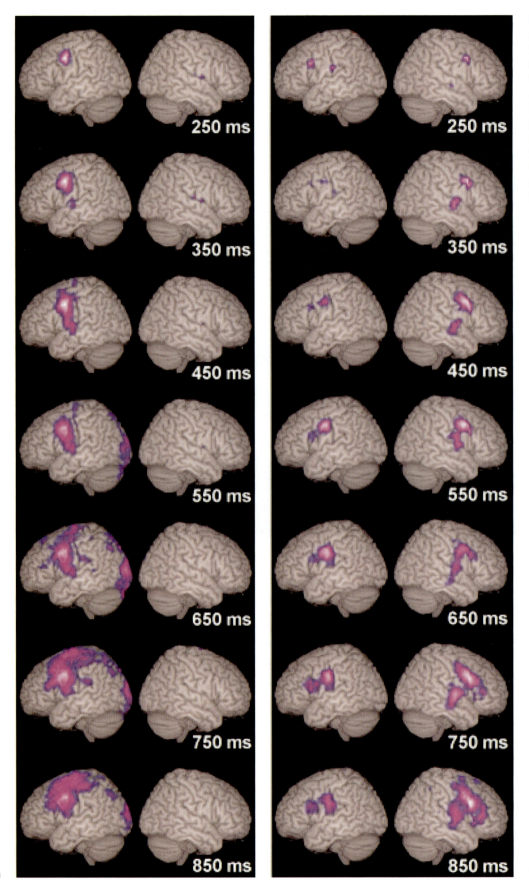

Fig. 8.4a,b Time course of average verb generation activations for **(a)** left-WADA patients and **(b)** right-WADA patients for the stimulus-locked condition. Activations were thresholded at half of the absolute maximum power value over the shown time course. Time windows of 650 through 850 ms for superior temporal and supramarginal gyrus were used in determining language laterality.

> **Pitfall**
>
> - Magnetoencephalographic imaging is primarily useful for measuring the function of cortical sources but has reduced sensitivity to deeper sources.

data were then validated against Wada test results. In a first cohort, the lateralization of language in each patient could be predicted with 100% certainty. Findings from prospective evaluation of the model in a second group showed that estimation of lateral language based on this examination correlated very highly with Wada results.

Functional Connectivity Imaging

The term *functional connectivity* essentially defines the complex functional interaction between local and more remote brain areas. This concept should be considered clinically as disturbances in these networks as abnormalities in functional connecting during resting state are observed primarily in brain tumor patients when compared to healthy controls.[51,52] Furthermore, neurocognitive effects are correlated with functional connectivity changes in brain tumor patients, especially in patients with low-grade gliomas.[53,54] Therefore, the mapping of functional connectivity may be an important component in surgical planning.[55]

Utilizing MEGI, the changes in the time-frequency space of functional connectivity in 15 brain tumor patients were compared to healthy controls[55] (**Fig. 8.5**). Mean imaginary coherence between brain voxels was calculated as an index for functional connectivity. When compared with healthy controls, all patients with brain tumors had diffuse brain areas with decreased alpha coherence. Decreased connectivity was seen around the lesion area in patients with lesion-induced neurologic deficits. In the resting connectivity in the delta and gamma frequency bands in patients with brain tumors, functional connectivity was decreased in patients with brain tumors and further decreased in left-sided versus right-sided tumors.[37,51] Specifically, there is a decrease in high-frequency bands for long distance connections and an increase in slower frequency bands for more local connections.[52]

A recent follow-up study demonstrated that these measures of functional connectivity can potentially be used to guide in-traoperative ECS mapping. Prospectively, we compared MEG functional connectivity maps with ECS maps of eloquent cortex in 57 brain tumor patients over a 9-month period. Maps of functional connectivity were generated from preoperative MEG recordings (**Fig. 8.5**). By comparing peritumoral regions against the corresponding regions in the contralateral hemisphere, we identified regions of altered connectivity. These maps were then compared with ECS-generated maps of language and motor function. Based on these comparisons, we determined the predictive value of the functional connectivity map. The negative predictive value of decreased connectivity was 87%, whereas the positive predictive value of increased connectivity was 64%. These results are highly encouraging, and demonstrate that MEGI of resting-state functional connectivity can be a useful adjunct to preoperative mapping in this patient population.

Conclusion

There are various complementary techniques available for preoperative functional brain mapping that have different spatial and temporal resolution capabilities. The best approach would be to combine these complementary methods during preoperative assessment. The problem of brain shift during surgery renders preoperatively acquired functional data inaccurate. Therefore, no method can completely replace the gold standard of direct intraoperative mapping. The combination of preoperative functional mapping, with diffusion tensor imaging, white-matter tractography, and intraoperative mapping can help maintain motor and language functions following surgical management of metastatic brain tumors.

However, the traditional approach to preoperative mapping assumes a static cortical functional organization. Although there is considerable individual functional variability, there also needs to be a consideration of cortical plasticity associated with the tumor. Cerebral plasticity is the short- to long-term remodeling of brain networks that has a critical role during ontogeny, learning, and recovery from lesions in the central nervous system or the peripheral nervous system. Brain plasticity due to the presence of a brain tumor and its surgical resection will impact tumor treatment strategies.[20] There needs to be a consideration of the dynamic interactions between the natural history of the tumor and the reactive process of cerebral adaptation to maximize tumor resection quality while minimizing the risk of irreversible postoperative deficits.

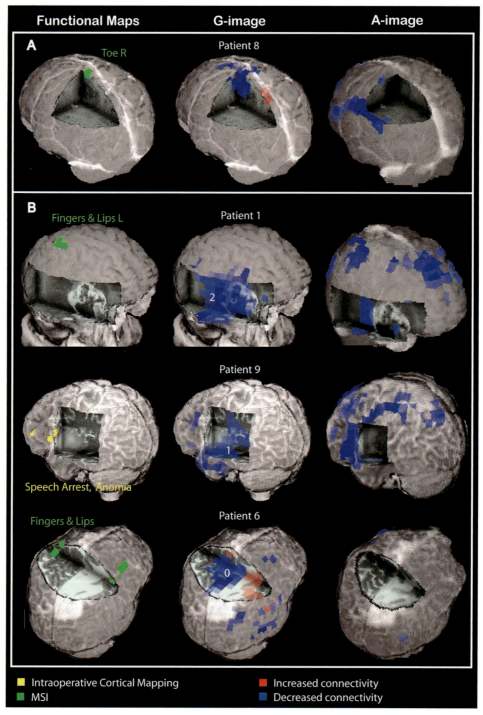

Functional Maps   **G-image**   **A-image**

A   Toe R   Patient 8

B   Fingers & Lips L   Patient 1

2

Patient 9

Speech Arrest, Anomia

1

Fingers & Lips   Patient 6

0

■ Intraoperative Cortical Mapping   ■ Increased connectivity
■ MSI   ■ Decreased connectivity

Fig. 8.5a,b Functional maps obtained with magnetic source imaging or intraoperative cortical mapping as well as two different kinds (L- and P- images) of functional connectivity in four patients with brain tumors superimposed over their 3D-rendered individual brain. The L-image is a lesion-specific image of connectivity, and the P-image is a patient-specific image of connectivity. **(a)** A 25-year-old woman with a central paresis of the right foot due to an astrocytoma (World Health Organization grade III) that infiltrated the left medial senso-rimotor cortex. Note that the L-image displays a corresponding decrease in functional connectivity in the sensorimotor cortex of the right foot. **(b)** The L-images of three tumor patients without presurgical functional deficits indicate functional disconnection (*in blue*) of different proportions of the corresponding tumor tissue (graded 0 to 2, with 0 indicating smallest proportion with discon-nection). In agreement with the L-images and the clinical status, functional cortex was mapped outside of disconnected (*blue*) areas by magnetic source imaging (MSI) and cortical mapping in all patients. In addition, L-images predicted the functional status after radical surgery; whereas patient 6 suffered from postsurgical sensible deficits in the left arm and leg, no deficits were observed in patients 1 and 9. P-images show diffuse or scattered areas with significantly lower connectivity estimates than a healthy control population, but these areas are unrelated to tumor location and brain regions with functional deficits.

Editor's Note

Currently there are a number of ways to functionally image the brain. These include PET, fMRI, and MEG. All of these techniques share the concept of activation of brain regions as a marker of functional activity. Each of these techniques differs in terms of how the information is obtained, but the information can be useful in a number of ways. The neurosurgeon can use this information to determine how close a resection could come to a functional region, along with determining when to use intraoperative functional mapping. The neuro-oncologist could utilize this information to determine critical aspects about quality of life and why patients are perhaps not doing as well as they would otherwise be expected to be doing at a given time during their treatment. The radiation oncologist could use this information to spare regions of the brain that could be injured with functional consequences as a result of the treatment. Perhaps the Holy Grail in this field will be to determine connectivity of various brain regions, which will have significant implications about the role that region plays in the overall particular function for that individual. These connectivity maps will become of greater value as the sensitivity and specificity of that test improves. (Berger)

Acknowledgments

This work was funded by National Institutes of Health grant R21 NS076171 and the National Science Foundation Cognitive Neuroscience Program. We thank our various collaborators, especially Drs. Sophia Vinogradov, Elliot Sherr, Pratik Mukherjee, Roland Henry, Kensuke Sekihara, Hagai Attias, John Houde, Marilu Gorno-Tempini, Steve Cheung, Robert Knight, Edward Chang, Nancy Byl, Elizabeth Disbrow, Elysa Marco, and Heidi Kirsch, for their invaluable help and contributions. Past and current members of the Biomagnetic Imaging Laboratory contributed significantly to this work, especially Anne Findlay, Susanne Honma, Mary Mantle, Danielle Mizuiri, Leighton Hinkley, Carrie Niziolek, Corby Dale, Tracy Luks, Adrian Guggisberg, Juan Martino, Phiroz Tarapore, Kamalini Wijesinghe, Kelly Westlake, Alex Herman, Julia Owen, David Wipf, Karuna Subramanium, Naomi Kort, Sarang Dalal, and Johanna Zumer.

References

1. Towle VL, Khorasani L, Uftring S, et al. Noninvasive identification of human central sulcus: a comparison of gyral morphology, functional MRI, dipole localization, and direct cortical mapping. Neuroimage 2003;19:684–697
2. Braun V, Dempf S, Tomczak R, Wunderlich A, Weller R, Richter HP. Functional cranial neuronavigation. Direct integration of fMRI and PET data. J Neuroradiol 2000;27:157–163
3. Castillo EM, Simos PG, Wheless JW, et al. Integrating sensory and motor mapping in a comprehensive MEG protocol: clinical validity and replicability. Neuroimage 2004;21:973–983
4. Kamada K, Houkin K, Takeuchi F, et al. Visualization of the eloquent motor system by integration of MEG, functional, and anisotropic diffusion-weighted MRI in functional neuronavigation. Surg Neurol 2003; 59:352–361, discussion 361–362
5. Kraus GE, Bernstein TW, Satter M, Ezzeddine B, Hwang DR, Mantil J. A technique utilizing positron emission tomography and magnetic resonance/computed tomography image fusion to aid in surgical navigation and tumor volume determination. J Image Guid Surg 1995; 1:300–307
6. Schiffbauer H, Berger MS, Ferrari P, Freudenstein D, Rowley HA, Roberts TP. Preoperative magnetic source imaging for brain tumor surgery: a quantitative comparison with intraoperative sensory and motor mapping. J Neurosurg 2002;97:1333–1342
7. Schiffbauer H, Berger MS, Ferrari P, Freudenstein D, Rowley HA, Roberts TP. Preoperative magnetic source imaging for brain tumor surgery: a quantitative comparison with intraoperative sensory and motor mapping. Neurosurg Focus 2003;15:E7. http://www.aans.org/education/journal/neurosurgi-cal/july03/15-1-7.pdf. Accessed September 5, 2006 [serial online]
8. Schiffbauer H, Ferrari P, Rowley HA, Berger MS, Roberts TP. Functional activity within brain tumors: a magnetic source imaging study. Neurosurgery 2001;49:1313–1320, discussion 1320–1321
9. Bittar RG, Olivier A, Sadikot AF, et al. Localization of somatosensory function by using positron emission tomography scanning: a comparison with intraoperative cortical stimulation. J Neurosurg 1999;90: 478–483
10. Reutens DC, Bittar RG, Tochon-Danguy H, Scott AM. Clinical applications of [(15)O] H(2)O PET activation studies. Clin Positron Imaging 1999;2:145–152
11. Bittar RG, Olivier A, Sadikot AF, Andermann F, Pike GB, Reutens DC. Presurgical motor and somatosensory cortex mapping with functional magnetic resonance imaging and positron emission tomography. J Neurosurg 1999;91:915–921
12. Reinges MH, Krings T, Meyer PT, et al. Preoperative mapping of cortical motor function: prospective comparison of functional magnetic resonance imaging and [15O]-H2O-positron emission tomography in the same co-ordinate system. Nucl Med Commun 2004;25:987–997
13. Buxton RB. Introduction to Functional Magnetic Resonance Imaging: Principles and Techniques. Cambridge: Cambridge University Press, 2002
14. Schreiber A, Hubbe U, Ziyeh S, Hennig J. The influence of gliomas and nonglial space-occupying lesions on blood-oxygen-level-dependent contrast enhancement. AJNR Am J Neuroradiol 2000;21:1055–1063
15. Schwindack C, Siminotto E, Meyer M, et al. Real-time functional magnetic resonance imaging (rt-fMRI) in patients with brain tumours: preliminary findings using motor and language paradigms. Br J Neurosurg 2005;19:25–32
16. Majos A, Tybor K, Stefańczyk L, Góraj B. Cortical mapping by functional magnetic resonance imaging in patients with brain tumors. Eur Radiol 2005;15:1148–1158
17. Kamada K, Todo T, Masutani Y, et al. Combined use of tractography-integrated functional neuronavigation and direct fiber stimulation. J Neurosurg 2005;102:664–672
18. Duffau H, Lopes M, Arthuis F, et al. Contribution of intraoperative electrical stimulations in surgery of low grade gliomas: a comparative study between two series without (1985–96) and with (1996–2003) functional mapping in the same institution. J Neurol Neurosurg Psychiatry 2005;76:845–851

19. Roessler K, Donat M, Lanzenberger R, et al. Evaluation of preoperative high magnetic field motor functional MRI (3 Tesla) in glioma patients by navigated electrocortical stimulation and postoperative outcome. J Neurol Neurosurg Psychiatry 2005;76:1152–1157

20. Duffau H. Lessons from brain mapping in surgery for low-grade glioma: insights into associations between tumour and brain plasticity. Lancet Neurol 2005;4:476–486

21. Voss J, Meier TB, Freidel R, et al. The role of secondary motor and language cortices in morbidity and mortality: a retrospective functional MRI study of surgical planning for patients with intracranial tumors. Neurosurg Focus 2013;34:E7

22. Kundu B, Penwarden A, Wood JM, et al. Association of functional magnetic resonance imaging indices with postoperative language outcomes in patients with primary brain tumors. Neurosurg Focus 2013;34:E6

23. Wood JM, Kundu B, Utter A, et al. Impact of brain tumor location on morbidity and mortality: a retrospective functional MR imaging study. AJNR Am J Neuroradiol 2011;32:1420–1425

24. Gallagher TA, Nair VA, Regner MF, et al. Characterizing the relationship between functional MRI-derived measures and clinical outcomes in patients with vascular lesions. Neurosurg Focus 2013;34:E8

25. Kamada K, Möller M, Saguer M, et al. A combined study of tumor-related brain lesions using MEG and proton MR spectroscopic imaging. J Neurol Sci 2001;186:13–21

26. Morioka T, Yamamoto T, Mizushima A, et al. Comparison of magnetoencephalography, functional MRI, and motor evoked potentials in the localization of the sensory-motor cortex. Neurol Res 1995;17:361–367

27. Gallen CC, Schwartz BJ, Bucholz RD, et al. Presurgical localization of functional cortex using magnetic source imaging. J Neurosurg 1995; 82:988–994 10.3171/jns.1995.82.6.0988

28. Kamada K, Takeuchi F, Kuriki S, Oshiro O, Houkin K, Abe H. Functional neurosurgical simulation with brain surface magnetic resonance images and magnetoencephalography. Neurosurgery 1993;33:269–272, discussion 272–273

29. Mäkelä JP, Kirveskari E, Seppä M, et al. Three-dimensional integration of brain anatomy and function to facilitate intraoperative navigation around the sensorimotor strip. Hum Brain Mapp 2001;12:180–192

30. Gaetz W, Cheyne D, Rutka JT, et al. Presurgical localization of primary motor cortex in pediatric patients with brain lesions by the use of spatially filtered magnetoencephalography. Neurosurgery 2009;64(3, Suppl)ons177–ons185, discussion ons186

31. Korvenoja A, Kirveskari E, Aronen HJ, et al. Sensorimotor cortex localization: comparison of magnetoencephalography, functional MR imaging, and intraoperative cortical mapping. Radiology 2006;241:213–222

32. Taniguchi M, Kato A, Ninomiya H, et al. Cerebral motor control in patients with gliomas around the central sulcus studied with spatially filtered magnetoencephalography. J Neurol Neurosurg Psychiatry 2004; 75:466–471

33. Ossenblok P, Leijten FS, de Munck JC, Huiskamp GJ, Barkhof F, Boon P. Magnetic source imaging contributes to the presurgical identification of sensorimotor cortex in patients with frontal lobe epilepsy. Clin Neurophysiol 2003;114:221–232

34. Rowley HA, Roberts TP. Functional localization by magnetoencephalography. Neuroimaging Clin N Am 1995;5:695–710

35. Lütkenhöner B, Krumbholz K, Lammertmann C, Seither-Preisler A, Steinsträter O, Patterson RD. Localization of primary auditory cortex in humans by magnetoencephalography. Neuroimage 2003;18:58–66

36. Plomp G, Leeuwen Cv, Ioannides AA. Functional specialization and dynamic resource allocation in visual cortex. Hum Brain Mapp 2010; 31:1–13

37. Schiffbauer H, Berger MS, Ferrari P, Freudenstein D, Rowley HA, Roberts TP. Preoperative magnetic source imaging for brain tumor surgery: a quantitative comparison with intraoperative sensory and motor mapping. Neurosurg Focus 2003;15:E7

38. Ishibashi H, Morioka T, Nishio S, Shigeto H, Yamamoto T, Fukui M. Magnetoencephalographic investigation of somatosensory homunculus in patients with peri-Rolandic tumors. Neurol Res 2001;23:29–38

39. Nagarajan S, Kirsch H, Lin P, Findlay A, Honma S, Berger MS. Preoperative localization of hand motor cortex by adaptive spatial filtering of magnetoencephalography data. J Neurosurg 2008;109:228–237 10.3171/JNS/2008/109/8/0228

40. Kirsch HE, Zhu Z, Honma S, Findlay A, Berger MS, Nagarajan SS. Predicting the location of mouth motor cortex in patients with brain tumors by using somatosensory evoked field measurements. J Neurosurg 2007;107:481–487 10.3171/JNS-07/09/0481

41. Rezai AR, Hund M, Kronberg E, et al. The interactive use of magnetoencephalography in stereotactic image-guided neurosurgery. Neurosurgery 1996;39:92–102

42. Kober H, Nimsky C, Möller M, Hastreiter P, Fahlbusch R, Ganslandt O. Correlation of sensorimotor activation with functional magnetic resonance imaging and magnetoencephalography in presurgical functional imaging: a spatial analysis. Neuroimage 2001;14:1214–1228

43. Cheyne D, Bakhtazad L, Gaetz W. Spatiotemporal mapping of cortical activity accompanying voluntary movements using an event-related beamforming approach. Hum Brain Mapp 2006;27:213–229 10.1002/hbm.20178

44. Papanicolaou AC, Simos PG, Castillo EM, et al. Magnetocephalography: a noninvasive alternative to the Wada procedure. J Neurosurg 2004; 100:867–876 10.3171/jns.2004.100.5.0867

45. Doss RC, Zhang W, Risse GL, Dickens DL. Lateralizing language with magnetic source imaging: validation based on the Wada test. Epilepsia 2009;50:2242–2248

46. Szymanski MD, Perry DW, Gage NM, et al. Magnetic source imaging of late evoked field responses to vowels: toward an assessment of hemispheric dominance for language. J Neurosurg 2001;94:445–453 10.3171/jns.2001.94.3.0445

47. Hirata M, Kato A, Taniguchi M, et al. Determination of language dominance with synthetic aperture magnetometry: comparison with the Wada test. Neuroimage 2004;23:46–53

48. Grummich P, Nimsky C, Pauli E, Buchfelder M, Ganslandt O. Combining fMRI and MEG increases the reliability of presurgical language localization: a clinical study on the difference between and congruence of both modalities. Neuroimage 2006;32:1793–1803

49. Kober H, Möller M, Nimsky C, Vieth J, Fahlbusch R, Ganslandt O. New approach to localize speech relevant brain areas and hemispheric dominance using spatially filtered magnetoencephalography. Hum Brain Mapp 2001;14:236–250

50. Hirata M, Goto T, Barnes G, et al. Language dominance and mapping based on neuromagnetic oscillatory changes: comparison with invasive procedures. J Neurosurg 2010;112:528–538

51. Bartolomei F, Bosma I, Klein M, et al. How do brain tumors alter functional connectivity? A magnetoencephalography study. Ann Neurol 2006;59:128–138 10.1002/ana.20710

52. Bartolomei F, Bosma I, Klein M, et al. Disturbed functional connectivity in brain tumour patients: evaluation by graph analysis of synchronization matrices. Clin Neurophysiol 2006;117:2039–2049

53. Bosma I, Douw L, Bartolomei F, et al. Synchronized brain activity and neurocognitive function in patients with low-grade glioma: a magnetoencephalography study. Neuro-oncol 2008;10:734–744

54. Bosma I, Stam CJ, Douw L, et al. The influence of low-grade glioma on resting state oscillatory brain activity: a magnetoencephalography study. J Neurooncol 2008;88:77–85 10.1007/s11060-008-9535-3

55. Guggisberg AG, Honma SM, Findlay AM, et al. Mapping functional connectivity in patients with brain lesions. Ann Neurol 2008;63:193–203 10.1002/ana.21224

Surgery

9   Perioperative Management

Jennifer Moliterno Gunel and Joseph M. Piepmeier

Optimizing the perioperative management of a patient with a brain tumor can have a profound effect on their surgical outcome. Attention to important details leads to better decisions and optimal patient recovery. This chapter addresses perioperative issues that are fundamental for appropriately managing patients undergoing surgical intervention for brain tumors. Although these principles can be generalized to every surgical patient, the importance of encompassing the needs of the individual patient should be emphasized.

■ Preoperative Considerations

History and Physical Examination

The three most important initial steps in evaluating a patient with a brain tumor are to obtain a comprehensive history of the patient's illness, carefully examine the patient, and obtain the appropriate imaging studies. These elements compose the foundation on which the perioperative assessment is established.

A detailed history can provide important clues regarding the likely underlying pathology, and, coupled with a thorough neurologic examination, can often reveal the lesion's location. Brain tumors come to clinical attention when they have reached a critical size or have caused sufficient brain swelling to result in headache, seizure, change in functional capacity (e.g., paresis, vision changes), or cognitive impairment.[1] The timing with which these problems arise is often inversely related to the aggressiveness of the tumor, such that the shorter the presentation and more rapid the onset of signs and symptoms, the more aggressive the underlying tumor pathology. Patients with malignant tumors, such as glioblastoma multiforme (GBM) or brain metastases, can often present with worsening focal neurologic deficits, occurring over days to weeks, or with the acute onset of seizure. In contrast, indolent lesions, such as low-grade glioma or meningioma, can remain clinically silent for years until they reach a critical size, at which time small changes in tumor volume or characteristics (e.g., hemorrhage) can generate neurologic symptoms.[1–3]

Because the temporal evolution of the history gives some indication of the anticipated growth rate of the tumor, it is important to inquire about signs and symptoms that may be considered by the patient to be unremarkable or unrelated. Partial epilepsy, for instance, is a common undetected sign of

> **Pearl**
>
> • A family history, when appropriate, can be of particular importance to identify families with germline mutations that predispose family members to cancer.

low-grade intrinsic brain tumors and can be unrecognized, often with a subtle history of progressively worsening difficulties at school or work, as well as unexplained learning disabilities. Such changes in function may be misinterpreted as the result of stress or inattention. In addition, the rapidity with which signs and symptoms evolve can also serve as a good indicator of how quickly intervention should be pursued, with more acute changes in functional capacity or altered consciousness necessitating a more urgent surgical intervention.

Although most neurosurgeons are comfortable with interpreting the results of a routine neurologic examination, this may prove to be inadequate to illustrate the impact of the tumor on cognitive abilities. Executive function can be further quantitatively assessed through psychometric testing.[4] Patients with tumors in the dominant mesial temporal lobe, for instance, are at risk for profound memory impairment with surgery, and preoperative memory testing can help determine the relative risk. In those patients who have memory loss of greater than two standard deviations from the mean, surgery typically does not result in a clinically significant further decline.[5] Although most right-handed patients maintain dominance for language and memory in the left hemisphere, long-standing lesions (e.g., low-grade glioma) as well as prior cortical injury can result in reorganization of function that is shifted to, or shared with, the right hemisphere. Such patients may benefit from investigation with preoperative functional studies to determine the localization of language and memory.

A family history can also be of importance. Immediate relatives with a history of brain tumors can raise the possibility of an inheritable predisposing condition (e.g., germline mutations) such as neurofibromatosis, von Hippel–Lindau disease, Turcot's syndrome, or Li-Fraumeni syndrome. Patients are often unaware of such familial risks, and a careful review of the family's medical history and a dedicated physical examination, including a search for café-au-lait macules in potential neurofibromatosis patients, can facilitate more frequent and thorough monitoring of the patient and family members.

■ Preoperative Imaging

Tumor location is one of the most important findings to consider in deciding on the type of surgical intervention, such as biopsy versus resection. The proximity of the tumor to motor, somatosensory, language, and visual areas, as well as to critical neurovascular structures, can help determine the relative risk of surgery (**Fig. 9.1**). The size of the lesion and its extension into the surrounding brain can also provide an estimate of the probability of achieving the surgical goals.

The most commonly used imaging modalities for evaluating a patient with a brain tumor are computed tomography (CT) and magnetic resonance imaging (MRI). MRI is superior for intrinsic tumors as it not only provides a high-resolution definition of normal anatomy but also better delineates tumor extension, invasion and displacement of normal structures. CT can be useful in cases with bone erosion or hyperostosis. Evaluating images in multiple planes aids in a three-dimensional understanding of the tumor and is crucial for surgical planning.

Specific imaging findings can be useful for establishing a probable diagnosis and offer insight into the likely pathology.

Low-grade gliomas are typically hypodense on CT and hyperintense on T2-weighted MRI—the majority being without appreciable contrast enhancement. Alternatively, most GBMs have a central nonenhancing region of necrosis surrounded by a ring of enhancement composed of tumor and neovascularity, along with a region of infiltrative tumor cells that can best be appreciated as abnormal T2-weighted signal extending into the surrounding brain. Contrast enhancement signifies an impaired blood–brain barrier with heterogeneous and homogeneous patterns typically displayed in high-grade tumors and meningiomas, respectively. The acquisition of contrast enhancement in a previously nonenhancing glioma is an indication that the tumor has evolved into a more anaplastic lesion.

The presence of contrast enhancement, however, lacks specificity for malignancy. Noninfiltrative low-grade gliomas, such as pilocytic astrocytoma and pleomorphic xanthoastrocytoma (PXA), display nodular enhancement. In addition, up to 25% of malignant gliomas may have faint or no detectable enhancement, whereas 30% of diffuse low-grade gliomas can demonstrate contrast enhancement.[6,7] Thus, interpretation of imaging must be made in the context of clinical information.

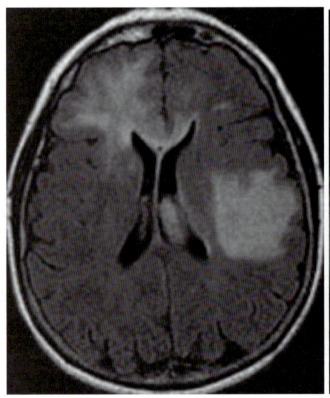
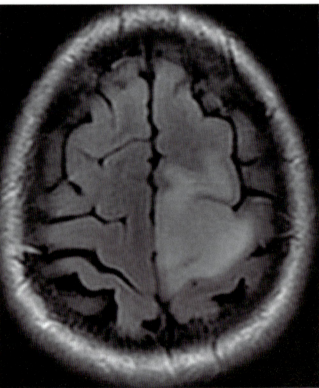

Fig. 9.1a,b **(a)** Axial fluid-attenuated inversion recovery (FLAIR) image of diffuse tumor infiltration into the left posterior frontal lobe and the right frontal lobe with involvement of the corpus callosum. These findings indicate a diffuse glioma. **(b)** Axial FLAIR image demonstrating a glioma within the left motor cortex. Both images show tumors that cannot be removed without serious neurologic sequelae and are best managed with a biopsy.

a

b

Pitfall

- The absence of contrast enhancement within a glioma on MRI does not exclude the possibility of a high-grade tumor. Restricted diffusion on DWI can indicate a highly cellular tumor or particularly cellular area of a tumor that can help direct biopsy.

Nonetheless, the risk of anaplasia in nonenhancing tumors increases with age.[8]

Imaging correlates of molecular tumor characteristics have been recognized. Oligodendrogliomas with deletions on chromosome 1p and 19q are usually hypointense compared with white matter and have indistinct borders on T1-weighted MRI, whereas tumors that lack such molecular features more commonly are sharply demarcated from surrounding brain. In addition, co-deleted oligodendrogliomas are characterized by signal heterogeneity on T1- and T2-weighted images with focal paramagnetic susceptibility effects likely related to calcium deposition within the tumor. Anaplastic tumors lacking 1p/19q deletions are characterized by ring enhancement.[9,10] Magnetic resonance imaging criteria have also been established for high-grade gliomas featuring overexpression of the epidermal growth factor receptor (EGFR).[11]

Diffusion-weighted imaging (DWI) delineates tissue characteristics based on the molecular motion of protons and can be quite useful. In a tumor of dense cellularity, such as GBM and lymphoma, the intracellular compartment is increased relative to the extracellular, and the diffusion signal is increased compared with normal brain. As a result, the signal of these tumors is often increased on DWI and correspondingly decreased on apparent diffusion coefficient (ADC) maps (**Fig. 9.2**). Diffusion-weighted imaging not only facilitates differential diagnosis of neoplasms and other structural lesions but also may be useful to identify a focus of increased cellularity and thus a favorable biopsy target, especially within a nonenhancing tumor. Areas of restricted diffusion in a nonenhancing low-grade glioma may reflect an early imaging sign of high-grade transformation.[12] Abscesses can lead to restricted diffusion, which once again underscores the need for considering the entire clinical picture.[13]

Functional Studies

Functional MRI (fMRI) can prove valuable for the surgical management of tumors located in or near eloquent cortical and subcortical anatomy.[14] The technique relies on focal changes in blood flow caused by a repetitive stereotypic activity to localize regions that subserve a specific function. Functional MRI is most often used to localize the primary motor and somatosensory cortex. Speech and language function are also commonly mapped with fMRI; however, the precision of this technique and the variability and complexity in localizing language function makes this less reliable. Tumors can invade or displace these critical regions, and functional anatomic imaging can help define anatomic relationships that direct surgical strategy.

Diffusion tensor imaging (DTI) takes advantage of preferential diffusion of water molecules in the direction of fiber bundles.[15] The distribution of major vectors in white matter (tractography) is commonly displayed using color-based maps

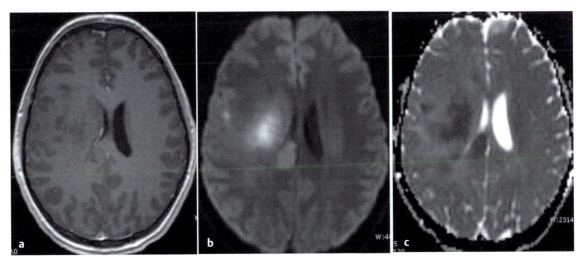

Fig. 9.2a–c **(a)** Axial T1-weighted MRI demonstrating a nonenhancing tumor in the right centrum. **(b)** Diffusion-weighted imaging of the same tumor showing areas of restricted diffusion (high cellularity), with **(c)** an apparent diffusion coefficient map of the same tumor, demonstrating dark regions matching the areas of restricted diffusion. These findings are suggestive of early anaplastic transformation of a low-grade glioma.

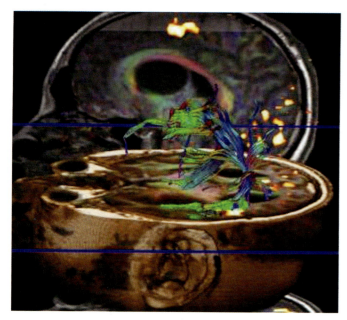

Fig. 9.3 Diffusion tensor imaging shows the arcuate fasciculus (*blue*) displaced by a large left frontal lobe glioma.

(**Fig. 9.3**). Displacement or invasion of these fiber tracts can be identified in patients with mass lesions in the brain, and this information can also be critical in avoiding major neurologic complications during tumor surgery.

Other Imaging Modalities

Proton magnetic resonance spectroscopy imaging (^{1}H-MRSI) has been utilized to map the infiltration of tumor cells into the brain by examining the relative concentration of choline (Cho), *N*-acetyl aspartate (NAA), and creatine (Cr).[16–18] The profile of each of these major metabolites in tumor tissue is distinct from the relative amounts found in normal brain. By examining their relative concentrations across a volume of tissue, metabolic maps of the extent of the tumor can be produced. The presence of lactate peaks on MRSI, for instance, often indicates anaerobic metabolism found in high-grade tumors. When the anatomic MRI presents an ambiguous lesion, MRSI can be useful for predicting the diagnosis of a glioma. The distribution of MRSI-identified tumor infiltration often extends beyond the volume identified by routine MRI.

p-[^{123}I]iodo-l-phenylalanine accumulates in tumors when imaged with single photon emission computed tomography (SPECT) and can help distinguish gliomas from nonneoplastic lesions.[19] Uptake of this radiolabeled amino acid does not require an altered blood–brain barrier, making it useful for preoperative evaluation of low-grade tumors, as well as anaplastic variants. Positron emission tomography (PET) images the uptake of 18-fluoro-2-deoxyglucose (FDG) and has been used to estimate tumor metabolism by imaging the relative level of uptake within the tumor in comparison with the contralateral

brain.[20] Higher FDG uptake has been reported to positively correlate with glioma grade. Positron emission tomography scanning has also been used preoperatively to better detect the most aggressive focus of a tumor in an effort to minimize the risk of sampling error from stereotactic biopsy. Likewise, PET can also be used following radiotherapy, to help differentiate radiation necrosis from recurrent tumor. It is accurate in predicting which tumors are low or high grade, but frequently provides false-negative images in heavily pretreated patients (i.e., hypometabolism in high-grade tumors).

■ Preoperative Medical Management Considerations

Patients with brain tumors can experience seizures and symptomatic cerebral brain edema. Medications to address these problems are often initiated preoperatively and adjusted peri- and postoperatively. In addition, the overall medical condition of the patient must be considered. It is helpful and often necessary to have input from primary care physicians and appropriate specialists prior to surgery to help optimize the patient's health. Conditions that could increase the risk of surgery such as bleeding problems, infections, or any other baseline comorbidities should be addressed and treated appropriately. Cancer patients are at high risk for venous thromboembolic events (VTEs), including deep venous thrombosis (DVT) and pulmonary embolus (PE), and should be carefully evaluated with preoperative diagnostic imaging such as lower extremity ultrasound when necessary. The finding of a DVT might necessitate placement of an inferior vena cava (IVC) filter, as anticoagulation would not be an option immediately prior to surgery.

Antiepileptic Medication Use

Antiepileptic drug (AED) treatment is uniformly initiated following a recognized seizure.[2,3] When the diagnosis of a seizure is obscure, electroencephalographic (EEG) monitoring may be helpful. The selection of an AED is typically dependent on the preferences of the surgeon or neuro-oncologist. Levetiracetam (Keppra) has gained increasing popularity over phenytoin (Dilantin) due to the fact that it is less sedating, has less frequent drug interactions, and does not require serum blood level monitoring.

Although the use of prophylactic AEDs in patients with brain tumors who have not had a seizure has been somewhat controversial, it is currently recommended that these patients not be placed on these medications.[21,22] The incidence of clinically significant and insignificant seizures has been reported as low as 3% and 8%, respectively, and randomized prospective studies have failed to show any benefit from prophylactic anticonvulsant treatment in brain tumor patients. Allergic reactions, poor compliance from medication side effects, and hepatic enzyme induction are some of the sequelae that can be avoided.

Cerebral Edema

Corticosteroids can be very helpful for providing relief from symptomatic mass effect caused by peritumoral vasogenic edema. Dexamethasone is the most common agent prescribed, and although the optimal dosage needs to be individualized, initial dosing of 16 mg/day in divided doses is typically used preoperatively. Improvement in edema-related neurologic signs and symptoms can begin within hours, but can take a few days to reach a maximal effect. The need for perioperative steroid use, however, must be balanced with the numerous and relatively common adverse effects, including gastritis, insomnia, weight gain, manic behavior, and hyperglycemia. Steroids can have an adverse effect on wound healing and increase the risk of postoperative infections. Patients with diabetes mellitus, in particular, require special attention. Preoperative use of corticosteroids should be avoided in patients with suspected brain lymphoma because rapid induction of lymphocytic apoptosis may render an inconclusive diagnosis. In such circumstances, steroids are often initiated in the operating room after a frozen section of biopsied tissue has been examined.

The preoperative use of steroids can significantly alter MRI findings as they can dramatically reduce the region of contrast enhancement. This steroid-induced effect is not specific and can be observed with various pathologies. Stereotactic biopsy targets, for instance, may be altered and a repeat scan the day of surgery is always prudent.

Pearl

- Preoperative use of corticosteroids should be avoided in patients with suspected brain lymphoma. In other patients, the lowest possible dexamethasone dose should be used to avoid common side effects.

■ Intraoperative Management Considerations

Surgical Planning

Surgical options include stereotactic biopsy, subtotal resection, and, in selected cases, aggressive surgical resection. The main goals of surgical resection are to safely obtain an accurate histological diagnosis, reduce tumor burden and mass effect, and improve or at least maintain the patient's neurologic status. Many factors are considered when making surgical decisions, including the patient's age, neurologic status, general medical condition, and likely diagnosis, as well as findings on imaging studies such as location, presence or absence of hydrocephalus, degree of mass effect, and extent of signal abnormality as an indicator of tumor invasion. Other important factors are prior treatments such as previous surgery, radiation, or chemotherapy, and potential wound healing issues.

Ultimately, the patient's understanding of the risks and benefits of surgery and possible alternatives is paramount. A thorough discussion with the patient and family is one of the most important steps in helping the patient make the best individualized decision and in planning future treatment. The risk of neurologic impairment with surgery must be balanced with the patient's lifestyle and wishes. A mild loss of motor control in the dominant hand may be acceptable for some patients, but not for others and this must be taken into account. In specific cases, transient postoperative neurologic impairment can be anticipated. For example, resection of tumors in the supplementary motor cortex often results in a period of paresis that can last for 2 to 3 weeks (**Fig. 9.4**). Furthermore, the anticipated risk of such an injury with surgery must also be weighed against the probability of that same problem arising if surgery is not performed. A candid presentation of the risks and benefits of treatment is necessary for informed consent and also facilitates planning of needs that may exist following surgery.

Special Consideration

- The decision on what specific type of surgical therapy is best for a particular patient is based on patient characteristics, tumor characteristics, and the patient's wishes.

Surgical Intervention

A discussion of the various surgical techniques and equipment used to facilitate brain tumor surgery is beyond the scope of this chapter. In general, brain relaxation from hyperventilation, osmotic diuretics, and cerebrospinal fluid (CSF) drainage via temporary placement of a lumbar or ventricular drain can be extremely useful for controlling intracranial pressure and avoiding unintended injury to normal brain, especially with

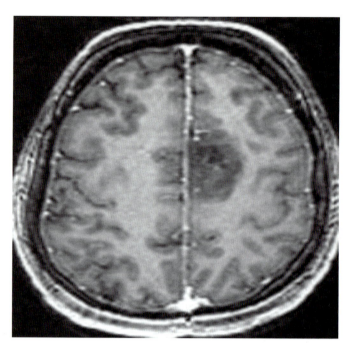

Fig. 9.4 Axial T1-weighted MRI of a glioma arising in the supplementary motor region. This patient is at risk for a superior mesenteric artery syndrome after tumor removal.

large tumors. Appropriate use requires planning and communication with the anesthesia team before surgery begins. A higher dose of dexamethasone (i.e., 10 mg) is often given in all cases except lymphoma, as well as antibiotic prophylaxis. Patient positioning is critical for gaining proper access to the tumor as well as patient safety. Sequential compression devices (SCDs) should be optimally used except on limbs with known DVTs. Patients undergoing motor or language mapping during awake craniotomy require specific attention to comfort and access so the appropriate information can be obtained.

It has become standard practice to perform a "time out" prior to the initiation of any elective neurosurgical procedure. This pause is used for verifying patient identification, marking the correct side and location for surgery, identifying potential problems, and confirming the type of operation to be performed. This checklist has gained wide acceptance as a method to reduce the potential for surgical error, and it markedly reduces the chance of wrong-site surgery. A preoperative time out is highly recommended as an effective way to improve patient safety.

Several surgical instruments and monitoring devices have been applied to tumor surgery to facilitate tumor identification, resection at the tumor margin with surrounding brain, and mapping primary motor, sensory, and language cortices.[23] Stereotactic localization by fixed-frame or frameless systems has gained wide acceptance for comparing intraoperative findings with preoperative imaging and can aid biopsy procedures. Neuronavigation, with registration of preoperative imaging, including functional and DTI information, is particularly helpful for localization in three-dimensional space, as well as for choosing the safest approach and avoiding critical neurovascular structures. Improved illumination and magnification provided by the microscope are helpful in identifying variations in color, texture, and vascularity that can distinguish tumor from brain. Additionally, intraoperative ultrasound is useful in localizing tumors obscured by the normal cortical surface, as well as deciphering obscured anatomy. The ultrasonic aspirator can be a particularly helpful instrument for actual tumor removal.

Intraoperative MRI (iMRI) is available at several major medical centers that treat large numbers of brain tumor patients (**Fig. 9.5**). This technology is expensive, but it enables the surgeon to assess the progress of the surgery, to examine the extent of resection, to address unanticipated complications, and to reregister frameless stereotactic coordinates for real-time volumetric tumor resection. It can be particularly useful during surgery for low-grade gliomas, as these tumors can be indistinguishable from normal white matter, thus limiting the surgeon's ability to identify the margins between the glioma and the brain. Following partial tumor resection, changes in anatomy can limit the reliability of preoperative stereotactic-guided images. Imaging during tumor removal will allow the surgeon to determine the location and amount of residual disease and to reregister updated stereotactic images for maximal tumor resection. The combination of stereotaxis, iMRI, and fMRI with DTI tractography provides the surgeon with detailed anatomic and functional images and the ability to plan tumor removal with real-time information that can produce better outcomes.

Fluorescence-guided surgery with 5-aminolevulinic acid for resection of malignant gliomas has also been demonstrated to increase the surgeon's ability to achieve a more aggressive tumor removal. 5-aminolevulinic acid is a nonfluorescent prodrug that leads to intracellular accumulation of fluorescent porphyrins in malignant gliomas. This can be detected through fluorescent filters attached to an operating microscope. Tumor fluorescence derived from 5-aminolevulinic acid enables more complete resections of contrast-enhancing tumor.[24]

Intraoperative neurophysiological monitoring with somatosensory evoked potentials for identification of the primary sensory cortex, rolandic sulcus, and motor cortex is commonly used for resection under general anesthesia of lesions

Pearl

- Surgical navigation or intraoperative imaging and awake craniotomy with cortical mapping, combined with standard microsurgical technique, are extremely useful tools for maximizing the effectiveness and safety of surgery for an intracranial tumor.

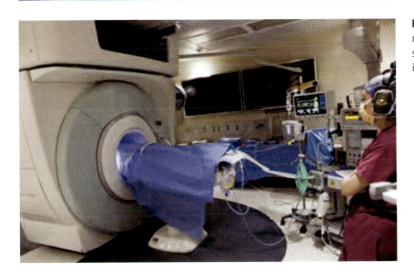

Fig. 9.5 Intraoperative 3-Tesla MRI utilized during the resection of a brain tumor. The patient is covered with a sterile drape and monitored by the anesthesiologist during imaging.

in such eloquent cortex.[23] Alternatively, direct motor stimulation can be used to confirm precise regions subserving control over hand, arm, face, and leg motor function. This monitoring can be performed with either general anesthesia or with neuroleptic agents in the absence of inhalation agents. Mapping language and other eloquent cortex requires local anesthesia and a cooperative patient who can understand the required tasks, but awake craniotomy can become very routine with good communication among team members and with the patient.[25] Careful preoperative instruction and education improves the patient's ability to provide appropriate responses needed for reliable testing. Likewise, the use of electrophysiological monitoring is also common practice for posterior fossa tumor surgery to help identify and minimize manipulation of cranial nerves.

Postoperative Management Considerations

The majority of patients who undergo an uncomplicated stereotactic biopsy for diagnosis can be monitored in the postanesthesia care unit until the anesthetic agents have dissipated and then transferred to a routine postoperative ward, or safely discharged home.[26] Patients who undergo craniotomy for tumor resection are traditionally observed at least overnight in an intensive care unit or neuro–critical care unit, although there are safe and less resource-intensive options for the management of such patients.[26] Those patients requiring longer monitoring or the presence of intracranial pressure monitoring devices or externalized lumbar or ventricular drains can remain in the critical care unit for an extended duration. Any patient with the onset of new neurologic signs and symptoms, during the immediate postoperative period, warrants immediate evaluation with imaging (typically CT scan) to rule out intracranial hemorrhage.

Surgery itself is generally well tolerated and mainly characterized by incisional pain that responds well to analgesics. Drugs that alter platelet function, such as nonsteroidal anti-inflammatory medications, should be avoided initially. The potential risk of postoperative neurologic deficits (e.g., superior mesenteric artery syndrome, increased motor/language problems) can usually be predicted based on the location of the lesion and the patient's preoperative neurologic status. In the majority of patients these problems can be transient, and recovery can be accelerated by early physical therapy and mobilization. Steroid utilization can also enhance recovery by minimizing edema, but dosing should be adjusted to the lowest dose required to improve function.

Patients with malignant primary and secondary brain tumors, as well as those with advanced age and preoperative motor deficits, are at increased risk for DVT and PE.[27] Routine use of prophylactic agents to reduce the risk of DVT is advised. Most surgeons prefer the use of low-dose heparin (5,000 U subcutaneously administered three times daily), but prophylactic low-molecular-weight heparins, such as enoxaparin, are also used.[28] Although symptomatic postoperative bleeding is relatively uncommon, it is still a reality, and judicious use of agents is advised. Subcutaneous heparin can typically be started the day after surgery. The presence of residual tumor or a particularly bloody resection with evidence of hemorrhage on postoperative MRI should be taken into consideration and may delay initiation. Nonetheless, SCDs can substantially decrease DVT risk alone and should be continued postoperatively while the patient is restricted to bed. Imaging of the deep leg veins is often performed on all immobilized patients. Compression boots should not be applied to limbs with known DVTs. Those patients with DVT or PE immediately postoperatively can be managed with insertion of an IVC filter, although anticoagulation is safe if there is no postoperative bleeding on CT. The timing of anticoagulation following surgery has not been adequately studied; however, most neurosurgeons are comfortable with its initiation or reinstitution within days of surgery if truly medically necessary. Long-term anticoagulation is generally preferable over filter placement due to thrombotic complications like IVC thrombosis that are frequently associated with the latter.

Depression is common in brain tumor patients and underrecognized by most physicians and can threaten quality of life substantially. Recognizing depression and addressing any concerns with patients should be part of the perioperative assessment, with referral to a psychiatrist or psychologist offered when needed.

Adjuvant Therapy and Follow-Up

The primary decision regarding the use of adjuvant therapies, such as radiation and chemotherapy, is largely dictated by the underlying histology. Often, however, the appropriate diagnosis of a primary brain tumor requires consideration of the clinical history and the imaging findings, as well as the morphological description of the tumor cells by the neuropathologist. In these specific cases, the history and imaging studies are critical in establishing a correct diagnosis.

Establishing the extent of tumor resection and evaluation for recurrence is best performed with serial MRIs. Surgical manipulation can induce enhancement at the resection margin, and although these postoperative changes are generally linear, and residual tumor tissue is most often nodular, the differentiation between the two can be difficult. It has been shown that surgically induced enhancement evolves over a few days, and in general this is minimal within the first 72 hours following an operation. Consequently, postoperative baseline imaging is most informative for staging when it is performed within the first 3 days after surgery. Early postoperative MRIs are also useful for newly appearing regions of ischemia. Such surgically induced infarcts may acquire contrast enhancement during the weeks after surgery and can mimic tumor progression. Perfusion-weighted imaging may also prove helpful in the assessment of brain tumors, particularly when the patient is undergoing adjuvant treatment. Foci of increased perfusion are suspicious for malignancy, whereas profoundly decreased perfusion may indicate a necrotic tumor area after irradiation.

Decisions regarding adjuvant therapy, surveillance for recurrence, and management of tumor-related issues such as

seizures and medications are best made in collaboration with a multidisciplinary tumor board that includes representation from neurosurgery, neuro-oncology, radiation oncology, neuroradiology, and neuropathology. This forum provides an opportunity for each of the related disciplines to interact in a collaborative manner with access to the pathological specimen, imaging studies, and relevant treatment history. Information from the tumor board can be collected and entered into a tumor data bank to generate longitudinal data for each patient and serve as a resource for evaluating therapies over the entire tumor patient population. In this way treating teams are able to critically evaluate management decisions.

■ Conclusion

The perioperative management of patients with brain tumors can often be challenging and requires input from multidisciplinary specialists. Careful attention can facilitate optimum decision making and help provide for the best possible outcome. Ultimately, a coordinated effort by each of the related disciplines will provide the ability to manage patients at all stages of their disease.

Pearl

- Postoperative imaging, if done to assess residual disease, should be performed within 72 hours of surgery to be most informative.

Editor's Note

Once a recommendation for surgery is proposed to a patient and accepted, a cascade of events transpires to maximize the chances of a successful surgery. For elective patients, which are the majority, most hospitals in North America and Europe use a same-day admission system in which the patient attends a preadmission clinic preoperatively and then presents to the hospital the morning of surgery, usually to have an MRI for up-to-date imaging and for use with the surgical navigation system. Medical treatment of cerebral edema, antibiotic prophylaxis, antiepileptics, and thromboembolism prophylaxis, when indicated, leads to a smooth perioperative period with fewer complications. The surgeon is central to this process, but many other members of the health care team are essential. Attention to detail is also essential postoperatively. Good pre-, intra-, and postoperative care are essential ingredients for as smooth a course as possible for the neuro-oncology patient. Answering patients questions and as full as possible disclosure of information about the entire process are also essential for improved patient satisfaction.[29,30] (Bernstein)

References

1. Byrne TPJ, Yoshida D. Imaging and clinical features of gliomas. In: Tindall G, Cooper P, Barrow D, eds. The Practice of Neurosurgery. Baltimore: Williams & Wilkins, 1995:637–648
2. Chang SM, Parney IF, Huang W, et al; Glioma Outcomes Project Investigators. Patterns of care for adults with newly diagnosed malignant glioma. JAMA 2005;293:557–564
3. Fransen P, de Tribolet N. Surgery of supratentorial tumors. Curr Opin Oncol 1993;5:450–457
4. Taphoorn MJ, Klein M. Cognitive deficits in adult patients with brain tumours. Lancet Neurol 2004;3:159–168
5. Cohen-Gadol AA, Westerveld M, Alvarez-Carilles J, Spencer DD. Intracarotid Amytal memory test and hippocampal magnetic resonance imaging volumetry: validity of the Wada test as an indicator of hippocampal integrity among candidates for epilepsy surgery. J Neurosurg 2004;101:926–931
6. Cohen-Gadol AA, DiLuna ML, Bannykh SI, Piepmeier JM, Spencer DD. Non-enhancing de novo glioblastoma: report of two cases. Neurosurg Rev 2004;27:281–285
7. Chaichana KL, McGirt MJ, Niranjan A, Olivi A, Burger PC, Quinones-Hinojosa A. Prognostic significance of contrast-enhancing low-grade gliomas in adults and a review of the literature. Neurol Res 2009; 31:931–939
8. Barker FG II, Chang SM, Huhn SL, et al. Age and the risk of anaplasia in magnetic resonance-nonenhancing supratentorial cerebral tumors. Cancer 1997;80:936–941
9. Megyesi JF, Kachur E, Lee DH, et al. Imaging correlates of molecular signatures in oligodendrogliomas. Clin Cancer Res 2004;10:4303–4306
10. Zlatescu MC, Tehrani-Yazdi A, Sasaki H, et al. Tumor location and growth pattern correlate with genetic signature in oligodendroglial neoplasms. Cancer Res 2001;61:6713–6715
11. Aghi M, Gaviani P, Henson JW, Batchelor TT, Louis DN, Barker FG II. Magnetic resonance imaging characteristics predict epidermal growth factor receptor amplification status in glioblastoma. Clin Cancer Res 2005;11(24 Pt 1):8600–8605
12. Baehring JM, Bi WL, Bannykh S, Piepmeier JM, Fulbright RK. Diffusion MRI in the early diagnosis of malignant glioma. J Neurooncol 2007;82: 221–225
13. Moffat BA, Chenevert TL, Lawrence TS, et al. Functional diffusion map: a noninvasive MRI biomarker for early stratification of clinical brain tumor response. Proc Natl Acad Sci U S A 2005;102:5524–5529
14. Roessler K, Donat M, Lanzenberger R, et al. Evaluation of preoperative high magnetic field motor functional MRI (3 Tesla) in glioma patients by navigated electrocortical stimulation and postoperative outcome. J Neurol Neurosurg Psychiatry 2005;76:1152–1157
15. Jena R, Price SJ, Baker C, et al. Diffusion tensor imaging: possible implications for radiotherapy treatment planning of patients with high-grade glioma. Clin Oncol (R Coll Radiol) 2005;17:581–590
16. Olsen KI, Schroeder P, Corby R, Vucic I, Bardo DM. Advanced magnetic resonance imaging techniques to evaluate CNS glioma. Expert Rev Neurother 2005;5(6, Suppl)S3–S11
17. Preul MC, Caramanos Z, Leblanc R, Villemure JG, Arnold DL. Using pattern analysis of in vivo proton MRSI data to improve the diagnosis and surgical management of patients with brain tumors. NMR Biomed 1998;11:192–200
18. Stadlbauer A, Moser E, Gruber S, et al. Improved delineation of brain tumors: an automated method for segmentation based on pathologic changes of 1H-MRSI metabolites in gliomas. Neuroimage 2004;23: 454–461
19. Vos MJ, Berkhof J, Postma TJ, Hoekstra OS, Barkhof F, Heimans JJ. Thallium-201 SPECT: the optimal prediction of response in glioma therapy. Eur J Nucl Med Mol Imaging 2006;33:222–227
20. Jacobs AH, Kracht LW, Gossmann A, et al. Imaging in neurooncology. NeuroRx 2005;2:333–347
21. Wu AS, Trinh VT, Suki D, et al. A prospective randomized trial of perioperative seizure prophylaxis in patients with intraparenchymal brain tumors. J Neurosurg 2013;118:873–883
22. Glantz MJ, Cole BF, Forsyth PA, et al; Report of the Quality Standards Subcommittee of the American Academy of Neurology. Practice parameter: anticonvulsant prophylaxis in patients with newly diagnosed brain tumors. Neurology 2000;54:1886–1893
23. Duffau H, Lopes M, Arthuis F, et al. Contribution of intraoperative electrical stimulations in surgery of low grade gliomas: a comparative study between two series without (1985-96) and with (1996-2003) functional mapping in the same institution. J Neurol Neurosurg Psychiatry 2005;76:845–851
24. Stummer W, Pichlmeier U, Meinel T, Wiestler OD, Zanella F, Reulen HJ; ALA-Glioma Study Group. Fluorescence-guided surgery with 5-aminolevulinic acid for resection of malignant glioma: a randomised controlled multicentre phase III trial. Lancet Oncol 2006;7:392–401
25. Serletis D, Bernstein M. Prospective study of awake craniotomy used routinely and nonselectively for supratentorial tumors. J Neurosurg 2007;107:1–6
26. Boulton M, Bernstein M. Outpatient brain tumor surgery: innovation in surgical neurooncology. J Neurosurg 2008;108:649–654
27. Chaichana KL, Pendleton C, Jackson C, et al. Deep venous thrombosis and pulmonary embolisms in adult patients undergoing craniotomy for brain tumors. Neurol Res 2013;35:206–211
28. Agnelli G, Piovella F, Buoncristiani P, et al. Enoxaparin plus compression stockings compared with compression stockings alone in the prevention of venous thromboembolism after elective neurosurgery. N Engl J Med 1998;339:80–85
29. Knifed E, July J, Bernstein M. Neurosurgery patients' feelings about the role of residents in their care: a qualitative case study. J Neurosurg 2008;108:287–291
30. Zener R, Bernstein M. Gender, patient comfort and the neurosurgical operating room. Can J Neurol Sci 2011;38:65–71

10 Imaged-Guided Surgery: Frame and Frameless

Michael W. McDermott, Roxanna M. Garcia, and Mark Bernstein

The development of image-guided techniques over the last 25 years has seen the progression from computed tomography (CT) frame-based stereotactic biopsy, to frameless image-guided surgical systems, to intraoperative real-time magnetic resonance imaging (MRI).

■ Stereotactic Brain Lesion Biopsy

Indications

Even with advances in modern brain imaging, optimal treatment still requires tissue diagnosis prior to recommending therapy in many cases. In certain situations one may entertain the possibility of forgoing biopsy particularly for the very elderly or medically infirm and initiate treatment based on imaging diagnosis. Other example situations include radiosurgery for vestibular schwannoma and metastases based on the fact that the differential diagnosis of such lesions is so narrow.

However, it is important to recognize that there is a substantial rate of unsuspected clinically significant diagnoses to be made when lesions are biopsied. This may be as high as 12 to 26% in some series, and includes pathologies such as multicentric glioma, infarct, infection, inflammation, benign cyst, and demyelination.[1,2] However, modern MRI techniques have now eliminated many of these surprising pathologies with the use of magnetic resonance spectroscopy (MRS), diffusion-weighted imaging, and regional or localized blood volume mapping.[3–5] Today, the biopsy of basal ganglia infarcts, demyelinating periventricular plaques, and encephalitis should be an extremely rare event.

The ideal lesion for stereotactic biopsy as opposed to craniotomy is a small, deep, contrast-enhancing lesion or one located in eloquent cortex for which the risk of craniotomy and excisional biopsy is felt to be too high (**Fig. 10.1**).

Considerations for Stereotactic Biopsy

- Lesion
  - Deep
  - Small
  - Eloquent location
  - Multiple lesions
  - Diffuse
- Patient
  - Too ill
  - Too old
  - Too well
  - Patient preference

Multifocal lesions, lesions that do not fit the clinical picture, and lesions that are diffuse are also suited to stereotactic biopsy. Contrast-enhancing lesions after intense focal therapies may create a diagnostic dilemma. Whether the image abnormality represents a treatment effect or recurrent tumor, stereotactic biopsy may be necessary to confirm or refute recurrent tumor and help direct subsequent therapies.

Although many clinicians would regard eloquent brain location such as primary motor cortex as a good indication for stereotactic biopsy, a surgeon should proceed in these situations with caution. Frequently, patients with mild neurologic deficit with lesions in eloquent cortex may experience a significant transient worsening of their neurologic condition even with small-core biopsies in the absence of a documented postoperative hemorrhage. For lesions in motor speech and primary motor cortex, open awake craniotomy with functional localization of tissue before cortical incision and biopsy remains an excellent treatment option.[6]

In the late 1980s and early 1990s, stereotactic biopsy had a significant role to play in the management of patients with human immunodeficiency virus (HIV) infection and AIDS.[7] Subsequently, patients with multiple contrast-enhancing lesions in the setting of HIV infection were prescribed empiric

---

Special Consideration

- It is good practice for a surgeon to review the diagnostic imaging with a neuroradiologist to confirm clinical impressions before proceeding with a surgical procedure.

Pearl

- After prior focal radiotherapy, biopsy may be necessary before proceeding with additional treatment to distinguish recurrent tumor from radiation necrosis.

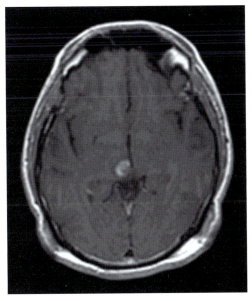
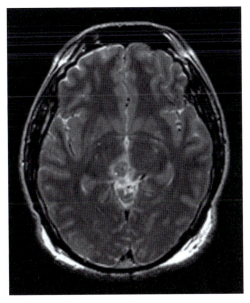

a   b

Fig. 10.1a,b (**a**) T1-weighted postcontrast MRI of a right thalamic tumor selected for frame-based stereotactic biopsy. Spinal imaging, cytology, serum, and cerebrospinal fluid (CSF) markers were nondiagnostic. (**b**) T2-weighted sequence showing low signal intensity of the core lesion, suggesting a high nuclear-to-cytoplasmic ratio. Two core biopsies were taken. The final diagnosis based on permanent section was germinoma.

Pitfall

- Dramatic reduction in the size of a contrast-enhancing lesion after steroids should raise consideration of the diagnosis of lymphoma. Biopsy in such settings will frequently result in nondiagnostic tissue.

antitoxoplasmosis therapy. Now this central nervous system (CNS) infection is a rare event, and stereotactic biopsy may be more important than empiric therapy. Lymphoma, bacterial infections, and progressive multifocal leukoencephalopathy remain other diagnostic considerations in this population. Care must be taken when previously obvious contrast-enhancing lesions are less intense after short courses of steroid medications, which may represent the early response of a lymphoma to steroids. Stereotactic biopsy in this setting is frequently nondiagnostic and reveals only the ghosts of cell membranes, requiring that steroid therapy be stopped and the patient observed until the lesions reappear and biopsy can be reconsidered (**Fig. 10.2**). One must keep in mind the high rate of complications in performing stereotactic biopsies in the HIV population, presumably related to their viral angiopathy.

General Technique of Stereotactic Biopsy

Stereotactic biopsy can currently be performed using frame-based technologies, image-guided surgical systems, or intra-operative MRI, and it is effectively done under local anesthesia with intravenous sedation. Operative times vary according to the technology used (**Table 10.1**).[8–11] The selection of anesthetic technique may affect the time to discharge and the health care costs associated with the procedure.

For frame-based procedures, the surgeon applies the frame with local anesthesia using four pins on posts. If there is a prominent skull defect, three-point fixation may be used. Positioning of the frame may be done with Velcro straps, manual handheld positioning, or the supplied ear bars, depending on the frame-based system to be used. The skin may be marked along the trajectory of the fixation pins, the frame temporarily removed, and then the scalp pin sites injected with a combination of Xylocaine (AstraZeneca, Westborough, MA) with epinephrine. Usually 1 to 2 cc at each pin site is adequate. The pins are then tightened manually using the thumb and index finger to the point where they cannot be tightened any further, and then a wrench is used. A torque wrench may be used to avoid overtightening and bending the frame.

Following frame application, the patient is taken to the imaging department where either CT or, more commonly now, MRI is done. Fiducial as well as target coordinates are then derived in the same axial imaging plane, and an entry point can be selected on coronal reconstructions to avoid structures such as the ventricle. Most biopsy needles have a side port opening of 9 to 10 mm in length and 1.2 mm in diameter. The target should be selected by placing the center of the biopsy needle port opening as close to the center of the target as possible or in the maximally enhancing area. For smaller di-

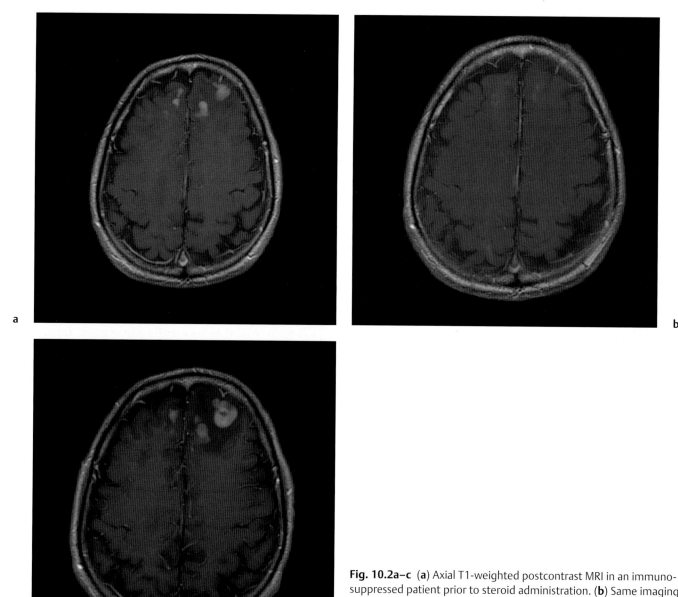

a

b

c

Fig. 10.2a–c (a) Axial T1-weighted postcontrast MRI in an immuno-suppressed patient prior to steroid administration. (b) Same imaging 5 days after starting steroids. The nonsurgical workup was negative for diagnosis. The planned biopsy was deferred. (c) Same imaging 14 days after discontinuation of steroids. Image directed an open bur hole biopsy confirmed the diagnosis of lymphoma.

ameter lesions, the tip of the biopsy needle should not extend past the deepest part of the lesion. If the first sample is non-diagnostic on frozen section, the depth can be advanced or shortened 2 to 3 mm in a sequential manner with the same trajectory.

In the operating room the surgeon uses either a twist drill or bur hole depending on whether the entry point is in hair-bearing or non–hair-bearing scalp and on personal preference. If a twist drill hole is performed, the dura can be opened by overdrilling by a few millimeters or with successively larger sizes of Kirschner wires (K-wires), so that the stereotactic bi-opsy needle can be passed through the dura without diffi-

culty. In both twist drill and bur hole situations, the standard brain biopsy needle with the side-cutting port is advanced to the target position. The needle is advanced with the side-cut-ting port closed and then opened at the target position to apply gentle suction, drawing tissue into the opening. While still applying gentle suction, the needle opening is closed by rotating the inner cannula 180 degrees. The entire needle, inner and outer cannula included, can then be gently rotated 360 degrees at the target position to ensure there is no resis-tance. If resistance is encountered, the needle may be opened briefly and then closed and rotated again to ensure it is free before removal. Surgeon preference will dictate whether the

Table 10.1 Comparisons of Operative Times for Frame-Based, Frameless, and Intraoperative MRI (iMRI) Biopsies

Authors	Year	System	Operative Time
Bernays et al[9]	2002	iMRI (low field)	73 minutes** (range 27–119)
Smith et al[8]	2005	Frame Frameless	114 ± 3 minutes* 185 ± 6 minutes*
Quinn et al[10]	2011	iMRI (low filed)	102 minutes*
Bekelis et al[11]	2012	Frameless (robotic)	44.6 minutes*

*Mean time.
**Median time.

inner cannula only is removed or whether the entire biopsy needle is removed for each sample obtained. Intraoperative frozen section examination of tissue is performed to ensure that sufficient pathological tissue has been obtained. The risk of hemorrhage rises with each biopsy sample taken.

Postoperative Management

Postoperatively, patients are monitored in a recovery room setting for a period of time until they return to their base neurologic status. In one study the clinical and economic consequences of early discharge of patients following supratentorial stereotactic brain biopsy was evaluated.[12] A total of 130 biopsies were performed and patient discharge status was defined as early discharge (< 8 hours) extended outpatient observation (≥ 8 eight hours but < 24 hours), and in-patient hospitalization (≥ 24 hours). All complications, of which five were serious, occurred within 6 hours after surgery. Intraoperative bleeding occurred in 12 patients (9.2%), but in only 40% of these cases did hemorrhage appear on postoperative CT scans. The authors concluded that early discharge of patients following stereotactic biopsy was safe in the absence of excessive intraoperative bleeding, development of new postoperative deficits, or demonstrated blood clot formation on a postoperative CT scan.

One group has prospectively assessed the feasibility of outpatient surgery, that is, discharge home 4 to 6 hours after stereotactic biopsy.[13,14] The authors started doing stereotactic biopsy on an outpatient basis in 1997, and published their pilot data in 2002 and an update in 2011. A total of 152 patients were in the intent-to-treat group and 94.1% were successfully discharged home without readmission. In the 5.9% protocol failure group two neurologic complications occurred (2.6%), and neither of these patients had hemorrhage on post-biopsy CT scans. The authors concluded that discharging patients home after 4 to 6 hours of observation and CT following stereotactic biopsy seemed to be safe and was expected to result in a savings of health care resources and costs, with a potential improvement in patient satisfaction and decreased complications because of the shorter hospital stay.

Controversy

• Stereotactic tumor biopsy can safely be done on an outpatient basis.

Complications

Although it is easy for neurosurgeons, and even for other physicians, to think of stereotactic biopsy as a simple minimally invasive procedure, one should resist this temptation. A thorough knowledge of the anatomy and of the trajectories to the target is necessary to avoid both intraoperative patient discomfort and postoperative disability. Should complications arise in the postoperative period, early recognition and treatment are necessary to maintain good patient outcomes. A comprehensive knowledge of these complications is essential to allow for their proper avoidance as well as informed discussion with the patient prior to the procedure.

Hemorrhage at the biopsy site, causing acute deterioration and new neurologic deficits, is the most feared complication of stereotactic brain biopsy. The incidence of neurologic morbidity and mortality, mostly due to hemorrhage, ranges from 0 to 5% in larger series (**Table 10.2**).[11][20] Clinically silent hemorrhage after stereotactic biopsy is very common. On CT scans obtained in 102 patients who underwent stereotactic biopsy, 59% of the scans exhibited hemorrhages.[21] In only six of the 61 patients were there clinical signs to suggest the patient may have suffered a hemorrhage, whereas in the remaining 55 the hemorrhage was clinically silent and unsuspected. The clinically silent hemorrhages ranged in size from less than 5 mm to between 30 and 40 mm. Of the 55 patients with clinically silent hemorrhages, only three demonstrated a new neurologic deficit, and all these occurred within 2 days of the procedure. All the patients with no hemorrhage on postoperative scans remained neurologically well and experienced no delayed deterioration. In a more recent series, hematoma at the biopsy site was seen in only 9% of patients, of whom four were symptomatic.[16] High-grade glioma was a risk factor for hematoma at the biopsy site but was not associated with a significant increase in morbidity.

All necessary steps should be taken preoperatively to help avoid hemorrhage, beginning with proper patient screening and obtaining a full hematological and coagulation profile when indicated. Patients are counseled to avoid nonsteroidal anti-inflammatories for 10 days prior to the planned procedure. Care should be taken to avoid targeting lesions in areas

Special Consideration

• If hemorrhage occurs during biopsy, it is best to leave the needle in place with the side port open so that blood can escape through the needle.

Table 10.2 Complication Rates in Recent Biopsy Series

Author	Year	No.	System	Mortality	Morbidity	Nondiagnostic Rate
Smith et al[8]	2005	213	FB	0.4%	4%	10%
McGirt et al[16]	2005	270	FB	1%	5%	7%
Woodworth et al[17]	2006	270	FL	1%	4%	10%
Kongkham et al[18]	2008	622	FB	1.3%	6.9%	1.6%
Shooman et al[24]	2010	134	FL	1.5%	2.2%	0.7%
Amin et al[19]	2011	48	FL	0%	4.1%	2%
Quinn et al[10]	2011	33	FL	0%	0%	3%
Bekelis et al[11]	2012	44	FL	0%	8%	4%
Ersahin et al[20]	2011	290	FB	0.8%	4.1%	4.5%

Abbreviations: FB, frame based; FL, frameless.

close to large arteries or veins such as the pineal region or perisylvian region, and superficial lesions near the pia-arachnoid. Avoidance of intraoperative complications calls for careful surgical technique while passing the needle to the biopsy site and taking the minimum number of samples necessary to satisfactorily obtain diagnostic tissue. If bleeding is encountered after the first biopsy, the first step is to leave the biopsy instrument in place with the side port open so that blood may exit through the needle. In patients who deteriorate neurologically in the operating room, the surgical team must be prepared to remove the stereotactic head frame rapidly should endotracheal intubation be necessary.

Postoperative management of suspected intraoperative bleeding involves close monitoring of the patient and then an early CT scan. If the patient's condition deteriorates quickly, emergency craniotomy may be required for more superficial lesions, whereas deep basal ganglia lesions may be managed with medical measures. In some cases, endoscopic or repeat stereotactic aspiration of hematomas may be of benefit. In certain cases in which the biopsy has shown a malignant neoplasm in an elderly patient who has developed a severe neurologic deficit due to a biopsy-induced hemorrhage, it may be appropriate after a thorough discussion with the patient's family to forgo craniotomy and provide only comfort measures. It is important to have such discussions with the patient and family prior to the procedure to determine their wishes.

Failed (Nondiagnostic) Biopsy

In most large clinical series, stereotactic biopsy results in nondiagnostic tissue sampling in less than 10% of cases.[17,22] Nondiagnostic tissue samples may be associated with nonneoplastic or nonenhancing lesions. Patients on prior steroid medications whose lesions are small at the time of stereotactic imaging may have lymphoma, which is extremely sensitive to steroid medications. Biopsy in this setting usually results in only necrotic tissue being obtained. Failed biopsies are more frequently associated with increased complications and failure to conduct an intraoperative pathological examination.

Pitfall

- Failure to use intraoperative frozen section will result in a higher rate of nondiagnostic biopsy.

The management of the failed biopsy begins in the operating room, where intraoperative examination of tissues is mandatory to ensure that diagnostic tissue is in fact obtained. Repeated sampling may increase the diagnostic yield, and the window of the side-cut needle can be changed in its orientation among 0, 90, 180, and 270 degrees for each sample. As well, the depth of the sampling point within the target lesion can be modified. If diagnostic tissue is not obtained, all parameters and measurements must be rechecked to ensure accurate localization, and then a repeat biopsy sample can be sent. If repeated samples do not provide diagnostic tissue, then the surgeon must weigh the risk of further attempts. Sending tissue for microbiological analysis as well as pathology must be considered for lesions that may be inflammatory or infectious.

Postoperatively an immediate CT scan can help localize the biopsy site, usually marked by a drop of air or blood to ensure that the appropriate location was sampled. With the use of image-guided systems, screen saves of the needle at the target position can be used as a record of correct target localization. If a final pathological examination is still not diagnostic, then the options include repeat biopsy, open biopsy, or empiric therapy.

Sampling Error

Stereotactic biopsy specimens provide tissues representative of only a small portion of the lesion. Frequently the target selected is based on static postcontrast MRI or CT, which may not be the best predictor of the most metabolically active component of a tumor. It is known that malignant gliomas have a great deal of heterogeneity within their volume, and surgeons must intentionally avoid areas of suspected non-enhancing necrotic tissue in selecting their target and avoiding cystic areas. In the latter case, draining the cyst first may change the morphology of the lesion before tissue is obtained, altering the intended target for sampling. With modern magnetic resonance (MR) techniques, MRS can help localize the area of greatest abnormality; MR perfusion techniques may have similar value in this regard.[3,5,23] In 29 patients with brain tumors who underwent high-resolution three-dimensional (3D) MRS before undergoing surgery, biopsies obtained at locations referenced on MRI were compared with MR spectral voxels centered on each of 79 biopsy locations, and metabolic levels were correlated with histological examinations of each specimen.[4] Elevated normalized choline ratios and low normalized *N*-acetylaspartase ratios were associated with viable tumor 90% of the time. Such spectroscopic information can be used particularly for low-grade, nonenhancing lesions to more accurately direct the biopsy target to the most abnormal area with elevated choline levels.

The question of whether intraoperative frozen section analysis should routinely be done has been addressed. Using one to three specimens from a single trajectory, 99.3% of biopsies done using a frameless system were diagnostic.[24] The single nondiagnostic case was a registration-trajectory error based on postoperative imaging. The authors estimated that not doing routine intraoperative neuropathology would save 67 hours of operating time for their 134 patients and over $100,000 in hospital costs. In addition, intraoperative frozen section would not have increased the diagnostic yield. Another option for future consideration is the use of fluorescent agents such as 5-aminolevulinic acid (5-ALA). Two cases were reported where biopsy specimens were evaluated under violet-blue light in the operating room, confirming fluorescence and pathological tissue.[25] However, these patients also require a low light environment for 72 hours after the administration of 5-ALA that may complicate postoperative management.

Specific Technical Considerations of Stereotactic Biopsy

Frame-Based Versus "Frameless" Systems

Currently both frame-based and image-guided (i.e., frameless stereotactic) systems are available for point localization and stereotactic biopsy. Although several types of frames have been used in the past, currently the most popular are the Leksell Stereotactic System (Elekta, Stockholm, Sweden) and the Cosman-Robert Wells (CRW) System (Integra Radionics, Burlington, MA). Both of these systems are target-centered devices that have two degrees of rotational freedom to allow adjustment of the entry point and trajectory to the target position. Both require imaging with a nine-rod fiducial localizing system applicable to both MRI and CT techniques.

Frameless stereotactic biopsies have been accomplished with several different navigational systems, and both articulated arm trajectory guides as well as skull-mounted trajectory guides can be used. Experience with 125 consecutive cases of stereotactic biopsy was reported using an infrared light–emitting diode navigational system and a stereotactic biopsy trajectory guide held over the entry point by a surgical arm mounted to the Mayfield Skull Clamp (Integra, Plainsboro, NJ).[1] Eighty-six procedures were MRI based and 39 were CT based. The mean diameter of biopsy lesions was 36 mm, and diagnostic tissue was obtained in 97.6% of cases. The mean operative time was 1.5 hours, and an average of six specimens was obtained for each procedure. Nondiagnostic tissue or "failed" biopsies occurred in three cases (2.4%). In 218 biopsies in 213 patients using either a sonic or optical digitizer and scalp-applied fiducial markers, 6.3% of biopsy specimens were diagnostic for lesions that had an average minimum dimension of 27.7 mm (range 5.4–62.7 mm).[26] There were five intracerebral hemorrhages, two of which required craniotomy.

Comparisons of frame-based and frameless stereotactic biopsy for single institutions have been reported. Data were collected on 213 consecutive stereotactic biopsies, 139 of which were frame-based and 74 frameless.[8] There were no significant differences between the frame-based and the frameless groups with regard to patient demographics, histopathology, nondiagnostic biopsy, and incidence of complications. General anesthesia was used for 6% of frame-based procedures and 95% of frameless biopsy cases. Frame-based biopsies required significantly less operating room time than frameless procedures (114 vs 185 minutes, $p < 0.0001$). Biopsy samples were nondiagnostic in 10% of the cases using either technique. There was no significant difference with regard to incidence of complications between frame-based and frameless biopsy groups. The authors concluded that frame-based stereotactic biopsy required significantly less anesthesia and less operating room time, and could still be considered a reasonable first approach for the surgical method to obtain a biopsy.

In another study a consecutive series of 110 frameless and 160 frame-based biopsies was evaluated.[17] The diagnostic yield was equivalent using both technologies, and complications, both transient and permanent, were equivalent. Symptomatic biopsy-site hemorrhage occurred with equal incidence in both techniques (4% frameless, 3% frame-based). Smaller and deep-seated lesions together were risk factors for nondiagnostic tissue biopsy. The authors concluded that the frameless technique for biopsy was comparable to frame-based procedures in terms of diagnostic yield and overall morbidity, but might allow for more efficient pathological diagnosis in cortical lesions. Of note, biopsies of brainstem lesions occurred without increased morbidity using image-guided stereotactic systems. Although this information provides support for both methods, to date there has been no prospective randomized trial of frame-based versus frameless techniques with regard to health care resource utilization, cost, safety, and patient satisfaction. Surgeons are encouraged to use the system with which they have the most experience, and to seek appropriate training prior to the use of new technologies. Over the last several years the trend in training residents and clinical practice has been to move away from frame-based systems.

Computed Tomographic versus Magnetic Resonance Localization

In modern-day neurosurgery, MRI is most often used for target localization. However, static magnetic-field distortions may influence the accuracy of target localization for biopsy. Appropriate quality assurance checks of field distortion should be done on every MRI unit before the system is used for stereotactic biopsy. A comparison of MR and CT coordinates found an overall discrepancy of about 2 mm that did not correlate with MR field strength.[27] For MR techniques, slice thickness, interscan spacing, phase encoding for image acquisition, and the imaging sequence are variables that can contribute to reduced accuracy. Some imaging sequences used for volumetric studies (spoiled gradient recall [SPGR]) may show less contrast enhancement than standard T1 sequences. Computed tomography imaging is not subject to such distortions, but it yields less eloquent anatomic detail of the target position. In addition, functional and metabolic studies cannot be acquired and superimposed on the image data to be used for biopsy with CT technologies.

Twist Drill Versus Bur Hole Skull Penetration

There is no evidence indicating superiority of one method over another. Typically in hair-bearing scalp, a bur hole provides better exposure of the cortical surface, allowing the surgeon to avoid superficial veins. In non–hair-bearing scalp, twist drill penetration may be preferred for cosmetic reasons. One factor to consider with twist drill methods is the angle of contact with the twist drill and the skull during penetration. Frameless systems allow for more options of patient positioning and trajectories that may avoid this problem. The surgeon must be careful not to apply too much pressure to the drill bit before the outer table is scored and penetrated by the lead edge of the bit. Otherwise, the drill bit may creep down the

skull before fully penetrating the outer table of the skull, which affects the final trajectory. The method of skull penetration is best left to surgeon preference.

Brainstem and Posterior Fossa Biopsy

Technical options for brainstem or posterior fossa biopsy include either a supratentorial trajectory or a transcerebellar infratentorial trajectory. The supratentorial trajectory may begin just in front of the coronal suture 3 to 4 cm lateral to the midline in order to avoid the ventricular system. Current planning software allows the surgeon to define the target as well as entry point, and then follow the course of the proposed trajectory through the depth of the brain along the trajectory path. For posterior fossa biopsies, brainstem lesions in the middle and upper pons can be accessed via a transcerebellar middle peduncle approach. When using frameless systems for biopsies in the posterior half of the cranium, scalp-based fiducial registration is used. Care must be taken during the registration to observe for shift of skin surface features and fiducials when the patient is positioned with the head rotated more than 90 degrees past the upright vertical. When biopsies are performed under local anesthesia with monitored anesthesia care, both the surgeon and the anesthesiologist should be aware of the lateral position of the descending trigeminal spinal tract, which may cause excruciating facial pain if this tract is disturbed by the needle trajectory.

Twist drill holes for posterior fossa biopsies limit the amount of muscle dissection and reduce the risk of air embolism. When a bur hole is made, the patient may be positioned prone and soft tissue closed over the bur hole site before proceeding with the stereotactic biopsy with the patient in the semi-sitting position. In one series with 13 frame-based transcerebellar brainstem biopsies, one patient experienced intraoperative air embolism after the placing of a suboccipital bur hole.[28] The patient then underwent successful transfrontal biopsy in the supine position without requiring replacement of the head frame. This was the only intraoperative complication in a series of 14 stereotactic procedures in 13 patients. One patient (8%) had a nondiagnostic tissue sample. Only five of the 12 diagnoses were consistent with what was predicted from preoperative MR images or CT scans. The diagnoses were glioma in five patients, metastasis in three, lymphoma in two, encephalitis in one, and inflammatory nonneoplastic gliosis in one. There was one new permanent neurologic deficit with sixth nerve palsy in a patient who had biopsy of a pontine mass, and this occurred just after passage of the needle into the pons. A postoperative CT scan did not reveal any hemorrhage.

Accuracy of Frame-Based Versus Frameless Stereotactic Techniques

Clinical studies have shown the utility of frameless stereotactic images achieving similar diagnostic rates as frame-based systems from the past. Complications rates are the same. There are differences in operating room time setup and usage for the two techniques. In an evaluation of the accuracy of frameless and frame-based localization in a skull model system using MRI, a light-emitting diode (LED) frameless stereotactic system using a skull-mounted trajectory guide was compared with an MR CRW localization system.[29] A mean localization error in the anteroposterior, lateral, and vertical planes were measured for both methods. Target vector errors were defined as the square root of the sum of the squares for the offset errors in all three planes and were not significantly different between the two methods of localization. Thus, there is evidence from both in vitro bench testing as well as from the clinic that these methods of stereotactic localization and biopsy have comparable accuracies.

◼ Image-Guided Craniotomy

Over the past two decades, surgical navigation systems have become a standard part of the operating room environment. The number of commercial vendors has been pared down, and the most common systems currently used involve LED systems using charge-coupled devices and magnetic field localizers. Although a variety of terms have been used to describe these individual technologies, all have in common the implementation of preoperative two-dimensional (2D) and 3D imaging information about normal and pathological anatomy of the brain that assists the surgeon in performing a more exact, efficient, and technically complete operation. None of these technologies is yet a replacement for the surgeon's knowledge of neuroanatomy, experience, skill, and intraoperative decision making, but rather is an adjunct to improve neurosurgery for both experienced surgeons and those starting out.

There are numerous potential sources of error at many steps, from preoperative imaging through registration, and intraoperative events when using surgical navigation systems.[30] System or mechanical accuracy refers to the precision with which the surgical navigation system (SNS) pointing device can bring its tip to a given point in stereotactic space as measured in a laboratory-type setting. Application accuracy refers to the precision with which the same device can bring its tip to a given point in anatomic space that corresponds to a point in imaging space. With respect to point localization, most systems have millimetric levels of application accuracy. Once the operation begins, however, the accuracy of this localization degrades in relation to a brain shift from tumor removal or cerebrospinal fluid (CSF) removal.[31] The greatest degree of displacement is in the direction of gravity, and tissue distortion tends to be maximum at the surface.[32] Surgeons should be aware that as the operation proceeds, the accuracy of the localization of anatomic structures degrades. The role of intraoperative imaging to perform re-registration is now being used in centers that have intraoperative MRI.

Table 10.3 Standard Fiducial Set for Imaging to Physical Space Registration

Position-Side	Number
Forehead: left, right center	3
Bregma, lambda	2
Mastoid tip: left, right	2
Parietal eminence: left, right	2
TOTAL	9

Preoperative Preparation

The decision to use surgical navigation systems for elective or urgent procedures is usually straightforward. In emergency situations such as trauma, these systems are not necessary and MR is usually not indicated. For adult patients who will be having elective image-guided surgical procedures, imaging may be done several days prior to the planned procedure with or without skin fiducials. In the past, skin surface markers were attached for the purpose of the registration, but now these are not necessary with surface-matching techniques, some of which rely on touch point and dragging techniques with a digitized probe, and others of which use infrared scanning instruments.

Whenever the patient is going to be positioned prone or three-quarter prone, skin-based fiducials are required because the face features are not available for tracer and surface registration. The standard fiducial image set includes a total of nine fiducials as listed in **Table 10.3**. The standardization of position has allowed radiology technicians to shave small patches of hair for placing fiducials at the vertex, parietal eminences, mastoid tip, as well as other non–hair-bearing sites. The skin visible through the center of each donut-shaped fiducial is marked with an indelible pen in case they come off prior to surgery. Placing fiducials over the medial two thirds of the occipital scalp should be avoided because supine positioning for imaging always deforms this area.

Fixation pins should be placed as far away from fiducials as possible to avoid stretching or deforming the skin adjacent to the fiducials and causing displacement from its image site. This would degrade the registration set and the accuracy of the anatomic localization. Reference LED or passive reflecting sets are usually attached to the skull fixation headrest to one side of the head or the other. The reference arc is usually

Pearl

- Surgical navigation systems are invaluable adjuncts for craniotomy for tumor—to locate the surface projection of the tumor and the resulting smallest scalp incision, to access it (usually linear), to locate and therefore avoid dural venous sinuses, and for other features.

brought out on the side opposite to which the scrub nurse is standing. The reference system should not be placed so as to interfere with the surgeon's movement or obstruct the line of sight. Hair removal and covering the eyes should be deferred until after the registration process is complete.

Imaging: Types and Physiological Data Overlay

The selection of imaging is crucial to providing the best information about the intracranial lesion to be approached. Decisions about the best type of imaging depend on whether or not the tumor is intra-axial, low or high grade, or extra-axial. For example, well-circumscribed, low-grade, superficial gliomas are best seen on T2-type fast spin echo (FSE) imaging as

opposed to T1 imaging. CT imaging may also be used and is best suited for skull-base lesions such as chordomas and chondrosarcomas. In this setting, both passive pointers and endoscopes that have been registered as objects can be used as the pointing device.

Although current software allows co-registration of two simultaneously obtained images (such as T1 and T2), usually only one set of images can be viewed at a time. Newer software platforms allow the viewing of magnetic resonance angiography (MRA) and magnetic resonance venography (MRV) images, which can be integrated into the 3D model and peeled away from the skin surface toward the center of the brain using the software application.

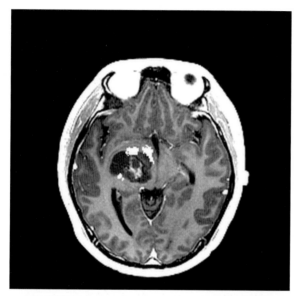

a

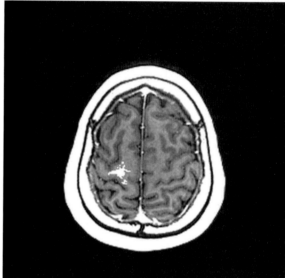

b

c

Fig. 10.3a–c (**a**) Axial T1-weighted postcontrast MRI of a pilocytic astrocytoma of basal ganglia with motor fibers seen on both the anterior and posterior aspects of the tumor cyst. (**b**) Axial image from the same study showing motor fiber projections to the primary motor cortex. (**c**) Axial image from the same patient 1 year after image-guided resection using catheter insertion through the middle temporal gyrus as a guide to cyst. No new deficit was found, and motor function improved after the total resection of the tumor.

Functional imaging data can now be overlaid fairly routinely on surgical navigation systems image sets. This includes data from magnetoencephalography (MEG), functional MRI (fMRI), and white matter fiber tracts from diffusion tensor imaging (DTI) (**Fig. 10.3**).[33,34] Initial efforts with functional mapping involved the overlay of MEG data.[35] Ten patients were studied preoperatively, and the position of the primary sensory cortex was determined using a biomagnetometer and overlaid on the T1-weighted images. This same image sequence was used for the surface reconstruction registration, and the position of the central sulcus could be seen only on MRI in three of the 10 patients and equivocally in two. At the time of surgery, motor mapping techniques were used to determine the exact position of the motor cortex, and this was compared with the estimated position of the sensory cortex from the intraoperative image-guided position of magnetic source imaging (MSI) somatosensory dipoles. In all 10 cases there was excellent spatial agreement about the position of the sensory motor cortex. Data from fMRI can also be used for regional changes in endogenous vascular paramagnetic deoxyhemoglobin, so-called blood oxygen level-dependent contrast imaging.[23,34] Echo planar imaging can be co-registered and used with 2D or 3D image sets and displayed during surgery. The relationship between motor localization using fMRI and pathology was described in 11 patients with infiltrating gliomas.[36] For grades II and III astrocytomas, fMRI motor activation was scattered and displaced, often intratumorally. For grade IV tumors, patterns of activation were more scattered and often intratumoral as well as displaced to the edges.

Diffusion tensor imaging is now routinely used to display the white matter fiber tracts for motor cortex descending from the surface, down through the subcortical white matter, through the peduncle and brainstem, and for visual fiber pathways (**Fig. 10.4**).[33,37] Software programs are currently available that allow seeding of selected sites of function of cortex with the display of white matter tracts emanating from or coming to these regions. Correlations between displayed DTI fiber tracts and subcortical motor mapping localization have confirmed the accuracy of fiber pathways as depicted on DTI imaging. In many cases where the DTI overlay shows fiber pathways more than 3 mm away from the lesion for planned resection, the surgeon has the option of proceeding without the necessity of intraoperative cortical and subcortical mapping to define motor fiber pathways.

Registration and Surgical Planning

Once the patient is positioned for surgery, the process of registering imaging to physical space is necessary for the navigation systems to work correctly. The process of registration assumes a solid body transformation taking into account translation, rotation, and scaling. Once completed and confirmed as being accurate using anatomic landmarks, the pre-

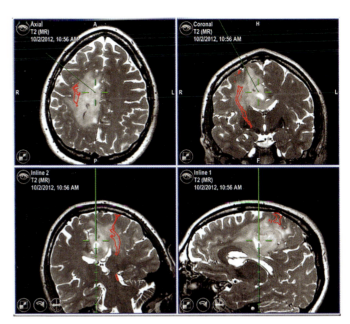

Fig. 10.4 T2 fast-spin echo (FSE) images for low-grade glioma surgery with descending motor fiber tracts superimposed in red.

operative imaging set can be used as the navigational image set for surgery.

The process of registration appears not to prolong significantly overall procedural time. In 125 matched pairs of image-guided and conventional operations, the mean surgery times were not significantly different between the two groups.[38] For a subgroup of 39 cases, times were examined in detail. The mean total time for the total use of intraoperative guidance was 7.0 minutes. During an early experience with a surgical navigation system, times from the end of patient positioning to the start of the operation and the registration times were recorded for 84 consecutive patients.[39] The mean/median times for patient registration were 13.2/10 minutes, with a learning curve evident by the fact that times were shorter in the second half of the patient experience than they were in the first (10.3 minutes versus 16.1 minutes). Subtracting registration time from the time duration from the end of patient positioning to the start of surgery indicated that about 15 to 20 minutes were spent attaching reference devices to the skull clamp, positioning the machine, and selecting the image set and 3D objects for registration.

For surgical planning, the common questions are where the lesion is and how best can the surgeon get there with as little tissue dissection as possible. With a planned surgical approach, one considers location of the lesion, where the skin and skull openings should be made, and what important structures need to be avoided. The anteroposterior and mediolateral boundaries of intracranial pathologies can be marked on the skin surface and the skin incisions planned appropriately.

Linear skin incisions can be used with confidence even for the exposure of large intracranial lesions. Once the skin is opened and the skull exposed, the boundaries can again be marked and the craniotomy flap planned. In addition, structures such as dural venous sinuses and air cell sinuses can also be noted on the skull.

The surgeon needs to recheck the accuracy using anatomic landmarks before the procedure begins to make sure that no shift has occurred between the initial registration and final operating room setup. Because preoperative imaging is used, the physical parameters change as tumor is removed and CSF is drained, such that there is a decline in the accuracy of anatomic localization as the operation proceeds. The decline in accuracy is worse at the surface of the brain than it is toward the center, and this has been confirmed with intraoperative ultrasound studies.[31]

Options for maintaining the accuracy of localization during tumor resection include placing image-directed catheters to the deep boundaries of tumors before debulking (so-called fence posting), re-registration of image sets using integrated ultrasound, and re-registration with intraoperative CT or MRI. The placement of image-directed boundary catheters is useful for intra-axial tumors (**Fig. 10.5**). Placement of the catheters with an image-guided stylet is done after opening of the dura and determining the extent of linear or surface corticectomy to be used. A radiopaque catheter(s) is then inserted to the deep boundary and cut at the surface. Tumor removal begins and the catheter is left in place until it is approached during the resection. Before removing the catheter, the position can be rechecked with the image-guided system to compare the localization with the initial placement. The catheter is removed and a cottonoid is used to mark this site as the margin guiding further resection.

Intraoperative Use

Gliomas

There is mounting evidence (none of it class I) that the extent of resection for malignant gliomas does improve survival, and there is a trend for low-grade gliomas that an increasing extent of resection improves survival and increases the time of tumor recurrence.[40–44] Image-guided systems enable this type of surgery to proceed more accurately and efficiently than in the past.

For tumor locations with the frontal, temporal, parietal, and occipital lobes, there are special considerations for the application of image-guided systems dependent on patient position. Extremes of position away from the chin-upright position will result in greater degrees of brain shift from the effects of gravity, and the brain shifts may be larger with larger skull openings.

Low-grade hemispheric gliomas with distinct margins on T2 FSE images often have reasonably distinct gross surgical borders with surrounding white matter and are ideal for surgical navigation systems (**Fig. 10.6**). There is little edema in the brain adjacent to the tumor, and as a result fewer problems with intraoperative swelling and brain displacement that might affect anatomic localization accuracy. In high-grade gliomas, the interface is less distinct and brain shift and edema are more of a problem. As the tumor is removed, the brain tends to return somewhat to its normal position; therefore, anatomic localization during the resection of larger malignant gliomas tends to be poorer. For this reason, the surgeon needs good surgical judgment and experience as to where the tumor ends.

Surgical options for removal of both grades of tumor depend on location, but there are two standard approaches: (1) limited corticectomy and internal debulking, and (2) superficial corticectomy with broad margin resection. With the former approach, surgical navigation systems help most with centering the corticectomy, and, with the latter, they help with defining the cortical margins for resection. When possible in noneloquent brain, a broad margin with resection is preferred. Newer methods of intraoperative visualization of the tumor borders using super-vital dyes are also being investigated, but they are not yet widely applied because the accuracy of registration deteriorates as the operation proceeds, related to the size of the craniotomy and to gravity.[32]

Metastases

Metastases are ideally suited to the application of navigational technology.[45] Pathologically, these tumors are well circumscribed, with distinct margins. Most metastases on which we now operate are tumors larger than 2 to 3 cm, with abundant vasogenic edema in patients who have controlled systemic disease. It should be noted that cystic tumors should not be drained before the margin of the solid tumors has been defined and dissected.

Meningiomas

Meningiomas are frequently benign dural-based tumors that arise from the arachnoid cap cells, and surgical approaches to these lesions are greatly aided by navigational systems.[46] Skin incisions and bone flaps can now be more accurately and precisely placed to deal with both the central globoid tumor as well as the dural tails. For small convexity, parasagittal and falcine tumors navigational systems are very useful. For skull-

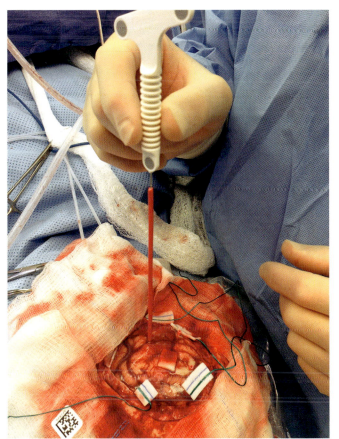

a

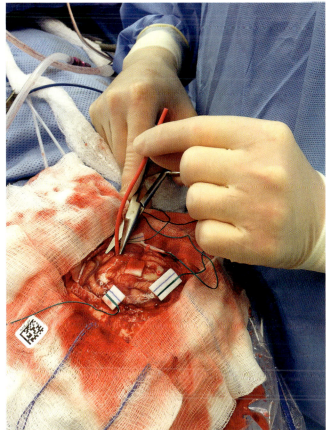

b

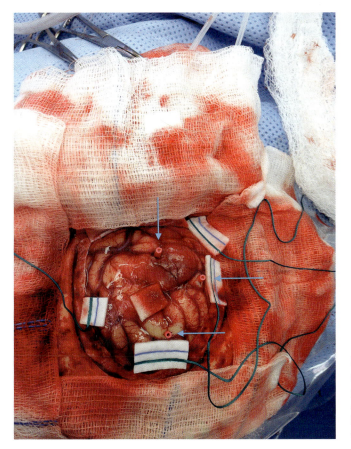

c

Fig. 10.5a–c (**a**) Image-guided stylet inserting a catheter to the deep margin of a malignant glioma before a corticectomy ("fence posting"). (**b**) The catheter is cut at the surface and left in place during tumor removal. (**c**) The surface of the brain showing three implanted catheters (*arrows*) used for defining deep margins of the tumor.

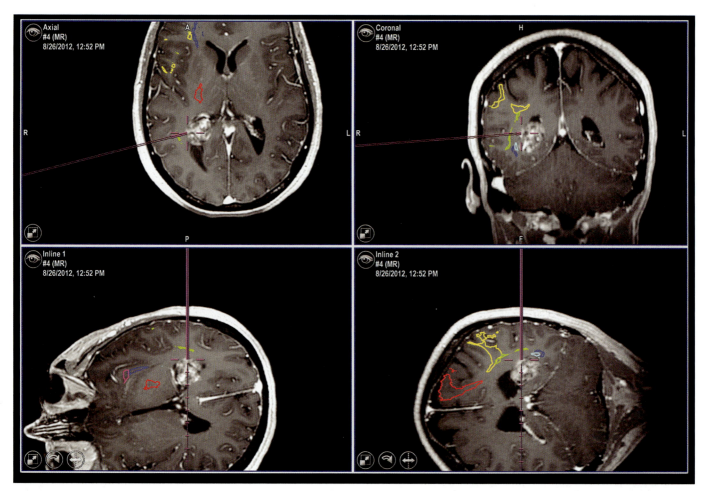

Fig. 10.6 Intraoperative screen images from surgery for an intraventricular tumor with visual fiber pathways in blue and motor pathways in red.

base meningiomas, which are not subject to the shift seen with intra-axial tumors, image-guided systems are invaluable in determining the extent of resection as the operation proceeds. Computed tomography imaging may also be useful when there is evidence of bony invasion and hyperostosis.

Skull-Base Tumors

With the increasing use of endoscopic approaches to skull-base tumors, image guidance has become an important adjunct for defining localization. A combination of CT and MR data sets can be used and merged or displayed separately in quadrants of the display screen. In addition, MRA or MRV images, obtained preoperatively, can be used to display the petrous and cavernous carotid and the internal jugular vein as colored 2D objects (**Fig. 10.7**). Registration in these cases is done with a skull-mounted reference array so that pin fixation of the head is not required. The increasing familiarity with these systems has for many surgeons obviated the need for intraoperative

fluoroscopy as a method of anatomic and instrumentation localization.

■ Conclusion

Image-guided surgery for brain tumors has undergone a quiet revolution in the last 20 years, with the addition of image-guided surgical systems that are now standard equipment for tumor biopsy and intracranial tumor surgery. Apart from anatomic image sets from CT and MRI, subcortical white matter tracts, functional imaging studies, and MRA/MRV data sets can be co-registered and used for intraoperative navigation. Additional development of robotic systems and the use of intraoperative MRI will likely drive the next wave of image-guided surgery. The cost of these technologies is not insignificant, and outcome studies are needed to evaluate their role in the management of patients with intracranial tumors.

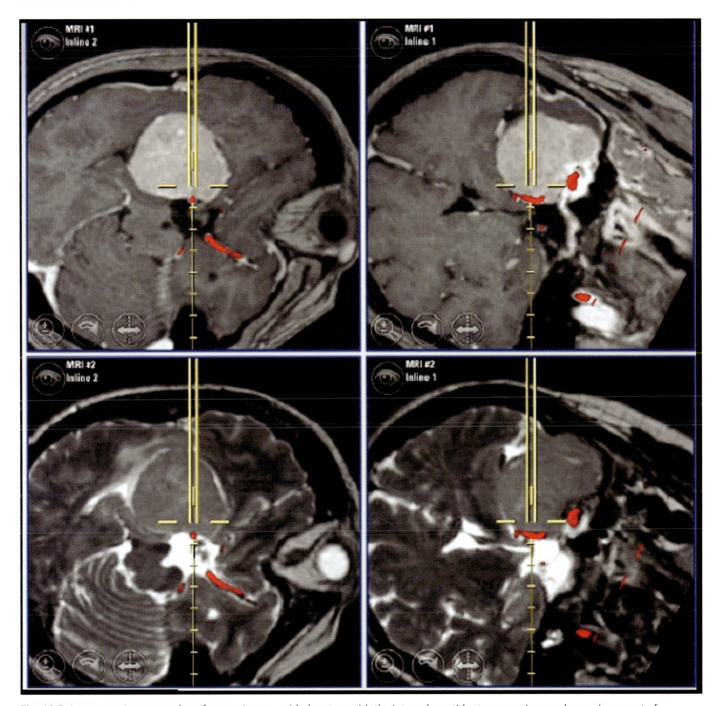

Fig. 10.7 Intraoperative screen shots from an image-guided system with the internal carotid artery superimposed on an image set of a skull-base meningioma as a two-dimensional red-colored object.

Editor's Note

The development of stereotactic frames many decades ago was an obvious but brilliant innovation. When positive imaging such as CT came along, accurate targeting of intracranial targets became incredibly reliable. This revolutionized the care of deep, small, or indistinct lesions by providing the means for accurate and fairly safe biopsy, cyst drainage, and the like. The evolution of frame-based stereotaxy to frameless stereotaxy was again obvious but brilliant.

In hospitals that are able to afford this technology, which is certainly the case in hospitals in North America, Europe and much of Asia, the use of frameless stereotaxy or surgical navigation should arguably be considered a standard of care for all patients undergoing an operation for biopsy or resection of a brain tumor (and most other cranial procedures). Besides helping find the tumor, it helps the surgeon avoid important normal structures such as venous sinuses, and additionally reduces to almost zero the small but finite risk of a devastating wrong-side error.[47] (Bernstein)

References

1. Paleologos TS, Dorward NL, Wadley JP, Thomas DG. Clinical validation of true frameless stereotactic biopsy: analysis of the first 125 consecutive cases. Neurosurgery 2001;49:830–835, discussion 835–837

2. Warnick RE, Longmore LM, Paul CA, Bode LA. Postoperative management of patients after stereotactic biopsy: results of a survey of the AANS/CNS section on tumors and a single institution study. J Neurooncol 2003;62:289–296

3. Cha S, Yang L, Johnson G, et al. Comparison of microvascular permeability measurements, K(trans), determined with conventional steady-state T1-weighted and first-pass T2*-weighted MR imaging methods in gliomas and meningiomas. AJNR Am J Neuroradiol 2006;27:409–417

4. Dowling C, Bollen AW, Noworolski SM, et al. Preoperative proton MR spectroscopic imaging of brain tumors: correlation with histopathologic analysis of resection specimens. AJNR Am J Neuroradiol 2001;22:604–612

5. McKnight TR. Proton magnetic resonance spectroscopic evaluation of brain tumor metabolism. Semin Oncol 2004;31:605–617

6. Serletis D, Bernstein M. Prospective study of awake craniotomy used routinely and nonselectively for supratentorial tumors. J Neurosurg 2007;107:1–6

7. Luzzati R, Ferrari S, Nicolato A, et al. Stereotactic brain biopsy in human immunodeficiency virus-infected patients. Arch Intern Med 1996;156:565–568

8. Smith JS, Quiñones-Hinojosa A, Barbaro NM, McDermott MW. Frame-based stereotactic biopsy remains an important diagnostic tool with distinct advantages over frameless stereotactic biopsy. J Neurooncol 2005;73:173–179

9. Bernays RL, Kollias SS, Khan N, Brandner S, Meier S, Yonekawa Y. Histological yield, complications, and technological considerations in 114 consecutive frameless stereotactic biopsy procedures aided by open intraoperative magnetic resonance imaging. J Neurosurg 2002;97:354–362

10. Quinn J, Spiro D, Schulder M. Stereotactic brain biopsy with a low-field intraoperative magnetic resonance imager. Neurosurgery 2011;68(1, Suppl Operative):217–224, discussion 224

11. Bekelis K, Radwan TA, Desai A, Roberts DW. Frameless robotically targeted stereotactic brain biopsy: feasibility, diagnostic yield, and safety. J Neurosurg 2012;116:1002–1006

12. Kaakaji W, Barnett GH, Bernhard D, Warbel A, Valaitis K, Stamp S. Clinical and economic consequences of early discharge of patients following supratentorial stereotactic brain biopsy. J Neurosurg 2001;94:892–898

13. Bhardwaj RD, Bernstein M. Prospective feasibility study of outpatient stereotactic brain lesion biopsy. Neurosurgery 2002;51:358–361, discussion 361–364

14. Purzner T, Purzner J, Massicotte EM, Bernstein M. Outpatient brain tumor surgery and spinal decompression: a prospective study of 1003 patients. Neurosurgery 2011;69:119–126, discussion 126–127

15. Bernstein M, Parent AG. Complications of CT-guided stereotactic biopsy of intra-axial brain lesions. J Neurosurg 1994;81:165–168

16. McGirt MJ, Woodworth GF, Coon AL, et al. Independent predictors of morbidity after image-guided stereotactic brain biopsy: a risk assessment of 270 cases. J Neurosurg 2005;102:897–901

17. Woodworth GF, McGirt MJ, Samdani A, Garonzik I, Olivi A, Weingart JD. Frameless image-guided stereotactic brain biopsy procedure: diagnostic yield, surgical morbidity, and comparison with the frame-based technique. J Neurosurg 2006;104:233–237

18. Kongkham PN, Knifed E, Tamber MS, Bernstein M. Complications in 622 cases of frame-based stereotactic biopsy, a decreasing procedure. Can J Neurol Sci 2008;35:79–84

19. Amin DV, Lozanne K, Parry PV, Engh JA, Seelman K, Mintz A. Image-guided frameless stereotactic needle biopsy in awake patients without the use of rigid head fixation. J Neurosurg 2011;114:1414–1420

20. Ersahin M, Karaaslan N, Gurbuz MS, et al. The safety and diagnostic value of frame-based and CT-guided stereotactic brain biopsy technique. Turk Neurosurg 2011;21:582–590

21. Kulkarni AV, Guha A, Lozano A, Bernstein M. Incidence of silent hemorrhage and delayed deterioration after stereotactic brain biopsy. J Neurosurg 1998;89:31–35

22. Soo TM, Bernstein M, Provias J, Tasker R, Lozano A, Guha A. Failed stereotactic biopsy in a series of 518 cases. Stereotact Funct Neurosurg 1995;64:183–196

23. Cha S. Update on brain tumor imaging: from anatomy to physiology. AJNR Am J Neuroradiol 2006;27:475–487

24. Shooman D, Belli A, Grundy PL. Image-guided frameless stereotactic biopsy without intraoperative neuropathological examination. J Neurosurg 2010;113:170–178

25. Moriuchi S, Yamada K, Dehara M, et al. Use of 5-aminolevulinic acid for the confirmation of deep-seated brain tumors during stereotactic biopsy. Report of 2 cases. J Neurosurg 2011;115:278–280

26. Barnett GH, Miller DW, Weisenberger J. Frameless stereotaxy with scalp-applied fiducial markers for brain biopsy procedures: experience in 218 cases. J Neurosurg 1999;91:569–576

27. Kondziolka D, Dempsey PK, Lunsford LD, et al. A comparison between magnetic resonance imaging and computed tomography for stereotac-

tic coordinate determination. Neurosurgery 1992;30:402–406, discussion 406–407

28. Sanai N, Wachhorst SP, Gupta NM, McDermott MW. Transcerebellar stereotactic biopsy for lesions of the brainstem and peduncles under local anesthesia. Neurosurgery 2008;63:460–466, discussion 466–468

29. Quiñones-Hinojosa A, Ware ML, Sanai N, McDermott MW. Assessment of image guided accuracy in a skull model: comparison of frameless stereotaxy techniques vs. frame-based localization. J Neurooncol 2006; 76:65–70

30. Maciunas R. Pitfalls. In: Roberts D, Barnett G, Maciunas R, eds. Image-Guided Neurosurgery. St. Louis: Quality Medical Publishing, 1998: 43–62

31. Keles GE, Lamborn KR, Berger MS. Coregistration accuracy and detection of brain shift using intraoperative sononavigation during resection of hemispheric tumors. Neurosurgery 2003;53:556–562, discussion 562–564

32. Roberts DW, Hartov A, Kennedy FE, Miga MI, Paulsen KD. Intraoperative brain shift and deformation: a quantitative analysis of cortical displacement in 28 cases. Neurosurgery 1998;43:749–758, discussion 758–760

33. Berman JI, Berger MS, Mukherjee P, Henry RG. Diffusion-tensor imaging-guided tracking of fibers of the pyramidal tract combined with intraoperative cortical stimulation mapping in patients with gliomas. J Neurosurg 2004;101.66–72

34. Henry RG, Berman JI, Nagarajan SS, Mukherjee P, Berger MS. Subcortical pathways serving cortical language sites: initial experience with diffusion tensor imaging fiber tracking combined with intraoperative language mapping. Neuroimage 2004;21:616–622

35. Roberts TP, Zusman E, McDermott M, Barbaro N, Rowley HA. Correlation of functional magnetic source imaging with intraoperative cortical stimulation in neurosurgical patients. J Image Guid Surg 1995;1: 339–347

36. Roux FE, Ranjeva JP, Boulanouar K, et al. Motor functional MRI for presurgical evaluation of cerebral tumors. Stereotact Funct Neurosurg 1997;68(Pt 1):106–111

37. Berger MS, Keles GE. Evolution of management strategies for cerebral gliomas: the effects of science and technology. Clin Neurosurg 2005; 52:292–296

38. Alberti O, Dorward NL, Kitchen ND, Thomas DG. Neuronavigation—impact on operating time. Stereotact Funct Neurosurg 1997;68(Pt 1): 44–48

39. McDermott MW, Binder DK, Kunwar S, Parsa AT, Berger MS. Surgical navigation systems for the resection of intracranial gliomas. In: Barnett GH, Maciunas RJ, Roberts DW, eds. Computer-Assisted Neurosurgery. New York: Taylor & Francis, 2006:179–193

40. Curran WJ Jr, Scott CB, Horton J, et al. Recursive partitioning analysis of prognostic factors in three Radiation Therapy Oncology Group malignant glioma trials. J Natl Cancer Inst 1993;85:704–710

41. Keles GE, Lamborn KR, Berger MS. Low-grade hemispheric gliomas in adults: a critical review of extent of resection as a factor influencing outcome. J Neurosurg 2001;95:735–745

42. Simpson JR, Horton J, Scott C, et al. Influence of location and extent of surgical resection on survival of patients with glioblastoma multiforme: results of three consecutive Radiation Therapy Oncology Group (RTOG) clinical trials. Int J Radiat Oncol Biol Phys 1993;26:239–244

43. Rostomily RC, Spence AM, Duong D, McCormick K, Bland M, Berger MS. Multimodality management of recurrent adult malignant gliomas: results of a phase II multiagent chemotherapy study and analysis of cytoreductive surgery. Neurosurgery 1994;35:378–388, discussion 388

44. Keles GE, Lamborn KR, Chang SM, Prados MD, Berger MS. Volume of residual disease as a predictor of outcome in adult patients with recurrent supratentorial glioblastomas multiforme who are undergoing chemotherapy. J Neurosurg 2004;100:41–46

45. Lang FF, Sawaya R. Surgical treatment of metastatic brain tumors. Semin Surg Oncol 1998;14:53–63

46. Palcologos TS, Wadley JP, Kitchen ND, Thomas DG. Clinical utility and cost-effectiveness of interactive image-guided craniotomy: clinical comparison between conventional and image-guided meningioma surgery. Neurosurgery 2000;47:40–47, discussion 47–48

47. Cohen FL, Mendelsohn D, Bernstein M. Wrong-site craniotomy: analysis of 35 cases and systems for prevention. J Neurosurg 2010;113: 461–473

11 Intraoperative Magnetic Resonance Imaging

Devon H. Haydon and Ralph G. Dacey, Jr.

Intraoperative magnetic resonance imaging (iMRI) first appeared in the neurosurgical operating room in the mid-1990s.[1] Initial designs were admittedly cumbersome, as the surgeon was forced to operate within the magnet itself. Such constrictions limited a surgeon's movements as well as the feasibility of additional intraoperative adjuncts, like the operating microscope. Image resolution was an added concern, as early models incorporated low-field-strength magnets such as the 0.2-tesla (T) magnet.

Such limitations hampered the widespread adoption of iMRI devices. However, new innovations such as ceiling-mounted units and high-field-strength magnets of 1.5 to 3 T strength are expanding iMRI's utility and efficiency (**Table 11.1**). As "next generation" iMRI suites emerge, the advantages of iMRI-guided craniotomies are increasingly recognized. Although iMRI has aided the surgical treatment of nonneoplastic disease,[2] by far the greatest benefits of this intraoperative aid have been witnessed in the field of neuro-oncology.

Extent of Resection

Maximal safe resection is a frequently, although not universally, accepted operative goal for many types of brain tumors. The primary benefit to iMRI-assisted surgery is the ability to identify residual pathological tissue in near real-time (**Fig. 11.1**). Such identification permits maximal resection of the lesion in question during the initial procedure. Maximal resections are thus achieved in addition to fewer secondary surgeries for residual disease.

Growing evidence, although mostly class 3, emphasizes the importance of extent of resection for both high- and low-grade glial tumors (**Fig. 11.2**). Critics often cite the absence of class 1 evidence (Oxford Centre of Evidence-Based Medicine, http://www.cebm.net/index.aspx?o=1025) in the neurosurgical literature to prove a survival advantage for greater surgical resection. However, one must also acknowledge the logistical and ethical limitations that likely preclude any future trial that randomizes solely on the basis of extent of resection. Would the neurosurgical community be willing to randomize an otherwise healthy 20-year-old patient with a suspected high-grade glioma of the right frontal pole to the biopsy arm of a surgical trial? Given these limitations, we are forced to rely upon well-controlled observational studies.

> **Controversy**
>
> - Observational studies suggest a correlation between extent of resection of gliomas and survival. However, randomized controlled studies, that is, class 1 evidence, do not exist to prove this view.

In 2001, a retrospective series of 416 histology-proven glioblastomas was published in which a 4.2-month overall survival advantage was found for patients who received at least a 98% extent of resection.[3] Interestingly, this study has been referenced by both sides of the extent of resection debate, as it contributed to the so-called all-or-nothing principle. Proponents of maximal resection note the statistically significant benefit for the greater extent of resection. Opponents emphasize that essentially only complete resections led to a survival advantage, which in turn lessened the study's clinical importance and relevance because a significant percentage of glioblastomas are not amenable to complete resection at presentation. Such lesions were frequently relegated to biopsy alone. Here, the notion of a maximal, albeit subtotal, resection is largely overlooked.

The only randomized clinical trial examining the extent of resection for high-grade gliomas randomized patients over 65 years of age with a suspected high-grade glial tumor to either stereotactic biopsy or craniotomy and resection.[4] The median survival of the surgical group was double the median survival of the biopsy arm. Despite the prospective, randomized design, a number of limitations restricted the study's findings, including a small sample size of only 30 patients as well as the inclusion of multiple pathologies.

The ALA-Glioma Study Group provided a unique opportunity to examine the effect of extent of resection on glioblastoma survival. The original study randomized patients to conventional microsurgery versus 5-aminolevulinic acid immunofluorescence-guided surgery.[5] Although not randomized to extent of resection, the study did provide well-controlled, prospective data. A post-hoc analysis demonstrated a survival advantage for greater resection even after confounders like age and eloquence were identified and controlled.[6] More recently, an extent of resection threshold for patients with newly diagnosed glioblastomas indicated that an extent of resection as low as 78% imparts a survival advantage.[7]

Table 11.1 Some Commonly Used IMRI Systems

System	Company	Field-Strength (Tesla)
PoleStar® Surgical MRI	Medtronic, Inc.	0.15
VISIUS® Surgical Theatre	IMRIS, Inc.	1.5–3
Brainsuite®	Brainlab	1.5–3
AIRIS®	Hitachi Medical Systems America, Inc.	0.3
Signa SP®	General Electric Medical Systems	0.5
Ingenia®	Philips Medical Systems	1.5–3

> **Pitfall**
>
> - Because of the strong feelings of surgeons and patients about the value of aggressive resection of gliomas, a proper randomized study can probably never be carried out to provide definitive proof.

A similar treatment paradigm emphasizing extent of resection should be considered in the management of low-grade glial tumors as well (**Fig. 11.3**). A series of 216 adults with low-grade hemispheric gliomas was reported in which improved outcome was predicted by a greater extent of resection.[8] Patients who underwent at least a 90% extent of resection experienced a 5-year overall survival of 97%, whereas those patients who underwent less extensive surgery had a 5-year survival of only 76%. Such evidence argues in favor of the value of optimizing the extent of resection when treating both low- and high-grade gliomas, even when a complete resection is prohibited by the proximity of eloquent structures, as this surgical parameter likely contributes to improved patient outcome.

Intraoperative Magnetic Resonance Imaging for Gliomas

Surgeons are notoriously poor judges of extent of resection during intracranial tumor resection. A recent study found that less than 25% of glioblastoma resections previously deemed

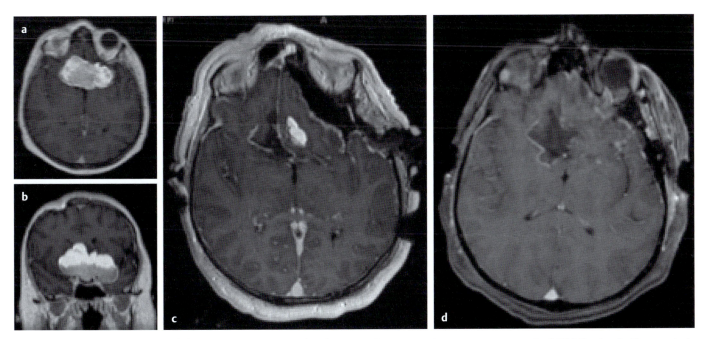

Fig. 11.1a–d Axial **(a)** and coronal **(b)** postcontrast, T1-weighted, preoperative magnetic resonance imaging (MRI) demonstrating a large teratoma of the anterior cranial fossa. **(c)** Intraoperative MRI demonstrating a small area of residual tumor. **(d)** No abnormal enhancement is seen on postoperative MRI following further surgical resection of the residual disease, thereby confirming a complete resection.

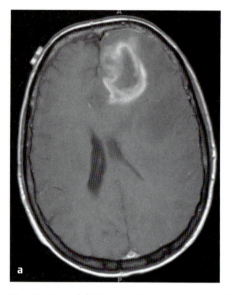
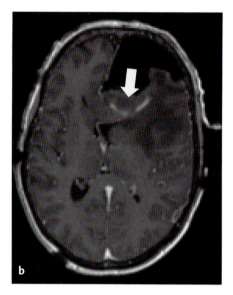
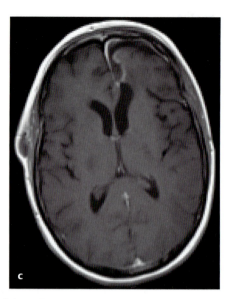

Fig. 11.2a–c **(a)** Preoperative, postcontrast, T1-weighted MRI demonstrating a large heterogeneously enhancing lesion of the left frontal lobe consistent with a glioblastoma. **(b)** Intraoperative MRI identified an area of nodular enhancement (*arrow*) of concern for residual disease. **(c)** Further surgery resulted in a complete resection confirmed by postoperative imaging.

"complete" by surgeon estimation were in fact confirmed by postoperative imaging.[9] Intraoperative MRI provides a more objective means to gauge extent of resection at a time when further intervention remains possible.

One experience with low-field strength iMRI for high-grade glioma resections was reported in 1999. Resections were initially performed with the assistance of neuronavigation to the point that all identifiable tumor was thought to have been removed. Intraoperative MRI subsequently identified residual enhancing tumor tissue in more than half of all cases. As a result of further resection post-iMRI, complete resections increased from 36 to 76%.[10] Soon after, another series of all intracranial glioma resections incorporating low-field-strength iMRI assistance was reported. Similar to the previous report, this study showed a decrease in the number of glioblastoma cases with identifiable residual tumor tissue on imaging after iMRI-assisted resections (from 62% to 33%).[11] Despite the limitations in image resolution accompanying low-field strength magnets, these early iMRI-guided craniotomies were still able to demonstrate improved surgical outcomes.

More recent studies advocate the utility of high-field-strength intraoperative magnets as well. An experience with

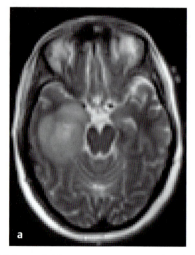
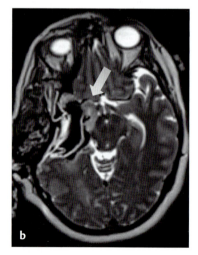
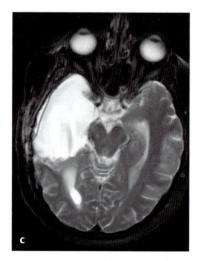

Fig. 11.3a–c **(a)** Preoperative, T2-weighted MRI of a low-grade glioma involving the right temporal lobe. **(b)** Intraoperative MRI confirmed the presence of residual tumor (*arrow*) along the medial resection margin. **(c)** Subsequent surgery yielded a complete resection, which was confirmed by postoperative MRI.

Pearl

- One randomized study provides class I evidence that intraoperative MRI can improve the extent of resection of gliomas.

all-grade supratentorial gliomas and iMRI-guided craniotomies was reported in 2006. The rate of complete resection at initial iMRI was only 27% of all cases but increased to 40% following further surgery.[12] More importantly, the rate of new permanent neurologic deficit following iMRI-guided surgery was less than 3%. A valid concern about iMRI-guided craniotomies is the possibility that the surgeon might be more aggressive during tumor resection as a result of iMRI findings, thereby leading to increased operative morbidity. However, studies have yet to validate this concern. Sound clinical and surgical judgment remains paramount during image interpretation of all imaging studies regardless of the timing of such studies. Strict adherence to this principle should avoid increased operative morbidity.

Another series of iMRI-guided craniotomies for glioma was analyzed using a volumetric analysis of the extent of resection. Overall extent of resection significantly increased from 76% to 96% as a result of further surgical resection following iMRI, with a 65% final rate of complete (i.e., 100%) resection.[13] Similarly, our own series noted an increased rate of complete resection for glioblastoma from 24% to 57% due to further surgery following high-field-strength iMRI.[14]

Although the majority of studies examining the effect of iMRI rely on observational data, in one study patients with a suspected intracranial glioma were randomly assigned to either conventional microsurgery or iMRI-guided surgery. Patients who received iMRI-guided surgery had a significantly higher rate of complete resection compared to the conventional surgery group (96% vs 68%, $p = 0.02$).[15] Again, no difference in the rate of new neurologic deficit was seen (13% vs 8%, $p = 1.0$). This study now provides class 1 evidence demonstrating iMRI's ability to safely improve the extent of resection for glial tumors.

Intraoperative Magnetic Resonance Imaging for Pituitary Tumors

The benefits of iMRI extend to multiple tumor pathologies in addition to multiple surgical approaches. In particular, iMRI assists the resection of pituitary adenomas via the transsphenoidal approach. With the exception of prolactinomas, surgical removal/debulking remains the primary treatment modality for most pituitary adenomas. Multiple iMRI systems have been used by various centers during pituitary surgery ranging from ultra-low-strength magnets to 3-T magnets.[16] Admittedly, ad-

equate intraoperative image resolution can be difficult with lower strength magnets, especially for sellar microadenomas. However, high-strength intraoperative systems consistently illustrate the advantages of this adjunct for pituitary and other sellar-based pathology (**Fig. 11.4**).

An increased rate of complete tumor removal from 58% to 82% following iMRI was noted in a series of 85 hormonally inactive pituitary macroadenomas for which complete removal was thought possible preoperatively.[17] Again, concerns regarding increased morbidity following more aggressive surgery must be addressed, especially given the unique risk of endocrinopathies following transsphenoidal surgery. However, studies continue to demonstrate the safety of iMRI-assisted transsphenoidal surgery.

A cohort of 60 hormonally inactive pituitary adenomas resected via an iMRI-assisted transsphenoidal technique was compared with 32 matched controls. The iMRI group not only enjoyed a superior rate of complete removal compared to the control group (85% vs 69%), but also experienced less postoperative hypopituitarism (29% vs 45%).[18]

Intraoperative Magnetic Resonance Imaging Criticism

Given the present reality of limited health care resources, a discussion of any surgical adjunct would be incomplete without considering financial implications. Neurosurgical suites with iMRI capabilities are expensive. Substantial initial capital investment is required to purchase these intricate machines. However, additional cost savings appear possible by minimizing the need for future surgical therapies via more complete primary procedures.

A decreasing trend in the need for early reoperation has been reported following craniotomies for tumor or focal cortical dysplasia in children. A higher rate of complete resections was noted with iMRI-guided resections compared to conventional surgery alone. The primary beneficiary of an iMRI-assisted craniotomy is, of course, the patient, who avoids the added risk and potential morbidity of a second surgical procedure. A supplementary cost analysis found potential savings of nearly $24,000 per case due the decreased need for further medical care.[19]

An additional criticism about iMRI-assisted surgery is the increased time required for such procedures. Intraoperative MRI acquisition and the subsequent resection following iMRI

Pitfall

- Intraoperative MRI is extremely expensive, which may make it relatively inaccessible especially in not-for-profit health care systems and in developing countries.

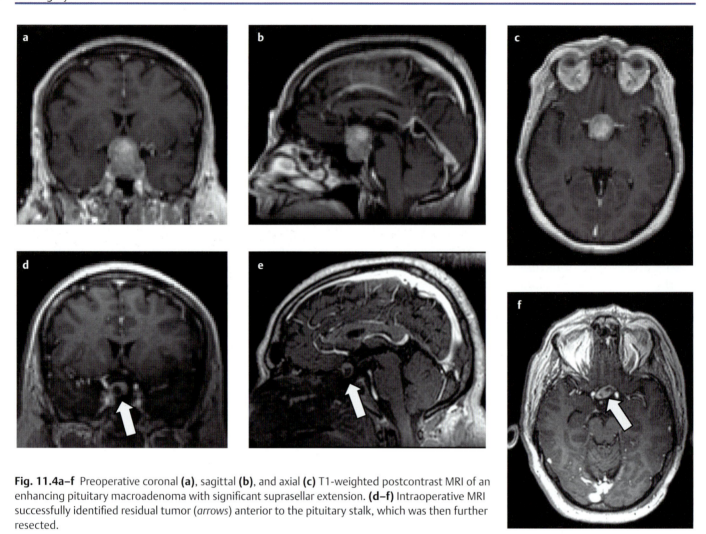

Fig. 11.4a–f Preoperative coronal **(a)**, sagittal **(b)**, and axial **(c)** T1-weighted postcontrast MRI of an enhancing pituitary macroadenoma with significant suprasellar extension. **(d–f)** Intraoperative MRI successfully identified residual tumor (*arrows*) anterior to the pituitary stalk, which was then further resected.

Pitfall

- Intraoperative MRI may increase the surgical time but this problem diminishes with experience.

interpretation add approximately 2 hours to a craniotomy for a high-grade glioma at our own institution. Numerous studies identify prolonged operative time as a risk factor for surgical morbidity. However, like most new intraoperative technologies, a learning curve exists for iMRI implementation. With increased experience, the time needed to complete an iMRI-guided resection decreases. Our own institution has witnessed an average decrease of 100 minutes for iMRI-guided glioma resections over the first 3 years of iMRI operation. Cumulative physician and nursing experience, anesthesia specialization, and equipment tray reorganization can all improve iMRI efficiency and operative workflow.

◼ Conclusion

Intraoperative MRI can be safely integrated into the neurosurgical operative suite. This tool is most widely used during the management and treatment of intracranial tumors, where it can be combined with additional techniques such as neuronavigation, awake craniotomy, and even laser interstitial thermal therapy.[20–22] Yet, iMRI has facilitated the treatment of a number of nonneoplastic diseases as well, including epilepsy and movement disorders. Like any novel intraoperative aid, iMRI lengthens operative time. However, improvements in efficiency are seen with accumulated experience.

The main advantage offered by iMRI is the accurate, near real-time assessment of the extent of resection. Following image interpretation and subsequent additional surgery, iMRI improves the extent of resection for multiple brain tumor types including both high- and low-grade gliomas as well as pituitary tumors. Mounting evidence indicates that these improvements in surgical outcome ultimately contribute to improved patient outcome as well. With "next generation" neurosurgical suites emerging that combine MRI, computed tomography, and angiographic capabilities, the full potential of iMRI for brain tumor management has likely yet to be seen.

Editor's Note

Intraoperative MRI is yet another in the string of ingenious neurosurgical innovations that have catapulted neuro-oncology forward over the last two or three decades. It has definite challenges, including the immense initial cost, logistic issues related to surgical instruments and patient flow, and increased operating time with its attendant risks. However, as increasing non–class I evidence suggests that

the extent of resection may really matter for both low- and high-grade glioma, tools to help improve the surgeon's "completeness" of resection will be invaluable, as surgeons' assessments of the extent of resection without such imaging are notoriously flawed. Intraoperative MRI is such a tool. It is hoped that the challenges outlined above will be partly or fully solved, resulting in more widespread availability and use by neurosurgeons everywhere. (Bernstein)

Disclosure

An unrestricted educational grant from IMRIS Inc. has helped establish and maintain a prospective iMRI database controlled by the Department of Neurological Surgery at Washington University School of Medicine.

References

1. Black PM, Moriarty T, Alexander E III, et al. Development and implementation of intraoperative magnetic resonance imaging and its neurosurgical applications. Neurosurgery 1997;41:831–842, discussion 842–845

2. Sommer B, Grummich P, Coras R, et al. Integration of functional neuronavigation and intraoperative MRI in surgery for drug-resistant extratemporal epilepsy close to eloquent brain areas. Neurosurg Focus 2013; 34:E4

3. Lacroix M, Abi-Said D, Fourney DR, et al. A multivariate analysis of 416 patients with glioblastoma multiforme: prognosis, extent of resection, and survival. J Neurosurg 2001;95:190–198

4. Vuorinen V, Hinkka S, Färkkilä M, Jääskeläinen J. Debulking or biopsy of malignant glioma in elderly people—a randomised study. Acta Neurochir (Wien) 2003;145:5–10

5. Stummer W, Pichlmeier U, Meinel T, Wiestler OD, Zanella F, Reulen HJ; ALA-Glioma Study Group. Fluorescence-guided surgery with 5-aminolevulinic acid for resection of malignant glioma: a randomised controlled multicentre phase III trial. Lancet Oncol 2006;7:392–401

6. Stummer W, Reulen HJ, Meinel T, et al; ALA-Glioma Study Group. Extent of resection and survival in glioblastoma multiforme: identification of and adjustment for bias. Neurosurgery 2008;62:564–576, discussion 564–576

7. Sanai N, Polley MY, McDermott MW, Parsa AT, Berger MS. An extent of resection threshold for newly diagnosed glioblastomas. J Neurosurg 2011;115:3–8

8. Smith JS, Chang EF, Lamborn KR, et al. Role of extent of resection in the long-term outcome of low-grade hemispheric gliomas. J Clin Oncol 2008;26:1338–1345

9. Orringer D, Lau D, Khatri S, et al. Extent of resection in patients with glioblastoma: limiting factors, perception of resectability, and effect on survival. J Neurosurg 2012;117:851–859

10. Knauth M, Wirtz CR, Tronnier VM, Aras N, Kunze S, Sartor K. Intraoperative MR imaging increases the extent of tumor resection in patients with high-grade gliomas. AJNR Am J Neuroradiol 1999;20:1642–1646

11. Wirtz CR, Knauth M, Staubert A, et al. Clinical evaluation and follow-up results for intraoperative magnetic resonance imaging in neurosurgery. Neurosurgery 2000;46:1112–1120, discussion 1120–1122

12. Nimsky C, Ganslandt O, Buchfelder M, Fahlbusch R. Intraoperative visualization for resection of gliomas: the role of functional neuronavigation and intraoperative 1.5 T MRI. Neurol Res 2006;28:482–487

13. Hatiboglu MA, Weinberg JS, Suki D, et al. Impact of intraoperative high-field magnetic resonance imaging guidance on glioma surgery: a prospective volumetric analysis. Neurosurgery 2009;64:1073–1081, discussion 1081

14. Haydon D, Chicoine M, Dacey R. The impact of high-field strength intraoperative magnetic resonance imaging on brain tumor management. Neurosurgery 2013;60:92–7

15. Senft C, Bink A, Franz K, Vatter H, Gasser T, Seifert V. Intraoperative MRI guidance and extent of resection in glioma surgery: a randomised, controlled trial. Lancet Oncol 2011;12:997–1003

16. Hlavica M, Bellut D, Lemm D, Schmid C, Bernays RL. Impact of ultra-low-field intraoperative magnetic resonance imaging on extent of resection and frequency of tumor recurrence in 104 surgically treated nonfunctioning pituitary adenomas. World Neurosurg 2013;79:99–109

17. Nimsky C, von Keller B, Ganslandt O, Fahlbusch R. Intraoperative high-field magnetic resonance imaging in transsphenoidal surgery of hormonally inactive pituitary macroadenomas. Neurosurgery 2006;59: 105–114, discussion 105–114

18. Berkmann S, Fandino J, Müller B, Remonda L, Landolt H. Intraoperative MRI and endocrinological outcome of transsphenoidal surgery for non-functioning pituitary adenoma. Acta Neurochir (Wien) 2012;154: 639–647

19. Shah MN, Leonard JR, Inder G, et al. Intraoperative magnetic resonance imaging to reduce the rate of early reoperation for lesion resection in pediatric neurosurgery. J Neurosurg Pediatr 2012;9:259–264

20. Leuthardt EC, Lim CC, Shah MN, et al. Use of movable high-field-strength intraoperative magnetic resonance imaging with awake craniotomies for resection of gliomas: preliminary experience. Neurosurgery 2011;69:194–205, discussion 205–206

21. Hawasli AH, Ray WZ, Murphy RK, Dacey RG Jr, Leuthardt EC. Magnetic resonance imaging-guided focused laser interstitial thermal therapy for subinsular metastatic adenocarcinoma: technical case report. Neurosurgery 2012;70(2, Suppl Operative):332–337, discussion 338

22. Bernstein M, Al-Anazi A, Kucharczyk W, Manninen P, Bronskill M, Henkelman N. Brain tumor surgery in the Toronto Open MRI system: preliminary results with 36 cases and analysis of advantages, weaknesses, and future prospects. Neurosurgery 2000;46:900–909

12 Other Intraoperative Aids

David W. Roberts and Pablo A. Valdes

Increasing evidence of the importance of accurate, reliable, and safe surgical resection of intracranial tumors has placed greater responsibility on the neuro-oncological surgeon. A wide variety of intraoperative technological advances have facilitated achievement of successful surgical resection, including co-registered image-guidance systems, intraoperative computed tomography (CT) and magnetic resonance imaging (MRI), as well as a number of other surgical adjuvant tools including intraoperative ultrasound and numerous optical imaging techniques. These other intraoperative technologies are the focus of this chapter. Some, such as intraoperative ultrasound, have a record of utilization over decades; others, such as confocal microscopy and optical coherence imaging, are relatively new to the operating room. All the technologies discussed here have been brought to clinical application, and their development is ongoing.

■ Intraoperative Ultrasound

Incorporation of ultrasound imaging into the operating room was begun more than three decades ago.[1,2] The ability of ultrasound to detect subcortical and deep objects of interest such as tumors, coupled with its ease of use, ready availability, and relatively low cost, led a number of practitioners to investigate its intraoperative utility and to report encouraging preliminary experiences.[1–3] The image quality in these early applications was low in comparison to today's technology, but guidance to tumors, the ventricular system, hematomas, and foreign objects was readily demonstrated. Perhaps overshadowed by the rapid adoption of image-guidance systems co-registering more intuitively appealing and higher quality preoperative CT and MRI data sets, wider utilization of intraoperative ultrasound was limited.

Integration of ultrasound into navigation systems that could show instrument location with respect to not just preoperative CT or MRI but also current ultrasound was soon forthcoming.[4] Using the digitizer technology of neuronavigation systems, the ability was acquired to track the location and orientation of the ultrasound transducer, and in turn, through a calibration step, that of the ultrasound image with respect to the surgical field and any other co-registered images (**Fig. 12.1**). Intraoperative two-dimensional (2D) ultrasound image, almost always double-oblique with respect to traditional imaging triplanar display, may be difficult for the surgeon to orient, but such co-registration enables simultaneous display of the more easily interpreted corresponding CT or MRI plane.

Two immediate advantages of such intraoperative imaging are the ability to determine the extent of ongoing tumor resection and the ability to demonstrate the amount of current intraoperative registration error resulting from brain deformation or shift. Systems have been promoted for utilizing the latter capability, although they have served more to point out registration error than to actually correct it. Corrective deformation of preoperative MRI using intraoperative ultrasound information has been pursued, however, and is in development.[5] As ultrasound itself improves sufficiently in image quality, navigating by the ultrasound image alone is becoming possible.

Further enabling such navigation are developments addressing the limitations of nonstandard, oblique image planes. Three-dimensional (3D) image data sets have been generated through acquisition of multiple 2D images that can then be registered to a common coordinate system and reformatted in axial, coronal, and sagittal planes. The challenges of such a strategy, including ensuring sufficient density of image data as well as the inefficiencies of acquiring such data sets, are not trivial, but they have been overcome by several groups. More recently, 3D ultrasound probes capable of acquiring full data sets more completely and efficiently have been utilized for such purposes.[6] A recent comparison of clinical experience with both a 3D ultrasound system integrated into a neuronavigation system (IGSonic, VectorVision; BrainLAB, Munich, Germany) and a nonintegrated 3D ultrasound system found that the latter was more time-efficient, but the spatial orientation enabled by navigation using reformatted images was superior.[7]

Progressive improvement in ultrasound image quality as well as integration into guidance systems has led to practical and effective clinical applications, and contemporary reports continue to raise the promise of inexpensive, accurate, updated intraoperative imaging. Use of an intraoperative 3D ultrasound integrated system (SonoWand, Trondheim, Norway)

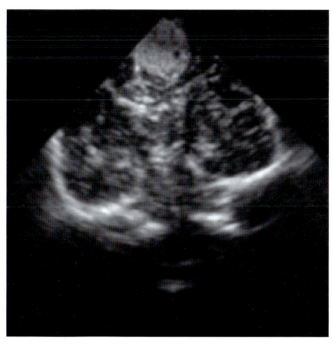
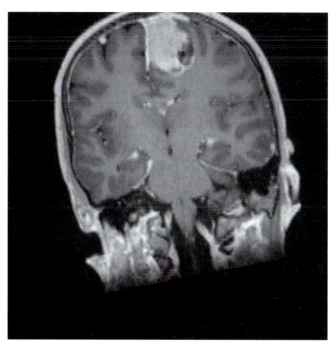

a b

Fig. 12.1a,b Co-registered ultrasound and magnetic resonance imaging (MRI). **(a)** Intraoperative ultrasound (coronal) image of a parasagittal meningioma. **(b)** Corresponding MRI plane.

has been reported in over 900 operations for intraparenchymal tumor as well as cavernoma, skull base tumor, and arteriovenous malformation. Advantages include portability among operating rooms, utilization of regular surgical instruments, little additional time required, and low cost.[8]

5-Aminolevulinic Acid–Induced Fluorescence

The preferential accumulation of the fluorophore protoporphyrin IX (PpIX) in tumor tissue following exogenous administration of the precursor 5-aminolevulinic acid (5-ALA) has generated excitement as a powerful intraoperative aid during glioma resection. An operating microscope adapted to enable illumination of the operative field with excitatory violet-blue light, and to optimize using filters for the perception of any resulting fluorescence, provides an intuitive, easy to use, and efficient platform for the elicitation of pink-red fluorescence in otherwise visibly indistinguishable tumor (**Fig. 12.2**). This was demonstrated in a C6 glioma rat brain tumor model[9] and then investigated in a single-institution clinical trial of 52 patients operated on for glioblastoma. Resection of fluorescent tissue when anatomic location safely allowed it resulted in complete resection of contrast-enhancing tumor on postoperative MRI in 63% of patients, with residual (unresectable) solid fluorescent tissue intraoperatively being a negative predictive factor for survival.[10]

Special Consideration

- There is high correlation between contrast-enhancement on MRI and 5-ALA–induced fluorescence. Fluorescence is also correlated with higher tumor grade, cellular proliferation, metabolic imaging, and capillary density.

This group then went on to carry out a landmark, multi-institutional prospective clinical trial randomizing patients with malignant gliomas to either 5-ALA–assisted tumor resection or conventional white-light microsurgery. Primary endpoints were the number of patients with residual contrast-enhancing tumor on postoperative MRI and 6-month progression-free survival. The study was terminated at interim analysis of 270 patients, 139 of whom received 5-ALA (20 mg/kg) orally 3 hours prior to surgery and 131 of whom were operated on under white light conditions only. Complete resection of MRI contrast-enhancing tumor was achieved in 90 patients (65%) in the 5-ALA group and in 47 patients (36%)

Special Consideration

- Fluorescence-guided resection of glioblastoma multiforme by using 5-ALA–induced porphyrins has been shown to provide higher levels of gross total resection.

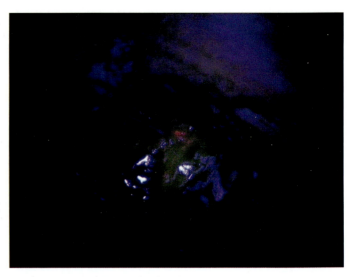

a

b

Fig. 12.2a,b 5-aminolevulinic acid (5-ALA)-induced protoporphyrin IX fluorescence. **(a)** White-light operating microscope view near the end of resection of a glioblastoma. The superposed green contours represent the tumor segmentation outline in the corresponding (preoperative) MRI plane. **(b)** Blue-light operating microscope image showing a small area of 5-ALA–induced protoporphyrin IX red fluorescence.

in the white light group. Six-month progression-free survival was 41% and 21.1%, respectively. Severe adverse events and adverse events within 7 days of surgery did not differ between groups.[11]

A subsequent supplemental analysis of this series focused on the potential trade-off of increased risks but potential later gains associated with more extensive resection. In the prospective, randomized trial, more frequent deterioration in the National Institutes of Health Stroke Scale (NIH-SS) score was seen in the 5-ALA cohort of patients, but there was no difference in Karnofsky Performance Scale scores. Those patients with neurologic deficits that had not been responsive to steroids were most at risk of postoperative decline. Over time, differences in NIH-SS scores between the two groups became nonsignificant, and the cumulative incidence of repeat surgery was significantly less in the 5-ALA group.[12]

Whether 5-ALA–induced fluorescence could help in the detection of anaplastic foci in diffusely infiltrating gliomas without significant contrast-enhancement on MRI was investigated in a series of 17 patients. Eight of nine patients whose histology was that of World Health Organization (WHO) grade III tumor had focal areas of fluorescence, whereas all eight patients with WHO grade II tumors did not. Focal areas of fluo-

> **Special Consideration**
>
> - Besides high-grade gliomas, relatively few low-grade gliomas, about 80% of meningiomas, and some metastatic tumors show visible 5-ALA fluorescence.

rescence were found to be topographically correlated with ^{11}C-methionine positron emission tomography (PET), and MIB-1 labeling index was significantly higher in fluorescing tissue.[13]

Increasing utilization of this PpIX fluorescence–guided technology has been associated with continued improvement in rates of complete resection of tumor. A recent report described no residual contrast-enhancing tumor > 0.175 cc in 51 of 53 patients (96%) and no residual enhancement in 89%,[14] results that certainly raise the bar. Another recent report focused on 52 patients with no residual contrast-enhancement on postoperative MRI and confirmed the favorable prognosis associated with no residual fluorescence at the close of surgery. Median survival in patients without residual fluorescence was 27 months, and that in patients with residual fluorescence was 17.5 months.[15]

All of the above series as well as most of the currently published data use subjectively assessed, visible fluorescence as visualized through one of two commercially available adapted microscopes. Quantitative measurement of PpIX levels in intracranial tumors has also been investigated. Intrinsic optical properties of tissue, including absorption and scattering, have major effects on visualization of fluorescence, and algorithms utilizing spectroscopic information can improve assessment

> **Pitfall**
>
> - Visual PpIX fluorescence tells the surgeon only about the exposed surface of the tumor; a tumor that is more than 0.25 mm below the surface or covered in blood will not be detected.

of intraoperative tissue. One series using such technology and a fiberoptic probe that could interrogate a focal region of the surgical field over several seconds demonstrated substantially improved diagnostic performance. In a group of 14 patients with diagnoses of low- or high-grade glioma, meningioma, or metastasis, significant differences in PpIX concentration were found in all tumor types compared with normal brain. Receiver operating characteristic (ROC) curve analysis showed a classification efficiency of 87% (area under the curve [AUC] = 0.95, specificity = 92%, sensitivity = 84%) using a quantitative probe versus a classification efficiency of 66% using conventional, qualitative fluorescence imaging (AUC = 0.73, specificity = 100%, sensitivity = 47%); 81% of quantitative measurements of tissue whose fluorescence was below the surgeon's visual perception were correctly classified in this series.[16]

More recently, more sensitive quantitative methodologies have been developed that employ wide-field imaging through the operating microscope, which is a more user-friendly and more efficient technology than the above probe. Such a methodology in which spectrally resolved data can be converted into images of absolute fluorophore concentration pixel by pixel across the surgical field has been shown to be linear, accurate, and precise relative to true values.[17] The ability to do this with multiple fluorophores simultaneously has intriguing potential as new fluorophores further develop.

Fluorescein Fluorescence

Although the last decade has seen great interest in fluorescence guidance for cranial tumor resection, particularly using ALA-induced PpIX fluorescence, the use of fluorescence for neurosurgical guidance dates back to the work in 1948 using a Wood's lamp for visualization of fluorescein in multiple tumor types including gliomas, meningiomas, and metastatic carcinomas.[18] Fluorescein is a visible fluorophore with a main excitation peak at approximately 490 nanometers (nm; visible range approximately 400 to 550 nm) and a main emission peak at approximately 520 nm (visible range approximately 480 to 650 nm) (**Fig. 12.3**). Patients usually receive a dose of 200 to 1,000 g of intravenous (IV) fluorescein. More recently, various groups have utilized surgical microscopes modified for fluorescein imaging. One group visualized fluorescein staining

of metastatic tumors under white light,[19] and another modified a Zeiss surgical microscope by adding a blue excitation filter and a long pass filter to enable visualization of green fluorescence from fluorescein in 10 patients with high-grade gliomas.[20] Various groups are using a commercial system (Zeiss OPMI, yellow 560 module) for excitation and visualization of green fluorescein fluorescence for resection of gliomas and metastases. These systems use a combination of excitation and long-pass emission filters, analogous to current clinical systems used for ALA-induced PpIX fluorescence, but optimized in the excitation and emission ranges of fluorescein.

Fluorescein accumulates in tissues via the enhanced permeability and retention (EPR) effect, and works as a blood pooling agent. As such, it is easily visualized in vasculature as well as in tissue with a broken blood–brain barrier (BBB). Nevertheless, the major biological limitation of fluorescein for tumor surgery is its nonspecific accumulation, such that areas of surgical injury with nonhomeostatic vessels will accumulate fluorescence, and edematous tissue has also been noted to accumulate green fluorescence.[21] Any region with blood pooling and a broken BBB will be similar. Optically, fluorescein requires excitation in the violet-blue range of the spectrum with emission in the green range. This means only superficial levels of fluorescein can be visualized as a result of limited penetration of excitation and emission of light through tissues.

Indocyanine Green

Indocyanine green (ICG) is a compound that is functionally similar to fluorescein, enabling effective visualization of blood flow. It binds plasma proteins and travels through the vascular compartments. Accumulation in tissue depends on the EPR effect and blood flow distribution, and as such, it encounters the same limitations in terms of specificity in tumor surgery. Furthermore, ICG is large enough that it does not freely cross the BBB, but rather accumulates in vessels and via the EPR effect in BBB-deficient tumors. Indocyanine green, unlike fluorescein or PpIX, is a solely near-infrared (NIR) agent, with a main excitation peak at 800 nm and a main emission peak at 830 nm. The NIR agents have the main advantage of allowing deeper visualization of tissue due to improved penetration of excitation and emission of light through tissue. Increased penetration results in decreased attenuation of light at the excitation and emission wavelengths. Nevertheless, NIR compounds cannot be visualized by the human eye and require camera detection for visualization.

Indocyanine green can be given as an IV dose of 25 mg in 5 mL of normal saline. Indocyanine green fluorescence contrast has been reported to aid in distinguishing normal brain from tumor tissues, specifically in malignant astrocytomas.[22] Others studies found ICG videoangiography particularly useful during tumor surgery (e.g., for meningiomas, gliomas, metastases) for delineation of major vessels, and suggested it as

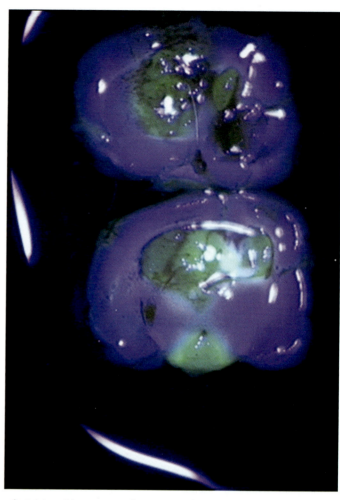

a

b

Fig. 12.3a,b Fluorescein fluorescence. **(a)** White light image through the operating microscope of a freshly prepared brain slice with a central nervous system-1 (CNS-1) tumor, from a rat that had been administered intravenous fluorescein. **(b)** The same field of view under blue light excitation, with readily distinguished tumor.

a possible alternative tool to Doppler or intraoperative angiography.[23,24] Some recent studies further exploited ICG accumulation in vessels to visualize 12 pituitary tumors, with mixed results.[25] Clinical studies have used both systems built in-house as well as readily available commercial systems (Zeiss OPMI Pentero 900).

To summarize, both ICG and fluorescein perform similar functions as nonspecific, nontargeted fluorescent agents for blood flow and blood pooling as well as EPR-dependent tissue accumulation. Further studies are required to fully characterize their diagnostic capabilities, yet an understanding of their biological mechanism may inform the neurosurgeon. The neurosurgeon can be critical regarding their use as "tumor targeting" agents, as advocated by some recent studies, as a result of the known limitations in specificity and positive predictive values.[21] Fluorescein functions as a visible fluorophore for imaging at the tissue surface, and ICG functions as an NIR agent for both superficial and deep imaging of tissue. More studies are required to further understand the role of these

Pitfall

- Both ICG and fluorescein perform similar functions as nonspecific, nontargeted fluorescent agents for blood flow, BBB, and blood pooling, but their clinical applicability in aiding tumor surgery has yet to be defined.

two compounds as surgical adjuncts for resection of brain tumors, with current justification of a role in blood flow and vessel assessment, but a less defined role, secondary to low specificity for tumor, as tumor-specific agents.

Confocal Fluorescence Imaging

The techniques for fluorescence guidance noted thus far utilize surgical microscopes, endoscopes, and point spectroscopy

Special Consideration

- The use of handheld confocal fluorescence probes for in vivo fluorescence imaging of tissue architecture at the cellular level is promising and may ultimately prove a useful adjunct to the neuropathologist in replacing frozen section diagnosis.

probes for macroscopic imaging and detection, with resolution of > 1 mm. A recent development is the use of handheld confocal fluorescence probes for in vivo fluorescence imaging of tissue architecture at the cellular level. Recent work has used a commercial handheld confocal microscope probe for both fluorescein[26] and ALA-induced PpIX fluorescence.[27] This embodiment of intraoperative confocal microscope scans approximately 1 frame per second [475 × 475 field of view (x,y)] with 488-nm excitation light enabling visualization of cellular architecture with micrometer resolution, compared to macroscopic fluorescence techniques using spectroscopy probes and surgical microscopes. The ability to acquire cellular-level images intraoperatively in living tissue is powerful, although using this technique generally requires the participation of a neuropathologist skilled in image interpretation. Experience and validation in interpretation of this image information is required. Limitations include the submillimeter field of view in both the (x,y) and z (i.e., depth) directions, requiring multiple single-point interrogations to examine a broad field of view. Unlike spectroscopic probes that perform spectrally resolved detection and as such can resolve multiple fluorophores simultaneously, current implementations of confocal probes can perform only single fluorophore detection using long-pass/bandpass filters. Nevertheless, the potential for this technology to complement and possibly replace conventional frozen section methodologies renders it of considerable interest.

Optical Spectroscopy Probes

The field of biomedical optics and optical engineering has for years exploited the diagnostic value of tissue optical properties (i.e., absorption and scattering). Light exhibits a well-known wavelength dependent attenuation in tissue. Various tissue components, including oxy- and deoxyhemoglobin, as well as cell density impact the degree and quality of light absorption and scattering observed in tissue. Pathophysiological changes that occur in tumor, such as angiogenesis, cellular proliferation, and hypoxia, impact the degree and intensity of intrinsic tissue optical properties (i.e., hemoglobin concentration and oxygen saturation). These optical properties have the potential to be used as a diagnostic biomarker(s).

Multiple optical spectroscopy probes have been used for diffuse reflectance detection. Briefly, tissue is interrogated with white light, and the diffusely reflected light is collected into a spectrometer, which enables spectrally resolved detection, that is, collection of full reflectance spectra at nanometer resolutions. The shape and magnitude of the diffusely reflected light will be a function of tissue optical properties (i.e., absorption and scattering). Spectroscopy probes have also combined spectrally resolved fluorescence and diffuse reflectance detection as tools for improved tumor surgery. Some work using both tissue autofluorescence and diffuse reflectance spectral information in an empirical algorithm to distinguish between tumor and normal parenchyma showed an overall decrease in the diffuse reflectance signal in tumors.[28] Subsequent work by the same group combined spectral information from tissue autofluorescence and diffuse reflectance with reported sensitivities and specificities > 80% for detecting brain tumor tissue in more than 20 patients with gliomas and 11 control temporal lobe epilepsy patients.[29] They also reported similar results in a pediatric brain tumor cohort.[30] Advanced multivariate signal analysis techniques such as neural networks have been utilized on empirical autofluorescence and diffuse reflectance spectral information to help improve diagnostic accuracy in tumor tissue identification to better than 90%.[31]

Nevertheless, these techniques are highly empirical in nature. These studies search for an optimal spectral peak or combination of peaks that provide the highest diagnostic accuracy in limited cohorts. A recent study collected in vivo fluorescence and diffuse reflectance spectroscopy data following administration of ALA in patients with low- and high-grade glioma.[32] Unlike the previous empirical studies, this work applied a light transport model algorithm to quantitatively extract the absolute values of optical biomarkers, including oxy- and deoxyhemoglobin (i.e., hemoglobin concentration and oxygen saturation), parameters of cellular density (scattering parameters), and porphyrin levels (i.e., PpIX and associated photoproducts). These multiple biomarkers are predictive of pathophysiological changes occurring in tissue, and one could exploit their combined predictive values for improved diagnostic assessment. A multivariate, machine learning algorithm that combined the various biomarkers significantly improved diagnostic accuracies of greater than 90% for distinguishing tumor versus normal tissue compared to the use of individual spectral peaks.

In summary, optical spectroscopy techniques have the advantage of collecting spectrally resolved data from either fluorescence or diffuse reflectance. In the case of fluorescence, this enables resolution of multiple fluorophores with overlapping fluorescence spectra. The diffuse reflectance spectra provide information regarding endogenous changes in tissue that depend on factors such as blood flow (e.g., hemoglobin concentration) and tissue oxygenation (e.g., oxygen saturation) (**Fig. 12.4**). Further, such information can be used to quantify in vivo biomarkers that are predictive of pathophysiological changes. Nevertheless, these techniques currently interrogate small regions of tissue (e.g., ~1 mm²). Furthermore, optical

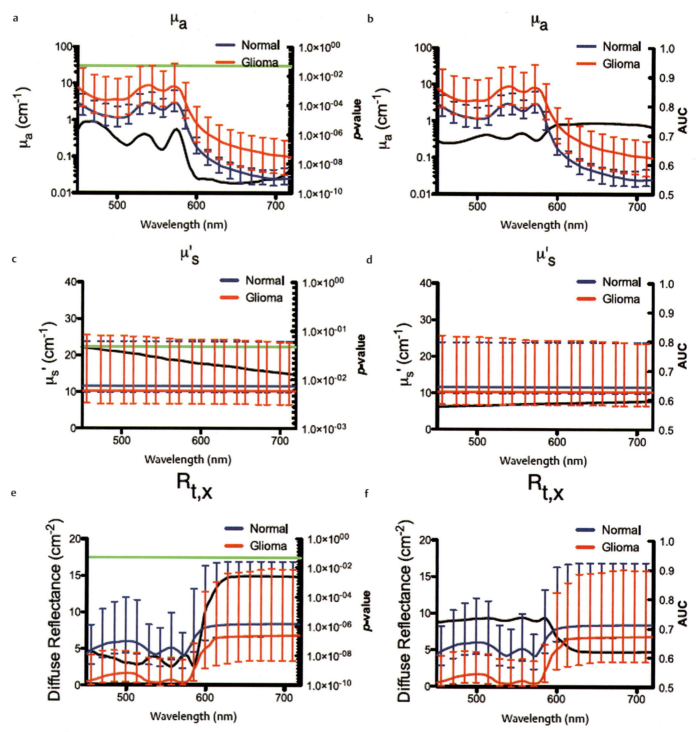

Fig. 12.4a–f Intraoperative diffuse reflectance spectroscopy spectra during glioma resection. An intraoperative probe was placed on tissue and the white light reflectance collected. A light transport model was applied to the white light reflectance to calculate the wavelength dependent **(a,b)** absorption ($\mu a(\lambda)$), **(c,d)** reduced scattering coefficients ($\mu s'(\lambda)$), and **(e,f)** model-fit diffuse reflectance ($Rt,x(\lambda)$) for tumor (*red*) and normal brain (*blue*). The median spectra for 264 spectra were calculated with error bars representing the interquartile range. Wavelength-specific *p*-values and receiver operating characteristic–derived area under the curve (AUC) values were calculated and shown in black. (From Valdés PA, Kim A, Leblond F, et al. Combined fluorescence and reflectance spectroscopy for in vivo quantification of cancer biomarkers in low- and high-grade glioma surgery. J Biomed Opt 2011;16:116007–7. Reproduced with permission.)

spectroscopy diagnostic studies have been performed on small patient cohorts, requiring additional validation of the diagnostic performance of these techniques.

Spatial Frequency Domain Imaging

Diffuse reflectance spectroscopy techniques take advantage of intrinsic tissue biomarkers that are predictive of physiological changes for surgical guidance, but as noted they have been limited by detection of a small area (~1 mm²). A recent development in biomedical optics is the use of spatial frequency domain or spatial light modulation imaging to quantify the same intrinsic optical biomarkers (hemoglobin, oxygen saturation, scattering parameters) across the full surgical field of view. This technique projects light at specific spatial frequencies and phases, collects the diffuse reflectance, and applies a model of light transport to quantify these markers.[33] Promising clinical results have been shown outside the brain, and a trial has been proposed for brain tumor surgical guidance.[34]

Near-Infrared Spectroscopy

Near-infrared spectroscopy (NIRS) is an optical technique that produces topographic 2D views of changes in cerebral cortex oxygenation. As such, it provides estimates of oxy- and de-oxyhemoglobin changes and total blood volume in tissue, similar to probe spectroscopy techniques. The difference lies in that this technique places multiple light sources and detectors on the patient's head. To enable sufficiently deep tissue penetration such as through skull, NIRS interrogates with near-infrared light (e.g., 780-, 805-, and 830-nm light sources). One study used NIRS as a means to monitor cortical oxygenation changes during cortical mapping, suggesting that it might serve a complementary role in monitoring physiological effects correlated with electrophysiological monitoring. This technique could also be used in conjunction with or complementary to functional magnetic resonance imaging (fMRI) and magnetoencephalography (MEG) for surgical planning,[35,36] as a noninvasive method to determine language lateralization,[37] or as an intraoperative method to further characterize gliomas.[38] This technique uses the same principles as diffuse reflectance spectroscopy in terms of biomarker optical contrast, but has the advantage that it can provide a 2D topographic view of blood flow and perfusion changes in vivo.

Infrared and Raman Spectroscopy and Imaging

Infrared (IR) and Raman techniques take advantage of the "vibrational fingerprints" intrinsic to the molecular milieu of

tissue. The physical basis for imaging contrast in IR techniques derives from absorption of IR electromagnetic radiation, which leads to vibrational energy changes in molecules that can be detected. Tumor tissue, which has a different molecular makeup than normal parenchyma, will have a distinct spectral signature in the IR spectrum. This difference derives from chemical structures with different vibrational energies both qualitatively and quantitatively.[39–41] For example, different electromagnetic bands in the IR spectra correlate with glycolipids, fatty acids, and lipid/protein ratios, and their intensities further correlate with the amount and proportion of these substances. Recent work on ex vivo brain tumors including gliomas and metastatic tumors[39–41] used multivariate analysis techniques (e.g., support vector machine [SVM], linear discriminant analysis [LDA]) to analyze IR spectra, achieving accuracies > 90%. These studies were limited in their ex vivo implementation, high acquisition time (> 5 minutes) per scan, and small field of view (cellular, micrometer level). Nevertheless, these are technological issues that could be optimized for intraoperative use. Further work would be required to better ascertain the diagnostic capabilities of these algorithms. Infrared spectroscopy provides yet another mode of optical contrast for tumor tissue identification that is in its infancy as an optical guidance technique.[42]

Raman techniques derive their contrast from scattering of light in which incident light induces a vibrational energy change in molecules and scattered light is emitted. Several ex vivo studies have used Raman techniques and multivariate analysis of data for diagnosis of multiple tumor types including pediatric tumors,[43] glioblastoma multiforme (GBM),[44] and meningioma.[45] This last study found a significant difference and contribution from nucleic acids in areas with more aggressive tumor cells. Similar to IR, Raman techniques have the potential to distinguish tissue based on intrinsic molecular makeup and "vibrational fingerprint." Currently, clinical applications are usually performed ex vivo, but recent developments in preclinical studies have demonstrated in vivo imaging.

Optical Coherence Tomography

Optical coherence tomography (OCT) is an optical imaging technique that uses back-scattered or back-reflected light from tissue as a means of imaging contrast, analogous to the use of sound waves in ultrasound.[46] In OCT, light is backscattered from tissue as a function of the endogenous optical properties of tissue structures. Contrast in OCT is sensitive to differences in the index of refraction of optical scattering, and because tissues are highly scattering, this limits OCT depths to a scale of millimeters. Optical coherence tomography enables in vivo, 3D, micrometer resolution images at the cellular level and can be done in real time. One study used in vivo OCT for microstructural imaging during brain tumor resection in nine patients.[47] Others have used handheld devices such as fiber optic probes, endoscopes, and modified neurosurgical microscopes.[48] This technique has the advantage of exploiting intrinsic optical contrast without the need for exogenous administration of drugs like ALA. It also provides physiological as well as micrometer architectural information, but is limited in its penetration depth and in the extent of molecular identification it can provide; thus, it does not provide molecular "fingerprints" like Raman or IR.

■ Electric Impedance

Electric impedance (EI) as a mode of contrast uses the principle of opposition to current flow in tissue, measured as the ratio of voltage over current flow, which depends on the makeup of brain tissue including myelin, fluid, and cell density, among other important factors. The utility of dynamic assessment of changes in EI has been suggested as a means to distinguish and localize tumor tissue.[49] Another study using CT-guided tumor biopsies and an EI probe noted the correlation of EI differences as a function of changing densities on CT. Low-density lesions like cystic areas demonstrated decreased impedance, whereas high-density lesions like ring-enhancing tumor demonstrated increased impedance. As such, monitoring of impedance changes would inform the neurosurgeon regarding tissue densities along a biopsy needle trajectory.[50] Electric impedance offers another mode of contrast that requires further development as a technique for tumor localization in neurosurgery.

■ Conclusion

There are numerous technologies employing a variety of modes of contrast that have been utilized or are in development for neurosurgical localization of brain tumors (**Table 12.1**). The majority of these techniques exploit principles of biomedical optics, including fluorescence, diffuse reflectance, IR, and Raman principles. All the techniques presented exploit endogenous sources of contrast like hemoglobin concentration, with the exception of fluorescence techniques, which

Table 12.1 Technologies of Differing Levels of Maturity and Tissue Scale that Have Been Utilized to Characterize and Differentiate Tissue Within the Operative Field

Technology	Resolution	Mode of Contrast	Mechanism/Biology	Ease of Use	Stage of Development
Ultrasound	Several mm	Acoustic	Tissue density	+	Mature
5-ALA	mm	Fluorescence	Substrate delivery and tissue metabolism	++	Adolescent
Fluorescein	mm	Fluorescence	Blood flow and enhanced permeability retention	++	Adolescent
ICG	mm	Fluorescence	Blood flow and enhanced permeability retention	+	Adolescent
Confocal	μm	Fluorescence	Dependent on fluorophore	+/−	Investigational
Optical spectroscopy	mm	Tissue optical properties	Chromophore levels, cellular density, etc.	+	Investigational
Spatial frequency domain	mm	Tissue optical properties	Chromophore levels, cellular density, etc.	+/−	Investigational
NIRS	Several mm–cm	Tissue optical properties	Oxy- and deoxyhemoglobin	−	Investigational
OCT	μm	Tissue optical properties	Chromophore levels, cellular density, etc.	+/−	Investigational
Infrared	μm	Electromagnetic vibrational absorption	Chemical composition	−	Investigational
Raman	μm	Electromagnetic vibrational scattering	Chemical composition	−	Investigational
Electrical impedance	mm	Electrical impedance	Tissue electrical properties	+	Investigational

Abbreviations: 5-ALA, 5-aminolevulinic acid; ICG, indocyanine green; NIRS, near-infrared spectroscopy; OCT, optical coherence tomography.

use either exogenous drug (e.g., ALA-induced PpIX, fluorescein), endogenous fluorophores (autofluorescence), or both. Additional work is required to validate and translate most of these techniques into daily neurosurgical practice, but with the computational resources available in the operating room environment today, active technological and investigative work is in progress.

Editor's Note

In the past, before the availability of surgical navigation based on archived imaging and ultimately real-time high-resolution intraoperative imaging, finding a tumor was generally a challenge for neurosurgeons. Thus, ultrasound represented an important innovation for neurosurgeons and their patients when it became available. It was another example of "necessity being the mother of invention" and also of the ingenuity of neurosurgeons. Now, with the marriage of ultrasound and navigation systems, it is still a valued tool for many surgeons. Another interesting such innovation is 5-ALA. If a surgeon is a strong believer in the real importance of radical resection of gliomas, and there is mounting non–class I evidence to support it, this is an important adjunct for a surgeon to have. The other modalities described in this chapter are in the experimental stage, and it will be interesting to see if they become clinically useful tools for helping the surgeon find the tumor edges and do as maximal a resection as possible. (Bernstein)

References

1. Dohrmann GJ, Rubin JM. Dynamic intraoperative imaging and instrumentation of brain and spinal cord using ultrasound. Neurol Clin 1985,3,425–437
2. Chandler WF, Knake JE. Intraoperative use of ultrasound in neurosurgery. Clin Neurosurg 1983;31:550–563
3. Grode ML, Komaiko MS. The role of intraoperative ultrasound in neurosurgery. Neurosurgery 1983;12:624–628
4. Koivukangas J, Louhisalmi Y, Alakuijala J, Oikarinen J. Ultrasound-controlled neuronavigator-guided brain surgery. J Neurosurg 1993;79:36–42
5. Ji S, Wu Z, Hartov A, Roberts DW, Paulsen KD. Mutual-information-based image to patient re-registration using intraoperative ultrasound in image-guided neurosurgery. Med Phys 2008;35:4612–4624
6. Unsgaard G, Rygh OM, Selbekk T, et al. Intra-operative 3D ultrasound in neurosurgery. Acta Neurochir (Wien) 2006;148:235–253, discussion 253
7. Bozinov O, Burkhardt JK, Fischer CM, Kockro RA, Bernays RL, Bertalanffy H. Advantages and limitations of intraoperative 3D ultrasound in neurosurgery. Technical note. Acta Neurochir Suppl (Wien) 2011;109:191–196
8. Unsgård G, Solheim O, Lindseth F, Selbekk T. Intra-operative imaging with 3D ultrasound in neurosurgery. Acta Neurochir Suppl (Wien) 2011;109:181–186
9. Stummer W, Stocker S, Novotny A, et al. In vitro and in vivo porphyrin accumulation by C6 glioma cells after exposure to 5-aminolevulinic acid. J Photochem Photobiol B 1998;45:160–169
10. Stummer W, Novotny A, Stepp H, Goetz C, Bise K, Reulen HJ. Fluorescence-guided resection of glioblastoma multiforme by using 5-aminolevulinic acid-induced porphyrins: a prospective study in 52 consecutive patients. J Neurosurg 2000;93:1003–1013
11. Stummer W, Pichlmeier U, Meinel T, Wiestler OD, Zanella F, Reulen HJ; ALA-Glioma Study Group. Fluorescence-guided surgery with 5-aminolevulinic acid for resection of malignant glioma: a randomised controlled multicentre phase III trial. Lancet Oncol 2006;7:392–401
12. Stummer W, Tonn JC, Mehdorn HM, et al; ALA-Glioma Study Group. Counterbalancing risks and gains from extended resections in malignant glioma surgery: a supplemental analysis from the randomized 5-aminolevulinic acid glioma resection study. Clinical article. J Neurosurg 2011;114:613–623
13. Widhalm G, Wolfsberger S, Minchev G, et al. 5-Aminolevulinic acid is a promising marker for detection of anaplastic foci in diffusely infiltrating gliomas with nonsignificant contrast enhancement. Cancer 2010;116:1545–1552
14. Schucht P, Beck J, Abu-Isa J, et al. Gross total resection rates in contemporary glioblastoma surgery: results of an institutional protocol combining 5-aminolevulinic acid intraoperative fluorescence imaging and brain mapping. Neurosurgery 2012;71:927–935, discussion 935–936
15. Aldave G, Tejada S, Pay E et al. Prognostic value of residual fluorescent tissue in glioblastoma patients after gross total resection in 5-ALA guided surgery. Neurosurgery 2013;72:915–921
16. Valdés PA, Leblond F, Kim A, et al. Quantitative fluorescence in intracranial tumor: implications for ALA-induced PpIX as an intraoperative biomarker. J Neurosurg 2011;115:11–17
17. Valdés PA, Leblond F, Jacobs VL, Wilson BC, Paulsen KD, Roberts DW. Quantitative, spectrally-resolved intraoperative fluorescence imaging. Sci Rep 2012;2:798
18. Moore GE, Peyton WT, et al. The clinical use of fluorescein in neurosurgery; the localization of brain tumors. J Neurosurg 1948;5:392–398
19. Okuda T, Kataoka K, Taneda M. Metastatic brain tumor surgery using fluorescein sodium: technical note. Minim Invasive Neurosurg 2007;50:382–384
20. Kuroiwa T, Kajimoto Y, Ohta T. Development of a fluorescein operative microscope for use during malignant glioma surgery: a technical note and preliminary report. Surg Neurol 1998;50:41–48, discussion 48–49
21. Stummer W. Fluorescein for vascular and oncological neurosurgery. Acta Neurochir (Wien) 2013;155:1477–1478 (Letter)
22. Haglund MM, Berger MS, Hochman DW. Enhanced optical imaging of human gliomas and tumor margins. Neurosurgery 1996;38:308–317
23. Kim EH, Cho JM, Chang JH, Kim SH, Lee KS. Application of intraoperative indocyanine green videoangiography to brain tumor surgery. Acta Neurochir (Wien) 2011;153:1487–1495, discussion 1494–1495
24. Ferroli P, Acerbi F, Albanese E, et al. Application of intraoperative indocyanine green angiography for CNS tumors: results on the first 100 cases. Acta Neurochir Suppl (Wien) 2011;109:251–257
25. Litvack ZN, Zada G, Laws ER Jr. Indocyanine green fluorescence endoscopy for visual differentiation of pituitary tumor from surrounding structures. J Neurosurg 2012;116:935–941

26. Eschbacher J, Martirosyan NL, Nakaji P, et al. In vivo intraoperative confocal microscopy for real-time histopathological imaging of brain tumors. J Neurosurg 2012;116:854–860

27. Sanai N, Snyder LA, Honea NJ, et al. Intraoperative confocal microscopy in the visualization of 5-aminolevulinic acid fluorescence in low-grade gliomas. J Neurosurg 2011;115:740–748

28. Lin WC, Toms SA, Johnson M, Jansen ED, Mahadevan-Jansen A. In vivo brain tumor demarcation using optical spectroscopy. Photochem Photobiol 2001;73:396–402

29. Toms SA, Lin WC, Weil RJ, Johnson MD, Jansen ED, Mahadevan-Jansen A. Intraoperative optical spectroscopy identifies infiltrating glioma margins with high sensitivity. Neurosurgery 2005;57(4, Suppl):382–391, discussion 382–391

30. Lin WC, Sandberg DI, Bhatia S, Johnson M, Oh S, Ragheb J. Diffuse reflectance spectroscopy for in vivo pediatric brain tumor detection. J Biomed Opt 2010;15:061709

31. Sivaramakrishnan A, Graupe D. Brain tumor demarcation by applying a LAMSTAR neural network to spectroscopy data. Neurol Res 2004;26:613–621

32. Valdés PA, Kim A, Leblond F, et al. Combined fluorescence and reflectance spectroscopy for in vivo quantification of cancer biomarkers in low- and high-grade glioma surgery. J Biomed Opt 2011;16:116007-7–116007-14

33. Konecky SD, Owen CM, Rice T, et al. Spatial frequency domain tomography of protoporphyrin IX fluorescence in preclinical glioma models. J Biomed Opt 2012;17:056008

34. Monitoring Neural Tissues Properties by Modulated Imaging (MI). ClinicalTrials.gov Identifier: NCT00555711. 2013 http://clinicaltrials.gov/ct2/show/NCT00555711

35. Hoshino T, Sakatani K, Katayama Y, et al. Application of multichannel near-infrared spectroscopic topography to physiological monitoring of the cortex during cortical mapping: technical case report. Surg Neurol 2005;64:272–275

36. Sakatani K, Murata Y, Fujiwara N, et al. Comparison of blood-oxygen-level-dependent functional magnetic resonance imaging and near-infrared spectroscopy recording during functional brain activation in patients with stroke and brain tumors. J Biomed Opt 2007;12:062110

37. Ota T, Kamada K, Kawai K, Yumoto M, Aoki S, Saito N. Refined analysis of complex language representations by non-invasive neuroimaging techniques. Br J Neurosurg 2011;25:197–202

38. Asgari S, Röhrborn HJ, Engelhorn T, Stolke D. Intra-operative characterization of gliomas by near-infrared spectroscopy: possible association with prognosis. Acta Neurochir (Wien) 2003;145:453–459, discussion 459–460

39. Bergner N, Romeike BF, Reichart R, Kalff R, Krafft C, Popp J. Tumor margin identification and prediction of the primary tumor from brain metastases using FTIR imaging and support vector machines. Analyst (Lond) 2013;138:3983–3990

40. Krafft C, Sobottka SB, Geiger KD, Schackert G, Salzer R. Classification of malignant gliomas by infrared spectroscopic imaging and linear discriminant analysis. Anal Bioanal Chem 2007;387:1669–1677

41. Krafft C, Thümmler K, Sobottka SB, Schackert G, Salzer R. Classification of malignant gliomas by infrared spectroscopy and linear discriminant analysis. Biopolymers 2006;82:301–305

42. Meyer T, Bergner N, Bielecki C, et al. Nonlinear microscopy, infrared, and Raman microspectroscopy for brain tumor analysis. J Biomed Opt 2011;16:021113

43. Leslie DG, Kast RE, Poulik JM, et al. Identification of pediatric brain neoplasms using Raman spectroscopy. Pediatr Neurosurg 2012;48:109–117

44. Krafft C, Belay B, Bergner N, et al. Advances in optical biopsy—correlation of malignancy and cell density of primary brain tumors using Raman microspectroscopic imaging. Analyst (Lond) 2012;137:5533–5537

45. Zhou Y, Liu CH, Sun Y, et al. Human brain cancer studied by resonance Raman spectroscopy. J Biomed Opt 2012;17:116021

46. Fujimoto JG, Pitris C, Boppart SA, Brezinski ME. Optical coherence tomography: an emerging technology for biomedical imaging and optical biopsy. Neoplasia 2000;2:9–25

47. Böhringer HJ, Lankenau E, Stellmacher F, Reusche E, Hüttmann G, Giese A. Imaging of human brain tumor tissue by near-infrared laser coherence tomography. Acta Neurochir (Wien) 2009;151:507–517, discussion 517

48. Böhringer HJ, Lankenau E, Rohde V, Hüttmann G, Giese A. Optical coherence tomography for experimental neuroendoscopy. Minim Invasive Neurosurg 2006;49:269–275

49. Organ L, Tasker RR, Moody NF. Brain tumor localization using an electrical impedance technique. J Neurosurg 1968;28:35–44

50. Bullard DE, Makachinas TT. Measurement of tissue impedence in conjunction with computed tomography-guided stereotaxic biopsies. J Neurol Neurosurg Psychiatry 1987;50:43–51

13 Endoscopic Approaches

Jennifer Moliterno Gunel, Mark M. Souweidane, and Theodore H. Schwartz

Over the last two decades, the use of the endoscope has become increasingly popular for approaching skull base and intraventricular tumors, as well as for serving as an adjunct and alternative for other intracranial tumor microsurgery. The endoscope increases the field of view of the microscope by advancing the lens and light source into the surgical cavity, permitting visualization around corners. Several factors have contributed to the growth and success of endoscopic surgery, including advances in available fiber optic equipment and specialized surgical instruments, as well as the fostering of collaborative efforts between rhinologic and neurologic surgeons.

Endoscopic Endonasal Skull Base and Pituitary Surgery

Intracranial tumors involving the skull base have been traditionally approached via transfacial and transcranial surgery and can be associated with relatively high morbidity and long recovery times. Although these approaches offer wide exposure and working space, performing brain retraction, neurovascular manipulation, sinus obliteration, and wound healing, and maintaining good cosmesis remain significant issues. The endoscope has enabled the transsphenoidal approach, as well as the advent of extended approaches, to serve as less invasive ways to manage a variety of intra- and extracranial neoplasms. The keys to performing successful endoscopic skull base surgery include an experienced surgical team, appropriate instrumentation, adequate operative resources (e.g., neuronavigation), and careful case selection. Stereotactic navigation is a standard in all endoscopic endonasal skull base surgeries.

The importance of careful case selection cannot be emphasized enough and is critical to ensuring the success of the operation. Pathology extending laterally over the orbits or behind and lateral to the carotid arteries, for instance, can be quite difficult to remove even with extended approaches. Likewise, lesions extending into or just behind the frontal sinus can prove difficult to reach even with angled scopes, and the closure of the resulting defects can be quite challenging. Although cavernous sinus invasion is not an absolute contraindication, it warrants careful preoperative evaluation of surgical goals. The surgeon may elect to enter the cavernous sinus to resect the tumor using a safer approach medial and posterior to the carotid artery or a riskier lateral and anterior

approach, understanding the additional risks to the neurovascular contents, or may opt for an intentional subtotal resection with planned stereotactic radiotherapy postoperatively, depending on the pathology. Finally, the differential diagnosis for masses of the sella can be quite vast, including pathology that would not benefit from endonasal surgery such as large cavernous segment aneurysms and exquisitely radiosensitive tumors. Such lesions can often be discovered preoperatively and may require a very different workup.

The endonasal skull base approaches can be classified based on which nasal sinus is opened to access the pathology and the ultimate target to be reached.[1] The available sinuses are the sphenoid, ethmoid, maxillary, and frontal. Each sinus can be utilized to access a different region of the midline and paramedian skull base, and these corridors can also be combined together for larger, multicompartmental tumors (**Table 13.1**). In addition, it is possible to merge the endonasal skull base approaches with the transcranial approaches for large multicompartmental tumors in either a combined or staged manner.

Transsphenoidal Corridor

The transsphenoidal corridor can be used to access the sella for pituitary tumors and small Rathke cleft cysts, and can also be extended superiorly, inferiorly, and laterally to reach the suprasellar cistern, the top one third of the clivus, and the medial cavernous sinus and medial optic canal, respectively. With these extended approaches, the range of suitable pathology increases to include craniopharyngiomas, meningiomas, chordomas, and chondrosarcomas. Pathology in this region can often remain clinically silent or cause symptoms of local mass effect on the brain or optic apparatus, commonly resulting in hypothalamic-pituitary dysfunction and visual deficits. Preoperative endocrinologic and ophthalmologic assessments are imperative in patients with parasellar pathology.

Table 13.1 Endonasal Skull Base Approaches

Corridor	Approach	Target
Transsphenoidal	Transsellar	Pituitary gland
	Transplanum, transtuberculum	Suprasellar cistern
	Transclival	Upper one third of clivus
	Transcavernous	Medial cavernous sinus
	Transcanalicular	Medial optic canal
Transnasal	Transcribriform	Olfactory groove
	Transclival	Lower two thirds of clivus and petrous apex
	Transodontoid	Craniovertebral junction
Transethmoidal	Transfovea ethmoidalis	Anterior fossa
	Transorbital	Medial orbit
	Transsphenoidal	Lateral cavernous sinus
Transfrontal	Transfrontal	Anterior fossa
Transmaxillary	Transpterygoidal	Pterygopalatine fossa
		Infratemporal fossa
		Lateral sphenoid sinus
		Lateral cavernous sinus
		Meckel's cave

Transsellar Approach

The transsellar approach is reserved for pituitary microadenomas, macroadenomas with minimal suprasellar or cavernous invasion (generally < 2.5 cm in diameter), and intrasellar Rathke cleft cysts. For intrasellar pathology, endoscopic endonasal approach (EEA) results are generally no better than those reported using transsphenoidal microscopic techniques, because the pathology is directly in front of the surgeon and the increased field of view offers no significant advantage. This is particularly true for microadenomas. A large review of 200 patients with micro- and macroadenomas demonstrated comparable rates of gross total resection (GTR) as measured against large historical microscopic series.[2] However, several studies have demonstrated that the use of endoscopy enables additional pituitary tumor removal following microscopic-assisted removal, indicating a clear role in increasing the extent of resection.[3] Similarly, for macroadenomas, the EEA clearly appears to increase the extent of resection.

Because the majority of hormone-producing adenomas are small, the results of EEA for hormone restoration are comparable to those achieved with a microscope. However, a study of 120 patients with functioning adenomas found the hypersecretion remission rate was significantly better in the EEA group (63%) than in the microsurgical group (50%).[4] Similarly, another large series reported 71% biochemical cure in growth hormone (GH)-secreting adenomas, in addition to 81% and 88% remission rates in Cushing's disease and prolactinomas, respectively.[5] Approximately 80 to 100% of patients with prolactinomas can be afforded endocrinologic remission (i.e., postoperative prolactin levels < 20 ng/mL in females or < 15 ng/mL in males).[6] Approximately 52 to 84% of patients

with acromegaly can also achieve endocrinologic cure with surgery.[6]

The EEA for Rathke cleft cysts (RCCs) has also shown excellent results. One study reported two recurrences in 23 symptomatic patients who underwent cyst drainage and partial wall resection.[7] All patients with visual impairments improved postoperatively with half of the patients experiencing improvement in preoperative pituitary dysfunction as well. Although the transsphenoidal approach currently remains the preferred approach for symptomatic RCCs, whether or not removal of the cyst wall is necessary remains debatable. Cyst wall excision increases the rate of diabetes insipidus and hypopituitarism but may decrease rates of recurrence when done safely.

Transplanum, Transtuberculum Approach

The transplanum, transtuberculum approach can be used to expose the suprasellar cistern to remove giant macroadenomas with significant suprasellar extent (> 1 cm above the jugum), as well as craniopharyngiomas and planum and tuberculum meningiomas. Harvesting a nasoseptal flap at the beginning of the operation is important because significant cerebrospinal fluid (CSF) leak is expected (see below). Placement of a lumbar drain at the start of the procedure has been shown to significantly prevent intraoperative CSF leaks.[8] Case selection is especially critical because tumors that extend lateral to the anterior clinoids and > 1 cm past the lateral wall of the carotid artery may not be suitable for EEA. Some practitioners have cautioned against endonasal resection of meningiomas that encase arteries or that are without evidence of a

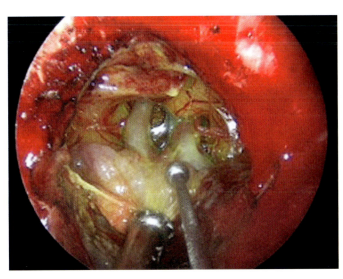

Fig. 13.1 An intraoperative image of the endoscopic removal of a planum meningioma, highlighting the dissection off the anterior communicating artery complex.

cortical cuff between the tumor and the anterior communicating artery,[9] but these are relative contraindications and can be overcome with advanced bimanual microsurgical dissection technique (**Fig. 13.1**). Another potential indication is the "hypophyseal transposition" or "hypophysopexy," whereby the pituitary gland is mobilized with a fat graft away from unresectable tumor in the cavernous sinus to protect the gland from the deleterious effects of stereotactic radiosurgery.[10]

Giant pituitary macroadenomas have generally been defined as > 4 cm in diameter, and more recently a 10 cm³ volumetric definition has been used.[11] A recent meta-analysis found significantly higher rates of GTR in patients with macroadenomas who underwent EEA resection compared to those who underwent transcranial or transsphenoidal microscopic surgery.[12] Specifically, GTR was achieved in 9.6% of patients undergoing open transcranial resection, with 82% of patients experiencing complications including permanent diabetes insipidus (9.1%), hypopituitarism (9.1%), CSF leak (7.1%), and cerebral infarcts (6.1%).[12] Conversely, GTR was achieved in 47.2% of patients undergoing EEA resection, and use of the endoscope was associated with a slightly lower overall complication rate (78.2%). A similar rate of GTR (40%) has also been reported in patients with the endoscopic removal of tumors greater than 10 cm³.[11] Compared to open and transsphenoidal microscopic surgery, respectively, EEA was associated with a significantly higher rate of improved visual outcomes (40% vs 34.8% vs 91.1%), lower recurrence rate (30% vs 20% vs 2.1%), and lower rate of hypopituitarism (9.1% vs 9.5% vs 1.06%).[12]

Craniopharyngiomas can be confined to the sella or can have significant suprasellar extension. The rates of GTR following EEA for craniopharyngiomas are, on average, 67%.[13] In a recent systematic review of the literature, endoscopic resection of craniopharyngiomas yielded significantly greater rates

of GTR than open surgery (66.9% vs 48.3%) and improved visual outcomes (56.2% and 33.1%). Recurrence rates were significantly lower in the transsphenoidal groups compared to open surgery. Although CSF leak rates were greater in the endoscopic (18.4%) and transsphenoidal microscopic (9%) groups compared with the open cohort (2.6%), more recent EEA series have reported rates of CSF leak of 3.8%.[14] Seizures, although absent in the endonasal groups, occurred in 8.5% of patients undergoing open surgery. The rate of permanent diabetes insipidus was significantly greater in the transcranial cohort (54.8%) compared to those patients who underwent endoscopic (27.7%) and transsphenoidal microscopic surgery (31.7%), whereas the rate of panhypopituitarism was lowest in the latter group.[13]

Meningiomas are perhaps the most controversial tumors removed by endonasal endoscopic surgeons. This arises from the widely held belief, based on Simpson grading, that the goal of meningioma surgery is complete resection (i.e., Simpson grade 1), including the removal of all involved dura and bone,[15] which some contend cannot be achieved via endonasal surgery.[16] Recent literature, however, suggests that the Simpson grade may not be a significant predictor of recurrence-free survival for skull base tumors in the modern neurosurgical era.[17] Nonetheless, advanced EEA techniques now permit more aggressive surgical removal of the planum sphenoidale, as well as opening of the medial optic canal to facilitate Simpson grade 1 results comparable to those achieved through a craniotomy.[18]

Results also vary based on the specific location of the meningioma. As recently demonstrated in a systematic review of the literature, the extent of resection is higher for planum and tuberculum tumors than for olfactory groove meningiomas, and thus the former location may be more suitable for EEA resection.[19] Meningiomas can characteristically cause hyperostosis in adjacent bone, and, in many such cases, invade the bone, often serving as the primary site of recurrence for anterior skull base meningiomas. One advantage of the EEA is that removal of any infiltrated or hyperostotic bone at the cranial base is integral to the approach. Another distinct advantage is the ability to devascularize the tumor early in the operation by controlling the ethmoidal arteries, which usually constitute the main blood supply. This is often not possible until later in the resection using transcranial approaches.

Perhaps the most significant advantage of the EEA for tuberculum and planum meningiomas is the ability to remove the tumor with minimal manipulation of the optic nerves.

Pearl

- Extension of the transsphenoidal EEA through the tuberculum sella and planum sphenoidale permits resection of larger masses with suprasellar extension that lie between the carotid arteries with excellent results.

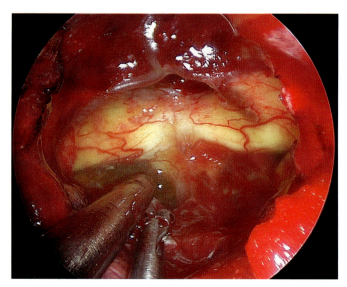

Fig. 13.2 An intraoperative image of the endoscopic removal of a meningioma. Note the optic nerve has been thinned from pressure against the anterior cerebral artery. The endonasal approach minimizes manipulation of the nerve.

The optic nerve lies directly in the transcranial trajectory and is often extremely thinned (**Fig. 13.2**). The EEA affords a better view of the medial optic canal (assuming it is opened) than a transcranial approach. A recent review of the published literature revealed that visual improvement occurred more frequently (69.1%) following EEA surgery compared with transcranial surgery (58.7%).[19] Tumor lateral to the optic nerve, however, cannot be removed endonasally. Although CSF leak rates reported in the literature for endonasal meningioma resection have been as high as 30%, more recent reports show that leak rates as low as 0% can be achieved with careful buttressed closure techniques.[18,19]

Transclival Approach

The clivus comprises the most ventral, midline posterior fossa skull base region, and thus surgical access can typically be quite difficult. Common neoplasms most commonly include chordomas, followed by chondrosarcomas, epidermoids/dermoids, and meningiomas. Various transfacial and transcranial approaches (i.e., subfrontal transbasal, anterior transfacial, subtemporal, transpetrosal or far lateral, transcondylar) have been described and can be used in combination during staged surgery.[20,21] Although a midline ventral approach to the clivus makes the most anatomic sense, the transfacial approach is morbid and cosmetically disfiguring. Lateral or paramedian approaches, on the other hand, require the surgeon to traverse cranial nerves, as well as the vertebrobasilar arteries, to reach the clival-based tumor. Collective results of these open approaches vary widely, with a GTR rate ranging from 44 to 83%, neurological morbidity rates of 0 to 80%, and CSF leak rates of 8.3 to 30%.

The extended EEA to this region has many advantages, including the utilization of natural apertures and corridors and the ability to look laterally with angled endoscopes that decrease the manipulation of critical neurovascular structures. With careful case selection, the endonasal approaches to the clivus have shown excellent results compared with open approaches, particularly for chordomas and chondrosarcomas, which arise extradurally in a midline and paramedian location (**Fig. 13.3**). A report of 20 patients who underwent an EEA for primary and recurrent chordomas demonstrated the overall mean extent of resection to be 90.85%, with nearly half of the patients undergoing GTR.[21] Extent of resection was significantly greater for primary chordomas (97.7%) compared with recurrent ones (81.8%). A consecutive case experience with seven patients who underwent EEA for clival chordomas similarly reported greater than 95% resection in 87% of patients, with greater extent of resection occurring in patients with smaller tumors (i.e., < 50 cm³).[20]

Transethmoidal Corridor

Malignant tumors involving the paranasal sinuses and anterior skull base, such as esthesioneuroblastoma and sinonasal undifferentiated carcinoma (SNUC), have long been treated with craniofacial surgery to achieve a goal of GTR with negative margins. Given the morbidity and often negative impact on quality of life, surgery has more recently been modified to a cranionasal approach with a combined EEA with bifrontal craniotomy when intracranial extension is evident (i.e., Kadish stage C). A purely EEA (without craniotomy), however, has become a reasonable alternative for achieving local control as long as the intracranial tumor does not extend lateral to the lamina papyracea.

A comparison of 120 patients with a wide variety of malignant sinonasal tumors who underwent a purely EEA ($n = 93$) versus cranionasal surgery ($n = 27$) showed that those patients with anterior skull base involvement and more extensive disease burden were more likely to undergo a combined cranionasal rather than purely endoscopic procedure.[22] Disease survival and recurrence, however, were not significantly different between the two groups. Overall postoperative CSF leak was 3% in both groups. A recent meta-analysis compared these different surgical approaches for esthesioneuroblastoma and found GTR was achieved in 98.1% after EEA surgery, compared to 81.3% of patients undergoing craniofacial resection. All patients undergoing cranionasal resection experienced GTR.[23] Negative margins were achieved in 93.8% of purely endoscopic cases, compared to 77.3% and 95.8% in patients who underwent craniofacial and cranionasal surgery, respectively. Similarly, the EEA group also had a significantly lower proportion of patients with intracranial tumor extension (i.e., Kadish stage C) compared with the other groups, suggesting the bias is still to treat intracranial disease with open transcranial surgery. Serious complications including meningitis and epidural hematoma were reported solely in the craniofacial group with

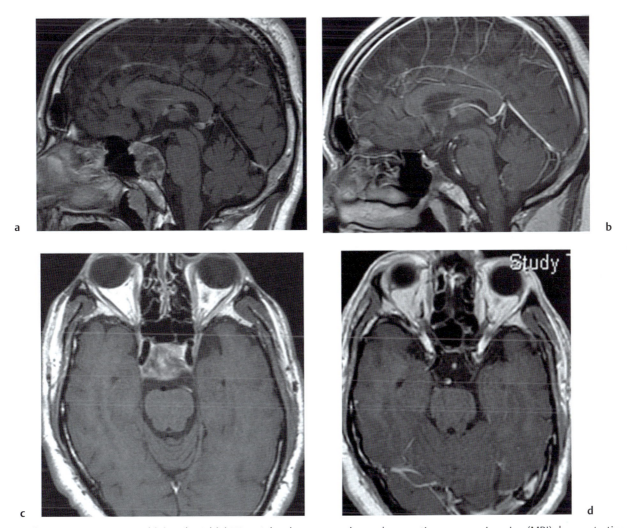

Fig. 13.3a–d A preoperative sagittal **(a)** and axial **(c)** T1-weighted contrast-enhanced magnetic resonance imaging (MRI) demonstrating a mass involving the clivus. The pathology was identified as a chordoma. **(b,d)** Postoperative images reveal gross total resection.

a corresponding perioperative mortality rate of 3.2% (compared to 0% in both endonasal groups). Nasal crusting was the major complication in the purely EEA group, and the CSF leak rate was 7.2%, which was lower than the 18.2% reported with cranionasal surgery.[23]

Benign tumors, such as olfactory groove meningiomas, can also be approached through the transethmoidal corridor.[24] Although a GTR can be achieved with reasonable rates of postoperative CSF leak, the literature on meningiomas in this region is still evolving and will likely take a few more years to sort out.[19]

Transmaxillary Corridor

Transpterygoidal Approach

Open surgical access to the pterygopalatine fossa (PPF) and the infratemporal fossa (ITF) can be limited laterally by the parotid gland, mandible, facial nerve, and masticator muscles.

Using a transmaxillary corridor extension, EEA access to these areas demonstrate the lateral infraorbital extent with access to the petrous apex down to the infratemporal fossa, therefore providing direct access to these regions with superior visualization, early identification, and preservation of neurovascular structures. This approach has been divided into subapproaches and zones using the petrous carotid artery as the key anatomic landmark.[25] It can be used for addressing lesions of the PPF, ITF, petrous apex, petroclival junction, and, in select cases, the lateral cavernous sinus, Meckel's cave, and the medial middle fossa. There is a vast differential for masses of the PPF and ITF with common benign lesions including inverted papillomas (IPs), juvenile nasal angiofibromas (JNAs), trigeminal schwannomas and neuromas, as well as malignant sinonasal tumors. The anatomy in this region of the skull base is particularly complex, and dense neurovascular contents render this approach more challenging than those involving the midline; however, successful endoscopic management with good long-term results has been reported in the literature.[26-29]

A comparison between patients with JNAs undergoing purely endoscopic resection and those undergoing conventional open surgery found that the former experienced significantly less intraoperative blood loss, lower occurrence of complications, shorter hospital stays, and lower rates of recurrence.[30] A study of six patients with solid petrous apex neoplasms, most commonly chondrosarcoma, reported 80% GTR (when attempted) following EEA surgery.[31]

Closure Techniques

The EEA was initially criticized for relatively high rates of postoperative CSF leak, initially occurring in 20 to 30% of patients who required repair of large (> 2 cm) skull base defects.[24] Inadequate reconstruction of the skull base can lead to persistent CSF leak, meningitis, pneumocephalus, and death. Such persistent leaks are of particular concern with use of the extended transsphenoidal approaches for the resection of larger tumors that require larger bony and dural openings, arachnoidal dissections, and occasional involvement of the third ventricle. Thus, preemptive measures to effectively reduce the incidence of residual CSF leak postoperatively are necessary to ensure the success of endoscopic skull base surgery.

Anticipating a CSF leak is extremely important, and surgeons should plan accordingly. Although some surgeons recommend placement of a lumbar drain, others feel it is not necessary.[32] Intrathecal fluorescein, injected at the beginning of the procedure, has been shown to be safe and effective in initially identifying CSF and ultimately ensuring that a watertight closure has been obtained.[33] In all cases, including those with purely intrasellar tumors, the abdomen should be prepped and draped for possible fat harvesting. For extended approaches in which a large skull base defect is anticipated, the thigh can also be prepped at the beginning of the procedure to harvest fascia lata. Additionally, a pedicled nasoseptal flap should be harvested early in such cases.[34] Since its advent in 2006,[35] the vascularized flap has become the repair method of choice for endoscopic skull base reconstruction, given its ease of use and low associated morbidity.

Closure techniques can be tailored based on the extent of leak during surgery. One option for a high-flow leak is a multilayer closure with inlays of synthetic material, onlay of fat, and a nasoseptal flap and a balloon buttress.[32] In cases with a large CSF leak, a "gasket seal" skull base closure can be used.[36]

> **Pitfall**
>
> • Failure to anticipate an intraoperative CSF leak can be problematic. The combination of a "gasket seal" closure, nasoseptal flap, and postoperative lumbar drainage can significantly reduce the rate of CSF leak following EEA surgery.

This involves onlay of a piece of fascia lata held in place with a countersunk Medpore buttress. Use of a bilayer fascia lata button has also been reported.[37] Finally, the construct is covered by a vascularized nasoseptal flap and Duraseal to complete the closure. In a recent systematic review of closure techniques used for reconstructing large skull base defects, the use of a vascularized flap was associated with a significantly lower rate of CSF leak (6.7%) than that associated with free grafts (15.6%).[38]

Complications

It is important to emphasize that endoscopic skull base surgery can be associated with significant complications, given the relatively small working environment and close proximity of critical neurovascular structures. Thus, it is imperative that EEA surgery be performed by experienced multidisciplinary teams. In addition to CSF leak and depending on the skull base approach used, complications from endoscopic endonasal skull base surgery can include (but are not limited to) infection (e.g., meningitis), bleeding, septal perforation, atrophic rhinitis, iatrogenic sinusitis, cranial nerve palsies, anosmia, pituitary dysfunction, diabetes insipidus, vision loss stroke, and death. Overall, the risk of CSF leak is most common, but has been significantly reduced with the improvement of the aforementioned closure techniques.

■ Endoscope-Assisted Transcranial Surgery

Although the microscope has improved illumination and visualization for intracranial tumor surgery, a good portion of light is disbursed, given the distance between the source and the incision. This can be particularly troublesome when working in deep locations, such as the cerebellopontine angle (CPA) and pineal gland region.[39] The aforementioned advancements in endoscopic instrumentation have enabled bimanual dissection with heightened illumination via the endoscope to become an increasingly popular alternative for guided resection of tumors in such deep areas of the brain, as well as resection of subcortical tumors.[40]

Endoscopes had been primarily used for assisting with open resection of vestibular schwannomas,[41] but more recently there have been reports of solely endoscopic surgery for these tumors.[42] Advantages of using the endoscope in this location include improved visualization around the tumor, to avoid blind dissection behind the facial nerve, and the ability to search for exposed air cells, to prevent CSF leak.[42] Tumor filling the prepontine cistern with brainstem compression is a contraindication to endoscope-assisted surgery as the traditional microscopic approach can enable the surgeon to open the cisterna magna early to relieve pressure. Likewise, authors have also suggested limiting endoscopic resection to hearing-preservation surgery only, as the preference is still for a translabyrinthine approach to improve facial nerve preservation when hearing is already lost.[39] A series of 527 fully endoscopically resected vestibular schwannomas via a "key-hole" retrosigmoid craniotomy reported a 94% GTR rate, with the remaining subtotal resection (STR) for hearing preservation.[42] Measureable hearing was preserved in 57% of cases, and the facial nerve was anatomically preserved in all patients, with 93% of patients maintaining excellent facial nerve function (House-Brackmann grades 1 and 2) 1-year postoperatively. No major complications were reported. These results are comparable to those for open surgery.

Another indication for endoscope-assisted posterior fossa surgery has been to access the pineal region. Although biopsy can be achieved through an endoscopic intraventricular surgery, complete resection requires a different approach.[43] Recently, a novel endoscope-guided supracerebellar infratentorial approach was described, and GTR or adequate cyst drainage was achieved in eight of nine cases.[43] This approach also facilitates management of hydrocephalus via concomitant endoscopic third ventriculostomies (ETVs) into the quadrigeminal cistern and can easily be converted to an open approach should it be needed.

Endoscopic Intraventricular Surgery

Endoscopic surgery for intraventricular tumors and cysts is a logical application of this technique, given the deep location of such lesions and the potential morbidity associated with conventional open neurosurgical approaches. The CSF affords excellent light and image transmission through the endoscope. Improvements in optics and incorporation of high definition, particularly through a rigid endoscope, have made visualization of, and approach to, complex lesions more feasible. In addition, the fact that most intraventricular lesions cause hydrocephalus greatly facilitates endoscopic surgery by providing a larger working corridor and less potential torque on the traversed cortical mantle. The inherent benefits of minimally invasive techniques, including reduced surgical time, improved cosmetic results, shortened hospital stay, and reduced cost, also factor into the appeal of neurosurgical endoscopy for managing intraventricular tumors.[44]

Endoscopic Fenestration

Septal fenestration and tumor cyst fenestration are two of the more widely performed endoscopic procedures owing to the typically avascular nature of these membranes. Fenestration of the septum pellucidum should be considered in a patient with a tumor mass situated in the anterior third ventricle or within the lateral ventricle at the foramen of Monro resulting in obstructive hydrocephalus. Shunt burden can be reduced in the former situation or eliminated in the latter by simply performing a septal fenestration to enable free communication of CSF between the two lateral ventricles.

Endoscopic fenestration of the septum pellucidum generally is performed via an entry site that lies more lateral than the conventional coronal bur hole, positioned at least 4 cm from the midsagittal plane. An alternative to a coronal approach is through an occipital route. This trajectory affords a longitudinal view of the septum and an enhanced potential for wide fenestrations with less manipulation of the endoscopic path. This trajectory also minimizes potential injury to the contralateral fornix and thalamus. It is critical to integrate navigational guidance when using a posterior approach. It is recommended that the site of septal fenestration be positioned between the larger tributaries of the septal veins and as superiorly directed away from the fornix. Generous fenestrations are made, typically with bipolar cautery. Compatible tissue shaving devices are also very effective for creating fenestrations in avascular membranes such as the septum pellucidum.

Duplicated septal leaflets can present some confusion if they are separated during the procedure. Confirmation of effective communication is established only by visualizing the contralateral ventricular landmarks such as the choroid plexus and ependymal veins. Angled endoscopes are also effective at visualizing the septum, particularly when the degree of hydrocephalus does not permit a very lateral entry trajectory. In these cases, identification of landmarks with a 0-degree endoscope, followed by transition to a 30-degree endoscope, usually permits excellent visualization of the superior septum pellucidum.

Tumor cyst fenestration is an important option when a patient's symptoms can be relieved by cyst decompression. This can obviate the need for aggressive tumor resection particularly when symptoms are caused by hydrocephalus or mass effect of the cystic tumor component. Craniopharyngiomas and hypothalamic/chiasmatic astrocytomas are the best examples of tumors that, although benign in histology, can produce large cystic regions causing obstruction of the ventricular system or symptoms by compression of the optic apparatus, fornix, hypothalamus, or infundibulum (**Figs. 13.4** and **13.5**).[45] For most cystic tumors causing obstructive hydrocephalus at the level of the third ventricle, a standard precoronal bur hole approach is an ideal trajectory. The transcavum interforniceal endoscopic approach[46] to the third ventricle is a further re-

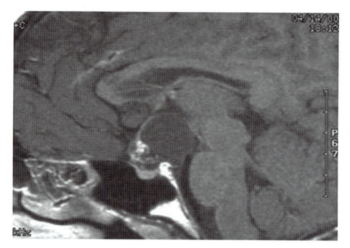

Fig. 13.4 A sagittal T1-weighted MRI obtained after gadolinium contrast administration shows a presumed craniopharyngioma in a patient presenting with a bitemporal hemianopia. Visual fields improved to normal after a transventricular endoscopic cyst decompression. The residual mass was treated with fractionated stereotactic radiotherapy.

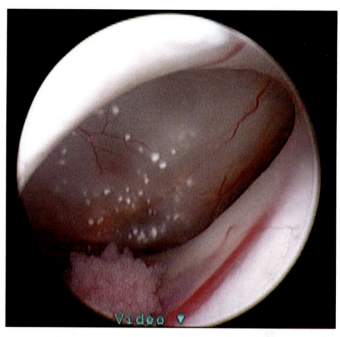

Fig. 13.5 An intraoperative image of a craniopharyngioma. Typical microcalcifications are evident on the craniopharyngioma surface.

finement of the technique for biopsy or fenestration of lesions within the third ventricle in patients with a large cavum vergae (i.e. the posterior extension of the septum pellucidum).

Tumor Biopsy with or Without Endoscopic Third Ventriculostomy

Endoscopic biopsy is a well-established method for sampling intraventricular brain tumors, particularly when surgical tumor removal may not be necessary or when the diagnosis would significantly alter the therapeutic approach. Examples of such situations include marker-negative germ cell tumors, Langerhans' cell histiocytosis, and infiltrative hypothalamic gliomas. Eligible patients should display overt intraventricular extension of tumor mass rather than a lesion that is entirely subependymal in location. T2-weighted magnetic resonance imaging (MRI) can often predict if the ependymal surface will have a discrete tumor or if a rim of thalamus or hypothalamus might preclude safe entry into the tumor. The diagnostic yield is high and the relative risk is low.[47] To maintain diagnostic accuracy it is imperative to avoid cauterizing the tumor prior to sampling, as samples are small and histological interpretation can be challenging even without superimposed artifact from cautery. If bleeding is encountered, continuous irrigation through the endoscope or an external catheter might be necessary until the CSF medium clears sufficiently to complete the biopsy or abort the remainder. Leaving a postoperative ventriculostomy is common, but often not necessary.

A majority of pineal region tumors may not require aggressive surgical resection due to radio- or chemoresponsiveness, but will require histological diagnosis. These tumors can often

result in obstructive hydrocephalus, and thus endoscopic tumor biopsy coupled with third ventriculostomy is a useful, dual-purpose procedure for such lesions. Notably, primary central nervous system germ cell tumors (GCTs), both pure germinomas and nongerminomatous GCTs, can be effectively treated without radical resection. Thus, patients who present with obstructive hydrocephalus with a pineal region tumor should always be considered for primary endoscopic management by way of ETV (**Fig. 13.6**) and tumor biopsy. Serum biochemical analysis for α-fetoprotein and human chorionic gonadotropin should always precede endoscopic biopsy because marker-positive GCT should be initially managed with neoadjuvant chemotherapy.[48]

When performing simultaneous ETV and tumor biopsy, the ETV should always be performed first given the fact that the patient's hydrocephalus is the more emergent clinical condition requiring treatment. Further, when tumor biopsy is performed, some intraventricular hemorrhage is expected that may obscure vision. Because the trajectories for ETV and pineal region tumor biopsy are different, two distinct entry sites are often used for performing these simultaneous procedures. The typical entry site for performing an ETV is at the

---

Pearl

- When performing simultaneous ETV and tumor biopsy, the ETV should always be performed first.

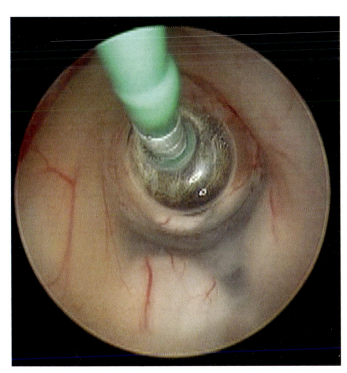

Fig. 13.6 An intraoperative image of the dilation of the endoscopic third ventriculostomy (ETV) stoma by inflating the balloon of a 3-French Fogarty embolectomy catheter.

coronal suture 2 cm off midline, whereas that for accomplishing a pineal region tumor biopsy is 4 to 6 cm precoronal. Alternatively, a single entry site that is midway between these has been shown to be successful. The optimal method for simultaneous tumor biopsy and ETV should be tailored to the individual patient based on the anatomic features of the tumor and third ventricular compartment.[49] The relationship of the anterior tumor mass with the interthalamic adhesion is critical in the decision making regarding a singular or dual route of simultaneous biopsy and ETV. Irrespective, in all circumstances navigational guidance is used such that a trajectory is chosen that best approximates a tangent with the roof of the third ventricle in a sagittal plane and bisects a path between the anterior pillar (column) of the fornix and the head of the caudate nucleus in an axial plane. Particular attention is applied to the trajectory as it relates to the interhemispheric sulci, most notably the callosal sulcus.

Solid Tumor Resection

Solid tumor removal can be challenging due to the lack of compatible instrumentation and the small caliber of current endoscopic portals. Undeniably, the success of endoscopic tumor resection is dictated by tumor characteristics including size, density, and vascularity. Tumors larger than 2 cm, those with calcification, and those that have significant subependy-

mal infiltration are currently not amenable to endoscopic removal.[50] The resection of solid tumors is principally achieved through aspiration with a variable, self-regulated suction catheter alternating with generous bipolar diathermy. It is important to note that aspiration is only used once the catheter tip is firmly and completely embedded within the tumor tissue so as to avoid rapid evacuation of CSF. The feasibility of endoscopic removal of solid tumors within the ventricular system is expected to improve with the advent of compatible instrumentation designed for tissue ablation, such as an ultrasonic aspirator and tissue-shaving devices.[51]

Colloid Cyst Removal

Colloid cysts of the third ventricle are ideally suited for endoscopic removal, largely due to their cystic nature (**Fig. 13.7**).[52] The deep central location within the ventricular compartment along with the associated complexity of standard microsurgical removal further favors endoscopic management. Similar to endoscopic skull base surgery, careful patient selection is critical, especially given that most patients are asymptomatic when diagnosed. Indications for surgical intervention include symptoms of increased intracranial pressure, ventriculomegaly (in the presence or absence of symptoms), and imaging evidence of increase in size of the ventricles or tumor mass. Less defined indicators include empiric resection to prevent clinical progression or sudden death, as well as young age at the time of diagnosis. The natural history is not clear but it is estimated that clinical progression occurs in about 8% of patients over 10 years.[53] The expectation of progression during a patient's lifetime is thus greater for younger patients. Variables that may precede clinical deterioration are ventriculomegaly, chronic headache, and cyst size (> 1 cm diameter). Offering surgery to avoid the possibility of acute neurologic deterioration must be balanced by a true estimation of operative risk to the patient, bearing in mind that many of the patients will have normal-sized ventricles.

A critical point of the operation is the trajectory selection by utilizing a frameless stereotaxy system. The nondominant side is selected, unless the colloid cyst appears to asymmetrically dilate the foramina of Monro and protrude into the dominant-side lateral ventricle (**Fig. 13.8**). The ideal trajectory has an entry point behind the hairline (or on a forehead skin crease), does not cross cortical sulci (including the cingulate sulcus at the medial surface of the hemisphere), does not violate cortical veins, is medial to the head of caudate, is tangential to the roof of the third ventricle, and, of course, targets the colloid cyst through the foramen of Monro. All these criteria are not always met to the fullest extent, and any compromises must be carefully weighed. A curvilinear skin incision, a bur hole, a dural incision, and a corticectomy are subsequently performed in a standard fashion. If ventriculomegaly is present, the endoscopic sheath with the obturator blocking the working channels is advanced into the lateral ventricle under

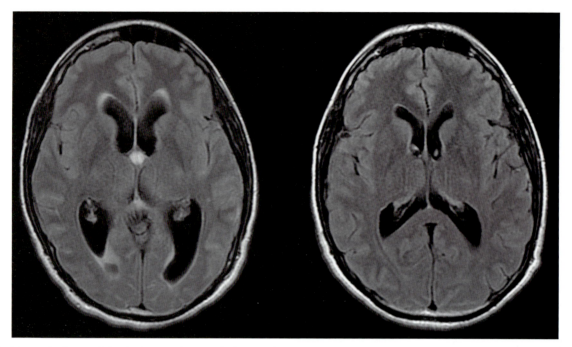

Fig. 13.7a,b **(a)** A colloid cyst of the third ventricle is an ideal tumor for endoscopic removal. **(b)** Postoperative imaging demonstrates resolution of preoperative hydrocephalus.

stereotactic guidance. When ventricular access is achieved, the obturator is replaced by the 0-degree endoscope (MINOP, Aesculap, Melsungen, Germany). In normal-sized ventricles, a ventricular catheter is first inserted under stereotactic guidance. Then, insufflation of the ventricular system with 5-cc

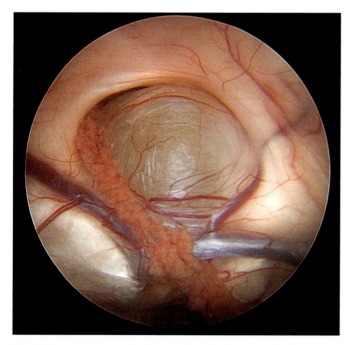

Fig. 13.8 An intraoperative image of a colloid cyst, occluding the right foramen of Monro.

aliquots of normal saline follows in order to increase the intraventricular working space. This step limits any injuries to the paraventricular neural structures by the insertion of the wider-in-diameter endoscopic sheath.[54]

Following the insufflation of the ventricular system, the endoscopic sheath with the endoscope in place is advanced along the previous tract of the ventricular catheter, under direct endoscopic visualization. Orientation and identification of the colloid cyst follows. A small area in the colloid cyst surface is coagulated and perforated by utilizing the bipolar cautery. A 6-French pediatric suction catheter (Kendall, Safe-T-Vac, Tyco Healthcare Group LP, Mansfield, MA) is inserted into the colloid cyst and the cyst contents are aspirated. A tissue-shaving device can prove helpful in cysts with a heavy mineralized core. Following the partial or complete evacuation of the cyst, the cyst membranes are drawn into the foramen with grasping forceps. Any adherent portions of choroid plexus to the cyst should be coagulated and sharply dissected. A rotary motion and slight traction are applied to the cyst membranes to achieve their dissection off the roof of the third ventricle. The cyst might separate from the third ventricle roof en bloc, and in that case it is removed from the ventricular system by simultaneously withdrawing the endoscopic sheath from the ventricular system. An attempt to remove the cyst through the working portal of the endoscopic sheath might lead to extrusion of cyst fragments because of the small diameter of the working channel compared to the cyst dimensions. If the colloid cyst does not separate en bloc, then cyst membranes remain adhered to the third ventricle roof and they should be generously coagulated and sharply dissected.

Some portions of the cyst wall may not be amenable to dissection due to adherence to venous structures and should be solely coagulated. Any small hematomas within the third ventricle are removed using aspiration applied directly to the clot. Based on the degree on intraventricular hemorrhage, an externalized ventricular drain might be placed. A standard fashion closure is performed by placing a small titanium plate over the bur hole.

Endoscopic resection of colloid cysts compares favorably with the main alternative surgical option, which is the microsurgical resection.[52] The rate of major complications is 5.45% versus 14.08% for the microsurgical approach; the postoperative shunt dependency is also lower in the endoscopic group (2.6% vs 11.35%). Although the recurrence rate is higher in the endoscopic group (12.3% vs 0.85%), it has been shown that the recurrence rate correlates with the extent of colloid cyst removal. The recurrence rate can be as high as 33.3% when coagulated cyst remnants are present, but it can also be as low as 2.2% in total colloid cyst resection.[55] Technical advancement and surgical experience has led to total resection rates of almost 90%,[56] so it is expected that the recurrence rate will tend to be lower in future case series of this technique.

■ Conclusion

Due to technological advancements and collaborative working efforts, the endoscope has become an essential tool for state-of-the-art neuro-oncological care. The endoscope has had a dramatic impact on anterior skull base and intraventricular surgery and is gaining popularity in a variety of other applications for improving visualization deep in the brain.

Editor's Note

Leave it to neurosurgeons to find new ways to be innovative in the operating room. It used to be for lesions involving the skull base, and, in particular the sellar and parasellar areas, that large morbid exposures were made to try to facilitate an aggressive resection. Enter the endoscope and the superb optical systems that are currently available for endoscopes that are even steerable around nooks and crannies. These systems have enabled surgeons to resect tumors through minimally invasive corridors to all aspects of not only the skull base but within the intraventricular system. This has changed the way in which these surgical procedures are now carried out, especially with regard to pituitary tumors and other lesions involving the midline skull base. The days of more radical open and very morbid procedures are waning; these procedures are being replaced with focused minimally invasive procedures that even with extended approaches still have a minimal degree of morbidity while allowing a maximal degree of resection. This is perhaps one of the most significant changes in all of neurosurgical oncology in the past decade, and we expect more and more lesions to be approached with these techniques. However, at the present time these approaches are not appropriate for intra-axial lesions that are not primarily within the ventricular system. It remains to be seen whether or not the endoscopes can be adapted for these types of tumors. Until then, for any skull base or intraventricular lesion, the endoscope should be considered first before considering more open and aggressive approaches. (Berger)

References

1. Schwartz TH, Fraser JF, Brown S, Tabaee A, Kacker A, Anand VK. Endoscopic cranial base surgery: classification of operative approaches. Neurosurgery 2008;62:991–1002, discussion 1002–1005
2. Dehdashti AR, Ganna A, Karabatsou K, Gentili F. Pure endoscopic endonasal approach for pituitary adenomas: early surgical results in 200 patients and comparison with previous microsurgical series. Neurosurgery 2008;62:1006–1015, discussion 1015–1017
3. McLaughlin N, Eisenberg AA, Cohan P, Chaloner CB, Kelly DF. Value of endoscopy for maximizing tumor removal in endonasal transsphenoidal pituitary adenoma surgery. J Neurosurg 2013;118:613–620
4. D'Haens J, Van Rompaey K, Stadnik T, Haentjens P, Poppe K, Velkeniers B. Fully endoscopic transsphenoidal surgery for functioning pituitary adenomas: a retrospective comparison with traditional transsphenoidal microsurgery in the same institution. Surg Neurol 2009;72:336–340
5. Dehdashti AR, Ganna A, Witterick I, Gentili F. Expanded endoscopic endonasal approach for anterior cranial base and suprasellar lesions: indications and limitations. Neurosurgery 2009;64:677–687, discussion 687–689
6. Hofstetter CP, Shin BJ, Mubita L, et al. Endoscopic endonasal transsphenoidal surgery for functional pituitary adenomas. Neurosurg Focus 2011;30:E10
7. Xie T, Hu F, Yu Y, Gu Y, Wang X, Zhang X. Endoscopic endonasal resection of symptomatic Rathke cleft cysts. J Clin Neurosci 2011;18:760–762
8. Mehta GU, Oldfield EH. Prevention of intraoperative cerebrospinal fluid leaks by lumbar cerebrospinal fluid drainage during surgery for pituitary macroadenomas. J Neurosurg 2012;116:1299–1303
9. Lindley T, Greenlee JD, Teo C. Minimally invasive surgery (endonasal) for anterior fossa and sellar tumors. Neurosurg Clin N Am 2010;21:607–620, v v.
10. Taussky P, Kalra R, Coppens J, Mohebali J, Jensen R, Couldwell WT. Endocrinological outcome after pituitary transposition (hypophysopexy) and adjuvant radiotherapy for tumors involving the cavernous sinus. J Neurosurg 2011;115:55–62
11. Hofstetter CP, Nanaszko MJ, Mubita LL, Tsiouris J, Anand VK, Schwartz TH. Volumetric classification of pituitary macroadenomas predicts outcome and morbidity following endoscopic endonasal transsphenoidal surgery. Pituitary 2012;15:450–463

12. Komotar RJ, Starke RM, Raper DM, Anand VK, Schwartz TH. Endoscopic endonasal compared with microscopic transsphenoidal and open transcranial resection of giant pituitary adenomas. Pituitary 2012; 15:150–159

13. Komotar RJ, Starke RM, Raper DM, Anand VK, Schwartz TH. Endoscopic endonasal compared with microscopic transsphenoidal and open transcranial resection of craniopharyngiomas. World Neurosurg 2012; 77:329–341

14. Leng LZ, Greenfield JP, Souweidane MM, Anand VK, Schwartz TH. Endoscopic, endonasal resection of craniopharyngiomas: analysis of outcome including extent of resection, cerebrospinal fluid leak, return to preoperative productivity, and body mass index. Neurosurgery 2012; 70:110–123, discussion 123–124

15. Simpson D. The recurrence of intracranial meningiomas after surgical treatment. J Neurol Neurosurg Psychiatry 1957;20:22–39

16. Mahmoud M, Nader R, Al-Mefty O. Optic canal involvement in tuberculum sellae meningiomas: influence on approach, recurrence, and visual recovery. Neurosurgery 2010;67(3,SupplOperative):ons108–ons118, discussion ons118–ons119

17. Sughrue ME, Kane AJ, Shangari G, et al. The relevance of Simpson Grade I and II resection in modern neurosurgical treatment of World Health Organization Grade I meningiomas. J Neurosurg 2010;113:1029–1035

18. Attia M, Kandasamy J, Jakimovski D, et al. The importance and timing of optic canal exploration and decompression during endoscopic endonasal resection of tuberculum sella and planum sphenoidale meningiomas. Neurosurgery 2012;71(1, Suppl Operative):58–67

19. Komotar RJ, Starke RM, Raper DM, Anand VK, Schwartz TH. Endoscopic endonasal versus open transcranial resection of anterior midline skull base meningiomas. World Neurosurg 2012;77:713–724

20. Fraser JF, Nyquist GG, Moore N, Anand VK, Schwartz TH. Endoscopic endonasal transclival resection of chordomas: operative technique, clinical outcome, and review of the literature. J Neurosurg 2010;112:1061–1069

21. Stippler M, Gardner PA, Snyderman CH, Carrau RL, Prevedello DM, Kassam AB. Endoscopic endonasal approach for clival chordomas. Neurosurgery 2009;64:268–277, discussion 277–278

22. Hanna E, DeMonte F, Ibrahim S, Roberts D, Levine N, Kupferman M. Endoscopic resection of sinonasal cancers with and without craniotomy: oncologic results. Arch Otolaryngol Head Neck Surg 2009;135:1219–1224

23. Komotar RJ, Starke RM, Raper DM, Anand VK, Schwartz TH. Endoscopic endonasal compared with anterior craniofacial and combined cranionasal resection of esthesioneuroblastomas. World Neurosurg 2013;80:148–159

24. Liu JK, Christiano LD, Patel SK, Tubbs RS, Eloy JA. Surgical nuances for removal of olfactory groove meningiomas using the endoscopic endonasal transcribriform approach. Neurosurg Focus 2011;30:E3

25. Kassam AB, Gardner P, Snyderman C, Mintz A, Carrau R. Expanded endonasal approach: fully endoscopic, completely transnasal approach to the middle third of the clivus, petrous bone, middle cranial fossa, and infratemporal fossa. Neurosurg Focus 2005;19:E6

26. DelGaudio JM. Endoscopic transnasal approach to the pterygopalatine fossa. Arch Otolaryngol Head Neck Surg 2003;129:441–446

27. Douglas R, Wormald PJ. Endoscopic surgery for juvenile nasopharyngeal angiofibroma: where are the limits? Curr Opin Otolaryngol Head Neck Surg 2006;14:1–5

28. Robinson S, Patel N, Wormald PJ. Endoscopic management of benign tumors extending into the infratemporal fossa: a two-surgeon transnasal approach. Laryngoscope 2005;115:1818–1822

29. Schlosser RJ, Mason JC, Gross CW. Aggressive endoscopic resection of inverted papilloma: an update. Otolaryngol Head Neck Surg 2001;125:49–53

30. Pryor SG, Moore EJ, Kasperbauer JL. Endoscopic versus traditional approaches for excision of juvenile nasopharyngeal angiofibroma. Laryngoscope 2005;115:1201–1207

31. Zanation AM, Snyderman CH, Carrau RL, Gardner PA, Prevedello DM, Kassam AB. Endoscopic endonasal surgery for petrous apex lesions. Laryngoscope 2009;119:19–25

32. Harvey RJ, Nogueira JF, Schlosser RJ, Patel SJ, Vellutini E, Stamm AC. Closure of large skull base defects after endoscopic transnasal craniotomy. Clinical article. J Neurosurg 2009;111:371–379

33. Placantonakis DG, Tabaee A, Anand VK, Hiltzik D, Schwartz TH. Safety of low-dose intrathecal fluorescein in endoscopic cranial base surgery. Neurosurgery 2007;61(3, Suppl):161–165, discussion 165–166

34. Eloy JA, Patel AA, Shukla PA, Choudhry OJ, Liu JK. Early harvesting of the vascularized pedicled nasoseptal flap during endoscopic skull base surgery. Am J Otolaryngol 2013;34:188–194

35. Hadad G, Bassagasteguy L, Carrau RL, et al. A novel reconstructive technique after endoscopic expanded endonasal approaches: vascular pedicle nasoseptal flap. Laryngoscope 2006;116:1882–1886

36. Leng LZ, Brown S, Anand VK, Schwartz TH. "Gasket-seal" watertight closure in minimal-access endoscopic cranial base surgery. Neurosurgery 2008;62(5, Suppl 2):E342–E343, discussion E343

37. Luginbuhl AJ, Campbell PG, Evans J, Rosen M. Endoscopic repair of high-flow cranial base defects using a bilayer button. Laryngoscope 2010;120:876–880

38. Harvey RJ, Parmar P, Sacks R, Zanation AM. Endoscopic skull base reconstruction of large dural defects: a systematic review of published evidence. Laryngoscope 2012;122:452–459

39. Pieper DR. The endoscopic approach to vestibular schwannomas and posterolateral skull base pathology. Otolaryngol Clin North Am 2012; 45:439–454, x x.

40. Kassam AB, Engh JA, Mintz AH, Prevedello DM. Completely endoscopic resection of intraparenchymal brain tumors. J Neurosurg 2009;110:116–123

41. Göksu N, Yilmaz M, Bayramoglu I, Aydil U, Bayazit YA. Evaluation of the results of endoscope-assisted acoustic neuroma surgery through posterior fossa approach. ORL J Otorhinolaryngol Relat Spec 2005;67:87–91

42. Shahinian HK, Ra Y. 527 fully endoscopic resections of vestibular schwannomas. Minim Invasive Neurosurg 2011;54:61–67

43. Uschold T, Abla AA, Fusco D, Bristol RE, Nakaji P. Supracerebellar infratentorial endoscopically controlled resection of pineal lesions: case series and operative technique. J Neurosurg Pediatr 2011;8:554–564

44. Cappabianca P, Cinalli G, Gangemi M, et al. Application of neuroendoscopy to intraventricular lesions. Neurosurgery 2008;62(Suppl 2):575–597, discussion 597–598

45. Delitala A, Brunori A, Chiappetta F. Purely neuroendoscopic transventricular management of cystic craniopharyngiomas. Childs Nerv Syst 2004;20:858–862

46. Souweidane MM, Hoffman CE, Schwartz TH. Transcavum interforniceal endoscopic surgery of the third ventricle. J Neurosurg Pediatr 2008;2:231–236

47. Luther N, Cohen A, Souweidane MM. Hemorrhagic sequelae from intracranial neuroendoscopic procedures for intraventricular tumors. Neurosurg Focus 2005;19:E9

48. Luther N, Edgar MA, Dunkel IJ, Souweidane MM. Correlation of endoscopic biopsy with tumor marker status in primary intracranial germ cell tumors. J Neurooncol 2006;79:45–50

49. Morgenstern PF, Souweidane MM. Pineal region tumors: simultaneous endoscopic third ventriculostomy and tumor biopsy. *World Neurosurg* 2013;79(2 Suppl):S18, e9–13

50. Souweidane MM. Endoscopic surgery for intraventricular brain tumors in patients without hydrocephalus. Neurosurgery 2005;57(4, Suppl):312–318, discussion 312–318

51. Qiao L, Souweidane MM. Purely endoscopic removal of intraventricular brain tumors: a consensus opinion and update. Minim Invasive Neurosurg 2011;54:149–154

52. Margetis K, Souweidane MM. Endoscopic treatment of intraventricular cystic tumors. World Neurosurg 2013;79(2, Suppl):e1–e11

53. Pollock BE, Huston J III. Natural history of asymptomatic colloid cysts of the third ventricle. J Neurosurg 1999;91:364–369

54. Margetis K, Souweidane MM. Endoscopic resection of colloid cyst in normal-sized ventricular system. Neurosurg Focus 2013;34(1, Suppl):8

55. Hoffman CE, Savage NJ, Souweidane MM. The significance of cyst remnants after endoscopic colloid cyst resection: a retrospective clinical case series. Neurosurgery 2013;73:233–237, discussion 237–239

56. Boogaarts HD, Decq P, Grotenhuis JA, et al. Long-term results of the neuroendoscopic management of colloid cysts of the third ventricle: a series of 90 cases. Neurosurgery 2011;68:179–187

14 Functional Mapping

Nader Sanai and Mitchel S. Berger

■ Basic Principles

Direct cortical stimulation has been employed in neurosurgery since 1930, first by Foerster,[1] and then later by Penfield.[2–4] In recent years, the technique of intraoperative cortical stimulation has been adopted for the identification and preservation of language function and motor pathways. Stimulation depolarizes a very focal area of cortex, which, in turn, evokes certain responses. Although the mechanism of stimulation effects on language are poorly understood, the principle is based on the depolarization of local neurons and also of passing pathways, inducing local excitation or inhibition, as well as possible diffusion to more distant areas by way of orthodromic or antidromic propagation.[5] Studies employing optical imaging of bipolar cortical stimulation in monkey and human cortex have shown precise local changes, within 2 to 3 mm, after the activation of cortical tissue.[6,7] With the advent of the bipolar probe, avoidance of local diffusion and more precise mapping have been enabled with an accuracy estimated to be approximately 5 mm.[6]

■ Rationale for Functional Mapping

Hemispheric gliomas are often located within or adjacent to functional areas (e.g., rolandic cortex, supplementary motor areas, corona radiata, internal capsule, and uncinate fasciculus). Because gliomas have a tendency to invade underlying white matter tracts, it is important to identify both cortical sites and their descending pathways for the motor and somatosensory systems. Although extensive resection of a tumor involving the nondominant temporal lobe may be achieved without functional consequences other than a quadrantanopia, surgical resections in the dominant temporal lobe are more challenging due to the variable localization of language. Thus, although traditional neurosurgical teaching restricts temporal lobe resections to within 4 cm of the temporal tip and limits the removal of the superior temporal gyrus, dominant temporal lobe resections can nevertheless be associated with permanent postoperative language deficits.

Thus, prediction of cortical language sites through classic anatomic criteria is inadequate, as there is significant individual variability of cortical organization,[8–11] distortion of cerebral topography from tumor mass effect, and functional reorganization through plasticity mechanisms.[12–14] A consistent finding of language stimulation studies has been the identification of significant individual variability among patients.[10] Speech arrest is variably located and can go well beyond the classic anatomic boundaries of Broca's area for motor speech. It typically involves an area contiguous with the face–motor cortex and, yet, in some cases is seen several centimeters from the sylvian fissure. This variability has also been suggested by studies designed to preoperatively predict the location of speech arrest based on the type of frontal opercular anatomy[15] or using functional neuroimaging.[16–22] Similarly, for temporal lobe language sites, one study of temporal lobe resections assisted by subdural grids demonstrated that the distance from the temporal pole to the area of language function varied from 3 to 9 cm.[23] Functional imaging studies have also corroborated such variability.[24] Furthermore, because functional tissue can be located within the tumor nidus,[25] the standard surgical principle of debulking tumor from within to avoid neurologic deficits is not always safe. Consequently, the use of intraoperative cortical and subcortical stimulation to accurately detect functional regions and pathways is essential for safely removing dominant hemisphere gliomas to the greatest extent possible.

It is recommended that, for any tumor involving the dominant temporal, mid- to posterior frontal, and mid- to anterior parietal lobes, an awake craniotomy should be employed to identify language sites before the tumor is removed. Functional magnetic resonance imaging (fMRI) may also provide preoperative assessment of sensory and motor pathways and has been shown to be valuable in determining the rolandic cortex. This method is not reliable, however, for identifying language sites and does not provide an adequate replacement for intraoperative stimulation mapping.

Preoperative Assessment

The patient's neurologic status should be assessed preoperatively to determine the extent of motor or language function impairment, if any. If the patient has severe hemiparesis or hemiplegia, motor mapping will often not be useful. However, if antigravity movements are present preoperatively, it is usually possible to stimulate both cortical and subcortical motor pathways intraoperatively. In children younger than 5 or 6 years of age, due to cortical electrical inexcitability, somatosensory evoked potentials (SSEPs) can be used to identify the central sulcus.

In addition to testing motor and sensory function, it is also imperative to assess the patient's language function intra-

Pearl

- Preoperative steroids or neoadjuvant chemotherapy may improve naming, reading, and motor speech significantly enough to allow a patient with difficulty in these functions to be successfully mapped.

operatively to determine if the baseline naming error rate is < 25%. Similarly, those patients who will undergo intraoperative mapping for language sites should be preoperatively tested for language errors by being presented a series of slides with common objects to be named. After confirming that the face–motor cortex and Broca's area are functional by asking the patient to protrude the tongue and count to 10, slides of common objects are shown. Each slide will start with a phrase such as "This is a . . ." or "These are . . ." to test reading and speech output. Patients must be able to name common objects with less than a 25% baseline error rate, based on presenting each slide three times.

In patients who have moderate to severe dysphasia in either comprehension or expression, successful language mapping will not be possible. Therefore, this group of patients may either be operated on asleep, without any attempt to do more than an internal decompression, or challenged with steroids for 7 to 10 days and reevaluated regarding their baseline error rate in naming. An alternative approach may be to biopsy the tumor, confirm histopathology, and then treat the lesion with chemotherapy to reduce its size and induce functional improvement that will subsequently allow for intraoperative mapping.

In 85% of the population, the left hemisphere is dominant for language, whereas language representation is bilateral in 9%, and right-side dominance is present in only 6%. The dominant hemisphere is on the left for 98 to 99% of right-handed individuals. When in doubt, cerebral dominance may be verified using Wada's (intracarotid amytal) test or estimated using fMRI or magnetic source imaging (MSI). On preoperative MRI, the central sulcus, and the motor strip that is located within the gyrus directly in front of it, is identified using the most cranial (rostral, superior) cuts of axial T2-weighted MRI. This landmark is a reliable marker for the motor cortex, regardless of mass effect, and allows one to predict where the functional motor region will be before surgery. On midsagittal and near-midsagittal MRI, the rolandic (i.e., somatosensory-motor) cortex is identified by following the cingulate sulcus posteriorly and superiorly to its termination point. These MRI landmarks serve as useful guides to preoperatively determine the proximity of the lesion to the motor cortex.

Intraoperative Preparation

The patient is brought to the operating room and placed in the position appropriate for the area to be exposed. Special care is given to padding and protecting all extremities. A Foley catheter is inserted regardless of the need for osmotic diuretics. The head is fixed in position using a Mayfield clamp and local analgesia. The area of the scalp around the incision is infiltrated with a local anesthetic consisting of a 1:1 ratio of lidocaine (0.5%) to Marcaine (0.25%), combined with bicarbonate. A heating blanket is used to keep the core temperature above 36.5°C. If the patient's temperature drifts too low, especially under general anesthesia, cortical stimulation mapping will be difficult due to cortical inhibition. An intravenous propofol drip maintains the sedative hypnotic anesthesia to keep the patient asleep. An alternative is dexmedetomidine, which lowers the risk of respiratory depression and therefore is advantageous for patients with potentially high intracranial pressure, although emergence from this agent is less rapid than from propofol. In case of a decrease in the arterial oxygen saturation, oxygen is administered through a nasal cannula. Prophylactic antibiotics are routinely used and given during the induction phase of anesthesia. Preoperative antiepileptics (e.g., 1 g fosphenytoin) are administered to minimize the risk of intraoperative seizures.

Intraoperative Stimulation of Cortical and Subcortical Pathways

In general, a limited craniotomy should expose the tumor and up to 2 cm of surrounding brain.

Prior to the dural opening, the patient should be awakened and encouraged to hyperventilate briefly in order to relax the brain. Using bipolar electrodes, cortical mapping is started at a low stimulus (1 mA per channel) and increased to a maximum of 6 mA, if necessary. A constant-current generator delivers biphasic square wave pulses (each phase, 1.25 ms) in 4-second trains at 60 Hz across 1-mm bipolar electrodes separated by 5 mm. Stimulation sites (approximately 10 to 20 per subject) can be marked with sterile numbered tickets. Throughout motor and language mapping, continuous electrocorticography should be used to monitor afterdischarge potentials and, therefore, eliminate the chance that speech or naming errors are caused by subclinical seizure activity.

This will abruptly stop the seizure activity originating from the irritated cortex without using short-acting barbiturates. The current necessary to evoke motor movement will vary depending on the anesthetic condition of the patient, with lower currents used under awake conditions. The motor strip is stimulated in the asleep patient with a starting current of

Pearl

- Because the dura is pain-sensitive, the area around the middle meningeal artery should be infiltrated with the lidocaine-Marcaine mixture to alleviate discomfort while the patient is awake.

2 mA per channel, and reduced to 1 mA when stimulating the awake patient. The amplitude of the per-channel current is adjusted in 1- to 2-mA increments until motor movements are identified. A total current above 16 mA (8 mA per channel) has never been necessary to evoke sensory or motor response. Most commonly, the inferior aspect of the rolandic cortex is first identified by eliciting responses in the face and hand. As the leg motor cortex is tucked away against the falx, a strip electrode may be inserted along the falx, and stimulation using the same current applied to the lateral cortical surface may be delivered through it to evoke leg motor movements. This maneuver is safe due to lack of bridging veins between the falx and the leg motor cortex. Similarly, if the craniotomy is near but not overlying the rolandic cortex, a subdural strip electrode may be inserted under the dural edge and stimulated to evoke the desired response.

Once the motor cortex is defined, the descending tracts may be found using similar stimulation parameters. Descending motor and sensory pathways may be followed into the internal capsule and inferiorly to the brainstem and spinal cord. This is especially recommended during resection of infiltrative glial tumors because functioning motor, sensory, or language tissue can be located within a grossly obvious tumor or surrounding infiltrated brain. The current spread associated with bipolar stimulation is limited to 2 or 3 mm. If the motor cortex is not identified under any circumstance by using a functional stimulator, an attempt to identify the subcortical pathway is made using a current between 5 and 10 mA. One of the potential reasons for failure to find functional cortical sites is the inability to open the dura overlying the cortex because of scar tissue. Another explanation could be the anesthetic regimen. A peripheral nerve stimulator is used to confirm a train of four muscle contractions before stimulating the cortex or subcortical white matter. If cortical sites of motor function are found and subcortical pathways cannot be identified, then repetitive stimulation of the cortical site is performed to ensure that the cortex and its descending pathways are intact. Tumor resection should be followed by a final

stimulation of cortical sites to confirm that the pathways are intact. Even if the patient's neurologic status is worse postoperatively, the presence of intact cortical and subcortical motor pathways implies that the deficit will be transient and resolve in days to weeks. Although SSEPs may be helpful in identifying the central sulcus, they do not help in localizing descending subcortical motor and sensory white matter tracts.

Determination of the subcortical pathways is important while removing a deeply located tumor within or adjacent to the corona radiata, internal capsule, insula, supplementary motor area, or thalamus. Because the current spread from the electrode contacts is minimal during bipolar stimulation, resection should be stopped when movement or paresthesia is evoked.

Identification of Language Sites

Speech arrest is based on blocking number counting without simultaneous motor response in the mouth or pharynx. Dysarthria can be distinguished from speech arrest by the absence of perceived or visible involuntary muscle contraction affecting speech. For naming or reading sites, cortical stimulation is applied for 3 seconds at sequential cortical sites during a slide presentation of line drawings or words, respectively. All tested language sites should be repeatedly stimulated at least three times. A positive essential site can be defined as an inability to name objects or read words in 66% or more of the testing per site. In all cases, a 1-cm margin of tissue should be measured and preserved around each positive language site in order to protect functional tissue from the resection.[26] The extent of resection is directed by targeting contrast-enhancing regions for high-grade lesions and T2-hyperintense areas for low-grade lesions. Some groups advocate the use of language mapping along subcortical white matter pathways as well.[27,28]

Despite the considerable evidence supporting the use of intraoperative cortical stimulation mapping of language function, the efficacy of this technique in preserving functional outcome following aggressive glioma resection remains poorly understood. Nevertheless, the long-term neurologic effects after using this technique for large, dominant-hemisphere gliomas are important to define in order to accurately advocate its use.[29]

There is no level I randomized trial for language mapping. Our experience with 250 consecutive dominant hemisphere glioma patients (World Health Organization [WHO] grades II to IV) suggests that functional language outcome following awake mapping can be favorable, even in the setting of an aggressive resection.[30] Overall, 159 of these 250 patients (63.6%) had intact speech preoperatively. At 1 week postoperatively, 194 (77.6%) remained at their baseline language function, whereas 21 (8.4%) worsened and 35 (14.0%) had new speech deficits. However, by 6 months, 52 (92.9%) of 56 patients with new or worsened language deficits returned to baseline or better, and the remaining four (7.1%) were left with a permanent deficit. Interestingly, among these patients, any additional language deficit incurred as a result of the surgery improved by 3 months or not all. Thus, using language mapping, only 1.6% (four of 243 surviving patients) of all glioma patients develop a permanent postoperative language deficit. One explanation for this favorable postoperative language profile may be our strict adherence to the "1-cm rule," first described in 1994, which demonstrated that, for temporal lobe tumors, a resection margin of 1 cm or more from a language site significantly reduces postoperative language deficits.[31]

Identification of Motor Sites

For patients with gliomas that are located within or adjacent to the rolandic cortex and, thus, the descending motor tracts, awake or asleep stimulation mapping of cortical and subcortical motor pathways enables the surgeon to identify these descending motor pathways during tumor removal and achieve an acceptable rate of permanent morbidity in these high-risk functional areas.[32–34] As with speech mapping techniques, no level I trial exists for motor mapping. The best evidence published comes from several level III studies over the last 15 years; all studies lack long-term survival data. In one study, new immediate postoperative motor deficits were documented in 59.3% of patients in whom a subcortical motor tract was identified intraoperatively and in 14.5% of those in whom subcortical tracts were not observed; permanent deficits were observed in 6.5% and 3.5% of patients (a nonsignificant difference), respectively.[32] In another study of subcortical motor pathways in 294 patients who underwent surgery for hemispheric gliomas, 14 patients (4.8%) had a persistent motor deficit after 3 months. Interestingly, in this study patients whose subcortical pathways were identified intraoperatively were statistically significantly more prone to develop an additional transient or permanent motor deficit (27.5% vs 13.1%).[34] In another study consisting of 60 patients (44 with glioma) with an 87% gross total or subtotal (< 10 cm³ residual) resection rate, the overall neurologic morbidity was 5% after using cortical motor mapping.[33] Thus, collectively the literature suggests that intraoperative cortical and subcortical motor mapping can safely identify corridors for resection, as well as define the limits of tumor resection.

Negative Mapping

In contrast to the classic mapping principles practiced in epilepsy surgery, where 95 to 100% of operative fields contain a positive language site, a paradigm shift is emerging in brain tumor language mapping, where positive language sites are not always found prior to resection. In our practice, because of our use of tailored cortical exposures, less than 58% of patients have essential language sites localized within the operative field. Our experience suggests that it is safe to employ a minimal exposure of the tumor and resect based on a negative language map, rather than rely on a wide craniotomy to

Controversy

- Limited cortical mapping without finding an essential functional site (i.e., negative mapping) can offer reliable data to proceed safely and efficiently with tumor removal. Negative mapping enables a tailored exposure of the tumor, rather than relying on a wider craniotomy to identify positive control sites.

find positive language sites well beyond the lesion. However, language mapping techniques such as this are generally more successful and safer at high-volume neurosurgical centers.

Negative language mapping, however, does not necessarily guarantee the absence of eloquent sites. Despite negative brain mapping, permanent postoperative neurologic deficits have been reported.[35] In our experience with 250 consecutive dominant hemisphere glioma patients, all four of our patients with permanent postoperative neurologic deficits had no positive sites detected prior to their resections. Other cases of unexpected postoperative deficits have also been attributed to progressive tumor infiltration into functional areas.[36] Furthermore, both intraoperative stimulation and functional imaging techniques have provided evidence of redistribution of functional neural networks in cases of stroke,[13,37,38] congenital malformations,[39,40] brain injury,[41] and tumor progression.[13,14,42] Not surprisingly, it has been hypothesized that brain infiltration by gliomas leads to reshaping or local reorganization of functional networks as well as neosynaptogenesis.[43,44] This would explain the frequent lack of clinical deficit despite glioma growth into eloquent brain areas,[13,42,45] as well as the transient nature of many postoperative deficits. In the case of language function located in the dominant insula, the brain's capacity for compensation of functional loss has also been associated with recruitment of the left superior temporal gyrus and left putamen.[45]

Postoperative Management

Following surgery, patients are managed in the intensive care unit for up to 48 hours. Antiepileptic levels are maintained above the upper limit for 3 to 5 days postoperatively, and then gradually lowered to the therapeutic range. A postoperative scan is obtained within 48 hours of surgery to avoid postoperative enhancement representing surgical trauma. Dexamethasone is maintained at the dose of 16 mg/d and tapered slowly depending on the remaining mass effect on the postoperative scan. Patients with a transient and resolving paresis or speech deficit may benefit from a short course of inpatient rehabilitation and speech therapy, although it is not necessary. Our current data indicate that for patients who started with no language deficit preoperatively, their new postoperative deficits resolve entirely by 3 months. For those with a preoperative language deficit, however, if they did not return to baseline by month 3, their deficit is likely permanent. When using stimulation mapping methods to identify subcortical pathways, the surgeon is able to achieve an acceptable risk of permanent motor deficits in a high-risk patient population, which consists of patients with gliomas that are within or adjacent to motor tracts. In this setting, if both cortical and subcortical sites are found with stimulation mapping, one can expect a 7.6% rate of permanent motor deficits postoperatively, of which only 2.3% of our patients had two-fifths strength or less. In cases in which subcortical pathways could not be identified but for whom the functionally intact status was confirmed by stimulation of the corresponding cortical sites, the incidence of permanent morbidity was 2.3%, and no patient had two-fifths function or less. Our results indicate that subcortical stimulation methods can be applied in patients whose tumors are located within or adjacent to functional motor pathways and will result in an acceptable rate of postoperative morbidity that is mostly transient.

■ Literature Review: Assessing the Value of Intraoperative Stimulation Mapping

In the literature, approximately 90 publications examine the utility of intraoperative stimulation mapping techniques in achieving greater extent of resection for gliomas while minimizing morbidity. Within these studies, cohorts varied between 20 and 648 patients, with a median of 50 patients per study. Nearly all these reports provide level III evidence in support of this microsurgical adjunct, with the exception of two randomized studies[46,47] that examined anesthetic or fluorescence-guided techniques to maximize extent of resection.

A recent meta-analysis of this growing literature included 8,091 patients and identified intraoperative cortical stimulation mapping as predictive of a twofold reduction (3.4% vs 8.2%) in late severe neurologic deficits in adult patients with supratentorial infiltrative gliomas.[48] Importantly, this additional benefit did not come at the expense of the extent of resection (75% gross total resection [GTR] with mapping vs 58% without mapping), even though lesions were more often located in eloquent locations (99.9% vs 95.8%). Typically, the observed transient neurologic deficits usually subsided within a few weeks to 3 months after resection and were due to the proximity of critical brain structures adjacent to the resection cavity. Ultimately, a randomized controlled trial to determine the impact of awake craniotomies and stimulation mappings will be necessary to control for all known and unknown confounders inherent to the existing observations studies.

■ Conclusion

Glioma resections using awake craniotomy and intraoperative stimulation mapping techniques are associated with fewer neurologic deficits and more extensive resection. Unlike motor function, speech and language are variably distributed and widely represented, thus emphasizing the utility of language mapping in this particular patient population. Using this approach, and in conjunction with standardized neuroanesthesia and neuromonitoring, the postoperative motor and language resolution profiles following glioma resection may be predictable. Specifically, any additional language deficit incurred as a result of the surgery will improve by 3 months or not at all. Our experience also emphasizes the value of negative language mapping in the setting of a tailored cortical exposure. Although the value of extent of resection remains less clear, the available literature for both low- and high-grade hemispheric gliomas demonstrates mounting evidence that a more extensive surgical resection is associated with a more favorable life expectancy for both low- and high-grade glioma patients. This objective should be cautiously pursued for all gliomas, even in the setting of eloquent location.

Editor's Note

Despite controversy over the past several decades it is now generally accepted that the extent of resection clearly affects both progression-free survival and overall survival for both low- and high-grade gliomas. In addition, for low-grade gliomas, the extent of resection also affects malignant transformation. Despite improvements in anatomic imaging, it is still imperative to functionally map the brain in vivo to determine the extent of potential tumor removal at the time of surgery based on the functional assessment of the tissue to be removed. In a very important meta-analysis that was published in 2012 in the *Journal of Clinical Oncology*,[48] it was determined that in reviewing the entire literature to date with or without stimulation mapping, the morbidity was 50% higher in patients who did not have stimulation mapping when attempting a resection of an intrinsic glioma. This points out the need to employ this methodology as the standard of care for all patients undergoing intra-axial tumor resection. Thus, in virtually every circumstance a radical resection should be attempted first before defaulting to a biopsy, and the best way to do this is with functional mapping to enhance the extent of resection and to maximize safety. (Berger)

References

1. Foerster O. The cerebral cortex in man. Lancet 1931;2:309–312
2. Penfield W, Bolchey E. Somatic motor and sensory representation in the cerebral cortex of man as studied by electrical stimulation. Brain 1937;60:389–443
3. Penfield W, Erickson TC. Epilepsy and Cerebral Localization. A Study of the Mechanism, Treatment, and Prevention of Epileptic Seizures. Springfield, IL: Charles C. Thomas, 1941
4. Penfield W, Rasmussen T. Secondary Sensory and Motor Representation. New York: Macmillan, 1950
5. Ranck JB Jr. Which elements are excited in electrical stimulation of mammalian central nervous system: a review. Brain Res 1975;98:417–440
6. Haglund MM, Ojemann GA, Blasdel GG. Optical imaging of bipolar cortical stimulation. J Neurosurg 1993;78:785–793
7. Haglund MM, Ojemann GA, Hochman DW. Optical imaging of epileptiform and functional activity in human cerebral cortex. Nature 1992;358:668–671
8. Herholz K, Thiel A, Wienhard K, et al. Individual functional anatomy of verb generation. Neuroimage 1996;3(3 Pt 1):185–194
9. Ojemann G, Ojemann J, Lettich E, Berger M. Cortical language localization in left, dominant hemisphere. An electrical stimulation mapping investigation in 117 patients. J Neurosurg 1989;71:316–326
10. Ojemann GA. Individual variability in cortical localization of language. J Neurosurg 1979;50:164–169
11. Ojemann GA, Whitaker HA. Language localization and variability. Brain Lang 1978;6:239–260
12. Ojemann JG, Miller JW, Silbergeld DL. Preserved function in brain invaded by tumor. Neurosurgery 1996;39:253–258, discussion 258–259
13. Seitz RJ, Huang Y, Knorr U, Tellmann L, Herzog H, Freund HJ. Large-scale plasticity of the human motor cortex. Neuroreport 1995;6:742–744
14. Wunderlich G, Knorr U, Herzog H, Kiwit JC, Freund HJ, Seitz RJ. Precentral glioma location determines the displacement of cortical hand representation. Neurosurgery 1998;42:18–26, discussion 26–27
15. Quiñones-Hinojosa A, Ojemann SG, Sanai N, Dillon WP, Berger MS. Preoperative correlation of intraoperative cortical mapping with magnetic resonance imaging landmarks to predict localization of the Broca area. J Neurosurg 2003;99:311–318
16. Dehaene S, Dupoux E, Mehler J, et al. Anatomical variability in the cortical representation of first and second language. Neuroreport 1997;8:3809–3815
17. Josse G, Hervé PY, Crivello F, Mazoyer B, Tzourio-Mazoyer N. Hemispheric specialization for language: Brain volume matters. Brain Res 2006;1068:184–193
18. Seghier ML, Lazeyras F, Pegna AJ, et al. Variability of fMRI activation during a phonological and semantic language task in healthy subjects. Hum Brain Mapp 2004;23:140–155
19. Steinmetz H, Seitz RJ. Functional anatomy of language processing: neuroimaging and the problem of individual variability. Neuropsychologia 1991;29:1149–1161
20. Turkeltaub PE, Eden GF, Jones KM, Zeffiro TA. Meta-analysis of the functional neuroanatomy of single-word reading: method and validation. Neuroimage 2002;16(3 Pt 1):765–780
21. Tzourio-Mazoyer N, Josse G, Crivello F, Mazoyer B. Interindividual variability in the hemispheric organization for speech. Neuroimage 2004;21:422–435
22. Tzourio N, Crivello F, Mellet E, Nkanga-Ngila B, Mazoyer B. Functional anatomy of dominance for speech comprehension in left handers vs right handers. Neuroimage 1998;8:1–16
23. Davies KG, Maxwell RE, Jennum P, et al. Language function following subdural grid-directed temporal lobectomy. Acta Neurol Scand 1994;90:201–206
24. FitzGerald DB, Cosgrove GR, Ronner S, et al. Location of language in the cortex: a comparison between functional MR imaging and electrocortical stimulation. AJNR Am J Neuroradiol 1997;18:1529–1539
25. Skirboll SS, Ojemann GA, Berger MS, Lettich E, Winn HR. Functional cortex and subcortical white matter located within gliomas. Neurosurgery 1996;38:678–684, discussion 684–685
26. Lacroix M, Abi-Said D, Fourney DR, et al. A multivariate analysis of 416 patients with glioblastoma multiforme: prognosis, extent of resection, and survival. J Neurosurg 2001;95:190–198
27. Duffau H, Capelle L, Denvil D, et al. Usefulness of intraoperative electrical subcortical mapping during surgery for low-grade gliomas located within eloquent brain regions: functional results in a consecutive series of 103 patients. J Neurosurg 2003;98:764–778
28. Duffau H, Capelle L, Sichez N, et al. Intraoperative mapping of the subcortical language pathways using direct stimulations. An anatomo-functional study. Brain 2002;125(Pt 1):199–214
29. Sanai N, Berger MS. Mapping the horizon: techniques to optimize tumor resection before and during surgery. Clin Neurosurg 2008;55:14–19
30. Sanai N, Mirzadeh Z, Berger MS. Functional outcome after language mapping for glioma resection. N Engl J Med 2008;358:18–27
31. Haglund MM, Berger MS, Shamseldin M, Lettich E, Ojemann GA. Cortical localization of temporal lobe language sites in patients with gliomas. Neurosurgery 1994;34:567–576, discussion 576
32. Carrabba G, Fava E, Giussani C, et al. Cortical and subcortical motor mapping in rolandic and perirolandic glioma surgery: impact on postoperative morbidity and extent of resection. J Neurosurg Sci 2007;51:45–51
33. Duffau H, Capelle L, Sichez J, et al. Intra-operative direct electrical stimulations of the central nervous system: the Salpêtrière experience with 60 patients. Acta Neurochir (Wien) 1999;141:1157–1167
34. Keles GE, Lundin DA, Lamborn KR, Chang EF, Ojemann G, Berger MS. Intraoperative subcortical stimulation mapping for hemispherical perirolandic gliomas located within or adjacent to the descending motor pathways: evaluation of morbidity and assessment of functional outcome in 294 patients. J Neurosurg 2004;100:369–375
35. Taylor MD, Bernstein M. Awake craniotomy with brain mapping as the routine surgical approach to treating patients with supratentorial intraaxial tumors: a prospective trial of 200 cases. J Neurosurg 1999;90:35–41
36. Berger MS. Lesions in functional ("eloquent") cortex and sub-cortical white matter. Clin Neurosurg 1993;41:443–463
37. Chollet F, DiPiero V, Wise RJ, Brooks DJ, Dolan RJ, Frackowiak RS. The functional anatomy of motor recovery after stroke in humans: a study with positron emission tomography. Ann Neurol 1991;29:63–71
38. Weder B, Seitz RJ. Deficient cerebral activation pattern in stroke recovery. Neuroreport 1994;5:457–460
39. Lewine JD, Astur RS, Davis LE, Knight JE, Maclin EL, Orrison WW Jr. Cortical organization in adulthood is modified by neonatal infarct: a case study. Radiology 1994;190:93–96
40. Maldjian J, Atlas SW, Howard RS II, et al. Functional magnetic resonance imaging of regional brain activity in patients with intracerebral arteriovenous malformations before surgical or endovascular therapy. J Neurosurg 1996;84:477–483
41. Grady MS, Jane JA, Steward O. Synaptic reorganization within the human central nervous system following injury. J Neurosurg 1989;71:534–537

42. Fandino J, Kollias SS, Wieser HG, Valavanis A, Yonekawa Y. Intraoperative validation of functional magnetic resonance imaging and cortical reorganization patterns in patients with brain tumors involving the primary motor cortex. J Neurosurg 1999;91:238–250

43. Duffau H, Capelle L, Denvil D, et al. Functional recovery after surgical resection of low grade gliomas in eloquent brain: hypothesis of brain compensation. J Neurol Neurosurg Psychiatry 2003;74:901–907

44. Thiel A, Herholz K, Koyuncu A, et al. Plasticity of language networks in patients with brain tumors: a positron emission tomography activation study. Ann Neurol 2001;50:620–629

45. Duffau H, Bauchet L, Lehéricy S, Capelle L. Functional compensation of the left dominant insula for language. Neuroreport 2001;12:2159–2163

46. Gupta DK, Chandra PS, Ojha BK, Sharma BS, Mahapatra AK, Mehta VS. Awake craniotomy versus surgery under general anesthesia for resection of intrinsic lesions of eloquent cortex—a prospective randomised study. Clin Neurol Neurosurg 2007;109:335–343

47. Stummer W, Pichlmeier U, Meinel T, Wiestler OD, Zanella F, Reulen HJ; ALA-Glioma Study Group. Fluorescence-guided surgery with 5-aminolevulinic acid for resection of malignant glioma: a randomised controlled multicentre phase III trial. Lancet Oncol 2006;7:392–401

48. De Witt Hamer PC, Robles SG, Zwinderman AH, Duffau H, Berger MS. Impact of intraoperative stimulation brain mapping on glioma surgery outcome: a meta-analysis. J Clin Oncol 2012;30:2559–2565

15 Complications of Surgery

Ronald E. Warnick and Michael J. Petr

Craniotomy for resection of intrinsic brain tumors is performed to provide a histological diagnosis, ameliorate neurologic symptoms, and help improve survival. Several studies have suggested a favorable association between cytoreductive surgery and survival in patients with low-grade astrocytoma, malignant glioma, and single brain metastasis.[1–4] During the same time period, there has been a significant evolution in the surgical management of these tumors, including the routine use of preoperative functional imaging, stereotactic navigation, cortical mapping, and intraoperative magnetic resonance imaging (MRI), all of which have improved our ability to localize and radically remove intrinsic brain tumors. For these reasons, there has been a renewed interest in understanding the risks of cytoreductive surgery to select appropriate candidates for aggressive tumor resection and to properly counsel patients regarding the expected outcomes of surgery. This chapter focuses on the complications associated with craniotomy for resection of intrinsic brain tumors (e.g., glioma, metastasis), with particular emphasis on the avoidance of these adverse events.

■ Defining a Complication

There is significant disagreement regarding what constitutes a complication. Everyone recognizes that an outcome must be unwanted to be considered a complication of surgery. Whether a particular event is undesirable may be different for the surgeon, patient, and patient's family. For example, a frontalis paresis developing after frontotemporal craniotomy would be considered an undesirable outcome by most neurosurgeons, whereas this deficit may go unnoticed by the patient. Another essential feature of a surgical complication is the unexpected nature of the outcome; in other words, the complication does not occur commonly. Most surgical procedures have a range of anticipated outcomes, and complications are those outcomes that deviate from this norm. However, classification of surgical outcomes is subjective. For example, a patient

> **Controversy**
>
> - If a patient develops an expected neurologic deficit after surgery, should it be classified as a complication? Does it make a difference whether it is transient or permanent?

> **Special Consideration**
>
> - The neurosurgeon must have an intimate knowledge of the complications and risk factors associated with craniotomy to counsel a patient regarding the optimal surgical option.

undergoing removal of a glioma located within the dominant supplementary motor area often experiences predictable postoperative neurologic deficits like hemiparesis that improve with time and rehabilitation. Should this be considered an expected, though undesirable, outcome of surgery or a neurologic complication? There is little consensus on this issue, although most surgical series document all adverse events without regard to whether they are expected.[5–9] In practice, however, the neurosurgeon must undertake careful discussions with the patient and family regarding expected, though undesirable, outcomes lest these be viewed as complications.

Classification of Complications

Various schemes have been introduced to classify surgical complications, and there is considerable overlap among them. Some authors view all complications as potentially avoidable and as resulting from three main causes: (1) lack of information (e.g., failure to recognize a preexisting medical condition); (2) incorrect judgment (e.g., suboptimal surgical approach); and (3) incorrect execution (e.g., excessive brain retraction).[10] Implicit in this classification system is the concept that complications are generally under the neurosurgeon's control, which certainly does not apply to most medical complications.

An alternative classification distinguishes among neurologic, regional, and systemic complications and provides a logical framework for discussing complications associated with craniotomy (**Table 15.1**).[7] In this system, *neurologic* complications are events that directly produce motor, sensory, language, or visual deficits (e.g., edema, vascular injury, hematoma). *Regional* complications are related either to the wound (e.g., infection, cerebrospinal fluid [CSF] leak) or to the brain (e.g., seizures, hydrocephalus) but are not associated with neurologic deficits. *Systemic* complications include more generalized medical conditions (e.g., thromboembolism, pneumonia). These main categories can be further subdivided on the basis of the degree of severity. *Major* complications include events that are permanent, significantly affect quality of life, or re-

Table 15.1 Complications Associated with Craniotomy

Neurologic	Regional	Systemic
Motor or sensory	Seizure	Deep vein thrombosis
Deficit	Hydrocephalus	Pulmonary embolus
Aphasia/dysphasia	Pneumocephalus	Pneumonia
Visual field deficit	Wound infection	Urinary infection
Caused by:	Meningitis	Sepsis
Direct brain injury	Brain abscess	Myocardial infarction
Brain edema	Cerebrospinal fistula	Gastrointestinal bleed
Vascular injury		Electrolyte disturbance
Hematoma		

Source: From Wolters Kluwer Health. Sawaya R, Hammoud M, Schoppa D, et al. Neurosurgical outcomes in a modern series of 400 craniotomies for treatment of parenchymal tumors. Neurosurgery 1998;42:1044–1056. Reprinted with permission.

quire surgical intervention. In contrast, *minor* complications are transient or permanent events without significant functional impact, and those that resolve without surgery.

Surgical Complications and Their Avoidance

General Considerations

The overall complication rate associated with craniotomy for intrinsic brain tumor ranges from 25 to 35% and includes all adverse events, expected and unexpected, regardless of severity.[5–7,9] The complication rate of a particular series depends on the authors' definition of a complication, the type of study (retrospective versus prospective), and the referral base of the institution. In general, higher complication rates are reported by those at tertiary neurosurgical centers that have prospectively analyzed complications and have included all adverse events, expected and unexpected.[7]

The key to minimizing complications is to thoroughly understand all potential adverse events associated with the procedure and to formulate a comprehensive plan to prevent their occurrence. The neurosurgeon must have an intimate understanding of the patient's history, neurologic findings, and diagnostic studies to determine an accurate preoperative diagnosis. The surgical approach must be individualized to each patient, and the neurosurgeon should either be familiar with the steps of the procedure or request the assistance of a

Pitfall

- Complication rates among neurosurgical centers may not be directly comparable because of differences in the classification of complications and data collection methods (retrospective versus prospective).

Special Consideration

- The key to complication avoidance is rigorous judgment, careful planning, and meticulous execution.

colleague. A complete understanding of the operative anatomy, which includes the structural and functional anatomy of the normal brain as well as any variations introduced by the tumor, is essential. The experienced neurosurgeon also mentally rehearses the entire operation and postoperative period to identify potential pitfalls and develop appropriate contingency plans.

Neurologic Complications

The risk of a new neurologic deficit, minor or major, after craniotomy for intrinsic tumor ranges from 10 to 25% in modern surgical series.[5–7,9] Risk factors shown to predict an adverse neurologic outcome include age > 60 years, Karnofsky Performance Scale (KPS) score< 60%, deep tumor location, and tumor proximity to eloquent brain areas.[5–8] Despite the concern that aggressive tumor resection might lead to greater neurologic morbidity, two studies have demonstrated the opposite, namely, that gross total resection of intrinsic tumors, particularly malignant glioma, is associated with fewer neurologic complications than is subtotal resection.[5,7] This finding is probably explained by the higher risk of postoperative edema and hemorrhage when a glioblastoma is incompletely removed.[11] Recognition of the preceding risk factors enables the neurosurgeon to estimate the risk of a neurologic complication for an individual patient.[7] In a clinical scenario, a 40-year-old patient with a normal neurologic examination and noneloquent tumor would have a predicted complication rate of about 5% (**Fig. 15.1a**). In contrast, a 65-year-old patient with a significant hemiparesis caused by a motor area glioblastoma would have a predicted complication rate as high as 26% (**Fig. 15.1b**).

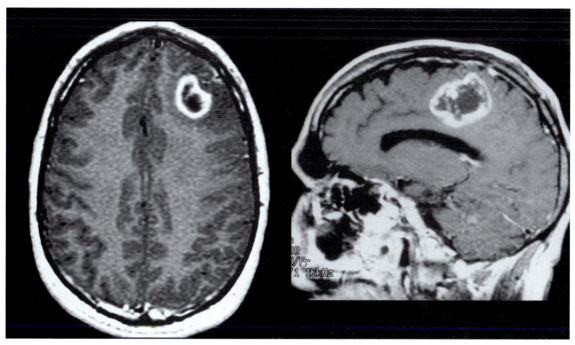

a   b

Fig. 15.1a,b (**a**) Contrast-enhanced magnetic resonance imaging (MRI) scan of a 40-year-old man who presented with a generalized seizure and normal neurologic examination. Craniotomy and resection of this left frontal tumor would be the procedure of choice for this patient, with a predicted complication rate of about 5%. (**b**) Contrast-enhanced MRI scan of a 65-year-old man who experi- enced progressive right-sided weakness over 6 weeks and was found to have an enhancing tumor within the left motor cortex. Open resection of this tumor would be associated with a predicted compli- cation rate of about 25% in this patient; therefore, stereotactic biopsy was recommended.

<table>
<tr><td>**Special Consideration**</td></tr>
</table>

- The surgical approach must be individualized to each patient based on factors related to the patient (age, neuro- logic status, preference) and the tumor (size, location, pre- sumed histology).

Injury to Normal Brain Structures

Neurologic complications result from one of the following eti- ologies: (1) direct injury to normal brain structures, (2) brain edema, (3) vascular injury, or (4) hematoma. Inadvertent in- jury to normal brain structures may occur because of incor- rect localization of the tumor in relation to adjacent eloquent brain areas. Avoidance of this problem begins with intimate knowledge of the normal structural and functional anatomy of the operative field and the relationship of the tumor bor- ders to adjacent critical brain structures. Functional MRI and diffusion tensor imaging can be used to determine tumor re- sectability and are powerful tools for surgical planning. For tumors located in the posterior frontal lobe, the motor strip can be identified by cortical mapping techniques and sub- cortical motor pathways preserved during tumor resection.[12]

Similarly, craniotomy using speech mapping with the patient awake allows the neurosurgeon to maximally resect dominant temporal lobe tumors while minimizing the risk of a postop- erative language deficit.[12]

The introduction of frameless stereotactic techniques has revolutionized the practice of neurosurgery by providing an easy, intuitive, and accurate method for intracranial naviga- tion. Frameless stereotaxis facilitates precise localization of superficial tumors and enables the neurosurgeon to plan op- timal trajectories to approach deeply seated tumors, thereby minimizing brain injury associated with dissection. Normal structures like motor cortex can be readily identified and pre- served. The information obtained from functional MRI and diffusion tensor imaging can be integrated into the frameless stereotactic system and used intraoperatively to maximize tumor resection while preserving neurologic function.[13] The intraoperative feedback provided by stereotactic navigation must, however, be integrated with conventional techniques to assess the extent of resection, including visual inspection, measurement of the tumor cavity, and identification of nor- mal adjacent structures (e.g., falx, skull base, sulci). More re- cently, intraoperative MRI has proven to be a useful adjunct by providing near real-time updates during the course of tumor surgery to overcome the problem of brain shift and maximize the degree of tumor resection.[14,15]

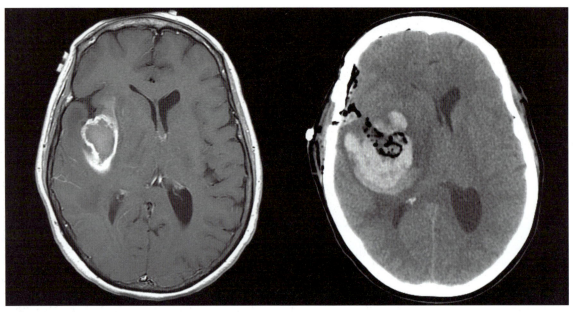

a   b

Fig. 15.2a,b **(a)** Preoperative contrast-enhanced MRI scan of a 62-year-old woman with a right insular glioblastoma. During surgery, the tumor was quite vascular and only a subtotal resection could be achieved. Four hours after surgery, the patient exhibited a sudden decline in level of consciousness with a left hemiplegia. **(b)** Noncon-trast computed tomography (CT) scan revealed a large parenchymal hemorrhage with edema and mass effect consistent with "wounded glioma" syndrome. She was returned to the operating room and underwent removal of the residual tumor and associated hemorrhage but did not achieve a functional recovery.

> **Pitfall**
>
> - The neurosurgeon should not rely too much on frameless stereotactic navigation to determine the extent of tumor resection because the accuracy of this information decreases when brain shifts occur during surgery. Intraoperative MRI provides near real-time updates that allow the surgeon to compensate for these changes.

Brain Edema

Brain edema is a common cause of neurologic morbidity and, in its extreme form, may result in herniation and death. Factors that contribute to postoperative edema include excessive brain retraction and subtotal resection of malignant tumors, especially glioblastomas. Retraction injury can be minimized by proper patient positioning, hyperventilation, high-dose corticosteroids, diuretics, and intermittent retractor placement. Stereotactic navigation can be used to determine the optimal surgical trajectory and to reduce the need for prolonged retraction. Most importantly, craniotomy and resection of malignant gliomas should be undertaken with the goal of either a gross total or radical subtotal resection. Internal debulking surgery leaves residual, vascular tumor that has the propensity to produce brain edema and intratumoral hemorrhage ("wounded glioma syndrome") (**Fig. 15.2**). There is some evidence that patients with malignant glioma who undergo a partial resection experience greater neurologic morbidity than do those who have a gross total resection.[5,7,11]

Injury to Vascular Structures

Injury to vascular structures is an infrequent complication of craniotomy but may have devastating neurologic consequences. The incidence of vascular injury has generally been reported to be 1 to 2%.[5] Major venous occlusion produces a hemorrhagic stroke, the onset of which is delayed by several days and from which the patient often recovers (**Fig. 15.3**). The risk of this complication can be reduced by early identification of major venous structures like the vein of Labbé, selective sacrifice of draining veins, protection of cortical veins during retraction, and intermittent application of retractors to allow reestablishment of venous flow. Videoangiography with indocyanine green (ICG) can be used to check the patency of draining veins during surgery.[16] When the viability of a major draining vein is questionable, a continuous mannitol drip (10 to 20 mL/h of 20% solution) and rehydration may improve the rheological profile sufficiently to prevent complete venous occlusion.

Arterial injury, in contrast, produces an immediate neurologic deficit that permanently affects the patient's quality of life (**Fig. 15.4**). To avoid this catastrophic complication, the neurosurgeon must have a clear understanding of the anatomic relationship between the tumor and the nearby arteries; this relationship is usually apparent on the preoperative MRI. Maintaining a subpial dissection plane is an important

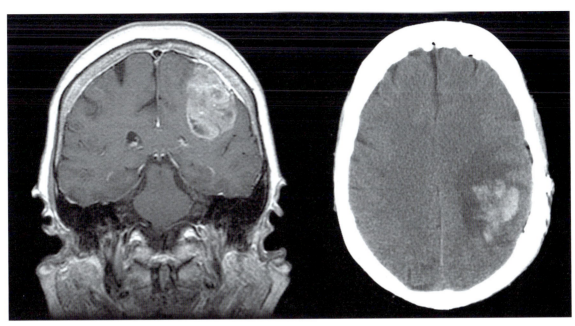

Fig. 15.3a,b **(a)** Preoperative contrast-enhanced coronal MRI scan of a 75-year-old woman with a left parietal glioblastoma. A large draining vein overlies the tumor. At the time of surgery, there was significant manipulation of the vein during tumor resection. Postoperatively, the patient was neurologically intact for 48 hours and then developed a progressive right hemiparesis. **(b)** Noncontrast CT scan revealed patchy hemorrhage and edema deep to the resection cavity consistent with venous infarction. The patient fully recovered over 3 months.

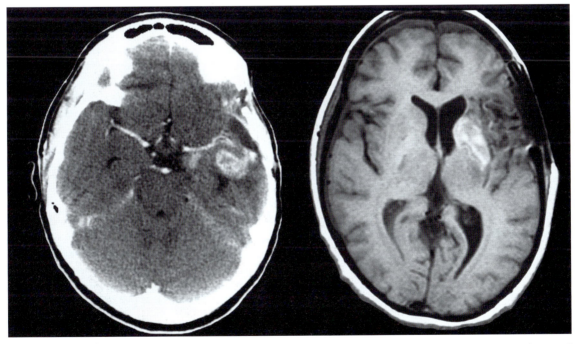

Fig. 15.4a,b **(a)** Preoperative contrast-enhanced CT scan of a 32-year-old woman with a recurrent left temporal glioblastoma abutting the sylvian fissure. During resection of the tumor using the ultrasonic aspirator, the pia-arachnoid of the sylvian fissure was traversed, causing injury to the middle cerebral artery. Postoperatively, the patient had a profound expressive aphasia and right hemiplegia. **(b)** Noncontrast MRI scan performed 2 months after surgery demonstrating infarction in the territory of the middle cerebral artery. Although the patient was left with a moderate expressive dysphasia and right arm weakness, she was able to ambulate.

strategy during tumor resection to avoid major arterial vessels, for example, the pericallosal artery during resection of a medial frontal lobe tumor. The greatest risk of arterial disruption occurs in the unusual circumstance of a malignant tumor that no longer respects the pial surfaces, such as a frontotemporal glioblastoma crossing the sylvian fissure and engulfing the middle cerebral artery. The ultrasonic aspirator must be used with care, and no artery should be sacrificed until it can be determined whether it is a tumor feeder or a vessel en passage. After the completion of tumor resection, exposed arteries should be covered with papaverine-soaked Gelfoam to reduce the risk of vasospasm.

Hematomas

Postoperative hematomas causing neurologic deficits occur in 1 to 5% of patients in recent surgical series.[5–7] These patients typically present in the early postoperative period with altered level of consciousness, focal neurologic deficits, and seizures. Early recognition and appropriate surgical intervention are essential to prevent permanent neurologic morbidity. Patients who have undergone a craniotomy and are slow to awaken or exhibit an unexpected neurologic deficit should undergo an urgent computed tomographic (CT) scan to rule out postoperative hemorrhage.

Most hematomas can be avoided by careful preoperative preparation, meticulous operative technique, and vigilant postoperative care. Careful questioning of the patient should reveal any history of bleeding diathesis or medication use (e.g., aspirin) that may alter hemostatic ability. Patients are generally screened preoperatively with a prothrombin time and partial thromboplastin time. A bleeding time or platelet aggregation studies can be obtained in patients with recent aspirin or nonsteroidal agent use to rule out significant platelet dysfunction. Intracerebral hematomas occur when tumor-bed hemostasis is incomplete or when vascular tumor remains (**Fig. 15.5**). As mentioned earlier, internal debulking of a glioblastoma may produce a "wounded glioma," with intratumoral hemorrhage and peritumoral edema leading to herniation and even death. The neurosurgeon must strive for complete removal of vascular tumor to avoid this complication. At the completion of tumor resection, all bleeding points must be precisely coagulated; most neurosurgeons use one of several hemostatic agents (e.g., Surgicel; Oxycel; FloSeal, Baxter, Deerfield, IL) to line the tumor cavity. Provocative testing using the Valsalva maneuver further tests the state of hemostasis.

Subdural hematomas are usually the result of torn bridging veins that have been stretched by brain shift. Factors contributing to brain shift include brain atrophy, the use of

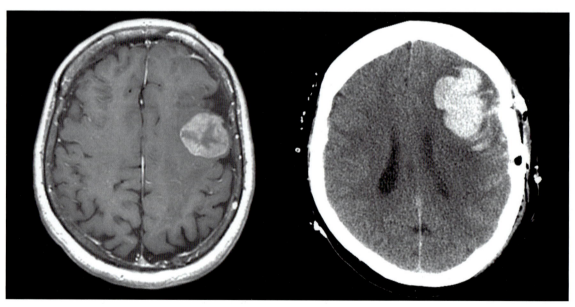

a   b

Fig. 15.5a,b (**a**) Contrast-enhanced MRI scan of a 43-year-old woman with a history of breast cancer who presented with a generalized seizure. She underwent resection of this left frontal metastatic tumor and was neurologically intact immediately after surgery. The next morning, the patient was noted to be lethargic, with an expressive dysphasia and a mild left hemiparesis. (**b**) Noncontrast CT scan showed a large hemorrhage filling the resection cavity and extending into the parenchyma. After return to the operating room for evacuation of the hematoma, she fully recovered neurologically.

diuretics, resection of large parenchymal tumors, and ventricular entry. When excessive brain shift is recognized during surgery, the anesthesiologist can gradually normalize the partial pressure of CO_2 and gently rehydrate the patient to facilitate brain reexpansion. The use of dural retention sutures along bone edges and centrally and waxing all bone edges may reduce the incidence of epidural hematomas. Some neurosurgeons also advocate the use of a hemostatic sponge (e.g., compressed Gelfoam, Biocol) over the dura and bone edges to prevent epidural bleeding; there is always the potential that the hemostatic agent may expand and form a compressive mass, however. The role of a subgaleal drain in preventing epidural hematomas is uncertain and a matter of individual preference. Lastly, effective prevention of hematomas continues well into the postoperative period. The anesthesiologist should be reminded to avoid arterial hypertension and the Valsalva maneuver (i.e., the patient resisting the endotracheal tube) in the early postoperative period, which could undo even the most meticulous hemostasis.

Regional Complications

Regional complications are events associated with the surgical site (e.g., infection, CSF leak) or the brain (e.g., seizures, hydrocephalus, pneumocephalus) but that do not result in neurologic deficits.[7] This type of complication occurs in 3 to 5% of patients undergoing craniotomy for removal of intrinsic brain tumors.[5–7,9] Regional complications are more common in elderly patients who are in poor neurologic condition. As one might expect, resection of parenchymal tumors located in the posterior fossa is associated with a higher risk of regional complications like pseudomeningocele, CSF fistula, and hydrocephalus.[7] The impact of previous surgery and radiotherapy on the risk of regional complications has not been clearly established in the literature. Reoperation has generally been associated with an increased risk of wound complications (e.g., infection, subgaleal collections, CSF fistula), especially in previously irradiated patients.[8] A prospective study failed, however, to demonstrate an increased risk of regional

complications in patients with a history of previous surgery or radiotherapy, or both.[7] This result may be explained by the fact that most experienced brain tumor surgeons recognize the increased risks inherent in reoperative neurosurgery and have modified their surgical techniques to reduce these complications to a level comparable with that of a first craniotomy.

Seizures

A seizure in the early postoperative period after craniotomy is a dramatic event that may have devastating effects on neurologic recovery. These events usually occur in the recovery room and may be focal or generalized or may even progress to status epilepticus if not treated in a timely fashion. The incidence of immediate seizures ranges from 0.5 to 10% after supratentorial craniotomy even with routine anticonvulsant use.[6,7,17,18] There are several known risk factors for seizures during the immediate postoperative period. A history of preoperative epilepsy and tumor proximity to the motor cortex are the strongest predictors of early seizures after craniotomy.[17] In general, the degree of cortical injury correlates with epileptogenic potential and increases with operations that involve prolonged retraction (e.g., transcortical approach to a deeply seated tumor) or when postoperative edema and hemorrhage complicate surgery (e.g., wounded glioma syndrome). Systemic factors such as hyponatremia or acidosis may also lower the threshold for postoperative seizures.

The efficacy of prophylactic anticonvulsants in preventing postcraniotomy seizures remains controversial. A small number of studies have demonstrated a lower frequency of seizures in patients who receive phenytoin either before or during a craniotomy.[19,20] However, a meta-analysis of 12 studies failed to demonstrate the efficacy of prophylactic anticonvulsant therapy.[21] A 2013 randomized trial examining the use of phenytoin for seizure prophylaxis did not show any reduction in the incidence of early postoperative seizures, and there was significantly higher rate of drug-related morbidity.[18]

The evidence-based approach would be not to start patients on antiepileptic medications unless they have already had a seizure. However, many neurosurgeons still routinely use anticonvulsants around the time of a craniotomy for resection of an intrinsic brain tumor. In these cases, the patient should receive an anticonvulsant (e.g., Keppra, UCB, Inc., Atlanta, GA) for several days prior to craniotomy. An additional dose is administered in the operating room to achieve a high therapeutic concentration by the time the patient emerges from anesthesia. Patients who present preoperatively with a focal seizure secondary to a motor area tumor may experience immediate postoperative seizures in spite of a therapeutic anticonvulsant concentration. In these patients, consideration should be given to double prophylaxis with Keppra and Ativan (Pfizer, New York, NY) during the perioperative period. Finally, postoperative seizures must be treated aggressively and patients should undergo a CT scan to rule out a structural cause such as edema, hemorrhage, or infarct.[22]

Infections

Postoperative infections at the site of craniotomy range from superficial cellulitis to deep infections that involve the bone flap, meninges, or resection cavity (**Fig. 15.6**). Studies have documented this risk to be about 1 to 2% after supratentorial craniotomy.[6,7,23] Most craniotomy infections result from contamination of the operative site by skin pathogens during surgery, although a superficial wound infection (e.g., suture abscess) may lead to a deep infection if untreated. The microbiological spectrum of craniotomy infections generally reflects the normal flora of the scalp, including *Staphylococcus aureus,* *Staphylococcus epidermidis,* and *Propionibacterium acnes;* however, nosocomial infections by gram-negative organisms also occur.[23] Most supratentorial craniotomies are considered clean cases and are associated with a postoperative infection rate of less than 1%.[23] Several factors increase the risk of infection, including proximity to paranasal sinuses (clean-contaminated), active CSF fistula (contaminated), foreign body, long surgery, and intensive corticosteroid use.[23] Previous surgery and cytotoxic therapy (e.g., radiation, chemotherapy) have been shown to increase the risk of craniotomy infection in some studies, but others have failed to demonstrate this association.[7,8,23]

Various strategies have been used to reduce the incidence of surgical-site infections. Patients should be screened for methicillin-resistant *S. aureus* using nasal swabs. Carriers should be decolonized with mupirocin ointment and chlorhexidine soap before surgery.[24] Several well-designed randomized trials have proven the efficacy of prophylactic antibiotics in preventing superficial and deep infections after craniot-

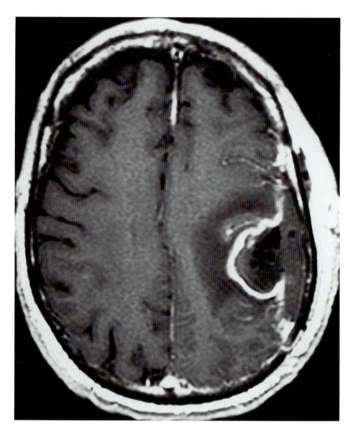

Fig. 15.6 Contrast-enhanced MRI scan of a 62-year-old man who underwent craniotomy and resection of a left parietal glioblastoma 1 month earlier. He then presented to the emergency room with fever, headache, and right-sided weakness. Because the craniotomy flap was full and erythematous, the patient underwent reexploration of the craniotomy with bone flap removal and evacuation of a subdural empyema that had extended into the resection cavity. The patient fully recovered after a course of intravenous antibiotics for *Staphylococcus aureus* infection.

omy.[25] Various drugs and administration schedules have been tested, but none has been found to be superior. In general, the antibiotic should be active against the common organisms causing craniotomy infections (i.e., skin pathogens) but does not need to cross the blood–brain barrier to be effective. Ideally, the infusion should be completed 30 to 60 minutes before making the skin incision to achieve an adequate blood concentration of antibiotic. Lastly, additional doses of the antibiotic are generally not necessary except during extended operations. In addition to antibiotic prophylaxis, meticulous wound closure and close vigilance after surgery minimize the risk of a superficial wound infection that could extend to the deep structures and lead to reoperation.

Systemic Complications

Medical complications occur in 5 to 10% of patients undergoing craniotomy and removal of an intrinsic brain tumor.[5–7,9] Analogous to the other categories, systemic complications pre-

Pearl

- Routine bedside Doppler studies should be used in post-craniotomy patients who are slow to ambulate or have a significant lower extremity paresis.

dominantly affect the elderly (> 60 years old) and those who are neurologically impaired (KPS < 60%).[7] In addition, pre-existing medical conditions also influence the risk of postoperative systemic complications. A wide range of medical complications occur after surgery, including deep vein thrombosis (DVT), pulmonary embolism, infection (pneumonia, urinary tract infection, sepsis), myocardial infarction, gastrointestinal hemorrhage, and electrolyte disturbance.

The most frequent systemic complication after craniotomy is DVT, with or without pulmonary embolism. The risk of DVT during the first month after craniotomy has been estimated to be 1 to 10%, although the cumulative risk increases to 20% during the 12 months following surgery.[5–8,26] Patients with glioblastoma or systemic cancer are at highest risk of thromboembolic complications, but other important predictors include age over 60 years, lower extremity paresis, prolonged bed rest, and long duration of surgery.[26]

Several preventive measures have been shown to reduce the risk of thromboembolic events after craniotomy. Patients should be out of bed and mobilized as soon as possible after surgery and encouraged to ambulate both in the hospital and during recovery at home. Elastic stockings and compression boots appear to be equally effective in reducing the risk of DVT when they are applied preoperatively and continued until the patient is ambulatory.[27] Both modalities enhance lower extremity venous return, whereas compression boots also increase general fibrinolytic activity and are therefore favored. Anticoagulation with "mini-dose" heparin (5,000 U) twice a day subcutaneously or low-molecular-weight heparin (LMWH) beginning 24 hours after craniotomy has been proven to reduce the risk of all thromboembolic events without affecting the frequency of intracranial hemorrhage.[28–30] Low-molecular-weight heparin has theoretical advantages over standard heparin, including less potent antithrombin activity and no significant effects on platelets, both of which should theoretically minimize the risk of bleeding diathesis. In a randomized, double-blind study, patients who received enoxaparin (Lovenox, Sanofi, Bridgewater, NJ) starting 1 day after surgery had a greater than 50% reduction in the frequency of proximal DVT compared with the placebo group, with no difference in hemorrhagic complications.[30] A prospective study using nadroparin (Fraxiparine, GlaxoSmithKline, Mississagua, Ontario, Canada) after cranial surgery showed that the incidence of postoperative intracranial bleeding was similar to patients not receiving anticoagulation therapy, whereas the risk of DVT was reduced.[31] The results of these studies favor the use of both perioperative mechanical prophylaxis and LMWH ther-

apy beginning within 1 day of craniotomy, assuming that the postoperative imaging study (CT or MRI) does not reveal significant intracranial hemorrhage.

Mortality Associated with Craniotomy

The mortality after craniotomy for intrinsic brain tumors has decreased steadily over the past three decades as a result of the significant evolution in the surgical management of these tumors.[5] The introduction of CT and MRI has allowed earlier detection and three-dimensional visualization of brain tumors. Advances in neuroanesthesia, including the perioperative administration of corticosteroids and diuretics, have reduced the morbidity and mortality previously associated with cytoreductive surgery. Finally, technical advances in neurosurgery, such as the preoperative functional imaging, stereotactic navigation, operating microscope, and cortical mapping, have improved the ability of neurosurgeons to aggressively resect most intrinsic brain tumors. The mortality rates reported by surgical series during this decade have ranged from 1.7 to 2.7%.[6–8] As expected, elderly patients with neurologic impairment have the highest 30-day mortality rate after a craniotomy. Most postoperative deaths result from neurologic complications such as hematoma, edema with herniation, or tumor progression, local or leptomeningeal. Most regional complications resolve with medical or surgical intervention and do not progress to death. Systemic complications account for the remainder of postoperative deaths and are evenly distributed among pulmonary embolism, myocardial infarction, and sepsis.

Special Consideration

- Elderly patients with poor neurologic function have the highest risk of morbidity and mortality; cytoreductive surgery should be used on a highly selective basis in this population.

Conclusion

Radical resection of intrinsic brain tumors can be performed in most patients with acceptable morbidity and mortality. This generalization includes tumors located near eloquent areas when appropriate techniques are used, such as stereotactic navigation, cortical mapping, and intraoperative MRI. The surgical approach needs to be individualized to each patient because the risk of postoperative complications varies greatly with patient age, neurologic status, and tumor location. The neurosurgeon should have intimate knowledge of the risk factors and predicted complication rates of craniotomy to select appropriate candidates for aggressive tumor resection and to properly counsel patients regarding the expected outcome of surgery. The majority of complications can be prevented by careful perioperative planning, meticulous technique, and the judicious use of prophylactic agents (e.g., anticonvulsants, antibiotics, LMWH). Neurosurgeons should regularly analyze the types and frequencies of complications within their practice and devise specific strategies to decrease their occurrence.

Editor's Note

Several factors are involved in the development of complications after brain tumor surgery. Attention to careful decision making, thorough pre- and postoperative care, and excellent technical execution of the procedure are obviously essential to minimizing harm. However, because of the tumor location, vascular supply, consistency, and intimacy with eloquent brain or vascular structures, many neurologic complications are unavoidable.

Much can be learned from studying the complications from one's own practice, and the first step in complication avoidance is complication recognition. Surgeons must be honest and open in tracking and discussing their complications. It is heartily recommended that surgeons keep a prospective database, from day 1, of their errors and complications and also be prepared to discuss them openly with peers and even consider publishing them.[32] Surgeons are deeply and intimately invested in their patients' welfare, and tend to take responsibility for their patients' outcomes, even when bad things happen beyond their direct control. They are sometimes embarrassed about discussing their complications, but it is the right thing to do to confront these issues head-on, both for the sake of honesty and to learn how to do things better in the future. (Bernstein)

References

1. Berger MS, Deliganis AV, Dobbins J, Keles GE. The effect of extent of resection on recurrence in patients with low grade cerebral hemisphere gliomas. Cancer 1994;74:1784–1791
2. Wood JR, Green SB, Shapiro WR. The prognostic importance of tumor size in malignant gliomas: a computed tomographic scan study by the Brain Tumor Cooperative Group. J Clin Oncol 1988;6:338–343
3. Patchell RA, Tibbs PA, Walsh JW, et al. A randomized trial of surgery in the treatment of single metastases to the brain. N Engl J Med 1990;322:494–500
4. Hardesty DA, Sania N. The value of glioma extent of resection in the modern neurosurgical era. Front Neurol 2012;3:E140
5. Fadul C, Wood J, Thaler H, Galicich J, Patterson RH Jr, Posner JB. Morbidity and mortality of craniotomy for excision of supratentorial gliomas. Neurology 1988;38:1374–1379
6. Cabantog AM, Bernstein M. Complications of first craniotomy for intra-axial brain tumour. Can J Neurol Sci 1994;21:213–218
7. Sawaya R, Hammoud M, Schoppa D, et al. Neurosurgical outcomes in a modern series of 400 craniotomies for treatment of parenchymal tumors. Neurosurgery 1998;42:1044–1055, discussion 1055–1056
8. Vorster SJ, Barnett GH. A proposed preoperative grading scheme to assess risk for surgical resection of primary and secondary intraaxial supratentorial brain tumors. Neurosurg Focus 1998;4:e2
9. Wong JM, Panchmatia JR, Ziewacz JE, et al. Patterns in neurosurgical adverse events: intracranial neoplasm surgery. Neurosurg Focus 2012;33:E16
10. Grossman RG. Preoperative and surgical planning for avoiding complications. In: Apuzzo MU, ed. Brain Surgery—Complication Avoidance and Management. New York: Churchill Livingstone, 1993:3–9
11. Ciric I, Ammirati M, Vick N, Mikhael M. Supratentorial gliomas: surgical considerations and immediate postoperative results. Gross total resection versus partial resection. Neurosurgery 1987;21:21–26
12. Berger MS, Ojemann GA, Lettich E. Neurophysiological monitoring during astrocytoma surgery. In: Rosenblum ML, ed. The Role of Surgery in Brain Tumor Management. Philadelphia: WB Saunders, 1990:65–80
13. Nimsky C, Ganslandt O, Hastreiter P, et al. Preoperative and intraoperative diffusion tensor imaging-based fiber tracking in glioma surgery. Neurosurgery 2005;56:130–137, discussion 138
14. Bohinski RJ, Kokkino AK, Warnick RE, et al. Glioma resection in a shared-resource magnetic resonance operating room after optimal image-guided frameless stereotactic resection. Neurosurgery 2001;48:731–742, discussion 742–744
15. Kuhnt D, Becker A, Ganslandt O, Bauer M, Buchfelder M, Nimsky C. Correlation of the extent of tumor volume resection and patient survival in surgery of glioblastoma multiforme with high-field intraoperative MRI guidance. Neuro-oncol 2011;13:1339–1348
16. Kim EH, Cho JM, Chang JH, Kim SH, Lee KS. Application of intraoperative indocyanine green videoangiography to brain tumor surgery. Acta Neurochir (Wien) 2011;153:1487–1495, discussion 1494–1495
17. Kvam DA, Loftus CM, Copeland B, Quest DO. Seizures during the immediate postoperative period. Neurosurgery 1983;12:14–17
18. Wu AS, Trinh VT, Suki D, et al. A prospective randomized trial of perioperative seizure prophylaxis in patients with intraparenchymal brain tumors. J Neurosurg 2013;118:873–883
19. Boarini DJ, Beck DW, VanGilder JC. Postoperative prophylactic anticonvulsant therapy in cerebral gliomas. Neurosurgery 1985;16:290–292
20. Lee ST, Lui TN, Chang CN, et al. Prophylactic anticonvulsants for prevention of immediate and early postcraniotomy seizures. Surg Neurol 1989;31:361–364
21. Glantz MJ, Cole BF, Forsyth PA, et al; Report of the Quality Standards Subcommittee of the American Academy of Neurology. Practice parameter: anticonvulsant prophylaxis in patients with newly diagnosed brain tumors. Neurology 2000;54:1886–1893
22. Fukamachi A, Koizumi H, Nukui H. Immediate postoperative seizures: incidence and computed tomographic findings. Surg Neurol 1985;24:671–676
23. Narotam PK, van Dellen JR, du Trevou MD, Gouws E. Operative sepsis in neurosurgery: a method of classifying surgical cases. Neurosurgery 1994;34:409–415, discussion 415–416
24. Savage JW, Anderson PA. An update on modifiable factors to reduce the risk of surgical site infections. Spine J 2013;13:1017–1029
25. Haines SJ. Antibiotic prophylaxis in neurosurgery: the controlled trials. In: Haines SJ, Hall WA, eds. Infections in Neurological Surgery. Philadelphia: WB Saunders, 1992:355–358

26. Brandes AA, Scelzi E, Salmistraro G, et al. Incidence of risk of thrombo-embolism during treatment high-grade gliomas: a prospective study. Eur J Cancer 1997;33:1592–1596

27. Bucci MN, Papadopoulos SM, Chen JC, Campbell JA, Hoff JT. Mechanical prophylaxis of venous thrombosis in patients undergoing craniotomy: a randomized trial. Surg Neurol 1989;32:285–288

28. Cerrato D, Ariano C, Fiacchino F. Deep vein thrombosis and low-dose heparin prophylaxis in neurosurgical patients. J Neurosurg 1978;49:378–381

29. Nurmohamed MT, van Riel AM, Henkens CM, et al. Low molecular weight heparin and compression stockings in the prevention of venous thromboembolism in neurosurgery. Thromb Haemost 1996;75:233–238

30. Agnelli G, Piovella F, Buoncristiani P, et al. Enoxaparin plus compression stockings compared with compression stockings alone in the prevention of venous thromboembolism after elective neurosurgery. N Engl J Med 1998;339:80–85

31. Gerlach R, Scheuer T, Beck J, Woszczyk A, Seifert V, Raabe A. Risk of postoperative hemorrhage after intracranial surgery after early nadroparin administration: results of a prospective study. Neurosurgery 2003;53:1028–1034, discussion 1034–1035

32. Stone S, Bernstein M. Prospective error recording in surgery: an analysis of 1108 elective neurosurgical cases. Neurosurgery 2007;60:1075–1080, discussion 1080–1082

IV Radiation

16 Fractionated Radiotherapy

Arjun Sahgal and Glenn S. Bauman

Radiotherapy is commonly used in the management of malignant and selected benign brain tumors. The majority of patients requiring radiotherapy are treated with fractionated external-beam photon beams, delivering 1.8 to 2.0 Gy per day, generated by linear accelerators (LINACs). Modern innovations in radiation treatment delivery technology (**Fig. 16.1**) have revolutionized radiation oncology treatments for brain tumor patients, and include near-rigid patient immobilization devices (**Fig. 16.2**), computed tomography (CT) and magnetic resonance imaging (MRI)-based simulation to allow for multimodal imaging-based target delineation, incorporation of on-board image guidance systems to ensure daily verification of the patient position prior to delivery, and precise beam shaping using multileaf collimators (MLCs) that also allow for modulation of the beam intensity during delivery (known as intensity modulated radiotherapy [IMRT]).[1] The potential benefits of these innovations include increasing tumor control by allowing safe dose-escalation, and decreasing risk of late radiation toxicity by minimizing the volume of brain exposed to collateral radiation dose.

■ Radiobiology and Physics

Radiation produces highly reactive free radicals in tissues. These free radicals damage nuclear DNA, resulting in reproductive cell death during cellular division or apoptotic cell death in response to the DNA injury.[2] There are three categories of radiation damage: (1) lethal damage, which is irreversible and leads to cellular death; (2) sublethal damage, which can be repaired unless additional sublethal damage is added; and (3) potentially lethal damage, which can be modified by environmental conditions.[2] The apparent radioresponsiveness of tissue depends on the inherent sensitivity of cells, the kinetics of the cell population, the microenvironment such as oxygen levels, and radiation parameters such as type of radiation, absorbed dose, and fractionation. Absorbed dose is the amount of energy deposited per unit mass at a point in tissue (measured in units of joules per kilogram, commonly referred to as a gray [Gy]).

Although photons (X-rays or gamma rays) are the most commonly used form of therapeutic radiation, charged particle therapies such as protons or other heavy particles like carbon or helium ions have also been used for the treatment of specific central nervous system (CNS) tumors such as chor-

domas.[3] Dose for charged particle beam therapy is typically quoted in cobalt gray equivalents (dose normalized for the relative biological effectiveness [RBE] of the particle versus cobalt gamma irradiation). For protons, the RBE is close to that of photons at 1.1, and can be considered biologically equivalent. The major benefit of a proton beam over a photon beam stems from the Bragg peak energy deposition that allows for sharp dose gradients at interfaces with critical structures, as the dose abruptly falls off at a depth in tissue specific to the energy of the proton beam.[4,5] This characteristic has resulted in protons being recognized as a standard of care, for the delivery of ultrahigh-dose radiation treatments for selected tumors of the brain and spine.[3,6,7] For example, historically, patients with clival chordoma and chondrosarcoma have been treated with protons with the aim of delivering doses in excess of 70 Gy, the reason being that the proximity of these tumors to critical structures like the brainstem, optic nerves, and chiasm limits the dose (tolerance typically 50 to 60 Gy depending on the fractionation) that can be safely delivered with conventional nonconformal radiation techniques.[8]

However, recent advances in photon beam delivery with IMRT and image-guided radiotherapy (IGRT) have improved the ability to deliver these high doses safely, and offer cost-effective and accessible alternatives to proton beam therapy.[3] Intensity modulated radiotherapy with subcentimeter leaf width MLCs can create steep dose gradients between the tumor and organs at risk (OAR) to permit the high-dose deposition (**Fig. 16.3**), and IGRT provides the security that the dose is delivered with submillimeter accuracy.[9] The drawback of IMRT lies in the increased exposure to the surrounding normal brain tissues to low-dose radiation (integral dose) as compared to protons.[5] This characteristic suggests protons may be justified for children with brain tumors, as it is assumed that less dose exposure to the healthy brain tissue would translate into a lower risk of a second malignancy and potentially other late effects such as neurocognitive impairment.

Controversy

- Particle beam accelerators are more expensive and complex than X-ray–based LINACs, and the cost-benefit analysis of charged particle therapy versus image-guided IMRT remains a major topic for debate.

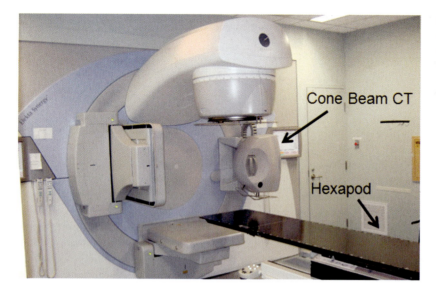

Fig. 16.1 The Elekta Synergy unit (Elekta AB, Stockholm, Sweden) currently in place at the University of Toronto equipped with a cone beam computed tomography (CT), a 4-mm multileaf collimator, and a Hexapod robotic couch allowing for six degrees of freedom in patient positioning.

Cone Beam CT

Hexapod

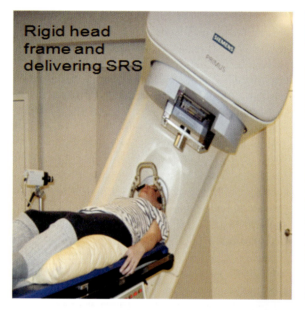

Rigid head frame and delivering SRS

a

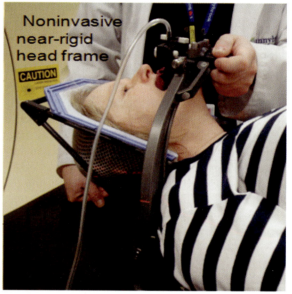

Noninvasive near-rigid head frame

CAUTION

b

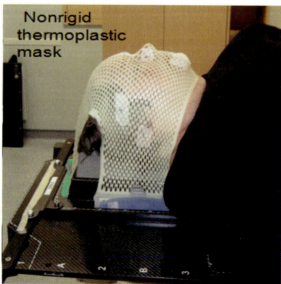

Nonrigid thermoplastic mask

c

Fig. 16.2a–c Three head frames commonly used for radiation delivery. **(a)** A patient with an invasive head frame receiving LINAC-based stereotactic radiosurgery (SRS). **(b)** A patient being fitted with a near-rigid relocatable head frame (aimed to replace the use of invasive frames), which is based on a head fixation device coupled to a bite block attached to a vacuum device via tubing that provides suction for the bite block to affix to the hard palate (Aktina system). **(c)** A nonrigid thermoplastic mask that is typically applied for fractionated daily radiotherapy and hypofractionated stereotactic radiotherapy when coupled to an image guidance system.

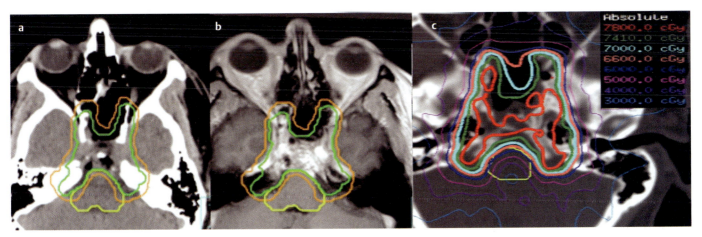

Fig. 16.3a–c An example of a postoperative chordoma patient treated with 78 Gy in 39 fractions. **(a,b)** The clinical target volume is in green and planning target volume in orange. **(c)** The dose-volume histogram and the isodose distribution with representative isodose lines as indicated. The highly conformal dose distribution and steep dose gradient at the brainstem is clearly appreciated.

Unlike protons, charged particles such as carbon ions are truly distinct from photons or protons, as the radiobiological effect is considerably larger than photons due to a greater linear energy transfer (LET) and higher efficiency in generating lethal DNA injury.[10] Although the physical properties of particle beams make them attractive for CNS irradiation, particle beam accelerators for heavy ion therapy are considerably more expensive and complex than X-ray linear accelerators, and there are still no data to support superiority with respect to clinical outcomes. Although protons are increasingly becoming available, carbon ions are available in only a few centers worldwide.

Radiation Fractionation

Radiation effects are manifest as cell attrition due to apoptosis or reproductive cell death. The brain is unique in that the normal parenchymal cell populations (neuronal, glial, and vascular) are either static or slowly dividing. Consequently, the clinical manifestations of radiation side effects within the normal brain usually do not appear until months to years after radiation is completed (i.e., late or delayed reaction). Normal CNS parenchyma is very sensitive to the size of individual doses or fractions of radiation, reflecting a large capacity for radiation repair with fractionated treatment. Tumor cells, for the most part, have less capacity for sublethal and potentially lethal damage repair, and are spared to a lesser degree at conventional fraction sizes compared with normal tissue. Other advantages to fractionation include the possibility of tumor cells undergoing re-assortment into more radiosensitive phases of the cell cycle and reoxygenation of hypoxic cells between fractions, as hypoxic cells are more radioresistant. Thus differences in radiosensitivity between normal and tumor cells can be exploited by fractionation to improve the

therapeutic ratio.[2] Most contemporary radiation treatments are fractionated on a once-a-day basis, Monday to Friday, over a period of 5 to 6 weeks (25 to 30 treatments), with total doses of 50 to 60 Gy.

Hyperfractionation and accelerated fractionation involve delivering multiple (usually two to three) fractions per day to allow an increase in the total dose, a reduction in late side effects (hyperfractionation), or a shorter overall treatment time to reduce the effects of tumor repopulation during treatment (accelerated fractionation).[2] Accelerated and hyperfractionation schemes have been explored in clinical trial settings for malignant supratentorial and brainstem gliomas and CNS lymphoma, but no significant clinical advantage over daily fractionation to conventional doses has been generally noted.[11] Conventional hypofractionation utilizes a larger dose per fraction, such as 3 to 5 Gy, to enable the delivery of therapeutic doses over shorter periods of time, and has been demonstrated to provide similar survival benefits when compared with conventionally fractionated treatments for patients with poor prognosis glioblastoma.[12] The use of altered fractionation schemes in other types of primary brain tumors has not been extensively explored.

Evidence is emerging that there is a separate mechanism of radiation response linked to the tumor microvasculature as a critical step in tumor death.[13,14] Work done on tumor response to single large doses of radiotherapy (8 to 10 Gy) suggests that damage to the tumor microvasculature takes place within 6 hours via activation of the acid sphingomyelinase (ASM) pathway.[13] Tumor cell death then follows secondary to vascular collapse. At the cellular level, membrane alterations caused by only high doses of ionizing radiation (> 8 Gy) result in ASM enzyme hydrolyzing sphingomyelin into ceramide, which then acts as an apoptosis messenger.[13] Because ASM is present 20-fold more in endothelial cells than in epithelial and tumor cells, this is a common pathway of apoptosis in the endothelium. This work supports the hypothesis that damage to tumor endothelial cells is strongly linked to tumor cell damage and is critical in the radiation response although this has yet to be definitely proven. This research may explain why radiosurgery has been so effective in tumor control despite sacrificing the potential benefits of re-assortment and reoxygenation that are present with longer fractionated course. The advent of modern radiation delivery systems has allowed the use of hypofractionated stereotactic radiotherapy (HSRT),[15] and HSRT with fraction sizes of ≥ 6 Gy is emerging as a common therapeutic modality for metastatic brain tumors.[16]

Stereotactic radiosurgery (SRS) refers to a single high dose of radiation delivered to a target localized in three-dimensions with technology that allows for submillimeter precision. The aim with SRS is to target only the visible tumor based on imaging, and to limit normal brain tissue exposure. Normal brain tissue is much less tolerant of high-dose radiation, with the consequence of radiation-induced edema and radiation necrosis.[17,18] Consequently, SRS is traditionally delivered with the use of an invasive head frame and a dedicated Gamma Knife (Elekta, AB, Stockholm, Sweden) or LINAC unit employing either multiple converging static beams or arcs.[1] The combination of rigid head immobilization, high precision collimation, and multiple beam trajectories afforded by these dedicated units ensures precision delivery and rapid dose falloff, maximizing brain sparing outside the target to be treated. The ability to spare the brain even with these dedicated units declines as lesions exceed 4 cm in size, and thus SRS is typically restricted to the treatment of smaller and well-circumscribed (noninvasive) lesions.

The role of SRS in the primary management of glioma is limited to small recurrent tumors.[19] The routine use of SRS boost in the primary treatment of malignant glioma has been investigated in a randomized trial which concluded no survival benefit.[20] Stereotactic radiosurgery is more often applied to brain metastases under 4 cm, and for selected small benign brain tumors such as acoustic neuroma and meningioma. In order to circumvent the size restriction inherent to SRS, HSRT is emerging as an alternative to SRS in the management of multiple tumor types and indications. Essentially, the approach refers to delivering two to five fractions of high dose per fraction radiation daily (> 5 Gy/fraction), with patients immobilized in a noninvasive head frame/mask. The benefits lie in that the size restriction associated with single-fraction SRS is relaxed by allowing for repair in between the fractions, and the lower dose per day is inherently less damaging both acutely and in the long term. Although it is necessary to reduce normal brain tissue exposure, the normal brain tissue can take a higher dose when exposed in this limited fractionated approach. Thus, rates of radiation necrosis are potentially reduced,[16] and larger or infiltrative lesions may be treated without the same risk of toxicity as SRS.[16]

As an example, the experience of using 30 Gy in five fractions as a salvage regimen for 24 patients with recurrent glioblastoma multiforme (GBM) in combination with bevacizumab has been reported.[19] Beyond the encouraging median overall survival rate of 12.5 months and a 1-year overall survival rate of 54%, no patient experienced radiation necrosis. It is likely that the bevacizumab yielded protective effects, mitigating the development of radiation necrosis; however, the fractionated approach of the radiation may also have helped lessen the risk of radiation necrosis.

In another series specific to brain metastases, 30 patients with surgically resected brain metastases were treated with 27.5 to 35 Gy in five fractions (median 30 Gy) to the postoperative surgical cavity using HSRT. The median planning target volumes (PTVs) were large, ranging from 24 to 35 cc and irregular, which would be prohibitive with single-fraction SRS due to the risk of radiation necrosis. The rates of local control were 79% and 100% at 1 year in those with no prior whole-brain radiation therapy (WBRT; 20 patients/21 cavities) and prior WBRT groups (10 patients/11 cavities), respectively. Importantly, no radiation necrosis was observed in the 21 surgical cavities treated in the no prior WBRT group. In a review of HSRT versus SRS for intact metastases, similar outcomes were noted for HSRT,[21] and another series indicated superior outcomes despite larger volumes treated when comparing HSRT to SRS.[16] As evidence supporting clinical equivalence continues to emerge, the advantages of HSRT[16] include the use of noninvasive head frames, less restriction by size of the target volume and proximity to OAR, and the ability to use conventional modern LINACs instead of specialized dedicated units, which suggests LINAC-based HSRT may become a modality of choice compared to traditional SRS.

■ Dose Selection

For primary infiltrative brain tumors, the most typical approach is to radiate with conventional fractionation of 1.8 to 2.0 Gy/day up to 50 to 60 Gy. This is the standard dose for the radical treatment of individuals with low- or high-grade glioma, either alone or in combination with chemotherapy. In the case of elderly patients or poor performance status patients with glioblastoma, results with conventionally fractionated radiotherapy have been disappointing,[22] and alternate radiation schedules have been investigated.[12] Shorter courses of radiation at 34 to 40 Gy in 10 to 15 fractions (2.67–3.4 Gy/d), designed to deliver similar biologically equivalent doses to 54 to 60 Gy in 30 fractions, have been shown to yield similar survival and toxicity rates as compared to more protracted schedules.[12,23]

When dealing with patients with a very poor performance status and an expected short survival, a more palliative approach to radiation may be justified. Short radiation schedules ranging from 20 to 30 Gy in five to 10 fractions can be given with the goal of temporizing the disease in the short-term, and minimizing radiation-induced side effects.[23]

For benign tumors such as meningioma, schwannoma, and craniopharyngioma doses of 50 to 54 Gy in 1.8- to 2.0-Gy fractions per day are commonly used.[24] If the tumors are small and amenable to SRS, this is a viable alternative with equivalent local control rates and more convenient for the patient. Use of HSRT is increasing in benign tumors but does not yet have the long track record of SRS.

Chemical Modifiers of Radiation Effect

Hypoxic cells have been demonstrated in vitro to exhibit up to a threefold decrease in radiosensitivity and may represent a radioresistant cell population, manifested clinically as tumors that have areas of central necrosis. Hypoxic cell sensitizers, high concentrations of oxygen (hyperbaric oxygen, carbogen), and hemoglobin modifiers have been utilized to address this issue.[2] Dose-limiting toxicity, poor drug delivery to tumor, and reoxygenation during standard fractionated treatment may account for the lack of therapeutic benefits observed in clinical trials to date. Halogenated pyrimidines are thymidine analogues, which are incorporated into the DNA of actively cycling cells and increase radiosensitivity in vitro. Clinical trials of these agents in malignant glioma have not resulted in improved survival.

Chemotherapeutic agents have the potential to interact with radiation to increase tumor cell death either additively (independent toxicity, spatial cooperation) or synergistically (by radiosensitization). Cisplatin, topotecan, tirapazamine, paclitaxel, and temozolomide are some of the chemotherapy agents that have shown synergistic effects against malignant glioma cells when combined with radiation in vitro. Clinically, temozolomide delivered concurrently with radiation has been demonstrated to yield significantly improved survival over radiation alone for patients with glioblastoma, and represents the most significant advance in the management of glioblastoma over the last 30 years.[25]

Agents such as efaproxiral, gadolinium texaphyrin, and temozolomide have demonstrated modest benefits in local control or preservation of neurologic function when used as radiosensitizers for patients with brain metastases, and are the subjects of ongoing trials; however, there is no conclusive evidence as of yet to support any agent in combination with WBRT or SRS for brain metastases. In fact, recent evidence suggests the potential for increased adverse effects,[26] and therefore at this time there is no evidence to support any drug therapy in combination with WBRT or SRS for the treatment of brain metastases outside of a clinical trial.

Most recently, antiangiogenic drugs have been a focus of clinical trials for glioma, and more specifically for glioblastoma. Bevacizumab has recently been investigated in phase 3 trials as an additional therapy to concurrent radiation and temozolomide as the backbone.[27] Bevacizumab is a humanized monoclonal antibody directed against vascular endothelial growth factor (VEGF), and as glioblastoma is a highly vascular tumor with elevated expression of VEGF, the rationale to inhibit this molecule was a reasonable target. However, preliminary data suggest no overall survival advantage. Additional clinical trials with new angiogenesis inhibitors are in progress, and time will tell if this class of drugs has a role in glioma.

With the experience of bevacizumab for brain tumors, it was postulated that this drug could be a therapeutic intervention for radiation necrosis. A small, randomized trial supports its role as a therapeutic intervention for necrosis, and it has become a first-line therapy for symptomatic necrosis.[28] This is a major advancement, as previous treatments with hyperbaric oxygen, pentoxifylline, and other agents have been largely disappointing, and often patients are subject to surgery. Furthermore, radiation necrosis can be a fatal adverse event.

Central Nervous System Radiotherapy: General Principles

Patient Assessment

A complete patient assessment by the radiation oncologist is essential prior to radiation treatment and includes a history and physical, with special attention paid to specific neurological signs and symptoms, the overall performance status, and the general health of the patient. Coexisting illnesses such as collagen vascular disease, uncontrolled hypertension, diabetes, or multiple sclerosis may be associated with a higher risk of late radiation effects, and are considered when deciding on the use of radiation as well as when selecting the technique and dose. A review of all surgical procedures, pathology reports, and diagnostic imaging is undertaken ideally in a multidisciplinary team setting with neurosurgical, neuropathology, neuro-oncology, neuro-radiology, and radiation oncology input.

In most cases, pathological confirmation is required prior to radiation and, at minimum, a stereotactic biopsy is usually possible with minimal morbidity for histological diagnosis. Empirical radiation without tissue confirmation is typically restricted to scenarios where the risk of misdiagnosis is minimized. Typical clinical situations include the patient with clinical symptoms and imaging consistent with a diffuse pontine glioma, the patient with a known history of cancer and imaging consistent with brain metastases, and patients in

Pearl

- Patient age, functional/neurologic performance status (Karnofsky Performance Scale), and tumor histology are strong prognostic factors for outcome and require consideration when counseling patients about treatment options and the expected benefits of radiation.

> **Pitfall**
>
> - Empirical radiation treatment of patients on the basis of imaging alone should generally be discouraged, but is appropriate in specific clinical circumstances.

whom the risk of biopsy is significant and imaging is consistent with glioblastoma.

Stereotaxis and Immobilization

Stereotaxis refers to identifying the precise location of the patient in a fixed three-dimensional (3D) coordinate system referenced to a point (the rotational isocenter of the treatment unit) in the treatment room. For the majority of patients receiving conventional fractionated radiotherapy, fixed axial, coronal, and sagittal lasers in the treatment room define the stereotactic coordinate space, and are used to align the patient using fiducial markers mounted on a custom thermoplastic immobilization shell (**Fig. 16.2**). Using room lasers and fiducial markers with a simple thermoplastic mask immobilization, a daily setup accuracy of 5 mm or less can be achieved (with IGRT this uncertainty can be reduced to 2 to 3 mm[29]). This level of accuracy is insufficient for SRS.

The increasing use of small-volume and highly conformal radiotherapy treatments, particularly for benign tumors, has increased the requirement for high precision localization for treatment. At one extreme, an invasive stereotactic frame rigidly attaches to the patient via screws penetrating the outer bone table of the skull (**Fig. 16.2**). Such devices can immobilize and localize points within the skull with submillimeter accuracy, and are typically used for single-fraction SRS. A disadvantage of invasive frame systems is the inability to use them for fractionated stereotactic radiotherapy or HSRT, because the frames are impractical to wear over an extended period of time.

For stereotactic radiotherapy applications, noninvasive localization/immobilization devices include fiducial bite block and reinforced thermoplastic mask-based systems that can reproducibly provide precision localization over the course of a multifraction treatment course (**Fig. 16.2**).[29–31] In addition, online image guidance systems can provide 3D localization capabilities through multiplanar fluoroscopy, or cross-sectional imaging, to facilitate precision radiotherapy without invasive frame systems.[29,30] Noninvasive systems can achieve stereotaxis with accuracy equal to or approaching that of invasive frame systems,[30] and allow single-fraction frameless SRS even for multiple metastases.[32]

Simulation and Target Definition

Once a radiation technique has been selected and custom immobilization/localization devices have been created, target localization and definition occur in preparation for treatment—a process that is called simulation. In the past, fluoroscopic simulation was used to delineate treatment fields based on the radiographic anatomy of the skull. Now treatment planning utilizes the acquisition of axial CT images through the head, acquired with the patient in the treatment position and immobilized. The acquisition of a volumetric CT study allows the physician to contour and reconstruct target volumes and normal structures in 3D (**Fig. 16.3**). The CT images are necessary to accurately calculate radiation dose distributions, and a planning CT is distinct from a diagnostic CT in that the entire surface has to be imaged to be able to model the entrance and exit of the beams (**Fig. 16.4**).

Depending on the type of tumor and tumor location, the CT images may be fused with MRI to better define tumor and normal tissue relationships. Dedicated CT simulators are routinely available in modern radiation oncology departments and incorporate tools for efficient target contouring and image manipulation such as image fusion. Methods for MRI-only simulation are being developed.[33] Fusion of metabolic imaging (positron emission tomography [PET], single photon emission computed tomography [SPECT], and magnetic resonance spectroscopy [MRS]) may become an important element of treatment planning in the future, by allowing better target definition based on tumor metabolism.

After imaging acquisition, the radiation oncologist defines the gross tumor volume (GTV) on the axial images and may choose to expand this volume to include other tissues at risk of tumor spread to generate the clinical target volume (CTV).[34] The necessary expansion is dependent on the disease to be treated and can range from 0 mm for a grade 1 meningioma to 1 to 2 cm for high-grade glioma. The final margin to be applied is the planning target volume (PTV), which is a margin that incorporates the technical uncertainties in delivery.[34] The exact amount is dependent on the particular stereotactic localization/immobilization system employed (typically, 0 mm for an invasive frame, 1.5 to 2 mm for near-rigid invasive frames, and 3 mm with a simple thermoplastic mask when combined with IGRT). A postoperative chordoma patient is illustrated in **Fig. 16.3**, and in this case there is no GTV as the tumor has been gross totally resected, the CTV incorporates the postoperative bed and any potential routes of spread based on the anatomy involved, and a 3-mm PTV is applied. This PTV margin was based on our evaluation of patients being immobilized in a thermoplastic mask, image guidance performed daily with cone-beam CT, and patient positioning corrected in all six degrees of freedom using the HexaPOD (Elekta, AB, Stockholm, Sweden) robotic couch top.[29]

Treatment Planning

Once the radiation oncologist has identified the critical structures and target volume to be treated, a radiation dosimetrist or physicist designs a plan according to the oncologist's instructions to deliver a uniform radiation dose to the PTV

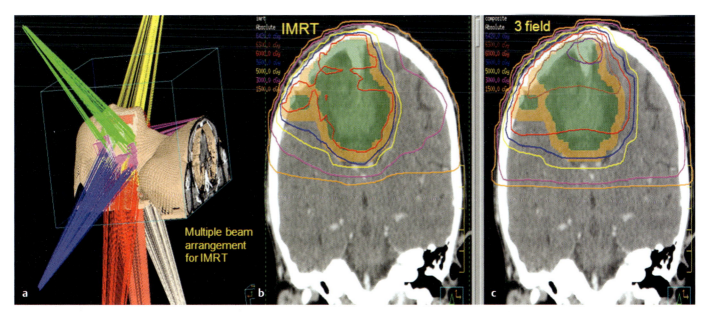

Fig. 16.4a–c (a) A depiction of five beams of radiation oriented around the patient's head, and multiple converging beam delivery is crucial for IMRT delivery. Typically, brain radiation was limited to two to three beams. **(b)** A coronal image of an IMRT dose distribution, and the shaping of the isodose lines (*red, blue, yellow, and pink*) around the planning target volume (*orange color wash*) is evident. One can appreciate that the treatment plan is based on maximizing coverage of the target while trying to spare the normal brain tissue. **(c)** The same patient but planned with the historic three-field technique. The dose distribution illustrates that although the target is covered, it is the normal brain tissue that is exposed to more high and intermediate doses of radiation due to the lack of beam shaping (compare the shape of the *red, blue, and yellow* isodose lines to the IMRT distribution).

while maximizing normal tissue sparing. Three-dimensional conformal radiotherapy (3D-CRT) seeks to minimize the high dose deposited outside the PTV by the use of multiple and converging radiation beams shaped or conformed to the configuration of the tumor as viewed along the beam trajectory ("beam's-eye view"). Three-dimensional CRT is now increasingly being replaced by IMRT, in which not just the shape of the beam but also the radiation fluence within a given beam shape is variably adjusted, providing even more flexibility to allow for "dose painting"[35,36] (**Fig. 16.4**). Rather than iterative manual "forward" optimization of beam arrangements with accompanying dose calculations required for 3D-CRT, IMRT utilizes an inverse planning process to generate the variable beam fluence patterns required for dose painting.[35] An example of the difference in the dose distribution from 3D-CRT to IMRT is illustrated in **Fig. 16.4.**

As part of the inverse planning process, the radiation oncologist specifies the desired dose distribution conforming to the target, as well as dose constraints for the organs at risk, and the back calculation analogous to the image reconstruction algorithms used by CT scanners, and then yields the appropriate beam delivery parameters to meet the radiation prescription requirements and constraints. Intensity modulated radiotherapy delivery offers potential benefits for the treatment of complex particularly concave tumor volumes and for the conformal avoidance of critical structures[37] (**Figs. 16.3** and **16.4**). In reality, inverse treatment planning still re-

quires considerable operator input in terms of comprehensive contouring to specify for the inverse planning engine all the critical organs in addition to the tumor volumes, and refining of the inverse planning objectives/dose-planning constraints. The generation of "optimized" plans, even with an inverse treatment planning system, may be an elusive and time-consuming goal, and poorly optimized IMRT plans may yield inferior results compared to forward-planned 3D-CRT plans.[38]

Pitfall

- Use of automatic computer contouring tools to generate the CTV and PTV through uniform margin expansion of imaged tumor volume (the GTV) may produce inappropriate margins. The radiation oncologist must inspect each volume slice by slice on the treatment planning CT to ensure that the margins take into account known pathways of tumor-specific types of spread, such as along white matter tracts or dura, and respect the normal anatomic barriers to tumor spread, such as skull and dural surfaces. Similarly, once the plan is achieved, the radiation oncologist must inspect the dose distribution slice by slice to appreciate the shape of the isodose lines and ensure appropriate coverage of the target volumes.

Treatment Delivery

Radical or curative radiation treatments for CNS tumors are typically delivered on a once-a-day basis, Monday to Friday, over a period of 5 to 6 weeks delivering 25 to 30 fractions. Treatment is usually performed with five to 10 static fields (**Fig. 16.4**), each conformally shaped by the multileaf collimator (MLC) to the individual beam's-eye view of the tumor. The MLCs have largely replaced those simple beam modifiers such as "wedges" or "compensators" that would have been used to selectively attenuate portions of the radiation beam to ensure that the dose was homogeneously distributed throughout the target volume. Intensity modulated radiotherapy using dynamic movement of the MLC can create highly conformal dose distributions suitable for treating complex target volumes in close proximity to critical structures (**Figs. 16.3** and **16.4**).

Although IMRT can provide a high degree of dose conformality, such treatments are inherently inhomogeneous in nature and require additional levels of quality assurance in planning and delivery to ensure that treatment goals (tumor treatment and normal tissue sparing) are met. For simple tumors, forward-planned 3D-CRT will often achieve treatment goals for many patients with brain tumors who are treated using conventional dose/fractionation schemes (**Fig. 16.4**), and IMRT may not yield any major clinical gains. However, it is clear that for complex tumors, such as large base of skull meningiomas or chordoma, IMRT is absolutely necessary to maximize target coverage and still respect normal tissue tolerance (**Fig. 16.3**).

Another major technical innovation is the introduction of in-room image guidance. The availability of on-board imaging devices mounted onto the LINAC allows the daily use of two-dimensional (2D) or 3D kilovoltage imaging for assistance in patient positioning and verification.[9,39,40] Combined with advanced noninvasive mask-based immobilization, 3D on-board imaging using helical or cone beam in-room CT allows the precise localization approaching the accuracy of invasive frame-based systems.[29,41]

As treatment planning and delivery complexity increases, treatment times have also become longer. New delivery technologies include volumetric modulated arc radiotherapy (VMAT) and flattening-filter-free (FFF) delivery, and these innovations were specifically designed to improve delivery efficiency. Volumetric modulated arc radiotherapy combines the principles of IMRT with arc-based delivery, moving the gantry during treatment to produce highly conformal plans that can be delivered in a time-efficient fashion.[36] For example, an image-guided five- to seven-static-field IMRT plan typically requires 20 to 30 minutes of delivery time per fraction, and with VMAT this time is reduced by approximately half. This is a major issue for busy centers where longer treatment times reduce total daily treatment capacity. Flattening-filter-free units are the most recent innovation and now allow for dose rates on the order of 1,400 to 2,400 monitor units per minute as opposed to 400 to 800. This has resulted in further

> **Pearl**
>
> - Most contemporary radiotherapy treatments are stereotactic, accurate, and effective, whether performed in one fraction suitable only for small targets or multiple fractions suitable for small or large targets. Simple opposed lateral radiation beam treatments for primary brain tumors are now uncommonly used due to the widespread availability of conformal planning and delivery tools.

dramatic reductions in treatment time, and, in combination with VMAT, delivery time is reduced to minutes.[42] Ultimately, through continued technical innovation, radiation oncology departments will be able to increase their capacity to offer highly conformal treatments to all patients, while maintaining overall patient throughput.

Side Effects of Radiotherapy

Early in the course of treatment, increased peritumoral edema due to transient increases in vascular permeability in response to radiation may exacerbate preexisting deficits. Most commonly, the patient experiences headache accompanied by nausea and vomiting, and requires institution of or adjustments in steroid dosage during treatment. This is not a foregone conclusion but common for patients with glioma, and patients should be warned of this potential complication. More commonly, patients experience less serious side effects that include fatigue, alopecia (temporary or permanent), radiation dermatitis (usually mild), otitis externa or serious otitis media (if the ear receives high doses of radiation), and changes in taste or decreased appetite.

Some techniques, such as craniospinal radiation, are much more apt to cause acute side effects (**Fig. 16.5**). Patients treated with craniospinal irradiation for germinoma[43] or medulloblastoma often experience fatigue, nausea, mucositis, esophagitis, hearing dysfunction, cough, and diarrhea due to the large volume irradiated and exit of the radiation through the oropharynx, mediastinum, and abdomen (**Fig. 16.5**). Fatigue and immunosuppression may be seen on treatment, especially when radiation is used concurrently with high-dose steroids or chemotherapy.

The acute side effects of radiation usually subside within 4 to 6 weeks postradiation. At 12 to 16 weeks postradiation, transient demyelination secondary to damage to oligodendroglial cells may occasionally result in return of fatigue sometimes accompanied by worsening clinical symptoms and imaging findings suggestive of early tumor progression.[44] Conservative management with steroids and repeat imaging in 4 to 6 weeks may be useful, because subacute side effects can be expected to improve over this time. Metabolic imaging (SPECT, PET, MSR) may be useful to differentiate between treatment

- Patients who are not on steroids prior to radiotherapy often require some steroid therapy during radiation due to radiation-induced edema. There is no evidence at this time to administer prophylactic steroid therapy if the patient has successfully tapered postsurgery. Even for SRS, there is no evidence to bolus a patient with dexamethasone prior to treatment delivery, although it is commonly practiced. Patients who are on steroids prior to the start of radiotherapy should be weaned off therapy to minimize the adverse events associated with dexamethasone, but in a careful manner, as exacerbation of edema is not uncommon.

effects or pseudo-progression[45] and tumor progression, although at this time there is no conclusive test.

Cranial irradiation can produce late neuropsychological changes as well as focal brain injury months to years after radiation.[44] Neurocognitive side effects are more frequent with high-dose treatment to large-volume brain irradiation, particularly with large doses per fraction (> 2.0 Gy). A serious late effect of radiotherapy is CNS parenchymal necrosis, which can produce symptoms from edema and focal deficits from tissue destruction, and occurs in 5 to 10% of patients. At the current time, the exact pathogenesis of CNS necrosis remains unclear, and it involves a complex interplay between vascular and glial injury and resulting neuroinflammatory responses leading to ongoing tissue injury.[46] Central nervous system necrosis may mimic tumor progression and is a diagnostic dilemma. Metabolic imaging (SPECT, PET, perfusion MRI) may help distinguish recurrent tumor from necrosis; however, the gold standard is surgical resection and tissue confirmation. Symptomatic necrosis is usually treated with steroids, hyperbaric oxygen, surgical debulking, and, as previously discussed, bevacizumab[28] is now a viable option to treat this adverse event. The caveat to the use of bevacizumab is that for a period of 6 to 8 weeks after its stoppage surgery should not be performed due to the increased risks of adverse surgical events.[47]

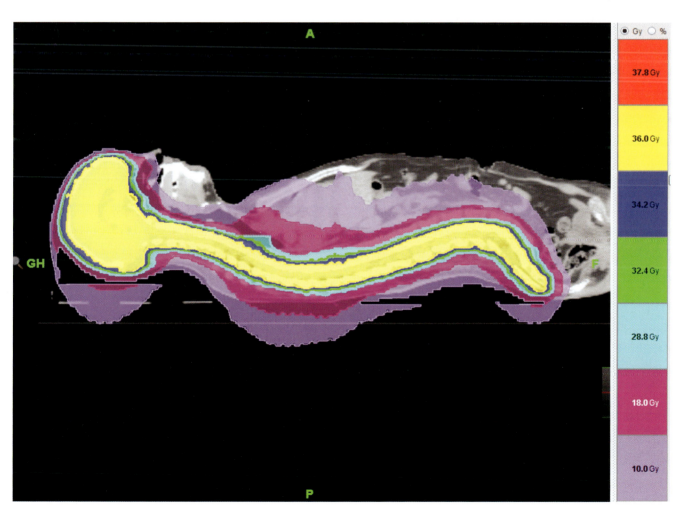

Fig. 16.5 An example of a craniospinal dose distribution where the entire craniospinal axis was treated with 36 Gy in 18 fractions. The conformality of the high dose is evident by the 36 Gy (*yellow*) and 28 Gy (*blue*) dose color wash, whereas the lower doses are shown to spill beyond the craniospinal axis as evident by the 18 Gy (*magenta*) and 10 Gy (*purple*) dose color wash.

A more diffuse leukoencephalopathy may be seen after combined treatment with chemotherapy, particularly methotrexate and radiation. The probability of the development of permanent cognitive dysfunction appears to be very low following stereotactic fractionated radiotherapy.[48]

In patients with low-grade or benign tumors, there are serious long-term sequelae of radiation that must be considered as the expected survival is prolonged. One of the most fearful is the risk of secondary malignancy, and although the risk is about 1% at 10 to 20 years,[49] the cancer can be fatal if a glioblastoma or sarcoma develops. Other major late effects are dependent anatomically on what tissues are exposed, and include pituitary dysfunction, stroke, cranial nerve injury, vision impairment from optic nerve neuropathy, retinopathy, brainstem necrosis, radiation myelopathy, and cataract. Lastly, for patients undergoing craniospinal radiation (CSI) (**Fig. 16.5**), issues regarding fertility must be discussed as the craniospinal fields extend into the pelvic region and contribute scatter radiation dose to the gonads.

■ Conclusion

Modern conventional radiotherapy represents the convergence of improvements in imaging, patient immobilization, and localization in radiation treatment planning and delivery. Highly conformal radiation treatment delivery, using stereotactic conformal radiotherapy techniques, is aimed at reducing the morbidity caused by radiation while maximizing tumor control. Further refinements in tumor volume delineation using advanced imaging and sophisticated beam delivery technology promise continued improvements in the outcome of patients requiring radiation for CNS tumors.

Editor's Note

Radiotherapy was the first modality for treating brain tumors to be properly assessed in a randomized controlled trial, in which it was proven to be of definitive value.[50] It has since been the core element of the standard care of many brain tumor patients, except for molecularly favorable oligodendrogliomas, which are treated with temozolomide. Further technological advances have improved the efficacy and decreased risks of radiation therapy for brain and spine tumors. One can argue that the positive therapeutic value may have been maximized, but minimizing of toxicity perhaps has not. In this light, there is, for example, a current trend on the part of both patients and clinicians away from the widespread use of WBRT for brain metastases, and simultaneous increased use of stereotactic radiosurgery for these patients. There is also more attention being paid to understanding and improving the quality of life, memory preservation, and overall cognitive function of brain tumor patients.[50] These are positive trends as long as the very beneficial value of radiation therapy is not overshadowed by the relatively uncommon complications. (Bernstein)

References

1. Sahgal A, Ma L, Chang E, et al. Advances in technology for intracranial stereotactic radiosurgery. Technol Cancer Res Treat 2009;8:271–280
2. Hall EJ. Radiobiology for the Radiologist, 5th ed. Philadelphia: Lippincott Williams & Wilkins, 2000:412–413
3. Combs SE, Laperriere N, Brada M. Clinical controversies: proton radiation therapy for brain and skull base tumors. Semin Radiat Oncol 2013;23:120–126
4. Verhey LJ, Smith V, Serago CF. Comparison of radiosurgery treatment modalities based on physical dose distributions. Int J Radiat Oncol Biol Phys 1998;40:497–505
5. Yoon M, Shin DH, Kim J, et al. Craniospinal irradiation techniques: a dosimetric comparison of proton beams with standard and advanced photon radiotherapy. Int J Radiat Oncol Biol Phys 2011;81:637–646
6. DeLaney TF, Liebsch NJ, Pedlow FX, et al. Phase II study of high-dose photon/proton radiotherapy in the management of spine sarcomas. Int J Radiat Oncol Biol Phys 2009;74:732–739
7. Rombi B, Ares C, Hug EB, et al. Spot-scanning proton radiation therapy for pediatric chordoma and chondrosarcoma: clinical outcome of 26 patients treated at Paul Scherrer Institute. Int J Radiat Oncol Biol Phys 2013;86:578–584
8. Terahara A, Niemierko A, Goitein M, et al. Analysis of the relationship between tumor dose inhomogeneity and local control in patients with skull base chordoma. Int J Radiat Oncol Biol Phys 1999;45:351–358
9. Hyde D, Lochray F, Korol R, et al. Spine stereotactic body radiotherapy utilizing cone-beam CT image-guidance with a robotic couch: intrafraction motion analysis accounting for all six degrees of freedom. Int J Radiat Oncol Biol Phys 2012;82:e555–e562
10. Ohno T. Particle radiotherapy with carbon ion beams. EPMA J 2013;4:9
11. Freeman CR, Krischer JP, Sanford RA, et al. Final results of a study of escalating doses of hyperfractionated radiotherapy in brain stem tumors in children: a Pediatric Oncology Group study. Int J Radiat Oncol Biol Phys 1993;27:197–206

12. Roa W, Brasher PM, Bauman G, et al. Abbreviated course of radiation therapy in older patients with glioblastoma multiforme: a prospective randomized clinical trial. J Clin Oncol 2004;22:1583–1588
13. Garcia-Barros M, Paris F, Cordon-Cardo C, et al. Tumor response to radiotherapy regulated by endothelial cell apoptosis. Science 2003;300: 1155–1159
14. El Kaffas A, Tran W, Czarnota GJ. Vascular strategies for enhancing tumour response to radiation therapy. Technol Cancer Res Treat 2012; 11:421–432
15. Sahgal A. Technological advances in brain and spine radiosurgery. Technol Cancer Res Treat 2012;11:1–2
16. Kim YJ, Cho KH, Kim JY, et al. Single-dose versus fractionated stereotactic radiotherapy for brain metastases. Int J Radiat Oncol Biol Phys 2011;81:483–489
17. Inoue HK, Seto KI, Nozaki A, et al. Three-fraction CyberKnife radiotherapy for brain metastases in critical areas: referring to the risk evaluating radiation necrosis and the surrounding brain volumes circumscribed with a single dose equivalent of 14 Gy (V14). J Radiat Res (Tokyo) 2013;54:727–735
18. Chin LS, Ma L, DiBiase S. Radiation necrosis following gamma knife surgery: a case-controlled comparison of treatment parameters and long-term clinical follow up. J Neurosurg 2001;94:899–904
19. Gutin PH, Iwamoto FM, Beal K, et al. Safety and efficacy of bevacizumab with hypofractionated stereotactic irradiation for recurrent malignant gliomas. Int J Radiat Oncol Biol Phys 2009;75:156–163
20. Souhami L, Seiferheld W, Brachman D, et al. Randomized comparison of stereotactic radiosurgery followed by conventional radiotherapy with carmustine to conventional radiotherapy with carmustine for patients with glioblastoma multiforme: report of Radiation Therapy Oncology Group 93-05 protocol. Int J Radiat Oncol Biol Phys 2004;60: 853–860
21. Rodrigues G, Zindler J, Warner A, Bauman G, Senan S, Lagerwaard F. Propensity-score matched pair comparison of whole brain with simultaneous in-field boost radiotherapy and stereotactic radiosurgery. Radiother Oncol 2013;106:206–209
22. Paszat L, Laperriere N, Groome P, Schulze K, Mackillop W, Holowaty E. A population-based study of glioblastoma multiforme. Int J Radiat Oncol Biol Phys 2001;51:100–107
23. Bauman GS, Gaspar LE, Fisher BJ, Halperin EC, Macdonald DR, Cairncross JG. A prospective study of short course radiotherapy in poor prognosis glioblastoma multiforme. Int J Radiat Oncol Biol Phys 1994;29: 835–839
24. Masson-Cote L, Masucci GL, Atenafu EG, et al. Long-term outcomes for adult craniopharyngioma following radiation therapy. Acta Oncol 2013;52:153–158
25. Stupp R, Mason WP, van den Bent MJ, et al; European Organisation for Research and Treatment of Cancer Brain Tumor and Radiotherapy Groups; National Cancer Institute of Canada Clinical Trials Group. Radiotherapy plus concomitant and adjuvant temozolomide for glioblastoma. N Engl J Med 2005;352:987–996
26. Sperduto PW, Wang M, Robins HI, et al. A phase 3 trial of whole brain radiation therapy and stereotactic radiosurgery alone versus WBRT and SRS with temozolomide or erlotinib for non-small cell lung cancer and 1 to 3 brain metastases: Radiation Therapy Oncology Group 0320. Int J Radiat Oncol Biol Phys 2013;85:1312–1318
27. Lee EQ, Nayak L, Wen PY, Reardon DA. Treatment options in newly diagnosed glioblastoma. Curr Treat Options Neurol 2013;15:281–288
28. Levin VA, Bidaut L, Hou P, et al. Randomized double-blind placebo-controlled trial of bevacizumab therapy for radiation necrosis of the central nervous system. Int J Radiat Oncol Biol Phys 2011;79:1487–1495
29. Lightstone AW, Tsao M, Baran PS, et al. Cone beam CT (CBCT) evaluation of inter- and intra-fraction motion for patients undergoing brain radiotherapy immobilized using a commercial thermoplastic mask on a robotic couch. Technol Cancer Res Treat 2012;11:203–209
30. Li G, Ballangrud A, Kuo LC, et al. Motion monitoring for cranial frameless stereotactic radiosurgery using video-based three-dimensional optical surface imaging. Med Phys 2011;38:3981–3994
31. Ruschin M, Nayebi N, Carlsson P, et al. Performance of a novel repositioning head frame for gamma knife perfexion and image-guided linac-based intracranial stereotactic radiotherapy. Int J Radiat Oncol Biol Phys 2010;78:306–313
32. Nath SK, Lawson JD, Simpson DR, et al. Single-isocenter frameless intensity-modulated stereotactic radiosurgery for simultaneous treatment of multiple brain metastases: clinical experience. Int J Radiat Oncol Biol Phys 2010;78:91–97
33. Wang C, Chao M, Lee L, Xing L. MRI-based treatment planning with electron density information mapped from CT images: a preliminary study. Technol Cancer Res Treat 2008;7:341–348
34. International Commission on Radiation Units. Report 50. Prescribing, recording, reporting photon beam therapy. Bethesda, MD: ICRU, 1993
35. Pirzkall A, Carol M, Lohr F, Höss A, Wannenmacher M, Debus J. Comparison of intensity-modulated radiotherapy with conventional conformal radiotherapy for complex-shaped tumors. Int J Radiat Oncol Biol Phys 2000;48:1371–1380
36. Davidson MT, Masucci GL, Follwell M, et al. Single arc volumetric modulated arc therapy for complex brain gliomas: is there an advantage as compared to intensity modulated radiotherapy or by adding a partial arc? Technol Cancer Res Treat 2012;11:211–220
37. Hermanto U, Frija EK, Lii MJ, Chang EL, Mahajan A, Woo SY. Intensity-modulated radiotherapy (IMRT) and conventional three-dimensional conformal radiotherapy for high-grade gliomas: does IMRT increase the integral dose to normal brain? Int J Radiat Oncol Biol Phys 2007; 67:1135–1144
38. Bauman GS, Shaw EG, Cha S, Barani IJ, McDermott M. Some like it hot . . . and others not! Int J Radiat Oncol Biol Phys 2009;74:1319–1322
39. Ma L, Sahgal A, Hossain S, et al. Nonrandom intrafraction target motions and general strategy for correction of spine stereotactic body radiotherapy. Int J Radiat Oncol Biol Phys 2009;75:1261–1265
40. Chuang C, Sahgal A, Lee L, et al. Effects of residual target motion for image-tracked spine radiosurgery. Med Phys 2007;34:4484–4490
41. Li W, Sahgal A, Foote M, Millar BA, Jaffray DA, Letourneau D. Impact of immobilization on intrafraction motion for spine stereotactic body radiotherapy using cone beam computed tomography. Int J Radiat Oncol Biol Phys 2012;84:520–526
42. Ong CL, Dahele M, Cuijpers JP, Senan S, Slotman BJ, Verbakel WF. Dosimetric impact of intrafraction motion during RapidArc stereotactic vertebral radiation therapy using flattened and flattening filter-free beams. Int J Radiat Oncol Biol Phys 2013;86:420–425
43. Foote M, Millar BA, Sahgal A, et al. Clinical outcomes of adult patients with primary intracranial germinomas treated with low-dose craniospinal radiotherapy and local boost. J Neurooncol 2010;100: 459–463
44. Schultheiss TE, Kun LE, Ang KK, Stephens LC. Radiation response of the central nervous system. Int J Radiat Oncol Biol Phys 1995;31:1093–1112
45. Sanghera P, Perry J, Sahgal A, et al. Pseudoprogression following chemoradiotherapy for glioblastoma multiforme. Can J Neurol Sci 2010; 37:36–42
46. Greene-Schloesser D, Robbins ME. Radiation-induced cognitive impairment—from bench to bedside. Neuro-oncol 2012;14(Suppl 4): iv37–iv44

47. Clark AJ, Lamborn KR, Butowski NA, et al. Neurosurgical management and prognosis of patients with glioblastoma that progresses during bevacizumab treatment. Neurosurgery 2012;70:361–370

48. Brown PD, Buckner JC, O'Fallon JR, et al. Effects of radiotherapy on cognitive function in patients with low-grade glioma measured by the Folstein Mini-Mental State Examination. J Clin Oncol 2003;21):2519–2524

49. Walter AW, Hancock ML, Pui CH, et al. Secondary brain tumors in children treated for acute lymphoblastic leukemia at St. Jude Children's Research Hospital. J Clin Oncol 1998;16):3761–3767

50. Walker MD, Green SB, Byar DP, et al. Randomized comparisons of radiotherapy and nitrosoureas for the treatment of malignant glioma after surgery. N Engl J Med 1980;303:1323–1329

17 Stereotactic Radiosurgery

Douglas Kondziolka

Over the past 25 years, stereotactic radiosurgery (SRS) has changed the management of most brain tumors. Through precise, conformal delivery of ionizing radiation to an imaging-defined target volume in a single procedure, the biological effect of radiosurgery can lead to cessation or inhibition of tumor cell division, cause neoplastic blood vessels to occlude, induce apoptosis or necrosis, and modify the blood–brain barrier around the tumor.[1-6]

Radiosurgery was conceived to destroy elements of brain circuits for functional disorders. The initial use preceded modern tumor imaging with computed tomography (CT), and thus utilization and acceptance was slow. The second-generation Gamma Knife unit (1975) incorporated a more spherical dose distribution that was better suited to neoplastic or vascular mass lesions. The third generation increased the number of sources and beam diameters, used greatly improved dose planning systems, and integrated CT and magnetic resonance imaging (MRI) for target definition. Later units facilitated cobalt reloading and added robotics. In 2006 the Perfexion® model (Elekta, Stockholm) expanded robotics, enlarged the potential treatment range, and eliminated helmet changes.[7,8] Although most published clinical and basic science research stems from studies using Gamma Knife® (Elekta, Stockholm) radiosurgery technique, modified linear accelerators and cyclotrons producing charged particles have been used for radiosurgery, including devices with robotics and image-based target localization (Cyberknife®, Accuray, Sunnyvale, California).[9-12]

Stereotactic radiosurgery for the management of tumors has been enhanced greatly by the introduction of MRI, which facilitated high-resolution brain tissue imaging and precise target delineation. In the 1980s, an increasing number of patients with benign tumors underwent radiosurgery, and, in the 1990s, treatment evolved to alter the management of malignant neoplasms. Stereotactic radiosurgery offered an alternative treatment modality with advantages over surgical intervention or radiation therapy. Typically radiosurgery has been used for smaller mass lesions. Older teaching noted that the "upper size limit" for radiosurgery was 3 cm in diameter. Although there was never such a specific cutoff, the teaching reflected the concept that larger tumor volumes, above 4 cm in diameter, would necessitate a dose reduction for safety. Such a dose reduction might be ineffective on the tumor. Although the generalization persists that radiosurgery has a lesser role for larger tumors, careful consideration of the clinical scenario including the degree of mass effect, tumor location, and the burden of systemic disease must also be considered. What also changed was the understanding that lower doses could be effective, and that brain location was critical. For example, a tumor located along a dural/skull surface has less circumferential radiation dose falloff into surrounding brain than the same tumor volume completely surrounded by brain.

As computer speed increased, so did the ability of radiosurgery clinicians to efficiently create highly conformal and selective volumetric dose plans for irregularly shaped lesions. The ability to do this is technology dependent. With the Gamma Knife delivery system, multiple isocenters using narrow radiation beams, or multiple delivery angles, are used to create a three-dimensional radiation volume that matches the imaging-defined tumor margin. The steep falloff of radiation into the surrounding normal structures maintains safety as radiation tolerance within the brain is location and volume dependent.

Because many targets are adjacent to critical brain and nerves, conformal radiosurgery is required to maintain low morbidity rates with high tumor control. In instances where a large decrease in dose is necessary to limit normal tissue toxicity, alternative modes of radiation delivery may be necessary. For instance, in proton radiosurgery, dose is delivered with a sharp beam profile and deposited at a determined depth with minimal exit dose, a radiobiological process termed the Bragg peak. What may suffer is the entrance dose, and the ability to create a truly conformal volume. Additionally, fractionated stereotactic radiotherapy (FSR) may be used in this scenario to provide a higher dose per fraction compared to conventional radiotherapy while maintaining some of the potential benefits of normal tissue repair observed with fractionated regimens.[13,14] As for any approach, "potential benefits" must be supported by actual clinical outcomes. It is clear that many aspects of radiobiological teaching proved to be unreliable when the real clinical outcomes of brain tumor radiosurgery were realized. Slowly responding tissue could respond to radiosurgery with tumor volume regression. The single-session radiobiological power of the procedure transcended the estimated radiobiological power of "equivalent" fraction-

---

Pearl

- The radiobiology of radiosurgery is different from that of fractionated radiation therapy.

ated doses that had never been used in patients, or delivered with imaging-based precision.

Vestibular Schwannoma

The evolution of SRS has impacted the management algorithm of cranial base tumors such as schwannomas, meningiomas, pituitary tumors, craniopharyngiomas, and other lesions. Rather than simply recommending surgical resection, observation, or fractionated radiation therapy, the multidisciplinary team can now offer radiosurgery as primary or in some cases as adjuvant care. Indeed, for some tumors this has become the preferred approach for many clinicians.

The goals of vestibular schwannoma radiosurgery are to prevent further tumor growth, to preserve cochlear and other cranial nerve function, to maintain or to improve the patient's neurologic status, and to avoid the risks associated with open surgical resection. Long-term results have established radiosurgery as an important minimally invasive alternative to microsurgery. Initially, radiosurgery was attractive to patients who were elderly or medically infirm, but was later offered to patients of all ages eligible for stereotactic frame fixation. We have found that the results have been consistent across age groups.[15,16]

During the past decade radiosurgery has emerged as an effective alternative to surgical removal of small to moderate-sized vestibular schwannomas. Initially, patients had radiosurgery as an alternative to microsurgical resection due to one or more of the following criteria: advanced patient age, poor medical condition for surgery, recurrent or residual tumor after prior surgery, neurofibromatosis type 2, or patient preference.[15,17,18] Currently, most patients select radiosurgery because the literature states that it has superior clinical outcomes that established its long-term safety and efficacy. Data from the University of Pittsburgh included the care of 1,500 patients with vestibular schwannomas using Gamma Knife stereotactic radiosurgery. The mean patient age was 57 years (range, 12 to 95). Eight percent had neurofibromatosis.[18,19] Symptoms before radiosurgery included hearing loss (92%), balance symptoms or ataxia (51%), tinnitus (43%), or other neurologic deficit (19.5%). Thirty-four percent of our patients had useful hearing, Gardner-Robertson grade I (speech discrimination score ≥ 70%; pure tone average ≤ 30 dB) or grade II (speech discrimination score ≥ 50%; pure tone average ≤ 50 dB).

Since 1992, the average dose prescribed to the tumor margin was 12.5 Gy, with the 50% isodose line being used in 90%

of patients. Lower or higher doses can be used depending on cranial nerve function, tumor volume, and clinical history. In the past decade or so, there has been increasing emphasis on dose to the cochlea in order to maximize hearing preservation. Techniques that reduce cochlear dose below 4 Gy appear to have higher rates of useful hearing preservation.[20,21] These can include beam blocking, use of the smallest collimators, or perhaps reducing the dose to the most lateral part of the tumor within the auditory canal.

Long-term follow-up documented a 98% clinical tumor control rate with no requirement for surgical intervention at 5 to 10 years.[17] Patients managed from 1992 to 1997 had a similar success rate.[15] Between 1987 and 1992 there were significant modifications in the technique of radiosurgery, including a change from CT- to MRI-based planning, improved computer workstations, conformal dose planning, the use of more isocenters of radiation, the use of smaller irradiation beams, and a reduction in the average margin dose to 12 to 13 Gy. Since modification of these techniques beginning in 1991, there has been a significant reduction in the morbidity of radiosurgery.[21,22] Currently, the risk for any grade delayed facial nerve dysfunction is below 1%.[21–23] Patients with useful hearing before radiosurgery continue to report an approximate 60 to 85% overall rate for maintenance of useful hearing, depending on tumor size.[24] For patients with intracanalicular tumors, the rate of hearing preservation is above 80%.[22,25] Radiosurgery has been shown to be a cost-effective, low risk, and an effective alternative to microsurgery for vestibular schwannoma patients.

For smaller tumors, it is likely that more patients now receive radiosurgery as primary management. Although there has not been a randomized trial providing level 1 evidence comparing radiosurgery with resection, and one is not likely to be performed, there are now five matched cohort studies. These studies reported on patients with similar-sized tumors, and evaluated clinical, imaging, and quality-of-life outcomes. All these reports consistently showed better results after radiosurgery for most clinical measures, similar results for the preoperative symptoms of tinnitus and imbalance, and similar freedom from tumor progression rates.[23,26–28] In some patients, there can be transient expansion of the tumor after irradiation, which usually can be observed without further treatment.[29,30] Based on these data, the remaining indications for surgical resection in a patient with a small to moderate-sized tumor are brainstem compression causing disabling imbalance, intractable trigeminal neuralgia or headache, hydrocephalus, an unclear diagnosis, or patient choice.

◼ Stereotactic Radiotherapy

Fractionated delivery of ionizing radiation is likely to result in radiobiological processes that are different from radiosurgery particularly from the standpoint of tissue repair. Fractionated stereotactic radiotherapy may or may not allow for a higher dose of conformal radiation to be delivered to the target in contrast to standard external beam techniques. It can allow for some degree of normal tissue sparing due to interfractional repair. Whether this makes a clinical difference remains to be documented. Fractionated regimens have varied from extended 20- to 30-fraction regimens, to 25.0 Gy provided in five fractions, and 21.0 Gy in three fractions to 18.0 Gy in three fractions. The Stanford group has reported their Cyberknife FSR experience with encouraging local control and hearing preservation.[31] The use of FSR may prove to be of value in the management of larger, asymptomatic lesions that are in close proximity to the vestibular or trigeminal system. A linear accelerator (LINAC)-based FSR and SRS comparison of 25.0 Gy provided in five fractions versus 12.5 Gy in one fraction demonstrated similar rates of local control but 5-year trigeminal nerve preservation in favor of the fractionated regimen, an outcome highly dependent on tumor volume.[32] Additional insight into the role of fractionated radiotherapy was established by a study of outcomes using stereotactic radiotherapy at a total dose of 50.4 or 46.8 Gy. Unfortunately, the hearing preservation results were not as good as those reported with other techniques, and the follow-up was relatively short (in patients with grades I or II hearing, the median follow-up was 65 weeks). At 3 years, the hearing preservation rate was 55 to 60%, and no patient with grade 2 hearing preserved it at the 50.0-Gy dose.[33] As dose becomes standardized in FSR and long-term results are obtained, comparisons between the differing delivery systems will be better appreciated. As with all forms of therapeutic radiation delivery, analysis of outcomes helps to refine techniques.

Although other intracranial schwannomas are less common, the value of stereotactic Gamma Knife radiosurgery has been evaluated in patients with facial, trigeminal, oculomotor, and jugular foramen region schwannomas (**Figs. 17.1** and **17.2**).

> **Pitfall**
>
> - Hearing outcomes after conventionally fractionated radiation therapy do not show improved outcomes when compared with radiosurgery.

◼ Meningioma

Radiosurgery has proven an effective strategy for patients with benign meningiomas. Initially, radiosurgery was only consid-

> **Pearl**
>
> - Meningiomas are especially suitable for radiosurgery because the tumors are usually well demarcated and rarely invade the brain. For benign tumors, the long-term control rate exceeds 90% in most studies.

ered for residual or recurrent tumors after prior resection.[34] Two decades ago the use of radiosurgery expanded to the care of patients with small to medium-sized tumors, where the risks of resection were high. Meningiomas are especially suitable for radiosurgery because the tumors are usually well demarcated and rarely invade the brain.[35] The steep radiation falloff can be directly conformed to the imaging-defined tumor margin while limiting the dose to normal tissue.[36] The problems of delayed tumor recurrence after surgery, surgical morbidity, and surgical mortality, especially in the elderly, increasingly led to consideration of radiosurgery as primary tumor management, particularly when a potentially curative grade 1 resection was not feasible.[37,38]

The University of Pittsburgh's 25-year experience included 1,500 intracranial meningiomas. In the last comprehensive analysis, 972 patients with 1,045 intracranial meningiomas were evaluated.[34] The series included 70% who were women, 49% who had undergone a prior resection, and 5% who received prior fractionated radiation therapy. The mean age was 57 years. Tumor locations included middle fossa ($n = 351$), posterior fossa ($n = 307$), convexity ($n = 126$), anterior fossa ($n = 88$), parasagittal region ($n = 113$), and other sites ($n = 115$). The mean tumor volume was 7.4 mL. Follow-up beyond 5, 7, 10, and 12 years was obtained in 327, 190, 90, and 41 patients, respectively.

The overall control rate for patients who had adjuvant radiosurgery for known World Health Organization (WHO) grade I meningiomas undergoing prior resection was 93%.[34] Primary radiosurgery patients (no prior histologic confirmation; $n = 482$), had a tumor control rate of 97%. The results were poorer for adjuvant radiosurgery used in patients with WHO grades II and III tumors. In those groups tumor control rates of 50% and 17%, respectively, were found. Recent studies indicate that there may be a dose–response relationship for these more aggressive tumors, with better control rates obtained using tumor margin doses above 15 Gy. At 10 years or more, adjuvantly treated grade I tumors were controlled in 91% ($n = 53$), and primary tumors, 95% ($n = 22$). No patient developed a radiation-induced tumor. Primarily treated patients had an unchanged or improved neurologic condition in 93%, whereas those with adjuvantly managed tumors were unchanged or improved in 91%. The overall morbidity rate was 7.7%, and symptomatic imaging changes developed in 4%, at an average of 8 months. Such changes were more common in parasagittal or convexity meningiomas. By 1992, a protocol was adopted that restricted the optic apparatus dose to ≤ 8 to

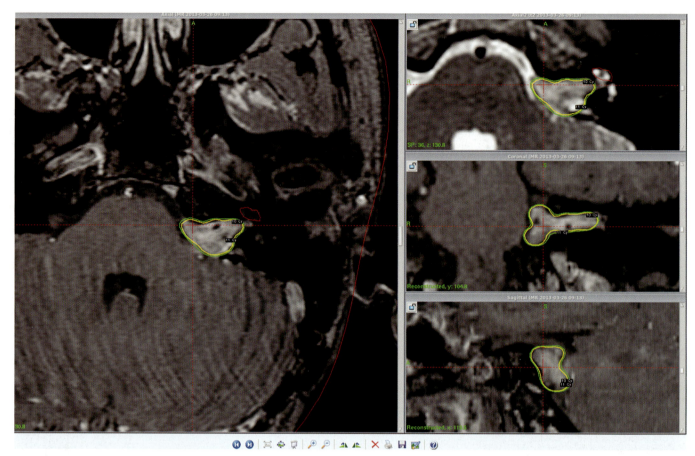

Fig. 17.1 Gamma Knife radiosurgery dose plan (magnetic resonance imaging, MRI) showing a left facial schwannoma. This 26-year-old woman had a partial resection and then radiosurgery at a margin dose of 11 Gy, using multiple small isocenters to this 0.88-cc tumor. The cochlea (*outlined*) was kept at a low dose (*upper right* long relaxation time image).

Pearl

- Although many clinicians aim to deliver < 8 Gy to the optic nerve or chiasm during radiosurgery, < 10 Gy may be a safe dose for most patients.

---

9 Gy using MRI to identify the optic nerve. By doing so, the risk of delayed radiation–related optic neuropathy is minimal. Indeed this dose prescription may have been too conservative, as others have reported visual safety at 9 and 10 Gy (**Fig. 17.3**).

Stereotactic radiosurgery has changed the way many neurosurgeons and radiation oncologists manage patients with meningiomas. Rather than performing a subtotal resection and "following the patient," postoperative radiosurgery to reduce the risk of delayed progression is a valuable option.[39] This strategy is particularly valuable for patients < 75 years of age. Several longitudinal studies have shown that untreated meningiomas under observation often continue to grow over time. Radiosurgery is also arguably the preferred option for a young patient with a critically located small meningioma. Observation may no longer be the best choice for such patients, especially if they are symptomatic, but strong evidentiary support is lacking.

Atypical or anaplastic/malignant meningiomas (WHO grade II or III) are best managed with complete resection followed by fractionated radiotherapy to 55 to 60 Gy because of their tendency to extend beyond the borders seen on imaging.[40] For nodular residual tumors, radiosurgery can be effective. The estimated risk of local recurrence following surgery alone is high particularly for grade III tumors where survival beyond 10 years is uncommon.[41] As a result, external beam radiotherapy is often recommended to improve local control. Radiotherapy planning is based on the pre- and postoperative MRI

Pitfall

- Tumor control rates for WHO grade II or III meningiomas are lower. For grade III tumors, use of fractionated radiation therapy plus radiosurgery should be considered.

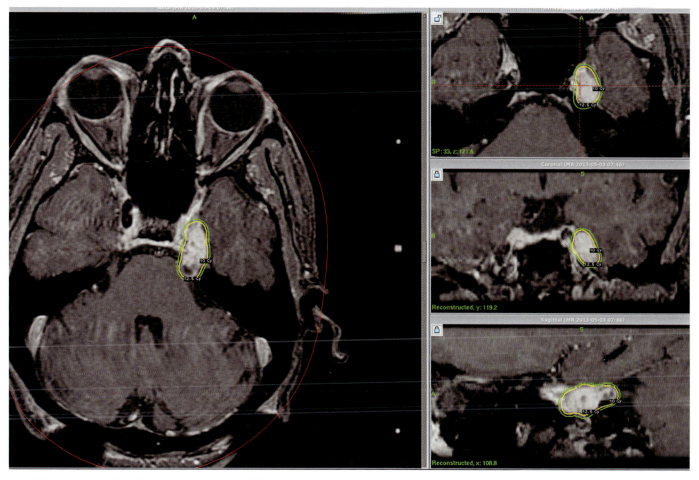

Fig. 17.2 Gamma Knife radiosurgery dose plan (MRI) showing a left trigeminal schwannoma. This 63-year-old woman presented with facial sensory loss. She underwent radiosurgery using a margin dose of 12.5 Gy, using multiple small isocenters to this 1.5-cc tumor.

with irradiation of the gross tumor volume (GTV) plus a margin of 1 to 2 cm.[42] Despite local control with resection alone, local and regional progression is still significant. This requires consideration of a multimodal approach that incorporates maximal surgical resection, fractionated radiation therapy, as well as a radiosurgery boost to residual gross disease. A current controversy is whether radiation should be used to the tumor bed after gross total resection of a grade II (atypical) meningioma. Recent data argue for close imaging follow-up in this situation. A tumor margin dose of ≥ 16 Gy should be used if possible for higher grade meningiomas.

included 290 patients with pituitary adenomas. In 41 patients who had radiosurgery for nonsecreting tumors, prior management included transsphenoidal resection, craniotomy and resection, or conventional radiation therapy. Endocrinologic, ophthalmologic, and imaging responses were evaluated. Typically, acromegaly patients respond best, with normalization of growth hormone hypersecretion in over 70% of patients and in approximately half of those with Cushing's disease. All patients with microadenomas and 97% of patients with macroadenomas had tumor control after radiosurgery. Recent work from the University of Virginia shows that patients who

Pituitary Adenoma

The goals of pituitary adenoma radiosurgery are to permanently control tumor growth; to maintain pituitary function; to normalize hormonal secretion in cases of functional adenomas; and to preserve neurologic function, especially vision.[43] Nonfunctioning pituitary adenomas comprise approximately 30% of all pituitary tumors. The University of Pittsburgh series

Special Consideration

- Radiosurgery has a lower rate of long-term pituitary insufficiency than fractionated radiation, although recent reports show that 15 to 25% of patients may develop some hormone deficiencies over time that may require medical replacement.

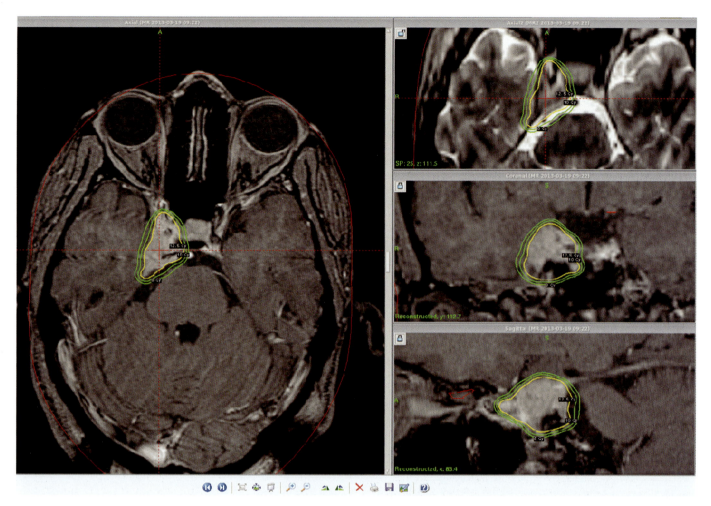

Fig. 17.3 Gamma Knife radiosurgery dose plan (MRI) showing a right cavernous sinus meningioma. This 44-year-old woman presented with diplopia. She underwent radiosurgery using a margin dose of 12.5 Gy, using multiple small isocenters to this 2.96-cc tumor. The maximum optic dose was 5.4 Gy.

Pearl

- Several studies show that cessation of hormone hypersecretion therapies (e.g., ketoconazole) for at least a month prior to radiosurgery, if possible, can lead to improved rates of hormone normalization.

---

undergo radiosurgery off ketoconazole can have faster reduction in hormone hypersecretion. Gamma Knife radiosurgery was essentially equally effective for control of adenomas with cavernous sinus invasion and suprasellar extension. Although endocrine deficits are less common after radiosurgery, recent reports show that 15 to 25% of patients may develop some hormone deficiencies over time that may require replacement. Advances in dose planning and dose selection facilitated tumor management even when the adenoma was adjacent to the optic apparatus or invaded the cavernous sinus (**Fig. 17.4**).

Even with optimal dose planning, lesions within close proximity to the optic pathway are limited to single fraction doses no higher than 8 to 10.0 Gy. As with optic nerve sheath meningiomas, fractionated therapies may be a safe and efficacious treatment. Using Cyberknife FSR and a dose of 25.0 Gy provided in five consecutive fractions, preservation or improvement of vision and imaging stabilization was observed in all 20 patients at approximately 30 months.[44]

Other Cranial Base Tumors

Tumor recurrence and progression of clinical symptoms often occurs in patients with malignant tumors of the skull base. Such tumors include chordomas, chondrosarcomas, nasopharyngeal carcinomas, or other adenocarcinomas or squamous cell carcinomas from regional structures. The North American Gamma Knife Consortium study reported 71 patients with chordoma.[45] The 5-year actuarial survival was 80%, and 93%

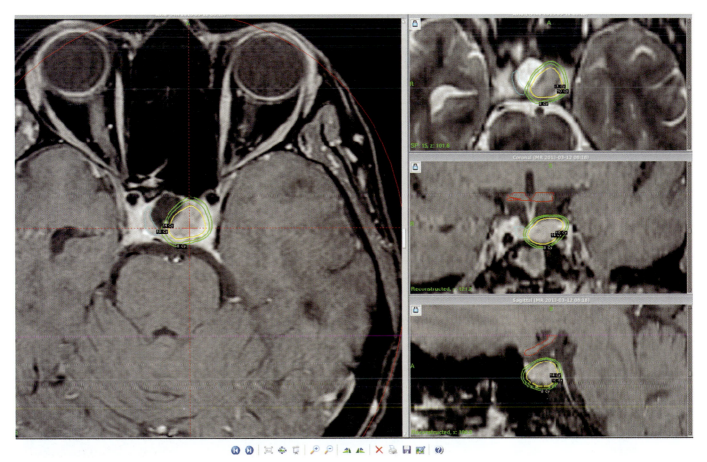

Fig. 17.4 Gamma Knife radiosurgery dose plan (MRI) showing a pituitary adenoma (prolactinoma) of the left sella and cavernous sinus wall. This 41-year-old woman had resection 5 years prior with regrowth. She underwent radiosurgery using a margin dose of 14 Gy, using seven isocenters to this 0.67-cc tumor. The maximum optic dose was 3.7 Gy.

for patients who had radiosurgery without prior radiotherapy. New techniques in cranial base microsurgery or endoscopic surgery coupled with new radiation approaches and stereotactic radiosurgery have improved long-term outcomes.

Radiosurgery is also used for residual or recurrent head and neck or metastatic cancers that invade the cranial base. The mean survival after radiosurgery was 10.5 months. There was no morbidity attributed to radiosurgery. Critical radiosurgical issues include optimal dose planning near the optic apparatus, tumor imaging (sometimes both CT and MRI may be helpful), and the use multiple small beam diameters to improve conformality and selectivity.

Because the radiation dose can be delivered in a single session and surrounding critical brain structures can be spared, radiosurgery has powerful radiobiological advantages over fractionated techniques or brachytherapy for malignant skull base tumors that can lead to an increased intratumoral cytotoxic effect as well as engagement of the tumor's vascular supply by inducing apoptosis. Further evaluation is necessary in larger series of patients to define the response of different tumor histologies.

■ Brain Metastases

Perhaps in no other tumor diagnosis has management changed so dramatically with radiosurgery as in the care of brain metastases.[46–56] Radiosurgery has emerged as a widely practiced treatment approach as the sole initial management, as a boost before or after whole-brain radiation therapy (WBRT), as a treatment for postoperative tumor bed, and as salvage of progressive/recurrent disease. The goal of radiosurgery without WBRT is to achieve brain control without the possible long-term neurotoxic or cognitive side effects of WBRT.[57,58] For decades, most patients with solitary or multiple brain metastases had been managed almost automatically with fractionated

Pearl
• Radiosurgery is the most cost-effective option for brain metastasis patients when compared to either resection or WBRT.

WBRT.[48] Hair loss, fatigue, and delayed cognitive deficits (in longer term survivors) are noted after WBRT and can adversely impact the patient's quality of life.[59] To achieve better clinical results, neurosurgeons and radiation oncologists have partnered in the evaluation of radiosurgery alone for solitary tumors, or radiosurgery plus WBRT for multiple tumors. Local control after radiosurgery generally exceeds 85% regardless of brain location. Radiosurgery is an attractive concept because it is minimally invasive, is done on an outpatient basis, provides excellent local control, palliates symptoms, avoids a craniotomy, and can be performed in the setting of multiple tumors (**Fig. 17.5**). To date, the results after radiosurgery plus WBRT appear to be as good as those after surgical resection plus WBRT for "resectable" tumors.[49] In three reports, radiosurgery has shown to be more cost-effective than any other option. It also can be used in any brain location. Radiosurgery is effective for tumors traditionally considered radiation-resistant, including melanoma and renal cell carcinoma.[54,56,60] Patient selection remains important as patients with large

Special Consideration

- The addition of WBRT to radiosurgery does not improve survival in patients with brain metastases, but can provide improved local control due to the additional radiation delivered to each tumor.

tumors causing mass effect and disabling symptoms should be considered for resection. However, over 50% of brain metastases are now identified in asymptomatic patients, and most are of smaller volume.

At the University of Pittsburgh and New York University, over 4,000 patients with brain metastases have been treated with SRS. Only 10% of these had undergone one or more prior resections. Early in this experience, most patients had already failed WBRT. More recently fewer patients have undergone WBRT before referral. The Karnofsky Performance Scale score

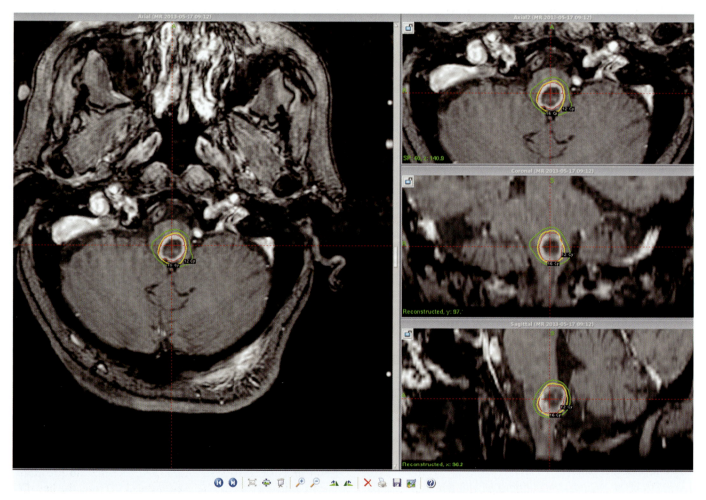

Fig. 17.5 Gamma Knife radiosurgery dose plan (MRI) showing a lung cancer metastasis within the medulla in a 75-year-old woman with multiple brain metastases. She underwent radiosurgery using a margin dose of 16 Gy and a maximum dose of 32 Gy, using 8- and 4-mm isocenters to this 0.97-cc tumor.

was 100 or 90 in over 90% of patients at presentation. The mean tumor volume was 1.7 mL (range, 0.1 to 27 mL). The range of tumor margin dose is 16 to 20 Gy; 20 Gy is used in most patients where radiosurgery is the initial treatment. The tumor margin isodose varies from 50 to 80% in most patients, depending on tumor volume.

Tumor control rates appear similar across histologies, although more volumetric regression is identified in breast cancer. The presence of active extracranial cancer activity has become the most important prognostic indicator for survival, not the presence of central nervous system (CNS) disease. Whole-brain radiation therapy improved local tumor control in lung cancer patients, a finding noted by others. For other tumor types, it affected neither survival nor local tumor control.

Radiosurgery is an excellent option for patients with multiple brain metastases who remain in good neurologic condition. Initially, this paradigm was considered controversial because conventional teaching was that the recognition of more than one metastasis heralded widespread subclinical micrometastases. This concept was proved incorrect once high-resolution MRI was able to show whether or not new tumors developed. In a randomized trial that compared radiosurgery plus WBRT with WBRT alone for patients with two to four brain metastases, improved tumor control was observed when patients received both radiosurgery and WBRT.[59] This study and others found that the presence of multiple metastases did not automatically herald the onset of more and more tumors. Thus, patients should continue to be managed aggressively if effective therapies remain for their extracranial cancer.[51] In one study, the survival expectation for patients with five to eight tumors was not significantly different for patients with two to four tumors, as long as the total tumor burden was less than 7.5 mL.[47] Recent work using SRS for patients with 10 or more tumors showed that outcomes in specific clinical scenarios could be similar to patients with limited numbers of brain tumors.[12] In addition, the toxicity of WBRT is being further characterized.[53] Randomized trials

that evaluate cognitive outcomes have shown the deleterious effects of WBRT, indicating that its use should be careful and judicious.[58]

Patient care needs to be individualized. Much was learned in the creation of the brain metastasis management guidelines, but care has moved quickly beyond those guidelines.[61] Brain metastases patients should not be managed as a homogeneous group. Tumor histologies differ widely with different responses to treatment. Molecular subcharacterizations of breast cancer, melanoma, and lung cancer have changed treatment and outcomes.[62] The focus on number of brain tumors, a key inclusion criteria for almost all prior clinical trials, may be largely irrelevant.

■ Glial Neoplasms

Malignant gliomas continue to represent one of the most serious challenges in neuro-oncology. Years ago the value of radiation was proven.[63] Radiation therapy continues to be an essential component in the multidisciplinary management of glioblastoma multiforme (GBM), with the current standard of care consisting of concurrent and adjuvant temozolamide.[64] However, nearly all patients will require salvage therapy to address recurrent disease within 2 years of diagnosis.[65] Radiosurgery can play a role in addressing this locally progressive disease, and therapeutic options have evolved to maximize the current advances in technology and treatment delivery.

With the majority of recurrences within the previously irradiated volume, there is an argument for dose escalation with the intention to improve primary local control. In order to maximize the benefits of radiation on intrinsic glial tumors of the brain, surgical procedures such as interstitial brachytherapy with temporary or permanent radioactive isotopes, intracavitary irradiation with colloidal isotopes, and balloon placement of radioactive isotopes have been used. Radiosurgery is a minimally invasive method to boost the radiation effect of fractionated radiotherapy for patients with malignant glial tumors.[66,67] Questions remain as to the optimum dose, target definition, and whether radiosurgery is best combined with other therapies.

Initially, radiosurgery was used mainly for carefully selected patients with residual or deep-seated malignant glial tumors < 3.5 cm in diameter as part of a multimodality approach. Typically, malignant glioma tumor volumes are small with a mean tumor volume of 3.5 mL. This is a form of selection bias. Radiosurgery is not for all patients who have completed fractionated radiotherapy. In comparison with patients who received radiotherapy alone, glioblastoma patients had significant prolongation of survival.[68] However, no prospective randomized trial has been completed to study the benefit of boost radiosurgery after radiation therapy for GBM. A randomized trial showed no benefit from upfront radiosurgery plus radiotherapy and carmustine, compared with radiotherapy and carmustine alone.[69] Radiosurgery is a useful concept for residual or recurrent smaller-volume malignant gliomas after completion of initial radiation therapy and chemotherapy. It may also provide tumor growth control in the setting of a later recurrence if other treatment options are limited.

By combining radiation therapy with targeted agents that engage the vascular component of tumors, which is also a proposed target of radiosurgery, future studies will focus on manipulating the signaling pathways that contribute to radioresistance as well as the pathogenesis of GBM.

The efficacy and safety of Gamma Knife stereotactic radiosurgery followed by bevacizumab combined with chemotherapy was recently evaluated in 11 patients with recurrent GBM who experienced tumor progression despite aggressive initial multimodality treatment.[70] At the time of radiosurgery, seven patients had a first recurrence and four had two or more recurrences (median interval from the initial diagnosis was 17 months [range, 5–34.5 months]). The median tumor volume was 14 cc (range, 1.2–45.1 cc) and the median radiosurgery margin dose was 16 Gy (range, 13–18 Gy). Following radiosurgery, bevacizumab was administrated with irinotecan in nine patients and with temozolomide in one patient. The outcomes were compared to 44 case-matched controls who underwent radiosurgery without additional bevacizumab.

At a median of 13.7 months (range, 4.6–28.3 months) after radiosurgery, tumor progression was evident in seven patients. The median progression-free survival (PFS) was 15 months. Compared with patients who did not receive bevacizumab, the patients who received bevacizumab had significantly prolonged PFS (15 months vs 7 months, $p = 0.035$) and overall survival (18 months vs 12 months, $p = 0.005$), and were less likely to develop an adverse radiation effect (9% vs 46%, $p = 0.037$). Thus, the combination of salvage radiosurgery followed by bevacizumab added potential benefit and little additional risk in a small group of patients with progressive glioblastoma. Further experience is needed to define the efficacy and long-term toxicity with this strategy.

Although the role of radiation therapy in the management of GBM is relatively well established, there are fewer available data on outcomes in low-grade gliomas.[71,72] Radiosurgery has

been reported for adults and children with pilocytic astrocytomas, fibrillary astrocytomas, mixed gliomas, and oligodendrogliomas.[73] Neurocytomas appear to regress in volume after radiosurgery.[74] Most patients had small-volume tumors in critical brain locations, or had residual tumors after prior resection. All had histological confirmation.

Radiosurgery also has been used as the sole radiation modality for the management of patients with small pilocytic astrocytomas in critical brain locations.[75,76] Fifty pediatric patients (28 boys and 22 girls) with juvenile pilocytic astrocytomas (JPA) underwent Gamma Knife SRS between 1987 and 2006. The most common brain location was the pons. The median patient age was 10.5 years (range, 4.2–17.9 years). Three patients had failed prior fractionated radiation therapy (RT) and two had failed RT and chemotherapy. The median radiosurgery target volume was 2.1 cc (range, 0.17–14.4 cc) and the median margin dose was 14.5 Gy (range, 11–22.5 Gy). At a median follow-up of 55.5 months (range, 6.0–190 months), one patient died and 49 were alive. The PFS after SRS (including tumor growth and cyst enlargement) for the entire series was 91.7%, 82.8%, and 70.8% at 1, 3, and 5 years, respectively. The best response was observed in small-volume residual solid tumors managed with early radiosurgery. Radiosurgery is also used as an alternative to fractionated radiation therapy in the management of patients with residual or recurrent ependymomas, or as additional treatment after tumor recurrence following radiation therapy.[77] Radiosurgery is also reported for recurrent medulloblastoma in patients who have failed radiotherapy and chemotherapy regimens.[78]

Future Considerations

Significant advances in brain tumor management have occurred over the past 25 years. Diagnostic imaging tools, molecular characterization, approaches and techniques of surgical resection, new drug-based treatments, and radiation-based approaches that include stereotactic radiosurgery have changed patient care. What has yet to occur are pharmacological modification strategies of the radiosurgery response, either for target sensitization or brain protection. These have been tested in animal models but have not yet reached clinical use.[1,2] Concomitant radiosurgery and bevacizumab may be the first foray into this area. Despite significant improvements in patient outcomes for certain tumor types, there is much work to be done.

Conclusion

Radiosurgery has changed neuro-oncology by allowing precise and effective management of brain tumors in any brain location. Clinical outcomes research continues to identify the optimum roles of the technique in comparison to other therapeutic options. Dose–response relationships are fairly well established, which should provide clinicians the confidence to perform radiosurgery as long as target accuracy, conformality, and selectivity are maintained.

Editor's Note

Stereotactic single-fraction radiosurgery is one of the truly monumental innovations in neuro-oncology; it enables treatment of patients who could not otherwise be treated. As well, it provides a treatment option for patients for whom other options exist that are more invasive and potentially morbid. It has revolutionized the treatment of multiple brain metastases or those in impossible locations, such as within the brainstem, and has facilitated the facile retreatment of recurrent tumors.[79] It has also revolutionized the treatment of benign tumors such as vestibular schwannoma, with arguably a much more satisfactory experience than with microsurgery.[80] Unfortunately, its efficacy for glial neoplasms is predictably unsatisfactory, for reasons obvious to all those involved in the care of glioma patients. The technology of radiosurgery has expanded its treatable regions from brain, to spine, and even to visceral lesions, and it is likely that the neuro-oncological indications of SRS will continue to grow. Practitioners are gaining experience with numerous excellent systems, including gamma knife, linear accelerator, cyberknife, and other new technologies. (Bernstein)

Acknowledgments

The author thanks his colleagues L. Dade Lunsford, John C. Flickinger, Ajay Niranjan, and Hideyuki Kano, together with the residents, fellows, and staff at the Center for Image-Guided Neurosurgery at the University of Pittsburgh, who participated in the research studies described in this report. He also thanks the staff at the Center for Advanced Radiosurgery at New York University Langone Medical Center, and the member sites of the North American Gamma Knife Consortium.

References

1. Kondziolka D, Lunsford LD, Claassen D, Maitz AH, Flickinger JC. Radiobiology of radiosurgery: Part I. The normal rat brain model. Neurosurgery 1992;31:271–279
2. Kondziolka D, Somaza S, Martinez AJ, et al. Radioprotective effects of the 21-aminosteroid U-74389G for stereotactic radiosurgery. Neurosurgery 1997;41:203–208
3. Kondziolka D, Lunsford LD, Flickinger JC. The radiobiology of radiosurgery. Neurosurg Clin N Am 1999;10:157–166
4. Kondziolka D, Lunsford LD, Witt TC, Flickinger JC. The future of radiosurgery: radiobiology, technology, and applications. Surg Neurol 2000; 54:406–414
5. Niranjan A, Gobbel GT, Kondziolka D, Flickinger JC, Lunsford LD. Experimental radiobiological investigations into radiosurgery: present understanding and future directions. Neurosurgery 2004;55:495–504, discussion 504–505
6. Witham TF, Okada H, Fellows W, et al. The characterization of tumor apoptosis after experimental radiosurgery. Stereotact Funct Neurosurg 2005;83:17–24
7. Niranjan A, Novotny J Jr, Bhatnagar J, Flickinger JC, Kondziolka D, Lunsford LD. Efficiency and dose planning comparisons between the Perfexion and 4C Leksell Gamma Knife units. Stereotact Funct Neurosurg 2009;87:191–198
8. Novotny J, Bhatnagar JP, Niranjan A, et al. Dosimetric comparison of the Leksell Gamma Knife Perfexion and 4C. J Neurosurg 2008;109(Suppl): 8–14
9. Chang SD, Adler JR Jr. Treatment of cranial base meningiomas with linear accelerator radiosurgery. Neurosurgery 1997;41:1019–1025, discussion 1025–1027
10. Chang SD, Gibbs IC, Sakamoto GT, Lee E, Oyelese A, Adler JR Jr. Staged stereotactic irradiation for acoustic neuroma. Neurosurgery 2005;56: 1254–1261, discussion 1261–1263
11. Friedman WA, Murad GJ, Bradshaw P, et al. Linear accelerator surgery for meningiomas. J Neurosurg 2005;103:206–209
12. Grandhi R, Kondziolka D, Panczykowski D, et al. Stereotactic radiosurgery using the Leksell Gamma Knife Perfexion unit in the management of patients with 10 or more brain metastases. J Neurosurg 2012;117: 237–245
13. Chan AW, Black P, Ojemann RG, et al. Stereotactic radiotherapy for vestibular schwannomas: favorable outcome with minimal toxicity. Neurosurgery 2005;57:60–70, discussion 60–70
14. Combs SE, Volk S, Schulz-Ertner D, Huber PE, Thilmann C, Debus J. Management of acoustic neuromas with fractionated stereotactic radiotherapy (FSRT): long-term results in 106 patients treated in a single institution. Int J Radiat Oncol Biol Phys 2005;63:75–81
15. Flickinger JC, Kondziolka D, Niranjan A, Lunsford LD. Results of acoustic neuroma radiosurgery: an analysis of 5 years' experience using current methods. J Neurosurg 2001;94:1–6
16. Flickinger JC, Kondziolka D, Niranjan A, Maitz A, Voynov G, Lunsford LD. Acoustic neuroma radiosurgery with marginal tumor doses of 12 to 13 Gy. Int J Radiat Oncol Biol Phys 2004;60:225–230
17. Kondziolka D, Lunsford LD, McLaughlin MR, Flickinger JC. Long-term outcomes after radiosurgery for acoustic neuromas. N Engl J Med 1998;339:1426–1433
18. Subach BR, Kondziolka D, Lunsford LD, Bissonette DJ, Flickinger JC, Maitz AH. Stereotactic radiosurgery in the management of acoustic neuromas associated with neurofibromatosis Type 2. J Neurosurg 1999;90:815–822
19. Mathieu D, Kondziolka D, Flickinger JC, et al. Stereotactic radiosurgery for vestibular schwannomas in patients with neurofibromatosis type 2: an analysis of tumor control, complications, and hearing preservation rates. Neurosurgery 2007;60:460–468, discussion 468–470
20. Baschnagel AM, Chen PY, Bojrab D, et al. Hearing preservation in patients with vestibular schwannoma treated with Gamma Knife surgery. J Neurosurg 2013;118:571–578
21. Kano H, Kondziolka D, Khan A, Flickinger JC, Lunsford LD. Predictors of hearing preservation after stereotactic radiosurgery for acoustic neuroma. J Neurosurg 2009;111:863–873
22. Niranjan A, Mathieu D, Flickinger JC, Kondziolka D, Lunsford LD. Hearing preservation after intracanalicular vestibular schwannoma radiosurgery. Neurosurgery 2008;63:1054–1062, discussion 1062–1063

23. Pollock BE, Driscoll CL, Foote RL, et al. Patient outcomes after vestibular schwannoma management: a prospective comparison of microsurgical resection and stereotactic radiosurgery. Neurosurgery 2006;59:77–85, discussion 77–85

24. Lunsford LD, Niranjan A, Flickinger JC, Maitz A, Kondziolka D. Radiosurgery of vestibular schwannomas: summary of experience in 829 cases. J Neurosurg 2005;102(Suppl):195–199

25. Niranjan A, Lunsford LD, Flickinger JC, Maitz A, Kondziolka D. Dose reduction improves hearing preservation rates after intracanalicular acoustic tumor radiosurgery. Neurosurgery 1999;45:753–762, discussion 762–765

26. Myrseth E, Møller P, Pedersen PH, Vassbotn FS, Wentzel-Larsen T, Lund-Johansen M. Vestibular schwannomas: clinical results and quality of life after microsurgery or gamma knife radiosurgery. Neurosurgery 2005;56:927–935, discussion 927–935

27. Pollock BE, Lunsford LD, Kondziolka D, et al. Outcome analysis of acoustic neuroma management: a comparison of microsurgery and stereotactic radiosurgery. Neurosurgery 1995;36:215–224, discussion 224–229

28. Régis J, Pellet W, Delsanti C, et al. Functional outcome after gamma knife surgery or microsurgery for vestibular schwannomas. J Neurosurg 2002;97:1091–1100

29. Hasegawa T, Kida Y, Yoshimoto M, Koike J, Goto K. Evaluation of tumor expansion after stereotactic radiosurgery in patients harboring vestibular schwannomas. Neurosurgery 2006;58:1119–1128, discussion 1119–1128

30. Pollock BE. Management of vestibular schwannomas that enlarge after stereotactic radiosurgery: treatment recommendations based on a 15 year experience. Neurosurgery 2006;58:241–248, discussion 241–248

31. Sakamoto GT, Blevins N, Gibbs IC. Cyberknife radiotherapy for vestibular schwannoma. Otolaryngol Clin North Am 2009;42:665–675

32. Meijer OW, Vandertop WP, Baayen JC, Slotman BJ. Single-fraction vs. fractionated linac-based stereotactic radiosurgery for vestibular schwannoma: a single-institution study. Int J Radiat Oncol Biol Phys 2003;56:1390–1396

33. Andrews DW, Werner-Wasik M, Den RB, et al. Toward dose optimization for fractionated stereotactic radiotherapy for acoustic neuromas: comparison of two dose cohorts. Int J Radiat Oncol Biol Phys 2009;74:419–426

34. Kondziolka D, Mathieu D, Lunsford LD, et al. Radiosurgery as definitive management of intracranial meningiomas. Neurosurgery 2008;62:53–58, discussion 58–60

35. Flickinger JC, Kondziolka D, Maitz AH, Lunsford LD. Gamma knife radiosurgery of imaging-diagnosed intracranial meningioma. Int J Radiat Oncol Biol Phys 2003;56:801–806

36. Kondziolka D, Flickinger JC, Perez B; Gamma Knife Meningioma Study Group. Judicious resection and/or radiosurgery for parasagittal meningiomas: outcomes from a multicenter review. Neurosurgery 1998;43:405–413, discussion 413–414

37. Kondziolka D, Levy EI, Niranjan A, Flickinger JC, Lunsford LD. Long-term outcomes after meningioma radiosurgery: physician and patient perspectives. J Neurosurg 1999;91:44–50

38. Kondziolka D, Nathoo N, Flickinger JC, Niranjan A, Maitz AH, Lunsford LD. Long-term results after radiosurgery for benign intracranial tumors. Neurosurgery 2003;53:815–821, discussion 821–822

39. Lee JY, Niranjan A, McInerney J, Kondziolka D, Flickinger JC, Lunsford LD. Stereotactic radiosurgery providing long-term tumor control of cavernous sinus meningiomas. J Neurosurg 2002;97:65–72

40. Condra KS, Buatti JM, Mendenhall WM, Friedman WA, Marcus RB Jr, Rhoton AL. Benign meningiomas: primary treatment selection affects survival. Int J Radiat Oncol Biol Phys 1997;39:427–436

41. Coke CC, Corn BW, Werner-Wasik M, Xie Y, Curran WJ Jr. Atypical and malignant meningiomas: an outcome report of seventeen cases. J Neurooncol 1998;39:65–70

42. Hug EB, Devries A, Thornton AF, et al. Management of atypical and malignant meningiomas: role of high-dose, 3D-conformal radiation therapy. J Neurooncol 2000;48:151–160

43. Sheehan JP, Niranjan A, Sheehan JM, et al. Stereotactic radiosurgery for pituitary adenomas: an intermediate review of its safety, efficacy, and role in the neurosurgical treatment armamentarium. J Neurosurg 2005;102:678–691

44. Killory BD, Kresl JJ, Wait SD, Ponce FA, Porter R, White WL. Hypofractionated CyberKnife radiosurgery for perichiasmatic pituitary adenomas: early results. Neurosurgery 2009;64(2, Suppl)A19–A25

45. Kano H, Iqbal FO, Sheehan J, et al. Stereotactic radiosurgery for chordoma: a report from the North American Gamma Knife Consortium. Neurosurgery 2011;68:379–389

46. Andrews DW, Scott CB, Sperduto PW, et al. Whole brain radiation therapy with or without stereotactic radiosurgery boost for patients with one to three brain metastases: phase III results of the RTOG 9508 randomised trial. Lancet 2004;363:1665–1672

47. Bhatnagar AK, Flickinger JC, Kondziolka D, Lunsford LD. Stereotactic radiosurgery for four or more intracranial metastases. Int J Radiat Oncol Biol Phys 2006;64:898–903

48. Flickinger JC, Kondziolka D. Radiosurgery instead of resection for solitary brain metastasis: the gold standard redefined. Int J Radiat Oncol Biol Phys 1996;35:185–186

49. Hasegawa T, Kondziolka D, Flickinger JC, Germanwala A, Lunsford LD. Brain metastases treated with radiosurgery alone: an alternative to whole brain radiotherapy? Neurosurgery 2003;52:1318–1326, discussion 1326

50. Hasegawa T, Kondziolka D, Flickinger JC, Lunsford LD. Stereotactic radiosurgery for brain metastases from gastrointestinal tract cancer. Surg Neurol 2003;60:506–514, discussion 514–515

51. Kondziolka D, Martin JJ, Flickinger JC, et al. Long-term survivors after gamma knife radiosurgery for brain metastases. Cancer 2005;104:2784–2791

52. Maesawa S, Kondziolka D, Thompson TP, Flickinger JC, Dade L. Brain metastases in patients with no known primary tumor. Cancer 2000;89:1095–1101

53. Monaco EA III, Faraji AH, Berkowitz O, et al. Leukoencephalopathy after whole-brain radiation therapy plus radiosurgery versus radiosurgery alone for metastatic lung cancer. Cancer 2013;119:226–232

54. Mori Y, Kondziolka D, Flickinger JC, Logan T, Lunsford LD. Stereotactic radiosurgery for brain metastasis from renal cell carcinoma. Cancer 1998;83:344–353

55. Peterson AM, Meltzer CC, Evanson EJ, Flickinger JC, Kondziolka D. MR imaging response of brain metastases after gamma knife stereotactic radiosurgery. Radiology 1999;211:807–814

56. Sheehan JP, Sun MH, Kondziolka D, Flickinger J, Lunsford LD. Radiosurgery in patients with renal cell carcinoma metastasis to the brain: long-term outcomes and prognostic factors influencing survival and local tumor control. J Neurosurg 2003;98:342–349

57. Chang EL, Wefel JS, Maor MH, et al. A pilot study of neurocognitive function in patients with one to three new brain metastases initially treated with stereotactic radiosurgery alone. Neurosurgery 2007;60:277–283, discussion 283–284

58. Chang EL, Wefel JS, Hess KR, et al. Neurocognition in patients with brain metastases treated with radiosurgery or radiosurgery plus whole-brain irradiation: a randomised controlled trial. Lancet Oncol 2009;10:1037–1044

59. Kondziolka D, Niranjan A, Flickinger JC, Lunsford LD. Radiosurgery with or without whole-brain radiotherapy for brain metastases: the

patients' perspective regarding complications. Am J Clin Oncol 2005; 28:173–179

60. Mathieu D, Kondziolka D, Cooper PB, et al. Gamma knife radiosurgery in the management of malignant melanoma brain metastases. Neurosurgery 2007;60:471–481, discussion 481–482

61. Linskey ME, Andrews DW, Asher AL, et al. The role of stereotactic radiosurgery in the management of patients with newly diagnosed brain metastases: a systematic review and evidence-based clinical practice guideline. J Neurooncol 2010;96:45–68

62. Kondziolka D, Kano H, Harrison GL, et al. Stereotactic radiosurgery as primary and salvage management for brain metastases from breast cancer. J Neurosurg 2011;114:792–800

63. Walker MD, Alexander E Jr, Hunt WE, et al. Evaluation of BCNU and/or radiotherapy in the treatment of anaplastic gliomas. A cooperative clinical trial. J Neurosurg 1978;49:333–343

64. Stupp R, Mason WP, van den Bent MJ, et al. European Organisation for Research and Treatment of Cancer Brain Tumor and Radiotherapy Groups; National Cancer Institute of Canada Clinical Trials Group. N Engl J Med 2005;352:987–996

65. Stupp R, Hegi ME, Mason WP, et al. RO; European Organisation for Research and Treatment of Cancer Brain Tumour and Radiation Oncology Groups. National Cancer Institute of Canada Clinical Trials Group: Lancet Oncol 2009;10:459–466

66. Larson DA, Gutin PH, McDermott M, et al. Gamma knife for glioma: selection factors and survival. Int J Radiat Oncol Biol Phys 1996;36: 1045–1053

67. Ulm AJ III, Friedman WA, Bradshaw P, Foote KD, Bova FJ. Radiosurgery in the treatment of malignant gliomas: the University of Florida experience. Neurosurgery 2005;57:512–517, discussion 512–517

68. Nagai H, Kondziolka D, Niranjan A, Flickinger J, Lunsford L. Results following stereotactic radiosurgery for patients with glioblastoma multiforme. Radiosurgery 2004;5:91–99

69. Souhami L, Seiferheld W, Brachman D, et al. Randomized comparison of stereotactic radiosurgery followed by conventional radiotherapy with carmustine to conventional radiotherapy with carmustine for patients with glioblastoma multiforme: report of Radiation Therapy Oncology Group 93-05 protocol. Int J Radiat Oncol Biol Phys 2004;60: 853–860

70. Park KJ, Kano H, Iyer A, et al. Salvage gamma knife stereotactic radiosurgery followed by bevacizumab for recurrent glioblastoma multiforme: a case-control study. J Neurooncol 2012;107:323–333

71. Hadjipanayis CG, Kondziolka D, Flickinger JC, Lunsford LD. The role of stereotactic radiosurgery for low-grade astrocytomas. Neurosurg Focus 2003;14:e15

72. Hadjipanayis CG, Niranjan A, Tyler-Kabara E, Kondziolka D, Flickinger JC, Lunsford LD. Stereotactic radiosurgery for well-circumscribed fibrillary grade II astrocytomas: an initial experience. Stereotact Funct Neurosurg 2002;79:13–24

73. Kano H, Niranjan A, Khan A, et al. Does radiosurgery have a role in the management of oligodendrogliomas? J Neurosurg 2009;110:564–571

74. Tyler-Kabara E, Kondziolka D, Flickinger JC, Lunsford LD. Stereotactic radiosurgery for residual neurocytoma. Report of four cases. J Neurosurg 2001;95:879–882

75. Kano H, Kondziolka D, Niranjan A, Flickinger JC, Lunsford LD. Stereotactic radiosurgery for pilocytic astrocytomas part 1: outcomes in adult patients. J Neurooncol 2009;95:211–218

76. Kano H, Niranjan A, Kondziolka D, et al. Stereotactic radiosurgery for pilocytic astrocytomas part 2: outcomes in pediatric patients. J Neurooncol 2009;95:219–229

77. Kano H, Niranjan A, Kondziolka D, Flickinger JC, Lunsford LD. Outcome predictors for intracranial ependymoma radiosurgery. Neurosurgery 2009;64:279–287, discussion 287–288

78. Germanwala AV, Mai JC, Tomycz ND, et al. Boost Gamma Knife surgery during multimodality management of adult medulloblastoma. J Neurosurg 2008;108:204–209

79. Klironomos G, Bernstein M. Salvage stereotactic radiosurgery for brain metastases. Expert Rev Neurother 2013;13:1285–1295

80. Clifford W, Sharpe H, Khu KJ, Cusimano M, Knifed E, Bernstein M. Gamma Knife patients' experience: lessons learned from a qualitative study. J Neurooncol 2009;92:387–392

18 Alternative Radiotherapy Approaches

Normand Laperriere and Penny K. Sneed

Although it is well established that radiotherapy has efficacy against brain tumors, it is also clear that standard radiotherapy has major shortcomings. Many brain tumors, including most malignant gliomas, recur or progress at some point following radiotherapy, and radiation dose and volume are limited by normal brain toxicity. This chapter describes alternative radiation approaches that have been investigated (mainly in malignant gliomas) to try to improve the results of radiotherapy: altered fractionation, particle therapy, radiation sensitizers, photodynamic therapy (PDT), boron neutron capture therapy (BNCT), brachytherapy, hyperthermia, and stereotactic body radiation therapy (SBRT) for spinal tumors.

Alternative Fractionation Schemes for Radiotherapy

Hyperfractionation

Hyperfractionation involves a larger number of smaller sized fractions to a total dose that is higher than with conventionally administered irradiation in the same overall treatment time. Normal glial and vascular cells limit the total amount of irradiation that can be administered. These cells divide very slowly and are better able to repair sublethal damage than are neoplastic cells. Consequently, there might be an advantage to administering multiple smaller sized fractions to a higher total dose, the theory being that the improved repair of sublethal damage at smaller sized fractions might allow a higher total dose to be associated with the same degree of late sequelae. Neoplastic cells are relatively rapidly dividing cells, and the increased number of daily fractions would increase the chance of radiating them at a more sensitive phase of their cell cycle. At smaller radiation doses per fraction, cell killing is less dependent on oxygen, which might be advantageous given the known areas of hypoxia in these tumors.

There have been six randomized studies of hyperfractionated radiotherapy compared with conventionally fractionated radiotherapy in patients harboring malignant gliomas.[1] Five of six studies demonstrated no benefit on the experimental arm, and one study showed a survival advantage for the hyperfractionated arm.[2] This latter study had a small number of patients per arm, and the median survival of 27 weeks for the conventionally fractionated arm was significantly worse

than all other published data for conventionally fractionated radiotherapy. The largest study on hyperfractionation clearly showed no benefit for the use of hyperfractionated radiotherapy in 712 patients with malignant gliomas.[3] In a pooled analysis of a systematic review of all published data on randomized studies of hyperfractionation in patients with malignant gliomas, no benefit of this approach was demonstrated.[1]

Accelerated Fractionation

The aim of accelerated fractionation is to reduce overall treatment time in an effort to reduce the possibility of tumor repopulation during treatment. This is achieved by delivering two or three normal-sized fractions per day. Accelerated fractionation has been evaluated in a randomized study conducted by the European Organization for Research on Treatment of Cancer (EORTC) in patients with malignant glioma.[4] In protocol 22803, 340 patients were randomly assigned to conventional radiotherapy or accelerated fractionation with or without misonidazole. Accelerated fractionation consisted of three fractions of 2 Gy per day with a 4-hour gap between fractions to deliver 30 Gy in 1 week. This treatment course was repeated after a 2-week break for a total of 60 Gy in 30 fractions in 4 weeks. There was no difference in survival among the three treatment groups and no increased toxicity with accelerated radiation.

In a randomized phase II dose-escalation study (Radiation Therapy Oncology Group [RTOG] 83–02), a subgroup of 305 patients received 1.6 Gy twice daily to total doses of 48 or 54.4 Gy.[5] The results demonstrated no significant survival difference among all dose schemes, and there was a low toxicity rate with accelerated fractionation. A single-arm study of accelerated radiation was reported in 211 patients with malignant astrocytomas.[6] Radiation treatment consisted of 55 Gy in 34 fractions (twice daily) delivered to the enhancing tumor

- Patients with glioblastoma multiforme are not the best population to assess the long-term effects of new fractionation schemes because of their short survival. It is possible that some of the hyperfractionated or accelerated schemes tried in this population would be associated with significant long-term complications if patients survived longer.

and a 3-cm margin. Median survival was 10 months, which was similar to a matched cohort of patients who had received 60 Gy in 30 fractions over 6 weeks. Two other small studies also found no improvement in survival or increased toxicity with accelerated fractionation schemes in malignant glioma.[7,8] One study evaluated 40 Gy in 20 fractions in 1 week as part of a randomized phase 2 study,[8] whereas the other evaluated 60 Gy in 16 days using a single-arm phase 2 design.[7]

A single-arm study was reported in which 10 patients with primary lymphoma of brain received 50 Gy delivered in 25 fractions of 2 Gy given twice a day with a minimum 6-hour gap between fractions.[9] Treatment was delivered on weekdays and weekend days, such that the total treatment (50 Gy) was delivered in 13 consecutive days (**Fig. 18.1**). There was no improvement in survival, with a reported median survival of 17 months. There was some evidence of increased toxicity, with autopsy evidence of radiation necrosis in the pons in one patient at 5 months. There was one long-term survivor at 69 months with evidence of radiation retinopathy and an undiagnosed degenerative neurologic condition.

Particle Therapy

Particle therapy refers to the use of subatomic particles as a form of treatment as opposed to photons. These particles include neutrons, protons, helium ions and heavier nuclei (carbon ions), and negative pi mesons (pions). The use of these particle beams offers two possible advantages over the use of photons: better physical dose localization to the tumor volume and greater biological effect.

Fast neutrons are usually produced in a cyclotron and at higher energies than the spectrum of energies associated with neutrons produced in a nuclear reactor; these latter neutrons are referred to as slow or thermal neutrons. Fast neutrons that have been studied have depth dose characteristics similar to those of a cobalt unit, and as such do not offer any improved dose localization effect but have been studied predominantly for their possible biological advantages over photons. Five randomized trials have evaluated particle therapy for gliomas.[10–14] None of these trials detected a significant survival benefit for particle therapy. The first four studies looked at neutrons, and the fifth study randomized 81 patients to either 60 Gy in 30 fractions with photons or pion therapy to 33.0 to 34.5 Gy where the median survival was 10 months in both groups.[14]

In the randomized, dose-searching study by the RTOG, autopsies were performed on 35 patients at all dose levels.[13] Some patients had both radiation damage to normal brain tissue and evidence of viable tumor. No evidence was found for a therapeutic window using this particular treatment regimen. Autopsies performed in the earlier RTOG study revealed actively growing persistent tumor in all photon-treated patients

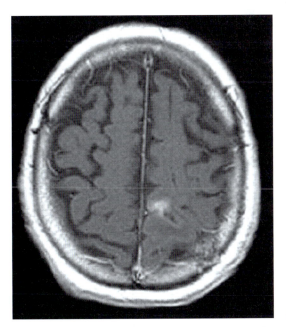

Fig. 18.1a,b **(a)** Axial T1-weighted gadolinium magnetic resonance imaging (MRI) of a 40-year-old man with a primary lymphoma of brain. **(b)** Axial T1-weighted gadolinium MRI of the same patient 1 month after having received accelerated radiation therapy of 5,000 cGy in 13 days, demonstrating a near-complete response.

compared with no evidence of actively growing tumor in the majority of neutron-treated patients.[12] In one study all patients who died had evidence of residual brain tumor.[11] None had signs of radiation-related morbidity. The subsequent trial by the same group was discontinued prematurely as a result of neutron morbidity.[10] In this study, four of nine patients treated by neutrons had evidence at autopsy of radiation-induced brain damage and all had residual malignant glioma.

An institutional phase 2 study was reported where 23 selected patients with glioblastoma were treated on an accelerated proton/photon scheme to cobalt 90-Gy equivalent.[15] One cannot comment on whether the median survival of 20 months represents an improvement in survival in such a selected cohort of patients, but it appears that most recurrences occurred in areas adjacent to the full 90-Gy volume and not in the 90-Gy volume, suggesting that the doses in the region of 90 Gy were high enough to control gross tumor.

One area where particle therapy may have been of some advantage is in the treatment of skull base tumors, particularly chordomas and low-grade chondrosarcomas. The management of these two neoplasms with higher doses of radiotherapy is associated with better local control rates and improved survival.[16] The challenge in delivering these higher doses lies in the critical structures that are immediately adjacent to or involved by these tumors, namely the brainstem, optic pathways, and cranial nerves and vessels. Improved local control and survival were seen in these tumors in the initial reports utilizing protons in the 1980s and 1990s where higher radiation doses in the 70-Gy range could be safely delivered compared with the photon techniques available during that era. However, in the last 15 years there have been significant advances in photon delivery technology, such that equivalent results are now seen with modern photon techniques in terms of local control and survival with the same low risk of toxicity as achieved with protons.[17,18]

Though photons are able to achieve the same high-dose volumes as with protons, the advantage of protons is in the intermediate- to low-dose volumes. As a result of this difference, protons and photons would be expected to achieve the same tumor control rates, but the potential advantage with protons over photons may lie in the expectation of a decrease

in the long-term effects of radiation related to cognition, hormonal deficiency, cerebral vascular events, and carcinogenicity. Children with primary central nervous system (CNS) neoplasms represent the group of patients with CNS neoplasms who might possibly benefit the most from the use of protons.

Boron-Neutron Capture Therapy

Boron-neutron capture therapy (BNCT) was developed in an effort to confine the damaging effects of particle therapy to tumor cells, sparing normal cells altogether. It involves the administration of a boron-containing chemical that theoretically would be preferentially taken up by tumor cells as opposed to normal cells. Boron has a large neutron capture cross section for slow or thermal neutrons, and these neutrons are present in abundance in nuclear reactors. They have an average energy of 0.025 electron volts (eV), far less than the 10 eV required to strip electrons from atoms and ionize tissue. When boron and these slow thermal neutrons interact, nuclear fission occurs, with the fragments sharing 2.4 MeV of energy in the following fashion:

$$^{10}B + {}^{1}n \rightarrow ({}^{11}B) \rightarrow {}^{7}Li + {}^{4}He + 2.4\ MeV$$

The lithium and helium fragments are heavy and travel at most 10 μm from the site of the capture reaction, which essentially limits the injury to the individual cell in which the reaction takes place. All other elements in tissue have a very low cross-section for neutron capture.

The first clinical experience was reported in 1954 when 10 patients with malignant brain tumors were treated.[19] The first group treated in this fashion in the United States included 17 patients with glioblastoma and one patient with a medulloblastoma; they were treated in 1960 and 1961.[20] No patient survived 1 year, and the average survival was 5.7 months. At autopsy, brain swelling, perivascular fibrosis, and cerebral necrosis were evident. The authors found that this was due to boron levels three to four times higher in blood vessels than in tumor, causing all subsequent work to cease at that point.

There has been a revival in studying this technology with the use of fast neutrons and newer boron-containing compounds.[21,22] Ongoing studies are being done in patients with glioblastoma, but further work will be required before this complex therapy becomes available outside of an experimental setting.

Radiation Sensitizers

Radiosensitizers are chemicals that increase the lethal effects of radiation. Many chemicals have been found to fit this definition; however, only those that have demonstrated a potential differential effect between tumor and normal tissues would warrant further investigation. The two major classes of compounds investigated to date are hypoxic cell sensitizers and halogenated pyrimidines.

Hypoxic Cell Sensitizers

Intraoperative in vivo measurements and examinations of patients using fluorine-18-fluoromisonidazole positron emission tomography (PET) have demonstrated the presence of hypoxic regions in glioblastomas.[23,24] It has been well established in the laboratory that hypoxic cells are significantly more resistant to radiation than are euoxic cells by an order of 2.5 to 3. Hypoxic cell sensitizers would thus sensitize the hypoxic tumor cells without increasing the radiation effect on the already well-oxygenated normal tissues. The first study reported a positive effect of metronidazole in a small randomized study in 1976.[25] However, the patient numbers were small, and the median survival of 4 months with radiation alone was considerably less than that seen in most other studies. Since then, there have been 11 additional randomized studies (involving 1,605 patients) that have not shown any benefit from the addition of nitroimidazoles to various combinations of radiotherapy and chemotherapy.[1]

Pitfall

- Hypoxic cell sensitizers may not be effective in malignant gliomas because sensitizing drugs may not add any additional effect over that achieved with the use of fractionated radiotherapy.

Halogenated Pyrimidines

The halogenated pyrimidines 5-bromodeoxyuridine (BUdR) and 5-iododeoxyuridine (IUdR) are similar to the normal DNA precursor thymidine, having a halogen substituted in place of a methyl group. These compounds are incorporated into DNA in place of thymidine in a competitive fashion, which leads to an increased sensitivity of cells incorporating these compounds to the effects of radiation and ultraviolet light. The rationale for using these compounds in the treatment of brain tumors is that mitotically active tumor cells are much more likely to incorporate these compounds than the slowly replicating glial and vascular cells in the normal brain. An increase in median survival was reported for anaplastic astrocytoma patients from 82 weeks in prior studies to 252 weeks in patients treated with radiation, BUdR, and chemotherapy.[26] There was no significant improvement seen with the use of BUdR for patients with glioblastoma. As a result of this observation, the RTOG embarked on a randomized study for patients with anaplastic astrocytoma: 60 Gy in 30 fractions with and without BUdR, both arms followed by a chemotherapy regimen known as PCV, consisting of procarbazine, chloroethylcyclo-

hexylnitrosourea (lomustine; CCNU), and vincristine. The study was closed prematurely when the initial 189 patients were analyzed. The 1-year survival rate for radiotherapy, PCV, and BUdR was 68% versus 82% for radiotherapy plus PCV, clearly a negative result.[27]

■ Photodynamic Therapy

5-Aminolevulinic acid (5-ALA) is the precursor for heme synthesis in mammalian cells, which is naturally metabolized to protoporphyrin-IX (Pp) prior to conversion to heme.[28] Malignant glial cells lack the ability to convert Pp to heme, and hence it accumulates in glial tumors selectively and not in normal glial or neuronal tissue, and Pp is a photoactive compound that absorbs violet blue light and emits red light, a quality that can be utilized to better appreciate the extent of the glioma at surgery and may help in achieving better resections.

Photodynamic therapy refers to the preoperative administration of a hematoporphyrin derivative generally 24 hours prior to taking the patient to the operating room, resecting as much tumor as safely achievable, and inserting a red light source into the center of the lipid-filled balloon expanded to fill the surgical cavity and expose the remaining glioma cells to this red light. When hematoporphyrin derivatives are exposed to red light, this creates singlet oxygen, which is cytotoxic to cells. As the hematoporphyrin selectively accumulate in malignant glial tissue, this should be a selective therapy that spares normal tissue.

As a result of the majority of patients with glioblastoma recurring locally, PDT has most extensively been investigated in this group of patients. There have been several uncontrolled single-arm phase II studies of the use of PDT in both newly diagnosed and recurrent glioblastomas with reported improvement in progression-free and overall median survival, but these uncontrolled reports must always be interpreted with caution as the result of the likelihood of selection of better prognostic patients for inclusion in the study.[29] Only one prospective randomized study of PDT only as an addition to surgery and radiotherapy has been performed in 43 patients in the PDT arm and 34 patients in the control arm.[30] There was an improvement in median survival from 8 months (95% confidence interval [CI], 3–10 months) to 11 months (95% CI, 6–14 months) for the PDT arm, but as the 95% CI overlapped, this was not a statistically significant result. There was a randomized trial of 5-ALA–guided resection and PDT in newly diagnosed patients presumed preoperatively to have high-grade gliomas, and there was an improvement in 6-month progression-free survival from 21% to 41% in the study arm, but no reported improvement in overall survival.[31]

Photodynamic therapy has been reported to be highly efficacious in superficial bladder, basal cell skin, and esophageal cancers, but the lack of efficacy in glial tumors of the brain and other solid tumors elsewhere is felt to be related to the lack of strong enough specificity of light sensitizer accumulation in tumor cells and to the inability to adequately reach all regions of tumor involvement with red light.[32]

■ Brachytherapy

Brachytherapy is performed using radioactive sources placed directly within a tumor. Dose decreases with the square of the distance away from a point source, and it is also attenuated by tissue, allowing delivery of a high dose to a tumor while sparing surrounding normal tissue. Furthermore, there are radiobiological advantages to low-dose-rate brachytherapy compared with external beam radiotherapy.[33]

Both interstitial and intracavitary brachytherapy techniques have been used for brain tumors. Temporary brain brachytherapy typically involves placing gamma-emitters such as iridium-192 or high-activity iodine-125 into catheters within the tumor or tumor bed, giving a dose of 50 to 60 Gy over 4 to 6 days at the edge of enhancement or with a small margin around enhancing tumor (**Fig. 18.2**). In contrast, permanent brain brachytherapy usually involves lining a resection cavity with multiple low-activity iodine-125 sources, giving 100 to 300 Gy over the lifetime of the sources at a depth of 5 to 10 mm. Iodine-125 sources have a mean energy of 28 KeV and a half-life of 60 days, whereas iridium-192 has a mean energy of 380 KeV and a half-life of 74 days. Intracavitary brachytherapy may be performed by injecting a radioactive solution into a tumor cyst, typically using a β-emitter such as phosphorus-32 (with a half-life of 14 days and a tissue half-value layer of 0.8 mm) or yttrium-90 (with a half-life of 2.7 days and a tissue half-value layer of 1.1 mm).[33] With the GliaSite (Cytyc Corp., Marlborough, MA) system, a 2-, 3-, or 4-cm-diameter balloon is inserted intraoperatively into a resection cavity and inflated with a radioactive iodine-125 solution to deliver 45 to 60 Gy over 3 to 5 days 0.5 to 1.0 cm from the balloon surface.[34]

The target for brachytherapy and other dose escalation techniques is usually the enhancing tumor on computed tomography (CT) or magnetic resonance imaging (MRI). However, newer functional imaging techniques show that the most active areas of high-grade glioma commonly lie outside of the enhancing region.[35] It is possible that results of brachytherapy could be improved by targeting the metabolically active region.

Controversy

- Radiation dose escalation may be of no benefit in malignant gliomas because of tumor cells infiltrating deeply into surrounding brain tissue. On the other hand, most malignant gliomas recur locally, and local control remains a fundamental challenge.

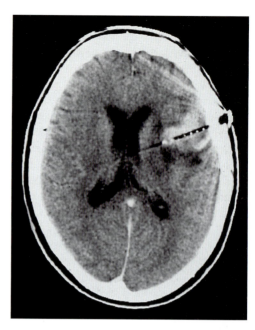

Fig. 18.2 Axial computed tomography (CT) image of an iodine-125 catheter inserted in a patient with a glioblastoma multiforme as a boost following prior external beam radiotherapy.

Common selection criteria for interstitial brachytherapy include a Karnofsky Performance Scale (KPS) score of at least 70, maximum tumor diameter less than 4 to 6 cm, and unifocal, circumscribed disease without leptomeningeal, subependymal, or corpus callosum involvement. Based on imaging studies and KPS, only 12 to 30% of patients with newly diagnosed glioblastomas are eligible for brachytherapy; furthermore, brachytherapy eligibility is associated with longer survival time after conventional therapy, biasing nonrandomized trials.[36,37]

The results of major brachytherapy trials are summarized in **Table 18.1** for newly diagnosed tumors[38–45] and in **Table 18.2** for recurrent tumors.[34,42,46–50] Nonrandomized trials of brachytherapy boost in conjunction with external beam radiation for glioblastoma yielded promising median survival times as high as 18 to 19 months, but with reoperation rates as high as 52 to 64% (**Table 18.1**). Pathological findings at the time of reoperation after brachytherapy may show tumor, necrosis, or both. Reoperation rates vary partially according to the aggressiveness of the center, but symptomatic radiation necrosis is a well-known complication of temporary brain brachytherapy; necrosis is much less common after permanent brachytherapy.

Disappointingly, two prospective, randomized trials failed to show a benefit of brachytherapy boost for malignant gliomas (**Table 18.1**). In the University of Toronto trial, malignant glioma patients received 50 Gy external beam radiation alone or followed by 60 Gy temporary brachytherapy. The median survival times, based on an intent-to-treat analysis, were 13.2 months for the control arm versus 13.8 months for the

Table 18.1 Major Trials of Brachytherapy Boost for Newly Diagnosed Brain Tumors

Reference	Number of Patients and Histology	Isotope and Technique	Median Age (Years)	Median KPS	Median Brachy Dose (Gy)	Median Volume (mL)	Median Survival (months)	Reoperation Rate (%)
Sneed et al[38]	159 GBM	Temporary [125]I	52	90	55	26	19	51
Wen et al[39]	56 GBM	Temporary [125]I	50	90	50	22	18	64
Videtic et al[40]	52 GBM	Permanent [125]I	57	90	104	15.5	16	–
Koot et al[41]	45 GBM	Temporary or Permanent [125]I	51	≥70	50–80	23	13 (17*)	9
	21 GBM	Temporary [192]Ir	54	≥70	40	48	16	33
Sneed et al[38]	52 AA	Temporary [125]I	40	90	50	21.5	36.3	67
Laperriere et al[43]	60 GBM/9 AA	Control arm	>50	90	0	–	13.2	33
	65 GBM/6 AA	Temporary [125]I	>50	90	60	42.3	13.8	31
Selker et al[44]	107 GBM/26 anaplastic	Control arm	>55	90	0	–	13.5	48
	123 GBM/14 anaplastic	Temporary [125]I	>55	90	~60	21	15.7	53
Kreth et al[45]	97 pilocytic	Temporary or permanent [125]I	28	90	60 (T)	14 (T)	–	–
	358 grade II				100 (P)	28 (P)	–	–
Sneed et al[†]	19 metastases	Permanent [125]I	58	80	400	13.6	12.0	21

*Subset analysis for patients > 30 years old with KPS at least 70 and non-midline tumor.
[†]Unpublished data.
Abbreviations. AA, anaplastic astrocytoma; GBM, glioblastoma multiforme, KPS, Karnofsky Performance Scale score.

brachytherapy arm ($p = 0.24$), but steroid requirements at 6 and 12 months were higher in the brachytherapy arm.[43] In the Brain Tumor Cooperative Group trial, brachytherapy was performed prior to external beam radiation to 60 Gy with bis-chloroethylnitrosourea (BCNU; carmustine), avoiding attrition due to tumor progression during radiotherapy. Median survival times were 13.5 months for the control arm versus 15.7 months for the brachytherapy arm ($p = 0.10$); a multivariate analysis adjusting for prognostic factors failed to show a benefit for brachytherapy.[44] Interestingly, reoperation rates were similar with or without brachytherapy in the two trials (31% vs 33% and 53% vs 48%).[43,44]

> **Special Consideration**
>
> - Results of brachytherapy may be limited by inadequate tumor targeting based on imaging appearance alone. Metabolic imaging techniques may be useful to identify more appropriate targets for focal high dose.

Brachytherapy for low-grade gliomas does not appear to be better than conventional radiotherapy. Five and 10-year survival probabilities of 85% and 83% have been reported for 97 pilocytic astrocytoma patients and 61% and 51% for 250

Table 18.2 Results of Brachytherapy for Recurrent Brain Tumors

Reference	Number of Patients and Histology	Isotope And Technique	Median Age (Years)	Median KPS	Median Brachy Dose (Gy)	Median Volume (mL)	Median Survival (Months)	Reoperation Rate (%)
Sneed et al[42]	66 GBM	Temporary [125]I	50	90	64	34	11.7	46
Bernstein et al[46]	32 GBM/12 AA	Temporary [125]I	46	80?	70.1	50.3	10.6	26
Shrieve et al[47]	32 GBM	Temporary [125]I	45	80	50	29	11.5	44
Chan et al[34]	24 GBM	GliaSite [125]I	48	80	53	15	9.1	8 necrosis
Gaspar et al[48]	37 GBM	Permanent [125]I	53	90	100	18.4	10.5	44
Larson et al[49]	38 GBM	Permanent [125]I	47	90	300	21	12.0	10
Patel et al[50]	40 GBM	Permanent [125]I	50	70	120–160	47.3	10.8	No necrosis
Sneed et al[42]	45 AA	Temporary [125]I	38	90	64	31	12.3	53
Sneed et al*	21 metastases	Permanent [125]I	59	80	300	19.2	7.3	14

*Unpublished data.
Abbreviations: AA, anaplastic astrocytoma; GBM, glioblastoma multiforme; KPS, Karnofsky Performance Scale score.

grade II astrocytoma patients treated with permanent brachytherapy to 100 Gy or low-dose-rate temporary brachytherapy to 60 Gy at 10 cGy/h or less[45] (**Table 18.1**).

Randomized trials of brachytherapy have not been performed for recurrent malignant gliomas. Retrospective series report median survival times of 9.1 to 11.7 months after temporary brachytherapy for recurrent glioblastoma,[34,42,46,47] 10.5 to 12.0 months after permanent brachytherapy for recurrent glioblastoma,[48-50] and 12.3 months after brachytherapy for recurrent anaplastic astrocytoma[42] (**Table 18.2**). Because of patient selection factors and the use of additional therapies after further disease progression, the value of brachytherapy for recurrent gliomas is difficult, if not impossible, to discern.

Interest in brachytherapy dropped drastically as noninvasive alternatives—radiosurgery and intensity-modulated radiotherapy—became widely available, as the problem of symptomatic radiation necrosis became more apparent, and after randomized trials in newly diagnosed tumors failed to show a benefit. However, there may still be a role for brachytherapy in selected cases such as focally recurrent tumors and resection cavities or margins at high risk for local recurrence, particularly for brain metastases and malignant or multiply recurrent meningiomas.[51] In addition, intracavitary brachytherapy may be useful to help control craniopharyngioma cysts.[52]

■ Hyperthermia

Hyperthermia kills cells as a function of time and temperature and sensitizes cells to radiation and many kinds of chemotherapy. It is also particularly effective against cells that tend to be resistant to radiation: S-phase cells and nutrient-deprived, low pH hypoxic cells.[53] An isoeffect formula allows different combinations of time and temperature to be translated into "equivalent minutes at 43°C" and thermal dose from separate hyperthermia treatments is summed up as "cumulative equivalent minutes at 43°C." Because heating within tumors is inevitably heterogeneous, thermal dose values are specified as to whether they are derived from the minimum, median, or maximum tumor temperatures or, for example, the 10th percentile (T_{90}) of the tumor temperature distribution.[54]

Common heating techniques include externally applied energy from microwave or ultrasound applicators for superficial tumors, regional heating using radiofrequency systems for deep-seated tumors, whole-body hyperthermia, or interstitially implanted microwave antennas, miniature tubular ultrasound transducers, radiofrequency electrodes, or hot sources for invasive heating.[55]

Numerous phase 1 and 2 trials in the 1980s attempting to heat superficial tumors to 41° to 45°C for an hour once or twice weekly in combination with radiation yielded complete response rates on the order of 35% for radiation alone versus 60% for radiation plus hyperthermia.[56] Two early phase 3 hyperthermia trials performed with inadequate tumor heating were negative, but later phase 3 hyperthermia trials have proven a significant benefit for hyperthermia in chest wall recurrence of breast cancer, melanoma, head and neck cancer, and cervical cancer.[57] Two more recent phase 3 trials of radiation with hyperthermia employed a test heat session so that only "heatable" tumors were randomized. In both trials, approximately 90% of tumors were "heatable." The complete response rates were 66% versus 42% for hyperthermia versus control in human superficial tumors (odds ratio 2.7; $p = 0.02$)[58] In pet dogs with sarcomas, multivariate analysis showed significantly longer local control in the higher versus lower thermal dose arm ($p = 0.023$).[59]

Brain hyperthermia poses special difficulties. The heat tolerance of normal brain tissue is quite limited. In canine brain, breakdown of the blood–brain barrier occurs with heat exposures of 42.8°C for 30 minutes or 42.4°C for 60 minutes and cerebral necrosis occurs with 44° to 44.3°C for 30 minutes or 42.8°C for 60 minutes.[60] Furthermore, brain hyperthermia is technically difficult to administer, usually requiring interstitially placed heat applicators if selective tumor heating is desired. Alternatively, fever-range brain heating can be accomplished via whole-body hyperthermia, though there is very little clinical experience with this approach.

Human brain hyperthermia trials were reviewed in 1995.[60] Phase 1 and 2 trials showed that brain hyperthermia could be accomplished successfully with various interstitial techniques, but complications were relatively common, including occasional surgical complications, generalized seizures, increased mass effect or intracranial pressure, and fairly frequent focal seizures and reversible neurologic changes (**Table 18.3**). There was a suggestion of benefit from a study of interstitial ferroseed hyperthermia for 60 minutes before and after iridium-192 brachytherapy to 26 to 41 Gy; 25 patients with primary malignant gliomas had significantly longer survival than a control group treated with radiation and brachytherapy without hyperthermia (median survival time 23.5 months vs 13.3 months; $p = 0.027$).[61] In another study, interstitial microwave hyperthermia was given for 30 minutes before and after iodine-125 brachytherapy to 60 Gy. Median survival time from the first hyperthermia treatment was 11.3 months for 25 patients with recurrent glioblastoma and 32.2 months for 16 patients with recurrent anaplastic astrocytoma.[62] T_{90} temperature of at least 41.2°C was associated with significantly longer survival time among the 25 glioblastoma patients ($p = 0.008$).[62]

In a phase 2 and 3 randomized trial patients with newly diagnosed glioblastoma were treated with partial brain radiotherapy to 59.4 Gy with hydroxyurea followed by 60 Gy temporary brachytherapy boost with or without interstitial microwave hyperthermia for 30 minutes before and after brachytherapy.[63] Of 112 eligible patients enrolled, 79 were randomized following external beam radiation and 68 actually underwent brachytherapy with or without hyperthermia. The most common reason for attrition was tumor progression. The median T_{90} thermal dose among heated patients was 14.1 cumulative equivalent minutes at 43°C. The addition of hyperthermia to brachytherapy was associated with a significant increase in toxicity (**Table 18.3**). Among all 79 randomized patients, the heat arm of the study had significantly longer freedom from progression ($p = 0.04$) and survival time ($p = 0.04$). Among the 68 patients who underwent brachytherapy the median freedom from progression was 49 versus 33 weeks ($p = 0.045$), median survival time 85 versus 76 weeks, and 18-month survival 59% versus 38% ($p = 0.02$) for heat versus no heat, with a reoperation rate of 69% versus 58%. A multivariate analysis of survival time adjusting for KPS score and age yielded a hazard ratio of 0.51 favoring the heat arm of the study ($p = 0.008$).

Despite the positive results of this randomized trial of hyperthermia for glioblastoma, there has been fairly limited further clinical use of brain hyperthermia. Enthusiasm was dampened by negative randomized brachytherapy trials, significant toxicity of brain brachytherapy and hyperthermia,

Table 18.3 Toxicities Related to Brachytherapy with or Without Hyperthermia[63]

Complication	Brachytherapy Only (33 Patients): Number of Patients	Brachytherapy with Hyperthermia (35 Patients): Number of Patients
Grade IV (meningitis)	1	1
Grade III (infection, neurological changes, generalized seizures)	1	6
Grade I–II (focal seizures)	3	7
Grade I–II (mild reversible neurological changes)	2	17

and the desirability of a treatment strategy for malignant gliomas that is more selective on a cellular basis, to address the problem of tumor cells infiltrating in normal brain tissue away from gross tumor.

Recently, there has been more interest in mild temperature hyperthermia in the range of 39° to 42°C, which enhances antitumor immune response and increases blood flow, tumor oxygenation, and vascular permeability, potentially improving delivery of chemotherapeutic, immunotherapeutic, and gene therapy agents.[64,65] Tumor reoxygenation is important in radiotherapy because hypoxic cells may be up to threefold more resistant to radiation than oxygenated cells. Brain hyperthermia needs to be reconsidered, combining mild heating with chemotherapy, molecular targeted therapy, immunotherapy, or gene therapy.

■ Stereotactic Body Radiation Therapy for Spinal Tumors

Metastatic disease in bone occurs in most primary cancers with dissemination, and represents the third most common site of metastatic disease behind lung and liver in approximately one third of all cancer patients.[66] Spinal radiotherapy is a commonly prescribed course of treatment for patients with vertebral metastases to help alleviate pain and possibly prevent the eventual progression to spinal cord compression that occurs in approximately 5 to 10% of cancer patients. Conventionally delivered radiotherapy delivers doses in the range from 8 Gy in one fraction to 20 Gy in five fractions or 30 Gy in 10 fractions, and is associated with a median duration of pain relief of 3 to 6 months irrespective of dose chosen.[66] With conventional radiotherapy, simple techniques of a single posterior field or anterior-posterior opposed parallel pairs of fields are utilized with the spinal cord receiving the same dose as the vertebral metastases and bone (**Fig. 18.3**). As a result of patients living longer with bony metastatic disease related to better systemic therapies available today, there has been an increased likelihood of recurrent painful vertebral metastases. This has led to two new issues: a need to dose escalate the initial course of palliative radiotherapy in hopes of achieving a longer time of pain relief, and an increased likelihood of having to reirradiate previously conventionally radiated regions of the spine.

Stereotactic body radiation therapy (SBRT) is a newly emerging technique that uses advanced techniques to deliver higher fraction sizes of radiotherapy to targets such as vertebral metastases with sparing of dose to the spinal cord/cauda equina. As with the use of radiosurgery in the brain, these techniques rely on excellent immobilization of the patient; treatment planning imaging utilizing CT, MRI, and occasionally CT myelography or conventional myelography to accurately delineate the target vertebral metastases and position of the intrathecal contents; sophisticated treatment planning computers to deliver highly conformal dose to bony metastases while sparing the intrathecal contents; and some form of image guidance or verification on the treatment unit and use of robotic couches with the ability to correct for six degrees of freedom to assess and correct patient position before and during treatment delivery.[67] The most commonly utilized techniques include linear accelerators capable of delivering intensity modulated radiation therapy (IMRT) or volumetric modified arc therapy (VMAT) and the use of cone beam CT on these units for image guidance, or less commonly utilizing a technology called CyberKnife® Robotic Radiosurgery (Accuray Inc., Sunnyvale, CA), in which a linear accelerator is mounted on a robotic arm capable of six degrees of freedom and delivers dose to a vol-

ume utilizing multiple isocenters. The doses vary from 18 to 20 Gy in a single fraction to 30 Gy in five fractions and include many variations in doses delivered between these two totals in two to four fractions (**Fig. 18.4**).

The management of spinal metastases requires a multidisciplinary approach involving spine surgeons to assess the need for surgery and radiation oncologists to advise on appropriate radiotherapy approach. As SBRT is a newly emerging approach, its current role in the management of vertebral metastases remains ill defined. However, it appears to be associated with longer pain relief and better progression-free intervals of the treated spinal sites following treatment than is conventional radiotherapy, but no upfront randomized comparisons have been undertaken to date.[68] Currently, SBRT seems a reasonable option in patients with expected longer survival with limited extent of metastatic disease, with a limited number of spinal vertebrae involved, possibly in patients with radiation-resistant histologies (sarcoma, melanoma, renal cell carcinoma), and as salvage treatment for previously conventionally radiated recurrent spinal metastases. The risk of spinal vertebral compression fractures following SBRT with

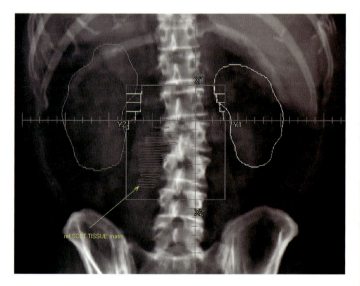

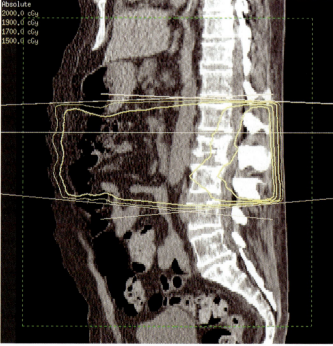

Fig. 18.3a,b (a) Digital reconstructed radiograph of a direct posterior field for the treatment of a patient with prostate cancer with metastatic disease L1–L3. **(b)** Radiation dose distribution for the same case for an anterior and posterior radiation fields to deliver 20 Gy in five daily fractions.

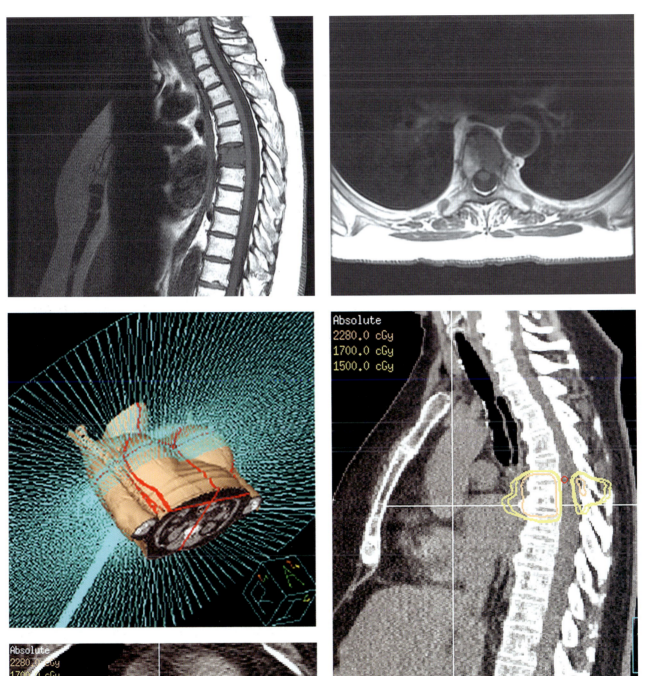

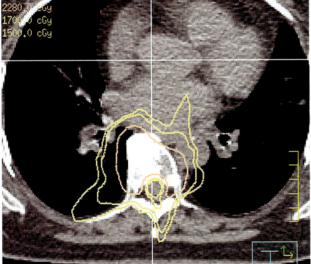

Fig. 18.4a–d **(a)** Sagittal (*left*) and axial (*right*) T1-weighted MRI of spine of a patient with metastatic breast cancer with involvement of T6 vertebral body. **(b)** Volumetric modified arc therapy (VMAT) of T6 vertebral body delivering 24 Gy in two daily fractions. **(c)** Radiation dose distribution on sagittal CT image demonstrating relative sparing of spinal cord to 15 Gy. **(d)** Radiation dose distribution on axial CT image demonstrating relative sparing of spinal cord to 15 Gy.

such high ablative doses was found to be 11% in one series and was related to the presence of kyphotic/scoliotic deformity and the presence of lytic tumor in a multivariate analysis.[69]

Stereotactic body radiation therapy is also being investigated for primary intradural, intramedullary, and extramedullary tumors of the spine.[70] The tumors typically treated in this fashion include meningiomas, schwannomas, hemangiomas, and only a very limited number of cases with limited follow-up have currently been reported, so the role of SBRT for this indication remains to be further elucidated. Surgery and conventionally fractionated radiotherapy remain the standard of care currently for these patients.

Conclusion

There have been many technical advances in the delivery of more precise radiotherapy for malignant brain tumors, but despite attempts at increasing total dose by altered fractionation, particle therapy, and brachytherapy, malignant gliomas continue to be incurable neoplasms. Particle therapy does offer the advantage of reduced dose to the adjacent normal tissues, and has the potential to lessen the long-term effects in children with brain tumors. Hypoxic cell sensitizers and halogenated pyrimidines have not proven effective, although it is likely that recent success with concurrent temozolomide during radiotherapy may in part be related to radiation sensitization.[71] Boron neutron capture therapy is a highly complex form of treatment that likely will continue in an experimental fashion for many years to come prior to being ready for any randomized studies. Photodynamic therapy remains an experimental approach that requires agents with greater affinity for tumor cells and light sources of greater penetration into brain. The greatest potential for improvements in the management of malignant gliomas lies in better understanding aberrant molecular pathways operational in these malignancies and combining radiation with new molecular therapies that may alter radiation response. Stereotactic body radiation therapy seems a promising approach for the palliative management of patients with vertebral metastases in selected cases, but its ultimate role in the overall management of patients with spinal metastases and primary benign spinal tumors will evolve over the next several years.

Editor's Note

The more prominent alternate radiotherapy approaches include alterations of size and temporal spacing of radiation fractions, radiation sensitizers, photodynamic therapy, boron neutron capture, particle therapy, brachytherapy, and hyperthermia. All these modalities have two overriding commonalities. The first is that they are backed up by strong theoretical scientific foundations, which made all of them promising to try, and they generated much excitement among radiation and other oncologists when they were introduced. The second is that they have essentially failed to live up to those expectations and make a positive impact on the disease they were primarily designed for—malignant glioma. The main reason is the challenge of delivery of destructive energy to every cell of a glioma without causing unreasonable toxicity to surrounding or intermingled functioning brain tissue. Although focal therapies for gliomas are certainly important, the current trend toward discovering therapies more targeted at cells and molecules as opposed to geographies may be more impactful. (Bernstein)

References

1. Laperriere N, Zuraw L, Cairncross G; Cancer Care Ontario Practice Guidelines Initiative Neuro-Oncology Disease Site Group. Radiotherapy for newly diagnosed malignant glioma in adults: a systematic review. Radiother Oncol 2002;64:259–273
2. Shin KH, Urtasun RC, Fulton D, et al. Multiple daily fractionated radiation therapy and misonidazole in the management of malignant astrocytoma. A preliminary report. Cancer 1985;56:758–760
3. Scott CB, Curran WJ, Yung WKA, et al. Long term results of RTOG 9006: a randomized study of hyperfractionated radiotherapy (RT) to 72.0 Gy and carmustine vs standard RT and carmustine for malignant glioma patients with emphasis on anaplastic astrocytoma (AA) patients. Proc ASCO 1998;17:A1546, 401a
4. Horiot JC, van den Bogaert W, Ang KK, et al. European Organization for Research on Treatment of Cancer trials using radiotherapy with multiple fractions per day. A 1978-1987 survey. Front Radiat Ther Oncol 1988;22:149–161
5. Werner-Wasik M, Scott CB, Nelson DF, et al. Final report of a phase I/II trial of hyperfractionated and accelerated hyperfractionated radiation therapy with carmustine for adults with supratentorial malignant gliomas. Radiation Therapy Oncology Group Study 83-02. Cancer 1996;77:1535–1543
6. Brada M, Sharpe G, Rajan B, et al. Modifying radical radiotherapy in high grade gliomas; shortening the treatment time through acceleration. Int J Radiat Oncol Biol Phys 1999;43:287–292
7. Keim H, Potthoff PC, Schmidt K, Schiebusch M, Neiss A, Trott KR. Survival and quality of life after continuous accelerated radiotherapy of glioblastomas. Radiother Oncol 1987;9:21–26
8. Simpson WJ, Platts ME. Fractionation study in the treatment of glioblastoma multiforme. Int J Radiat Oncol Biol Phys 1976;1:639–644
9. Laperriere NJ, Wong CS, Milosevic MF, Whitton AC, Wells WA, Patterson B. Accelerated radiation therapy for primary lymphoma of the brain. Radiother Oncol 1998;47:191–195
10. Duncan W, McLelland J, Jack WJ, et al. Report of a randomised pilot study of the treatment of patients with supratentorial gliomas using neutron irradiation. Br J Radiol 1986;59:373–377
11. Duncan W, McLelland J, Jack WJ, et al. The results of a randomised trial of mixed-schedule (neutron/photon) irradiation in the treatment of

supratentorial grade III and grade IV astrocytoma. Br J Radiol 1986; 59:379–383

12. Griffin TW, Davis R, Laramore G, et al. Fast neutron radiation therapy for glioblastoma multiforme. Results of an RTOG study. Am J Clin Oncol 1983;6:661–667

13. Laramore GE, Diener-West M, Griffin TW, et al; Radiation Therapy Oncology Group. Randomized neutron dose searching study for malignant gliomas of the brain: results of an RTOG study. Int J Radiat Oncol Biol Phys 1988;14:1093–1102

14. Pickles T, Goodman GB, Rheaume DE, et al. Pion radiation for high grade astrocytoma: results of a randomized study. Int J Radiat Oncol Biol Phys 1997;37:491–497

15. Fitzek MM, Thornton AF, Rabinov JD, et al. Accelerated fractionated proton/photon irradiation to 90 cobalt gray equivalent for glioblastoma multiforme: results of a phase II prospective trial. J Neurosurg 1999; 91:251–260

16. Hug EB, Loredo LN, Slater JD, et al. Proton radiation therapy for chordomas and chondrosarcomas of the skull base. J Neurosurg 1999;91: 432–439

17. Combs SE, Laperriere N, Brada M. Clinical controversies: proton radiation therapy for brain and skull base tumors. Semin Radiat Oncol 2013;23:120–126

18. Potluri S, Jefferies SJ, Jena R, et al. Residual postoperative tumour volume predicts outcome after high-dose radiotherapy for chordoma and chondrosarcoma of the skull base and spine. Clin Oncol (R Coll Radiol) 2011;23:199–208

19. Farr LE, Sweet WH, Robertson JS, et al. Neutron capture therapy with boron in the treatment of glioblastoma multiforme. Am J Roentgenol Radium Ther Nucl Med 1954;71:279–293

20. Asbury AK, Ojemann RG, Nielsen SL, Sweet WH. Neuropathologic study of fourteen cases of malignant brain tumor treated by boron-10 slow neutron capture radiation. J Neuropathol Exp Neurol 1972;31:278–303

21. Barth RF, Coderre JA, Vicente MG, Blue TE. Boron neutron capture therapy of cancer: current status and future prospects. Clin Cancer Res 2005;11:3987–4002

22. Barth RF, Vicente MGH, Harling OK, et al. Current status of boron neutron capture therapy of high grade gliomas and recurrent head and neck cancer. Radiat Oncol 2012;7:146

23. Rampling R, Cruickshank G, Lewis AD, Fitzsimmons SA, Workman P. Direct measurement of pO2 distribution and bioreductive enzymes in human malignant brain tumors. Int J Radiat Oncol Biol Phys 1994; 29:427–431

24. Valk PE, Mathis CA, Prados MD, Gilbert JC, Budinger TF. Hypoxia in human gliomas: demonstration by PET with fluorine-18-fluoromisonidazole. J Nucl Med 1992;33:2133–2137

25. Urtasun R, Band P, Chapman JD, Feldstein ML, Mielke B, Fryer C. Radiation and high-dose metronidazole in supratentorial glioblastomas. N Engl J Med 1976;294:1364–1367

26. Phillips TL, Prados MD, Bodell WJ, Levin VA, Uhl V, Gutin PH. Rationale for and experience with clinical trials of halogenated pyrimidines in malignant gliomas: the UCSF/NCOG experience. In: Dewey WC, Edington M, Fry RJM, Hall EJ, Whitmore GF, eds. Radiation Research: A Twentieth-Century Perspective, vol 2: Congress Proceedings. San Diego: Academic Press, 1992:601–606

27. Prados MD, Scott C, Sandler H, et al. A phase 3 randomized study of radiotherapy plus procarbazine, CCNU, and vincristine (PCV) with or without BUdR for the treatment of anaplastic astrocytoma: a preliminary report of RTOG 9404. Int J Radiat Oncol Biol Phys 1999;45:1109–1115

28. Yang VXD, Muller PJ, Herman P, Wilson BC. A multispectral fluorescence imaging system: design and initial clinical tests in intra-operative Photofrin-photodynamic therapy of brain tumors. Lasers Surg Med 2003;32:224–232

29. Eljamel S. Photodynamic applications in brain tumors: a comprehensive review of the literature. Photodiagn Photodyn Ther 2010;7: 76–85

30. Muller P, Wilson B. A randomized two arm clinical trial of protoporphyrin PDT and standard therapy in high grade gliomas. Phase III trial. In: Proceedings of the 6th International PDT Symposium, 2006

31. Stepp H, Beck T, Pongratz T, et al. ALA and malignant glioma: fluorescence-guided resection and photodynamic treatment. J Environ Pathol Toxicol Oncol 2007;26:157–164

32. Wilson BC, Patterson MS. The physics, biophysics and technology of photodynamic therapy. Phys Med Biol 2008;53:R61–R109

33. McDermott MW, Berger MS, Kunwar S, Parsa AT, Sneed PK, Larson DA. Stereotactic radiosurgery and interstitial brachytherapy for glial neoplasms. J Neurooncol 2004;69:83–100

34. Chan TA, Weingart JD, Parisi M, et al. Treatment of recurrent glioblastoma multiforme with GliaSite brachytherapy. Int J Radiat Oncol Biol Phys 2005;62:1133–1139

35. Pirzkall A, McKnight TR, Graves EE, et al. MR-spectroscopy guided target delineation for high-grade gliomas. Int J Radiat Oncol Biol Phys 2001;50:915–928

36. Curran WJ Jr, Scott CB, Weinstein AS, et al. Survival comparison of radiosurgery-eligible and -ineligible malignant glioma patients treated with hyperfractionated radiation therapy and carmustine: a report of Radiation Therapy Oncology Group 83-02. J Clin Oncol 1993;11:857–862

37. Florell RC, Macdonald DR, Irish WD, et al. Selection bias, survival, and brachytherapy for glioma. J Neurosurg 1992;76:179–183

38. Sneed PK, Prados MD, McDermott MW, et al. Large effect of age on the survival of patients with glioblastoma treated with radiotherapy and brachytherapy boost. Neurosurgery 1995;36:898–903, discussion 903–904

39. Wen PY, Alexander E III, Black PM, et al. Long term results of stereotactic brachytherapy used in the initial treatment of patients with glioblastomas. Cancer 1994;73:3029–3036

40. Videtic GM, Gaspar LE, Zamorano L, Stitt LW, Fontanesi J, Levin KJ. Implant volume as a prognostic variable in brachytherapy decision-making for malignant gliomas stratified by the RTOG recursive partitioning analysis. Int J Radiat Oncol Biol Phys 2001;51:963–968

41. Koot RW, Maarouf M, Hulshof MC, et al. Brachytherapy: results of two different therapy strategies for patients with primary glioblastoma multiforme. Cancer 2000;88:2796–2802

42. Sneed PK, Larson DA, Gutin PH. Brachytherapy and hyperthermia for malignant astrocytomas. Semin Oncol 1994;21:186–197

43. Laperriere NJ, Leung PM, McKenzie S, et al. Randomized study of brachytherapy in the initial management of patients with malignant astrocytoma. Int J Radiat Oncol Biol Phys 1998;41:1005–1011

44. Selker RG, Shapiro WR, Burger P, et al; Brain Tumor Cooperative Group. The Brain Tumor Cooperative Group NIH Trial 87-01: a randomized comparison of surgery, external radiotherapy, and carmustine versus surgery, interstitial radiotherapy boost, external radiation therapy, and carmustine. Neurosurgery 2002;51:343–355, discussion 355–357

45. Kreth FW, Faist M, Warnke PC, Rossner R, Volk B, Ostertag CB. Interstitial radiosurgery of low-grade gliomas. J Neurosurg 1995;82:418–429

46. Bernstein M, Laperriere N, Glen J, Leung P, Thomason C, Landon AE. Brachytherapy for recurrent malignant astrocytoma. Int J Radiat Oncol Biol Phys 1994;30:1213–1217

47. Shrieve DC, Alexander E III, Wen PY, et al. Comparison of stereotactic radiosurgery and brachytherapy in the treatment of recurrent glioblastoma multiforme. Neurosurgery 1995;36:275–282, discussion 282–284

48. Gaspar LE, Zamorano LJ, Shamsa F, Fontanesi J, Ezzell GE, Yakar DA. Permanent 125 iodine implants for recurrent malignant gliomas. Int J Radiat Oncol Biol Phys 1999;43:977–982

49. Larson DA, Suplica JM, Chang SM, et al. Permanent iodine 125 brachytherapy in patients with progressive or recurrent glioblastoma multiforme. Neuro-oncol 2004;6:119–126

50. Patel S, Breneman JC, Warnick RE, et al. Permanent iodine-125 interstitial implants for the treatment of recurrent glioblastoma multiforme. Neurosurgery 2000;46:1123–1128, discussion 1128–1130

51. Ware ML, Larson DA, Sneed PK, Wara WW, McDermott MW. Surgical resection and permanent brachytherapy for recurrent atypical and malignant meningioma. Neurosurgery 2004;54:55–63, discussion 63–64

52. Hasegawa T, Kondziolka D, Hadjipanayis CG, Lunsford LD. Management of cystic craniopharyngiomas with phosphorus-32 intracavitary irradiation. Neurosurgery 2004;54:813–820, discussion 820–822

53. Dewey WC, Freeman ML, Raaphorst GP, et al. Cell biology of hyperthermia and radiation. In: Meyn RE, Withers HR, eds. Radiation Biology in Cancer Research. New York: Raven Press, 1980:589–621

54. Dewey WC. Arrhenius relationships from the molecule and cell to the clinic. Int J Hyperthermia 1994;10:457–483

55. Stauffer PR. Evolving technology for thermal therapy of cancer. Int J Hyperthermia 2005;21:731–744

56. Sneed PK, Phillips TL. Combining hyperthermia and radiation: how beneficial? Oncology (Williston Park) 1991;5:99–108, discussion 109–110, 112

57. Dewhirst MW, Sneed PK. Those in gene therapy should pay closer attention to lessons from hyperthermia. Int J Radiat Oncol Biol Phys 2003;57:597–599, author reply 599–600

58. Jones EL, Oleson JR, Prosnitz LR, et al. Randomized trial of hyperthermia and radiation for superficial tumors. J Clin Oncol 2005;23:3079–3085

59. Thrall DE, LaRue SM, Yu D, et al. Prospective application of thermal dose is related to duration of local control in canine sarcomas treated with hyperthermia and radiation. Clin Cancer Res 2005

60. Seegenschmiedt MH, Klautke G, Grabenbauer GG, Sauer R. Thermoradiotherapy for malignant brain tumors: review of biological and clinical studies. Endocurie Hyperthemia Oncol 1995;11:201–221

61. Stea B, Rossman K, Kittelson J, Shetter A, Hamilton A, Cassady JR. Interstitial irradiation versus interstitial thermoradiotherapy for supratentorial malignant gliomas: a comparative survival analysis. Int J Radiat Oncol Biol Phys 1994;30:591–600

62. Sneed PK, Gutin PH, Stauffer PR, et al. Thermoradiotherapy of recurrent malignant brain tumors. Int J Radiat Oncol Biol Phys 1992;23:853–861

63. Sneed PK, Stauffer PR, McDermott MW, et al. Survival benefit of hyperthermia in a prospective randomized trial of brachytherapy boost +/– hyperthermia for glioblastoma multiforme. Int J Radiat Oncol Biol Phys 1998;40:287–295

64. Calderwood SK, Theriault JR, Gong J. How is the immune response affected by hyperthermia and heat shock proteins? Int J Hyperthermia 2005;21:713–716

65. Song CW, Park HJ, Lee CK, Griffin R. Implications of increased tumor blood flow and oxygenation caused by mild temperature hyperthermia in tumor treatment. Int J Hyperthermia 2005;21:761–767

66. Bhatt AD, Schuler JC, Boakye M, Woo SY. Current and emerging concepts in non-invasive and minimally invasive management of spine metastasis. Cancer Treat Rev 2013;39:142–152

67. Lo SS, Sahgal A, Wang JZ, et al. Stereotactic body radiation therapy for spinal metastases. Discov Med 2010;9:289–296

68. Lo SS, Lutz ST, Chang EL, et al; Expert Panel on Radiation Oncology-Bone Metastases. ACR Appropriateness Criteria® spinal bone metastases. J Palliat Med 2013;16:9–19

69. Cunha MVR, Al-Omair A, Atenafu EG, et al. Vertebral compression fracture (VCF) after spine stereotactic body radiation therapy (SBRT): analysis of predictive factors. Int J Radiat Oncol Biol Phys 2012;84: e343–e349

70. Sahgal A, Chou D, Ames C, et al. Image-guided robotic stereotactic body radiotherapy for benign spinal tumors: the University of California San Francisco preliminary experience. Technol Cancer Res Treat 2007;6: 595–604

71. Stupp R, Mason WP, van den Bent MJ, et al; European Organisation for Research and Treatment of Cancer Brain Tumor and Radiotherapy Groups; National Cancer Institute of Canada Clinical Trials Group. Radiotherapy plus concomitant and adjuvant temozolomide for glioblastoma. N Engl J Med 2005;352:987–996

V Systemic Therapy

19 Systemic Chemotherapy

Rebecca DeBoer and Michael D. Prados

The Challenge

The use of systemic chemotherapy for central nervous system (CNS) tumors presents a significant challenge for neuro-oncologists. These tumors represent a biologically diverse group of diseases with unique growth characteristics and variable response to treatment. Inherent or acquired mechanisms of resistance play an important limiting role in drug development and clinical trial design. Drug delivery is especially problematic, particularly to areas of microscopic invasive disease distant from the main tumor bed. Assessment of the response to treatment is difficult due to the limited ability of imaging to specifically distinguish tumor from areas of injured brain tissue, or to identify microscopic tumor within normal-appearing brain. In addition to these inherent biological, pharmacological, and radiological challenges, the perceived lack of successful treatment in the setting of recurrent malignant glioma often contributes to the nihilistic approach of many physicians caring for these patients, with the result that few patients enter clinical trials.

Despite these problems, however, a concerted effort continues in this field of research that is now largely based on scientific models rather than on the empiricism of the past. Clinical trials serve as the cornerstone of the research effort in neuro-oncology. In recent years several new approaches to trial design have been developed to enhance the traditional model of phase 1, 2, and 3 investigations. New strategies such as the continual reassessment method and "phase 0" testing may optimize early-phase evaluation of dosing and toxicity. Randomized phase 2 trials and adaptive randomization may improve later-phase evaluation of antitumor efficacy. This chapter reviews the principles of traditional clinical trial design and highlights these new approaches.

Progress in the development of effective chemotherapy for CNS tumors has been modest. The use of systemic chemotherapy for CNS tumors first entered routine clinical practice in the late 1960s. Numerous types of cytotoxic chemotherapy agents were used initially, and favored regimens became the standard of care based largely on empiric observation, with some input from prospective trials. In the late 1970s the nitrosoureas became the first cytotoxic chemotherapy agents approved for use in malignant glioma by the United States Food and Drug Administration (FDA). The nitrosoureas remained the most widely used agents in brain tumors until temozolomide was approved by the FDA in 2005 and subsequently became the most commonly used first-line agent. More recently, molecularly targeted agents such as monoclonal antibodies and small molecular tyrosine kinase inhibitors have demonstrated promise in CNS tumors, as in other cancers; however, their role in standard treatment remains to be established. In 2008, the FDA gave accelerated approval status to bevacizumab (a monoclonal antibody) for recurrent glioblastoma based on an uncontrolled randomized phase 2 trial, although final approval is pending subsequent phase 3 trials, and its approval status can be reversed if these trials are not positive. At the time of this writing, it is not clear whether bevacizumab will remain FDA approved.

Aside from bevacizumab, the only approved agents for malignant glioma are the cytotoxic agents (temozolomide and the nitrosoureas). There are no FDA-approved drugs for adult low-grade glioma, but nitrosoureas and temozolomide are frequently used off-label. There is one approved agent (everolimus or RAD-001) for a rare pediatric low-grade glioma called subependymal giant cell astrocytoma (SEGA). There are no approved agents for primitive neuroectodermal tumors (PNETs) or medulloblastomas, although by consensus and based on phase 3 studies, children with newly diagnosed PNET and high-grade glioma typically receive adjuvant chemotherapy, most commonly using multiple agents with or without nitrosoureas or temozolomide. Chemotherapy is also frequently used in ependymoma, although in general it has not proven to be effective. This chapter highlights major clinical issues surrounding the use of cytotoxic chemotherapy in CNS tumors and briefly describes the types of commonly used drugs, including the FDA-approved agents (**Table 19.1**) and several other classes that are frequently used in the "off-label" setting. A description of newer molecularly targeted agents (monoclonal antibody and small molecular tyrosine kinase inhibitors) is presented in Chapter 22; these agents are not discussed here.

Goals and Structure of Clinical Trials

One goal of clinical trials is to measure response to therapy. Response may be an assessment of drug toxicity or some direct or surrogate measure of antitumor efficacy. Phase 1 studies are done to establish a maximum tolerable drug dose as well as describe pharmacokinetic aspects of the drug in

Table 19.1 Chemotherapy Agents Approved by the U.S. Food and Drug Administration for Central Nervous System Tumors

Drug	Class	Indication
Lomustine	Nitrosoureas	• 1970s: newly diagnosed GBM and recurrent glioma
Polifeprosan 20 with carmustine implant	Nitrosoureas	• 1997: newly diagnosed GBM and recurrent glioma
Temozolomide	Methylating agent	• 1999: recurrent grade 3 astrocytoma • 2005: newly diagnosed GBM
Bevacizumab	Monoclonal Ab to VEGF	• 2008: recurrent GBM
Everolimus	mTOR inhibitor	• 2010: subependymal giant cell astrocytoma

Abbreviations: GBM, glioblastoma multiforme; mTOR, mammalian target of rapamycin; VEGF, vascular endothelial growth factor.

Pearl

- Phase 1 trials that test cytostatic or biological therapies with minimal or no expected toxicity may require the use of surrogate biological or pharmacological end points.

---

question. A specific goal is to establish a favorable starting dose for later phase 2 trials based on the maximum toxicity and pharmacokinetics of the drug. Thus these studies emphasize toxicity as an important treatment end point. In most cases, patients enter into these trials having previously failed standard treatment regimens or prior phase 2 or 3 studies.

Because a treatment benefit is not the primary goal of these early phase 1 studies, they may present an ethical challenge to the physician treating the patient and a difficult dilemma for the patients and their families. Often these patients are desperate for any treatment and may not recognize the true intent of the study and the risks associated with drug escalation schemas. Patients who enroll early in the studies will probably have little chance of any potential therapeutic benefit because of the very low initial starting doses. Traditional phase 1 studies enroll small numbers of patients into each dose level in an attempt to minimize the number of patients exposed to either too low or too high a dose of the drug. As a consequence, these studies are at best an estimate of expected toxicity or therapeutic benefit.

Novel phase 1 trial strategies are being developed, such as continual reassessment method (CRM), that may allow even smaller numbers of patients to be enrolled in the lower drug dose levels and larger numbers in the likely phase 2 drug dose level. Newer agents that do not generate the traditional cytotoxic end points of myelosuppression or end-organ damage, such as cytostatic or biological agents, pose a challenge in phase 1 design and determination of study end points. Several new agents have been in phase 1 testing for long periods of time because either toxicity does not occur despite a very high drug dose, or anticipated biological end points are not reached. In these settings, the phase 2 dose is estimated based on preclinical models. Pharmacological or biologically predetermined surrogate end points are being developed to address

this problem. In a new model of early-phase testing called "phase 0," an extremely low dose of an investigational drug is administered purely for the purpose of determining a pharmacodynamic end point, including specific interaction with a known molecular target such as a tumor-specific cell surface receptor.[1] Evaluation of therapeutic efficacy or toxicity in the traditional sense is not the goal of these phase 0 studies. Few patients are needed, the risks are assumed to be very low, and long-term exposure to the agent is not typically planned so that subsequent treatment with other agents can be used in a short time interval.

Phase 2 studies apply the dosing information gathered from phase 1 trials and attempt to measure response to the agent in a larger group of patients. Ideally, patients who enter into these trials will be homogeneous relative to important prognostic clinical factors such as age, performance status, and tumor histology. Unfortunately, many phase 2 trials treat small sample sizes of only 30 to 50 patients, and response is estimated based on a best- or worst-case response scenario without tight confidence intervals around the observed end point. In some studies a drug is deemed worthy of further phase 2 or 3 testing if an "observed" response rate of 20 to 30% is seen. The "true" response rate may be greater or less than the observed response rate because of the limited number of patients available for assessment of response. In addition, patient selection factors may significantly influence this early look at observed response. Younger, healthier patients with good performance status are often overrepresented in these trials because of investigator or patient bias.

When larger cohort, less-selective patient entry occurs in later phase 2 or 3 trials, the "true" response rate will often be significantly less than that observed in early pilot phase 2 testing. One way to mitigate this bias is to conduct a randomized phase 2 trial comparing patients treated with the investiga-

---

Controversy

- A treatment benefit is not the specific goal of phase 1 research trials and may pose an ethical challenge for physicians who conduct these studies.

tional agent to a matched control group treated concurrently with the standard of care. The sample size needed for a randomized phase 2 trial is smaller than that needed for a more definitive phase 3 study and inadequately powered to prove superior efficacy. Thus, although there is a strong tendency to assume the best arm in these smaller phase 2 trials should become the new standard of care, a subsequent phase 3 trial still must be conducted. Another new strategy for phase 2 trials called adaptive randomization uses data gathered from patients treated early in the trial to inform decision making for subsequent patients as the trial proceeds. With this iterative approach, several hypotheses can be tested within the context of a single study, using multiple agents or combinations of drugs. As with the continual reassessment method for earlier phase studies, adaptive randomization requires real-time statistical analysis as the trial proceeds, rather than after the trial ends.

If an investigational agent shows promise in phase 2 trials, a phase 3 study is often considered to be the definitive next step for drug development. The hallmark of phase 3 trials is randomized comparison of the new agent with the standard treatment. Where a standard does not exist, a placebo-controlled, double-blind study is preferable to an open-label study. Randomization must successfully balance patient selection factors in both arms of a phase 3 trial in order to minimize bias that may influence the final results. Intention-to-treat analysis is critical because patients will often opt out of standard treatment or observation-only arms following randomization, particularly if the standard therapy is perceived as inadequate and early phase 2 data are published demonstrating promise in the new agent. Intention-to-treat analysis avoids the misleading effects of patient dropout and crossover by analyzing results based on initial treatment assignment rather than treatment actually received.

■ Assessment of Response to Chemotherapeutic Drugs

The major goal of phase 2 and phase 3 clinical trials using chemotherapy is to measure the antitumor response of a treatment. The end point in phase 3 studies is typically survival time, whereas antitumor response in phase 2 is usually assessed using magnetic resonance imaging (MRI). Other end points for response could include progression-free survival, duration of objective response, median time to tumor pro-

gression, improvement in patient-reported symptoms, overall change in quality of life, or pharmacodynamic end points such as modulation of a known tumor-specific molecular target. Correlation between these surrogate end points and overall survival requires confirmation in subsequent phase 3 trials.

Objective assessment of tumor response is difficult because the actual extent of a tumor is not always clear on MRI, either in the setting of newly diagnosed disease or in disease subjected to treatment. This is particularly true following high-dose radiation therapy such as interstitial brachytherapy or radiosurgery. It may also be true following various forms of systemic high-dose chemotherapy or surgically implanted polymer-based chemotherapy placed directly into surgically created cavities or directly into tumor. Contrast-enhanced T1 and the various T2 MRI sequences are only indirect measures of tumor location or overall tumor burden and are neither specific nor sensitive enough for the investigator to be 100% confident that a positive biological change seen after treatment is caused by that treatment. Fortunately, most MRI measures of assessment are at least adequate enough to provide reasonable assurance that the extremes of a very bad or very good response to investigational treatment are measurable.[2] Newer MRI sequences or nuclear imaging may overcome some of the difficulties surrounding standard MRI sequence based assessment, but until they are validated, standard MRI is the imaging of choice for assessment of response. Section II of this book describes these newer imaging modalities as they relate to end point determination, as well as new consensus approaches to assessment of response and progression.

Currently, response to treatment is often arbitrarily defined by the degree of reduction in tumor volume, with 50% or greater reduction usually signifying response. However, limiting the definition of response to large changes in tumor volume risks deeming a chemotherapy drug inadequate or not worthy of further investigation when in fact it has antitumor activity. Alternative measures of treatment success or failure that depend somewhat less on imaging nuances include time-dependent patient variables, such as the interval of clinically stable disease or overall survival. Death, defined as disease-specific or treatment-related, is the least controversial measure of a treatment effect. Progression-free survival is more problematic because a robust clinical and imaging methodology is required to determine when tumor progression occurs. The diagnosis of progression may be biased simply by the interval of MRI scanning as well as the specific definition of clinical and radiographic progression. Some clinical trials require a certain volume change to declare treatment failure, yet few malignant gliomas are well-circumscribed lesions that are easily measured, even with sophisticated volumetric software systems. Until specific, reliable neuroimaging tools are verified, the assessment of response to treatment will have some degree of subjectivity.

A final caveat in clinical trials of systemic chemotherapy is the now well-studied observation that patients with brain tumors demonstrate unique drug metabolism, primarily due to the concurrent use of steroids and anticonvulsant medications. These drugs may alter hepatic metabolism through various pathways, including via cytochrome P-450, such that standard dosing based on experience in other cancers will often be inadequate. Several phase 2 studies in malignant glioma have had to revert to a phase 1 study design because the expected dose based on results in other cancers did not produce significant or anticipated toxicity in patients with malignant glioma. For example, phase 2 studies of irinotecan were conducted in patients with malignant glioma using the phase 2 dose established in colon cancer patients, and minimal activity and toxicity were noted because the standard use of anticonvulsant medications altered drug metabolism. A subsequent phase 1 trial determined that the recommended phase 2 dose for patients with glioma was more than twice the dose expected for colon cancer patients.[3]

The same experience has been noted with the use of paclitaxel, erlotinib, and several other investigational agents. Detailed pharmacokinetic studies confirmed the altered metabolism, typically with more rapid clearance rates seen for patients on enzyme-inducing anticonvulsants. The converse may also be true; drug interactions may dangerously increase the serum level of drugs used in clinical trials. Newer pharmacogenomic assessment of patient-specific genome-based alterations in metabolic pathways is currently being used in some drug studies and may minimize risks for the rare patient with those alterations. For instance, identifying variations in UGT1A1 genotypes can be used to individually tailor irinotecan dosing. These examples of variables related to drug metabolism raise the concern that previous studies using a pharmacologically inadequate (or excessive) dose could have resulted in a potentially active drug being abandoned for further testing. Most phase 1 and many phase 2 clinical trials now account for these potential metabolic pathway differences and require pharmacokinetic or pharmacogenomic testing.

■ The Role of Chemotherapy in a Multimodality Approach

A multimodality approach that includes surgery, radiation therapy, and chemotherapy is the most common strategy used to treat patients with malignant gliomas. In most cases, a drug or drug combination is used with radiation (concurrent) or as an adjuvant to (following) radiation, or both. Unless adequate patient controls exist in the context of a clinical trial, it is often impossible to know with certainty whether concurrent or adjuvant chemotherapy provides added benefit for an individual patient. During the interval of what appears to be radiographically stable disease, it is possible that adjuvant chemotherapy may only be adding to patient toxicity and not to tumor cell kill. As described earlier, because of the nonspecificity of MRI, actual tumor progression may occur with minimal change in the appearance of the MRI scan until more dramatic increases in tumor burden are finally unambiguous on imaging. This phenomenon is particularly relevant following maximal surgical resection when no apparent residual disease is seen on MRI. It is also virtually impossible to assess response to chemotherapy when the tumor type has a very slow growth potential, such as low-grade glioma. These patients normally have a prolonged disease-free interval following initial treatment that is measured in years. The tumor burden is actually reflected by total cell loss as opposed to cell gain. Tumor cell turnover rates may be so slow that changes in the radiographic appearance of the lesion may take years to manifest.

Phase 3 trials done in the 1960s and early 1970s appeared to demonstrate a survival benefit for patients with malignant astrocytoma when chemotherapy was added as an adjuvant to surgery and radiation therapy.[4] However, when patient variables that are known to be predictive for survival are accounted for, such as age, performance status, and extent of resection (biopsy vs resection), the survival impact of chemotherapy becomes less pronounced, particularly in some patient groups.[5] For instance, older patients with glioblastoma multiforme who are neurologically impaired and only undergo a surgical biopsy will derive no survival benefit from the addition of chemotherapy in a multimodality approach. Conversely, younger, healthier patients with lower grade tumors appear to have a greater survival benefit with the use of adjuvant chemotherapy. This perceived benefit, however, may be confounded by the favorable biological behavior of tumors in younger patients. Unfortunately, the numbers of patients enrolled in these older studies were inadequate to confidently evaluate the survival benefit of chemotherapy for smaller subgroups.

More recent phase 3 studies do account for these subgroups by prospective stratification with sample sizes sufficient to resolve any differences in patient selection factors that could favorably or unfavorably bias the study. The influential phase 3 study in glioblastoma of radiation alone versus radiation plus temozolomide, for instance, did show a survival benefit of temozolomide in all patient subgroups that were treated.[6] Older patients were excluded from that trial, however, and the benefit of chemotherapy in the older population remains unproven. A survival benefit from the addition of chemotherapy to radiotherapy has also not been proven in grade 2 or grade 3 astrocytic tumors, with the exception of patients with anaplastic oligodendroglioma who have co-deletion of chromosome 1p and 19q. These patients do show a survival benefit when combined modality treatment is used. Predictive biomarkers (those that predict a response to a particular therapy) unfortunately are still rare in these diseases, whereas prognostic biomarkers (those that predict survival) are more common. Currently agreed upon prognostic biomarkers include the recently described mutations in the *IDH-1* gene, promoter methylation of the *MGMT* gene, and chromosome deletions found in some types of oligodendroglioma. Prognostic biomarkers must be accounted for in the design of large phase 3 studies, and should be addressed in smaller phase 2 trials as well.

Chemotherapeutic Drug Delivery

Chemotherapy may be given systemically by enteral or intravenous delivery, or directly by intra-arterial injection, placement into a tumor cavity, or interstitial delivery into the tumor. Chapter 21 describes the various drug delivery options in more detail. An important limitation of systemic drug delivery is the blood–brain barrier, which excludes large-molecule, water-soluble agents from entry into the brain substance.[7]

The blood–brain barrier is a network of tight junctions between endothelial cells. Molecules larger than approximately 40 kd are unlikely to penetrate the intact barrier, and drugs with low lipid solubility and tight protein binding also have limited drug delivery. The blood–brain barrier is often altered in the setting of malignant glioma, particularly in regions that include the contrast-enhancing tumor volume. Although these areas of altered blood–brain barrier do allow entrance of some drugs that may not normally gain access to the tumor bed, the concentration of these drugs may not be adequate for efficient tumor cell kill. Moreover, in this altered blood–brain or blood–tumor environment, tumor cells will infiltrate regions of brain adjacent to the dominant tumor volume, and these

Special Consideration

- An important limitation of systemic drug delivery is the blood–brain barrier.

tumor cells are largely protected by an intact blood–brain barrier. Intra-arterial, intracavitary, and interstitial drug delivery strategies are used in an attempt to circumvent this limitation to systemic chemotherapy and increase drug concentrations to the entire tumor. Although progress has been made in the development of these techniques, much more work is needed to achieve this goal.

Basic Principles of Chemotherapy

Numerous types of cytotoxic chemotherapy agents are used to treat patients with brain tumors. These include alkylating and methylating agents, antimetabolites, topoisomerase inhibitors, and taxanes, to name a few classes of drugs. Newer small-molecule agents are also being studied (see Chapter 22). Drugs may be used as single agents or in combination. Very few drug combinations have thus far proved to be effective for treatment of patients with CNS tumors. One prominent exception is the combination of procarbazine, chloroethylcyclohexylnitrosourea (CCNU; lomustine), and vincristine (PCV) for anaplastic oligodendroglioma tumors that are 1p19q codeleted. Often, the decision to use combinations of drugs is based on knowledge of different mechanisms of action of each drug and nonoverlapping toxicity. In the past the decision to use these drugs in combination was largely empirical rather than the consequence of scientific results from in vitro or in vivo models.

Most drugs used in clinical trials now are subject to intense laboratory research evaluation prior to clinical testing. Potential new drugs are initially screened in standard human tumor cell lines using in vitro systems.[8] Active agents then go on to in vivo testing in animals, usually inserted into the flank (subcutaneously) or brain (orthotopically) of an athymic nude mouse model bearing human tumors of interest. Drugs known to be active in vivo are then tested further in more formal toxicity and pharmacology studies. An understanding of the toxicity and pharmacokinetics of the drug, as well as its cellular mechanism of action, is now a minimum requirement of animal testing that must be met prior to human testing. It is only after this preclinical testing that phase 1 studies are undertaken in healthy human volunteers or patients with recurrent tumors. With careful laboratory investigations and some knowledge of mechanisms of action, phase 1 and phase 2 studies can be more rationally designed. Although an improvement over past approaches, further research is needed to establish more effective screening models to test cytotoxic as well as biological or cytostatic agents.

Resistance to Chemotherapeutic Drugs

Unfortunately, many drugs that are effective in the laboratory are not effective in patients. One of the many problems seen with the use of systemic chemotherapy (in addition to drug delivery and metabolism, as previously mentioned) is the problem of intrinsic or acquired resistance.[9] Genetic, epigenetic, kinetic, and local host factor-mediated events are mechanisms of resistance that may occur, altering resistance or sensitivity to chemotherapy drugs. An example of resistance mediated by a local host factor is the observation that relatively hypoxic or nutrient-deprived tumor cells have a decreased capacity to enter chemosensitive periods of the cell cycle. As the tumor grows, it may become increasingly hypoxic, with a decreased growth rate. Thus, chemotherapy drugs that normally have a greater cytotoxic effect during the S phase of the cell cycle will not be as active if the tumor cell remains in phase G_0.

As tumor cells mutate over time, genetic instability may also occur and ultimately cause a change in the sensitivity of the tumor cells to drugs that were once effective. These changes may be due to several factors, including changes in protein synthesis and repair processes. Tumor cells may overcome the effects of drug therapy by various mechanisms of repair of DNA damage. The alkylating agents, for instance, produce some of their antitumor effects through the formation of crosslinks with DNA at the O6 or N7 positions on guanine. As a consequence of these crosslinks, DNA replication is halted and tumor cells die. Repair of this damage is possible via O6-alkylguanine-DNA alkyltransferase (O6-AGAT), a repair protein found in normal cells as well as in many human brain tumors.[10] Thus, the tumor has a mechanism to repair DNA

damage produced by various alkylating agents. The more repair protein present, the less likely it is that the alkylating agent will cause cell death. Other specific mechanisms of resistance exist, such as p-glycoprotein, an energy-dependent efflux pump, and other enzyme systems such as glutathione, glutathione S-transferase, metallothionein, and aldehyde dehydrogenase. All of these may be implicated in the accelerated degradation of chemotherapy agents. Modulation of these mechanisms of resistance is an area of intense research.

Chemotherapeutic Drugs

Nitrosoureas

The nitrosoureas are bifunctional alkylating agents that were previously the most widely used drugs for patients with brain tumors. In recent years, a methylating agent temozolomide has become more frequently used as initial treatment (described later). The nitrosoureas alkylate DNA in multiple locations, primarily on guanine but also on adenine and cytosine, as well as carbamylate amino groups through isocyanate products.[11] The resultant DNA crosslinks produce single- or double-strand breaks, as well as depletion of glutathione, causing inhibition of DNA repair and RNA synthesis. The most commonly used nitrosoureas are lomustine (CCNU), an oral agent, and carmustine (bischloroethylnitrosourea [BCNU]), an intravenous agent. Both of these drugs are lipid soluble. A third nitrosourea, nimustine (3-[(4-amino-2-methyl-5-pyrimidinyl)methyl]-1-(2-chloroethyl)-1-nitrosourea hydrochloride) ; ACNU), is used commonly in Europe and Japan. It is unique in that it is water soluble and has been used both systemically and intraventricularly.

Bischloroethylnitrosourea can now be delivered in the form of a biodegradable wafer called polifeprosan 20 (Gliadel, MGI Pharma, Inc., Bloomington, MN); FDA approval was given for the use of polifeprosan 20 in both newly diagnosed glioblastoma multiforme and recurrent malignant glioma based on phase 3 studies.[12,13] In one of the phase 3 studies, patients with newly diagnosed malignant glioma (grade 3 and grade 4 tumors) were randomized to receive the biodegradable wafer with BCNU or a placebo wafer at the time of initial surgical resection. All patients were then treated with radiation. The group treated with the BCNU wafer had a slight but statistically significant improvement in survival (13.9 months) compared with the placebo groups (11.6 months). A similar placebo-controlled phase 3 study in recurrent malignant glioma also showed a slight survival increase (8 weeks).

All of the nitrosoureas have the dose-limiting side effect of prolonged myelosuppression, and also cause nausea and emesis. Pulmonary fibrosis may occur with prolonged, high-dose exposure. The drugs are used as single agents or in combination with other drugs, such as vincristine, procarbazine, and the platinum drugs. High-dose chemotherapy regimens have also been tested using the nitrosoureas in the setting of autologous bone marrow or peripheral stem cell transplants. Both ACNU and BCNU have been used as intra-arterial agents, but prospective trials have largely been negative with this delivery strategy. BCNU is most commonly used as adjuvant chemotherapy following radiation therapy, but may also be given during radiation in an effort to induce radiosensitization. However, it is unlikely to have this impact when given at intervals of 6 weeks, as it is currently used. The nitrosoureas have activity in the treatment of glioblastoma multiforme, anaplastic gliomas (including oligodendroglioma and mixed tumors), medulloblastomas, and other PNETs, as well as various low-grade gliomas. They have minor activity against ependymoma.

Temozolomide, Procarbazine, and Dacarbazine

Temozolomide, procarbazine, and dacarbazine [(dimethyltriazeno)imidazole carboxamide (DTIC)] are methylating agents. They are also sometimes considered alkylating agents. They produce cytotoxicity by causing single-strand breaks in tumor cell DNA.

Temozolomide (Temodar; Schering-Plough, Kenilworth, NJ) has become the most commonly used chemotherapy agent for high-grade glioma and has received FDA approval for both recurrent anaplastic astrocytoma and newly diagnosed glioblastoma multiforme.[6,14] Temozolomide is an imidazotetrazine derivative of DTIC. It has good oral bioavailability with minimal myelotoxicity. It has been shown to produce objective responses in the setting of newly diagnosed and recurrent malignant tumors. A single-arm phase 2 study in grade 3 anaplastic astrocytoma patients at the time of first tumor progression resulted in a high objective response rate (8% complete response, 27% partial response) with prolonged progression-free survival (46%) at 6 months.[14] The results in recurrent glioblastoma were more modest, with only a 5% complete response rate and 6-month progression-free survival rate of 21%.[15] As a consequence of these initial studies, temozolomide became the first oral agent approved for use in recurrent anaplastic glioma in this country in many decades. Additional successful phase 2 and phase 3 testing of this agent in newly diagnosed glioblastoma has resulted in FDA approval of temozolomide in this patient population as well. Temozolomide has been used in combination with many agents now, including BCNU, irinotecan, thalidomide, erlotinib, imatinib, gefitinib, cis-retinoic acid, and other drugs, and is also being extensively studied in low-grade gliomas. Side effects include modest myelosuppression, nausea, constipation, and fatigue.

Procarbazine is a water-soluble alkylating agent that is nonspecific to cell cycle. It is a methylhydrazine derivative and appears to inhibit DNA, RNA, and protein synthesis. Procarbazine is readily absorbable by mouth and is given as a daily drug for 2 to 3 weeks. The major toxicity includes myelosuppression, nausea, fatigue, and rash. It is also a monoamine oxidase inhibitor and can interact with drugs and food that contain tyramine, causing hypertension and neurotoxic effects such as agitation and hallucinations. Although it can be used as a single agent, it is most commonly used in combination with other chemotherapy drugs, such as in the combination of procarbazine, CCNU, and vincristine (the PCV regimen). It is active against a wide variety of CNS tumors, including glioblastoma multiforme, anaplastic gliomas, medulloblastomas, and other PNETs, primary CNS lymphoma, and various low-grade gliomas.

Dacarbazine (DTIC) is metabolized by the liver to MTIC [5-(3-methyl-1-triazeno)imidazole-4-carboxamide], which can inhibit nucleoside incorporation.[16] Toxicity includes myelosuppression, nausea and emesis, and rare cases of hepatic vein thrombosis. It is not routinely used as a single agent. It has been used in combination with the nitrosoureas in the treatment of malignant gliomas and low-grade glioma.

Platinum Compounds

Carboplatin and cisplatin produce DNA toxicity via chelation and the formation of intrastrand DNA crosslinks.[17] These are water-soluble alkylating agents that are given via intravenous or intra-arterial routes. Penetration into the brain is significantly limited by an intact blood–brain barrier; however, in the setting of a malignant glioma, the blood–brain barrier is at least partially disrupted, accounting for the modest objective responses seen with this group of drugs. Cisplatin is usually given in combination with other chemotherapy drugs, often with BCNU and other alkylating agents, particularly in childhood tumors. Its major dose-limiting toxicity is renal failure, and it can also produce hearing loss and peripheral neuropathy. Little to no myelosuppression occurs, making this an attractive drug to use with myelosuppressive drugs. Carboplatin can be used as a single agent or in combination with other agents. It is often used in high-dose chemotherapy regimens with stem cell support. Its major dose-limiting toxicity is myelosuppression as well as nausea and emesis. Allergic reactions to carboplatin and cisplatin are possible. These drugs are occasionally used in the treatment of glioblastoma multiforme and anaplastic gliomas, and more frequently in medulloblastomas and other PNETs, ependymomas, and germ cell tumors.

Vinca Alkaloids and Epipodophyllotoxins

The vinca alkaloids, vincristine and vinblastine, act on tubulin, the basic subunit of microtubules.[18] They inhibit microtubule assembly by depolymerization, ultimately producing mitotic arrest. They do affect nonproliferating cells in the G_1 phase of the cell cycle; however, cells appear to be most sensitive when in the S phase. Resistance to these agents is at least partially due to the multidrug resistance (MDR) phenotype mediated by the P-170 membrane glycoprotein efflux pump.[19] Although vinblastine is infrequently used in the management of CNS tumors, vincristine is widely used, particularly in pediatric tumors such as PNET, medulloblastoma, and low-grade glial tumors of childhood. Vincristine causes neurologic toxicity, particularly peripheral neuropathy, which can be dose limiting. The peripheral neuropathy initially manifests as symmetrical sensory impairment and can eventually lead to motor weakness. Constipation may also occur as a consequence of its effect on autonomic function; severe toxicity can include paralytic ileus and urinary retention. The only route of drug delivery is intravenous. The drug is a vesicant and can cause tissue necrosis if extravasation occurs during treatment. Vincristine is rarely used as a single agent. It is given in combination with CCNU and procarbazine as part of the PCV regimen, and in combination with carboplatin for low-grade glioma. It is also used in combination for the treatment of medulloblastoma and PNET.

The epipodophyllotoxins, such as etoposide, cause an irreversible blockade of cells in the premitotic phases of the cell cycle, leading to accumulation of cells in late G_2 or S phase.[20] The inhibitory effects appear to be a consequence of the interaction of these agents with the topoisomerase II enzyme, with stabilization of the cleavage enzyme–DNA complex. Single-strand DNA breaks occur, and cell death. The most commonly used topoisomerase II inhibitor in CNS tumors is etoposide. Etoposide may be given either intravenously or by oral administration. The major toxicity is myelosuppression, which can be dose limiting. Nausea and emesis may occur. Rarely used as a single agent, it is commonly given in combination with drugs such as cisplatinum, carboplatin, ifosfamide, and vincristine. It is frequently used in pediatric brain tumor patients to treat malignant gliomas, medulloblastomas and other PNETs, ependymomas, and low-grade gliomas.

Taxanes

The taxanes affect microtubule assembly by stabilization of microtubule dynamics.[21] Two taxanes are commercially available: paclitaxel (Taxol, Bristol-Meyers Squibb, New York, NY) and docetaxel (Taxotere, Sanofi-Aventis, Bridgewater, NJ). They bind to the b-subunit on the microtubule and produce polymerization. Inhibition of depolymerization ultimately causes a mitotic block and, most likely, apoptotic cell death. The taxanes are given by intravenous injection, and various schedules have been evaluated. Myelosuppression, alopecia, neurotoxicity, cardiac arrhythmia, and hypersensitivity reactions are reported toxicities. Hypersensitivity may be related to the vehicle used to solubilize the drug Cremophor, and is largely prevented by premedication with dexamethasone, diphenhydramine, and histamine H_2 antagonists such as cimetidine. Paclitaxel and docetaxel have been used as single agents for malignant glioma and have also been evaluated as radiosensitizers. Hepatic cytochrome P-450 mixed-function oxidases are important in the metabolism of paclitaxel and must be considered for patients who are using enzyme-inducing drugs such as anticonvulsant medications.

Topoisomerase I Inhibitors

As mentioned above, topoisomerase is a critical enzyme in cellular growth regulation. Inhibition of this enzyme system can lead to DNA strand breaks. Etoposide inhibits topoisomerase II; the camptothecins inhibit topoisomerase I. Camptothecin, the first topoisomerase I inhibitor, was found to be highly toxic.[22] Various other inhibitors of topoisomerase I were subsequently developed, including topotecan, 9-amino-camptothecin (9AC), and irinotecan (Camptosar, CPT-11; Pfizer Inc., New York, NY). Topotecan and irinotecan are semisynthetic derivatives of camptothecin with less toxicity and greater activity in vitro and in vivo against several glioma cell lines. Topoisomerase I functions normally during DNA replication to cause transient breaks in the single strand of DNA, releasing the torsional strain caused by synthesis of a new strand of DNA or RNA around a double helix.[23] Topotecan and irinotecan target this topo I-DNA complex, stabilizing it and inhibiting reannealing of the parent DNA. Ultimately, double-strand DNA breaks occur when the advancing replication fork collides with the camptothecin-topo I-DNA complex. Both drugs are given intravenously in various schedules. The dose-limiting toxicity of irinotecan is diarrhea; myelosuppression may occur with topotecan. Significant modulation of the pharmacokinetics of irinotecan occurs when used in combination with enzyme-inducing anticonvulsants, which must be taken into account when prescribing this drug. These drugs have modest activity when used as single agents.[24] Topotecan has also undergone testing as a radiation sensitizer.[25] Their spectrum of activity awaits further clinical research, primarily in combination strategies.

New Chemotherapeutic Drugs

It is clear that newer systemic agents need to be tested. Unfortunately, the literature is full of negative studies. Better understanding of the molecular biology of tumor cells and their environment, along with better model systems, however, give promise to the many new agents now in preclinical and early clinical testing.

To illustrate the difficulty of research in this area, one example of an approach that turned out to be negative was the use of an agent to modify resistance to the nitrosoureas and temozolomide, the only FDA-approved cytotoxic drugs. As discussed earlier, one of the DNA repair enzymes, O^6-AGAT, mediates the repair of the alkylation products of nitrosoureas.[10] Inhibition of this repair protein was the subject of several clinical trials using O^6-benzylguanine, a methylating agent.[26] This drug is nontoxic even in very high doses and had been tested in phase 1 and phase 2 trials in combination with BCNU and temozolomide. The hope was that O^6-benzylguanine would enhance BCNU or temozolomide cytotoxicity and potentially allow a reduction of the dose of either agent needed for therapy. In the initial studies, O^6-benzylguanine was given to patients with malignant gliomas prior to surgical resection.[27] The dose that was found to completely inhibit the repair enzyme most effectively, as measured in the removed tumor tissue, was used in combination with BCNU or temozolomide. More than 70% of tumors have high levels of O^6-AGAT, and thus any strategy that inhibits this protein should have been helpful in increasing response rates to BCNU or temozolomide chemotherapy. One early report did suggest some modest activity of the combination in nitrosourea-resistant tumors.[28] Unfortunately, because the drug also causes enhanced toxicity to bone marrow, the final dose of the active agent (BCNU or temozolomide) had to be reduced so much that tumor efficacy was impacted negatively, and this strategy is rarely or no longer used.

In addition to serving as potential drug targets, DNA repair mechanisms may serve as biomarkers of potential clinical benefit. In terms of temozolomide chemotherapy, preliminary evidence suggested that levels of O^6-methylguanine-DNA methyltransferase (MGMT) would predict benefit from this agent.[29] High levels of MGMT in tumor cells confirms resistance to temozolomide; conversely, low levels may predict susceptibility to the drug. MGMT activity may be silenced at the gene level by methylation of the gene promoter, which can now be measured. Many recent studies have suggested that MGMT promoter methylation status is a predictive biomarker for temozolomide sensitivity as well as a stronger prognostic biomarker for longer survival. Modern clinical trials use MGMT expression, or its methylation status, as a selection factor for patients who are otherwise candidates for temozolomide treatment.

Other new treatment strategies include the use of drugs that inhibit or modify cellular growth and proliferation, apoptosis, angiogenesis, or invasion (described in detail in Chapter 22). These include specific molecularly targeted drugs or multitargeted agents. Cellular targets of interest include various cell surface regulating growth factors and angiogenic protein kinases, transcription factors, proapoptotic pathways, and regulatory components of the immune system. New therapeutic chemotherapy strategies are being developed using monoclonal antibodies or small-molecule tyrosine-kinase inhibitors. Specific inhibitors of substrates regulated by polyamine biosynthesis, or inhibition or blockage of cell surface receptors, such as the wild-type or mutant epidermal growth factor

receptor, platelet-derived growth factor, and the vascular endothelial growth factor and its receptor, are being studied. Alteration of cell signaling is also an important arena of research using newer agents that target various pathways, including the phosphatidylinositol 3-kinase (PI3K) and Akt pathways, and the mitogen-activated protein kinase and farnesyltransferase pathways. Because of the complexity of tumor cell biology, it is likely that combination approaches will ultimately be required. Each of these strategies is appropriate for clinical research and, it is hoped, will soon become part of standard therapy for patients with brain tumors.

Editor's Note

Chemotherapy continues to be a very challenging area for the treatment of gliomas in particular. Most of the progress has been made with the introduction of temozolomide, which has largely replacement the alkylating agents such as BCNU and CCNU. Although there are many drugs evaluated through phase 1 and phase 2 clinical trials most of these studies are done in small groups of patients, and typically only a small benefit is seen with any of these agents administered alone. This is especially true in neuro-oncology since temozolomide was the last chemotherapy agent approved by the FDA for brain tumors in the recurrent as well as the newly diagnosed setting. The only other agents to gain approval are targeted therapies such as bevacizumab and everolimus for recurrent glioblastoma and subependymal giant cell astrocytoma, respectively.

Currently when patients demonstrate methylation of the MGMT promoter region, and, they are given Temodar, there is a 46% chance of a 2-year survival and a 10 to 15% chance of a survival greater than 5 years, which is a significant improvement since the BCNU era. It appears that Temodar given concomitantly with radiation followed by Temodar chemotherapy will be the platform for which all other agents will be judged in a phase 3 setting. It is hoped that some of the other targeted therapies will demonstrate efficacy in phase 1 and phase 2 studies, enabling them onto be added on the Temodar platform for future therapies. (Berger)

References

1. Hunsberger S, Rubinstein LV, Dancey J, Korn EL. Dose escalation trial designs based on a molecularly targeted endpoint. Stat Med 2005; 24:2171–2181
2. Galanis E, Buckner JC, Maurer MJ, et al. Validation of neuroradiologic response assessment in gliomas: measurement by RECIST, two-dimensional, computer-assisted tumor area, and computer-assisted tumor volume methods. Neuro-oncol 2006;8:156–165
3. Prados MD, Yung WKA, Jaeckle KA, et al; North American Brain Tumor Consortium study. Phase 1 trial of irinotecan (CPT-11) in patients with recurrent malignant glioma: a North American Brain Tumor Consortium study. Neuro-oncol 2004;6:44–54
4. Fine HA, Dear KB, Loeffler JS, Black PM, Canellos GP. Meta-analysis of radiation therapy with and without adjuvant chemotherapy for malignant gliomas in adults. Cancer 1993;71:2585–2597

5. Curran WJ Jr, Scott CB, Horton J, et al. Recursive partitioning analysis in three Radiation Therapy Oncology Group malignant glioma trials. J Natl Cancer Inst 1993;85:704–710

6. Stupp R, Mason WP, van den Bent MJ, et al; European Organisation for Research and Treatment of Cancer Brain Tumor and Radiotherapy Groups; National Cancer Institute of Canada Clinical Trials Group. Radiotherapy plus concomitant and adjuvant temozolomide for glioblastoma. N Engl J Med 2005;352:987–996

7. Greig NH. Optimizing drug delivery to brain tumors. Cancer Treat Rev 1987;14:1–28

8. Boyd MR. Status of the NCI preclinical antitumor drug discovery screen. Principles and Practice of Oncology Updates 1989;3:1–12

9. Phillips PC. Antineoplastic drug resistance in brain tumors. Neurol Clin 1991;9:383–404

10. Wiestler O, Kleihues P, Pegg AE. O6-alkylguanine-DNA alkyltransferase activity in human brain and brain tumors. Carcinogenesis 1984;5:121–124

11. Levin VA. Pharmacokinetics and central nervous system chemotherapy. In: Hellmann K, Carter SK, eds. Fundamentals of Cancer Chemotherapy. New York: McGraw-Hill, 1986:28–40

12. Westphal M, Hilt DC, Bortey E, et al. A phase 3 trial of local chemotherapy with biodegradable carmustine (BCNU) wafers (Gliadel wafers) in patients with primary malignant glioma. Neuro-oncol 2003;5:79–88

13. Brem H, Piantadosi S, Burger PC, et al; The Polymer-brain Tumor Treatment Group. Placebo-controlled trial of safety and efficacy of intraoperative controlled delivery by biodegradable polymers of chemotherapy for recurrent gliomas. Lancet 1995;345:1008–1012

14. Yung WK, Prados MD, Yaya-Tur R, et al; Temodal Brain Tumor Group. Multicenter phase II trial of temozolomide in patients with anaplastic astrocytoma or anaplastic oligoastrocytoma at first relapse. J Clin Oncol 1999;17:2762–2771

15. Yung WK, Albright RE, Olson J, et al. A phase II study of temozolomide vs. procarbazine in patients with glioblastoma multiforme at first relapse. Br J Cancer 2000;83:588–593

16. Skibba JL, Ramirez G, Beal DD, Bryan GT. Metabolism of 4(5)-(3,3-dimethyl-1-triazeno)-imidazole-5(4)-carboxamide to 4(5)-aminoimidazole-5(4)-carboxamide in man. Biochem Pharmacol 1970;19:2043–2051

17. Heiger-Bernays WJ, Essigmann JM, Lippard SJ. Effect of the antitumor drug cis-diamminedichloroplatinum(II) and related platinum complexes on eukaryotic DNA replication. Biochemistry 1990;29:8461–8466

18. Jordan MA, Thrower D, Wilson L. Mechanism of inhibition of cell proliferation by Vinca alkaloids. Cancer Res 1991;51:2212–2222

19. Moscow JA, Cowan KH. Multidrug resistance. J Natl Cancer Inst 1988;80:14–20

20. Loike JD. VP16-213 and podophyllotoxin. A study on the relationship between chemical structure and biological activity. Cancer Chemother Pharmacol 1982;7:103–111

21. Rowinsky EK, Cazenave LA, Donehower RC. Taxol: a novel investigational antimicrotubule agent. J Natl Cancer Inst 1990;82:1247–1259

22. Potmesil M. Camptothecins: from bench research to hospital wards. Cancer Res 1994;54:1431–1439

23. Hsiang YH, Lihou MG, Liu LF. Arrest of replication forks by drug-stabilized topoisomerase I-DNA cleavable complexes as a mechanism of cell killing by camptothecin. Cancer Res 1989;49:5077–5082

24. Friedman HS, Keir ST, Houghton PJ. The emerging role of irinotecan (CPT-11) in the treatment of malignant glioma in brain tumors. Cancer 2003;97(9, Suppl):2359–2362

25. Mattern MR, Hofmann GA, McCabe FL, Johnson RK. Synergistic cell killing by ionizing radiation and topoisomerase I inhibitor topotecan (SK&F 104864). Cancer Res 1991;51:5813–5816

26. Friedman HS, Keir S, Pegg AE, et al. O6-benzylguanine-mediated enhancement of chemotherapy. Mol Cancer Ther 2002;1:943–948

27. Friedman HS, Kokkinakis DM, Pluda J, et al. Phase I trial of O6-benzylguanine for patients undergoing surgery for malignant glioma. J Clin Oncol 1998;16:3570–3575

28. Quinn JA, Pluda J, Dolan ME, et al. Phase II trial of carmustine plus O(6)-benzylguanine for patients with nitrosourea-resistant recurrent or progressive malignant glioma. J Clin Oncol 2002;20:2277–2283

29. Hegi ME, Diserens AC, Gorlia T, et al. MGMT gene silencing and benefit from temozolomide in glioblastoma. N Engl J Med 2005;352:997–1003

20 Intratumoral Chemotherapy

Kaisorn L. Chaichana, Jon D. Weingart, and Henry Brem

The infiltrative nature of malignant glioma is one of the greatest hurdles to effective therapy. These tumors are primarily a regional disease, and 80% of recurrences are within 2 cm of the initial resection field.[1] Thus, improving local disease control may significantly affect overall survival. Surgery is limited by the increased risk of removing tumor-infiltrated functional brain tissue, resulting in significant neurologic sequelae. Similarly, doses of radiation that would be optimal for tumor eradication may cause damage to the surrounding brain. Thus improving chemotherapeutic control of these tumors is necessary to improve overall survival. Physiological and pathological barriers within the central nervous system (CNS) limit the efficacy of systemic chemotherapy for brain tumors. As a result, systemic administration of antineoplastic agents by oral or intravenous routes has failed to achieve effective drug concentrations into the target site even at systemically toxic doses. A major limiting factor for adjuvant systemic therapies is the blood–brain barrier (BBB), which restricts entry of drugs into the brain.

Several approaches to improving drug delivery have been investigated (**Fig. 20.1**). This chapter focuses on the options to overcome the limitations of systemic therapy by using local delivery. The goal of these therapies is to provide sustained tumoricidal doses of drug intratumorally or peritumorally while avoiding systemic toxicity. Three systems have been utilized clinically: direct injection, convection-enhanced delivery (CED), and implantation of a drug-loaded polymeric matrix within the tumor.

■ Direct Injection

Direct injection of drug, into either the tissue or the ventricle, was one of the earliest local delivery systems. Catheter implants into the tumor cavity or ventricle, connected to an Ommaya reservoir, have been used to deliver intermittent bolus injections of both chemotherapeutic[2–4] and biological agents.[5,6] There are anecdotal case reports indicating successful outcomes using the Ommaya system or direct injection of various agents, but there have been no successful large-scale clinical trials proving their efficacy. One main limitation to these systems is poor drug distribution into solid brain or tumor tissue. With small molecules, depth of distribution with a concentration-based gradient is often limited to several millimeters, with an exponential decay in concentration from the

point source. Thus, distribution of therapeutic concentrations of drug is limited to a small volume of tissue around the injection site, often with high and sometimes toxic concentrations of drug at the point source.

Direct injection is being clinically used for the distribution of carmustine (bischloroethylnitrosourea [BCNU]) dissolved in absolute ethanol (DTI-015).[5] Preliminary studies using direct injection of viral agents have been performed with adeno associated virus containing p53 transcript or the herpes simplex virus thymidine kinase gene. Unfortunately, studies have shown good local distribution and gene expression in the injected tissue at distances of only a few millimeters.[7,8]

■ Convection-Enhanced Delivery

Convection-enhanced delivery is a drug delivery method in which macromolecules are distributed into brain parenchyma using a positive pressure gradient. Whereas diffusion uses a concentration gradient to distribute molecules, the use of a pressure gradient facilitates the distribution of a homogeneous concentration of small and large molecules over large distances by bulk displacement of the extracellular fluid with the infusate. The therapeutic agent is delivered into the parenchyma via a microcatheter inserted into the tissue with infusion rates of 0.5 to 10 µL/min. The distribution from a single point source creates an elliptical to spherical distribution with 2 to 3 cm diameter, resulting in a linear relationship between infusion volume and distribution volume. Distribution of macromolecules by CED results in a large improvement over conventional forms of drug delivery. For example, 200 µL of radiolabeled albumin injected into the brain distributes to less than a 2-mm radius into the adjacent brain tissue after 4 hours (diffusion), whereas microinfusion of the same volume of albumin results in distribution of 1.5 cm radius.[9,10]

The efficacy of CED is based on the half-life, surface characteristics, and size of the macromolecules to be delivered, as well as the delivery catheter and infusion characteristics. Convection-enhanced delivery into gray and white matter has

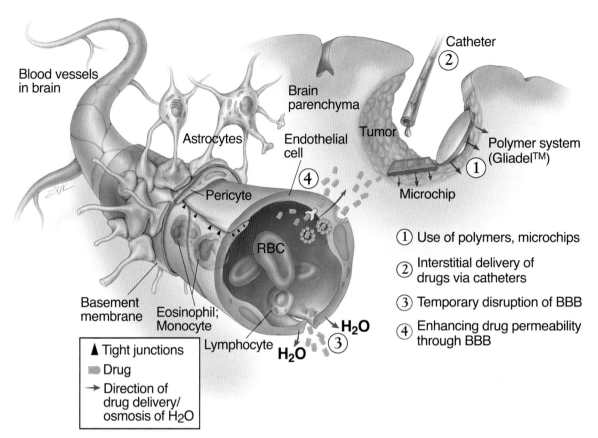

Fig. 20.1 Illustration of the main approach for drug delivery to the central nervous system. Local delivery via controlled-release enhancement of drug permeability is depicted (*4*). BBB, blood-brain barrier; RBC, red blood cells. (From Raza SM, Pradilla G, Legnani FG, et al. Local delivery of antineoplastic agents by controlled-release polymers for the treatment of malignant brain tumours. Expert Opin Biol Ther 2005;5:477–494. Illustration by I. Suk. Reprinted with permission of Informa Healthcare.)

shown reproducible distributions to a large volume of tissue with homogeneous drug concentration of macromolecules, including immunoglobulin G (IgG) (180 kd).[9,10] A key element for effective large-scale distribution of a molecule or nanoparticle is a stable half-life of the agent in the extracellular space. The distribution of lipophilic molecules such as BCNU is severely limited by transvascular export through blood vessels leading to a high efflux of drug. Other molecules may be prone to degradation from peptidases located in the extracellular space of the brain parenchyma.

Another critical determinant for distribution is the surface characteristic of the macromolecule. Binding of the agent to extracellular matrix or surface receptors may limit distribution of drug. Although binding to cell surface receptors may be overcome by saturating receptor binding, adherence to heparin sulfate proteoglycan in the extracellular matrix has limited distribution of growth factors.[11] Co-infusion of heparin or fibroblast growth factor has overcome this limitation and enables reproducible large volumes of distribution.[12]

The size of the molecule also affects volume of distribution. Initially, 180 kd was felt to be the upper limit to pass through the extracellular space. Recently, adeno-associated virus (40 nm) and liposomes (50 to 200 nm) have been distributed to large volumes of brain tissue.[13,14] Both agents, however, require modification of the surface (pegylation with liposomes and heparin co-infusion to saturate heparin sulfate proteoglycan binding with adeno-associated virus). In addition, the volume of distribution is also affected by retrograde movement of fluid along the outside of the catheter (backflow) (**Fig. 20.2**). The distance of retrograde flow along the catheter is determined by catheter diameter, infusion rate, and tissue density. The larger the diameter of the catheter, the greater the backflow along the catheter. If the retrograde flow of fluid around the catheter reaches low pressure zones (necrosis, cerebrospinal fluid [CSF] space), the fluid will inadvertently be lost into the CSF space. This leads to the accumulation of drug in the region of necrosis, or loss of drug into the intrathecal space. Finally, increasing the infusion rate can increase the overall volume of distribution; however, this will also increase the backflow distance, potentially shunting fluid away from the target volume. Parameters affecting the distribution of infusate are described in the text box below.

Although the physical parameters influencing optimal drug delivery by CED have not been finalized, the potential of ob-

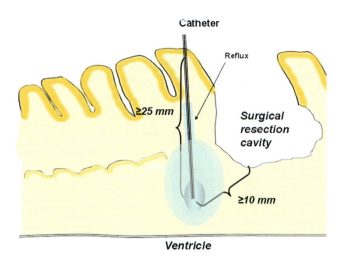

Fig. 20.2 Catheter position guidelines.

taining significantly high concentrations of a therapeutic agent over large volumes of brain tissues has led to several clinical trials in patients with neurodegenerative disorders and malignant gliomas. Therapeutic studies for malignant gliomas have focused on distributing targeted macromolecules (chimeric toxins) or currently available small-molecule drugs. A phase 1 study of CED of topotecan consisting of 16 patients established a maximum tolerable dose of 0.1 mg/mL.[15] A phase 2 study of intratumoral CED of paclitaxel showed some preliminary positive results but was associated with some

Key Convection-Enhanced Delivery Parameters Affecting Infusate Distribution

- Catheter
  - Configuration
  - Location of port
  - Size
  - Trajectory
  - Depth of positioning
- Drug
  - Surface characteristics
  - Tissue half-life
  - Size
- Target tissue
  - Microanatomy
  - Tissue density
  - Location of cerebrospinal fluid spaces
    - § Ventricles
    - § Virchow-Robin spaces
    - § Sulci
- Drug administration
  - Flow rate
    - § Presence of air bubbles

nonspecific toxicity including meningitis, infection, and transient neurologic deterioration.[16] More recently, CED of topotecan was used in two pediatric patients with diffuse intrinsic pontine gliomas, and this study demonstrated that CED was possible for brainstem tumors but that only lower infusion rates were tolerated (< 0.4 mL/h).[17] Some ongoing studies are designed to de-escalate the drug concentration.

TransMID (Transferrin-CRM107)

The first CED clinical study was of TransMID-107 (Xenova Group, Berkshire, United Kingdom), which is a thioether conjugation of human transferrin and a mutant form of diphtheria toxin known as CRM-107.[18] TransMID targets tumor cells by binding to the transferrin receptor, which is overexpressed on rapidly dividing cells. In a phase 2 multicenter, open-label, single-arm study, 44 patients received intratumoral CED of TransMID at 0.67 ng/mL.[18] The results confirmed the safety and tumor response data from the early studies. A phase 3 multicenter, randomized study in recurrent, nonresectable glioblastoma multiforme (GBM) is currently open with the best available standard treatment as the control arm.

NBI-3001 (IL4-PE)

IL4-PE (NBI-3001, Neurocrine, San Diego, California) is another recombinant toxin composed of interleukin-4 (IL-4) and a truncated form of the *Pseudomonas* exotoxin.[19] A phase 1 study of intratumoral CED of IL4-PE started at a concentration of 2 ng/mL and was dose escalated to determine the maximum tolerated dose.[20] Drug-related grade 3 or 4 CNS toxicity was seen in a total of 39% of patients in all groups, and no systemic toxicity was seen. A phase 2, multicenter, randomized study of intratumoral IL4-PE followed by tumor resection between 2 and 7 days after the completion of toxin infusion enrolled a total of 30 adult patients. The accrual was completed in 2003, but no final published results of the study were made available. There are no plans for a phase 3 study.

TP38

TP38 (TEVA, Inc., PA) is a recombinant toxin composed of transforming growth factor-α, a native epidermal growth factor receptor (EGFR) ligand, and a 38-kd fragment of the *Pseudomonas* exotoxin. TP38 binds to EGFR, and, once internalized, enzymatically arrests protein synthesis. A phase 1 study of intratumoral and peritumoral infusion of TP38 was performed in patients with recurrent malignant glioma with a concentration escalation of 0.025 to 0.1 μg/mL.[21] Two catheters were initially placed during tumor resection, and then a total volume of 40 mL was infused. The TP38 was well tolerated and a maximum tolerated dose was not established. At the completion of the study, four patients had no recurrence of tumor at 55 to 116 weeks after treatment. The overall median survival for all patients after treatment was 23 weeks.

A phase 2 multicenter randomized study was conducted in adults with recurrent GBM. Patients were randomized to two groups treated with peritumoral CED of 0.05 or 0.1 ng/mL of TP38. The total volume infused was approximately 40 mL. Postinfusion magnetic resonance imaging (MRI) changes were seen 1 to 4 months after treatment, near the site of catheter placement. These changes usually resolved by 20 weeks post-treatment. There were no grade 3 or 4 toxicities related to TP38. Further clinical trials are pending the final evaluation of the phase 2 data.

Cintredekin Besudotox (IL13-PE38)

Cintredekin besudotox is a recombinant toxin consisting of human interleukin-13 (IL-13) with the same 38-kd fragment of the *Pseudomonas* exotoxin. IL-13 receptors have been found in more than 90% of glioblastoma cells in vitro and in situ, whereas expression in the brain is not present or expressed at low levels.[22] Intratumoral and peritumoral CED of IL13-PE38 has been investigated with four separate phase 1 studies. In the largest peritumoral phase 1 study, a maximum tolerated concentration of 0.5 μg/mL was observed.[23] In this four-stage study, histological efficacy, maximum tolerated concentration, and maximum infusion time were assessed. The final stage explored the stereotactic placement of catheters after the tumor resection to improve the targeting of catheters into the peritumoral brain tissue. With the implementation of steroid guidelines, all patients tolerated the volume of infusion of 40 mL in two to three catheters. The median survival of all patients treated with peritumoral CED of IL13-PE38 ($n = 44$) was 44 weeks.[24] Catheter placement was noted to be variable in the early portion of the study, with some catheter tips placed in the ventricle or other CSF spaces.

A retrospective review of catheter placement demonstrated a correlation with survival when at least two or more catheters had been placed optimally to minimize loss of drug into the CSF compartment. The 27 GBM patients with two or more optimally placed catheters had a median survival of 55.6 weeks, with 18.5% of patients surviving beyond 2 years after a single treatment (**Fig. 20.3**). There were no grade 3 or 4 adverse events associated with drug infusion at concentrations less than 0.5 μg/mL, and no systemic toxicities were observed. Delayed radiographic changes were observed in some patients 2 to 4 months after therapy, which responded to steroids and may represent an inflammatory response or non-specific activity.[25]

A phase 3 multicenter, randomized study (known as the PRECISE study) was initiated in patients with first-time recurrent GBM. The patients were randomized 2:1 to surgery followed by peritumoral infusion of IL13-PE38 versus surgery and Gliadel wafer (MGI Pharma, Inc., Bloomington, MN) implant; 296 patients were enrolled from 52 centers, and there

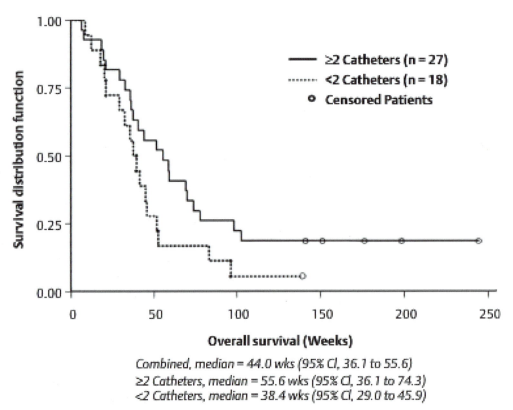

Fig. 20.3 Kaplan-Meier estimates for recurrent glioblastoma multiforme patients by catheter positioning in three phase 1 studies. CI, confidence interval.

was no difference in survival and the adverse events profile between the Cintredekin besudotox group and the Gliadel wafer group ($p = 0.31$), with the exception that pulmonary embolism was higher in the Cintredekin besudotox group.[24] In a separate study of these same patients, there was no difference in outcome in respect to catheter positioning.[26]

Future Directions

Convection-enhanced delivery of chemotherapeutic molecules has shown considerable promise in preclinical, and now phase 1 and phase 2 clinical, trials in patients with recurrent malignant gliomas; however, only limited phase 3 results are available. The use of more targeted macromolecules enables either intratumoral or peritumoral treatment. The optimal treatment design remains uncertain. The increased interstitial pressures within the tumor resulting in widely dispersed edema may help facilitate drug distribution to larger volumes of brain tissue. However, the chaotic pressure gradients formed by fibrosis and necrosis within the tumor may result in unpredictable distribution of drug. Furthermore, the presence of a disrupted BBB within the contrast-enhancing mass may increase the efflux of drug out of the CNS.

Even within the peritumoral margins, targeting infiltrating tumor cells may be limited by the normal anisotropy of the brain tissue, resulting in the preferential flow of fluid away from the intended target. In addition, the potency of these recombinant toxins may lead to nonspecific activity, potentially injuring normal tissue. This was seen with IL4-PE, which started at an infusion concentration 2000 times greater than the active concentration against receptor-bearing tumor cells. Despite these limitations, significant responses have been observed in all of the CED studies. Better understanding of the drug distribution will become a critical part of evaluating future studies involving CED.

Recently, diffusion tensor imaging (DTI) has been used to predict the hydraulic conductivity within the peritumoral brain tissue. This can then be used to predict distribution of drug from a point source within a specific region of brain. Iflow (BrainLAB, Munich, Germany) is currently approved by the Food and Drug Administration (FDA) to help in catheter planning. This predictive software will estimate the distribution of drug based on MRI and DTI data from a given patient and will help the surgeon plan the optimal catheter trajectory and tip placement to best cover the target volume. Additionally, real-time monitoring of drug distribution by CED in non-

human primates and dogs using MRI-based surrogate tracers has been developed.[27] Once we have a better understanding of drug distribution, other unsolved questions, including optimal catheter design and placement, duration of infusion, and the benefit of repeat infusions, can be addressed. Beyond drug distribution, the potential benefit of targeting multiple molecules by combining recombinant toxins, or combining these agents with other chemotherapies, remains unknown. The CED-based therapies continue to evolve, with a need for additional preclinical and clinical research. In fact, more recently it has been shown that the use of nanoparticles as large as 114 nm coated with poly(ethylene glycol) can diffuse through ex vivo brain tissue.[28] This larger size will enable diffusion of larger drug delivery system, which may enhance the efficacy of CED.

Implantable Polymers

Surgically implanted polymers loaded with chemotherapeutic agents provide another approach to intratumoral drug delivery. The polymer enables sustained delivery of active drug at the site of the residual tumor. For BCNU, which has a serum half-life of < 15 minutes, delivery with a sustained-release polymer results in intracranial tumoricidal concentrations of BCNU for up to 21 days in animal models.[29] The theoretical advantage of polymer-based delivery over catheter technology is that polymers are not subject to clogging. Once the polymer is implanted, there are no maintenance requirements. Furthermore, drug delivery to an irregular postoperative cavity may be more effective with multiple polymers.

Polymer Technology

To effectively deliver drugs to the brain using an implantable polymer, several characteristics are necessary. First, the polymer matrix needs to be biocompatible and biodegradable so that it does not need to be removed. Second, it needs to release drug in a dependable, reproducible rate over a sustained time period. Third, incorporated drug within the polymer matrix must be protected from degradation by the surrounding environment so that active drug continues to be released. Fourth, incorporation of drug into the matrix must occur under conditions that will maintain the bioactivity of the drug. Finally, the physical character of the polymer must allow for surgical handling and manipulation.

The polyanhydride poly[1,3-bis (carboxyphenoxy) propane-co-sebacic-acid] (PCPP-SA) matrix is an example of a biodegradable polymer that is useful in treating brain tumors. Because the matrix degrades at a steady rate, the drug can be released over an extended period of time with a relatively steady concentration. Biodegradable polyanhydrides prevent hydrolytic breakdown of the chemotherapeutic agent, thus maintaining its desired cytotoxic effects. The rate of drug re-

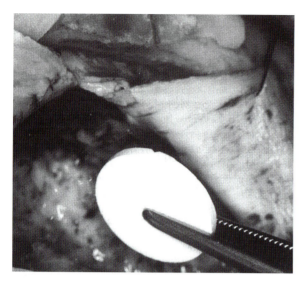

Fig. 20.4 Carmustine-impregnated polymer wafers are surgically implanted in the tumor resection cavity.

lease by these polymers can be controlled by changing the relative ratios of monomers in the copolymer matrix. Consequently, the drug can be delivered over weeks, months, or years, as needed. The polyanhydride polymers degrade as they release the drug, so surgical removal is not necessary. Because of these characteristics, PCPP-SA has been used to deliver BCNU (Gliadel) in clinical trials (**Fig. 20.4**).

There are currently several polymeric systems designed to optimize local delivery. They have been tested only in the laboratory. A second polyanhydride, the fatty acid dimmer–sebacic acid (FAD-SA) copolymer, has been developed to deliver hydrophilic agents such as platinum drugs.[30] The introduction of the poly(lactide-co-glycolide) polymer allows chemotherapeutic agents as well as larger molecules to be incorporated into microspheres that can be stereotactically injected into the brain.[31] Polyethylene glycol-coated liposomes that encapsulate anthracyclines show promise as delivery agents that both decrease systemic side effects and improve the therapeutic indices of these drugs.[32] Also, poly(lactide-co-glycolide) nanospheres can be covalently linked to a polyethylene glycol coating that reduces opsonization and elimination by the immune system before drug release.[33] Finally, gelatin microspheres have been shown to release cytokines in vivo.[34]

Clinical Trials

Based on encouraging preclinical data, clinical trials were initiated using a BCNU polymer formulation. Following a phase 1 study that evaluated escalating doses of BCNU loaded in PCPP-SA polymer for treatment of recurrent glioma,[35] a randomized, placebo-controlled, double-blinded, prospective phase 3 clinical trial to evaluate the efficacy of 3.8% BCNU in polyanhydride polymer was performed for patients with recurrent gliomas for whom standard therapy had failed.[36] A

total of 222 patients from 27 medical centers in the United States and Canada were entered. Enrolled patients received either BCNU-loaded polymer or "empty" placebo polymers implanted on the surface of the resected tumor cavity. The patients were equally distributed between the two groups for all known prognostic factors (e.g., median age, neurologic function, prior treatment, median interval from first operation, number of previous operations, and tumor grade). Most patients (65.5% for the BCNU-loaded polymer group and 65.2% for the placebo group) had GBM. Before enrollment, 52.7% of the BCNU group and 48.2% of the control group had undergone previous systemic chemotherapy, and all patients had received conventional external beam whole-brain radiation therapy. A few patients had received experimental immunotherapy or brachytherapy. Postoperatively, approximately 25% of patients underwent additional systemic chemotherapy (equally distributed in treatment and control groups).

For these 222 patients, all of whom had failed prior therapy, those who received BCNU-loaded polymer had an additional median survival of 31 weeks compared with 23 weeks for the control group. Use of a Cox proportional hazards model that adjusts for patient age, prior treatment, and tumor grade gave a hazard ratio of 0.67 ($p = .007$) (**Fig. 20.5**). When the results for patients with GBM were analyzed separately, the 6-month survival improved by 50%. Of importance, no significant local or systemic adverse reactions were attributable to the BCNU-loaded polymer. This study established that BCNU delivered via polyanhydride polymers is a safe, effective treatment for patients with recurrent malignant gliomas. This study provided the basis of the FDA approval of BCNU-loaded polymer as a treatment for patients with recurrent glioma.[33]

The encouraging results with controlled-release polymers for patients with recurrent gliomas led to the development of these treatments for newly diagnosed gliomas. A phase 1 study with 22 patients newly diagnosed with malignant glioma (21 with GBM) was conducted to evaluate the overall safety of BCNU-loaded polymer and the safety of receiving it with concurrent standard external beam radiation therapy.[37] No neurotoxicity or systemic toxicity was attributable to the locally released BCNU in conjunction with radiation therapy, and it appeared to be safe and well tolerated for this group.

To evaluate further the effectiveness of BCNU-loaded polymer in the initial therapy of malignant gliomas, a prospective, randomized, double-blinded phase 3 clinical trial enrolled 32

Special Consideration

- Patients who had been treated with intravenous BCNU in the course of their treatment before receiving the BCNU-loaded polymer were just as likely to benefit as the patients who had not been treated previously with chemotherapy.

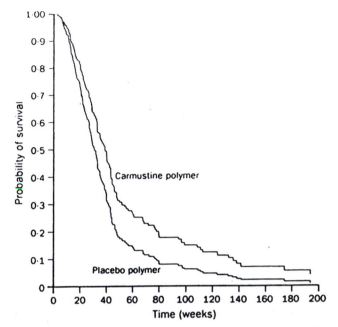

Fig. 20.5 Overall survival by treatment group after adjustment for prognostic factors. The curves illustrate the treatment effect expected if all patients were approximately age 48, white, had performance status > 70, underwent > 75% resection, had local irradiation, had not previously been exposed to nitrosoureas, and had glioblastomas pathologically classified as active. (From Brem H, Piantadosi S, Burger PC, et al. Placebo-controlled trial of safety and efficacy of intraoperative controlled delivery by biodegradable polymers of chemotherapy for recurrent gliomas. The Polymer-Brain Tumor Treatment Group. Lancet 1995;345:1008–1012. Reprinted with permission from Elsevier.)

patients at the time of initial surgical resection.[38] All patients had subsequent radiation therapy. Median survival was 58 weeks for the BCNU treatment group versus 40 weeks for the placebo group ($p = 0.001$). When patients with glioblastoma, the largest subgroup, were evaluated separately, median survival was 53 weeks with BCNU-loaded polymer (11 patients) and 40 weeks with placebo implants (16 patients) ($p = 0.0083$). At 1 year, 63% of the BCNU-loaded polymer patients were alive versus 19% of the control group. At 2 years, 31% of the BCNU-loaded polymer patients were alive versus only 6% of the control group. At 3 years, 25% of the BCNU-loaded polymer group were alive (three GBM, one anaplastic astrocytoma) compared with 6% (one GBM) of the control group. Overall, patients treated with BCNU polymers ($n = 16$) had a 73% reduction in the risk of death ($p = 0.006$). This study establishes that polymer technology is a safe, effective treatment for patients initially presenting with malignant gliomas.

A third, larger, randomized, prospective, placebo-controlled study randomized 240 patients with newly diagnosed malignant glioma and treated with BCNU polymers or control polymers.[39,40] All patients were then treated with radiation therapy.[39] Overall survival showed a 29% reduction in the risk of death ($p = 0.03$, log rank statistic) in the BCNU-polymer

- The BCNU-loaded polymer used as an initial treatment is well tolerated and effective at prolonging survival. There is a fivefold increase in the proportion of patients surviving 3 to 4 years. Furthermore, the prolonged survival is achieved without the severe systemic complications usually associated with chemotherapy, and treatment is additive to the benefit of radiation therapy.

treated group. Fifty-nine percent of the patients treated with BCNU polymer versus 49% of the placebo-polymer patients survived 1 year. The median survival of the BCNU-polymer group was 13.8 months in contrast to 11.6 months for the control group. There was a consistent and durable survival advantage for more than 3 years that was statistically significant ($p = 0.01$)[40] (**Fig. 20.6**). There is an approximate fivefold increase in the proportion of patients surviving 3 to 4 years after BCNU polymer implantation.

In 2003, the FDA approved expanded use of BCNU polymers for initial surgery, as well as recurrence, and for all malignant gliomas. In 2004, European approval was given for initial therapy and the U.S. Centers for Medicare and Medicaid Services (CMS) created a new diagnosis-related group (DRG) for patients treated with chemotherapy polymer implants.

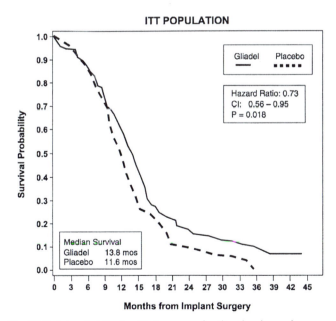

Fig. 20.6 Extended Kaplan-Meier curves for the placebo and carmustine wafer–treated patients for all 240 patients enrolled in the study, including the data from long-term follow-up. (From Springer Science Business Media. Westphal M, Ram Z, Riddle V, Hilt D, Bortey E. On behalf of the Executive Committee of the Gliadel Study Group. Gliadel wafer in initial surgery for malignant glioma: long-term follow-up of a multicenter controlled trial. Acta Neurochir (Wien) 2006;148:269–275. Reprinted with permission.)

More recently, a retrospective study was conducted in 26 centers in France, where 83 (51%) and 80 (49%) patients underwent BCNU wafer placement for newly diagnosed and recurrent GBM, respectively.[41] The median survival in the newly diagnosed GBM group was 17 months, which is among the highest reported survival rates among phase III clinical trials.[41] Additionally, carmustine wafers have also been used for other intracranial pathologies including metastatic brain cancer[42] and anaplastic ependymomas.[43]

Clinical Principles Associated with the Use of BCNU-Loaded Polymer

As the clinical experience with BCNU-loaded polymer has increased, several important lessons have been learned. The therapeutic advantage of interstitial chemotherapy is to treat the infiltrating cells at the margin of the tumor where the tumor cells are intermingled in brain that is potentially still functional. Furthermore, released chemotherapeutic agent, which kills residual tumor cells, can result in localized increased intracranial pressure from cerebral edema. The mass effect and additional brain edema from tumor that is being treated and becoming necrotic can result in symptoms of increased intracranial pressure. Therefore, it is important to achieve maximal tumor debulking to create room for any brain edema resulting from release of BCNU.

Because the effective release of BCNU into the brain can cause edema in the surrounding brain, high doses of corticosteroids are recommended in all patients receiving BCNU-loaded polymer. For the average patient, 16 to 20 mg per day of dexamethasone is adequate. In patients in whom edema is of particular concern or in whom there is postoperative neurologic deficit, supraphysiological corticosteroid doses (as high as 120 mg of dexamethasone per day) can be used, and then the dose can be slowly tapered as clinically indicated. There appear to be minimal deleterious effects of extremely high corticosteroid doses administered for short periods of time. Blood sugar should be carefully monitored during administration.

In retrospective analyses, BCNU-loaded polymers, when combined with temozolomide chemotherapy and radiation, were associated with prolonged survival as compared with patients with BCNU polymers and radiation alone for patients with primary GBM (21.3 vs 12.4 months, $p = 0.005$).[44] This combinatorial use of Gliadel and temozolomide was not associated with increased complications.[44,45] The enhanced survival with combinatorial therapy has also been shown in

---

xenograft mammalian models.[46] Therefore, although clinical trials do not exist, the use of Gliadel wafers does not preclude the use of temozolomide and radiation adjuvant therapy. Moreover, in patients older than 65 years, the use of Gliadel was associated with prolonged survival in a case-control series (8.7 vs 5.5 months, $p = 0.007$).[47]

In assessing the adverse effects of BCNU-loaded polymer in clinical trials, it was found that intracranial or wound infections occurred more commonly in patients who received BCNU (4/110 patients who received BCNU-loaded polymer vs 1/112 patients receiving placebo).[36] Although this difference was not found to be statistically significant, high doses of local BCNU can adversely affect wound healing. All patients who had a serious infection were found to have a prior CSF leak; therefore, aggressive wound care is recommended for these patients.

Clinical studies have shown that postoperative seizures overall are not more common in patients receiving BCNU-loaded polymer, but they occur with greater frequency in the immediate postoperative period.[36] This underscores the need to initiate anticonvulsant therapy in all patients preoperatively and to pay particular attention to serum drug levels, especially because corticosteroids can affect the anticonvulsant dose.

Preclinical studies in rabbits did not demonstrate a risk of direct exposure of the ventricle to BCNU-loaded polymer. However, small openings in the ventricle do not preclude the use of the polymer. If there is a large opening of the ventricle, the polymer wafer itself could theoretically enter the ventricle system and cause mechanical obstruction of CSF pathways, possibly leading to acute hydrocephalus. In this circumstance, BCNU-loaded polymer is not indicated, and other adjuvant therapies should be considered.

Postoperative imaging studies can remain abnormal related to the local release of BCNU for up to 3 months after implantation. Rim enhancement around the tumor cavity that may not have been present on the immediate postoperative MRI may develop and remain over the first 3 months. This effect on the BBB is similar in appearance to that seen after radiation therapy. Despite an MRI that shows new enhancement, patients who are clinically stable on fixed or decreasing steroid doses should be followed for another 2 months and have the MRI repeated at that time. A cause for concern is when patients develop signs or symptoms of increased brain edema and intracranial pressure and then require that their steroids be increased sequentially. These patients should be treated either medically or surgically for increased intracranial pressure because of expanding mass. Other adjuvant therapies should be considered for these patients at this time.

Animal studies demonstrating that higher doses of BCNU prolonged survival and distribution of drug while remaining well tolerated[29,48] formed the basis of a clinical trial evaluating higher intracranial doses for patients. A National Institutes of Health (NIH)-funded open-label, multicenter, dose-escalating study demonstrated the safety of BCNU-loaded polymer wafers containing up to 20% BCNU in patients with recurrent glioma and defined the true maximum tolerated dose. This study showed that patients tolerated up to (but not more than) five times the currently clinically used dose.[49]

The BCNU-loaded polymer is also being evaluated for both safety and efficacy as a therapy for radioresistant metastatic brain tumors. In patients with systemic cancer, current therapies have limited ability to control CNS disease, and many die of intracranial metastases. Furthermore, as improved systemic therapies become available, intracranial relapse may become more common. Therefore, the BCNU-loaded polymer may become a useful additional to the armamentarium available for the treatment of CNS metastases. Two multi-institutional trials are under way to evaluate BCNU-loaded polymer in patients with brain metastases. Several clinical trials are under way to evaluate the safety and effectiveness of combining direct treatment of the brain tumor by BCNU using BCNU-loaded polymer together with a variety of systemic chemotherapeutic agents such as carboplatin, temozolomide, and CPT-11.

Microchips

Microchips represent a relatively new technology for local chemotherapeutic delivery. Microchips enable pulsatile release of various types of chemotherapeutic agents using various micrometer-sized pumps, valves, and channels, where the release can be controlled by time-dependent biodegradation[50] or regulated degradation by electrochemical dissolution.[51] This release can involve single or multiple agents.[50] A study of temozolomide-loaded microchips in a rodent gliosarcoma model showed that the flow rates from the microchips were predictable and led to prolonged survival compared to rodents that underwent oral temozolomide therapy.[52] Human GBM clinical trials have yet to be established, but microchips have been used in humans with osteoporosis.[53] These microchips were implanted into eight postmenopausal women, and release of parathyroid hormone was under wireless control.[53] These women all showed increased bone density without any adverse effects.[53]

◼ Conclusion

As more effective drugs or delivery strategies become available for local delivery, whether alone or in combination, the challenge will be to improve on these initial results and develop treatment strategies that further enhance patient survival and quality of life. With the development of experimental therapies such as novel chemotherapeutic agents, immunotherapy, or virus-mediated gene therapy, local delivery with biodegradable polymers or catheters will play an increasing role in the management of patients with malignant brain tumors.

Editor's Note

The concept of intratumoral chemotherapy is intriguing. It makes a great deal of sense to try to get the therapeutic agent directly into the tumor as opposed to giving it systemically. Thus, there is a lot of appeal with this technique, yet unfortunately it has not been successful in its many different forms. The state of the art of this type of therapy currently lies with CED and polymer delivery of chemotherapy. Convection enhanced delivery has had some very interesting and intriguing results, but unfortunately the delivery technique leaves a lot to be desired because the distribution within the tumor is sporadic in terms of reflux around the catheter. However, new catheter designs are improving the ability to target the tumor to a greater degree without the reflux present. We believe that this technique will have a resurgence in the very near future, especially in the area of nanoparticle delivery.

The other strategy has been to load polymers with various chemotherapies such as BCNU in the form of wafers.

This has been studied in various clinical trials in the United States and abroad, and the bottom line is that there is some, albeit modest, survival benefit for polymer delivered chemotherapy. Certainly this method could be improved with better agents placed in the polymers, and ongoing studies in preclinical models continue to explore this as a potential therapeutic strategy for patients with high-grade tumors. (Berger)

References

1. Sneed PK, Gutin PH, Larson DA, et al. Patterns of recurrence of glioblastoma multiforme after external irradiation followed by implant boost. Int J Radiat Oncol Biol Phys 1994;29:719–727

2. Patchell RA, Regine WF, Ashton P, et al. A phase I trial of continuously infused intratumoral bleomycin for the treatment of recurrent glioblastoma multiforme. J Neurooncol 2002;60:37–42

3. Voulgaris S, Partheni M, Karamouzis M, Dimopoulos P, Papadakis N, Kalofonos HP. Intratumoral doxorubicin in patients with malignant brain gliomas. Am J Clin Oncol 2002;25:60–64

4. Walter KA, Tamargo RJ, Olivi A, Burger PC, Brem H. Intratumoral chemotherapy. Neurosurgery 1995;37:1128–1145

5. Bodell WJ, Giannini DD, Singh S, Pietronigro D, Levin VA. Formation of DNA adducts and tumor growth delay following intratumoral administration of DTI-015. J Neurooncol 2003;62:251–258

6. Rainov NG. A phase III clinical evaluation of herpes simplex virus type 1 thymidine kinase and ganciclovir gene therapy as an adjuvant to surgical resection and radiation in adults with previously untreated glioblastoma multiforme. Hum Gene Ther 2000;11:2389–2401

7. Hadaczek P, Mirek H, Berger MS, Bankiewicz K. Limited efficacy of gene transfer in herpes simplex virus-thymidine kinase/ganciclovir gene therapy for brain tumors. J Neurosurg 2005;102:328–335

8. Lang FF, Bruner JM, Fuller GN, et al. Phase I trial of adenovirus-mediated p53 gene therapy for recurrent glioma: biological and clinical results. J Clin Oncol 2003;21:2508–2518

9. Bobo RH, Laske DW, Akbasak A, Morrison PF, Dedrick RL, Oldfield EH. Convection-enhanced delivery of macromolecules in the brain. Proc Natl Acad Sci U S A 1994;91:2076–2080

10. Lieberman DM, Laske DW, Morrison PF, Bankiewicz KS, Oldfield EH. Convection-enhanced distribution of large molecules in gray matter during interstitial drug infusion. J Neurosurg 1995;82:1021–1029

11. Saito R, Krauze MT, Noble CO, et al. Tissue affinity of the infusate affects the distribution volume during convection-enhanced delivery into rodent brains: implications for local drug delivery. J Neurosci Methods 2006;154:225–232

12. Nguyen JB, Sanchez-Pernaute R, Cunningham J, Bankiewicz KS. Convection-enhanced delivery of AAV-2 combined with heparin increases TK gene transfer in the rat brain. Neuroreport 2001;12:1961–1964

13. Cunningham J, Oiwa Y, Nagy D, Podsakoff G, Colosi P, Bankiewicz KS. Distribution of AAV-TK following intracranial convection-enhanced delivery into rats. Cell Transplant 2000;9:585–594

14. Saito R, Bringas JR, McKnight TR, et al. Distribution of liposomes into brain and rat brain tumor models by convection-enhanced delivery monitored with magnetic resonance imaging. Cancer Res 2004;64:2572–2579

15. Bruce JN, Fine RL, Canoll P, et al. Regression of recurrent malignant gliomas with convection-enhanced delivery of topotecan. Neurosurgery 2011;69:1272–1279, discussion 1279–1280

16. Lidar Z, Mardor Y, Jonas T, et al. Convection-enhanced delivery of paclitaxel for the treatment of recurrent malignant glioma: a phase I/II clinical study. J Neurosurg 2004;100:472–479

17. Anderson RC, Kennedy B, Yanes CL, et al. Convection-enhanced delivery of topotecan into diffuse intrinsic brainstem tumors in children. J Neurosurg Pediatr 2013;11:289–295

18. Weaver M, Laske DW. Transferrin receptor ligand-targeted toxin conjugate (Tf-CRM107) for therapy of malignant gliomas. J Neurooncol 2003;65:3–13

19. Puri RK, Hoon DS, Leland P, et al. Preclinical development of a recombinant toxin containing circularly permuted interleukin 4 and truncated Pseudomonas exotoxin for therapy of malignant astrocytoma. Cancer Res 1996;56:5631–5637

20. Weber F, Asher A, Bucholz R, et al. Safety, tolerability, and tumor response of IL4-Pseudomonas exotoxin (NBI-3001) in patients with recurrent malignant glioma. J Neurooncol 2003;64:125–137

21. Sampson JH, Akabani G, Archer GE, et al. Progress report of a Phase I study of the intracerebral microinfusion of a recombinant chimeric protein composed of transforming growth factor (TGF)-alpha and a mutated form of the Pseudomonas exotoxin termed PE-38 (TP-38) for the treatment of malignant brain tumors. J Neurooncol 2003;65:27–35

22. Husain SR, Puri RK. Interleukin-13 receptor-directed cytotoxin for malignant glioma therapy: from bench to bedside. J Neurooncol 2003;65:37–48

23. Kunwar S. Convection enhanced delivery of IL13-PE38QQR for treatment of recurrent malignant glioma: presentation of interim findings from ongoing phase 1 studies. Acta Neurochir Suppl (Wien) 2003;88:105–111

24. Kunwar S, Chang S, Westphal M, et al; PRECISE Study Group. Phase III randomized trial of CED of IL13-PE38QQR vs Gliadel wafers for recurrent glioblastoma. Neuro-oncol 2010;12:871–881

25. Parney IF, Kunwar S, McDermott M, et al. Neuroradiographic changes following convection-enhanced delivery of the recombinant cytotoxin interleukin 13-PE38QQR for recurrent malignant glioma. J Neurosurg 2005;102:267–275

26. Mueller S, Polley MY, Lee B, et al. Effect of imaging and catheter characteristics on clinical outcome for patients in the PRECISE study. J Neurooncol 2011;101:267–277

27. Murad GJ, Walbridge S, Morrison PF, et al. Real-time, image-guided, convection-enhanced delivery of interleukin 13 bound to pseudomonas exotoxin. Clin Cancer Res 2006;12:3145–3151

28. Nance EA, Woodworth GF, Sailor KA, et al. A dense poly(ethylene glycol) coating improves penetration of large polymeric nanoparticles within brain tissue. Sci Transl Med 2012;4:ra119

29. Fung LK, Ewend MG, Sills A, et al. Pharmacokinetics of interstitial delivery of carmustine, 4-hydroperoxycyclophosphamide, and paclitaxel from a biodegradable polymer implant in the monkey brain. Cancer Res 1998;58:672–684

30. Olivi A, Ewend MG, Utsuki T, et al. Interstitial delivery of carboplatin via biodegradable polymers is effective against experimental glioma in the rat. Cancer Chemother Pharmacol 1996;39:90–96

31. Menei P, Capelle L, Guyotat J, et al. Local and sustained delivery of 5-fluorouracil from biodegradable microspheres for the radiosensitization of malignant glioma: a randomized phase II trial. Neurosurgery 2005;56:242–248, discussion 242–248

32. Gabizon A, Isacson R, Libson E, et al. Clinical studies of liposome-encapsulated doxorubicin. Acta Oncol 1994;33:779–786

33. Gref R, Minamitake Y, Peracchia MT, Trubetskoy V, Torchilin V, Langer R. Biodegradable long-circulating polymeric nanospheres. Science 1994;263:1600–1603

34. Rhines LD, Sampath P, DiMeco F, et al. Local immunotherapy with interleukin-2 delivered from biodegradable polymer microspheres combined with interstitial chemotherapy: a novel treatment for experimental malignant glioma. Neurosurgery 2003;52:872–879, discussion 879–880

35. Brem H, Mahaley MS Jr, Vick NA, et al. Interstitial chemotherapy with drug polymer implants for the treatment of recurrent gliomas. J Neurosurg 1991;74:441–446

36. Brem H, Piantadosi S, Burger PC, et al; The Polymer-brain Tumor Treatment Group. Placebo-controlled trial of safety and efficacy of intraoperative controlled delivery by biodegradable polymers of chemotherapy for recurrent gliomas. Lancet 1995;345:1008–1012

37. Brem H, Ewend MG, Piantadosi S, Greenhoot J, Burger PC, Sisti M. The safety of interstitial chemotherapy with BCNU-loaded polymer followed by radiation therapy in the treatment of newly diagnosed malignant gliomas: phase I trial. J Neurooncol 1995;26:111–123

38. Valtonen S, Timonen U, Toivanen P, et al. Interstitial chemotherapy with carmustine-loaded polymers for high-grade gliomas: a randomized double-blind study. Neurosurgery 1997;41:44–48, discussion 48–49

39. Westphal M, Hilt DC, Bortey E, et al. A phase 3 trial of local chemotherapy with biodegradable carmustine (BCNU) wafers (Gliadel wafers) in patients with primary malignant glioma. Neuro-oncol 2003;5:79–88

40. Westphal M, Ram Z, Riddle V, Hilt D, Bortey E; Executive Committee of the Gliadel Study Group. Gliadel wafer in initial surgery for malignant glioma: long-term follow-up of a multicenter controlled trial. Acta Neurochir (Wien) 2006;148:269–275, discussion 275

41. Menei P, Metellus P, Parot-Schinkel E, et al; Neuro-oncology Club of the French Society of Neurosurgery. Biodegradable carmustine wafers (Gliadel) alone or in combination with chemoradiotherapy: the French experience. Ann Surg Oncol 2010;17:1740–1746

42. Abel TJ, Ryken T, Lesniak MS, Gabikian P. Gliadel for brain metastasis. Surg Neurol Int 2013;4:289–293

43. Sardi I, Sanzo M, Giordano F, et al. Intracavitary chemotherapy (Gliadel) and oral low-dose etoposide for recurrent anaplastic ependymoma. Oncol Rep 2008;19:1219–1223

44. McGirt MJ, Than KD, Weingart JD, et al. Gliadel (BCNU) wafer plus concomitant temozolomide therapy after primary resection of glioblastoma multiforme. J Neurosurg 2009;110:583–588

45. McGirt MJ, Brem H. Carmustine wafers (Gliadel) plus concomitant temozolomide therapy after resection of malignant astrocytoma: growing evidence for safety and efficacy. Ann Surg Oncol 2010;17:1729–1731

46. Recinos VR, Tyler BM, Bekelis K, et al. Combination of intracranial temozolomide with intracranial carmustine improves survival when compared with either treatment alone in a rodent glioma model. Neurosurgery 2010;66:530–537, discussion 537

47. Chaichana KL, Zaidi H, Pendleton C, et al. The efficacy of carmustine wafers for older patients with glioblastoma multiforme: prolonging survival. Neurol Res 2011;33:759–764

48. Sipos EP, Tyler B, Piantadosi S, Burger PC, Brem H. Optimizing interstitial delivery of BCNU from controlled release polymers for the treatment of brain tumors. Cancer Chemother Pharmacol 1997;39:383–389

49. Olivi A, Grossman SA, Tatter S, et al; New Approaches to Brain Tumor Therapy CNS Consortium. Dose escalation of carmustine in surgically implanted polymers in patients with recurrent malignant glioma: a New Approaches to Brain Tumor Therapy CNS Consortium trial. J Clin Oncol 2003;21:1845–1849

50. Richards Grayson AC, Choi IS, Tyler BM, et al. Multi-pulse drug delivery from a resorbable polymeric microchip device. Nat Mater 2003;2:767–772

51. Santini JT Jr, Cima MJ, Langer R. A controlled-release microchip. Nature 1999;397:335–338

52. Scott AW, Tyler BM, Masi BC, et al. Intracranial microcapsule drug delivery device for the treatment of an experimental gliosarcoma model. Biomaterials 2011;32:2532–2539

53. Farra R, Sheppard NF Jr, McCabe L, et al. First-in-human testing of a wirelessly controlled drug delivery microchip. Sci Transl Med 2012;4: 22ra21

21 Targeted Therapies for Gliomas

Barbara J. O'Brien, W. K. Alfred Yung, and John F. de Groot

Since the publication of the previous edition of this book in 2008, our understanding of glioma tumor biology and associated molecular pathways and cellular alterations continues to progress rapidly. A more comprehensive understanding of the molecular basis of glioma initiation, progression, and treatment failure is emerging.[1] The Cancer Genome Atlas established a comprehensive catalog of genomic alterations driving gliomagenesis, and identified several distinct molecular subtypes of glioblastoma that share common genetic mutations, methylation profiles, and molecular pathway activation. However, this growing insight into the molecular biology of glioma has not yet translated into effective therapies.[2] Ongoing and future studies will evaluate specific inhibitors of these molecular targets, moving the field toward the development of personalized cancer therapy by which tumors with specific molecular alterations will be treated with agents inhibiting these activated pathways. These approaches will complement other strategies, such as targeting angiogenesis, glioma stem-like cells, and the immune response, with the ultimate goal of improving the outcome of patients with malignant gliomas.

■ The Rationale for Targeted Therapy

Several molecular alterations are thought to be important drivers of glioma tumorigenesis, growth, and treatment resistance, and provide the basis of the development of targeted therapies.[3] Pharmacological inhibitors and modulators of these alterations have been tested in clinical trials, and further trials are ongoing. Most of these targeted therapies have been directed at receptor tyrosine kinases and their intracellular signaling pathways, identified preclinically as important for supporting tumor growth, proliferation, and angiogenesis.[1] Despite these strategies, little has been accomplished in prolonging patient survival. Challenges include the genetic heterogeneity, inherent genetic instability, and rapid development of resistance pathways of gliomas, which make single-agent tar-

> **Pitfall**
>
> - Combination therapy consisting of multiple targeted agents can be associated with markedly increased toxicity because of coexpression of multiple targets in normal cells.

> **Pearl**
>
> - Combination therapy consisting of targeted small-molecule inhibitors and cytotoxic therapy may provide a therapeutic advantage.

geted therapies ineffective.[1] Strategies including combination-agent targeted therapies and targeting multiple pathways are under design and evaluation, although treatment-related toxicity is a dose-limiting concern.[1]

■ Subclassification of Glioblastoma and Implications for Treatment

Studies of gene expression and DNA methylation have identified multiple glioma subtypes, with some studies identifying an association between glioma subtype and survival.[4–6] The Cancer Genome Atlas (TCGA) analysis confirmed three subtypes of high-grade glioma—proneural, mesenchymal, and proliferative—and identified the neural and classic subtypes.[4–6] The proneural and mesenchymal subtypes are consistently identified and are the best characterized. The proneural subtype is more frequently identified in younger patients, and is associated with platelet-derived growth factor receptor (*PDGFR*) amplification and isocitrate dehydrogenase (*IDH*) 1 mutation.[5] The mesenchymal subtype is associated with neurofibromatosis type 1 (*NF1*) gene loss or mutation, and mesenchymal markers, such as *MET*.[5] The neural subtype is associated with expression of neuronal markers,[5] while the classic subtype is associated with phosphatase and tensin homolog (*PTEN*) loss, a distinct lack of *TP53* mutation, and a high level of epidermal growth factor receptor (*EGFR*) alterations, found in over 95% of samples with this subtype.[1,5] Grade II and III gliomas are predominantly of the proneural subtype, whereas glioblastomas can be of any subtype.[5] Although one series suggested patients with proneural glioblastoma survive longer than those with mesenchymal glioblastoma, another study found no difference.[5] Neural and classic subtypes are not clearly associated with different survival outcomes.[1] Aggressive treatment with radiation with concurrent and adjuvant temozolomide chemotherapy significantly improved survival in classic and mesenchymal subtypes. A statistically nonsignificant association is observed in the neural subtype, but no significant effect on survival was observed in the proneural subtype.[5] This subclassification of glioblastoma provides a foundation for a better molecular understanding of gliomagenesis and glioma signaling pathways and may be important for enriching clinical trials with patients screened for participation based on tumor molecular profile.[1,5]

Critical Pathways in Gliomagenesis

The mutation spectrum of glioblastoma, as described by TCGA, reveals that the majority of glioblastoma have aberrations in the TP53 pathway, RB pathway, or receptor tyrosine kinase (RTK) with downstream signaling through the Ras or phosphatidylinositol 3-kinase (PI3K) pathways.[3,5] The majority of tumor samples analyzed had alterations in all three pathways, suggesting that dysregulation of these three pathways is key to gliomagenesis,[7] although other pathways may also play critical roles[3] (**Fig. 21.1**). In the TCGA cohort, inactivation of the p53 pathway occurred, for instance, in the form of ARF deletions, MDM amplifications, and mutations of *p53* itself.[7] Dysregulation of the RB pathway most commonly occurred with deletion of the *CDKN2A/CDKN2B* locus on chromosome 9p21, followed by *CDK4* locus amplification.[7] In the RTK/PI3K pathway, *PTEN* deletions and mutations were frequent, as were aberrations in *EGFR, ERBB2, PDGFRA,* and *MET*.[7] Clearly, molecular heterogeneity and redundancy of molecular pathway activation will require careful selection of tumors for treatment with agents targeting the main drivers of tumor growth.

Tumor Biomarkers

Identifying and validating biomarkers are critical components of the development and evaluation of targeted therapies. Insight into glioma signaling pathways has helped uncover biomarkers that predict response to treatment and outcome in patients with glioma.[3] Prognostic markers include O-6-methylguanine DNA-methyltransferase (*MGMT*) promoter methylation (epigenetic marker in glioblastoma, correlating with better prognosis), chromosomes 1p and 19q co-deletion (associated with better prognosis with treatment with radiotherapy plus chemotherapy), and *IDH1* and *IDH2* gene mutations (indicating better prognosis in gliomas). *MGMT* methylation may be predictive of response to alkylating chemotherapies, although this may be related to its strong prognostic effect. However, a lack of meaningful response with this potential predictive biomarker may relate to tumor heterogeneity of signaling pathway activation at a regional, subpopulation, or individual cell level.[3] The somewhat recent discovery of *IDH1* and *IDH2* mutations in glioma enables a reproducible prognostic biomarker as well as a therapeutic target.[1] *IDH* mutations have a significant positive statistical association with overall survival, and in low-grade gliomas, anaplastic gliomas, and glioblastomas, *IDH* mutation status appears to be the most important prognostic factor.[1,8]

Proneural glioblastoma with *IDH* mutations seem to segregate almost exclusively into a distinct CpG island hypermethylator phenotype (G-CIMP).[1,9] This G-CIMP signature may be in fact the most robust prognostic indicator in glioblastoma, although the complexity and cost of determining G-CIMP status currently limit its utility as a routine prognostic test.[1] There appears to be an almost complete overlap between

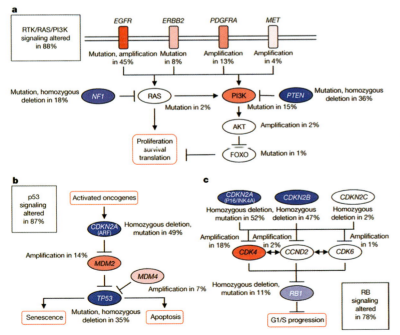

Fig. 21.1a–c Frequent genetic alterations in three critical signaling pathways. Primary sequence alterations and significant copy number changes for components of the (**a**) RTK/RAS/PI3K, (**b**) p53, and (**c**) RB signaling pathways are shown. Red indicates activating genetic alterations. Blue indicates inactivating alterations. The nature of the alteration and the percentage of affected tumors affected are indicated. Blue boxes contain the final percentages of glioblastoma with alterations in at least one known component gene of the designated pathway. (From Nature Publishing Group. Comprehensive genomic characterization defines human glioblastoma genes and core pathways. The Cancer Genome Atlas Research Network, Fig. 5. Nature 2008;455:1061–1068. Reprinted with permission.)

G-CIMP status and *IDH1/2* mutation status, which likely relates to the role of *IDH* mutations on the accumulation of epigenetic events leading to the hypermethylation phenotype.[10] Although there is currently no alternative treatment for patients with a favorable or unfavorable molecular profile, incorporating these biomarkers is critical for patient stratification in clinical trials. Prospective identification of targets and genetic profiles of tumor tissue from patients who respond to specific treatments are now being introduced into clinical trials.

The Ideal Target

Ideally a target has all of the following characteristics: it is highly expressed on cancer cells; it is specific to tumor cells; it is causally related to tumor cell growth, proliferation, or invasion (tumor phenotype); and it is involved in tumor initiation (gliomagenesis). Gliomas have a multitude of genetic aberrations, and thus the most critical oncogenic target(s) and pathways that must be interrupted for cell death need to be identified. In addition, because tumors utilize multiple cellular pathways in a redundant manner, therapies targeted to a single molecule or pathway are likely to be ineffective.

> **Special Consideration**
>
> - Ideally, the target must be highly expressed in the tumor, the target must be active, and this activity must contribute to tumor growth, proliferation, and survival.

Molecular Targets in Gliomas

As described above, specific genetic alterations identified in gliomas regulate several key pathways controlling cell growth, proliferation, invasion, and resistance to cell death. These highly complex processes involve signaling between multiple interrelated pathways. Key regulators of gliomagenesis include growth factor and growth factor receptors and their downstream effectors (i.e., molecules that mediate signal transduction and contribute to the transformed phenotype). Redundant and overlapping signaling pathways may explain, in part, the extreme resistance of these tumors to treatment. That is, attempts to inhibit a specific pathway within a tumor may result in the activation of a compensatory pathway or induce other cellular mechanisms that ultimately enable the tumor cells to survive. Nonetheless, some of the genetic alterations important in signal transduction pathways may be amenable to targeted therapy. Additionally, certain tumor suppressor genes such as *PTEN* and *TP53* may also be important in determining tumor responsiveness to a specific molecular therapy, even though they may not represent a target for therapy.

> **Pitfall**
>
> - Single-agent therapy aimed at one target is unlikely to be effective in the treatment of gliomas because these tumors contain highly heterogeneous cell populations with multiple compensatory growth pathways.

> **Special Consideration**
>
> - The oncologist must have a working knowledge of glioma biology in order to understand the distribution and expression of the target in tumor and normal tissues and thus to anticipate the potential toxicities of molecular targeted therapies.

Specific Therapeutic Targets and Relevant Clinical Trials

Cell Surface Growth Factor Receptors

Several growth factor receptors frequently overexpressed in gliomas are oncogenes believed to "drive" glioma formation and progression, and therefore are major targets of drug development.[11,12] These receptors, which predominantly act through receptor tyrosine kinases, are located on the cell surface, where they interact with effector molecules, second messengers, and other intracellular signaling pathway mediators, including the Ras/Raf/mitogen-activated protein kinase (MAPK) and PI3K pathways.[12] These secondary pathways then activate additional downstream effectors, ultimately leading to enhanced cell survival, proliferation, migration and invasion, evasion of apoptosis, angiogenesis, and resistance to treatment.[12] Growth factor pathways involved in glioma formation and progression include those mediated by EGFR, PDGFR, vascular endothelial growth factor (VEGF), transforming growth factor receptor (TGFR)-α and -β, and fibroblast growth factor receptor (FGFR)[11] (**Fig. 21.2**). Glioma cells are also known to secrete growth factors for these receptors, which are overexpressed on the cell surface, thus establishing autocrine and paracrine growth stimulatory loops. The dominant role of these growth factors and their overexpression on glial tumors has made them central in the search for effective targeted therapeutic agents.

Epidermal Growth Factor Receptor

Epidermal growth factor receptor, a receptor tyrosine kinase that plays a fundamental role in the growth and transformation of primary glioblastoma, is a prime target for therapy.[13]

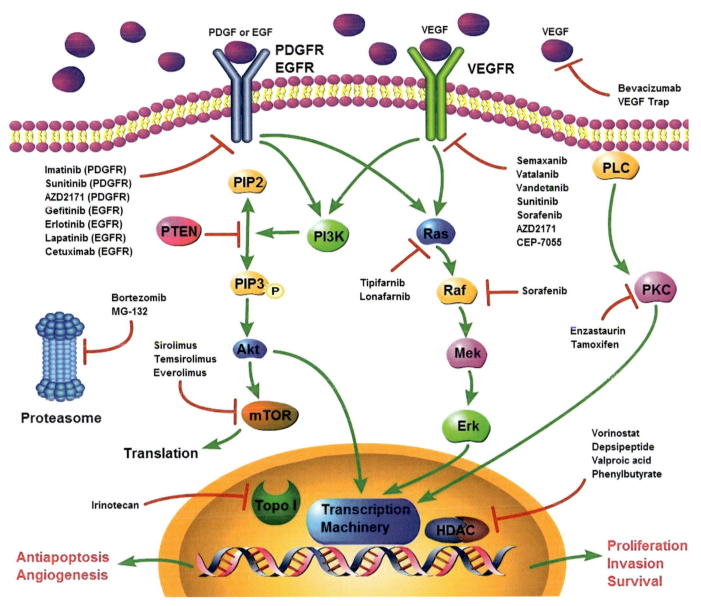

Fig. 21.2 Molecular genetic aberrations and molecularly targeted therapies for malignant glioma. Growth factor receptors and intracellular signaling pathways are activated in glioblastoma and have been implicated in gliomagenesis. Downstream effects of these mutated pathways affect tumor survival, invasiveness, proliferation, evasion of apoptosis, avoidance of immune surveillance, and ability to form and sustain new blood vessels. Several constituents of these pathways are targets for molecularly targeted therapies. (From Thaker NG, Pollack IF. Molecularly targeted therapies for malignant glioma: rationale for combinatorial strategies. Expert Rev Neurother 2009;9:1815–1836. Reprinted with permission.)

Indeed, by far the most frequent oncogenic alteration in gliomas is the overexpression, amplification, or mutation of *EGFR*, identified in approximately 60% of primary glioblastoma.[13,14] *EGFR* expression has been associated with increased tumor cell proliferation, increased cellular migration and invasion, and increased resistance to chemotherapy. Aberrant EGFR signaling is less common in low-grade glioma and secondary glioblastoma that arise from lower grade tumors. Glioblastoma with the amplified *EGFR* gene are enriched in the classic subtype and are frequently associated with deletion of the *CDKN2A* gene locus.[13]

The EGFR pathway can be activated through multiple mechanisms, and initiates signal transduction through major pathways such as the MAPK cascade and PI3K/Akt[13] to promote cell proliferation and survival. Some glioblastoma express EGFR and can also secrete the ligands EGF and TGF-α, thereby establishing autocrine and paracrine loops that effect the constitutive activation of the receptor and its downstream pathways. The most common *EGFR* mutation in glioblastoma is the intragenic deletion of exons 2 to 7, resulting in loss of the extracellular ligand-binding domain and constitutive activation of the receptor. This mutant receptor, referred to as EGFRvIII, is present in approximately 40% of tumors with EGFR amplification.[11,14] EGFRvIII may be an independent prognostic factor for poor survival, as excessive activation of EGFR may provide cells with a growth advantage.[11]

There are several reasons why EGFR and its downstream pathways are ideal targets for therapy. First, as noted above, EGFR is highly expressed in gliomas. Second, EGFR overexpression correlates with poor patient prognosis (decreased survival time and shorter time to progression). Third, EGFR plays no critical physiological role in healthy adults.

The first-generation single-agent small-molecule tyrosine kinase inhibitors (TKIs) used in clinical trials targeting EGFR in glioblastoma were gefitinib (ZD1839; Iressa) and erlotinib (OSI-779; Tarceva). Although the drugs were well tolerated with mild side-effect profiles, no treatment benefit was found.[13] It should be noted that these trials were offered to unselected patients with glioblastoma and the pharmacokinetics of these EGFR inhibitors were in some cases likely altered by the concurrent use of enzyme-inducing antiepileptic drugs.[13] Independent trials did not confirm a benefit in patients with EGFRvIII expression and PTEN loss,[15] as was previously reported.[16] Failure of the first-generation EGFR inhibitors in glioma clinical trials may have been related to inadequate drug levels in the tumor, the inability to turn off the receptor for a sufficient period of time, and the rapid activation of resistance pathways. Future trials will attempt to minimize the confounding impact of these important factors when evaluating newer agents.

Limited efficacy was observed with cetuximab (Erbitux, ImClone Systems), a monoclonal antibody against EGFR and lapatinib (GW572016, GlaxoSmithKline USA, Philadelphia, PA), a TKI targeting HER1 and HER2 (Tan). Cetuximab has limited penetration across the blood–brain barrier, which may have been responsible for its limited clinical activity.[11] Preclinical studies have identified lapatinib as an irreversible inhibitor of EGFR, which may confer greater therapeutic benefit over previous TKIs such as erlotinib.[16] Ongoing studies with lapatinib will determine if intermittent high-dose (pulsed-dosing) strategies can improve the efficacy of EGFR inhibition. Next-generation TKIs, such as afatinib, dacomitinib, and nimotuzumab, which have reversible EGFR inhibition, are under development and testing.[3]

Combining erlotinib with other therapies, including radiation therapy, cytotoxic chemotherapy, and other small-molecule therapies, failed to improve its efficacy. A phase 2 trial of EGFR and mammalian target of rapamycin (mTOR) inhibition was ineffective, but patients were not stratified for a specific molecular signature. Several studies have shown a response typically in tumors with EGFR amplification and low levels of Akt or expression of the EGFRvIII variant and preservation of PTEN, suppressing constitutive Akt activation, providing rationale for stratifying patients.

The basic principle of targeted therapy is that tumors expressing the target will respond to a particular drug designed to inhibit that target. However, although the concept is simple, realizing this clinically has not proved to be straightforward. Molecular testing of glioblastoma tissue of patients under treatment has established drug concentrations in the tissue, and has helped further our understanding of the effects on pathway signaling.[13] However, few or no responders in these clinical trials of EGFR inhibitors suggests that there is not a "signature" that will inform efficacy. Vaccination approaches targeting the EGFRvIII mutant with a tumor-specific antigen are ongoing in randomized phase 3 clinical trials.[13]

Platelet-Derived Growth Factor Receptor

Similar to EGFR, the stimulation of PDGFR activates downstream signaling cascades involving Ras/Raf/MAPK and PI3K/Akt pathways, and is involved in promoting cell survival, proliferation, invasion, and resistance to apoptosis. In addition, similar to other receptor tyrosine kinases, both the ligand (PDGF) and its receptor (PDGFR) are overexpressed in primary brain tumors, suggesting that autocrine and paracrine growth stimulatory loops result in the constitutive activation of this receptor.[17] Both low- and high-grade astrocytomas overexpress PDGF and PDGFR, supporting the notion that PDGFR is important for the development of glial tumors in general. Further, PDGFR amplification is a marker of the proneural subtype of glioblastoma, and so subtype may be a starting point for patient selection when developing clinical trials with inhibitors of PDGFR, in combination with other agents.

Several targeted agents, including imatinib (STI-571; Gleevec; Novartis Pharmaceuticals, East Hanover, NJ), inhibit PDGFR. Although imatinib showed some activity in preclinical testing in glioma cell lines, it has shown only minimal activity in both single-agent and combination therapy.[3,18,19] Second-generation TKIs with better central nervous system (CNS) penetration, such as tandutinib and dasatinib, are under evaluation in clinical trials. Preliminary results are not encouraging, suggesting that targeting PDGFR in glioblastoma might not be effective and that the understanding of this pathway's role in glioma may warrant further investigation.[3]

Fibroblast Growth Factor Receptor

Dysregulation of fibroblast growth factor receptor signaling via overexpression or genetic modification may occur, and inhibition of FGFR signaling may block angiogenesis.[20] FGFR dysregulation ultimately leads to upregulation of both the (Ras-dependent) Ras/MAPK pathway and the (Ras-independent) PI3K/Akt pathway.[20] Although FGFR is thus a rational therapeutic target, it is unclear how to select patients whose tumors will likely respond, and there is the potential concern of toxicity, as FGFR is also intimately involved in many normal biological processes.[20] However, recent studies identified a FGFR-TACC fusion protein that appears to be a central driver of the malignant glioma phenotype in a small subset of glioblastoma patients (estimated to be < 3%).[21] Some small-molecule agents targeting FGFR are brivanib, dovitinib, ponatinib, and nintedanib.[20] Although the activity of most of these agents against FGFR is weak, newer agents with high specificity for FGFR are entering clinical trial. Studies in development will select patients based on a high level of *FGFR* amplification or expression of the FGFR-TACC fusion. Other possible treatment approaches include monoclonal anti-FGFR antibodies and FGF-ligand trap approaches.[20]

Receptor Tyrosine Kinase Signaling and Downstream Effectors

The activation of cell-surface receptor tyrosine kinases (growth factor receptors) initiates a complex series of intracellular signaling cascades. Receptor tyrosine kinases such as EGFR or PDGFR are activated by binding of appropriate ligands (growth factors), or in response to the constitutive activation of a mutant receptor. The basic objective of signal transduction is to translate and amplify an extracellular stimulus into signals interpreted at the cellular level. Signals are transduced by the receptor through several common pathways, such as Ras/MAPK and PI3K/Akt, and information is eventually relayed to downstream intracellular effectors such as mTOR and protein kinase C, which modulate tumor growth, proliferation, angiogenesis, and apoptosis.[11] Inhibiting receptor tyrosine kinases or intermediate and downstream effectors may interfere with processes that promote tumor growth.

Special Consideration

- Because receptor tyrosine kinases can activate distinct signaling cascades or simultaneously activate multiple growth-promoting pathways, there are overlapping signaling mechanisms and crosstalk between pathways. This adds a layer of complexity to targeted therapy for gliomas.

Ras/Mitogen-Activated Protein Kinase

Ras is an important signal transduction effector of the receptor tyrosine kinases EGFR and PDGFR. Oncogenic mutations in Ras lead to its overactivation in 25% of cancers.[22] However, increased Ras activity has been observed in up to 88% of glioblastomas,[23] and this is thought to be due to multiple genetic events: activation of receptor tyrosine kinases, mutation or homozygous deletion of *NF1* (18%), mutation or homozygous deletion of *PTEN* (35%), mutation of PIK3CA (15%), *RAS* mutation (2%), amplification of *AKT* (2%), and mutation of *FOXO* (1%).[11]

Ras must be farnesylated, catalyzed by the farnesyltransferase enzyme, to become activated and hence recruited to the plasma membrane. Ras then activates a number of downstream molecules, including Raf, which activates several MAPKs. The Ras/MAPK pathway enhances cell proliferation and plays a role in cell migration.

There are several reasons why Ras is a good therapeutic target in gliomas. First, it is activated by many receptor tyrosine kinases. Second, it is activated in gliomas. Third, inhibiting Ras dramatically decreases glioma growth. The approach taken in the pharmacological inhibition of Ras activity is indirect. That is, it is the farnesyltransferase, rather than Ras per se, that is inhibited. Although initial studies of Tipifamib (R115777, Zarnestra, Johnson & Johnson, New Brunswick, NJ), a farnesyltransferase inhibitor (FTI) of Ras farnesylation with antiproliferative activity, seemed promising as a potential therapy for glioblastoma, only modest activity against glioblastoma has been seen.[11] Initial studies of lonafarnib (SCH66336, SARASAR, Schering Plough, Kenilworth, NJ), another FTI, were also encouraging, and further evaluation will be needed to determine efficacy against gliomas.[11]

The MAPK cascade involves multiple protein kinases, including Raf, which phosphorylate and activate MEK, which subsequently activates MAPK.[11,24] Sorafenib (BAY43-9006; Bayer, Wayne, NJ) is a Raf kinase inhibitor, as well as a VEGF receptor (VEGFR) inhibitor, and is a component of past and ongoing combination studies in gliomas.[11,25,26] Results from clinical trials targeting Raf have thus far been discouraging.

PI3-Kinase/Akt

As well as bringing about the overactivation of the Ras/MAPK pathway, activation of receptor tyrosine kinases such as EGFR results in the activation of the PI3K pathway, which acts through a complex second-messenger signaling cascade to activate several molecules, including Akt and mTOR.[27] Like the Ras/MAPK pathway, the PI3K pathway regulates cancer cell growth, proliferation, and apoptosis, and activation of this pathway is associated with poor prognosis in glioma.[11,28,29] The activation of Akt via PI3K is a major pathway in growth factor receptor signaling.[11]

Because of its ability to antagonize PI3K, the tumor suppressor phosphatase and tensin homologue (*PTEN*) is an important regulator of the EGFR pathway. PTEN function is lost in at least 35% of glioblastomas, leading to constitutive activation of the PI3K pathway.[11] PTEN loss in turn correlates with higher activated Akt levels in glioma cells. Akt activates additional downstream targets that play a role in cell survival and growth signaling (e.g., Bad, mTOR, and forkhead transcription factor).[11,30-32]

Because Akt has a central role in numerous biological processes, it has been difficult to translate a strategy for inhibiting Akt into clinical use for the treatment of cancer. The Akt inhibitor perifosine and the PI3K inhibitor LY294002 looked promising in preclinical studies, but have poor toxicity profiles.[11] Alternate approaches to inhibiting Akt have been designed, including inhibiting upstream and downstream targets within the PI3K/Akt pathway, including inhibitors directly targeting PI3K and mTOR. Recently, blood–brain barrier penetrant inhibitors of PI3K have been developed including BKM120 (Novartis) and GNE-317 (Genentech, Mahwah, NJ). These agents are in phase 1 and 2 clinical trials in patients with recurrent glioblastoma. Some trials are selecting patients based on biomarker expression in tumor tissue such as *PIK3CA* mutations or *AKT* overexpression.

mTOR, which is activated by both Akt and Ras pathways, transduces proliferative signals mediated by PI3K/Akt activating downstream effectors. Overexpression of growth factors or deletion of *PTEN* increases mTOR activation. mTOR inhibitors include rapamycin (sirolimus, Rapamune, Wyeth, Collegeville, PA), temsirolimus (CCI-779, Wyeth), AP23573 (Ariad, Cambridge, MA), and everolimus (Rad-001, Certican, Novartis). These agents inhibit glioblastoma proliferation in glioma cell lines.[11] As might be expected from a cytostatic therapy, using these drugs as a single agent in patients with recurrent glioblastoma or in combination with EGFR TKIs has been ineffective.[11,33,34] However, mTOR inhibitors may benefit a subpopulation of patients with glioblastoma who possess high tumor levels of a downstream activator of mTOR signaling.[3,33] Inhibitors of mTORC1 such as rapamycin have been associated with a paradoxical increase in activation of Akt, which is now known to be due to inhibition of a negative feedback loop.[35,36] Newer agents known to inhibit both mTORC1 and mTORC2 may be more effective than mTORC1 inhibitors.[36] Furthermore, agents with a theorized larger range of activity are under study in clinical trials, including BKM-120, a pan-PI3K inhibitor.[3] Finally, recent studies identified the PML protein as a potential mediator of resistance following mTOR inhibition. Studies are in development to combine mTOR inhibitors with arsenic trioxide, an inhibitor of PML.[37]

Protein Kinase C

Protein kinase C (PKC) is a family of protein tyrosine kinases that are downstream signaling pathway components of several receptor tyrosine kinases such as EGFR and PDGFR. Like Ras, the overactivity of PKC has not been linked to mutations in PKC, but rather results from the activation of upstream kinases. Protein kinase C has also been shown to be important in angiogenesis and in glioma growth and proliferation and to contribute to the malignant progression of tumors, including gliomas.[38–40] Activation of PKC induces phosphorylation of other effectors, such as Raf and MAPK, as well as Ras activation.[11,38,41]

Until recently, the ability to clinically target PKC in glioblastoma has been limited. Tamoxifen, an antiestrogen drug

that also inhibits PKC, unfortunately failed to show benefit in clinical studies.[11,42,43] Enzastaurin (LY317615, Eli Lilly, Indianapolis, IN) is a PKC inhibitor with antiangiogenic and antitumor activity in glioma cell lines,[11,44] inhibiting signaling through the PI3K/Akt pathway. Despite initially encouraging results, a phase 3 study was terminated early given clinical inefficacy.[11]

TP53

TP53 constitutes another key signaling pathway in glioblastoma. Loss of *p53* function via mutation or homozygous deletion provides a tumor growth advantage, and thus clonal expansion of glioma cells and brain tumor progression.[45] Inactivation of the p53 pathway occurs as mutation of *p53* itself, or as *ARF* deletion (55%), or as amplifications of *MDM2* (11%) and *MDM4* (4%).[7] The *TP53* tumor-suppressor gene encodes a protein that causes cell-cycle arrest in the G_1 or G_2 phase of the cell cycle, and promotes apoptosis following DNA damage.[3,45,46]

Rb Signaling

The cell cycle is kept in check by the RB protein until phosphorylated by cyclin D, CDK4, and CDK66.[3] Rb constitutes another key signaling pathway in glioblastoma. PD 0332991, a CDK4 and CDK6 inhibitor, is one agent under investigation in recurrent glioblastoma with known Rb-pathway alterations.

■ Vascular Endothelial Growth Factor Receptor and Angiogenesis

Rapidly growing tumors outstrip their blood supply unless new blood vessels form. As they grow, tumors therefore release growth factors that promote new blood vessel formation, a process called angiogenesis. Vascular endothelial growth factor is a growth factor involved in cellular proliferation and in new vessel formation resulting from remodeling of the primary vascular network or from sprouting from existing vessels. Angiogenesis has an essential role in the development and maintenance of solid tumors, including malignant gliomas. Vascular endothelial growth factor is released by glioma cells and the microenvironment, which then activates VEGF tyrosine kinase receptors on vascular endothelial cells, lead-

Controversy

- Bevacizumab may improve 6-month PFS for glioma patients, but treatment response is difficult to assess with standard imaging methodology, and the optimal dose and length of treatment are unclear.

ing to the activation of an intracellular signaling cascade through stimulation of the PI3K/Akt and Ras/MAPK pathways, culminating in endothelial cell proliferation, migration, and survival.[3,47] Indeed, vascular proliferation is one diagnostic criterion for the histological classification of glioblastoma, and VEGF has been linked to the high proliferation rate of high-grade astrocytoma.

Antiangiogenic therapy is attractive because of the prominent role of angiogenesis in glioblastoma growth and proliferation, the lack of VEGF-mediated processes in adult human tissues, and the accessibility of VEGFR on endothelial cells, which overcomes the challenge of delivering the drug to the tumor itself. In the development of antiangiogenic targeted therapy, efforts so far have focused on using small molecules that target the VEGF receptor tyrosine kinase and humanized monoclonal antibodies (or antibody fragments) that bind to and neutralize VEGF. Other mediators of angiogenesis in glioblastoma are PDGF, the angiopoietins (ang1 and ang2), and their receptor (Tie-2), bFGH, HIF-1α, and HGF,[3,48] and the Notch signaling pathway.[3,49]

Bevacizumab (Avastin), a humanized monoclonal antibody to VEGF, received accelerated FDA approval for recurrent glioblastoma in 2009 due to improved 6-month progression-free survival (PFS) over historic controls.[3,50] Bevacizumab is the only antiangiogenic agent currently approved for the treatment of glioblastoma. Complicating factors with bevacizumab treatment include the difficulty of accurately assessing tumor response, unclear optimal dosing and length of treatment, and concerns that bevacizumab may increase glioblastoma invasion. Recent phase 3 studies of bevacizumab for patients with newly diagnosed glioblastoma failed to show increased overall survival.[51,52]

Although bevacizumab has limited activity when used alone, it may be more effective when combined with cytotoxic chemotherapy or other targeted therapies. Recent clinical trials of bevacizumab with lomustine showed additive benefit versus bevacizumab alone.[53] Clinical trials are currently under way to examine additional combinations, although previous results have been discouraging. For instance, bevacizumab, when combined with erlotinib in a phase 2 study, did not improve survival compared to bevacizumab alone.[3,54]

A phase 1 trial with biomarker studies of vatalanib (PTK787), a VEGFR antagonist in patients with newly diagnosed glioblastoma treated with standard radiation and temozolomide, found that the drug was well tolerated.[55] Although a European Organization for Research on Treatment of Cancer (EORTC) study of vatalanib also demonstrated feasibility and safety, the planned randomized phase 2 trial was discontinued due to an industry decision not to further develop this agent.[56] Another approach was taken with VEGF-Trap (aflibercept), designed as a "decoy receptor" for the VEGF ligand. As its name implies, this agent traps VEGF, and placental growth factor, before the ligand can bind to its native receptors. Although initial studies of aflibercept in glioblastoma showed promising results, further study showed single-agent therapy to be

associated with moderate toxicity, and there was minimal evidence of single-agent activity in unselected patients with recurrent malignant glioma.[57]

Treatment with cediranib, a pan-VEGF tyrosine kinase inhibitor with additional activity against PDGFR and c Kit, was associated with improved 6-month PFS compared to historical controls in a phase 2 trial of patients with recurrent glioblastoma. Unfortunately, it failed to show significant improvement in PFS in a randomized controlled phase 3 trial, as a single agent or in combination with lomustine, over lomustine alone.[3] Another antiangiogenic agent, cilengitide, was found to have modest activity against recurrent glioblastoma, with a 6-month PFS of 15%, but it is no longer in development due to negative phase 3 clinical trials.[3,58] CENTRIC, the phase 3 trial in glioblastoma with *MGMT* methylation, did not meet its primary endpoint of increasing overall survival, and CORE, a phase 1–2 trial in glioblastoma without *MGMT* methylation, is ongoing.[3] Other VEGFR tyrosine kinase inhibitors, such as sunitinib, vandetanib, and cabozantinib (XL 184), have been evaluated in clinical studies, with limited benefit in unselected patients.[3,59–61]

■ Combination Strategies

Single-agent molecularly targeted therapies have not been effective.[11] Given the molecular heterogeneity of gliomas and the complexity and redundancy of signaling pathways, resistance to targeted agents is expected and has been a barrier to the development of effective therapies. Therefore, combinations of multiple targeting agents or single agents targeting multiple receptor tyrosine kinases may be better strategies for effective therapy.[11,62] However, there is some concern regarding increased toxicity with these combinations. For example, a study combining erlotinib and temsirolimus in recurrent glioblastoma showed treatment-limiting toxic effects.[11,63]

Multiple receptor tyrosine kinases are coactivated by redundant inputs, which maintain downstream signaling and limits efficacy of single agents. Parallel processing of signaling pathways and activation of compensatory pathways also occur, as do constitutive activation either of downstream molecules or receptor tyrosine kinases, and secondarily acquired mutations.[11]

Multi-targeting kinase inhibition with single agents is another potential strategy for the treatment of glioblastoma. The combination of sorafenib, a multi-agent TKI that inhib-

Special Consideration

- Rational combination therapy trial design must include an understanding of the major mechanisms of tumor resistance, which include tumor heterogeneity and redundancy.

its EGFR, PDGFR, VEGFR, and Raf, and temsirolimus, which inhibits mTOR, was moderately well tolerated, but without significant activity against glioblastoma.[11] A phase 2 trial assessing the combination of erlotinib and sorafenib was recently completed and reported only modest antitumor activity[64] Despite its status as a multi-target agent, sorafenib has unfortunately not yet proved effective as a single agent or in combination therapy for either upfront or recurrent glioblastoma.[3,26,65]

Other Molecularly Targeted Therapies

Histone Deacetylase Inhibition

Alterations of gene expression by epigenetic changes may influence tumor growth.[11] Histone proteins organize DNA into nucleosomes and histone deacetylases (HDACs) that play an important part in regulating gene expression.[11,66] Histone processing may be altered in gliomas, and inhibition of histone deacetylases has been another target of glioma therapy.[3,11] HDAC inhibitors include LBH589, valproic acid, depsipeptide, and suberoylanilide hydroxamic acid (SAHA) (vorinostat).[11] Both LBH589 and vorinostat in combination with bevacizumab are undergoing evaluation in recurrent glioblastoma.[3,60] Vorinostat has shown mixed results,[67,68] and an ongoing phase 2 trial of vorinostat plus temozolomide is being completed within the North Central Cancer Treatment Group (NCCTG).

Isocitrate Dehydrogenase 1

Cytosolic isocitrate dehydrogenase 1 (IDH1) mutations are present in about 70% of diffuse astrocytomas and secondary glioblastomas, but in less than 10% of primary glioblastomas.[8] The presence of mutant IDH results in increased levels of 2-hydroxyglutarate (2-HG), which then alters a number of downstream cellular activities.[69] This mutation is a favorable prognostic factor in patients with glioma, and the prognostic power of this mutation exceeds that of other markers.[8] Patients with IDH mutations have a better outcome than those with wild-type IDH gliomas. Although the role of IDH1 mutation in tumorigenesis is under study,[8,70] it may play an im-

portant part in tumor maintenance, in addition to its ability to promote transformation in certain cellular contexts.[16]

Small-molecule IDH1-mutant–specific inhibitors are under development for secondary glioma. For instance, a selective mutant R132H-IDH1 inhibitor (AGI-5198) was found to block the ability of mutant IDH1 to produce R-2-hydroxyglutarate (R-2HG). The mutant IDH1 inhibitor induced expression of genes associated with gliogenic differentiation, and the blockade of mutant IDH1 impaired the growth of IDH1-mutant glioma cells, and suggested that mutant IDH1 may promote glioma growth through mechanisms beyond epigenetic effects.[71] Eligible patients for a trial of mutant IDH1 inhibitors should be selected based on tumor IDH mutation status.

Glioma Stem Cell Signaling

Glioma stem-like cells (GSCs) are distinguished by self-renewal, multi-lineage differentiation, and tumorigenicity.[3] GSCs have improved the understanding of glioma treatment resistance mechanisms and associated pathways.[72] Sonic hedgehog (SHH) and Notch are key GSC regulators. SHH binds to a transmembrane receptor that releases a membrane protein, Smoothened homolog, which activates Gli proteins, which in turn modulate target genes such as MYC and CCND1.[72] Notch signaling is likely involved in GSC proliferation and self-renewal.[73] Other signaling pathways, such as Wnt/Beta-catenin and the RTK-mediated pathways are also likely critical.[72] Glioblastomas of the mesenchymal subtype overexpress genes associated with a GSC phenotype.[74] GSCs are by nature resistant to both radiotherapy and chemotherapy, and this may account for a proportion of patients with poor response to standard upfront treatment of glioblastoma. Treatment targeting pathways that regulate GSC phenotypes, such as STAT3 and TGF-β, may prove more effective in this population.[75,76] RO4929097, a gamma-secretase inhibitor with a role in Notch signaling, and vismodegib, a small molecule targeting the signaling of sonic hedgehog, are under investigation.

Conclusion

Glioblastomas are difficult tumors to treat because of their location within the brain and because they are highly resistant to conventional therapies. However, with our greatly increased understanding of these tumors over the last two decades, and the resultant dramatic improvement in our knowledge of the role of receptor tyrosine kinases and the molecular pathways they activate in promoting tumor growth, future patients with this tumor are likely to fare better. Further determining the oncogenic signals that drive tumor survival and proliferation will enable the development of therapies targeted at the "Achilles' heel" of the tumor. A greater understanding of these molecular alterations has already led to the development of pharmacological inhibitors and modulators currently being tested in clinical trials in patients with gliomas.

Recent genome-wide molecular classifications have provided a better understanding of the molecular genetics of glioblastoma, and research has focused on molecularly targeted therapies that specifically target unique tumor aberrations.[11] These targeted therapies are directed at receptor tyrosine kinases and their intracellular signaling pathways such as EGFR, PDGFR, mTOR, and VEGF, all of which have been identified as being important for sustaining glioma growth, proliferation, and angiogenesis. Clinical trials are gleaning important information about the biology and characteristics of tumors that respond to particular therapies. However, single-agent targeted therapies have not been effective, and further efforts must concentrate on combination therapies, as well as other novel targets such as angiogenesis, and on glioma stem-like cells.

Editor's Note

We learned from the important foundations of The Cancer Genome Atlas study that the vast majority of high-grade gliomas have molecular alterations in three critical pathways, namely p53, RB, and Ras or PI3K. In fact, over 80% of glioblastomas have defects in these three pathways, which

suggests that therapeutic targets can be developed to alter these pathways and suppress the growth promoting capabilities of various components of these pathways. Yet to date, this information has been more for diagnosis and prognosis than for a beneficial effect with regard to therapy. The reason for this is that no one pathway holds the key to success, and it certainly appears as if neuro-oncologists will have to target several of these components simultaneously, which could result in increased toxicity. That said, it appears that the field continues to make significant progress with our understanding of glioma biology as it relates to potential new therapeutic targets.

The latest critical pathway in the glioma field has to do with the IDH mutation and its metabolic consequences, which alter the biology of certain gliomas. Whether or not blocking the by-product of the IDH mutation, namely hydroxyglutarate, can have a beneficial effect on slowing growth or preventing transformation, remains to be seen. Certainly at the present time the overarching benefit in neuro-oncology has been in the ability to better classify on a molecular basis these tumors and enable us to better predict how these lesions will behave. Despite the early disappointment with targeted therapies, this is a field that will dominate neuro-oncology in the next several decades and should be very exciting to watch. (Berger)

References

1. Theeler BJ, Yung WK, Fuller GN, De Groot JF. Moving toward molecular classification of diffuse gliomas in adults. Neurology 2012;79:1917–1926
2. Westermark B. Glioblastoma—a moving target. Ups J Med Sci 2012;117:251–256
3. Tanaka S, Louis DN, Curry WT, Batchelor TT, Dietrich J. Diagnostic and therapeutic avenues for glioblastoma: no longer a dead end? Nat Rev Clin Oncol 2013;10:14–26
4. Liang Y, Diehn M, Watson N, et al. Gene expression profiling reveals molecularly and clinically distinct subtypes of glioblastoma multiforme. Proc Natl Acad Sci U S A 2005;102:5814–5819
5. Verhaak RG, Hoadley KA, Purdom E, et al; Cancer Genome Atlas Research Network. Integrated genomic analysis identifies clinically relevant subtypes of glioblastoma characterized by abnormalities in PDGFRA, IDH1, EGFR, and NF1. Cancer Cell 2010;17:98–110
6. Phillips HS, Kharbanda S, Chen R, et al. Molecular subclasses of high-grade glioma predict prognosis, delineate a pattern of disease progression, and resemble stages in neurogenesis. Cancer Cell 2006;9:157–173
7. Cancer Genome Atlas Research Network. Comprehensive genomic characterization defines human glioblastoma genes and core pathways. Nature 2008;455:1061–1068
8. Hartmann C, Hentschel B, Wick W, et al. Patients with IDH1 wild type anaplastic astrocytomas exhibit worse prognosis than IDH1-mutated glioblastomas, and IDH1 mutation status accounts for the unfavorable prognostic effect of higher age: implications for classification of gliomas. Acta Neuropathol 2010;120:707–718
9. Noushmehr H, Weisenberger DJ, Diefes K, et al; Cancer Genome Atlas Research Network. Identification of a CpG island methylator phenotype that defines a distinct subgroup of glioma. Cancer Cell 2010;17:510–522
10. Turcan S, Rohle D, Goenka A, et al. IDH1 mutation is sufficient to establish the glioma hypermethylator phenotype. Nature 2012;483:479–483
11. Thaker NG, Pollack IF. Molecularly targeted therapies for malignant glioma: rationale for combinatorial strategies. Expert Rev Neurother 2009;9:1815–1836
12. Kleihues P, Cavenee WK, and International Agency for Research on Cancer. Pathology and Genetics of Tumours of the Nervous System. World Health Organization Classification of Tumours. Lyon: IARC Press, 2000:314
13. Hegi ME, Rajakannu P, Weller M. Epidermal growth factor receptor: a re-emerging target in glioblastoma. Curr Opin Neurol 2012;25:774–779
14. Wong AJ, Bigner SH, Bigner DD, Kinzler KW, Hamilton SR, Vogelstein B. Increased expression of the epidermal growth factor receptor gene in malignant gliomas is invariably associated with gene amplification. Proc Natl Acad Sci U S A 1987;84:6899–6903
15. van den Bent MJ, Brandes AA, Rampling R, et al. Randomized phase II trial of erlotinib versus temozolomide or carmustine in recurrent glioblastoma: EORTC brain tumor group study 26034. J Clin Oncol 2009;27:1268–1274
16. Mellinghoff IK, Wang MY, Vivanco I, et al. Molecular determinants of the response of glioblastomas to EGFR kinase inhibitors. N Engl J Med 2005;353:2012–2024

17. Hermanson M, Funa K, Hartman M, et al. Platelet-derived growth factor and its receptors in human glioma tissue: expression of messenger RNA and protein suggests the presence of autocrine and paracrine loops. Cancer Res 1992;52:3213–3219

18. Wen PY, Yung WK, Lamborn KR, et al. Phase I/II study of imatinib mesylate for recurrent malignant gliomas: North American Brain Tumor Consortium Study 99-08. Clin Cancer Res 2006;12:4899–4907

19. Reardon DA, Dresemann G, Taillibert S, et al. Multicentre phase II studies evaluating imatinib plus hydroxyurea in patients with progressive glioblastoma. Br J Cancer 2009;101:1995–2004

20. Brooks AN, Kilgour E, Smith PD. Molecular pathways: fibroblast growth factor signaling: a new therapeutic opportunity in cancer. Clin Cancer Res 2012;18:1855–1862

21. Singh D, Chan JM, Zoppoli P, et al. Transforming fusions of FGFR and TACC genes in human glioblastoma. Science 2012;337:1231–1235

22. Burgart LJ, Robinson RA, Haddad SF, Moore SA. Oncogene abnormalities in astrocytomas: EGF-R gene alone appears to be more frequently amplified and rearranged compared with other protooncogenes. Mod Pathol 1991;4:183–186

23. Guha A, Feldkamp MM, Lau N, Boss G, Pawson A. Proliferation of human malignant astrocytomas is dependent on Ras activation. Oncogene 1997;15:2755–2765

24. Freed E, Symons M, Macdonald SG, McCormick F, Ruggieri R. Binding of 14-3-3 proteins to the protein kinase Raf and effects on its activation. Science 1994;265:1713–1716

25. Jane EP, Premkumar DR, Pollack IF. Coadministration of sorafenib with rottlerin potently inhibits cell proliferation and migration in human malignant glioma cells. J Pharmacol Exp Ther 2006;319:1070–1080

26. Wilhelm SM, Carter C, Tang L, et al. BAY 43-9006 exhibits broad spectrum oral antitumor activity and targets the RAF/MEK/ERK pathway and receptor tyrosine kinases involved in tumor progression and angiogenesis. Cancer Res 2004;64:7099–7109

27. Engelman, JA. Targeting PI3K signalling in cancer: opportunities, challenges and limitations. Nat Rev Cancer 2009;9(8):550–562

28. Chakravarti A, Zhai G, Suzuki Y, et al. The prognostic significance of phosphatidylinositol 3-kinase pathway activation in human gliomas. J Clin Oncol 2004;22:1926–1933

29. Newton HB. Molecular neuro-oncology and development of targeted therapeutic strategies for brain tumors. Part 2: PI3K/Akt/PTEN, mTOR, SHH/PTCH and angiogenesis. Expert Rev Anticancer Ther 2004;4: 105–128

30. Cardone MH, Roy N, Stennicke HR, et al. Regulation of cell death protease caspase-9 by phosphorylation. Science 1998;282:1318–1321

31. Cross DA, Alessi DR, Cohen P, Andjelkovich M, Hemmings BA. Inhibition of glycogen synthase kinase-3 by insulin mediated by protein kinase B. Nature 1995;378:785–789

32. Vivanco I, Sawyers CL. The phosphatidylinositol 3-Kinase AKT pathway in human cancer. Nat Rev Cancer 2002;2:489–501

33. Galanis E, Buckner JC, Maurer MJ, et al; North Central Cancer Treatment Group. Phase II trial of temsirolimus (CCI-779) in recurrent glioblastoma multiforme: a North Central Cancer Treatment Group Study. J Clin Oncol 2005;23:5294–5304

34. Kreisl TN, Lassman AB, Mischel PS, et al. A pilot study of everolimus and gefitinib in the treatment of recurrent glioblastoma (GBM). J Neurooncol 2009;92:99–105

35. Sun SY, Rosenberg LM, Wang X, et al. Activation of Akt and eIF4E survival pathways by rapamycin-mediated mammalian target of rapamycin inhibition. Cancer Res 2005;65:7052–7058

36. Dunn GP, Rinne ML, Wykosky J, et al. Emerging insights into the molecular and cellular basis of glioblastoma. Genes Dev 2012;26:756–784

37. Iwanami A, Gini B, Zanca C, et al. PML mediates glioblastoma resistance to mammalian target of rapamycin (mTOR)-targeted therapies. Proc Natl Acad Sci U S A 2013;110:4339–4344

38. Couldwell WT, Uhm JH, Antel JP, Yong VW. Enhanced protein kinase C activity correlates with the growth rate of malignant gliomas in vitro. Neurosurgery 1991;29:880–886, discussion 886–887

39. Yoshiji H, Kuriyama S, Ways DK, et al. Protein kinase C lies on the signaling pathway for vascular endothelial growth factor-mediated tumor development and angiogenesis. Cancer Res 1999;59:4413–4418

40. da Rocha AB, Mans DR, Regner A, Schwartsmann G. Targeting protein kinase C: new therapeutic opportunities against high-grade malignant gliomas? Oncologist 2002;7:17–33

41. Marais R, Light Y, Mason C, Paterson H, Olson MF, Marshall CJ. Requirement of Ras-GTP-Raf complexes for activation of Raf-1 by protein kinase C. Science 1998;280:109–112

42. Brandes AA, Ermani M, Turazzi S, et al. Procarbazine and high-dose tamoxifen as a second-line regimen in recurrent high-grade gliomas: a phase II study. J Clin Oncol 1999;17:645–650

43. Spence AM, Peterson RA, Scharnhorst JD, Silbergeld DL, Rostomily RC. Phase II study of concurrent continuous Temozolomide (TMZ) and Tamoxifen (TMX) for recurrent malignant astrocytic gliomas. J Neurooncol 2004;70:91–95

44. Graff JR, McNulty AM, Hanna KR, et al. The protein kinase Cbeta-selective inhibitor, Enzastaurin (LY317615.HCl), suppresses signaling through the AKT pathway, induces apoptosis, and suppresses growth of human colon cancer and glioblastoma xenografts. Cancer Res 2005; 65:7462–7469

45. Sidransky D, Mikkelsen T, Schwechheimer K, Rosenblum ML, Cavanee W, Vogelstein B. Clonal expansion of p53 mutant cells is associated with brain tumour progression. Nature 1992;355:846–847

46. Vousden KH, Lane DP. p53 in health and disease. Nat Rev Mol Cell Biol 2007;8:275–283

47. Gomez-Manzano C, Fueyo J, Jiang H, et al. Mechanisms underlying PTEN regulation of vascular endothelial growth factor and angiogenesis. Ann Neurol 2003;53:109–117

48. Norden AD, Drappatz J, Wen PY. Antiangiogenic therapies for high-grade glioma. Nat Rev Neurol 2009;5:610–620

49. Kerbel RS. Tumor angiogenesis. N Engl J Med 2008;358:2039–2049

50. Friedman HS, Prados MD, Wen PY, et al. Bevacizumab alone and in combination with irinotecan in recurrent glioblastoma. J Clin Oncol 2009;27:4733–4740

51. Gilbert M, et al. RTOG 0825: Phase III double-blind placebo-controlled trial evaluating bevacizumab (Bev) in patients (Pts) with newly diagnosed glioblastoma (GBM). J Clin Oncol 2013;31:3

52. Henriksson R, et al. Progression-free survival (PFS) and health-related quality of life (HRQoL) in AVAglio, a phase III study of bevacizumab (Bv), temozolomide (T), and radiotherapy (RT) in newly diagnosed glioblastoma (GBM). J Clin Oncol 2013;31: (suppl; abstr 2005^)

53. Taal W, Annemiek ME, Walenkamp L, et al. A randomized phase II study of bevacizumab versus bevacizumab plus lomustine versus lomustine single agent in recurrent glioblastoma: the Dutch BELOB study. J Clin Oncol 2013;31(Suppl; abstr)

54. Sathornsumetee S, Desjardins A, Vredenburgh JJ, et al. Phase II trial of bevacizumab and erlotinib in patients with recurrent malignant glioma. Neuro-oncol 2010;12:1300–1310

55. Gerstner ER, Eichler AF, Plotkin SR, et al. Phase I trial with biomarker studies of vatalanib (PTK787) in patients with newly diagnosed glioblastoma treated with enzyme inducing anti-epileptic drugs and standard radiation and temozolomide. J Neurooncol 2011;103:325–332

56. Brandes AA, Stupp R, Hau P, et al. EORTC study 26041-22041: phase I/II study on concomitant and adjuvant temozolomide (TMZ) and radiotherapy (RT) with PTK787/ZK222584 (PTK/ZK) in newly diagnosed glioblastoma. Eur J Cancer 2010;46:348–354

57. de Groot JF, Lamborn KR, Chang SM, et al. Phase II study of aflibercept in recurrent malignant glioma: a North American Brain Tumor Consortium study. J Clin Oncol 2011;29:2689–2695

58. Reardon DA, Fink KL, Mikkelsen T, et al. Randomized phase II study of cilengitide, an integrin-targeting arginine-glycine-aspartic acid peptide, in recurrent glioblastoma multiforme. J Clin Oncol 2008;26:5610–5617

59. De Groot JF, et al. A phase II study of XL184 in patients (pts) with progressive glioblastoma multiforme (GBM) in first or second relapse. J Clin Oncol 2009;27

60. Drappatz J, Norden AD, Wong ET, et al. Phase I study of vandetanib with radiotherapy and temozolomide for newly diagnosed glioblastoma. Int J Radiat Oncol Biol Phys 2010;78:85–90

61. Neyns B, Sadones J, Chaskis C, et al. Phase II study of sunitinib malate in patients with recurrent high-grade glioma. J Neurooncol 2011;103:491–501

62. Stommel JM, Kimmelman AC, Ying H, et al. Coactivation of receptor tyrosine kinases affects the response of tumor cells to targeted therapies. Science 2007;318:287–290

63. Chang S, et al. Phase I/II study of erlotinib and temsirolimus for patients with recurrent malignant gliomas (MG) (NABTC 04–02). J Clin Oncol 2009;27:15s

64. Peereboom DM, Ahluwalia MS, Ye X, et al; New Approaches to Brain Tumor Therapy Consortium. NABTT 0502: a phase II and pharmacokinetic study of erlotinib and sorafenib for patients with progressive or recurrent glioblastoma multiforme. Neuro-oncol 2013;15:490–496

65. Hainsworth JD, Ervin T, Friedman E, et al. Concurrent radiotherapy and temozolomide followed by temozolomide and sorafenib in the first-line treatment of patients with glioblastoma multiforme. Cancer 2010;116:3663–3669

66. Gray SG, Ekström TJ. The human histone deacetylase family. Exp Cell Res 2001;262:75–83

67. Friday BB, Anderson SK, Buckner J, et al. Phase II trial of vorinostat in combination with bortezomib in recurrent glioblastoma: a north central cancer treatment group study. Neuro-oncol 2012;14:215–221

68. Phuphanich S, Supko JG, Carson KA, et al. Phase 1 clinical trial of bortezomib in adults with recurrent malignant glioma. J Neurooncol 2010;100:95–103

69. Prensner JR, Chinnaiyan AM. Metabolism unhinged: IDH mutations in cancer. Nat Med 2011;17:291–293

70. Yan, H, et al. IDH1 and IDH2 mutations in gliomas. N Engl J Med, 2009;360(8):765–773

71. Rohle D, Popovici-Muller J, Palaskas N, et al. An inhibitor of mutant IDH1 delays growth and promotes differentiation of glioma cells. Science 2013;340:626–630

72. Dietrich J, Diamond EL, Kesari S. Glioma stem cell signaling: therapeutic opportunities and challenges. Expert Rev Anticancer Ther 2010;10:709–722

73. Hovinga KE, Shimizu F, Wang R, et al. Inhibition of notch signaling in glioblastoma targets cancer stem cells via an endothelial cell intermediate. Stem Cells 2010;28:1019–1029

74. Colman H, Zhang L, Sulman EP, et al. A multigene predictor of outcome in glioblastoma. Neuro-oncol 2010;12:49–57

75. Anido J, Sáez-Borderías A, Gonzàlez-Juncà A, et al. TGF-b Receptor Inhibitors Target the CD44(high)/Id1(high) Glioma-Initiating Cell Population in Human Glioblastoma. Cancer Cell 2010;18:655–668

76. Carro MS, Lim WK, Alvarez MJ, et al. The transcriptional network for mesenchymal transformation of brain tumours. Nature 2010;463:318–325

22 Immunobiology and Immune Therapy

Bryan D. Choi, Peter E. Fecci, and John H. Sampson

Glioblastoma multiforme (GBM) is the most common and most aggressive primary malignant brain tumor. Despite numerous advances in therapy, including image-guided surgical resection, high-dose external beam radiotherapy, antiangiogenic treatments, and chemotherapy, patients with GBM generally live less than 15 months from the time of diagnosis.[1] Moreover, these treatments are often nonspecific and result in incapacitating damage to surrounding normal brain and systemic tissues. A promising alternative is the use of the immune system, which has the theoretical capacity to eliminate neoplastic cells while leaving healthy cells intact. Although first proposed over a century ago, the concept of antitumor immunotherapy has historically struggled to successfully translate effective treatments for patients with cancer. This changed dramatically in 2010 after pivotal approvals by the Food and Drug Administration for immune-based cancer treatments, sipuleucel-T and ipilimumab,[2] in the treatment of hormone-refractory prostate cancer and metastatic melanoma, respectively. Moreover, in human brain tumors, several novel tumor-specific antigens have been identified,[3–7] lending further credence to the advancement of immunotherapy as a standard-of-care treatment for GBM. A number of approaches are currently in development toward this end, and a broad understanding of their applications, particularly in the context of intracerebral tumors, represents an emerging priority.

Pearl

- After several decades, the long-standing goal of activating the immune system for therapeutic benefit in cancer has recently been proven in clinical trials to yield significant survival benefits in patients with malignant disease.

■ Central Nervous System Immune Privilege

One of the most prominent challenges that has hampered the successful translation of immunotherapies for intracerebral tumors is that of central nervous system (CNS) immune privilege. The notion of limited immune surveillance in the CNS was suggested by several studies in the early 20th century, and was perhaps most clearly demonstrated in 1948 by Sir Peter Medawar, who showed that allogeneic tissue grafts were not rejected following transplantation into the brains of exper-

imental animals. Over the decades that followed, additional work would suggest that these findings were likely due to several characteristics now commonly attributed to the CNS—namely, the presence of a specialized blood–brain barrier (BBB), the lack of conventional lymphatics or resident antigen-presenting cells, and generally low expression of human leukocyte antigens (HLAs) in the brain.

Although the CNS certainly exhibits aspects of immune privilege to some degree, a growing body of literature suggests that CNS isolation from the immune system is not as complete as was once believed. It is now known, for example, that CNS antigen egress occurs along cerebrospinal fluid compartments toward cervical lymph nodes, and that several resident glial cells have the capacity to mediate HLA-restricted antigen presentation as surrogate antigen-presenting cells in the brain. Moreover, despite the BBB, both antibodies[8] and immune cells have been shown to penetrate and contribute to routine immune surveillance throughout the CNS. Intracerebral immune access is perhaps most convincingly demonstrated by the presence of tumor-infiltrating lymphocytes in patients with GBM and the positive association between intratumoral T cells and clinical outcome.[9] Importantly, deterioration of the BBB has also been well documented in the setting of glioma, which may contribute to the freer penetration of immune cells, especially in areas of frank neural inflammation.

As alluded to above, large molecules such as antibodies have also been shown to localize to intracerebral tumors.[8] In addition to tumor-mediated BBB disruption, one leading explanation for this phenomenon is the emerging "antigen-sink hypothesis," which states that antibodies and other macromolecules can accumulate beyond the BBB in the proximity of their cognate antigen, if and only if this cognate antigen is not also expressed in other tissues outside the CNS. Because basal levels of nonspecific peripherally circulating antibodies can be detected in the CNS under normal conditions (between 0.1% and 1% of that found in serum), it is thought that, in the absence of cross-reactivity with systemic antigens, small amounts of highly tumor-specific proteins will penetrate the CNS through passive diffusion, and be retained there over time to reach therapeutically relevant quantities. This theory has been corroborated by studies in which systemic infusion with a monoclonal antibody against a tumor-specific mutant of the epidermal growth factor receptor, EGFRvIII, resulted in elevated levels of intracerebral uptake in patients with GBM compared to antibodies possessing cross-reactivity against systemic antigen (**Fig. 22.1**).[10] Moreover, vaccine-induced humoral immunity to EGFRvIII has been shown to lead to com-

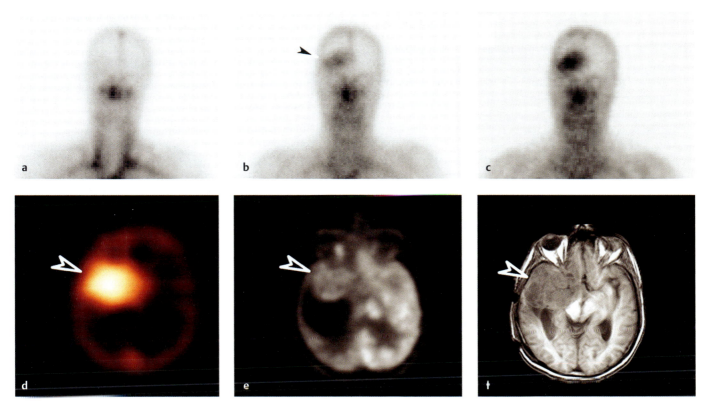

Fig. 22.1a–f Targeting of glioma by radiolabeled chimeric monoclonal antibody directed against the EGFRvIII tumor antigen. (**a–c**) Planar images of the head and neck obtained on (**a**) day 0, (**b**) day 3, and (**c**) day 7 after infusion of ^{111}In-ch806. Initial blood pool activity is seen on day 0, and uptake of ^{111}In-ch806 in an anaplastic astrocytoma in the right frontal lobe is evident by day 3 (*arrow*) and increases by day 7. (**d–f**) Tumor-specific uptake of ^{111}In-ch806 (*arrow*) is demonstrated in (**d**) a single photon emission computed tomography (SPECT) image of the brain, (**e**) ^{18}F-fluorodeoxyglucose positron emission tomography, and (**f**) magnetic resonance imaging (MRI). (From Scott AM, Lee FT, Tebbutt N, et al. A phase I clinical trial with monoclonal antibody ch806 targeting transitional state and mutant epidermal growth factor receptors. Proc Natl Acad Sci U S A 2007; 104:4071–4076. Reprinted with permission from Macmillan Publishers Ltd.)

Pearl

- Despite conventional notions of CNS immune privilege, growing evidence suggests that both immune cells and antibodies have the capacity to penetrate and treat tumors in the brain.

---

plete elimination of EGFRvIII expression in recurrent tumors of patients with GBM,[11] providing further evidence of the capacity of antibody responses in the periphery to mediate therapeutic effects beyond the BBB.

■ Glioma-Induced Immune Suppression

Gliomas are also known to potentiate a hostile environment that can antagonize the development of efficacious antitumor immune responses. Immune suppression in patients with

GBM is manifested by several metrics including low peripheral lymphocyte counts, depressed skin reactivity to recall antigens, and impaired T-cell function with a counterproductive Th2 cytokine skew. A number of pathways have been shown to contribute to the development of this pro-tumorigenic milieu. Like other cancers, gliomas secrete immunosuppressive cytokines including prostaglandin E_2 (PGE$_2$), transforming growth factor-β (TGF)-β, and interleukin-10 (IL-10), leading to potentiation of immune resistance through downregulation of major histocompatibility complex (MHC) expression and suppression of both normal T-cell proliferation and dendritic cell (DC) maturation.

The catabolic enzyme indoleamine 2,3-dioxygenase (IDO) has also been shown to possess immunosuppressive and tolerogenic effects in cancer, in part through the depletion of essential tryptophan stores.[12] In addition to modulation of soluble factors, specific subsets of immune regulatory cells have been cited as central mediators of tumor-associated immune suppression. Among these are tumor-associated myeloid-derived suppressor cells (MDSCs) and macrophages, as well as a subset of T cells known as regulatory T cells (T$_{regs}$), which perhaps have been most frequently implicated. Not only

Pearl

- Successful translation of immunotherapy for GBM will have to carefully account for the complex interplay among the several immune suppressive mechanisms, including tumor-secreted factors (e.g., TGF-β), cell-surface proteins (e.g., B7-H1), immunoregulatory leukocytes (e.g., T_{regs}, MDSCs), and cell-signaling pathways (e.g., STAT3), in these patients.

Table 22.1 Conserved Tumor-Specific Mutations in Brain Tumors

Protein	Mutation	Function
EGFR[10]	EGFRvIII	Constitutively activated form of EGFR, promotes cell proliferation, inhibits apoptosis, resistance to radiation and chemotherapy
BRAF[10,49]	f-BRAF	Promotes cell proliferation, differentiation, and survival
H3.3[5]	K27M, G34R/V	Implicated in chromatin remodeling and telomere architecture
IDH1[4]	R132H	Central metabolism, oxidative decarboxylation of isocitrate to 2-oxoglutarate

have T_{regs} been shown to be present in increased proportions in both the peripheral blood and tumors of patients with GBM,[13,14] but also their presence has been correlated with the overall malignant behavior of these tumors.[15] T_{regs} are known to suppress effector T-cell responses, specifically by restricting IL-2 production and inducing T-cell anergy. Importantly, T_{reg} depletion has been positively associated with enhanced immunity in patients with GBM,[16] and in vivo impairment in tumor-bearing mice has been shown to prolong survival.

Gliomas not only possess low levels of surface MHC, but also are known to express co-stimulatory inhibitory molecules that may lead to direct inhibition of immune responses.[17] These interactions may be manipulated by GBM cells to unfavorably alter signaling through immune checkpoints such as programmed cell death (PD)-1 and cytotoxic T-lymphocyte antigen (CTLA)-4. Importantly, CTLA-4 blockade has been demonstrated as an effective therapy in murine models of GBM[18] as well as in patients with melanoma brain metastases.[19] Other areas of investigation have underscored the role of signal transducer and activator of transcription-3 (STAT3) in regulating inflammatory responses. Interestingly, the STAT3 pathway in both immune cells and tumor cells has been shown to potentiate immune suppression, leading to generalized impairment of effector responses. As such, therapies designed to modulate STAT3 as well as co-stimulatory signaling[18] to enhance antitumor immune responses are among many promising therapies for GBM under current investigation.

◼ Glioma-Associated Tumor Antigens

It is likely that as immunotherapies become more potent, the risk of adverse immune side effects may increase. This is especially true for immunotherapeutic platforms designed to target glioma-associated antigens that are shared with normal, healthy brain tissue; active immunization against these antigens could escalate the risk of uncontrolled CNS autoimmunity, similar to what has been observed in preclinical models of experimental allergic encephalomyelitis (EAE). Importantly, following vaccination with tissue derived from human gliomas, lethal EAE or EAE-like toxicity has been documented both in nonhuman primates as well as in human

studies of immunotherapy for brain tumors. These results are to some degree expected, given that gliomas are known to express both normal adult and fetal brain antigens, and because several preclinical protocols are already known to produce EAE upon immunization with CNS tissue.

The risk of autoimmune toxicity represents an ongoing concern for tumor vaccines that are not carefully selected for tumor specificity. However, this issue can be avoided to some extent by redirecting immune responses against antigens that are expressed solely in gliomas and completely absent from all normal tissues. To date, a number of such antigens have been characterized (**Table 22.1**). Among these are the tumor-specific mutant protein, EGFRvIII,[10] as well as frequent and homogeneous mutations associated with isocitrate dehydrogenase 1 (IDH1).[4] More recently, conserved tumor-specific mutations in H3.3[5] and BRAF[3,20] have also been isolated as potential targets in pediatric GBM and pilocytic astrocytomas, respectively. Also notable are viral antigens unique to human cytomegalovirus (CMV), which have been shown to be expressed in a high percentage of GBM tumors but not surrounding normal brain.[21] Interestingly, although the presence of CMV proteins (e.g., IE1, pp65, gB) in gliomas has been confirmed by several independent groups, there have been occasional reports of failure to detect CMV antigen as well, likely owing to methodological differences and the low levels of CMV antigen expression associated with these tumors.[22]

In addition, several nonrecurrent tumor-specific mutations have been identified, particularly in pediatric GBM; these in-

Pitfall

- Although immunotherapeutic targeting of single tumor-specific mutations holds promise, the inherent heterogeneity of malignant gliomas may require implementation of broader approaches, which in turn must be balanced against the risk of autoimmunity against normal tissues.

clude sporadic variants in ATRX/DAXX,[5,6] TP53,[5] NF1,[7] and PDGFRA.[7] Almost certainly, advances in high-throughput genomic screening technologies will continue to reveal additional antigens that may serve as tumor-specific targets, the discovery of which would represent a potential boon for the further development of safe, effective immunotherapies for glioma.

Glioblastoma Vaccines and Immunotherapeutic Approaches

The overall goal of tumor immunotherapy is to develop or enhance immune responses against established disease, even in cases where natural immune surveillance has either failed or been rendered less effective by mechanisms of tumor-associated immune evasion. To date, a wide range of immune-based strategies have been developed toward this end. Among these are passive infusion with antibodies as well as adoptive transfer of tumor-reactive lymphocytes, cytokine-based stimulatory treatments, and an array of active immunization methods in the form of vaccines administered to elicit host immunity against tumor cells. The following subsections introduce the basic principles of several of these modalities, with a focus on major advances that have emerged from representative clinical trials.

Active Immunotherapy

Active immunotherapies seek to achieve priming of host immunity and immunologic memory against tumors through the use of vaccines (**Fig. 22.2**). Over the years, approaches to establishing active immunotherapy against brain tumors have varied widely, and in some cases have led to successful advancement toward phase III randomized studies.

Autologous Tumor Cell Vaccines

One of the oldest methods of active immunization for cancer consists of direct vaccination with tumor cells, which in some cases have been modified to increase immunogenicity. In this approach, autologous tumor cells are resected during surgery and, following inactivation by radiation, are incorporated into a vaccine to elicit immune reactivity in the individual from whom the tumor was isolated. Early clinical studies have been performed with tumor cells that have been genetically modified to enhance biological activity through increased secretion of immune-potentiating cytokines including IL-4,[23] IL-12,[24] and granulocyte-macrophage colony-stimulating factor (GM-CSF). Overall, approaches using autologous tumor cell vaccines have been shown to elicit antitumor immune responses and to be well tolerated without severe adverse events.

Compared to other methods, vaccination with whole tumor material has a distinct advantage of eliciting immune responses that are tailored to each individual tumor, thereby accounting for the broad interpatient variability and heterogeneous antigen expression associated with gliomas. However, for the same reasons, whole tumor vaccines are conversely hampered by a certain lack of methodological standardization across trials and in a technical sense, owing to the need for a significant amount of tumor tissue. Other disadvantages of using whole tumor cells include the theoretical dilution of tumor antigens by normal cellular components, and difficulties associated with isolating and characterizing antigen-specific immune responses following vaccination.

Peptide Vaccines

Peptide vaccines comprise delivery of the tumor antigen itself, often in conjunction with an immune-stimulating adjuvant. Peptide vaccines represent an especially attractive platform for active immunotherapy, given that they are relatively easy to manufacture, can be tailored to individual or mixed antigens, and can be standardized in formulations across multiple institutions. Several groups have demonstrated that peptide vaccines can be administered in the setting of malignant glioma to achieve tumor-specific immune responses in clinical trials. One notable peptide vaccine, the EGFRvIII-specific PEP-3-KLH (CDX-110) formulation, has been shown to elicit EGFRvIII-specific immune responses, leading to subsequent elimination of EGFRvIII-expressing tumor cells.[11]

Although phase 2 clinical studies of peptide vaccines against EGFRvIII and Wilms' tumor 1 (WT1)[25] have yielded encouraging results, one concern is that targeting single antigens may inadequately address the diverse and heterogeneous nature of malignant gliomas, leading to eventual outgrowth of antigen-negative recurrence and immune escape. As such, personalized vaccines in the form of several peptide combinations have been attempted, which have also demonstrated the capacity to develop specific immunity and favorable responses in clinical trials.[26] One variation on this theme is the use of vaccines composed of heat shock protein peptide complexes (HSPPCs), which are thought to deliver an array of tumor-specific antigenic peptides in a form that facilitates interaction with antigen-presenting cells. One recent HSPPC-based vaccine demonstrated promise in early clinical studies, where treatment resulted in safe immunization and extended median survival in responding patients, consistent with focal immune cell infiltration on biopsies of brain tissue.[27]

Dendritic Cell Vaccines

Dendritic cells (DCs) are antigen-presenting cells whose main function is to modulate immune responses through the processing and presenting of antigenic material to effector T cells. Given recent advances in their *ex vivo* generation and manipulation, DCs have emerged as a vaccine platform with great potential for patients with GBM. To manufacture a DC vaccine, autologous DCs are harvested from peripheral blood or bone

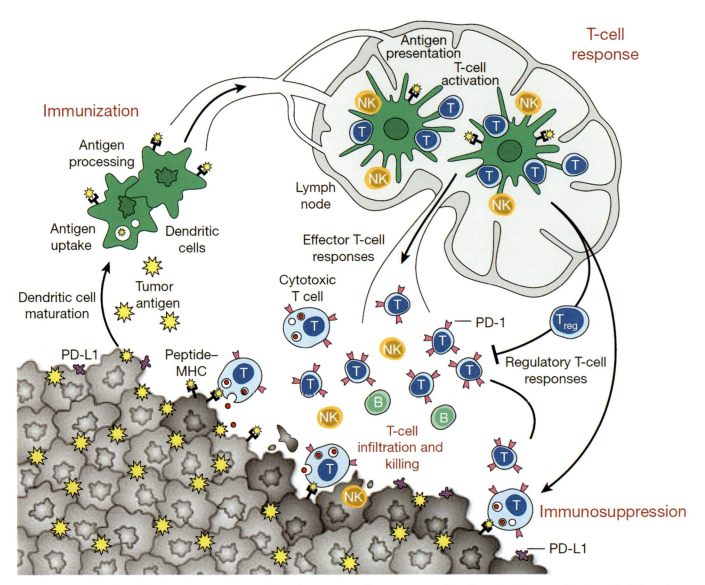

Fig. 22.2 Understanding the events in generating and regulating antitumor immunity suggests at least three sites for therapeutic intervention: promoting the antigen presentation functions of dendritic cells, promoting the production of protective T-cell responses, and overcoming immunosuppression in the tumor bed. Antitumor immune responses must begin with the capture of tumor-associated antigens by dendritic cells, either delivered exogenously or captured from dead or dying tumor cells. The dendritic cells process the captured antigen for presentation or cross-presentation on major histocompatibility complex (MHC) class II or class I molecules, respectively, and migrate to draining lymph nodes. If capture and presentation occurred in the presence of an immunogenic maturation stimulus, dendritic cells will elicit anticancer effector T-cell responses in the lymph node; if no such stimulus was received, dendritic cells will instead induce tolerance, leading to T-cell deletion, anergy, or the production of T_{reg} cells. In the lymph node, antigen presentation to T cells will elicit a response depending on the type of dendritic cell maturation stimulus received and on the interaction of T-cell co-stimulatory molecules with their surface receptors on dendritic cells. Thus, interaction of CD28 or OX40 with CD80/86 or OX40L will promote potentially protective T-cell responses, whereas interaction of CTLA4 with CD80/86 or PD-1 with PD-L1/PD-L2 will suppress T-cell responses, and possibly promote T_{reg} formation. Antigen-educated T cells (along with B cells and natural killer [NK] cells) will exit the lymph node and enter the tumor bed, where a host of immunosuppressive defense mechanisms can be produced by tumors (or infiltrating myeloid cells) that oppose effector T-cell function. These include the upregulation of PD-L1/L2 on the cancer cell surface, release of prostaglandin E_2 (PGE$_2$), arginase, and indoleamine 2,3-dioxygenase (IDO), which are all T-cell suppressors, and the release of vascular endothelial growth factor (VEGF) (triggered in part by intratumoral hypoxia), which inhibits T-cell diapedesis from the vasculature, and thus infiltration into the tumor bed. (From Mellman I, Coukos G, Dranoff G. Cancer immunotherapy comes of age. Nature 2011;480:480–489. Reprinted with permission from Macmillan Publishers Ltd. Copyright 2011.)

marrow and exposed in vitro to tumor antigens in the form of tumor homogenate, peptides, or even genetic material encoding antigens of interest, prior to injection back into the patient. Several clinical trials have demonstrated that DCs loaded with tumor homogenate or lysate are well tolerated,[28,29] and may be complemented by certain adjuvant therapies (e.g., Toll-like receptor agonists)[30] to produce antitumor T-cell responsiveness. In addition, recent efforts to integrate tumor-pulsed DC vaccines with standard postoperative care have met with early success.[31]

Instead of whole tumor lysate, peptides have also been used as an alternative source of antigenic material for the DC vaccine platform. One notable peptide-based DC vaccine targeting EGFRvIII has successfully demonstrated the capacity to elicit EGFRvIII-specific immune responses without serious adverse events.[10] Other studies of peptide-pulsed DC vaccines include DCs loaded with multi-epitope antigen formulations either through the use of acid-eluted, tumor-associated MHC class I peptides[32,33] or synthetic peptide combinations; recent examples of the latter have targeted glioma-associated antigens including HER2, TRP-2, EphA2, IL-1Rα2, AIM-2, YKL-40, and gp100,[34,35] in one case administered in a formulation with polyinosinic-polycytidylic acid stabilized by lysine and carboxymethylcellulose (poly-ICLC).[35] Lastly, efforts have also been developed to elicit antitumor immune responses using DCs loaded with autologous, tumor-antigen–encoding RNA; early clinical trials using this strategy have demonstrated safety and feasibility, particularly in the setting of pediatric brain cancers.[36,37]

Adoptive Immunotherapy

In general, adoptive immunotherapy refers to the ex vivo activation and expansion of immune cells, which are then administered to treat patients through intratumoral or intravenous infusion. To date, the most encouraging results for CNS tumors have been achieved in the setting of melanoma brain metastases, where adoptive transfer of either autologous tumor-infiltrating lymphocytes (TILs) or T-cells genetically modified to target tumor antigens resulted in complete response rates of 41% and 22%, respectively.[38] In addition, chimeric antigen receptors (CARs), which consist of surface-expressed antibody-derived fragments translated in tandem with intracellular T-cell signaling domains, have also been shown to mediate antitumor activity against intracranial neuroblastoma.[39] Despite this promise, adoptive transfer therapies for high-grade glioma have not yet realized this level of success.

Historically, clinical trials of adoptive immunotherapy for glioma have attempted transfer of various cell types including lymphokine-activated killer (LAK) cells as well as cytotoxic T lymphocytes (CTLs) that have been isolated from expanded tumor-infiltrating lymphocytes (TIL) or lymph nodes from vaccinated patients. Although several groups have demonstrated

> **Special Consideration**
>
> - Several strategies that seek to induce potent antitumor immune responses are currently under evaluation for CNS malignancies. These include passive administration of antibodies, adoptive transfer of tumor-specific lymphocytes, and active immunotherapy platforms that rely on endogenous responses to tumor antigen in the form of tumor lysate, peptides, and cell-based vaccines.

the general feasibility of these approaches, therapeutic outcomes have been relatively modest, especially when taking into account the high levels of antitumor cytotoxicity observed during corresponding preclinical studies in vitro. As such, current efforts seek to elucidate additional factors that may refine the translation of adoptive transfer therapies in vivo; among them are the identification of specific effector cell phenotypes predictive of antitumor responses, as well as improvements to enhance persistence of infused cells, either through host-conditioning lymphodepletive regimens or the concomitant use of homeostatic cytokines (e.g., IL-7, IL-15).

Clinical Trial Design

One challenge in the translation of antitumor immunotherapy has been the absence of a methodological framework specifically designed for early-phase clinical studies of immune-based treatments. Interestingly, clinical trials in immunotherapy have historically followed paradigms similar to those that have been established for chemotherapy. However, this is probably inappropriate, given the vast dissimilarities between the two forms of treatment with regard to their respective mechanisms of action and other pharmacodynamic properties. For instance, unlike chemotherapy, immune-based antitumor vaccines often do not have an identifiable maximum tolerated dose (MTD); instead, they frequently seek to identify a maximum *feasible* dose, based on the amount of "drug" that can be manufactured from limited biological material. On a practical level, it should also be noted that when using standard dose-escalation designs (e.g., classical 3 + 3 study), the probability of dose escalation exceeds 90% even when potential toxicity rates are approximately 10%.[40] Thus, the chance of dose escalation is exceedingly high in immunotherapy trials, wherein limiting toxicity is seldom observed at elevated rates. This should be considered along with the finding that administered doses in immunotherapy typically do not ostensibly correlate with clinical efficacy or magnitude of antitumor immune responses. Together, these factors support the emerging idea that traditional dose-escalation designs in phase I studies may not provide the most appropriate approach for obtaining relevant early-phase clinical data in the setting of immunotherapy.[40]

Assessing Response to Immunotherapy

It is also evident that methods by which clinical outcomes are assessed following immunotherapy add another layer of complexity to the accurate interpretation of clinical trial data. This is partly due to the fact that, in this setting, clinical outcomes can be delayed and in some cases may occur even after imaging evidence of tumor progression. Along these lines, a notable observation in immunotherapy trials has been the seemingly incongruous finding in some patients of unaltered time to progression, yet improved overall survival.[41] Because this scenario is considered unusual for chemotherapies and other directly cytotoxic therapies, World Health Organization (WHO) or Response Evaluation Criteria in Solid Tumors (RECIST) criteria have traditionally mandated such outcomes should be labeled progressive disease (PD), which, due to certain conventions has become synonymous with drug failure. However, in the setting of immune therapy, these assessments may be suboptimal, not only because they have the potential to dilute observed therapeutic effects but also to completely cease experimental therapy that might otherwise yield objective clinical benefit. One example showcasing this discrepancy between overall survival and PD is the randomized placebo-controlled phase 3 trial of sipuleucel-T, which initially failed to meet its primary end point of progression-free survival yet demonstrated evidence of improved overall survival (25.8 months versus 21.7 months; $p = 0.032$), and which was ultimately confirmed in a follow-up study.[42] Similarly, a randomized controlled phase 3 trial of ipilimumab for metastatic melanoma also led to improved overall survival in the absence of concomitantly prolonged time to progression.[2]

These inconsistencies are further confounded by the fact that quantifying imaging changes in patients with brain tumors has proven to be technically challenging owing both to irregularities intrinsic to resection cavities[43] as well as to the criteria by which these changes have traditionally been assessed.[44,45] It has become apparent, for instance, that metrics relying heavily on contrast-enhancing components of tumor do not accurately portray transient changes associated with pseudoprogression, and in addition, fail to account for non-enhancing components of tumor frequently observed upon treatment with antiangiogenic agents. Standardization of response assessment criteria continues to be an active area of research,[46] and ongoing discussions draw greater attention to whether assessment of immune-based treatments might be adjusted to better detect significant responses.[47]

In an effort to collectively reconcile these potential issues, groups such as the Cancer Immunotherapy Consortium of the Cancer Research Institute have designed and implemented more appropriate immune-response criteria to be applied specifically during immunotherapy trials. Importantly, in order to foster more accurate alignment between clinical outcome (i.e., overall survival) and radiographic metrics of tumor progression, these new criteria broaden the types of observed patterns in tumor growth that might qualify a significant re-

Controversy

- Recent clinical trial data for sipuleucel-T and ipilimumab demonstrated discrepancies wherein benefits in overall survival were achieved despite unaltered time to progression. Thus, systematic frameworks for assessing immune-related responses are currently being developed and seek to capture additional response patterns—even those that occur after initial evidence of tumor progression—beyond those originally described by WHO or RECIST.

sponse to therapy. Although not yet universally accepted, these criteria continue to expand in recognition and use.

Considerations for Immune Monitoring

Owing to the inherent variability associated with survival end points, clinical studies of immunotherapy for glioma have historically focused on measures of immunity as surrogates for objective clinical response. Several immunologic assays have been employed for this purpose, including delayed-type hypersensitivity (DTH) reactions, enzyme-linked immunosorbent spot (ELISpot), tetramer analysis, lymphoproliferative assays, intracellular cytokine staining (ICS), and an array of in vitro cytotoxicity assays thought to be predictive of antitumor efficacy in vivo. Although they have certainly provided valuable insight, none of these metrics have been universally validated to date, largely due to their inability to consistently correlate with clinical outcomes. Numerous efforts are underway to establish alternative markers for antitumor immunotherapy; however, until these parameters are fully validated, care should be taken to avoid overinterpretation of immunologic surrogate data.

It is reasonable to speculate that given current shortcomings, immune monitoring will likely transition from a predominant focus on T-cell responses to a broader, more global view of host immunity. For instance, increasing attention may be placed on previously neglected immune cell types including monocytes, natural killer cells, and other effectors that may favorably contribute to antitumor immunity. Moreover, efforts to assess the immunologic status of the brain tumor microenvironment—as opposed to analyses limited to cells present in peripheral blood—may also reveal predictive data that have been underappreciated to date.

Importantly, it should be noted that past failures in immune monitoring may be as much a result of technical limitations as they are a result of incomplete scientific understanding. That is to say, currently available immune assays (e.g., ELISpot, ICS, etc.) have been shown to suffer from significant methodological inconsistencies between laboratories, leading to a state of generalized variability and unreliability in the interpretation of immune response data.[48] To address this issue, recent studies have developed tools for assay harmonization that would implement widespread adoption of standard operating procedures; such efforts have been shown to significantly mitigate several of these inconsistencies[49] and thus should be strongly considered for integration into future plans for clinical development.

Translation Through Phase 2 Clinical Trials

Translation of immunotherapies beyond early phase 1/2 studies for malignant brain tumors has yet to enjoy widespread success. Perhaps one of the greatest barriers to the development of novel therapeutics is the current fiscal climate of the pharmaceutical industry, which has increasingly favored drugs that not only can be sold at extraordinarily high prices but also can be recommended for use in large patient populations. Unfortunately, these factors have contributed to the notion that developing drugs or biologics solely for patients with GBM may be less attractive. Moreover, financial pressures from investors are similarly causing pharmaceutical companies to shift their focus away from early drug discovery and development, placing the onus on investigators to accrue the necessary capital for expensive, randomized clinical studies to attract stakeholders capable of sponsoring phase 3 trials. Unfortunately, current funding levels from the National Institutes of Health have generally not been sufficient to enable investigators to complete investigational new drug applications and adequately powered early-phase clinical trials, which together often require an excess of $1 million, excluding costs associated with manufacture of the therapeutic agent itself. Thus, the development of alternative methods to subsidize and support effective translation for brain tumor therapies should be an emergent priority.

◾ Conclusion

Given recent progress toward approval for other tumors, the use of immunotherapy to treat malignant glioma may provide a promising option for future study, where the need for safer, more effective treatment is great. In order to continue to advance immune-based treatments for patients with brain tumors, it will be necessary to broadly address a number of limitations that pertain especially to the treatment of tumors in the CNS. Among these are aspects of drug delivery, glioma-induced immune suppression, and methodological inconsistencies in clinical trial design. Lastly, special consideration will have to be dedicated to the use of vaccines and other immune-based treatment in the context of standard-of-care treatments, including radiation and chemotherapy. Successful treatment of these devastating CNS tumors will likely require a combinatorial, multipronged approach, and further studies will seek to elucidate the ways in which immune-based therapy might complement or even work synergistically with these existing strategies.

Editor's Note

The concept of the brain being immunologically privileged has been challenged in the last several years, and we now know that there is a reasonable degree of immune surveillance throughout the CNS. Especially considering the fact that the BBB is often disrupted in high-grade tumors, one has to consider the fact that immune cells can gain access to tumors and that an inflammatory process often ensues. Perhaps one of the most significant advances in this field is our understanding of glioma-induced immune suppression, which is a formidable foe for those interested in immune modulation and immunotherapy of gliomas. Regulatory T cells act as important immunosuppressing components, and these clearly have been shown to be capable of modulation, thus improving the inflammatory response. The other confounding variable is that there are numerous glioma-associated tumor antigens, thus making it difficult to use one specific antigen to produce the ultimate vaccine or immunotherapy. There have been a number of different types of glioma immunotherapy trials developed involving active immunotherapy, such as autologous tumor cell vaccines, peptide vaccines, and dendritic cell vaccines. The other approach is to utilize adoptive immunotherapy to expand an immune population of cells and then administer that to patients either intravenously or directly into the tumor. (Berger)

References

1. Stupp R, Mason WP, van den Bent MJ, et al; European Organisation for Research and Treatment of Cancer Brain Tumor and Radiotherapy Groups; National Cancer Institute of Canada Clinical Trials Group. Radiotherapy plus concomitant and adjuvant temozolomide for glioblastoma. N Engl J Med 2005;352:987–996

2. Hodi FS, O'Day SJ, McDermott DF, et al. Improved survival with ipilimumab in patients with metastatic melanoma. N Engl J Med 2010;363: 711–723

3. Jones DT, Kocialkowski S, Liu L, et al. Tandem duplication producing a novel oncogenic BRAF fusion gene defines the majority of pilocytic astrocytomas. Cancer Res 2008;68:8673–8677

4. Yan H, Parsons DW, Jin G, et al. IDH1 and IDH2 mutations in gliomas. N Engl J Med 2009;360:765–773

5. Schwartzentruber J, Korshunov A, Liu XY, et al. Driver mutations in histone H3.3 and chromatin remodelling genes in paediatric glioblastoma. Nature 2012;482:226–231

6. Heaphy CM, de Wilde RF, Jiao Y, et al. Altered telomeres in tumors with ATRX and DAXX mutations. Science 2011;333:425

7. Verhaak RG, Hoadley KA, Purdom E, et al; Cancer Genome Atlas Research Network. Integrated genomic analysis identifies clinically relevant subtypes of glioblastoma characterized by abnormalities in PDGFRA, IDH1, EGFR, and NF1. Cancer Cell 2010;17:98–110

8. Scott AM, Lee FT, Tebbutt N, et al. A phase I clinical trial with monoclonal antibody ch806 targeting transitional state and mutant epidermal growth factor receptors. Proc Natl Acad Sci U S A 2007;104:4071–4076

9. Lohr J, Ratliff T, Huppertz A, et al. Effector T-cell infiltration positively impacts survival of glioblastoma patients and is impaired by tumor-derived TGF- β. Clin Cancer Res 2011;17:4296–4308

10. Choi BD, Archer GE, Mitchell DA, et al. EGFRvIII-targeted vaccination therapy of malignant glioma. Brain Pathol 2009;19:713–723

11. Sampson JH, Heimberger AB, Archer GE, et al. Immunologic escape after prolonged progression-free survival with epidermal growth factor receptor variant III peptide vaccination in patients with newly diagnosed glioblastoma. J Clin Oncol 2010;28:4722–4729

12. Choi BD, Fecci PE, Sampson JH. Regulatory T cells move in when gliomas say "I Do". Clin Cancer Res 2012;18:6086–6088

13. Fecci PE, Mitchell DA, Whitesides JF, et al. Increased regulatory T-cell fraction amidst a diminished CD4 compartment explains cellular immune defects in patients with malignant glioma. Cancer Res 2006;66: 3294–3302

14. El Andaloussi A, Lesniak MS. An increase in CD4+CD25+FOXP3+ regulatory T cells in tumor-infiltrating lymphocytes of human glioblastoma multiforme. Neuro-oncol 2006;8:234–243

15. Heimberger AB, Kong LY, Abou-Ghazal M, et al. The role of tregs in human glioma patients and their inhibition with a novel STAT-3 inhibitor. Clin Neurosurg 2009;56:98–106

16. Sampson JH, Schmittling RJ, Archer GE, et al. A pilot study of IL-2Ra blockade during lymphopenia depletes regulatory T-cells and correlates with enhanced immunity in patients with glioblastoma. PLoS ONE 2012;7:e31046

17. Parsa AT, Waldron JS, Panner A, et al. Loss of tumor suppressor PTEN function increases B7-H1 expression and immunoresistance in glioma. Nat Med 2007;13:84–88

18. Fecci PE, Ochiai H, Mitchell DA, et al. Systemic CTLA-4 blockade ameliorates glioma-induced changes to the CD4+ T cell compartment without affecting regulatory T-cell function. Clin Cancer Res 2007;13:2158–2167

19. Margolin K, Ernstoff MS, Hamid O, et al. Ipilimumab in patients with melanoma and brain metastases: an open-label, phase 2 trial. Lancet Oncol 2012;13:459–465

20. Schindler G, Capper D, Meyer J, et al. Analysis of BRAF V600E mutation in 1,320 nervous system tumors reveals high mutation frequencies in pleomorphic xanthoastrocytoma, ganglioglioma and extra-cerebellar pilocytic astrocytoma. Acta Neuropathol 2011;121:397–405

21. Mitchell DA, Xie W, Schmittling R, et al. Sensitive detection of human cytomegalovirus in tumors and peripheral blood of patients diagnosed with glioblastoma. Neuro-oncol 2008;10:10–18

22. Sampson JH, Mitchell DA. Is cytomegalovirus a therapeutic target in glioblastoma? Clin Cancer Res 2011;17:4619–4621

23. Okada H, Pollack IF, Lotze MT, et al. Gene therapy of malignant gliomas: a phase I study of IL-4-HSV-TK gene-modified autologous tumor to elicit an immune response. Hum Gene Ther 2000;11:637–653

24. Ehtesham M, Kabos P, Kabosova A, Neuman T, Black KL, Yu JS. The use of interleukin 12-secreting neural stem cells for the treatment of intracranial glioma. Cancer Res 2002;62:5657–5663

25. Izumoto S, Tsuboi A, Oka Y, et al. Phase II clinical trial of Wilms tumor 1 peptide vaccination for patients with recurrent glioblastoma multiforme. J Neurosurg 2008;108:963–971

26. Yajima N, Yamanaka R, Mine T, et al. Immunologic evaluation of personalized peptide vaccination for patients with advanced malignant glioma. Clin Cancer Res 2005;11:5900–5911

27. Crane CA, Han SJ, Ahn B, et al. Individual patient-specific immunity against high-grade glioma after vaccination with autologous tumor derived peptides bound to the 96 KD chaperone protein. Clin Cancer Res 2013;19:205–214

28. Wheeler CJ, Black KL, Liu G, et al. Vaccination elicits correlated immune and clinical responses in glioblastoma multiforme patients. Cancer Res 2008;68:5955–5964

29. De Vleeschouwer S, Fieuws S, Rutkowski S, et al. Postoperative adjuvant dendritic cell-based immunotherapy in patients with relapsed glioblastoma multiforme. Clin Cancer Res 2008;14:3098–3104

30. Prins RM, Soto H, Konkankit V, et al. Gene expression profile correlates with T-cell infiltration and relative survival in glioblastoma patients vaccinated with dendritic cell immunotherapy. Clin Cancer Res 2011; 17:1603–1615

31. Ardon H, Van Gool S, Lopes IS, et al. Integration of autologous dendritic cell-based immunotherapy in the primary treatment for patients with newly diagnosed glioblastoma multiforme: a pilot study. J Neurooncol 2010;99:261–272

32. Yu JS, Wheeler CJ, Zeltzer PM, et al. Vaccination of malignant glioma patients with peptide-pulsed dendritic cells elicits systemic cytotoxicity and intracranial T-cell infiltration. Cancer Res 2001;61:842–847

33. Liau LM, Prins RM, Kiertscher SM, et al. Dendritic cell vaccination in glioblastoma patients induces systemic and intracranial T-cell responses modulated by the local central nervous system tumor microenvironment. Clin Cancer Res 2005;11:5515–5525

34. Phuphanich S, Wheeler CJ, Rudnick JD, et al. Phase I trial of a multiepitope-pulsed dendritic cell vaccine for patients with newly diagnosed glioblastoma. Cancer Immunol Immunother 2013;62:125–135

35. Okada H, Kalinski P, Ueda R, et al. Induction of CD8+ T-cell responses against novel glioma-associated antigen peptides and clinical activity by vaccinations with alpha-type 1 polarized dendritic cells and polyinosinic-polycytidylic acid stabilized by lysine and carboxymethylcellulose in patients with recurrent malignant glioma. J Clin Oncol 2011;29:330–336

36. Caruso DA, Orme LM, Neale AM, et al. Results of a phase 1 study utilizing monocyte-derived dendritic cells pulsed with tumor RNA in children and young adults with brain cancer. Neuro-oncol 2004;6:236–246

37. Caruso DA, Orme LM, Amor GM, et al. Results of a Phase I study utilizing monocyte-derived dendritic cells pulsed with tumor RNA in children with Stage 4 neuroblastoma. Cancer 2005;103:1280–1291

38. Hong JJ, Rosenberg SA, Dudley ME, et al. Successful treatment of melanoma brain metastases with adoptive cell therapy. Clin Cancer Res 2010;16:4892–4898

39. Pule MA, Savoldo B, Myers GD, et al. Virus-specific T cells engineered to coexpress tumor-specific receptors: persistence and antitumor activity in individuals with neuroblastoma. Nat Med 2008;14:1264–1270

40. Heimberger AB, Sampson JH. Immunotherapy coming of age: what will it take to make it standard of care for glioblastoma? Neuro-oncol 2011; 13:3–13

41. Tuma RS. Immunotherapies in clinical trials: do they demand different evaluation tools? J Natl Cancer Inst 2011;103:780–781

42. Kantoff PW, Higano CS, Shore ND, et al; IMPACT Study Investigators. Sipuleucel-T immunotherapy for castration-resistant prostate cancer. N Engl J Med 2010;363:411–422

43. Kanaly CW, Ding D, Mehta AI, et al. A novel method for volumetric MRI response assessment of enhancing brain tumors. PLoS ONE 2011;6: e16031

44. Sorensen AG, Batchelor TT, Wen PY, Zhang WT, Jain RK. Response criteria for glioma. Nat Clin Pract Oncol 2008;5:634–644

45. van den Bent MJ, Vogelbaum MA, Wen PY, Macdonald DR, Chang SM. End point assessment in gliomas: novel treatments limit usefulness of classical Macdonald's Criteria. J Clin Oncol 2009;27:2905–2908

46. Wen PY, Macdonald DR, Reardon DA, et al. Updated response assessment criteria for high-grade gliomas: response assessment in neuro-oncology working group. J Clin Oncol 2010;28:1963–1972

47. Wolchok JD, Hoos A, O'Day S, et al. Guidelines for the evaluation of immune therapy activity in solid tumors: immune-related response criteria. Clin Cancer Res 2009;15:7412–7420

48. Hoos A, Britten CM, Huber C, O'Donnell-Tormey J. A methodological framework to enhance the clinical success of cancer immunotherapy. Nat Biotechnol 2011;29:867–870

49. Hoos A, Eggermont AM, Janetzki S, et al. Improved endpoints for cancer immunotherapy trials. J Natl Cancer Inst 2010;102:1388–1397

23 Gene Therapy for Gliomas

Joseph H. Miller and James M. Markert

Malignant gliomas are aggressive neoplasms that cannot be completely resected and result in high mortality rates even with aggressive adjuvant therapy. Despite the evolution of treatment paradigms, less than 10% of patients with high-grade gliomas survive more than 5 years.[1-3] Gliomas are infiltrative tumors within the brain parenchyma but they rarely metastasize to distant locations.[4] Local inoculation of gene therapy vectors that exhibit tropism for the central nervous system (CNS) thus may be ideally suited for these tumors, and also avoids the systemic toxicity associated with current chemotherapeutic regiments.[5] A burgeoning understanding of the molecular and genetic features of gliomas has produced novel targeted gene therapies. The combined failure of the current standard of care along with promising preclinical studies has resulted in hope for discovering a clinically effective glioma gene therapy.

Initial gene therapy clinical trials began in the 1990s using retrovirus as a vector to transfect glioma cells with the herpes simplex virus type 1 (HSV1) gene thymidine kinase (TK).[4] HSV1-TK is an example of suicide gene therapy. The HSV1-TK protein phosphorylates peripherally administered ganciclovir (GCV) and, following further phosphorylation by the cellular kinase, a highly cytotoxic GCV-triphosphate (GCV-TP) is produced. This GCV-TP is highly cytotoxic as it (1) inhibits DNA polymerases, thus resulting in DNA damage and cell death; (2) is antiangiogenic; and (3) has a strong immunostimulatory effect.[6] Since gene therapy was initially attempted using this approach, numerous strategies using both viral and non-viral vectors to deliver suicide, tumor suppressor, apoptotic, and toxic genes have been employed (**Table 23.1**). Viruses have also been utilized in direct oncolytic and immunogene therapy. The successful treatment of glioblastoma multiforme (GBM) will likely require a multifaceted approach (**Fig. 23.1**).

the production of cytokines by mononuclear cells that infiltrate the tumor following HSV-TK therapy. The bystander effect was demonstrated to produce significant tumor cell death despite less than 10% transfection rates.[7] A multicenter phase 3 study randomized 248 patients with newly diagnosed GBM to receive surgical resection and radiotherapy or surgical resection, radiotherapy, and retroviral delivered HSV-TK followed by peripherally administered GCV. Unfortunately, this study found no difference in survival, safety, or time to tumor progression.[8]

The initial failures of gene therapy trials demonstrate the importance of having both an effective vector and gene therapy target. The failure of retrovirus as a vector and HSV1-TK in initial clinical trials was likely secondary to low transduction rates (a nonreplicating virus was used, and producer cells likely were rejected shortly after implantation) and low catalytic activity of HSV1-TK on GCV.[9] In a comparison of transduction rates, *lac*Z-expressing adenovirus (Ad) was found to have much higher transduction rates (11%) than the retrovirus (~4%) in a murine model of human glioma.[10] In a head-to-head clinical trial comparing Ad to retrovirus delivery of HSV-TK, a significant increase in survival was found in patients treated with adenoviral HSV-TK (15 months) versus retroviral delivered HSV-TK (7.4 month).[11] Subsequent clinical trials demonstrated the safety of HSV-TK adenoviral vectors in doses up to 2.0×10^{11} plaque-forming units (pfu, active viral particles). Above this dose, patients had severe adverse reactions, including hyponatremia, altered mental status, increased intracranial pressure, and seizure activity. Although many of these clinical trials resulted in the occasional long-term survivor and evidence of increased long-term survival,

■ Suicide Gene Therapy

Gene therapy for treatment of gliomas was pioneered by suicide gene-prodrug therapies such as the aforementioned GCV-TP. The first of these clinical trials employed a nonreplicating retrovirus to express HSV-TK. Histological studies of these early trials demonstrated low levels of transduction (< 5% of tumor cells) with improved survival confined only to the smallest tumors. The antitumor effect was hypothesized to result, at least in part, from a bystander effect mediated by

Pitfalls

- Suicide gene therapy appears to require transduction rates to be effective, but those rates have not been achieved in vivo.
- Gene catalytic activity on prodrugs requires further optimization.
- Certain preclinical models (e.g., C6 glioma) may result in artificially high antitumor immune responses.
- More than 15 suicide gene therapy trials (phases 1 to 3) have demonstrated no definitive increase in median survival.

Table 23.1 Overview of Gene Therapies

Strategy	Examples of Genes	Mechanism
Suicide gene	HSV-TK, cytosine deaminase	Gene encodes an enzyme that converts a prodrug into a toxin
Restoring apoptotic pathways	p53, retinoblastoma p16, phosphatase and tensin homologue (PTEN)	Corrects mutations in apoptotic pathways in tumor cells
Immunotherapy	GM-CSF, TNF-α, interleukins, interferons, B-7, sFlt-3-L, ICAM	Enhanced presentation of tumor antigens, and cytokines resulting in activation of tumor-killing immune cells

Abbreviations: HSV-TK, herpes simplex virus thymidine kinase; TNF, tumor necrosis factor; GM-CSF, granulocyte-macrophage colony-stimulating factor; ICAM, intercellular adhesion molecule.

no phase 3 trial has definitively shown a significant improvement in survival and tumor progression.[4,12–15] The majority of side effects were due to inflammation and malignant edema. Inflammation produced by Ad particles was at least partially responsible for the tumor response seen in these trials.[15]

The *HSV1-TK* gene used in previous human trials required a very high dose of GCV to be administered. The near-immunosuppressive doses of GCV may have offset some of the immunostimulatory effects of the *HSV1-TK* suicide gene. The mutant gene *HSV1-sr39TK* exerts a 14-fold higher catalytic

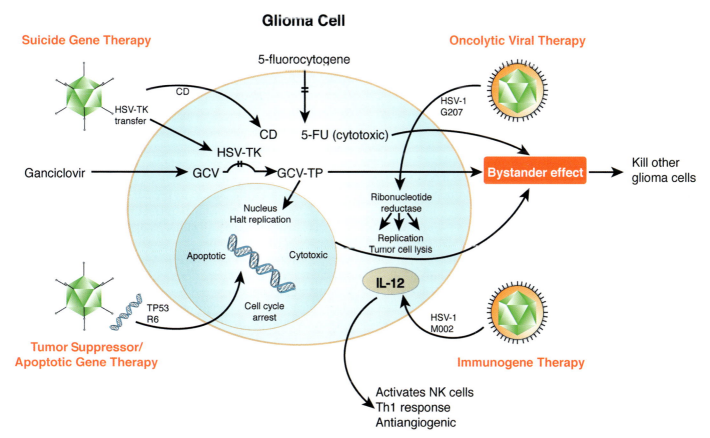

Fig. 23.1 Viral gene therapeutic approaches for gliomas fall within four categories. Suicide gene therapy (*top left*) involves HSV-TK converting peripherally administered GCV into cytotoxic GCV-TP. Tumor suppressor/apoptotic gene therapy (*bottom left*) can insert suppressor genes such as *TP53* into the nucleus. This results in cell-cycle arrest and even apoptosis. Oncolytic viral therapy using HSV-1 G207 (*top right*) leads to tumor cell lysis through viral replication, enabled by the presence of cellular ribonucleotide reductase present in trans. Immunogene (*bottom right*) therapy produces an inflammatory response through interleukins (e.g., IL-12) that can result in both cell death and, in the case of IL-12, a decrease in angiogenesis. Additionally, peripheral administered medications (prodrugs) (*top center*) can be metabolized by microbial enzymes introduced into the cell through gene therapy, allowing the local (rather than systemic) creation of a cytotoxic intermediate (5-fluorouracil [5-FU]). This schematic illustrates multiple targets within glioma cells that can be synergistically attacked to result in local and bystander cell death.

response than *HSV1-TK,* allowing for lower dosing of GCV. Pre-clinical studies in a C6 glioma model have demonstrated a stronger therapeutic efficacy. Further refinement of both the viral vector and gene may yield promising results in future clinical trials.

Cytosine deaminase (CD)-5FC is another example of a suicide gene therapy. CD is not found in mammalian cells but is expressed in certain bacteria and fungi. The enzyme has been shown to deaminate 5-fluorocytosine (5-FC) to 5-fluorouracil (5-FU), an antimetabolite that interrupts RNA and DNA synthesis. This approach may have some advantages over the HSV-TK approach because fewer cells must be transfected, as 5-FU is a small molecule that passively diffuses between cells and has enhanced cytotoxic effect on surrounding cells (bystander effect). In comparison, GCV-TP is a large molecule and is dependent on connexins for transport to adjacent cells.[16] The CD model has demonstrated effectiveness in preclinical glioma models, and a clinical trial is currently underway (clinicaltrials.gov, trial NCT01156584).[17] The vector under study, Toca 511, has important advantages, utilizing a retroviral replicating vector encoding an optimized CD, and has demonstrated a threefold prodrug catalyzation in infected cells.[18] Data available for the first three patients have not demonstrated any adverse reactions.[17]

Tumor Suppressor and Apoptotic Gene Therapy

Glioblastoma multiforme has undergone the most extensive genetic profiling of any cancer, and therapies aimed at specific mutations may result in clinically significant improvements in survival.[19,20] *TP53, RB1, NF1,* and *PTEN* are tumor suppressor genes implicated in GBM. Various vectors have been used in an attempt to repair these oncogenic mutations. These repairs are aimed at restoring apoptotic pathways and intrinsic cell-cycle regulation. Mutations of the *TP53* gene are seen in 30 to 40% of GBM patients and the TP53 pathway is involved in upwards of 80% of tumors. As a result, the *TP53* gene and pathway have been a primary target in attempts to restore normal cell-cycle regulation. A phase 1 clinical trial testing an Ad-p53 vector in 15 patients did not show significant toxicity but demonstrated transduction in only a small portion of the tumors. No significant increase in survival was noted.[21] Another study of 18 patients demonstrated improvements in both survival and 6-month Karnofsky Performance Scale scores in the treatment group compared to the surgery-alone group ($n = 20$).[22]

Adenoviral vectors have also been used to transfer the Rb tumor suppressor gene to malignant gliomas. In vitro studies were promising, but transfection of tumor cells with Rb during in vivo studies was ineffective.[23–25] The heterogeneity of genetic mutations in gliomas will likely restrict the utility of restoration therapy.[26]

Nonviral Vectors

Nonviral vectors could potentially be a safer method of delivering genetic material than viral vectors as they are nonpathogenic and nonimmunogenic.[27,28] In an early gene therapy trial, a patient with partial ornithine transcarbamylase deficiency died when the adenoviral vector spread beyond the liver, producing a vigorous immune response and multiple system organ failure.[29] Concerns over the oncogenic potential of some viral vectors, recombination of viral vectors to virulent forms, and the insertion of viral genes into gametes have been raised.[27] However, to date few adverse events and no deaths have occurred in glioma gene therapy trials as a result of viral vectors.[8,15,21,30]

Nonviral vectors range from naked DNA to complex chemical carriers to stem cells. The delivery of naked DNA into cells has extremely low transduction efficiency, but certain mechanical methods may increase gene uptake. These techniques include electroporation, gene gun delivery, ultrasound, and hydrodynamic (high-pressure) injection. Mechanical augmentation has improved gene transfer in systemic organs but is not yet practical for CNS use with the exception of convection-enhanced delivery.

The ability to customize cationic lipids and polymers for delivery of genes to specific tissues has dramatically improved the efficiency of this approach. Lipoplexes are DNA-liposomal complexes that have been widely used for gene delivery. Nonviral vectors have met with moderate success in glioma animal models. One study delivered an antisense RNA molecule directed at the epidermal growth factor receptor (EGFR).[28] To overcome the blood–brain barrier, injections of bradykinin were given with the vector. To further increase efficiency of transfection, two monoclonal antibodies were bound to the vehicle: one for human insulin receptor and the other for murine transferrin receptor. This treatment resulted in a 95% suppression of EGFR function and an 88% increase in the survival times.[28] Nonviral vectors have been implemented in immunotherapy for glioma as well. Interferon (IFN)-β delivered with a cationic liposome by stereotactic injection into an intracranial mouse model produced a significant increase in survival time and histologically produced an increased T-cell lymphocyte infiltrate. Of the mice receiving IFN-β gene therapy, 40 to 50% had complete cures, and upon rechallenge did not develop tumors over a 50-day period.[31]

The relatively low transfection rates of nonviral vectors and the susceptibility of plasmids to degradation led to the development of a *Sleeping Beauty* transposon-based vector to insert genes into nuclear DNA in the tumor cell, potentially

---

Pearl

- Nonviral vectors may avoid the antiviral immune response and potential toxicity of viral vectors.

resulting in long-term expression of the gene product, even after tumor cell mitosis. Such stable long-term production of protein would be ideal for antiangiogenic therapy. The failure of endostatin and other antiangiogenic trials was thought to be due to the relatively transient effect of antiangiogenic therapies. Two vectors were produced that delivered genes for soluble endothelial growth factor receptor (sFlt-1) and angiostatin-endostatin (statin-AE) fusion protein.[32] Long-term production of these proteins was achieved by combining them with the Sleeping Beauty transposable element, and delivery was augmented by convection-enhanced delivery. sFlt-1 and statin-AE combined produced a significant increase in survival compared to controls and either gene alone.[32,33]

Nonviral vectors require the manufacture of a vehicle that can attach to a target cell's surface, be internalized, escape from endosomes, enter the nucleus, and initiate transcription.[27] The ability to engineer chemical carriers that can more efficiently accomplish these goals has been remarkable and promising.[34] However, at present nonviral vectors are 1,000 to 50,000 times less efficient at transfecting gliomas when compared with adenoviral vectors.[27] This low transfection rate has prevented the emergence of a successful nonviral, acellular vector for clinical use.

Nonviral Cellular Vectors: Neural and Mesenchymal Stem Cells

Recent work suggests that stem cells are responsible for driving continued cell growth in many cancers, including GBM. These stem cells (also called glioma progenitor cells or glioma-initiating cells) are thought to constitute less than 5% of the tumor, are resistant to traditional therapy, and thus are largely responsible for recurrence.

Stem cells not only may be responsible for tumorigenesis but also may provide an avenue for treatment. Neural and mesenchymal stem cells have been used as gene therapy vectors. The promise of stem cells in treating gliomas was first realized when it was demonstrated that they exhibit tropism for sites of CNS injury. It was then demonstrated that neural stem cells exhibit tropism for gliomas.[5] Obtaining neural stem cells can be difficult, and so mesenchymal stem cells, which are easily collected from bone marrow or adipose tissue, have been extensively studied. Several investigators have demonstrated that mesenchymal stem cells also localize to gliomas.[35] The implications of selective tropism for gliomas enable these cellular vectors to potentially deliver a wide variety of therapies including the aforementioned gene therapies, IFN-β, secretable tumor necrosis factor-related apoptosis-inducing ligand (S-TRAIL), microRNA, and oncolytic viruses.[35] Stem cells can potentially target the infiltrating tumor margins that have been resistant to traditional therapies.

The tumor selective tropism of bone-marrow–derived human mesenchymal stem cells (BM-hMSCs) for gliomas was recently found to be associated with transforming growth factor-β (TGF-β).[36] BM-hMSCs have TGF-β receptors that respond to TGF-β secreted from glioma cells. BM-hMSCs also exhibit tropism for glioma stem cells that, as mentioned previously, are likely responsible for the majority of treatment failures and recurrences.[36] Finally, BM-hMSC were shown to be an effective in vivo vector for the oncolytic Delta-24-RGD Ad when intravascularly delivered.

Mesenchymal stem cells enable the study of novel gene therapies that require a vector. For example, micro-RNAs (miRNAs) are small noncoding RNAs that can regulate proliferation, apoptosis, cell-cycle regulation, invasion, glioma stem cell function, and angiogenesis by augmenting or down-regulating gene expression.[37] Certain miRNAs appear to be attractive targets for glioma gene therapy.

Oncolytic Viral Therapy

Replication-incompetent viral vectors are inefficient and have not produced clinically significant improvements in survival during clinical trials to date. As a result, conditionally replicating viral vectors have been engineered to selectively replicate in tumor cells. These vectors can kill tumor cells from direct tumor cell lysis and from amplification of therapeutic genes (**Table 23.2**). Oncolytic viruses currently being studied in antiglioma clinical trials include oncolytic herpes simplex virus (oHSV), conditionally replicating Ad (CRAd), reovirus, poliovirus, vaccinia virus, measles virus, and Newcastle virus.[38]

Herpes Simplex Virus

A genetically engineered HSV-1 that conditionally replicated in tumor cells was created using a virus constructed with a deletion of the thymidine kinase (tk) gene, and it was effec-

Table 23.2 Overview of Viral Vectors

Virus	Replicating Ability	Genes Delivered (examples)
Retrovirus	Nonreplicating and replicating	HSV-TK, IL-2 (NR); CD (R)
Adenovirus	Nonreplicating/oncolytic	HSV-TK, CD, IL-2, IL-4, IL-12, GM-CSF, IFN-β p53
Herpesvirus	Nonreplicating/oncolytic	IL-2, IL-4, IL10, IL-12, GM-CSF
Reovirus	Oncolytic	N/A

Abbreviations: CD, cytosine deaminase; GM-CSF, granulocyte-macrophage colony-stimulating factor; HSV-TK, herpes simplex virus thymidine kinase; IL, interleukin; NR, nonreplicating; R, replicating.

tive in animal glioma models. This virus was never taken to human trials because the deletion of the *tk* gene rendered the virus resistant to acyclovir.[39] The HSV-1 G207 was constructed, containing two mutations initially created in two separate viral constructs. The two mutations were combined in anticipation of clinical trials to prevent a potential in-situ recombination event from restoring a wild-type phenotype. G207 contains the deletions present in the γ_1 34.5 region and a disabling *lacZ* insertion at the U_L39 locus. U_L39 encodes the large subunit of the viral ribonucleotide reductase that is necessary for the synthesis of nucleotides in postmitotic cells.[40] Ribonucleotide reductase is necessary for viral replication and is present in trans in actively dividing cells. γ_1 34.5-deleted HSVs replicate at lower levels than wild-type viruses, but these replication deficits can be significantly overcome by the administration of ionizing radiation shortly after virus inoculation.[41,42] Radiation increases late viral protein production via activation of p38l; this increases viral replication and spread of infection. The increase in replication does not appear to result in an increase in toxicity.

Additionally, the virus has been shown to be hypersensitive to acyclovir and ganciclovir, drugs already in clinical use.[43] G207 was examined extensively in a variety of preclinical murine and primate models and was demonstrated to be both safe and effective at doses up to 10^9 pfu.[44]

Subsequently, a phase 1 trial of G207 in patients with recurrent malignant glioma was conducted. This dose-escalating study enrolled 21 patients with the maximum dose reached of 3×10^9 pfu. No major toxicities were noted that could be attributed to G207, and some patients demonstrated reduction in tumor volume after treatment.[30] Two patients survived 5 years or more, and a third patient died of an unrelated stroke with no residual tumor found at autopsy. A maximum-tolerated dose was not reached.

To determine if there was an immune component to the response, as had been demonstrated in preclinical studies, a follow-up trial was designed; six patients were enrolled.[45,46] The trial was designed to include an initial inoculation of virus followed by tumor resection and reinoculation of the virus into the tumor bed. There was evidence using reverse-transcriptase polymerase chain reaction (RT-PCR) and documentation of late viral proteins indicating that viral replication was taking place within tumor cells. The patient with the longest survival had the highest detectable amount of HSV RNA and the smallest degree of lymphocytic infiltration, perhaps suggesting that patients with the least amount of antiviral immune response may survive the longest.

These promising results have led to the development of a follow-up phase 1 clinical trial. Nine patients with malignant recurrent gliomas had the G207 virus stereotactically inoculated into multiple sites of the tumor margin. On postoperative day 1, patients underwent treatment with a single fraction of 5 Gy radiation. Although publication of this study is pending, the approach demonstrates promise for future trials of combination treatments.

Adenovirus

An early application of oncolytic viral therapy was the delivery of wild-type Ad to patients with cervical cancer in 1956.[47] Since that time, the development of genetic techniques has facilitated the production of conditionally replicating Ad that can be utilized in the treatment of brain tumors. Ad has produced the widest variety of oncolytic viruses for glioma therapy, including the ONYX-015, 01/PEME, and the previously mentioned Delta-24-RGD virus.[48]

The wild-type Ad genome encodes five transcription units, E1A, E1B, E2, E3, and E4, whose products regulate viral DNA replication, gene expression, and capsid packaging.[49] These important early transcription units have been manipulated in various ways to generate targeted oncolytic therapies.

ONYX-015 is an Ad with a deletion in the E1B region that was originally thought to produce selective replication in tumor cells with a defect in the p53 pathway. It was shown that the selective replication of ONXY-015 is independent of p53 activity, and that the role of E1B-55 kd protein in viral RNA export was responsible for selective replication in tumor cells. The deletion of E1B-55 kd leads to the induction of p53 but not its activation. Thus ONXY-015 was able to replicate in tumor cells expressing wild-type p53. However, tumor cells are able to efficiently export late viral RNA in the absence of E1B-55 kd protein, whereas normal cells lack this ability.[50] The completion of a phase 1 trial has demonstrated the safety of ONYX-015. The trial enrolled 24 patients with malignant gliomas in a dose-escalation study. The virus was injected into 10 sites within the tumor bed immediately following resection of the tumor. No adverse reactions were attributed to viral treatment, although adverse events related to tumor progression or standard therapy did occur. Although not a trial of efficacy, no significant antitumor activity for high-grade gliomas was found.

Although the virus appears safe, the deletion of E1B protein results in decreased expression of late viral proteins. This may explain the limited response of cancers to ONYX-015 to date.[51] Currently, no phase 2 or 3 trials have been completed using E1B gene-deleted Ad for gliomas.

The *E1A* gene's interaction with pRb has also been exploited to create oncolytic adenoviruses. Most gliomas contain mutations of the pRb/p16 pathway that arrest the cell cycle and prevent progression from the G_1 phase to the S phase.[52] The E1A region contains two evolutionary conserved regions (CRs); CR1 and CR2 are essential for binding to pRb. By inactivating these CRs, adenoviruses have been engineered that selectively replicate in neoplastic cells with a mutation in the pRb pathway. Several viruses, dl922–947 and Delta 24 RGB (δ24), contain mutations in the CR2 region.[25,52] The δ24 construct has demonstrated efficacy in several glioma xenograft models and is currently being studied in a phase 1/2 clinical trial.[25,53,54] The δ24 virus has been shown to kill glioma stem cells, with induction of autophagy, as demonstrated through upregulation of Atg5, a critical protein in the autophagy pathway. Oncolytic viruses such as δ24 may represent an effective treatment for the resistant brain tumor stem cell population.

Another strategy to produce tumor-selective viral replication has been to target specific receptors expressed on tumor cells. Many neoplastic cells lack coxsackievirus and adenovirus receptors (CARs). Glioma cell explants have been shown to exhibit decreased cell surface expression of CARs compared with glioma cell lines, a potential impediment to effective treatment. By incorporating an arginine-glycine-aspartate sequence into the capsid of a δ24 virus, investigators were able to create a virus that selectively binds integrins, which are commonly expressed by glioma cells and not in normal brain. The strategy was to create a virus that not only selectively replicated in malignant cells but also had increased ability to infect tumor cells. In vitro studies and a xenograft model exhibited this new δ24-RGD virus's increased oncolytic activity.[55] This virus is currently under study in a clinical trial

(F. Lang, personal communication). Adenoviruses have provided the widest range of selectively replicating viruses and demonstrate the importance of developing an intimate knowledge of viral gene expression and tumor biology to construct effective oncolytic viruses.

Reovirus

Reovirus is a nonenveloped, double-stranded RNA virus that has a lytic replication cycle and induces cell apoptosis in cells with mutations of the Ras signaling pathway. An intact Ras-PKR pathway prevents viral protein synthesis and replication. Mutations or overproduction of Ras permit reovirus protein synthesis and replication, making it an ideal agent for oncolytic therapy.[56] Gliomas commonly possess mutations that result in the overexpression of Ras, for example, EGFR and platelet-derived growth factor receptor mutations. Additionally, reovirus therapy has the advantage of needing no genetic manipulation, and this may avoid the reduced replication capacity that has been noted in attenuated HSV and adenoviruses. One disadvantage of reovirus is that it is relatively more difficult to engineer to express additional foreign genes.

In one study, reovirus successfully lysed 20 of 24 glioma cell lines and furthermore cured subcutaneous and intracerebral tumors in severe combined immunodeficiency disease (SCID) nonobese diabetic (NOD) xenograft models. This study, however, produced toxicity in these severely immunocompromised models.[57] It was thought that such toxic infections were unlikely in humans with relatively intact immune systems. A dose escalation phase 1 clinical trial of 12 recurrent malignant glioma patients found that reovirus (REOLYSIN™, Oncolytics Biotech Inc., Calgary, Alberta, Canada) intratumoral injections were well tolerated.[58] Another phase 1 trial treated 15 patients with recurrent malignant glioma with a 72-hour intratumoral reovirus infusion.[59] Further clinical trials will be needed to determine efficacy.

Other Oncolytic Viruses

Newcastle disease virus (NDV) is another naturally attenuated virus that has been proposed for viral therapy in various tumors.[60] It is an avian paramyxovirus that causes a fatal infection in birds but produces relatively innocuous infections in humans with flulike symptoms, conjunctivitis, and laryngitis. The ability of NDV to selectively replicate in neoplastic cells arises from its ability to usurp the Ras pathway much like reovirus.[61] NDV has been used in a variety of tumors.[60] An intriguing use of NDV can be found in the case report of a single 14-year-old boy diagnosed with GBM. This patient had undergone a resection, developed a recurrence, and received repeated intravenous injections of NDV in 1996. Between 1996 and 1998 the tumor decreased in size on imaging, and the patient remained alive in 1999 following discontinuation of his regimen in 1998.[62]

Special Considerations

- The native adenovirus receptor CAR has been shown to be markedly downregulated in glioma cells in vivo compared with in vitro cell lines. Such potential differences between in vivo tumors and in vitro cells need to be taken into account when engineering viruses for glioma therapy.
- Approximately 85% of adults exhibit systemic immunity against Ad secondary to naturally occurring infections. Generation of vectors lacking transcriptionally active adenoviral regions mitigates the risk of anti-adenovirus immune system activation and enables long-term transgene expression.

Poliovirus is a well-known neuropathic picornavirus that causes paralytic poliomyelitis. The neuropathic properties of poliovirus have been mapped to the internal ribosome entry sites (IRES). Through the replacement of the polio IRES region with the human rhinovirus type 2 IRES, the PVI(RIPO) mutant was constructed, which is attenuated but retains its ability to replicate in nonneuronal cells.[63] Preclinical studies have supported its safety and efficacy as a therapy for glioma, and a clinical trial in malignant glioma is currently underway.

Vaccinia virus is a member of the Poxviridae family of viruses that has been used as a smallpox vaccine and more recently as a tumor vaccine.[64] Both attenuated and nonattenuated vaccinia viruses have been applied as oncolytic viruses and vectors. The oncolytic effects of vaccinia were found to be enhanced by the expression of interleukin-2 (IL-2) and IL-12.[65] The construction of a vaccinia virus expressing wild-type p53 induced apoptosis in several human glioma cell lines and in C6 rat glioma models.[66] This effect was enhanced by the subsequent delivery of radiation.[67] Vaccinia virus has shown the most promise as a tumor vaccine, but its potential as an oncolytic therapy has yet to be fully explored.[68]

Immunogene Therapy

The CNS has traditionally been viewed as an immune-privileged location, but increasing evidence points to a critical role for the immune response in gene therapy. Primary CNS cancers display several adaptations to escape an effective immunologic response. Details of such adaptations can be found in Chapter 22.

The immune system plays an important and complex role in most gene therapy protocols even when the therapy is not directly targeting the immune system. Viral vectors have become the most popular means of delivering genetic material and are key factors in the interplay between the immune system and gene therapy.

The immune response to HSV as a vector has been studied in detail in rodents. The immune response both aids and hinders the viral mediate destruction of tumors. The initial response to the virus through the innate immune system hinders viral spread through the tumor.[69,70] Following viral infection there is a rapid immune response mediated by neutrophils, natural killer (NK) cells, macrophages, and microglia.[69,71] This influx of cells is quickly followed by the re-lease of the proinflammatory cytokines tumor necrosis factor-α (TNF-α), IL-1β, IFN-γ, adhesion molecules, and chemokines, which may reduce viral spread but also initiate an adaptive immune response.[71] Although the immune system may reduce viral replication and spread initially, the memory T-lymphocyte response of the adaptive system is essential for viral-mediated destruction of tumors.[72] The importance of an intact immune system in viral therapy was demonstrated in an intracranial melanoma murine model, using the construct HSV-1716. The cohorts in this experiment included knockout mice with deletions that produced general immunodeficiency and specific knockouts for CD-4+ and CD-8+ T cells and NK cells. Immunodeficient cohorts had no prolongation of survival, whereas those with an intact immune system had increased survival times.[72]

In a previous study, high-dose cyclophosphamide rendered mice immune deficient and eliminated any benefit of oncolytic viral therapy. Another group of investigators demonstrated that oHSV expressing an immunosuppressive cytokine produced no survival advantage, whereas oHSV expressing an immunoactivating cytokine did.[70,73] The adaptive immune response induced by HSV therapy can thus be specific for tumor antigens as well as viral antigens. Proliferation of CD-4+ T cells induces destruction of tumor cells by NK cells and macrophages; a TH$_1$ memory response against tumors may also develop and produce tumor cell killing after viral replication has ended.[72]

To enhance the immune response to tumors treated with viral therapy, several viruses have been engineered to deliver cytokines. Both HSV vectors and Ad vectors have been produced that express IL-4, which is produced primarily by CD4+ T cells and induces expression of major histocompatibility complex (MHC) class II antigen expression and CD8+ T cell infiltration and proliferation.[73,74] Interleukin-12 has been inserted in Ad, HSV, and vaccinia vectors. It may have advantages over IL-4 by promoting NK and cytotoxic T cell activity.[75,76] M002, an oHSV that expresses IL-12, seeks to take advantage of the virus's oncolytic properties as well as IL-12's ability to induce an immune response to the tumor.[76] Interleukin-12 may also produce an antiangiogenic response, augmenting the antitumor efficacy of the virus.[77] A humanized variant of M002, M032, has received investigational new drug (IND) status from the Food and Drug Administration (FDA) to allow testing in clinical trials (J.M. Markert, personal communication). TNF-α and IL-2 have been delivered by Ad and vaccinia vectors, respectively, as well. Delivery of IL-2, IL-4, IL-12, and

TNF-α has demonstrated an enhanced immune response and prolonged survival in various animal models.[74–76]

The first clinical trial for glioma of cytokine delivery by viral vector was disappointing. One study constructed a non-replicating Ad that expressed IFN-β. IFN-β has multiple antitumor effects: it produces cell-cycle arrest of tumor cells in the S phase; it is an immune system activator, causing increased expression of MHC I, heightened cytotoxic lymphocyte activity, amplified generation of CD4+ T lymphocytes, and enhanced activity of macrophages and NK cells; and it has antiangiogenic effects.[78] The construct caused remission of tumors and increased survival times in preclinical testing. However, the phase 1 clinical trial for this therapy was closed before reaching its accrual goals, and there is no plan to reopen the study.[79] Other reports of IL-2 and B7-2/granulocyte-macrophage colony-stimulating factor (GM-CSF) immunogene therapy appear as isolated reports or lack final clinical trial publications.

Cyclophosphamide (CPA) in high doses that deplete leukocytes has been shown to render oncolytic HSV therapy ineffective.[70] However, lower dose CPA has been shown to improve survival times in preclinical oHSV studies. Low-dose CPA causes a temporary immunosuppression of monocytes and associated cytokines that appears to allow for increased viral replication.

To date, however, the complex nature of the interaction of the immune system and gene therapy has not been fully elucidated. Clearly, further study resulting in a better understanding of the intricacies of the immune system and its complex interaction with tumor cells will be essential to maximize effectiveness of gene therapy for gliomas.

Delivery of Gene Therapy Agents

Gene therapy is limited by the inability to disperse vector throughout a targeted tumor. Secreted proteins, oncolytic viruses, and immunotherapy have sought to overcome the limited distribution of vector within a tumor through biochemical means. However, viral replication is restricted by the immune system, and secreted proteins and immunotherapy require a critical volume of tumor cells to be infected to be effective.[79,80] Clinical trial delivery systems have remained primitive and rely heavily on diffusion.[80] Convection-enhanced delivery (CED) improves the distribution of molecules within the CNS. CED utilizes a syringe pump to infuse solute through a catheter, creating a pressure gradient that induces bulk flow within tissue. It achieves high concentrations of particles through large volumes of tissue. This delivery method may be ideal to maximize the number of cells transfected by vector.

Suicide gene therapy could potentially benefit greatly from CED, because this therapy requires a large portion of the tumor to become infected to be effective. Although a by-

> **Pearl**
>
> - Convection-enhanced delivery may increase the distribution of viral and nonviral vectors within a tumor and thereby overcome low transfection rates.

stander effect has been shown to spread tumor destruction beyond transfected cells in suicide gene treatments, greater than 50% of the tumor may require transfection to achieve significant effects. CED of an adenoassociated virus vector used to deliver the *HSV-TK* gene achieved transfection rates of 39% and significant increases in survival time in intracranial U87 glioma animal models.[81] A liposomal vector for the delivery of *HSV-TK* gene has completed a phase 1/2 clinical trial. This vector was administered via infusion into eight patients with recurrent gliomas and resulted in no increased morbidity or mortality. Two of the eight patients exhibited a 50% tumor reduction as measured by methionine uptake on positron emission tomography.

The inability for CED to produce a dramatic improvement in initial gene therapy trials is due to the physical characteristics of the vectors employed in gene therapy. When comparing Ad and adenoassociated virus to charged nanospheres, the 80- to 90-nm Ad achieved areas of distribution that far exceeded adenoassociated virus (23 nm) and 20-nm nanospheres. The difference was attributed to specific and nonspecific binding to tissues. Further improvements in the use of CED for gene therapy will occur once the key variables of vector change, molecular interactions, and size are better understood.[80] Coadministration with other agents, such as heparin and albumin, may further increase the volume of distribution of some vectors by interfering with undesirable viral attachment to tumor cells immediately adjacent to the catheter tip.[80,81]

Conclusion

Gene therapy alone may or may not provide a cure for malignant glioma. The heterogeneity of these tumors and the unique environment of the CNS make the eradication of a glioma by a single therapy unlikely. However, gene therapy provides an approach to glioma treatment that is uniquely targeted at tumor cells and may induce cell death through multiple mechanisms with a single treatment, avoiding many of the current mechanisms of therapeutic resistance prevalent in glioma. The continued improvement of vectors and integration of new delivery show great promise for improving outcome. The timely advance of effective gene therapies into pivotal phase 3 trials is necessary to provide sorely needed adjuvant treatment for these aggressive neoplasms.

Editor's Note

Initial clinical trials primarily involving suicide gene therapy have demonstrated no significant difference in survival for patients with high-grade gliomas, yet interest remains extremely high to develop new avenues to pursue in this field. It is possible that nonviral vectors could play an even greater role in the success of gene therapy trials, although this remains to be seen; yet nonviral vectors have the advantage of being nonpathogenic. We have seen in the past from experimental models that neural, as well as mesenchymal, stem cells can be carriers for various viral vectors and have the potential to infiltrate tumors as well as cells throughout the margin of the tumor. At the present time, mesenchymal stem cells seem to have a slight advantage based on the experimental models created thus far and can be delivered from the intravascular route. Oncolytic viral therapy is yet another mechanism to be engineered so that it can selectively replicate in tumor cells, and several of these viral types are currently being examined. There are other oncolytic viruses such as Newcastle and polio virus as well as vaccinia that could be quite effective. One of the keys to this field is to somehow regulate the immune response in a patient so that the gene construct can be effective and not be neutralized by the immune system. Thus, this remains a very exciting field and we anticipate a significant amount of progress in the upcoming years. (Berger)

References

1. Schulder M, Loeffler JS, Howes AE, Alexander E III, Black PM. Historical vignette: the radium bomb: Harvey Cushing and the interstitial irradiation of gliomas. J Neurosurg 1996;84:530–532 10.3171/jns.1996.84.3.0530
2. Stupp R, Hegi ME, Mason WP, et al; European Organisation for Research and Treatment of Cancer Brain Tumour and Radiation Oncology Groups; National Cancer Institute of Canada Clinical Trials Group. Effects of radiotherapy with concomitant and adjuvant temozolomide versus radiotherapy alone on survival in glioblastoma in a randomised phase III study: 5-year analysis of the EORTC-NCIC trial. Lancet Oncol 2009;10:459–466 10.1016/S1470-2045(09)70025-7
3. Stewart LA. Chemotherapy in adult high-grade glioma: a systematic review and meta-analysis of individual patient data from 12 randomised trials. Lancet 2002;359:1011–1018
4. Immonen A, Vapalahti M, Tyynelä K, et al. AdvHSV-tk gene therapy with intravenous ganciclovir improves survival in human malignant glioma: a randomised, controlled study. Mol Ther 2004;10:967–972 10.1016/j.ymthe.2004.08.002
5. Aboody KS, Brown A, Rainov NG, et al. Neural stem cells display extensive tropism for pathology in adult brain: evidence from intracranial gliomas. Proc Natl Acad Sci U S A 2000;97:12846–12851 10.1073/pnas.97.23.12846
6. Marsh JC, Goldfarb J, Shafman TD, Diaz AZ. Current status of immunotherapy and gene therapy for high-grade gliomas. Cancer Contr 2013;20:43–48
7. Freeman SM, Ramesh R, Shastri M, Munshi A, Jensen AK, Marrogi AJ. The role of cytokines in mediating the bystander effect using HSV-TK xenogeneic cells. Cancer Lett 1995;92:167–174
8. Rainov NG. A phase III clinical evaluation of herpes simplex virus type 1 thymidine kinase and ganciclovir gene therapy as an adjuvant to surgical resection and radiation in adults with previously untreated glioblastoma multiforme. Hum Gene Ther 2000;11:2389–2401 10.1089/104303400750038499
9. Li L-Q, Shen F, Xu X-Y, Zhang H, Yang X-F, Liu W-G. Gene therapy with HSV1-sr39TK/GCV exhibits a stronger therapeutic efficacy than HSV1-TK/GCV in rat C6 glioma cells. Scientific World J 2013;2013:951343
10. Puumalainen AM, Vapalahti M, Agrawal RS, et al. Beta-galactosidase gene transfer to human malignant glioma in vivo using replication-deficient retroviruses and adenoviruses. Hum Gene Ther 1998;9:1769–1774 10.1089/hum.1998.9.12-1769
11. Sandmair AM, Loimas S, Puranen P, et al. Thymidine kinase gene therapy for human malignant glioma, using replication-deficient retroviruses or adenoviruses. Hum Gene Ther 2000;11:2197–2205 10.1089/104303400750035726
12. Chiocca EA. Gene therapy: a primer for neurosurgeons. Neurosurgery 2003;53:364–373, discussion 373
13. Germano IM, Fable J, Gultekin SH, Silvers A. Adenovirus/herpes simplex-thymidine kinase/ganciclovir complex: preliminary results of a phase I trial in patients with recurrent malignant gliomas. J Neurooncol 2003;65:279–289
14. Smitt PS, Driesse M, Wolbers J, Kros M, Avezaat C. Treatment of relapsed malignant glioma with an adenoviral vector containing the herpes simplex thymidine kinase gene followed by ganciclovir. Mol Ther 2003;7:851–858
15. Trask TW, Trask RP, Aguilar-Cordova E, et al. Phase I study of adenoviral delivery of the HSV-tk gene and ganciclovir administration in patients with current malignant brain tumors. Mol Ther 2000;1:195–203 10.1006/mthe.2000.0030
16. Huang Q, Liu X-Z, Kang C-S, Wang G-X, Zhong Y, Pu P-Y. The anti-glioma effect of suicide gene therapy using BMSC expressing HSV/TK combined with overexpression of Cx43 in glioma cells. Cancer Gene Ther 2010;17:192–202 10.1038/cgt.2009.64
17. Pertschuk D, Cloughesy T, Gruber HE. Ascending dose trials of the safety and tolerability of Toca 511, a retroviral replicating vector encoding cytosine deaminase, in patients with recurrent high-grade glioma. Chicago, 2012
18. Perez OD, Logg CR, Hiraoka K, et al. Design and selection of Toca 511 for clinical use: modified retroviral replicating vector with improved stability and gene expression. Mol Ther 2012;20:1689–1698 10.1038/mt.2012.83
19. Dunn GP, Rinne ML, Wykosky J, et al. Emerging insights into the molecular and cellular basis of glioblastoma. Genes Dev 2012;26:756–784 10.1101/gad.187922.112
20. Zalatimo O, Zoccoli CM, Patel A, Weston CL, Glantz M. Impact of genetic targets on primary brain tumor therapy: what's ready for prime time? Adv Exp Med Biol 2013;779:267–289 10.1007/978-1-4614-6176-0_12

21. Lang FF, Bruner JM, Fuller GN, et al. Phase I trial of adenovirus-mediated p53 gene therapy for recurrent glioma: biological and clinical results. J Clin Oncol 2003;21:2508–2518

22. Zhu JX, Li ZM, Geng FY, et al. [Treatment of recurrent malignant gliomas by surgery combined with recombinant adenovirus-p53 injection]. Zhonghua Zhong Liu Za Zhi 2010;32:709–712

23. Fueyo J, Gomez-Manzano C, Yung WK, et al. Suppression of human glioma growth by adenovirus-mediated Rb gene transfer. Neurology 1998;50:1307–1315

24. Jiang H, Gomez-Manzano C, Lang FF, Alemany R, Fueyo J. Oncolytic adenovirus: preclinical and clinical studies in patients with human malignant gliomas. Curr Gene Ther 2009;9:422–427

25. Fueyo J, Gomez-Manzano C, Alemany R, et al. A mutant oncolytic adenovirus targeting the Rb pathway produces anti-glioma effect in vivo. Oncogene 2000;19:2–12 10.1038/sj.onc.1203251

26. Li H, Alonso-Vanegas M, Colicos MA, et al. Intracerebral adenovirus-mediated p53 tumor suppressor gene therapy for experimental human glioma. Clin Cancer Res 1999;5:637–642

27. Thomas M, Klibanov AM. Non-viral gene therapy: polycation-mediated DNA delivery. Appl Microbiol Biotechnol 2003;62:27–34 10.1007/s00253-003-1321-8

28. Zhang Y, Zhang Y-F, Bryant J, Charles A, Boado RJ, Pardridge WM. Intravenous RNA interference gene therapy targeting the human epidermal growth factor receptor prolongs survival in intracranial brain cancer. Clin Cancer Res 2004;10:3667–3677 10.1158/1078-0432.CCR-03-0740

29. Marshall E. Gene therapy death prompts review of adenovirus vector. Science 1999;286:2244–2245

30. Markert JM, Medlock MD, Rabkin SD, et al. Conditionally replicating herpes simplex virus mutant, G207 for the treatment of malignant glioma: results of a phase I trial. Gene Ther 2000;7:867–874 10.1038/sj.gt.3301205

31. Natsume A, Mizuno M, Ryuke Y, Yoshida J. Antitumor effect and cellular immunity activation by murine interferon-beta gene transfer against intracerebral glioma in mouse. Gene Ther 1999;6:1626–1633 10.1038/sj.gt.3300990

32. Ohlfest JR, Lobitz PD, Perkinson SG, Largaespada DA. Integration and long-term expression in xenografted human glioblastoma cells using a plasmid-based transposon system. Mol Ther 2004;10:260–268 10.1016/j.ymthe.2004.05.005

33. Ohlfest JR, Demorest ZL, Motooka Y, et al. Combinatorial antiangiogenic gene therapy by nonviral gene transfer using the sleeping beauty transposon causes tumor regression and improves survival in mice bearing intracranial human glioblastoma. Mol Ther 2005;12:778–788 10.1016/j.ymthe.2005.07.689

34. Tzeng SY, Guerrero-Cázares H, Martinez EE, Sunshine JC, Quiñones-Hinojosa A, Green JJ. Non-viral gene delivery nanoparticles based on poly(β-amino esters) for treatment of glioblastoma. Biomaterials 2011;32:5402–5410 10.1016/j.biomaterials.2011.04.016

35. Doucette T, Rao G, Yang Y, et al. Mesenchymal stem cells display tumor-specific tropism in an RCAS/Ntv-a glioma model. Neoplasia 2011;13:716–725

36. Shinojima N, Hossain A, Takezaki T, et al. TGF-β mediates homing of bone marrow-derived human mesenchymal stem cells to glioma stem cells. Cancer Res 2013;73:2333–2344 10.1158/0008-5472.CAN-12-3086

37. Lee HK, Finniss S, Cazacu S, et al. Mesenchymal stem cells deliver synthetic microRNA mimics to glioma cells and glioma stem cells and inhibit their cell migration and self-renewal. Oncotarget 2013;4:346–361

38. Tobias A, Ahmed A, Moon K-S, Lesniak MS. The art of gene therapy for glioma: a review of the challenging road to the bedside. J Neurol Neurosurg Psychiatry 2013;84:213–222 10.1136/jnnp-2012-302946

39. Martuza RL, Malick A, Markert JM, Ruffner KL, Coen DM. Experimental therapy of human glioma by means of a genetically engineered virus mutant. Science 1991;252:854–856

40. Goldstein DJ, Weller SK. Herpes simplex virus type 1-induced ribonucleotide reductase activity is dispensable for virus growth and DNA synthesis: isolation and characterization of an ICP6 lacZ insertion mutant. J Virol 1988;62:196–205

41. Bradley JD, Kataoka Y, Advani S, et al. Ionizing radiation improves survival in mice bearing intracranial high-grade gliomas injected with genetically modified herpes simplex virus. Clin Cancer Res 1999;5:1517–1522

42. Weichselbaum RR, Kufe DW, Advani SJ, Roizman B. Molecular targeting of gene therapy and radiotherapy. Acta Oncol 2001;40:735–738

43. Mineta T, Rabkin SD, Martuza RL. Treatment of malignant gliomas using ganciclovir-hypersensitive, ribonucleotide reductase-deficient herpes simplex viral mutant. Cancer Res 1994;54:3963–3966

44. Hunter WD, Martuza RL, Feigenbaum F, et al. Attenuated, replication-competent herpes simplex virus type 1 mutant G207: safety evaluation of intracerebral injection in nonhuman primates. J Virol 1999;73:6319–6326

45. Todo T, Rabkin SD, Sundaresan P, et al. Systemic antitumor immunity in experimental brain tumor therapy using a multimutated, replication-competent herpes simplex virus. Hum Gene Ther 1999;10:2741–2755 10.1089/10430349950016483

46. Markert JM, Liechty PG, Wang W, et al. Phase Ib trial of mutant herpes simplex virus G207 inoculated pre-and post-tumor resection for recurrent GBM. Mol Ther 2009;17:199–207 10.1038/mt.2008.228

47. Huebner RJ, Rowe WP, Schatten WE, Smith RR, Thomas LB. Studies on the use of viruses in the treatment of carcinoma of the cervix. Cancer 1956;9:1211–1218

48. Chiocca EA, Abbed KM, Tatter S, et al. A phase I open-label, dose-escalation, multi-institutional trial of injection with an E1B-Attenuated adenovirus, ONYX-015, into the peritumoral region of recurrent malignant gliomas, in the adjuvant setting. Mol Ther 2004;10:958–966 10.1016/j.ymthe.2004.07.021

49. Barcia C, Jimenez-Dalmaroni M, Kroeger KM, et al. One-year expression from high-capacity adenoviral vectors in the brains of animals with pre-existing anti-adenoviral immunity: clinical implications. Mol Ther 2007;15:2154–2163 10.1038/sj.mt.6300305

50. O'Shea CC, Johnson I, Bagus B, et al. Late viral RNA export, rather than p53 inactivation, determines ONYX-015 tumor selectivity. Cancer Cell 2004;6:611–623 10.1016/j.ccr.2004.11.012

51. Ramachandra M, Rahman A, Zou A, et al. Re-engineering adenovirus regulatory pathways to enhance oncolytic specificity and efficacy. Nat Biotechnol 2001;19:1035–1041 10.1038/nbt1101-1035

52. Heise C, Hermiston T, Johnson L, et al. An adenovirus E1A mutant that demonstrates potent and selective systemic anti-tumoral efficacy. Nat Med 2000;6:1134–1139 10.1038/80474

53. Alonso MM, Jiang H, Gomez-Manzano C, Fueyo J. Targeting brain tumor stem cells with oncolytic adenoviruses. Methods Mol Biol 2012;797:111–125 10.1007/978-1-61779-340-0_9

54. Safety Study of Replication-Competent Adenovirus. (Delta-24-rgd) in Patients with Recurrent Glioblastoma. http://clinicaltrials.gov/ct2/show/NCT01582516. Accessed May 6, 2013

55. Suzuki K, Fueyo J, Krasnykh V, Reynolds PN, Curiel DT, Alemany R. A conditionally replicative adenovirus with enhanced infectivity shows improved oncolytic potency. Clin Cancer Res 2001;7:120–126

56. Coffey MC, Strong JE, Forsyth PA, Lee PW. Reovirus therapy of tumors with activated Ras pathway. Science 1998;282:1332–1334

57. Wilcox ME, Yang W, Senger D, et al. Reovirus as an oncolytic agent against experimental human malignant gliomas. J Natl Cancer Inst 2001;93:903–912

58. Forsyth P, Roldán G, George D, et al. A phase I trial of intratumoral administration of reovirus in patients with histologically confirmed recurrent malignant gliomas. Mol Ther 2008;16:627–632 10.1038/sj.mt.6300403

59. Kicielinski KP, Chiocca EA, Yu JS, Gill GM, Markert JM. Phase 1 clinical trial of intratumoral reovirus infusion for the treatment of recurrent malignant gliomas in adults. Mol Ther 2014;22:1056–1062

60. Pecora AL, Rizvi N, Cohen GI, et al. Phase I trial of intravenous administration of PV701, an oncolytic virus, in patients with advanced solid cancers. J Clin Oncol 2002;20:2251–2266

61. Lorence RM, Katubig BB, Reichard KW, et al. Complete regression of human fibrosarcoma xenografts after local Newcastle disease virus therapy. Cancer Res 1994;54:6017–6021

62. Csatary LK, Bakács T. Use of Newcastle disease virus vaccine (MTH-68/H) in a patient with high-grade glioblastoma. JAMA 1999;281:1588–1589

63. Gromeier M, Alexander L, Wimmer E. Internal ribosomal entry site substitution eliminates neurovirulence in intergeneric poliovirus recombinants. Proc Natl Acad Sci U S A 1996;93:2370–2375

64. McCart JA, Ward JM, Lee J, et al. Systemic cancer therapy with a tumor-selective vaccinia virus mutant lacking thymidine kinase and vaccinia growth factor genes. Cancer Res 2001;61:8751–8757

65. Chen B, Timiryasova TM, Andres ML, et al. Evaluation of combined vaccinia virus-mediated antitumor gene therapy with p53, IL-2, and IL-12 in a glioma model. Cancer Gene Ther 2000;7:1437–1447 10.1038/sj.cgt.7700252

66. Timiryasova TM, Chen B, Haghighat P, Fodor I. Vaccinia virus-mediated expression of wild-type p53 suppresses glioma cell growth and induces apoptosis. Int J Oncol 1999;14:845–854

67. Gridley DS, Andres ML, Li J, Timiryasova T, Chen B, Fodor I. Evaluation of radiation effects against C6 glioma in combination with vaccinia virus-p53 gene therapy. Int J Oncol 1998;13:1093–1098

68. Wallack MK, Sivanandham M, Balch CM, et al. Surgical adjuvant active specific immunotherapy for patients with stage III melanoma: the final analysis of data from a phase III, randomized, double-blind, multicenter vaccinia melanoma oncolysate trial. J Am Coll Surg 1998;187:69–77, discussion 77–79

69. McKie EA, Brown SM, MacLean AR, Graham DI. Histopathological responses in the CNS following inoculation with a non-neurovirulent mutant (1716) of herpes simplex virus type 1 (HSV 1): relevance for gene and cancer therapy. Neuropathol Appl Neurobiol 1998;24:367–372

70. Miller CG, Fraser NW. Role of the immune response during neuro-attenuated herpes simplex virus-mediated tumor destruction in a murine intracranial melanoma model. Cancer Res 2000;60:5714–5722

71. Olschowka JA, Bowers WJ, Hurley SD, Mastrangelo MA, Federoff HJ. Helper-free HSV-1 amplicons elicit a markedly less robust innate immune response in the CNS. Mol Ther 2003;7:218–227

72. Miller CG, Fraser NW. Requirement of an integrated immune response for successful neuroattenuated HSV-1 therapy in an intracranial metastatic melanoma model. Mol Ther 2003;7:741–747

73. Andreansky S, He B, van Cott J, et al. Treatment of intracranial gliomas in immunocompetent mice using herpes simplex viruses that express murine interleukins. Gene Ther 1998;5:121–130 10.1038/sj.gt.3300550

74. Yoshikawa K, Kajiwara K, Ideguchi M, Uchida T, Ito H. Immune gene therapy of experimental mouse brain tumor with adenovirus-mediated gene transfer of murine interleukin-4. Cancer Immunol Immunother 2000;49:23–33

75. Liu Y, Ehtesham M, Samoto K, et al. In situ adenoviral interleukin 12 gene transfer confers potent and long-lasting cytotoxic immunity in glioma. Cancer Gene Ther 2002;9:9–15 10.1038/sj.cgt.7700399

76. Parker JN, Gillespie GY, Love CE, Randall S, Whitley RJ, Markert JM. Engineered herpes simplex virus expressing IL-12 in the treatment of experimental murine brain tumors. Proc Natl Acad Sci U S A 2000;97:2208–2213 10.1073/pnas.040557897

77. Wong RJ, Chan M-K, Yu Z, et al. Angiogenesis inhibition by an oncolytic herpes virus expressing interleukin 12. Clin Cancer Res 2004;10:4509–4516 10.1158/1078-0432.CCR-04-0081

78. Qin X-Q, Tao N, Dergay A, et al. Interferon-beta gene therapy inhibits tumor formation and causes regression of established tumors in immune-deficient mice. Proc Natl Acad Sci U S A 1998;95:14411–14416

79. Eck SL, Alavi JB, Judy K, et al. Treatment of recurrent or progressive malignant glioma with a recombinant adenovirus expressing human interferon-beta (H5.010CMVhIFN-beta): a phase I trial. Hum Gene Ther 2001;12:97–113 10.1089/104303401451013

80. Chen MY, Hoffer A, Morrison PF, et al. Surface properties, more than size, limiting convective distribution of virus-sized particles and viruses in the central nervous system. J Neurosurg 2005;103:311–319 10.3171/jns.2005.103.2.0311

81. Hadaczek P, Mirek H, Berger MS, Bankiewicz K. Limited efficacy of gene transfer in herpes simplex virus-thymidine kinase/ganciclovir gene therapy for brain tumors. J Neurosurg 2005;102:328–335 10.3171/jns.2005.102.2.0328

VI Specific Tumors

24 Low-Grade Gliomas

Hugues Duffau

Supratentorial infiltrative grade II glioma, as defined by the current World Health Organization (WHO) classification system (diffuse low-grade glioma [LGG]), is a complex and heterogeneous entity in adults, accounting for about 15% of all gliomas.[1] Management of LGG patients has long been a matter of debate, for many reasons.

First, for a long time, the natural course of this disease was poorly studied. Indeed, in the classic literature, the vast majority of authors considered LGG as a "stable" and "benign" brain tumor. Therefore, the "wait and see" approach was advocated for many years, especially because LGG usually affects young adults (in the fourth decade of life) enjoying a normal life with no or only a mild deficit on a standard neurologic examination, even if they were taking antiepileptic drugs for seizures, as were 80 to 90% of patients.[2]

Second, it was traditionally thought that this infiltrative tumor cannot be removed without generating functional consequences, in particular when LGG is located in or close to so-called eloquent areas, as is commonly observed.

Third, mainly based on the subjective estimation of the extent of resection by the neurosurgeon, it was argued that surgical removal had no impact on the natural history of LGG. Thus, it was common to perform only a biopsy in order to obtain samples for neuropathological examination, and then to choose between a single follow-up or radiotherapy according to the morphological criteria established by the WHO classification (see below). Of note, the clinical results were evaluated in the majority of series on only few parameters, such as progression-free survival (PFS), overall survival (OS), and eventually Karnofsky Performance Scale (KPS) score.

Interestingly, recent technical and conceptual advances in genetics, cognitive neurosciences, imaging, and treatment revolutionized our knowledge of LGG, leading to the seminal principle of *personalized management*. Indeed, it is now well known that these aggressive tumors grow continuously, migrate along the white matter pathways, and inevitably progress to a higher grade of malignancy, leading to neurologic disability and ultimately to death. Furthermore, a better understanding of cerebral processing enables us to take into consideration interaction between the disease (the glioma) and the host (the brain), namely, mechanisms of neuroplasticity.[3] As a result of this reorganization of cerebral networks, in parallel with developments in brain-mapping techniques, the benefit–risk ratio of surgery dramatically increased in the past decade. Such an improvement of the onco-functional balance of surgical resection should result in a paradigmatic shift in LGG, by switching from a traditional "wait and see" approach to an early and maximal resection based on functional-mapped guided resection. Moreover, a multistage surgical approach integrated in an individualized multimodal therapeutic strategy should be more systematically considered, with the ambitious aim of increasing the median survival as well as improving the quality of life (QoL)—that is, to solve the classic dilemma opposing OS against preservation of neurologic functions.[4]

In this setting, this chapter reviews the behavior and management of diffuse LGG in light of new insights provided by the recent literature.

■ Pathology and Genetics: Toward a Molecular Classification of Low-Grade Glioma?

The WHO classification recognizes grade II astrocytomas, oligodendrogliomas, and oligoastrocytomas. Morphological features distinguish astrocytomas from oligodendrogliomas, but the diagnosis of oligoastrocytomas may pose difficulties and may be prone to neuropathologist subjectivity. Among WHO grade II astrocytomas, cellularity is moderately increased and nuclear atypia is occasional, but mitoses, endothelial proliferation, and necrosis are not present (although rare mitotic activity is permitted in a large specimen). Diffuse astrocytomas include fibrillary (the most common), gemistocytic, and protoplasmic variants. Of note, gemistocytic astrocytomas are more prone to malignant progression. The Ki-67/MIB-1 labeling index in diffuse astrocytomas usually is < 4%. The best immunohistochemical marker is glial fibrillary acidic protein, which is expressed in both tumor cells and astrocytic processes. In oligodendrogliomas, the nuclei are round and regular, and clear perinuclear haloes are present in most paraffin-embedded specimens ("fried-eggs"). They are moderately cellular and have a dense network of capillaries and frequently

> **Pitfall**
>
> - The World Health Organization classification for LGGs is based on criteria that are highly subjective to individual pathologist interpretation and not reproducible.

contain calcifications. Occasional mitoses and a Ki-67/MIB-1 labeling index up to 5% are compatible with WHO grade II oligodendrogliomas. There is no immunohistochemical marker specific for oligodendrogliomas.

However, the WHO classification suffers from several limitations. First, it is not reproducible. This lack of reproducibility among pathologists is proven (or even when the same observer was asked to reinterpret the same histological preparations a few weeks later), with a difference of interpretation between reaction cells and tumor cells, and between astrocytes and oligodendrocytes. The interobserver discordance may reach 48% (recently reviewed elsewhere[5]). In addition, some elements are too subjective concerning the grading, such as the notion of anaplasia or cell density. Furthermore, the WHO classification does not distinguish tumoral cells from infiltrated residual brain parenchyma, and it considers the tumor to be homogeneous. Nonetheless, one frequently finds heterogeneous households on a background of diffuse LGG, corresponding to foci of increased cell density, possibly with cytonuclear atypical more pronounced than expected in LGG, which is why the term *intermediate diffuse glioma* was suggested for those cases in which the presence of these foci may lead to a faster evolution toward anaplasia.[5]

Advances in genetics brought new insights into the comprehension of LGG biology. The most frequent molecular alteration is the *IDH1/2* mutation, which occurs at a very early stage and is reported in about 80% of LGGs. Thus, development of an *IDH1-R132H* mutation-specific antibody (H09) greatly assists in the diagnosis of astrocytomas, oligodendrogliomas, and oligoastrocytomas, and distinguishes these diffuse tumors from other lower grade gliomas. About 60% of diffuse astrocytomas carry *TP53* mutations, which constitute a prognostic marker for shorter survival; gemistocytic astrocytomas carry *TP53* mutations in > 80%, whereas combined 1p/19q deletion is rare. The molecular profile of oligodendrogliomas is the combined loss of 1p/19q occurring in 70 to 80% of these tumors, which is associated with longer survival, whereas *TP53* mutations are encountered in only 5%. Most oligoastrocytomas carry either 1p/19q loss or *TP53* mutations, with a tendency for these aberrations to be present in both tumor compartments.

Thus, since the vast majority (> 90%) of WHO grade II diffuse gliomas carry at least one of these alterations, the development of a molecular classification has been proposed that complements and eventually replaces histological typing. Interestingly, the molecular profile of LGG based on *IDH1/2* mutations, *TP53* mutations, and 1p/19q loss seems to provide a more objective classification that correlates well with patient survival.[6] Additional genetic markers and molecular signatures have recently been proposed to refine the prognosis.[7]

■ Clinical Presentation

As mentioned, LGG usually affects young adults who enjoy a normal life. After an asymptomatic period that lasts several years (as demonstrated in incidentally found LGG), seizures are the most common presentation and may be partial or generalized. They occur in about 80 to 90% of patients and are intractable in 50%, especially in Rolandic, mediotemporal, and insular/paralimbic locations. Seizures are mainly due to cortical invasion, and are more frequently associated with oligodendroglial tumors. There is no clear association between severity of epilepsy and behavior of the tumor. Focal neurologic deficits due to mass effect, hemorrhage, and intracranial hypertension are not common presenting features. Indeed, neurologic deficits are rare, even if these tumors are frequently located within "eloquent areas," because of cerebral plasticity mechanisms. This phenomenon is explained by the fact that LGG is a slow-growing tumor, giving the brain many years to accomplish functional remapping, with a recruitment of perilesional or remote areas within the ipsilesional hemisphere or of contrahemispheric homologous areas.[8]

Cognitive deficits, nonetheless, are often observed when objective neuropsychological assessments are performed at the time of diagnosis, despite a normal social and professional life, challenging the traditional view that LGG patients have a normal examination.[9] Indeed, many LGG patients experience disorders of executive functions, attention, concentration, working memory, or emotion. These deficits can be attributed to the tumor itself, to seizures, and to antiepileptic drugs. Thus, a systematic assessment of higher functions and health-related QoL is now recommended before any oncological treatment for the following purposes: (1) to search for possible subtle neuropsychological deficits not identified by a classic neurologic examination; (2) to decide on a treatment strategy based on these individual results (e.g., decision of surgery first versus neoadjuvant chemotherapy in cases of very diffuse LGG-inducing important cognitive disturbances); (3) to adapt the surgical methodology to the results of this assessment (e.g., to perform functional mapping under local anesthesia even in the right hemisphere in right-handers in cases of preoperative language deficits, or to participate in the selection of optimal tasks to administer during awake surgery); (4) to provide a pretherapeutic baseline enabling a comparison with the posttherapeutic evaluation; and (5) to plan a specific functional rehabilitation following the surgical resection, which can induce a transient neurologic worsening.

■ Imaging

On magnetic resonance imaging (MRI), LGG is characteristically homogeneously isointense to hypointense on T1-weighted images and hyperintense on T2/fluid-attenuated inversion recovery (FLAIR)-weighted images (**Fig. 24.1**). When a nodular contrast enhancement is present, it indicates generally a focal area of malignant transformation, although patchy enhancement may remain stable over time in some tumors. However, one should be aware that this conventional structural MRI does not show the whole disease. Indeed, LGG invades the brain beyond the abnormalities visible on imaging,

with tumoral cells present at a distance of 10 to 20 mm of the glioma boundaries defined by MRI.[10]

Recent advances in MRI sequence development and use provided a new conceptual approach to diagnosis and follow-up of LGG based on a multiparametrical and dynamic study of metabolism enabled by spectroscopy (even multinuclear) and perfusion-weighted imaging, namely, oncological biometabolic imaging. Proton magnetic resonance spectroscopy measures major metabolites in tumoral tissue. The typical (but not specific) spectrum of an LGG shows elevated choline, reflecting increased membrane turnover and decreased N-acetyl aspartate (reflecting neuronal loss). The presence of lactate and lipids is correlated to a more aggressive tumor.[11] Dynamic susceptibility contrast MRI (DSC-MRI) enables the measurement of relative cerebral blood volume (rCBV), which is associated with vascularity. In astrocytoma, increase in rCBV in LGG predicts malignant transformation before contrast enhancement occurs. Diffusion-weighted imaging with calculation of apparent diffusion coefficient and positron emission tomography (PET) imaging (especially with ^{11}C-methionine (MET) or ^{18}F-fluoro-L-thymidine, which is a

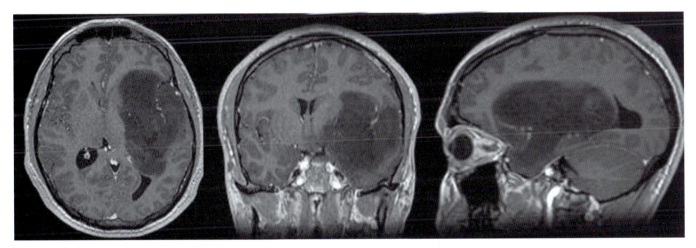

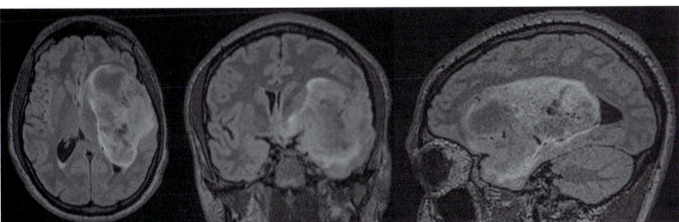

Fig. 24.1a,b Typical magnetic resonance imaging (MRI) of a low-grade glioma (LGG), involving the left paralimbic system, with enhanced (**a**) T1-weighted and (**b**) fluid-attenuated inversion recovery (FLAIR)-weighted MRI in a patient enjoying a normal life.

proliferation marker) can also be performed in LGG. Finally, metabolic imaging may be useful in guiding a biopsy to an area of high-grade activity.

From a functional point of view, advances in functional neuroimaging, for example, functional MRI (fMRI), magneto-encephalography, diffusion tensor imaging (DTI), and, more recently, transcranial magnetic stimulation, have enabled us to perform a noninvasive mapping of the whole brain. These techniques estimate the location of the eloquent areas (e.g., regions involved in sensorimotor, language, visual, and even higher cognitive functions) in relation to the glioma, and provide information with regard to the hemispheric language lateralization. Yet, it is crucial to emphasize that functional neuroimaging methods are not yet reliable enough *at the individual scale*, despite constant efforts for their improvement, mainly because they are based on biomathematical reconstruction; that is, their results may change according to the model used. Correlations with intraoperative electrophysiology have recently demonstrated that the sensitivity of fMRI is currently 59 to 100% for language (specificity, 0% to 97%).[12]

Diffusion tensor imaging enables the identification of the tractography of the main fiber bundles. This new method needs to be validated, especially by intraoperative electrophysiological techniques, before it can be used routinely for surgical planning. Indeed, comparison between distinct fiber tracking software tools found different results, showing that neurosurgeons have to be cautious about applying tractography results intraoperatively, especially when dealing with an abnormal or distorted fiber tract anatomy.[13] Correlations between DTI and intrasurgical subcortical stimulation demonstrated that, despite a good correspondence in 82% of cases, DTI is not yet optimal to map language tracts in patients. Negative tractography does not rule out the persistence of a fiber tract, especially when invaded by a glioma.[14] Moreover, DTI enables the study of the sole anatomy of the subcortical pathways, but not of their function.

■ New Insights into the Natural Course of Low-Grade Glioma

Contrary to what was claimed in the classic literature, there is no stable LGG. Objective calculation of growth rate (based on at least two MRIs spaced 3 months apart before any treatment) showed that all LGGs had a constant growth during their premalignant phase, with a linear increase of the mean diameter (computed from the volume) of about 4 mm/year.[15] This growth was observed not only in symptomatic patients but also in incidentally discovered LGG.[16] Thus, the concept of PFS is meaningless in LGG before any treatment or after an incomplete surgical resection because, in essence, all LGGs are continuously growing (whereas this end point would be unambiguous after a total resection or generally could be defined under adjuvant treatment such as chemotherapy/radiotherapy). In this context, the traditional imaging criteria, as initially proposed by MacDonald or more recently by the Response Assessment in Neuro-Oncology (RANO) group,[17] are not appropriate to monitor LGG kinetics. Furthermore, there is an inverse correlation between growth rates and survival in LGG, showing that the mean velocity of diametric expansion is a better prognostic factor than the neuropathological examination performed according to the current WHO classification.[15]

These tumors are migrating along the white matter tracts (U fibers, association, projection, and commissural pathways). Thus, LGG is not a "tumor mass," but is in fact an infiltrating chronic disease progressively invading the central nervous system, especially the subcortical connectivity. Such a diffusion of glioma cells may induce cognitive disorders, probably due (at least partly) to a "disconnection syndrome."[18]

Finally, LGGs inescapably become malignant. Such malignant transformation leads to functional deficits, with a worsening of QoL, and ultimately to death. In two European Organization for Research on Treatment of Cancer (EORTC) randomized multicenter trials with more than 600 patients, in the subgroup of patients with a favorable prognostic score, the OS was 7.7 years, whereas in the subgroup of patients with a poor prognostic score, the OS was only 3.2 years.[19] Recently, a study comparing early resection versus single biopsy demonstrated that the OS was 5.8 years in the biopsy group.[20] Thus, these data show that LGG cannot be considered any more as a "benign" tumor but rather as a cancerous disease.

■ Spontaneous Prognostic Factors

A number of retrospective and a few prospective series have evaluated clinical, radiological, pathological, and molecular variables of potential prognostic significance in patients with LGG.[19] Some of these factors have been fully validated. Clinically, age > 40 years, presence of neurologic deficits, absence of seizures at onset, and low performance status (KPS score < 70) are associated with a poorer outcome. Larger tumors, tumors crossing the midline, and rapid growth rate are also adverse prognostic factors. There are conflicting reports as to whether contrast enhancement is associated with a worse prognosis. A low CBV and low uptake of ^{11}C-MET seem to correlate with longer OS. Histologically, oligodendrogliomas have a better prognosis than astrocytomas, whereas oligoastrocytomas have an intermediate outcome. Among molecular markers, 1p-19q co-deletion and *IDH1* mutation are the most important prognostic factors.[21]

The Impact of Surgical Resection in Low-Grade Glioma

Comprehensive reviews suggest that a more extensive resection of LGG was correlated with a more favorable OS.[22] An analysis of 10 studies since 1990[23] showed that the OS increased from 61.1 to 90.5 months with a greater extent of resection (EOR), that is, gross total versus subtotal resection. However, the main problem explaining discrepancies in the older literature is related to the fact that, in the vast majority of series, EOR was not objectively assessed on postoperative MRI, but was based solely on the subjectivity of the surgeons or on a single computed tomography (CT) scan, with no volume measurement of the residue. Due to the invasive features of LGG, the residual tumor was doubtlessly underestimated in numerous studies, resulting in erroneous conclusions about the benefit of surgery. In fact, T2/FLAIR-MRI is the only way to actually calculate the postsurgical volume of (possible) residual tumor.

The Modern Literature

In all the recent series based on an objective postoperative evaluation of EOR on T2/FLAIR-MRI, a more aggressive resection predicted a significant improvement in OS compared with a simple debulking. These studies confirmed that when no signal abnormality was visible on control MRI ("complete resection"), patients had a significantly longer OS compared with patients having any residual abnormality. In a series examining 216 LGGs, after adjusting for the effects of age, KPS score, tumor location, and tumor subtype, EOR remained a significant predictor of OS (hazard ratio [HR], 0.972; 95% confidence interval [CI], 0.960–0.983; $p < 0.001$), with 98% of patients with complete resection having an OS of 8 years.[24] In another series of 156 LGGs, patients who underwent incom-

plete resection were at 4.9 times the risk of death relative to patients with total resection.[25] A third series of 222 LGGs found a significant correlation between complete resection and OS.[26] One study demonstrated that, in multivariate analysis performed in a consecutive series with 93 LGGs, EOR and postoperative KPS score showed independent prognostic significance for OS rates.[27] Another study observed that grosstotal resection versus subtotal resection was independently associated with increased OS (HR, 0.36; 95% CI, 0.16–0.84; $p = 0.017$).[28]

In a study of 130 LGGs, extended surgery was shown to significantly prolong OS.[29] It was also reported that, in an experience with 314 LGG patients, adverse prognostic factors for OS identified by multivariate analysis were tumor size 5 cm or larger, presentation with sensory motor symptoms, pure astrocytoma histology, Kernohan grade 2, and less than subtotal resection.[30] In 190 LGGs, it was demonstrated that patients with an EOR of 90% or greater had an estimated 5-year OS rate of 93%, those with EOR between 70% and 89% had a 5-year OS rate of 84%, and those with EOR less than 70% had a 5 year OS rate of 41% ($p < 0.001$).[31] Recently, one study investigated survival in population-based parallel cohorts of LGGs from two Norwegian university hospitals with different surgical treatment strategies.[20] The study found that treatment at a center that favored early surgical resection was associated with better OS (median survival not reached) than treatment at a center that favored biopsy and watchful waiting (median survival 5.9 years; 95% CI, 4.5-7.3). Finally, the French Glioma Network published the largest surgical series of LGG ever reported, 1,097 patients, and found that EOR as well as the postsurgical residual volume were independent prognostic factors significantly associated with a longer OS.[32]

Even in incomplete tumor removal, patients with a greater percentage of resection had a significantly longer OS. The survival was significantly better, with at least 90% EOR compared with less than 90% EOR, whereas EOR of at least 80% remained a significant predictor of OS.[24] The postoperative tumor volume is also a predictor of survival, with a significantly longer OS when the residue is less than 10 cc ("subtotal resection") compared with more than 10 cc ("partial resection"). In a subgroup of 122 LGG patients who underwent surgery with intraoperative functional mapping, one study reported that, with a median follow-up of 4 years, 20.6% of patients with more than 10 cc of residue died, whereas only 8% of patients with less than 10 cc of residue died, and that no patients with complete resection died ($p = 0.02$).[26]

Such an impact on OS is due to the fact that surgery delayed histological upgrading, because the volume of residual tumor serves as a predictor of malignant transformation. In a recent series, after adjusting for the effects of age, KPS score, tumor location, and subtype, EOR remained a significant predictor of PFS (HR, 0.983; 95% CI, 0.972–0.995; $p = 0.005$).[24] In 191 consecutive LGGs, one study showed that total resection was an independent factor associated with malignant trans-

- Early and maximal resection is the first therapeutic option to consider for patients with LGG. It is associated with greater overall survival, better seizure control, and better quality of life.

formation (relative risk [RR], 0.526; 95% CI, 0.221–1.007; p = 0.05).[33]

To summarize, early and maximal surgical resection is the first therapeutic option to consider in LGG, as recommended by the European Federation of Neurological Societies guidelines.[21] Finally, beyond its oncological interest, surgery also has a positive impact on seizure control and thus on QoL. The factors associated with postoperative freedom from seizures are gross-total resection, preoperative seizure history of less than 1 year, and non–simple partial seizure type.[34]

Toward a Supratotal Resection of Low-Grade Glioma (Fig. 24.2)

As already mentioned, biopsy samples within and beyond MRI-defined abnormalities showed that imaging underestimated the spatial extent of LGG, because tumoral cells were present around the area of MRI signal abnormalities, up to 20 mm. Therefore, a recent series reported that a "supratotal" resection, that is, resection extending beyond the area of MRI signal abnormalities, performed in 15 patients with a LGG within non-eloquent brain regions avoided malignant transformation with a mean follow-up of 35.7 months (range, 6–135 months).[10] This series was compared with a control group of 29 patients who had only complete resection for a LGG; malignant transformation was observed in seven cases in the control group but in no cases in the series of patients who underwent supratotal resection (p = 0.037). Furthermore, adjuvant treatment was administrated in 10 patients in the control group, whereas only one patient who underwent supracomplete resection had adjuvant treatment (p = 0.043). However, four of 15 patients with supracomplete resection experienced recurrence, probably due to the fact that it was not possible to take 20 mm of margin all around the tumor in all patients due to functional limitations. Thus, the goal of supratotal resection is to delay malignant transformation and the administration of adjuvant therapy, without claiming to cure LGG patients.

The Value of Reoperation

Because relapse is possible after total or even supratotal resection, and because continuous growth of the residual tumor is ineluctable after incomplete resection, the impact of a second surgery was investigated. In 40 patients reoperated for recurrent LGG without other intervening therapy between sur-

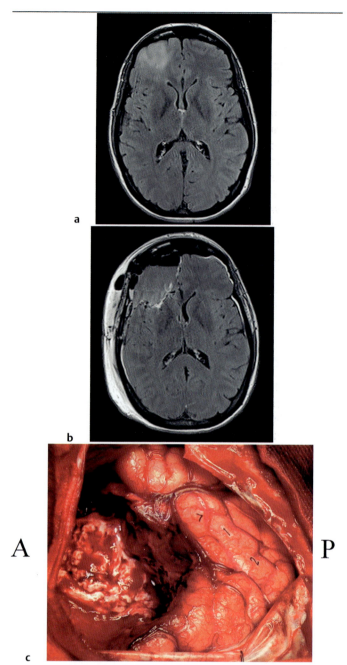

Fig. 24.2a–c Supratotal resection of a right frontal LGG in a left-handed patient, demonstrated by comparing (**a**) preoperative FLAIR MRI and (**b**) immediate postoperative FLAIR MRI. (**c**) The resection was performed with the patient in the awake condition according to functional boundaries identified both at cortical and subcortical levels (*number tags*). A, anterior; P, posterior.

geries, gross-total resection was associated with an increased time to repeated surgery.[35] In another series of 130 LGGs, extended resection for nonmalignant relapse (a total resection could be achieved in 53.1% of recurrent tumors) prolonged the OS significantly.[29] In the French Glioma Network series, subsequent surgical resection was an independent prognostic factor significantly associated with a longer OS.[32] One study also reported a consecutive series of 19 patients who underwent a second surgery for recurrent LGG in eloquent areas.[36] A total or subtotal resection was achieved in 73.7% of patients during the reoperation, despite an involvement of functional areas. Such a multistage surgical approach, with an initial maximal function-guided resection, followed by a period of several years, and then a second surgery with optimization of EOR while preserving QoL, is possible thanks to mechanisms of brain plasticity induced both by the tumor (re)growth as well as by the first resection itself.[37] The median time between surgeries was 4.1 years and the median follow-up from initial diagnosis was 6.6 years with no death during this period. Thus, the authors suggested considering reoperation in all recurrent LGGs. Nonetheless, due to a high rate of malignant transformation, histologically proven to be 57.9% at reoperation, it was proposed that "over-indicating" an early reintervention was preferable to performing a late surgery when malignant transformation had already occurred.[36]

The Limited Role of Biopsy in Low-Grade Glioma

Currently, the indications for biopsy are very limited in LGG. Indeed, by combining clinical and imaging data, the diagnosis of glioma is typical in the vast majority of cases. Thus, the main goal of neuropathological examination is to give the actual grade of the glioma. However, there is a high risk of sampling error. Overgrading of WHO grade I gliomas occurs in approximately 11% of cases and undergrading of WHO grade III gliomas occurs in 28%.[38] Conversely, maximal LGG resection provides a more extensive amount of tumoral tissue, and thus increases the reliability of the histological diagnosis and grading.[22]

Furthermore, biopsy has no therapeutic impact. Therefore, because the risk of permanent deficit after MRI-guided stereotactic biopsy is still around 2%, its indication for presumed LGG is essentially a contraindication for surgery. Beyond patients who do not want or who are unable to undergo surgical resection for medical reasons, biopsy can be mainly considered in diffuse lesions, such as gliomatosis, or when a subtotal resection is not possible a priori. Such a presurgical prediction can be optimized by the use of a probabilistic map of postoperative residue, based on the computation of residual gliomas resected according to functional boundaries; this atlas enables a preoperative estimation of the expected EOR with a success rate of 82%.[39]

Special Consideration

- The use of biopsy in LGG is very limited. It may be used in the setting of a diffuse lesion or when subtotal resection is not possible.

From an Image-Guided Surgery Toward a Functional Mapping-Guided Resection

Because of a great interindividual anatomofunctional variability, even though anatomic landmarks remain essential during cerebral surgery, they are definitely not enough. The aim is to continue the removal of the brain invaded by LGG until crucial eloquent structures have been encountered, at both the cortical and subcortical levels, with no margin around these functional boundaries.[40] As mentioned, the data provided by fMRI and DTI are not the absolute truth. Their results may change according to the biomathematical model used, which explains their lack of reliability at the individual level, especially regarding cognitive functions such as language. Neuroimaging cannot differentiate areas crucial for brain functions from regions that could be functionally compensated. Thus, there is a double risk (1) of not selecting a patient for LGG surgery because fMRI activations are visible very near or within the tumor, whereas it was in fact possible to remove it with no permanent deficit (thus, a lost opportunity from an oncological point of view), or (2) of inducing a permanent deficit due to a false negative.

Intraoperative electrostimulation mapping in awake patient is actually the more reliable method to identify eloquent regions. The goal here is not to detail the methodology of direct electrical stimulation (DES), extensively described in previous reports.[41] This is an easy, safe, inexpensive, reliable, and reproducible technique enabling the identification of crucial (nonfunctionally compensable) structures at the level of the cortex, white matter pathways, and deep gray nuclei, and thus enabling performing real-time anatomofunctional correlations throughout the resection.

In the past decade, brain mapping has led to an impressive improvement of both functional and oncological outcomes in LGG surgery. First, patients who were historically not selected for surgery, on the basis of pure anatomic criteria (e.g., gliomas involving Broca's area), can now benefit from resection with no dogmatic evidence against the surgical feasibility due to tumor location. The use of intrasurgical DES enabled a significant increase of the surgical indications for LGG involving so-called eloquent areas, when compared with a control group of patients who underwent resection under general anesthesia with no mapping.[26] For example, surgical resection is possible with no permanent neurologic worsening for LGGs in Broca's area, Wernicke's area, the insula, the left dominant inferior parietal lobule, the retrocentral area, and even the precentral region[4] (**Fig. 24.3**).

Furthermore, awake mapping has significantly decreased the rate of permanent neurologic deficits to less than 2% in series using DES.[42,43] This rate is highly reproducible among the teams using awake mapping worldwide. Indeed, a recent meta-analysis studying 8,091 patients who underwent surgical resection for a brain glioma demonstrated that the use of intrasurgical mapping enabled a statistically significant reduction of permanent deficit, despite an increased rate of resection within eloquent areas.[44]

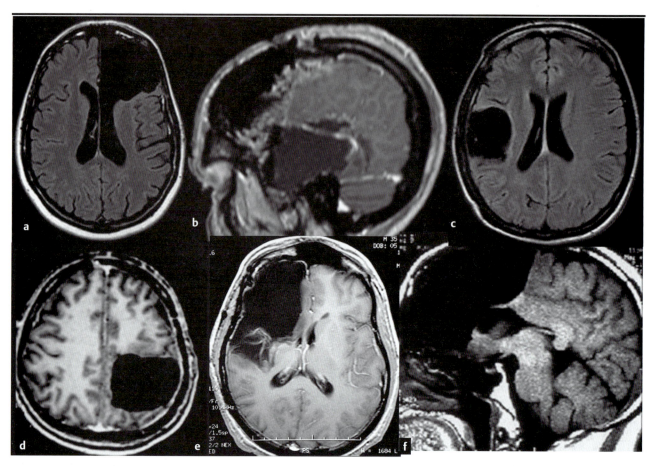

Fig. 24.3a–f Maximal surgical resections of LGGs in eloquent areas (e.g., Broca's area, Wernicke's area, Rolandic area, insula, corpus callosum) with no functional consequences owing to mechanisms of brain plasticity.

This meta-analysis also showed that EOR was increased. This is in line with a recent series in which nine patients underwent two consecutive surgeries for a LGG; the first resection was performed in a traditional way, that is, under general anesthesia and without mapping, whereas the subsequent surgery was done in a maximal way, in awake patients using DES. Following the reoperation, postoperative MRI showed that the resection was improved in all cases compared with the first surgery ($p = 0.04$), with no permanent neurologic worsening.[45] Finally, a series of 281 patients demonstrated that the use of functional mapping-guided resection of LGG in presumed eloquent areas enabled not only a maximization of EOR but also a significant improvement of OS.[46]

In this era of dramatic improvement of functional outcomes, performing early and radical surgical resections in incidental LGG has recently been suggested. A higher rate of total and supratotal resections have been achieved, due to the fact that the tumors were smaller. However, microfoci of malignant transformation were observed, even in asymptomatic patients. Interestingly, in a series of incidental LGGs involving eloquent areas that were operated on with awake mapping, the rate of permanent deficit was zero. These preliminary results support the development of a "prophylactic functional neuro-oncological surgery" in LGG.[47,48]

■ Adjuvant therapy

Although watchful waiting should be the rule following a complete or supratotal resection for LGG, adjuvant therapy could be considered in high-risk patients—those with partial resection (with a residual volume > 10–15 cc) or with rapid progression calculated on regular postoperative MRIs per-

> **Pearl**
>
> • DES enables reliable delineation of true functional and non-functional regions and should be universally implemented as standard of care for glioma surgery.

formed every 6 months (or every 3 months in LGGs with foci of malignant transformation on pathological examination). Postoperative intractable seizures can also be an indication for adjuvant treatment.

Chemotherapy

Chemotherapy has shown clinical benefits against tumor progression for patients who cannot be operated or reoperated on due to a diffuse involvement of eloquent structures by the tumor. Procarbazine, chloroethylcyclohexylnitrosourea (CCNU; lomustine), and vincristine (PCV) and temozolomide (TMZ) yield similar objective response rates on MRI, with more than 90% of patients experiencing initial decrease of the mean tumor diameter.[49] However, a toxicity profile favors TMZ in terms of better tolerability (reduced myelotoxicity) and QoL.

> **Pearl**
>
> - Adjuvant chemotherapy may be useful for shrinking a tumor prior to surgery and enabling a more extensive resection.

Patients more likely to respond have oligodendroglial tumors, but mixed or astrocytic tumors may respond as well. Beyond this initial chemosensitivity, which is almost constant in LGG, chemotherapy may also result in a control of epilepsy and thus may enable an improvement of cognition and QoL. When chemotherapy was discontinued in the absence of tumor progression, a majority of LGGs resumed their progressive growth within 1 year,[49] whereas a tumor volume decrease can be delayed longer.[50] The response rate after chemotherapy is higher and the duration of response is longer in patients with 1p/19q loss. A stronger role for chemotherapy with surgery has been discussed more recently in unresectable tumors, by allowing glioma shrinkage due to neoadjuvant chemotherapy and thus making surgery (with total or at least subtotal removal) possible.[51]

Radiotherapy

Two phase 3 randomized trials demonstrated no advantage for high versus low radiation doses, with increased toxicity for higher doses (EORTC 22844 and North Central Cancer Treatment Group [NCCTG]). Regarding the timing of radiotherapy (RT), one study demonstrated that early RT had no impact on overall survival (despite an improved PFS; EORTC 22845).[52] In addition, although RT may participate in seizure control, it was shown that patients who had a neuropsychological follow-up at a mean of 12 years and were free of tumor progression maintain their cognitive status if not irradiated, whereas patients receiving RT do worse with regard to their

> **Pearl**
>
> - Radiotherapy, because of its potential delayed neurotoxicity and the equivalent results in terms of survival whatever the timing of the treatment (early or late), is increasingly offered to patients with unresectable tumors (or tumor that cannot be reoperated) and in cases of progression after chemotherapy, but not as a first therapeutic option.

attentional and executive functioning as well as information processing speed.[53] Recently, Radiation Therapy Oncology Group (RTOG) trial 9802 compared RT alone with RT plus PCV. The PFS, but not the OS, improved. However, on post hoc analysis, for 2-year survivors ($n = 211$), the addition of PCV to RT conferred a survival advantage, suggesting a delayed benefit for chemotherapy. Indeed, the probability of OS for an additional 5 years was 74% with RT + PCV versus 59% with RT alone (HR, 0.52; 95% CI, 0.30–0.90; log-rank $p = 0.02$).[54]

▓ Individualized Multistage Therapeutic Strategies in Low-Grade Glioma

An optimal strategy should be adapted to the complex biological course of LGG at the individual level (**Fig. 24.4**). Indeed, in the traditional literature, the vast majority of studies investigated the role of only one specific treatment (e.g., impact of surgery, impact of radiotherapy, or impact of chemotherapy) without a global view of treatment. The goal is now to switch to a more holistic view, based on the anticipation of a personalized and long-term multistage therapeutic approach, with an online adaptation of the management over years through the feedback provided by clinical, radiological, and pathologico-molecular monitoring at the individual scale. This dynamic strategy challenges the traditional attitude regarding different factors: by proposing earlier therapy; by repeating treatments (e.g., two to four surgical resections spaced by several years, or periods of 6 to 12 months of chemotherapy spaced by periods of single follow-up); and by reversing the traditional order of therapies (e.g., neoadjuvant chemotherapy followed by surgery after tumor shrinkage, and no early radiotherapy), with the ultimate goal of increasing both OS and QoL. To this end, beyond the benefit-to-risk ratio of each isolated treatment, the impact of the whole therapeutic strategy on the cumulative time with QoL versus time to malignant transformation (and not solely on survival independent of the functional status of the patient) should be taken into account. In other words, new individualized management strategies should deal with the chronic interactions among the natural

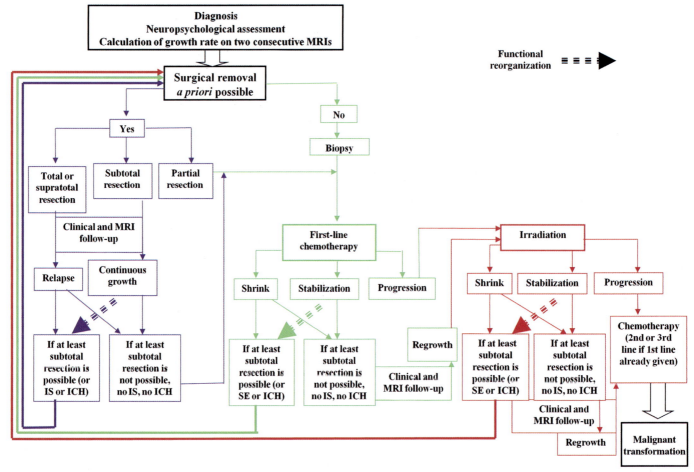

Fig. 24.4 Multistage and plurimodal therapeutic strategies in LGG. ICH, intracranial hypertension; IS, intractable seizure; SE, seizure. (Adapted from Duffau H. Diffuse Low-Grade Gliomas in Adults: Natural History, Interaction with the Brain, and New Individualized Therapeutic Strategies. London: Springer, 2013.)

course of the LGG, the reactional brain remapping, and the onco-functional modulation elicited by serial treatments.[4]

■ Conclusion

The current philosophy for treatment of LGG patients is to anticipate (before neurologic or even cognitive worsening) a personalized, multimodal, and long-term management approach from the diagnosis to the malignant stage of the disease, with online treatment adjustment over time on the basis of regular functional feedback and radiological monitoring. The ultimate aim is not (yet) to cure this tumor but nonetheless to be preventive by delaying malignant transformation as longer as possible while preserving an optimal QoL. To this end, a multidisciplinary discussion is crucial at every stage of the glioma, allowing evaluation of new strategies and open discussions between medical and surgical neuro-oncologists. Such an attitude has already enabled a significant improvement of both functional and oncological outcomes in the past

decade. The goal is now to use this new state of mind to challenge the old dogmas, in order to continue to elaborate and validate original strategies through national and international networks, with the goal of giving LGG patients the best QoL, including long-term projects such as pregnancy.

Editor's Note

In spite of the growing evidence supporting early and aggressive resection of LGGs in adults, the evidence is not class 1. The "wait and see" approach consisting of periodic monitoring with MRI and clinical status without intervention upfront may still be appropriate, particularly for those patients with eloquently situated or indistinct tumors and minimal symptoms, such as having only one seizure. Of course, at signs of progression on the MRI, usually first seen on FLAIR, surgery that is as aggressive as safely possible is indicated.

A recent German survey found that about 50% of centers in that country use the "wait and see" approach routinely for patients with suspected LGG.[55] Another current study used qualitative research methodology to discover that patients treated with a "wait and see" approach did not experience undue anxiety while waiting.[56]

This is a group of tumors with variable biology, and many are extremely indolent and even quiescent. Until class I evidence demonstrates definitive superiority of aggressive early surgery for LGG, the "wait and see" approach, which among other things defers risk, still must be considered part of the armamentarium for some patients. (Bernstein)

References

1. Rigau V, Zouaoui S, Mathieu-Daudé H, et al; Société Française de Neuropathologie (SFNP), Société Française de Neurochirurgie (SFNC); Club de Neuro-Oncologie of the Société Française de Neurochirurgie (CNO-SFNC); Association des Neuro-Oncologues d'Expression Française (ANOCEF). French brain tumor database: 5-year histological results on 25 756 cases. Brain Pathol 2011;21:633–644

2. Smits A, Duffau H. Seizures and the natural history of World Health Organization grade II gliomas: a review. Neurosurgery 2011;68:1326–1333

3. Duffau H. Lessons from brain mapping in surgery for low-grade glioma: insights into associations between tumour and brain plasticity. Lancet Neurol 2005;4:476–486

4. Duffau H. Diffuse Low-Grade Gliomas in Adults: Natural History, Interaction with the Brain, and New Individualized Therapeutic Strategies. London: Springer, 2013

5. Rigau V. Histological classification. In Duffau H, ed. Diffuse Low-Grade Gliomas in Adults: Natural History, Interaction with the Brain, and New Individualized Therapeutic Strategies. London: Springer, 2013

6. Kim YH, Nobusawa S, Mittelbronn M, et al. Molecular classification of low-grade diffuse gliomas. Am J Pathol 2010;177:2708–2714

7. Rème T, Hugnot JP, Bièche I, et al. A molecular predictor reassesses classification of human grade II/III gliomas. PLoS ONE 2013;8:e66574

8. Desmurget M, Bonnetblanc F, Duffau H. Contrasting acute and slow-growing lesions: a new door to brain plasticity. Brain 2007;130(Pt 4):898–914

9. Klein M, Duffau H, De Witt Hamer PC. Cognition and resective surgery for diffuse infiltrative glioma: an overview. J Neurooncol 2012;108:309–318

10. Yordanova YN, Moritz-Gasser S, Duffau H. Awake surgery for WHO grade II gliomas within "noneloquent" areas in the left dominant hemisphere: toward a "supratotal" resection. Clinical article. J Neurosurg 2011;115:232–239

11. Guillevin R, Menuel C, Taillibert S, et al. Predicting the outcome of grade II glioma treated with temozolomide using proton magnetic resonance spectroscopy. Br J Cancer 2011;104:1854–1861

12. Giussani C, Roux FE, Ojemann J, Sganzerla EP, Pirillo D, Papagno C. Is preoperative functional magnetic resonance imaging reliable for language areas mapping in brain tumor surgery? Review of language functional magnetic resonance imaging and direct cortical stimulation correlation studies. Neurosurgery 2010;66:113–120

13. Duffau H. The dangers of magnetic resonance imaging diffusion tensor tractography in brain surgery. World Neurosurg 2013; In press

14. Leclercq D, Duffau H, Delmaire C, et al. Comparison of diffusion tensor imaging tractography of language tracts and intraoperative subcortical stimulations. J Neurosurg 2010;112:503–511

15. Pallud J, Blonski M, Mandonnet E, et al. Velocity of tumor spontaneous expansion predicts long-term outcomes for diffuse low-grade gliomas. Neuro-oncol 2013;15:595–606

16. Pallud J, Fontaine D, Duffau H, et al. Natural history of incidental World Health Organization grade II gliomas. Ann Neurol 2010;68:727–733

17. van den Bent MJ, Wefel JS, Schiff D, et al. Response assessment in neuro-oncology (a report of the RANO group): assessment of outcome in trials of diffuse low-grade gliomas. Lancet Oncol 2011;12:583–593

18. Duffau H. The "frontal syndrome" revisited: lessons from electrostimulation mapping studies. Cortex 2012a;48:120–131

19. Pignatti F, van den Bent M, Curran D, et al; European Organization for Research and Treatment of Cancer Brain Tumor Cooperative Group; European Organization for Research and Treatment of Cancer Radiotherapy Cooperative Group. Prognostic factors for survival in adult patients with cerebral low-grade glioma. J Clin Oncol 2002;20:2076–2084

20. Jakola AS, Myrmel KS, Kloster R, et al. Comparison of a strategy favoring early surgical resection vs a strategy favoring watchful waiting in low-grade gliomas. JAMA 2012;308:1881–1888

21. Soffietti R, Baumert BG, Bello L, et al; European Federation of Neurological Societies. Guidelines on management of low-grade gliomas: report of an EFNS-EANO Task Force. Eur J Neurol 2010;17:1124–1133

22. Sanai N, Chang S, Berger MS. Low-grade gliomas in adults. J Neurosurg 2011;115:948–965

23. Sanai N, Berger MS. Glioma extent of resection and its impact on patient outcome. Neurosurgery 2008;62:753–764, discussion 264–266

24. Smith JS, Chang EF, Lamborn KR, et al. Role of extent of resection in the long-term outcome of low-grade hemispheric gliomas. J Clin Oncol 2008;26:1338–1345

25. Claus EB, Horlacher A, Hsu L, et al. Survival rates in patients with low-grade glioma after intraoperative magnetic resonance image guidance. Cancer 2005;103:1227–1233

26. Duffau H, Lopes M, Arthuis F, et al. Contribution of intraoperative electrical stimulations in surgery of low grade gliomas: a comparative study between two series without (1985–96) and with (1996–2003) functional mapping in the same institution. J Neurol Neurosurg Psychiatry 2005;76:845–851

27. Yeh SA, Ho JT, Lui CC, Huang YJ, Hsiung CY, Huang EY. Treatment outcomes and prognostic factors in patients with supratentorial low-grade gliomas. Br J Radiol 2005;78:230–235

28. McGirt MJ, Chaichana KL, Attenello FJ, et al. Extent of surgical resection is independently associated with survival in patients with hemispheric infiltrating low-grade gliomas. Neurosurgery 2008;63:700–707, author reply 707–708

29. Ahmadi R, Dictus C, Hartmann C, et al. Long-term outcome and survival of surgically treated supratentorial low-grade glioma in adult patients. Acta Neurochir (Wien) 2009;151:1359–1365

30. Schomas DA, Laack NN, Rao RD, et al. Intracranial low-grade gliomas in adults: 30-year experience with long-term follow-up at Mayo Clinic. Neuro-oncol 2009;11:437–445

31. Ius T, Isola M, Budai R, et al. Low-grade glioma surgery in eloquent areas: volumetric analysis of extent of resection and its impact on overall survival. A single-institution experience in 190 patients: clinical article. J Neurosurg 2012;117:1039–1052

32. Capelle L, Fontaine D, Mandonnet E, et al. Spontaneous and therapeutic prognostic factors in adult hemispheric WHO grade II gliomas: a series of 1097 cases. J Neurosurg 2013;118:1157–1168

33. Chaichana KL, McGirt MJ, Laterra J, Olivi A, Quiñones-Hinojosa A. Recurrence and malignant degeneration after resection of adult hemispheric low-grade gliomas. J Neurosurg 2010;112:10–17

34. Englot DJ, Berger MS, Barbaro NM, Chang EF. Predictors of seizure freedom after resection of supratentorial low-grade gliomas. A review. J Neurosurg 2011;115:240–244

35. Schmidt MH, Berger MS, Lamborn KR, et al. Repeated operations for infiltrative low-grade gliomas without intervening therapy. J Neurosurg 2003;98:1165–1169

36. Martino J, Taillandier L, Moritz-Gasser S, Gatignol P, Duffau H. Reoperation is a safe and effective therapeutic strategy in recurrent WHO grade II gliomas within eloquent areas. Acta Neurochir (Wien) 2009; 151:427–436, discussion 436

37. Gil Robles S, Gatignol P, Lehéricy S, Duffau H. Long-term brain plasticity allowing multiple-stages surgical approach for WHO grade II gliomas in eloquent areas: a combined study using longitudinal functional MRI and intraoperative electrical stimulation. J Neurosurg 2008; 109:615–624

38. Muragaki Y, Chernov M, Maruyama T, et al. Low-grade glioma on stereotactic biopsy: how often is the diagnosis accurate? Minim Invasive Neurosurg 2008;51:275–279

39. Mandonnet E, Jbabdi S, Taillandier L, et al. Preoperative estimation of residual volume for WHO grade II glioma resected with intraoperative functional mapping. Neuro-oncol 2007;9:63–69

40. Gil-Robles S, Duffau H. Surgical management of World Health Organization Grade II gliomas in eloquent areas: the necessity of preserving a margin around functional structures. Neurosurg Focus 2010;28:E8

41. Duffau H. Brain Mapping: From Neural Basis of Cognition to Surgical Applications. New York: Springer, 2011

42. Duffau H, Gatignol P, Mandonnet E, Capelle L, Taillandier L. Contribution of intraoperative subcortical stimulation mapping of language pathways: a consecutive series of 115 patients operated on for a WHO grade II glioma in the left dominant hemisphere. J Neurosurg 2008; 109:461–471

43. Sanai N, Mirzadeh Z, Berger MS. Functional outcome after language mapping for glioma resection. N Engl J Med 2008;358:18–27

44. De Witt Hamer PC, Robles SG, Zwinderman AH, Duffau H, Berger MS. Impact of intraoperative stimulation brain mapping on glioma surgery outcome: a meta-analysis. J Clin Oncol 2012;30:2559–2565

45. De Benedictis A, Moritz-Gasser S, Duffau H. Awake mapping optimizes the extent of resection for low-grade gliomas in eloquent areas. Neurosurgery 2010;66:1074–1084, discussion 1084

46. Chang EF, Clark A, Smith JS, et al. Functional mapping-guided resection of low-grade gliomas in eloquent areas of the brain: improvement of long-term survival. Clinical article. J Neurosurg 2011;114:566–573

47. Duffau H. Surgery of low-grade gliomas: towards a 'functional neuro-oncology'. Curr Opin Oncol 2009;21:543–549

48. Duffau H. Awake surgery for incidental WHO grade II gliomas involving eloquent areas. Acta Neurochir (Wien) 2012b;154:575–584, discussion 584

49. Ricard D, Kaloshi G, Amiel-Benouaich A, et al. Dynamic history of low-grade gliomas before and after temozolomide treatment. Ann Neurol 2007;61:484–490

50. Peyre M, Cartalat-Carel S, Meyronet D, et al. Prolonged response without prolonged chemotherapy: a lesson from PCV chemotherapy in low-grade gliomas. Neuro-Oncol 2010;12:1078–1082

51. Blonski M, Taillandier L, Herbet G, et al. Combination of neoadjuvant chemotherapy followed by surgical resection as a new strategy for WHO grade II gliomas: a study of cognitive status and quality of life. J Neurooncol 2012;106:353–366

52. van den Bent MJ, Afra D, de Witte O, et al; EORTC Radiotherapy and Brain Tumor Groups and the UK Medical Research Council. Long-term efficacy of early versus delayed radiotherapy for low-grade astrocytoma and oligodendroglioma in adults: the EORTC 22845 randomised trial. Lancet 2005;366:985–990

53. Douw L, Klein M, Fagel SS, et al. Cognitive and radiological effects of radiotherapy in patients with low-grade glioma: long-term follow-up. Lancet Neurol 2009;8:810–818

54. Shaw EG, Wang M, Coons SW, et al. Randomized trial of radiation therapy plus procarbazine, lomustine, and vincristine chemotherapy for supratentorial adult low-grade glioma: initial results of RTOG 9802. J Clin Oncol 2012;30:3065–3070

55. Seiz M, Freyschlag CF, Schenkel S, et al. Management of patients with low-grade gliomas—a survey among German neurosurgical departments. Cent Eur Neurosurg 2011;72:186–191

56. Hayhurst C, Mendelsohn D, Bernstein M. Low grade glioma: a qualitative study of patients' perspectives on the wait and see approach. Can J Neurol Sci 2011;38:256–261

25 Malignant Gliomas

Richard G. Everson and Linda M. Liau

Over 23,000 new cases of primary nervous system tumors are diagnosed in the United States every year, resulting in nearly 14,000 deaths annually.[1,2] Although primary intrinsic malignant brain tumors occur less frequently than either extra-axial tumors or metastatic disease to the central nervous system (CNS), they are disproportionately lethal.[3] Despite significant advances in diagnostic neuroimaging and in techniques for surgical resection and for the delivery of chemotherapy and radiation over the past 50 years in neuro-oncology, improvements in the survival of glioblastoma multiforme (GBM), the most common type of malignant glioma, remain modest. As such, innovative translational research and clinical trials of novel therapeutics continue to be actively pursued for this disease.

Gliomas are tumors of neuroepithelial origin derived from glial cells or cell precursors.[4] The designation *malignant* refers to the abnormal proliferation, invasion, and metastatic potential of the cells forming these tumors. Glioma is a more inclusive classification encompassing two major basic histopathological subtypes: astrocytoma and oligodendroglioma. Current treatment consists of surgical resection, postoperative radiation, and chemotherapy, and has been found to provide a slight increase in overall survival.[5]

■ Tumor Types

World Health Organization Classification

Several different systems of classification of malignant gliomas based on survival, histological, and molecular data have been used. Today, the main system of classification of malignant gliomas is the World Health Organization (WHO) system.[6] The system divides astrocytomas into four grades: grade I, pilocytic astrocytomas; grade II, diffuse low-grade astrocytomas; grade III, anaplastic astrocytomas; and grade IV, glioblastomas. Although grade III and IV tumors are commonly designated as the "malignant" varieties, grade II astrocytomas could also be considered as such, given the high rate of malignant degeneration and ultimate fatality of low-grade astrocytomas. The WHO system designates those tumors with nuclear atypia alone as grade II, those with higher degrees of mitosis and nuclear atypia as grade III, and reserves a grade IV designation for those exhibiting microvascular proliferation or necrosis (**Fig. 25.1**).

Oligodendrogliomas and oligoastrocytomas are classified by morphological appearance, with the term *anaplastic* added to those with a high incidence of mitoses and nuclear atypia.

Molecular Classification

Glioblastoma was one of the first tumor types studied in the large-scale National Institutes of Health (NIH) effort, The Cancer Genome Atlas (TCGA) project, which seeks to systematically and robustly characterize the molecular alterations found in cancer. Gene expression profiling of GBM found four distinct molecular subtypes of primary glioblastomas (classical, proneural, mesenchymal, and neural) that correlate with genomic abnormalities, bear prognostic significance, and may predict benefit of therapy.[7]

The classical GBM group is characterized by overexpression of epidermal growth factor receptor (EGFR), as well as the absence of *TP53* mutations. Clinically, the classical group survived the longest of the subgroups in response to aggressive treatment.

Proneural tumors make up the largest proportion of GBMs and frequently harbor mutations of *TP53, PDGFRA,* and *IDH1*. Patients with the proneural type tended to be significantly younger than the other subgroups and survive longer, but did not appear to benefit significantly from aggressive treatment.

Mesenchymal GBMs are categorized by *NF1* mutations, as well as by having frequent mutations in *PTEN* and *TP53*. Patients in the mesenchymal subgroup had the worst prognosis; although they appeared to realize a benefit from aggressive chemotherapy, the benefit not as much as that seen in the classical subgroup of GBM.

The neural group did not have significant rates of unique genetic alterations.

With an increasing number of studies validating the above classification scheme, future treatments for malignant gliomas may become more tailored to molecular genetic subgroups.

■ Epidemiology

Gliomas constitute 29% of all primary brain tumors, and 54% of gliomas are glioblastoma, by far the most common subtype. The reported incidence of grade III anaplastic astrocytomas (AAs) varies widely from 10 to 30% of all the gliomas.[1,3] In

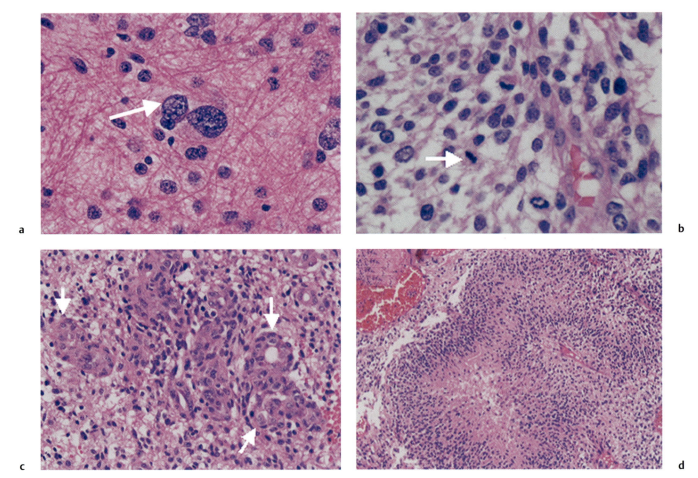

Fig. 25.1a–d Pathological features and grading of malignant gliomas (WHO grades III to IV). (**a**) Nuclear atypia (*arrow*). (**b**) Mitotic figures (*arrow*). (**c**) Neovascular proliferation (*arrows*). (**d**) Pseudopalisading necrosis.

the pediatric population, AA and GBM constitute only a minority (< 10%) of all intracranial tumors.[8]

Glioblastoma (WHO grade IV) is rare in patients younger than 30 years of age, and most frequent between the ages of 45 and 65. The male-to-female ratio is 1.6:1. Anaplastic astrocytoma (WHO grade III AA) tends to occur in middle age (35 to 55 years), generally a decade before GBM appears.[6] The annual incidence of malignant gliomas is approximately 5 cases per 100,000 people.[3] Anaplastic oligodendroglioma (AO) commonly occurs around the fourth decade of life. The incidence of these tumors has increased slightly over the past two decades, especially in the elderly, likely as a result of improved diagnostic imaging.[9]

Special Consideration

- Malignant gliomas tend to spread or recur in adjacent brain regions along white matter tracts. Spread outside the central nervous system (CNS) is extremely rare.

Approximately 60% of gliomas are located in one of the cerebral hemispheres, with the frontal lobe most common (25.6%), followed by the temporal lobe (19.6%) and parietal lobe (12.6%). Glioblastoma multiforme is uncommon in the region of the third ventricle (< 1%) and rarely occurs in the posterior fossa. Although most GBMs are centered in the deep white matter, approximately 10% may present on the surface with an epicenter at the gray-white junction in the brain.[3]

Malignant gliomas are believed to occur spontaneously, with the majority of cases having no genetic or environmental cause identified. Genetic syndromes including neurofibromatosis types 1 and 2 and Li-Fraumeni and Turcot's syndromes, are putatively responsible for around 5% of these tumors, and these patients often have a positive family history.[10] Ionizing radiation is the only well-established risk factor, whereas the evidence for head injury, foods, occupational exposures, electromagnetic fields, and cellular telephones as causative agents is inconclusive.[11,12] Aspects of the immune system may play a protective role, as patients with a history of asthma, eczema, allergies, and high levels of immunoglobulin E (IgE) have been found to have a decreased risk of gliomas.[13]

Clinical Presentation

Patients with malignant gliomas present with a variety of symptoms, depending on the size, location, and relative mass effect of their tumors. Initial symptoms most commonly include headaches, seizures, focal neurologic deficits, confusion, memory loss, and personality changes. There are no clinical findings unique to the various tumor types (anaplastic astrocytomas vs anaplastic oligodendrogliomas vs glioblastomas); however, more aggressive, rapidly progressing lesions tend to have a more rapid onset and severity of symptoms, whereas lower grade tumors have a more insidious course. In recent years, the interval from symptom onset to diagnosis is diminishing, given the increasingly widespread availability of neurodiagnostic imaging. Classically, the headache associated with mass lesions causing increased intracranial pressure is worse in the morning after awakening from sleep and decreases throughout the day. However, most patients experience headaches that are indistinguishable from other, nonmalignant causes of headaches.[14] When severe, the headaches may be associated with nausea and vomiting, indicating increased intracranial pressure. Tumors located in the posterior fossa are associated with a higher incidence of obstructive hydrocephalus and can have the additional findings of ataxia, dizziness, and incoordination.[1]

Special Consideration

- Clinical presentation is determined mostly by anatomic location, mass effect, and growth rate, but not necessarily histology. Tumors in eloquent locations that cause mass effect, regardless of size, can present with rapid onset of symptoms, whereas very large tumors in non-eloquent areas (e.g., right frontal lobe) may be clinically silent for a long time. Similarly, seizure activity does not correlate with tumor grade, but may be related to *IDH1* mutational status and correlated with 2-hydroxyglutarate production.

Imaging Studies

The initial study that is appropriate for diagnosing a malignant glioma is usually either a head computed tomography (CT) or brain magnetic resonance imaging (MRI) scan. On CT, AAs may appear as low- or mixed-density lesions with indistinct borders that cause mass effect and edema with variable amounts of enhancement.[15] A GBM typically displays more heterogeneous density and can have areas of hemorrhage, necrosis, or cysts. Oligodendrogliomas are also hypodense and often contain areas of calcification.[16]

Currently, MRI is the imaging modality of choice for malignant gliomas, as assessment of the size and extent of gliomas

Special Consideration

- The differential diagnoses of contrast-enhancing "butterfly" lesions crossing the corpus callosum into both hemispheres includes CNS lymphoma, oligodendroglioma, and glioblastoma. These lesions should be biopsied to avoid misdiagnosis, as CNS lymphomas and oligodendrogliomas with 1p19q deletions may be more responsive to adjuvant therapies than glioblastomas and have a significantly different prognosis.

is more accurate based on MRI than on CT. On MRI, both AA and GBM display considerable heterogeneity. Most tumors of both types enhance with gadolinium contrast, but there is variability, with some studies finding that 30 to 50% of AAs do not enhance, whereas only around 5% of GBMs do not.[17] The GBMs also more commonly display a ring-enhancing appearance due to areas of central necrosis as well as spread across white matter tracts, including the corpus callosum or anterior and posterior commissures. Such spread across the midline in a classic "butterfly" appearance is more common in glioblastoma.

However, the appearance of malignant gliomas on contrast-enhanced MRI does not fully represent the extent of tumor, which is often highly infiltrative. Tumor cells are often clearly seen on microscopic histopathological analysis infiltrating into brain tissue that appears as uninvolved, nonenhancing areas on MRI. Owing to this fact, surgeons often attempt a maximal safe resection into areas of T2/fluid-attenuated inversion recovery (FLAIR) signal suggestive of nonenhancing tumor. The current standard of care is for radiation oncologists to treat a 2-cm margin around the imaging-defined tumor. These strategies are validated by autopsy studies, where diffusely infiltrative cells are identified well beyond areas of contrast enhancement, often distantly into the opposite hemisphere.[18]

Newer imaging modalities are being increasingly used to help with neurosurgical planning and resection, as well as to define and monitor responses to treatment. When tumor resection in or near an eloquent area is planned, surgeons now use functional MRI (fMRI) and diffusion tensor imaging (DTI) to better delineate areas that can be safely removed from critical eloquent areas, such as speech and motor cortex and associated fiber tracts, where removal may lead to unacceptable

Pitfall

- Despite being "malignant," 30 to 50% of anaplastic astrocytomas and 5% of glioblastomas may lack contrast enhancement on either CT or MRI, leading to a false imaging diagnosis of a low-grade glioma.

neurologic deficit.[19] Intraoperative MRI (iMRI) guidance is being used increasingly to aid resection.[20]

Magnetic resonance spectroscopy (MRS) can help differentiate areas of tumor from necrosis or benign lesions by measuring the relative concentration of several metabolites. Malignant gliomas typically show a relative increase in choline (Cho), which is associated with cell membrane synthesis, and a decrease in N-acetyl aspartate (NAA), which is typically reflective of neurons. Other metabolites, such as lipids and lactate, are useful in differentiating entities such as abscess, radiation necrosis, and pseudoprogression from true tumor.[21] Positron-emission tomography (PET) using various tracers (FDG, FLT, DOPA) is similarly being used to help diagnose tumors and shed light on their malignant potential; aid in guiding resection, stereotactic biopsy, and radiotherapy targets; as well as in monitoring response to therapy.[22]

■ Natural History and Survival

Prior to the last decade, progress in the treatment of malignant gliomas had remained relatively stagnant compared to successes in the treatment of other types of brain tumors, including medulloblastomas and meningiomas. More recently, data from the 2012 Surveillance Epidemiology and End Results (SEER) population analysis revealed an encouraging trend for malignant glioma patients. Patients in the years 2000 to 2008 exhibited a statistically significantly improved overall survival compared to patients diagnosed in the decades earlier.[1] This suggests that new developments in diagnostics, surgical technique, and radiotherapy and chemotherapy have led to some realized benefits for patients.

■ Prognostic Factors

Several prognostic factors, including age, Karnofsky Performance Scale (KPS) score, extent of surgical resection, postoperative radiation treatment, degree of necrosis within the resection pathology, and the degree of enhancement on preoperative and postoperative MRI, have been observed to influence outcome in malignant glioma patients.[23–25] Patients under 40 years of age tend to survive longer than those 40 and over, independently of their improved ability to tolerate treatments such as chemotherapy and surgery.[24] However, this may be due to the fact that patients under 40 are more likely to have the "proneural" subtype of GBM, which is associated with longer survival.[26] The KPS is also a strong independent predictor of outcome in clinical trials, with a cutoff value of 70 stratifying patients into groups with large differences in survival.[27]

Age, Performance Score, and Extent of Resection

Since its initial development in the early 1990s, the Radiation Therapy Oncology Group (RTOG) recursive partitioning analysis (RPA) classification system has proved useful and has been validated in multiple clinical trials.[28–31] It has served as a historical control to compare findings from phase 1/2 clinical trials before phase 3 studies are begun. It also identified relatively homogeneous patient subgroups that may benefit most from a particular experimental approach, thereby sparing other patients from unnecessary treatment. The findings of a recent simplification of the RPA classes for glioblastoma are shown in (**Table 25.1**).[28] The median survival for AO is 3.9 years, with 5- and 10-year survival being 41% and 20%, respectively. For AA, RPA analysis found median survivals of 13, 9, 5.5, and 2.25 years, respectively, from the lowest to the highest RPA risk groups.

Histology

Histologically, AA and GBM both contain pleomorphic nuclei, hypercellularity with mitotic figures, and endothelial prominence (**Fig. 25.1**). Macroscopically, glioblastomas typically

Table 25.1 Simplified RPA Model for the Expanded RTOG GBM Database

RPA Class for Glioblastoma	Defining Variables	Median Survival Time (Months)	Overall Survival (1 Year, 3 Years, 5 Years)
RPA III	< 50 y and KPS ≥ 90	17.1	70%, 20%, 14%
RPA IV	< 50 y and KPS < 90; ≥ 50 y, KPS ≥ 70, resection and working	11.2	46%, 7%, 4%
RPA V + VI	≥ 50 y, KPS ≥ 70, resection and not working; ≥ 50 y, KPS ≥ 70 biopsy only; ≥ 50 y, KPS < 70	7.5	28%, 1%, 0%

Abbreviations: GBM, glioblastoma multiforme; KPS, Karnofsky Performance Scale score; RPA, recursive partitioning analysis; RTOG, Radiation Therapy and Oncology Group.

Special Consideration

- Proliferation index (i.e., Ki-67/MIB-1), immunohistochemical staining, and molecular genetic tests are increasingly being used as adjuvant studies for tumor classification and prognostication of malignant gliomas.

Pearl

- Molecular biomarkers have yielded new insights into the biology of malignant gliomas and their expected clinical course. Patients with tumors harboring methylguanine methyltransferase (MGMT) methylation, *IDH* mutation, and 1p19q deletion may have a significantly better prognosis than those without these genetic alterations.

show areas of necrosis and hemorrhage. Differentiating them from AA, glioblastomas typically display what is termed "glomeruloid" vascular endothelial proliferation as well as pseudopalisading necrosis. The designation *multiforme,* no longer used in the most recent WHO system, was reflective of the extreme pleomorphism of tumor cells, ranging from small and tightly packed to enormous and bizarrely shaped.[6]

Oligodendrogliomas have the characteristic microscopic appearance of round nuclei with sharply defined membranes and inconspicuous chromatin. Formalin fixation yields perinuclear clear halos with the characteristic "fried egg" appearance as well as an array of fine, hexagonal capillaries, which are commonly described as a "chicken wire" pattern. Grade III or anaplastic oligodendrogliomas are distinguished from grade II oligodendrogliomas by the presence of areas of hypercellularity and increased proliferative activity. Oligoastrocytomas display both astrocytic and oligodendroglial components (**Fig. 25.2**).

Molecular Markers

Although cellular morphology has formed the foundation of brain tumor classification since the days of Cushing and Bailey in the 1920s, and remains the standard for diagnosis in the current WHO scheme, considerable variability in biological behavior and clinical course remains even within individual histological grades. This inherently denotes that a greater degree of complexity on the molecular level than can be appreciated by conventional histopathology underlies the behavior of these tumors. Discoveries related to underlying molecular abnormalities in these tumors have begun to generate new paradigms for understanding how these neoplasms develop and are diagnosed, and how they might be more effectively

treated. Currently, the most actively researched individual molecular markers in neuro-oncology are 1p/19q co-deletion in oligodendroglial tumors, alterations in the EGFR and associated signaling pathway genes in glioblastomas, hypermethylation of the *MGMT* gene promoter in gliomas, and mutations in the *IDH1/2* genes in low- and high-grade diffuse gliomas.[32]

1p/19q Chromosomal Co-Deletion

The 1p/19q co-deletion seen in tumors with an oligodendroglial component appears to confer a significant survival advantage and improved response to chemotherapy. This co-deletion results from an unbalanced centromeric translocation of t(1;19)(q10;p10) and can be detected by fluorescence in-situ hybridization (FISH) or polymerase chain reaction (PCR)-based strategies for the detection of loss of heterozygosity. It is frequently seen in oligodendroglial tumors and is present in 80 to 90% oligogdendrogliomas, 60% of anaplastic oligodendrogliomas, and 30 to 50% of oligoastrocytomas.[32] This translation appears to have a strong association with classic histological features of round, uniform nuclei with perinuclear halos and a "chicken-wire" vascular pattern. Early studies of patients with this marker found that its presence predicts a better response to chemotherapy with the procarbazine, chloroethylcyclohexylnitrosourea (CCNU; lomustine), and vincristine (PCV) regimen and longer survival in patients with anaplastic oligodendroglioma as well as response to treatment with the alkylating drug temozolomide (TMZ) and radiotherapy.[33] However, other retrospective studies have shown benefit regardless of therapy modality, and the marker may therefore be prognostic rather than predictive.[34] Recent findings indicate

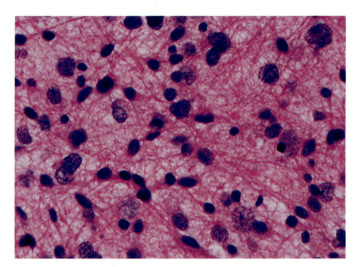
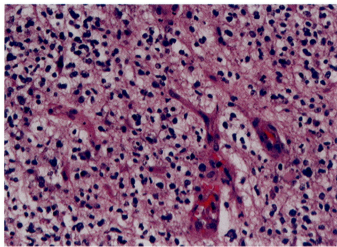

Fig. 25.2a–b Astrocytomas and oligodendrogliomas. (**a**) Typical astrocytoma with bizarre astrocytes on a fibrillary background. (**b**) Oligodendroglioma displaying the typical "fried egg" appearance of perinuclear halos on a "chicken-wire" capillary background.

that the *CIC* and *FUBP1* genes at these chromosomal sites may play a role in oligodendroglioma pathology.[35]

0⁶ Methylguanine Methyltransferase (MGMT) Methylation

Up to 50% of glioblastomas show decreased levels of MGMT protein, which could make them more susceptible to the effects of the chemotherapy drug TMZ. TMZ, which has now become standard of care for treatment of malignant gliomas, acts primarily to methylate the O^6 position of the nucleotide guanine, which ultimately results in cell death. The DNA repair enzyme MGMT irreversibly transfers this methyl group from the O^6 position of the modified guanine to a cysteine residue of the MGMT protein, thereby disrupting the cytotoxic effects of chemotherapy.[36] However, the activity of this enzyme is limited stoichiometrically; after the reaction, the active enzyme is not regenerated after it is alkylated. The primary mechanism whereby MGMT expression is downregulated in glioblastomas appears to be methylation of the *MGMT* gene promoter.[37] Several studies suggest such a correlation in glioblastoma, including those in pediatric and elderly patients, as well as in lower grade gliomas.[37–39] In a pivotal study of 106 TMZ-treated patients, 46% of patients with MGMT methylated tumors were alive at 2 years versus only 22% of patients with tumors with unmethylated MGMT.[40] However, other trials found methylated MGMT conferred a prognostic benefit that did not predict the response to therapy specifically with alkylating agents, as the improved survival with MGMT methylation was seen in patients treated with radiotherapy alone as well.[41]

Epidermal Growth Factor Receptor Amplification

Gliomas harbor numerous alterations in growth factor signaling pathways. One of the most frequently amplified and over-expressed gene identified in primary glioblastomas (40–60%) is *EGFR*. Increased activity of this pathway usually indicates an aggressive malignancy, especially in younger patients. A constitutively active variant of *EGFR*, *EGFRvIII*, is also found in 20 to 30% of primary glioblastomas and 50 to 60% of those with *EGFR* amplification, and may be associated with a poorer response to radiation and chemotherapy.[42]

Given the prevalence of *EGFR* overexpression and mutation in glioblastomas, numerous EGFR-targeted agents have been tested against glioblastoma. However, the clinical benefit of EGFR inhibitors has been rather disappointing, possibly owing to alterations in downstream signaling factors such as Akt, Phosphatase and TENsin homolog (PTEN), and phosphatidylinositol 3-kinase (PI3K).[43]

Isocitrate Dehydrogenase (IDH) Mutations

Mutant forms of *IDH1* and *IDH2* in malignant gliomas are associated with markedly improved survival. Genome sequencing screens identified mutations in *IDH1* in 60 to 90% of WHO grades II and III diffuse gliomas, as well as in the secondary glioblastomas (WHO grade IV) that developed from these lower grade tumors.[44] *IDH2* mutations were found in another 5% of low-grade gliomas. Although glioblastomas with mutant forms of *IDH1/2* comprise only approximately 12% of all GBMs, they are notable for their markedly improved survival relative to nonmutants. Patients with *IDH* mutant GBMs had a median overall survival of 31 months versus 15 months for nonmutants, and in AAs, *IDH* mutants reached a median survival of 65 months versus 20 months in nonmutants.

The underlying biology accounting for this difference has yet to be elucidated. Mechanistic studies indicate that these mutations lead to epigenetic alterations in the expression of genes, which correlate with invasion, angiogenesis, and survival of tumors. *IDH* mutations may also confer an enzymatic gain of function, to catalyze the reduced nicotinamide adenine dinucleotide phosphate (NADPH)-dependent reduction of a-ketoglutarate to 2-hydroxyglutarate (2-HG), which may alter response to oxidative stress.[45]

Interestingly, *IDH1* mutations appear in secondary glioblastomas but are rare in primary GBMs and are completely absent in (grade I) pilocytic astrocytomas.[46] *IDH* mutations are frequently found in oligodendrogliomas and often coexist with 1p/19q deletion, suggesting that they may have a common cell of origin. *IDH1* and *IDH2* mutations are not found in nonneoplastic conditions that can histologically mimic gliomas (e.g., reactive gliosis, radiation changes, viral infections, infarcts, demyelinating conditions, etc.), allowing for improved diagnostic accuracy of suboptimal brain biopsies.[45] Additionally, 2-hydroxyglutarate is detectable on MRS of *IDH1*-mutant gliomas, which may enabler a noninvasive imaging-based biopsy to detect this genetic marker in such tumors.[47]

Treatment of Malignant Glioma

Surgery

Surgery for Newly Diagnosed Malignant Glioma

Although surgery is a mainstay of treatment, it has long been understood that malignant gliomas are not surgically curable. In the 1920s, Walter Dandy attempted radical hemispherectomies on patients with GBM, but all ultimately succumbed to the disease. Although extensive surgical resection fails to cure malignant glioma, it does improve the quality of life for many patients and increases the duration of survival for selected patients. Along with survival, rapid and sustained improvement in neurologic status can be achieved after extensive resection. Without treatment, 95% of patients with GBM die within 3 months. The goal of surgery in glioblastoma treatment is to provide maximal safe tumor resection with preservation or restoration of neurologic function. The rationale for surgical resection of malignant gliomas is listed below.

Practical Considerations for Surgical Resection of Malignant Gliomas

- **Rationale for surgery**
  - Obtain tissue diagnosis
  - Improve symptoms
  - Delay onset of new symptoms
  - Increase survival
  - Allow time for adjuvant treatments
  - Decrease steroid doses

Recent SEER data found increased survival in patients receiving resections compared to those who did not, but did not evaluate extent of resection (EOR).[1] A recent report that evaluated the EOR on 500 patients found statistically significant survival advantages for patients who had an EOR as little as

---

78%. Those with 100%, 90%, 80%, and 78% EOR had overall survival times of 16, 13.8, 12.8, and 12.5 months, respectively.[48] These findings corroborated an earlier report that demonstrated that increased EOR was associated with improved survival in a retrospective cohort of over 1,000 patients.[49]

The criteria for extensive surgical resection reflect a complex series of decisions based on individual patient circumstances and include patient age, KPS score, proximity of the tumor to eloquent regions of the brain, feasibility of resection (including number and location of satellite lesions), and the medical condition of the patient.

Partial resection of glioblastoma carries significant risk of postoperative hemorrhage or the development of severe cerebral edema termed "wounded glioma syndrome," with risk of herniation. In that sense, a better outcome with extensive resection is likely because of reduction in mass, thereby providing space for postoperative brain swelling. The benefit of a subtotal resection is unclear. Surgical excision should be considered when gross total removal is feasible. Therefore, elderly patients (usually those > 80 years old) or with KPS scores < 70, and those whose tumors are multifocal, involve both hemispheres (e.g., butterfly gliomas), or extensively involve the dominant hemisphere are usually not deemed candidates for surgical resection and may be better served by image-guided needle biopsy, either frameless or frame-based.[50]

Using careful surgical technique, employing up-to-date intraoperative neuronavigational imaging and brain mapping adjuncts, and attempting with corticosteroids to decrease cerebral edema preoperatively and postoperatively, the neurologic morbidity is less than 10% and mortality less than 5% for malignant glioma surgery.[51] Recent advances, such as intraoperative cortical and subcortical stimulation mapping and intraoperative MRI-guided tumor resection, have added to the surgical armamentarium for malignant gliomas.

Refinement of neurosurgical technique has enabled safer operations with more aggressive outcomes. One cornerstone

---

Pitfall

- Because a neurosurgeon's impression of the amount of tumor resected is generally inaccurate, a contrast-enhanced MRI should be obtained within 24 to 48 hours of surgery to more accurately assess the extent of resection.

Controversy

- The use of intraoperative MRI has not been conclusively shown to improve overall survival in patients undergoing surgery for malignant gliomas. The true clinical value and cost/benefit of intraoperative MRI is still controversial.

of modern-day practice is the utilization of intraoperative electrocortical stimulation (ECS) mapping. Using awake craniotomy techniques, ECS can be used to identify critical motor and language pathways.[19] Given the individual variability of cortical language localization, such awake language mapping is essential to minimize language deficits following tumor resection. Experience suggests that cortical and subcortical language mapping is a safe and efficient adjunct to optimize tumor resection while preserving essential language sites, even in the setting of negative mapping data.

Neuronavigation and intraoperative MRI (iMRI) are other tools that are being used for glioma surgery. A systematic review of 12 studies on the use of iMRI found evidence that iMRI-guided surgery is more effective than conventional neuronavigation-guided surgery in increasing the extent of tumor resection in patients with glioblastoma.[20] However, the true clinical benefit of the use of iMRI in terms of improving quality of life and overall survival in malignant glioma patients has yet to be proven.

Surgery for Recurrent Malignant Glioma

For recurrent malignant gliomas, repeat surgical resection is undertaken for several reasons. First, gross tumor debulking can reduce mass effect and thereby improve symptoms and quality of life for patients, and add the associated benefits of reduced steroid doses.[52] Second, reoperation may increase overall survival in patients with recurrent malignant gliomas by 2 to 5 months.[53] Finally, reduced disease burden also theoretically could improve the efficacy of additional adjuvant therapies being considered.

Special Consideration

- Reoperation alone is of limited value for patients with recurrent glioblastoma. Surgical resection of recurrent malignant gliomas should be undertaken as part of a comprehensive plan for further adjuvant postoperative treatment or enrollment into clinical trials.

A recently devised scale identifies which patients will benefit from repeat surgery.[54] The scale assigns points if the KPS score is 80 or less, the tumor volume is 50 cm³ or greater, or if certain eloquent brain regions are involved. Patient survival after surgery can be stratified based on the total score, ranging from 0 to 3. Good (0 points), intermediate (1 to 2 points), and poor (3 points) prognostic groups were found to have postoperative survival times of 10.8, 4.5, and 1.0 months, respectively.

Radiotherapy

Newly Diagnosed Malignant Glioma

Standard radiotherapy (RT) for malignant glioma utilizes three-dimensional conformal external-beam radiation for up to a total of 60 Gy in 30 fractions of 200 cGy each, given 5 days a week.[55] Alternative fractionation techniques currently being trialed, such as hyper- or hypofractionated radiotherapy, enable either higher cumulative doses or shorter treatment times, respectively, and may be tailored to the tolerance of individual patients. RT is administered to the area encompassing the tumor plus an extra margin, which usually involves areas of T2/FLAIR hyperintensity thought to represent nonenhancing locations of tumor infiltration. This margin may be limited in eloquent brain areas.

Radiotherapy can increase survival of patients with malignant glioma, regardless of whether or not the patient underwent surgical resection, or the extent of resection.[1] Immediate response to RT correlates very well with survival both in a univariate analysis after correction for age and KPS, and in multivariate analyses. Several other modalities of radiation delivery have been studied, including stereotactic radiosurgery, fractionated stereotactic RT, brachytherapy, and intensity-modulated RT (IMRT), but none has overtaken conventional external beam RT as the standard of care for malignant glioma.[56,57] RT is recommended for almost all patients with malignant gliomas, except for infants, young moribund children, and elderly adults with poor functional status.

Complications from radiotherapy can occur both acutely and over the long term. Acute side effects occur during treatment and include increased cerebral edema leading to focal neurologic deficits requiring treatment with steroids; other acute side effects are nausea, vomiting, dysphagia, and transient demyelination causing other cerebral or cerebellar dysfunction. In the long term, radiation necrosis becomes the most prominent complication. Occurring in 10 to 15% of brain tumor patients who received RT, radiation necrosis can mimic symptomatic tumor recurrence by exhibiting mass effect and cerebral edema and take on the contrast-enhancing appearance of tumor on MRI, also known as "pseudoprogression."[58] Newer imaging modalities such as MRS or diffusion-perfusion MRI are increasingly being utilized to help differentiate the two.[59] Management of patients with presumed radiation necrosis consists of diagnostic tissue biopsy, resection of the necrotic tissue, the use of high-dose steroids, or a combination of these.[58] Therapy with hyperbaric oxygen is controversial, but often considered as an adjunctive treatment. Recently, bevacizumab has emerged as promising treatment for severe radiation necrosis.[60]

Stereotactic radiosurgery (SRS) focuses multiple beams of ionizing radiation to converge from multiple origins with high precision at an intracranial target, delivering a high dose of radiation, while exposing adjacent healthy tissue to a much smaller level of radiation than conventional radiotherapy. Radiosurgery using linear accelerator (Linac) or gamma knife has been considered for the treatment of newly diagnosed glioblastoma. However, evidence for the efficacy of its use has been limited.[61] The limited efficacy of this very precisely targeted therapy may be due to the diffusely infiltrative nature of gliomas. Radiosurgery is limited primarily to the treatment of lesions that are < 3 cm in diameter and by the risk of radiation necrosis with radiosurgery, which is about 15%.[57] A prospective randomized trial by the RTOG failed to show improvements in survival or quality of life with the addition of radiosurgery to conventional established treatment modalities.[61] Further studies investigating the role of radiosurgery for primary brain tumors are in progress, but the current guidelines for the initial treatment of malignant gliomas do not recommend SRS.[62]

Brachytherapy using stereotactically implanted iodine-125 seeds or intracavitary delivery using a balloon catheter system (e.g., GliaSite®, IsoRay Medical, Inc., Richland, WA) enables local delivery of high-dose radiation and has been used for the treatment of malignant gliomas.[63] However, initial optimism about the technique was tempered by the results of two prospective trials of implanted iodine-125 in which brachytherapy groups did not show any survival improvements and had more side effects.[64]

Recurrent Malignant Glioma

For recurrent malignant gliomas, further delivery of radiation is often limited to additional focal treatments with stereotactic radiotherapy (SRT), because patients with malignant gliomas already receive a full course of external beam irradiation as part of their initial treatment. Combined data from over 300 patients receiving palliative reirradiation regimens without additional chemotherapy demonstrated 6-month progression-free survival (PFS) of 28 to 39% and 1-year survival of 18 to 48%, as well as clinical improvements, reduction in steroid

dependency, and low occurrence of toxicity.[65] This compares favorably with targeted systemic therapies that have been evaluated for recurrent GBM. As discussed above, the use of radiosurgery is limited to small tumors (< 3 cm in diameter) and is not indicated for newly diagnosed malignant gliomas. However, SRS may have a potential role in recurrence, if the patient is otherwise not a candidate for reoperation.

Chemotherapy

Prior to the advent of TMZ era, there was considerable debate about whether chemotherapy was useful in the treatment of malignant gliomas at all. The primary agents used were the nitrosoureas, carmustine (bischloroethylnitrosourea [BCNU]) or lomustine (CCNU), chosen for their confirmed ability to cross the blood–brain barrier (BBB). These agents were combined with the DNA alkylator, procarbazine, and the microtubule disruptor, vincristine, to comprise the PCV regimen for malignant gliomas. No single study conclusively defined the effectiveness of these agents for glioblastoma, but a meta-analysis combining data on over 3,000 patients from 12 randomized trials documented a slight increase in 1-year survival from 40 to 46% with chemotherapy.[66] However, there has been a revival of interest in these agents as the results of several long-term studies of patients with lower grade lesions such as AA and oligodendroglioma treated with PCV have demonstrated marked improvements in survival, particularly for those with the 1p/19q co-deletion, suggesting that this chromosomal co-deletion may somehow render susceptibility to this regimen independent of the improved prognosis discussed above.[67,68]

Temozolomide

Temozolomide is an atypical alkylating chemotherapeutic agent that was approved by the Food and Drug Administration (FDA) for the treatment of newly diagnosed glioblastoma in 2005.[69] A landmark phase 3 study published in 2005 led to this approval and established TMZ as the current standard of care.[55] In this study, patients were randomized to either post-resection RT alone or postresection RT with TMZ. The RT with concurrent TMZ group demonstrated a statistically significant improved median survival of 14.6 versus 12.1 months as well as improved 2-year survival rates of 26.5% versus 10.4%. In the 5-year follow-up analysis of the trial, the benefit of TMZ was confirmed in all clinical prognostic subgroups receiving the drug.[70] Overall survival at 5 years was 9.8% in the RT plus TMZ group compared with 1.9% in the radiotherapy alone group. Standard dosing for concomitant TMZ therapy is 75 mg/m^2/d given daily during RT followed by 150 to 200 mg/m^2/d for 5 days every 28 days for a total of six cycles.[55] Temozolomide is usually well tolerated with myelosuppression as the most commonly reported toxicity. Grade III or IV events occurred in around 15% of patients receiving TMZ. As discussed above, MGMT methylation may further impact the efficacy of TMZ therapy.

Gliadel BCNU Wafers

Implantation of biodegradable carmustine (BCNU) wafers (Gliadel®, Arbor Pharmaceuticals, Atlanta, GA) is an FDA-approved therapeutic option for patients with newly diagnosed and recurrent malignant gliomas. These wafers are implanted into the resection cavity at the time of surgery and the agent diffuses into surrounding, tumor-infiltrated, brain tissue over the subsequent weeks at over 100-fold the concentration that could be achieved with systemic administration. Their use in malignant gliomas was established by a multicenter, placebo-controlled trial for recurrent GBMs, which showed survival improvements.[71] In phase 3 clinical trials including 240 patients, Gliadel improved the overall survival (OS) of patients undergoing initial surgery for malignant gliomas in a statistically significant manner (13.9 vs 11.6 months).[72] However, subgroup analysis failed to show significant benefit in glioblastoma patients.

Although Gliadel has shown safety and efficacy in large trials and is FDA approved, the clinical adoption of its use as first-line therapy has not become universal.[73] As seen in phase 3 studies, the wafers have several side effects that some surgeons argue outweigh the marginal survival benefits, including increased wound breakdown, cerebral edema requiring prolonged steroids, and increased frequency of seizures.

Bevacizumab

Bevacizumab is a monoclonal antibody that inhibits vascular endothelial growth factor A (VEGF-A), a growth factor that is involved in angiogenesis. In 2009, bevacizumab (Avastin®, Genentech, South San Francisco, CA) received FDA approval for recurrent glioblastoma based on phase 2 trials that demonstrated increased time to tumor progression and impressive responses on imaging.[74] A meta-analysis of 548 patients in 15 studies reviewed the efficacy of bevacizumab treatment in patients with recurrent glioblastoma. Median OS, 6-month PFS, and 6-month OS were 9.3 months, 45%, and 76%, respectively.[75] Although requiring confirmation in further clinical trials, the analysis found no difference in bevacizumab dose-response benefit among 5, 10, and 15 mg/kg. Bevacizumab has also been used in phase 1 trials of intra-arterial delivery with no distinctive advantage. Bevacizumab has several potential side effects including intracranial hemorrhage and throm-

Pitfall

- Infection rate and wound dehiscence may be higher in re-operation surgery following treatment with bevacizumab. Bevacizumab should be stopped at least 4 weeks prior to and held for 4 weeks after surgery. Furthermore, the value of bevacizumab in prolonging life for patients with malignant glioma is questionable.

botic events, deep venous thrombosis, pulmonary embolus, and ischemic stroke.[76]

Recently, two large multicenter trials reported at the 2013 meeting of the American Society for Clinical Oncology (ASCO) failed to demonstrate improvements in OS in patients treated with the addition of bevacizumab (Avastin) to standard chemoradiation. In one trial, the RTOG 0825 trial investigators randomized 637 patients to TMZ-based chemoradiation with or without bevacizumab. Patients in the bevacizumab arm started the agent 4 weeks into the radiation therapy protocol and continued for 6 to 12 cycles of maintenance therapy. The results showed a median overall survival of 15.7 months with the addition of bevacizumab and 16.1 months without the targeted agent. PFS improved slightly in the bevacizumab arm (10.7 vs 7.3 months), but the difference did not meet a pre-specified level of statistical significance. Results from the larger, AVAglio™ (Roche, Indianapolis, IN) trial, which involved 921 patients, similarly showed no benefit to overall survival with the addition of bevacizumab to standard radiation and TMZ chemotherapy. Although these results are discouraging for newly diagnosed disease, the role of bevacizumab in the recurrent setting remains unclear.

■ Conclusion

Decades of research have led to advances in diagnostic modalities, optimization of surgical techniques, and refinement of radiation and chemotherapeutic regimens for the treatment of malignant gliomas. Surgery can address mass effect and reduce disease burden, and advances in surgical tools and techniques have made surgery safe not just for initial resection, but also in the management of recurrent disease. Conformal external beam radiation therapy has earned a well-established role in the initial treatment of malignant gliomas, and newer modalities such as SRS show some promise in the recurrent setting. With the advent of TMZ, the usefulness of chemotherapy in the management of malignant gliomas is no longer debated as it was prior to 2005.

Despite these advances, the diagnosis of malignant glioma still carries a death sentence for the overwhelming majority of patients. This is partly due to the infiltrative growth patterns of malignant gliomas, which disperse into the surrounding brain parenchyma by the time of presentation, rendering surgical resection and local treatments only capable of addressing the gross, bulk disease. The delivery of chemotherapeutic agents is limited by the relative impermeability of the BBB, limited macromolecular diffusion within the CNS, and lack of tumor specificity. Therefore, new treatment avenues must be developed in the laboratory and clinically translated.

New insights into glioma biology have transformed our understanding of the molecular pathogenesis of the disease and informed our prognostic ability. These insights have paved the way for the development of many novel therapies that have shown promise in the preclinical setting and await clinical translation. Growth factor signaling pathways continue to be an area of active exploration, with more targets and inhibitors identified as our understanding of their role in the development/progression of these tumors increases. Immunotherapy, which attempts to train the immune system to specifically recognize and reject cancer cells, is emerging as another promising adjuvant for glioma therapy. Oncolytic viruses and gene therapy have garnered much interest as a way to "infect" tumor precisely while leaving normal brain unharmed. Viruses can be programmed to either kill the cells themselves or deliver lethal payloads. Several such agents are undergoing clinical trials. Additionally, other forms of gene therapy, drugs targeting glioma "cancer stem cells," modulators of angiogenesis, the tumor microenvironment, epigenetic modifying agents, and the use of convection enhanced delivery to infuse these and other antitumor agents, remain actively pursued. Informing patients about the development of these new therapeutic options and their eligibility for clinical trials is critical for providing hope and excellent care for the individual patient, as well as advancing our scientific knowledge toward a cure for malignant gliomas.

Editor's Note

Malignant gliomas are arguably the number one challenge in all of neuro-oncology, and arguably in all of oncology. Randomized trial data exist in radiation oncology, and in medical neuro-oncology, but not in surgery. Despite all the failures and the few successes, much research is being done by dedicated people exploring scientifically sound and promising hypotheses. Interestingly, malignant gliomas represent the ideal neoplasm for clinical study for two main reasons: (1) the course is shorter than in most other malignant tumors, so results can be obtained in a few years, not many years or decades; (2) the disease does not usually spread outside the brain, so there is no contaminant of metastatic disease, and these tumors therefore represent the archetypal challenge in obtaining local control. Unfortunately, the role of aggressive surgery will almost certainly never be solved by proper randomized controlled trials, but much great work is going on in the laboratory and in the clinic, and all members of the neuro-oncology team should take heart in the fact that nihilism has not supplanted hope. (Bernstein)

References

1. Thumma SR, Fairbanks RK, Lamoreaux WT, et al. Effect of pretreatment clinical factors on overall survival in glioblastoma multiforme: a Surveillance Epidemiology and End Results (SEER) population analysis. World J Surg Oncol 2012;10:75
2. Siegel R, Naishadham D, Jemal A. Cancer statistics, 2013. CA Cancer J Clin 2013;63:11–30
3. Dolecek TA, Propp JM, Stroup NE, Kruchko C. CBTRUS statistical report: primary brain and central nervous system tumors diagnosed in the United States in 2005-2009. Neuro-oncol 2012;14(Suppl 5):v1–v49
4. Vogel H. Nervous system. New York: Cambridge University Press, 2009
5. Brem SS, Bierman PJ, Black P, et al; National Comprehensive Cancer Network. Central nervous system cancers: Clinical Practice Guidelines in Oncology. J Natl Compr Canc Netw 2005;3:644–690
6. Louis DN, Ohgaki H, Wiestler OD, et al. The 2007 WHO classification of tumours of the central nervous system. Acta Neuropathol 2007;114:97–109
7. Cancer Genome Atlas Research Network. Comprehensive genomic characterization defines human glioblastoma genes and core pathways. Nature 2008;455:1061–1068
8. Gajjar A, Packer RJ, Foreman NK, Cohen K, Haas-Kogan D, Merchant TE; COG Brain Tumor Committee. Children's Oncology Group's 2013 blueprint for research: central nervous system tumors. Pediatr Blood Cancer 2013;60:1022–1026
9. Fisher JL, Schwartzbaum JA, Wrensch M, Wiemels JL. Epidemiology of brain tumors. Neurol Clin 2007;25:867–890, vii vii.
10. Hottinger AF, Khakoo Y. Neurooncology of familial cancer syndromes. J Child Neurol 2009;24:1526–1535
11. Braganza MZ, Kitahara CM, Berrington de González A, Inskip PD, Johnson KJ, Rajaraman P. Ionizing radiation and the risk of brain and central nervous system tumors: a systematic review. Neuro-oncol 2012;14:1316–1324
12. Corle C, Makale M, Kesari S. Cell phones and glioma risk: a review of the evidence. J Neurooncol 2012;106:1–13
13. Linos E, Raine T, Alonso A, Michaud D. Atopy and risk of brain tumors: a meta-analysis. J Natl Cancer Inst 2007;99:1544–1550
14. Iacob G, Dinca EB. Current data and strategy in glioblastoma multiforme. J Med Life 2009;2:386–393
15. Osborn AG. Osborn's Brain: Imaging, Pathology, and Anatomy. Salt Lake City: Amirsys, 2013
16. Zulfiqar M, Dumrongpisutikul N, Intrapiromkul J, Yousem DM. Detection of intratumoral calcification in oligodendrogliomas by susceptibility-weighted MR imaging. AJNR Am J Neuroradiol 2012;33:858–864
17. Scott JN, Brasher PM, Sevick RJ, Rewcastle NB, Forsyth PA. How often are nonenhancing supratentorial gliomas malignant? A population study. Neurology 2002;59:947–949
18. Yamahara T, Numa Y, Oishi T, et al. Morphological and flow cytometric analysis of cell infiltration in glioblastoma: a comparison of autopsy brain and neuroimaging. Brain Tumor Pathol 2010;27:81–87

19. Garrett MC, Pouratian N, Liau LM. Use of language mapping to aid in resection of gliomas in eloquent brain regions. Neurosurg Clin N Am 2012;23:497–506

20. Kubben PL, ter Meulen KJ, Schijns OE, ter Laak-Poort MP, van Overbeeke JJ, van Santbrink H. Intraoperative MRI-guided resection of glioblastoma multiforme: a systematic review. Lancet Oncol 2011;12:1062–1070

21. Martínez-Bisbal MC, Celda B. Proton magnetic resonance spectroscopy imaging in the study of human brain cancer. Q J Nucl Med Mol Imaging 2009;53:618–630

22. Petrirena GJ, Goldman S, Delattre JY. Advances in PET imaging of brain tumors: a referring physician's perspective. Curr Opin Oncol 2011;23:617–623

23. Barnholtz-Sloan JS, Maldonado JL, Williams VL, et al. Racial/ethnic differences in survival among elderly patients with a primary glioblastoma. J Neurooncol 2007;85:171–180

24. Siker ML, Wang M, Porter K, et al. Age as an independent prognostic factor in patients with glioblastoma: a Radiation Therapy Oncology Group and American College of Surgeons National Cancer Data Base comparison. J Neurooncol 2011;104:351–356

25. Kuhnt D, Becker A, Ganslandt O, Bauer M, Buchfelder M, Nimsky C. Correlation of the extent of tumor volume resection and patient survival in surgery of glioblastoma multiforme with high-field intraoperative MRI guidance. Neuro-oncol 2011;13:1339–1348

26. Freije WA, Castro-Vargas FE, Fang Z, et al. Gene expression profiling of gliomas strongly predicts survival. Cancer Res 2004;64:6503–6510

27. Adamson C, Kahn OO, Mehta AI, et al. Glioblastoma multiforme: a review of where we have been and where we are going. Expert Opin Investig Drugs 2009;18:1061–1083

28. Li J, Wang M, Won M, et al. Validation and simplification of the Radiation Therapy Oncology Group recursive partitioning analysis classification for glioblastoma. Int J Radiat Oncol Biol Phys 2011;81:623–630

29. Paravati AJ, Heron DE, Landsittel D, et al. Radiotherapy and temozolomide for newly diagnosed glioblastoma and anaplastic astrocytoma: validation of Radiation Therapy Oncology Group-Recursive Partitioning Analysis in the IMRT and temozolomide era. J Neurooncol 2011;104:339–349

30. Scott JG, Bauchet L, Fraum TJ, et al. Recursive partitioning analysis of prognostic factors for glioblastoma patients aged 70 years or older. Cancer 2012;118:5595–5600

31. Park CK, Lee SH, Han JH, et al. Recursive partitioning analysis of prognostic factors in WHO grade III glioma patients treated with radiotherapy or radiotherapy plus chemotherapy. BMC Cancer 2009;9:450

32. Jansen M, Yip S, Louis DN. Molecular pathology in adult gliomas: diagnostic, prognostic, and predictive markers. Lancet Neurol 2010;9:717–726

33. Erdem-Eraslan L, Gravendeel LA, de Rooi J, et al. Intrinsic molecular subtypes of glioma are prognostic and predict benefit from adjuvant procarbazine, lomustine, and vincristine chemotherapy in combination with other prognostic factors in anaplastic oligodendroglial brain tumors: a report from EORTC study 26951. J Clin Oncol 2013;31:328–336

34. Brandes AA, Tosoni A, Cavallo G, et al; GICNO. Correlations between O6-methylguanine DNA methyltransferase promoter methylation status, 1p and 19q deletions, and response to temozolomide in anaplastic and recurrent oligodendroglioma: a prospective GICNO study. J Clin Oncol 2006;24:4746–4753

35. Bettegowda C, Agrawal N, Jiao Y, et al. Mutations in CIC and FUBP1 contribute to human oligodendroglioma. Science 2011;333:1453–1455

36. Esteller M, Garcia-Foncillas J, Andion E, et al. Inactivation of the DNA-repair gene MGMT and the clinical response of gliomas to alkylating agents. N Engl J Med 2000;343:1350–1354

37. Gerstner ER, Yip S, Wang DL, Louis DN, Iafrate AJ, Batchelor TT. Mgmt methylation is a prognostic biomarker in elderly patients with newly diagnosed glioblastoma. Neurology 2009;73:1509–1510

38. Everhard S, Kaloshi G, Crinière E, et al. MGMT methylation: a marker of response to temozolomide in low-grade gliomas. Ann Neurol 2006;60:740–743

39. Pollack IF, Hamilton RL, Sobol RW, et al. O6-methylguanine-DNA methyltransferase expression strongly correlates with outcome in childhood malignant gliomas: results from the CCG-945 Cohort. J Clin Oncol 2006;24:3431–3437

40. Hegi ME, Diserens AC, Gorlia T, et al. MGMT gene silencing and benefit from temozolomide in glioblastoma. N Engl J Med 2005;352:997–1003

41. Rivera AL, Pelloski CE, Gilbert MR, et al. MGMT promoter methylation is predictive of response to radiotherapy and prognostic in the absence of adjuvant alkylating chemotherapy for glioblastoma. Neuro-oncol 2010;12:116–121

42. Del Vecchio CA, Li G, Wong AJ. Targeting EGF receptor variant III: tumor-specific peptide vaccination for malignant gliomas. Expert Rev Vaccines 2012;11:133–144

43. Taylor TE, Furnari FB, Cavenee WK. Targeting EGFR for treatment of glioblastoma: molecular basis to overcome resistance. Curr Cancer Drug Targets 2012;12:197–209

44. Parsons DW, Jones S, Zhang X, et al. An integrated genomic analysis of human glioblastoma multiforme. Science 2008;321:1807–1812

45. Schaap FG, French PJ, Bovée JV. Mutations in the isocitrate dehydrogenase genes IDH1 and IDH2 in tumors. Adv Anat Pathol 2013;20:32–38

46. Korshunov A, Meyer J, Capper D, et al. Combined molecular analysis of BRAF and IDH1 distinguishes pilocytic astrocytoma from diffuse astrocytoma. Acta Neuropathol 2009;118:401–405

47. Pope WB, Prins RM, Albert Thomas M, et al. Non-invasive detection of 2-hydroxyglutarate and other metabolites in IDH1 mutant glioma patients using magnetic resonance spectroscopy. J Neurooncol 2012;107:197–205

48. Sanai N, Polley MY, McDermott MW, Parsa AT, Berger MS. An extent of resection threshold for newly diagnosed glioblastomas. J Neurosurg 2011;115:3–8

49. McGirt MJ, Chaichana KL, Gathinji M, et al. Independent association of extent of resection with survival in patients with malignant brain astrocytoma. J Neurosurg 2009;110:156–162

50. Kongkham PN, Knifed E, Tamber MS, Bernstein M. Complications in 622 cases of frame-based stereotactic biopsy, a decreasing procedure. Can J Neurol Sci 2008;35:79–84

51. Wong JM, Panchmatia JR, Ziewacz JE, et al. Patterns in neurosurgical adverse events: intracranial neoplasm surgery. Neurosurg Focus 2012;33:E16

52. Barbagallo GM, Jenkinson MD, Brodbelt AR. 'Recurrent' glioblastoma multiforme, when should we reoperate? Br J Neurosurg 2008;22:452–455

53. Bloch O, Han SJ, Cha S, et al. Impact of extent of resection for recurrent glioblastoma on overall survival: clinical article. J Neurosurg 2012;117:1032–1038

54. Park JK, Hodges T, Arko L, et al. Scale to predict survival after surgery for recurrent glioblastoma multiforme. J Clin Oncol 2010;28:3838–3843

55. Stupp R, Mason WP, van den Bent MJ, et al; European Organisation for Research and Treatment of Cancer Brain Tumor and Radiotherapy Groups; National Cancer Institute of Canada Clinical Trials Group. Radiotherapy plus concomitant and adjuvant temozolomide for glioblastoma. N Engl J Med 2005;352:987–996

56. Amelio D, Lorentini S, Schwarz M, Amichetti M. Intensity-modulated radiation therapy in newly diagnosed glioblastoma: a systematic re-

view on clinical and technical issues. Radiother Oncol 2010;97:361–369

57. Koga T, Saito N. Efficacy and limitations of stereotactic radiosurgery in the treatment of glioblastoma. Neurol Med Chir (Tokyo) 2012;52:548–552

58. Siu A, Wind JJ, Iorgulescu JB, Chan TA, Yamada Y, Sherman JH. Radiation necrosis following treatment of high grade glioma—a review of the literature and current understanding. Acta Neurochir (Wien) 2012;154:191–201, discussion 201

59. Alexiou GA, Tsiouris S, Voulgaris S, Kyritsis AP, Fotopoulos AD. Glioblastoma multiforme imaging: the role of nuclear medicine. Curr Radiopharm 2012;5:308–313

60. Sadraei NH, Dahiya S, Chao ST, et al. Treatment of Cerebral Radiation Necrosis With Bevacizumab: The Cleveland Clinic Experience. Am J Clin Oncol 2013;Jun:24

61. Souhami L, Seiferheld W, Brachman D, et al. Randomized comparison of stereotactic radiosurgery followed by conventional radiotherapy with carmustine to conventional radiotherapy with carmustine for patients with glioblastoma multiforme: report of Radiation Therapy Oncology Group 93-05 protocol. Int J Radiat Oncol Biol Phys 2004;60:853–860

62. Buatti J, Ryken TC, Smith MC, et al. Radiation therapy of pathologically confirmed newly diagnosed glioblastoma in adults. J Neurooncol 2008;89:313–337

63. Liu BL, Cheng JX, Zhang X, Zhang W. Controversies concerning the application of brachytherapy in central nervous system tumors. J Cancer Res Clin Oncol 2010;136:173–185

64. Laperriere NJ, Leung PMK, McKenzie S, et al. Randomized study of brachytherapy in the initial management of patients with malignant astrocytoma. Int J Radiat Oncol Biol Phys 1998;41:1005–1011

65. Nieder C, Astner ST, Mehta MP, Grosu AL, Molls M. Improvement, clinical course, and quality of life after palliative radiotherapy for recurrent glioblastoma. Am J Clin Oncol 2008;31:300–305

66. Stewart LA. Chemotherapy in adult high-grade glioma: a systematic review and meta-analysis of individual patient data from 12 randomised trials. Lancet 2002;359:1011–1018

67. Cairncross G, Wang M, Shaw E, et al. Phase III trial of chemoradiotherapy for anaplastic oligodendroglioma: long-term results of RTOG 9402. J Clin Oncol 2013;31:337–343

68. van den Bent MJ, Brandes AA, Taphoorn MJ, et al. Adjuvant procarbazine, lomustine, and vincristine chemotherapy in newly diagnosed anaplastic oligodendroglioma: long-term follow-up of EORTC brain tumor group study 26951. J Clin Oncol 2013;31:344–350

69. Cohen MH, Johnson JR, Pazdur R. Food and Drug Administration Drug approval summary: temozolomide plus radiation therapy for the treatment of newly diagnosed glioblastoma multiforme. Clin Cancer Res 2005;11(19 Pt 1):6767–6771

70. Stupp R, Hegi ME, Mason WP, et al; European Organisation for Research and Treatment of Cancer Brain Tumour and Radiation Oncology Groups; National Cancer Institute of Canada Clinical Trials Group. Effects of radiotherapy with concomitant and adjuvant temozolomide versus radiotherapy alone on survival in glioblastoma in a randomised phase III study: 5-year analysis of the EORTC-NCIC trial. Lancet Oncol 2009;10:459–466

71. Brem H, Piantadosi S, Burger PC, et al; The Polymer-brain Tumor Treatment Group. Placebo-controlled trial of safety and efficacy of intraoperative controlled delivery by biodegradable polymers of chemotherapy for recurrent gliomas. Lancet 1995;345:1008–1012

72. Westphal M, Hilt DC, Bortey E, et al. A phase 3 trial of local chemotherapy with biodegradable carmustine (BCNU) wafers (Gliadel wafers) in patients with primary malignant glioma. Neuro-oncol 2003;5:79–88

73. Nagpal S. The role of BCNU polymer wafers (Gliadel) in the treatment of malignant glioma. Neurosurg Clin N Am 2012;23:289–295, ix ix.

74. Vredenburgh JJ, Desjardins A, Herndon JE II, et al. Bevacizumab plus irinotecan in recurrent glioblastoma multiforme. J Clin Oncol 2007;25:4722–4729

75. Wong ET, Gautam S, Malchow C, Lun M, Pan E, Brem S. Bevacizumab for recurrent glioblastoma multiforme: a meta-analysis. J Natl Compr Canc Netw 2011;9:403–407

76. Higa GM, Abraham J. Biological mechanisms of bevacizumab-associated adverse events. Expert Rev Anticancer Ther 2009;9:999–1007

26 Pilocytic Astrocytomas and Other Indolent Tumors

Robert P. Naftel and Ian F. Pollack

By definition, indolent tumors are slow to grow or progress and present with an insidious onset of symptoms over a period of months to years. Generally, such tumors are World Health Organization (WHO) grade I neoplasms with low proliferative potential and may be amenable to cure following resection alone.[1] The most prevalent indolent tumor is pilocytic astrocytoma (PA); however, this chapter also discusses other WHO grade I intra-axial neoplasms, categorized as astrocytic tumors, neuronal and mixed neuronal-glial tumors, and ependymal tumors (see Text Box), focusing first on general considerations in therapeutic management, and then on specific considerations relevant to individual tumor subgroups.

Indolent, WHO Grade 1, Intra-Axial Brain Tumors Included in This Chapter

- Astrocytic Tumors
  - Pilocytic astrocytoma (PA)
  - Subependymal giant cell astrocytoma (SEGA)
- Neuronal or mixed neuronal-glial tumors
  - Ganglioglioma and gangliocytoma
  - Desmoplastic infantile ganglioglioma (DIG) and astrocytoma (DIA)
  - Dysembryoplastic neuroepithelial tumor (DNT)
  - Papillary glioneuronal tumor
  - Lhermitte-Duclos disease (dysplastic gangliocytoma of the cerebellum)
- Ependymal tumors
  - Subependymoma

Researchers have identified patient populations that are at risk of developing some of these tumors,[2–4] and increasingly, genetic mutations associated with these tumors are being identified.

Pearl

- Some patient populations, such as those with neurofibromatosis type 1 (NF1), tuberous sclerosis complex (TSC), and Cowden disease, are at particular risk of developing indolent tumors.

Special Consideration

- Increasingly, researchers are discovering molecular alterations associated with each of these tumors, which is providing a basis for logical strategies in molecularly targeted therapy.

General Management Considerations

Because each neoplasm has unique characteristics and the mode of presentation can vary substantially, the evaluation and treatment of these patients is often individualized. Some lesions present with subtle neurologic symptoms, others with seizures, and still others are incidentally detected. Magnetic resonance imaging (MRI) with and without gadolinium contrast enhancement is the imaging modality of choice to define the location and growth characteristics of the tumor and to guide subsequent management.

A fundamental determination is whether surgery is warranted in a given case and, if so, the timing of the operative intervention. Children with relatively large lesions and significant local mass effect who are minimally symptomatic are scheduled for surgery on the next available operating day, and corticosteroids are generally begun upon diagnosis. In contrast, smaller lesions presenting with seizures and minimal or no mass effect are treated electively or, in some cases, monitored closely with serial imaging, particularly if the growth course of the tumor is uncertain and the lesion location presents a high risk of surgical morbidity. This expectant management approach may also be appropriate for small, indolent lesions that are identified incidentally. For small lesions that are considered to be appropriate for removal, corticosteroids, if warranted, are deferred until surgery, and, in such cases, are typically tapered over 3 to 7 days if significant tumor debulking has been achieved.

Pearl

- If resection is felt to be warranted, the major predictor for a favorable oncological outcome is achieving GTR of the indolent tumor.

In treating indolent tumors, the primary predictor of favorable oncological outcome is achieving gross total resection (GTR) of the tumor.[5,6] If the initial operation was undertaken with the goal of achieving a GTR and postoperative imaging reveals residual tumor, another attempt at GTR may be a reasonable option before considering adjuvant therapeutic modalities. Additionally, because many indolent tumors are also associated with epilepsy, outcomes are also measured by improvement in seizure control, and multiple preoperative and operative adjuncts may assist with this.[7]

Multiple surgical adjuncts can assist with preoperative and intraoperative planning. Stereotactic guidance systems allow the surgeon to plan an operative approach that minimizes manipulation of eloquent brain and optimizes the extent of maximum safe resection; however, the limitations of this technology must be recognized.

Cortical stimulation techniques,[8] which may be applied extraoperatively, using previously inserted grid or strip electrodes, or intraoperatively, at the time of the planned tumor resection, are useful for identifying speech and motor areas. Additionally, functional MRI and diffusion tensor imaging can localize critical cortical and subcortical areas and pathways to assist with surgical planning.[9,10] These functional studies can be fused with stereotactic guidance imaging to precisely delineate relevant loci around the tumor. In patients with intractable epilepsy in association with cortical lesions, electrocorticography can discriminate whether the seizures originate from the lesion alone or if there is additional epileptogenic cortex.[8]

Astrocytic Tumors

Pilocytic Astrocytomas

Pilocytic astrocytomas are WHO grade I neoplasms accounting for 5 to 6% of all gliomas, primarily affecting children and young adults with no gender predilection.[1] They are the most common type of glioma in children, and although they can be located anywhere in the central nervous system (CNS), most are located in the cerebellum (67%).[11] Presenting symptoms typically result from tumor mass effect causing focal neurologic signs or seizures. Some patients have nonlocalizing signs due to raised intracranial pressure or hydrocephalus.[12] On imaging, PAs are infrequently calcified and often exhibit well-defined borders with enhancement of a mural nodule or a uniform, ring-like pattern (**Fig. 26.1**).[13] In rare cases, such as optic pathway glioma in patients with NF1, in whom such tumors are relatively common, the MRI appearance is sufficient to establish the diagnosis without requiring surgical biopsy. PAs associated with NF1 are considered to be even more indolent than sporadic PAs.[2]

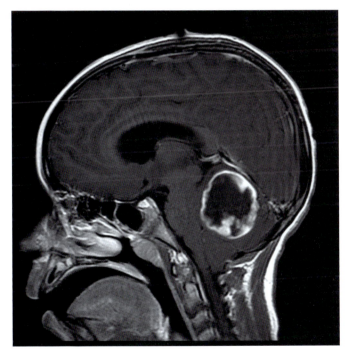

Fig. 26.1 A 7-year-old boy presenting with severe headaches, nausea, and vomiting due to hydrocephalus was found to have this posterior fossa tumor. This sagittal T1-weighted contrast-enhanced magnetic resonance imaging (MRI) scan reveals a cerebellar pilocytic astrocytoma with a mural nodule and enhancing cyst capsule. He underwent suboccipital craniotomy for resection of the nodule and enhancing cyst wall.

Histologically, regions with compact bipolar astrocytes are interspersed with loosely packed multipolar cells containing microcysts. Eosinophilic granular bodies and Rosenthal fibers are also seen. Although not believed to adversely affect prognosis, occasional mitotic figures, leptomeningeal infiltration, vascular proliferation, and necrosis may be noted.[1] Recently, PAs were noted to characteristically demonstrate changes in the *BRAF* gene.[14–16]

The observation of recurring abnormalities in *BRAF* or other elements in its signaling pathway has provided insight into strategies for molecularly targeted therapies for PAs. There are ongoing clinical trials of MEK inhibitors, RAF/multiple tyrosine kinase inhibitors such as Sorafenib, and mammalian target of rapamycin (mTOR) inhibitors for tumors not amenable to complete resection or those recurring after resection or initial adjuvant chemotherapy or radiotherapy.[17]

Because PAs are generally well circumscribed, they are amenable to GTR. The extent of resection has correlated closely with outcome.[5,6] Generally, the cyst wall does not need to be excised unless it is enhancing.[18] Adjuvant therapy is usually not employed after a GTR because recurrences are infrequent.

Even though at least half of patients after STR will progress within 5 years, overall survival rates exceed 90%.[5,6] The observation that PAs may remain quiescent after an incomplete resection suggests that tumors can exhibit decelerated growth kinetics over time, which fits with observations that tumor cells with *BRAF* alterations may undergo senescence after an initial period of growth.[19] Because of this biological variability, many neuro-oncologists prefer to expectantly follow patients with small amounts of residual tumor, only administering additional therapy in the event of tumor progression. In such cases, reoperation for GTR is sometimes feasible[6,20,21]; if not, adjuvant therapy, including chemotherapy or radiotherapy (RT), may then be employed. Typically, RT is reserved for older children or those who have failed chemotherapy because of

the adverse effects of radiation on the developing brain.[22,23] A variety of agents and regimens have been observed to delay tumor regrowth and delay or avoid the need for radiation, including carboplatin/vincristine, 6-thioguanine/procarbazine/chloroethylcyclohexylnitrosourea (CCNU)/vincristine, and vinblastine, among others.

An attempt at determining the role of RT for incompletely resected low-grade gliomas in the Children's Cancer Group-9891/Pediatric Oncology Group-8930 study failed because of difficulties in patient recruitment. Nonrandomized single-center series suggest that although irradiation significantly increases progression-free survival after incomplete resection, there is no significant impact on overall survival, in part attributed to their increased likelihood of developing malignant lesions within the treatment fields.[6,24] Later studies have focused on conformal irradiation with narrow peritumoral margins using three-dimensional image-based treatment planning.[25]

Rarely, PAs can seed the neuraxis, typically from tumors in the hypothalamic-chiasmatic location.[26] PAs have been reported to undergo malignant transformation; however, it is unclear whether this is secondary to radiation-induced changes.[24]

Pilomyxoid astrocytomas (PMAs) were once classified as PAs, but they are more aggressive tumors, classified as WHO grade II.[1] They typically affect infants with a median age at presentation of 10 months. They are most commonly located in the hypothalamic-chiasmatic region.[27] Histologically, there is a mucoid matrix with monomorphous bipolar cells radiating around vessels. Ordinarily, there are no Rosenthal fibers or eosinophilic granular bodies.[1] These tumors are more aggressive than PAs, with more frequent local recurrence and cerebrospinal spread.[28]

Subependymal Giant Cell Astrocytomas

Subependymal giant cell astrocytomas are WHO grade I tumors, arising near the midline in close proximity to the foramen of Monro, and develop in 5 to 15% of patients with TSC.[29,30] Most commonly, SEGAs develop in the first two decades of life with a mean age at presentation of 11 years.[31]

Due to their deep location and proximity to the foramen of Monro, patients often develop symptoms from either hydrocephalus or direct compression of the deep nuclei.[32] With the increasing use of MRI for screening children with TSC, such tumors are often diagnosed before symptoms develop. On imaging, SEGAs can be difficult to differentiate from subependymal nodules, but if a lesion is larger than 12 mm, enhances, and is near the foramen of Monro, it is likely to be a SEGA (**Fig. 26.2**).[33]

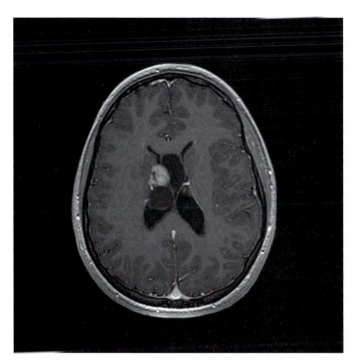

Fig. 26.2 A 13-year-old girl presenting with frequent headaches and syncopal events was found to have this subependymal giant cell astrocytoma (SEGA) causing obstructive hydrocephalus. On this axial T1-weighted contrast-enhanced MRI scan, the enhancing, cystic, intraventricular lesion is noted. She underwent a transcallosal resection of the tumor.

Histologically, the tumors consist of large cells resembling astrocytes and are often calcified. Nuclear pleomorphism and multinucleated cells are often present, and there can be increased mitotic activity. Immunoreactivity for both glial and neuronal markers may be noted.[1] On molecular analysis, dysregulation of mTOR signaling has been found to underlie the development of SEGAs in TSC.[34,35]

Surgery has been first-line therapy for SEGAs, which is curative with GTR.[33] Typically, a transcallosal or transcortical approach is used for tumor removal; however, purely endoscopic approaches also have been described.[36] When complete resection is not feasible, patients typically experience slow growth of the residual tumor, necessitating additional treatment.[37] Stereotactic single-dose RT has been used in both primary and adjuvant treatments, but the outcomes have not been consistently positive.[38,39] Recent advances in pharmacological therapy for SEGAs have taken advantage of mTOR pathway inhibition, using rapamycin (sirolimus), its prodrug CCI-779 (temsirolimus), or its analogue RAD001 (everolimus)

Pearl

- Surgery has been the treatment of choice for SEGAs, which is curative with complete resection.

Controversy

- The role of mTOR inhibitors in the long-term treatment of SEGAs has not been clearly established. Possibly, there are clinical scenarios that will be managed using mTOR inhibitors as either a neoadjuvant therapy or for residual or surgically unresectable lesions.

to halt the uncontrolled mTOR pathway.[31] This treatment strategy is still under clinical investigation, but published findings indicate that the majority of patients experienced significant reduction in the size of their tumors. However, the reduction was not durable after cessation of treatment, raising questions about whether therapy will need to be maintained indefinitely to prevent tumor regrowth.[34,35,40]

Neuronal and Mixed Neuronal-Glial Tumors

Gangliogliomas and Gangliocytomas

These WHO grade I tumors account for 1.3% of all brain tumors, with gangliogliomas being far more prevalent than gangliocytomas. Patients most commonly present in the second, third, or fourth decades of life.[1] The tumors can be located anywhere within the CNS, but they have a propensity for the temporal lobe.[41]

The presenting complaint is frequently long-standing partial complex seizures.[42] Signs of increased intracranial pressure and focal neurologic deficits are infrequent. On imaging, these enhancing tumors can be solid or cystic, occasionally with calcification, and may resemble PAs or other low-grade gliomas (**Fig. 26.3**).[43]

Histologically, gangliocytomas contain neoplastic mature ganglion cells alone, and gangliogliomas contain both neoplastic mature ganglion cells and neoplastic glial cells. Gangliogliomas contain neoplastic neurons with binucleation and atypia in a background of neoplastic astrocytes.[1] The genetic mutations associated with gangliogliomas have not been fully elucidated, but many have $BRAF^{v600E}$ mutations, rather than the $BRAF-KIAA$ translocation mutations that are common in PAs.[44]

Similar to PAs, gangliogliomas are usually amenable to GTR, and long-term progression-free survival is dependent

Pearl

- Patients with ganglioglioma often present with partial complex seizures that in many cases are refractory to anticonvulsant medications. Often, seizures have been present for years before diagnosis of the tumor.

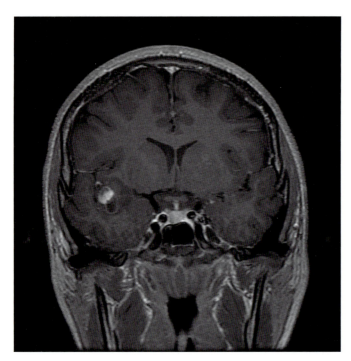

Fig. 26.3 A 15-year-old boy presenting with medically refractory epilepsy localized to his right temporal region. A coronal T1-weighted contrast-enhanced MRI scan shows an enhancing mixed cystic and solid tumor in the inferior portion of the right insula. He underwent a grid-based resection of the lesion and epileptogenic cortex. Pathology confirmed ganglioglioma.

on the extent of resection.[45] The 5-year survival rate exceeds 90%.[5,42] The role of irradiation after STR remains unclear. Due to their indolence, adjuvant therapy is used only when there is evidence of progression.[46]

Because epilepsy is often present, patients often undergo preoperative and intraoperative measures to localize and resect the epileptogenic cortex to improve epilepsy outcomes.[47] Seizure freedom is dependent on the extent of resection, the duration of seizures before resection, and the presence of generalized seizures. In temporal lobe surgery, there appears to be a benefit to the resection of the medial structures.[7]

Anaplastic gangliogliomas, WHO grade III neoplasms, exhibit more aggressive behavior and have worse outcomes. They may develop after RT to gangliogliomas.[1,48]

Special Consideration

- Because many gangliogliomas are associated with intractable epilepsy, preoperative and intraoperative measures to localize and resect epileptogenic foci in the vicinity of the tumor may have a role in improving ultimate seizure control.

Desmoplastic Infantile Gangliogliomas and Astrocytomas

Desmoplastic infantile gangliogliomas (DIGs) and astrocytomas (DIAs) are WHO grade I neoplasms with similar clinical presentation, imaging findings, and prognosis. Originally described as occurring only in the first 18 months of life, cases in older children have since been reported[49]; however, they most frequently occur within the first year of life. They are notable for the young age of affected patients, the large size of the lesion, and the presence of a pronounced desmoplastic histological component.[1] Most frequently, they are located supratentorially with a preference for the frontal and parietal lobes.[1,50]

Because DIGs and DIAs are large and typically arise during infancy, children frequently present with signs of increased intracranial pressure.[50] They can also present with seizures, especially in children older than 2 years.[49] On imaging, these tumors are characterized by their large size, superficial location, and frequent involvement of the leptomeninges. The tumors are partially cystic and have a densely enhancing solid component (**Fig. 26.4**).[51] On computed tomography (CT) and plain films, suture diastasis is often seen.

Histologically, DIGs and DIAs are characterized by three components: a desmoplastic leptomeningeal component, a

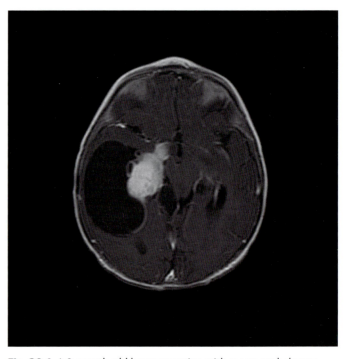

Fig. 26.4 A 9-month-old boy presenting with macrocephaly was found on this axial T1-weighted contrast-enhanced MRI scan to have a right medial temporal tumor with a large enhancing nodule and associated cyst. He underwent a subtotal resection of the desmoplastic infantile ganglioglioma (DIG).

poorly differentiated neuroepithelial component, and a cortical component. DIGs and DIAs are differentiated by the presence of neuronal cells in DIGs; calcification is not usually seen. Mitotic activity, microvascular proliferation, and necrosis are uncommon.[1] Molecular and genetic analysis is limited.

When feasible, the goal of treatment is GTR, including the affected leptomeninges, which is associated with a favorable prognosis for long-term progression-free survival.[52,53] Special precautions must be taken with surgery, including special attention directed to obtaining adequate hemodynamic monitoring and intravenous access before beginning the resection and ensuring appropriate blood and clotting factor replacement.[54] In view of the large size and profuse vascularity of these lesions, subtotal resection or staged resection may be necessary in select cases. Because residual disease frequently progresses, some neuro-oncologists have favored administering adjuvant chemotherapy after STR.[54] This issue is controversial, however, and other groups advocate expectant management and reexploration in the event of tumor progression because spontaneous regression of the residual tumor has sometimes been observed.[55,56] Cerebrospinal fluid (CSF) dissemination has been reported but is not common.[57]

Dysembryoplastic Neuroepithelial Tumors

Dysembryoplastic neuroepithelial tumors (DNTs) are WHO grade I tumors that typically present with seizures before the age of 20 years.[1] Occurring almost exclusively in the supratentorial compartment, DNTs have a predilection for the temporal lobe.[58,59] The incidence of DNTs is difficult to estimate because of changing diagnostic criteria and because many are operated on for epilepsy resections rather than as oncological procedures. Increased prevalence has been noted in patients with NF1 and XYY genotype.[1]

Dysembryoplastic neuroepithelial tumors predominantly present with refractory partial complex epilepsy. In many cases, seizures have been present for years before diagnosis.[58]

Signs of increased intracranial pressure and focal neurologic deficits are infrequent. On imaging, the tumors are well-demarcated, superficial lesions that are hypodense on CT, hypointense on T1-weighted MRI, and hyperintense on T2-weighted MRI. Lesions have no mass effect or surrounding edema (**Fig. 26.5**). Enhancement, if present, is slight and true cyst formation is uncommon.[60] The leptomeninges are generally not involved.[1,61]

Histologically, there is a "specific glioneuronal element" described as columns oriented perpendicular to the cortical surface, and without an intact specimen, pathologist may not be able to recognize this specific architecture.[1] DNTs are notable for their cortical location and multinodular structure with neoplastic oligodendrocytes, neurons, and astrocytes. Between nodules there is a neuroglial component, with neurons in a background of oligodendroglial cells. In many cases the DNT is associated with cortical dysplasia.[1,62] There is both a

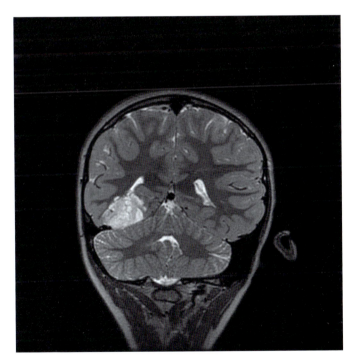

Fig. 26.5 A 7-year-old boy presenting with medically refractory epilepsy that localized to his right posterior temporal region. A T2-weighted coronal MRI sequence demonstrated a lesion without surrounding edema, and upon contrast administration there was no enhancement. He underwent grid based resection of this dysembryoplastic neuroepithelial tumor (DNT) and epileptogenic cortex.

simple and complex form of this histology; the latter is associated with other grade I tumor components, such as PA.[1]

Like the other indolent lesions, DNTs have a favorable long-term oncological outcome. These tumors are generally well circumscribed and amenable to GTR. However, even after an STR long-term progression-free survival is common, and adjuvant therapy is often deferred.[63] For favorable epilepsy outcomes, it is recommended that the associated cortical dysplasia also be resected.[60] Risk factors associated with the development of recurrent or continued seizures are incomplete resection, associated cortical dysplasia, and long duration of epilepsy.[1,64] Malignant degeneration has been reported, although it is infrequent, and may be promoted by the use of cytotoxic therapies.[1]

Papillary Glioneuronal Tumors

Originally considered a variant of a ganglioglioma, this WHO grade I neoplasm is rare with only several dozen having been reported. The age distribution is wide, but most patients present before the age of 30 years.[1,65] Typically presenting with headaches and seizures,[1] the tumors are commonly found in the temporal lobe.[66] On CT and MRI they appear as well-circumscribed lesions that are cystic with an enhancing mural nodule (**Fig. 26.6**). Calcification can be present and surrounding edema is rare.[66]

Histologically, they are characterized by a pseudopapillary architecture. There can be a single or pseudostratified layer of small, cuboidal glial cells surrounding hyalinized blood vessels and interpapillary sheets of neurocytes and occasional ganglion cells.[1] A common molecular genetic mutation has not been identified.[66]

Although this is a rare tumor, GTR without adjuvant therapy is believed to offer good long-term progression-free survival.[1,66] However, because this is a recently defined entity, long-term follow-up information on these patients is sparsely available.

Lhermitte-Duclos Disease (Dysplastic Gangliocytoma of the Cerebellum)

Because it is unclear whether Lhermitte-Duclos disease (LDD) is a neoplastic or hamartomatous process, no WHO grade has

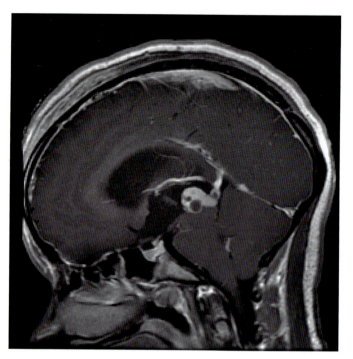

Fig. 26.6 A 16-year-old girl presenting with headaches and papilledema was found to have hydrocephalus due to a posterior third ventricular tumor. A T1-weighted sagittal MRI sequence with contrast demonstrated a mixed cystic and solid enhancing tumor. After treatment of her hydrocephalus, she underwent a transcallosal, interforniceal approach to the posterior third ventricle for resection of the tumor. Pathology revealed that it was a papillary glioneuronal tumor.

been officially assigned, although the slow growth over time suggests that this is a neoplastic disorder, albeit an indolent one. LDD is a benign mass of the cerebellum formed by ganglion cells. It can affect all ages but most commonly presents in the third through fifth decades of life.[1] Often, LDD is associated with Cowden disease, and development of LDD in adulthood meets diagnostic criteria for Cowden disease.[4] It is an autosomal dominant disorder with age-dependent penetrance that is associated with the formation of hamartomas and multiple types of neoplasms.[67]

Patients typically present with cerebellar signs including dysmetria or ataxia.[1] Hydrocephalus or focal brainstem signs can develop.[4] Classically, LDD affects only one hemisphere, but it can be bilateral. On MRI the abnormality is best visualized on T2-weighted images with hyperintense gyral striations and enlargement of the cerebellar folia. Upon contrast administration, there is no enhancement.[4]

Histologically, there is diffuse thickening of the molecular and internal granular layers of the cerebellum. The cerebellar architecture is relatively preserved with affected layers hypertrophied. Genetically, *PTEN* mutations, which are the responsible abnormalities for 80% of Cowden disease cases, have been identified in all adult-onset cases. In affected children without Cowden disease, *PTEN* mutations may be absent, but downstream mutations have been identified in the mTOR pathway.[4] The *PTEN* tumor suppressor gene was mapped to chromosome 10q23.[68]

Untreated, LDD slowly progresses, and, historically, outcomes have been uniformly poor.[69] Surgical resection is the treatment of choice; however, achieving GTR can be challenging because the abnormal tissue blends with normal tissue. Radiation therapy has been used without benefit.[69] Patients with hydrocephalus often require spinal fluid diversion.[69,70] Because Cowden disease can lead to different forms of cancer, patients diagnosed with LDD should be screened for tumors associated with Cowden disease.[1,4]

Ependymal Tumors

Subependymomas

Subependymomas are WHO grade I tumors normally presenting in middle-aged or elderly patients with a male predilection.[1] The incidence is believed to be 0.2 to 0.7% of all intracranial tumors, but it is difficult to estimate because patients can be asymptomatic and lesions may go undetected until they are incidentally discovered at autopsy.[71] Subependymomas can occur in proximity to any ventricle; most develop in the fourth ventricle (50 to 60%), followed by the lateral ventricles (30 to 40%). Rarely, they can occur in the third ventricle or in the spinal cord.[1] Clinically, these tumors can present with symptoms and signs of hydrocephalus due to ventricular obstruction. They can also be incidentally diagnosed on imaging that is performed for other reasons.[71] On MRI, they are well-demarcated tumors that are hypointense to isointense on T1-weighted images, and hyperintense on T2-weighted images, with minimal to moderate enhancement.[71]

Histologically, these lesions are characterized by clusters of isomorphic nuclei within a dense fibrillary matrix of glial cell processes, and mitoses are rare.[1] Although there are rare familial cases, a genetic linkage has not been identified.[72]

Because of their indolent course, asymptomatic patients may be observed with serial imaging. For symptomatic patients or patients in whom there is suspicion for a more aggressive tumor, surgery is indicated. GTR without adjuvant therapy is usually curative. Recurrences are reported after subtotal resection.[1,71] No definitive role for RT has been established.[71]

Conclusion

Pilocytic astrocytomas and other indolent tumors are often treated surgically, with generally favorable outcomes, although a subset of tumors that are small, asymptomatic, and in deep or eloquent locations may be carefully observed with serial imaging. Complete surgical resection is often curative in patients with accessible tumors. Surgery goals should also include treating epilepsy, if this is a component of the presenting symptomatology. Ongoing research into the molecular genetics of several of these tumors is providing insight into potential targeted therapies for those lesions not amenable to complete resection.

Editor's Note

A brain tumor diagnosis is a devastating event in a person's life, often heralding in their mind the beginning of the end. Fortunately, many indolent species exist, particularly in children, who respond even better than adults to brain tumor surgery and other modalities for a variety of reasons. Generally when such a lesion is found in a child, surgery is recommended. In adults, we may assume that the lesion has been there a long time and we can safely observe the patient with periodic imaging, especially if the lesion is in eloquent cortex, and given that imaging is quite reliable at excluding a more ominous diagnosis.

Fortunately, the indolent, largely neuroectodermal, neoplasms such as pilocytic astrocytoma have excellent prognoses, even if resection has to be incomplete due to anatomic and other factors. New variants have been described over the last several decades, some of which are a little worse than their "progenitor," such as the pilomyxoid variant of pilocytic astrocytoma, which may require radiation therapy. Another new variant is the rosette-forming glioneuronal tumors of the posterior fossa, which are often not completely resectable because of their diffuseness or their involvement of the brainstem.[73] (Bernstein)

References

1. Louis DN, International Agency for Research on Cancer. WHO Classification of Tumours of the Central Nervous System, 4th ed. Lyon: International Agency for Research on Cancer, 2007

2. Pollack IF, Mulvihill JJ. Special issues in the management of gliomas in children with neurofibromatosis 1. J Neurooncol 1996;28:257–268

3. Curatolo P, Bombardieri R, Jozwiak S. Tuberous sclerosis. Lancet 2008; 372:657–668

4. Robinson S, Cohen AR. Cowden disease and Lhermitte-Duclos disease: an update. Case report and review of the literature. Neurosurg Focus 2006;20:E6

5. Wisoff JH, Sanford RA, Heier LA, et al. Primary neurosurgery for pediatric low-grade gliomas: a prospective multi-institutional study from the Children's Oncology Group. Neurosurgery 2011;68:1548–1554, discussion 1554–1555

6. Pollack IF, Claassen D, al-Shboul Q, Janosky JE, Deutsch M. Low-grade gliomas of the cerebral hemispheres in children: an analysis of 71 cases. J Neurosurg 1995;82:536–547

7. Englot DJ, Berger MS, Barbaro NM, Chang EF. Factors associated with seizure freedom in the surgical resection of glioneuronal tumors. Epilepsia 2012;53:51–57

8. Berger MS, Kincaid J, Ojemann GA, Lettich E. Brain mapping techniques to maximize resection, safety, and seizure control in children with brain tumors. Neurosurgery 1989;25:786–792

9. Schneider W, Noll DC, Cohen JD. Functional topographic mapping of the cortical ribbon in human vision with conventional MRI scanners. Nature 1993;365:150–153

10. Moshel YA, Elliott RE, Monoky DJ, Wisoff JH. Role of diffusion tensor imaging in resection of thalamic juvenile pilocytic astrocytoma. J Neurosurg Pediatr 2009;4:495–505

11. Ohgaki H, Kleihues P. Population-based studies on incidence, survival rates, and genetic alterations in astrocytic and oligodendroglial gliomas. J Neuropathol Exp Neurol 2005;64:479–489

12. Clark GB, Henry JM, McKeever PE. Cerebral pilocytic astrocytoma. Cancer 1985;56:1128–1133

13. Fulham MJ, Melisi JW, Nishimiya J, Dwyer AJ, Di Chiro G. Neuroimaging of juvenile pilocytic astrocytomas: an enigma. Radiology 1993;189: 221–225

14. Bar EE, Lin A, Tihan T, Burger PC, Eberhart CG. Frequent gains at chromosome 7q34 involving BRAF in pilocytic astrocytoma. J Neuropathol Exp Neurol 2008;67:878–887

15. Jones DT, Kocialkowski S, Liu L, et al. Tandem duplication producing a novel oncogenic BRAF fusion gene defines the majority of pilocytic astrocytomas. Cancer Res 2008;68:8673–8677

16. Korshunov A, Meyer J, Capper D, et al. Combined molecular analysis of BRAF and IDH1 distinguishes pilocytic astrocytoma from diffuse astrocytoma. Acta Neuropathol 2009;118:401–405

17. Jones DT, Gronych J, Lichter P, Witt O, Pfister SM. MAPK pathway activation in pilocytic astrocytoma. Cell Mol Life Sci 2012;69:1799–1811

18. Beni-Adani L, Gomori M, Spektor S, Constantini S. Cyst wall enhancement in pilocytic astrocytoma: neoplastic or reactive phenomena. Pediatr Neurosurg 2000;32:234–239

19. Raabe EH, Lim KS, Kim JM, et al. BRAF activation induces transformation and then senescence in human neural stem cells: a pilocytic astrocytoma model. Clin Cancer Res 2011;17:3590–3599

20. Hirsch JF, Sainte Rose C, Pierre-Kahn A, Pfister A, Hoppe-Hirsch E. Benign astrocytic and oligodendrocytic tumors of the cerebral hemispheres in children. J Neurosurg 1989;70:568–572

21. Bowers DC, Krause TP, Aronson LJ, et al. Second surgery for recurrent pilocytic astrocytoma in children. Pediatr Neurosurg 2001;34:229–234

22. Merchant TE, Conklin HM, Wu S, Lustig RH, Xiong X. Late effects of conformal radiation therapy for pediatric patients with low-grade glioma: prospective evaluation of cognitive, endocrine, and hearing deficits. J Clin Oncol 2009;27:3691–3697

23. Ater JL, Zhou T, Holmes E, et al. Randomized study of two chemotherapy regimens for treatment of low-grade glioma in young children: a report from the Children's Oncology Group. J Clin Oncol 2012;30: 2641–2647

24. Dirks PB, Jay V, Becker LE, et al. Development of anaplastic changes in low-grade astrocytomas of childhood. Neurosurgery 1994;34:68–78

25. Merchant TE, Kun LE, Wu S, Xiong X, Sanford RA, Boop FA. Phase II trial of conformal radiation therapy for pediatric low-grade glioma. J Clin Oncol 2009;27:3598–3604

26. Pollack IF, Hurtt M, Pang D, Albright AL. Dissemination of low grade intracranial astrocytomas in children. Cancer 1994;73:2869–2878

27. Fernandez C, Figarella-Branger D, Girard N, et al. Pilocytic astrocytomas in children: prognostic factors—a retrospective study of 80 cases. Neurosurgery 2003;53:544–553, discussion 554–555

28. Tihan T, Fisher PG, Kepner JL, et al. Pediatric astrocytomas with monomorphous pilomyxoid features and a less favorable outcome. J Neuropathol Exp Neurol 1999;58:1061–1068

29. Franz DN, Bissler JJ, McCormack FX. Tuberous sclerosis complex: neurological, renal and pulmonary manifestations. Neuropediatrics 2010; 41:199–208

30. Adriaensen ME, Schaefer-Prokop CM, Stijnen T, Duyndam DA, Zonnenberg BA, Prokop M. Prevalence of subependymal giant cell tumors in patients with tuberous sclerosis and a review of the literature. Eur J Neurol 2009;16:691–696

31. Beaumont TL, Limbrick DD, Smyth MD. Advances in the management of subependymal giant cell astrocytoma. Childs Nerv Syst 2012;28: 963–968

32. Fuller GN, Scheithauer BW. The 2007 Revised World Health Organization (WHO) Classification of Tumours of the Central Nervous System: newly codified entities. Brain Pathol 2007;17:304–307

33. Cuccia V, Zuccaro G, Sosa F, Monges J, Lubienieky F, Taratuto AL. Subependymal giant cell astrocytoma in children with tuberous sclerosis. Childs Nerv Syst 2003;19:232–243

34. Krueger DA, Care MM, Holland K, et al. Everolimus for subependymal giant-cell astrocytomas in tuberous sclerosis. N Engl J Med 2010;363: 1801–1811

35. Lam C, Bouffet E, Tabori U, Mabbott D, Taylor M, Bartels U. Rapamycin (sirolimus) in tuberous sclerosis associated pediatric central nervous system tumors. Pediatr Blood Cancer 2010;54:476–479

36. Souweidane MM, Luther N. Endoscopic resection of solid intraventricular brain tumors. J Neurosurg 2006;105:271–278

37. de Ribaupierre S, Dorfmüller G, Bulteau C, et al. Subependymal giant-cell astrocytomas in pediatric tuberous sclerosis disease: when should we operate? Neurosurgery 2007;60:83–89, discussion 89–90

38. Wang LW, Shiau CY, Chung WY, et al. Gamma Knife surgery for low-grade astrocytomas: evaluation of long-term outcome based on a 10-year experience. J Neurosurg 2006;105(Suppl):127–132

39. Park KJ, Kano H, Kondziolka D, Niranjan A, Flickinger JC, Lunsford LD. Gamma knife surgery for subependymal giant cell astrocytomas. Clinical article. J Neurosurg 2011;114:808–813

40. Franz DN, Leonard J, Tudor C, et al. Rapamycin causes regression of astrocytomas in tuberous sclerosis complex. Ann Neurol 2006;59: 490–498

41. Blümcke I, Wiestler OD. Gangliogliomas: an intriguing tumor entity associated with focal epilepsies. J Neuropathol Exp Neurol 2002;61: 575–584

42. Haddad SF, Moore SA, Menezes AH, VanGilder JC. Ganglioglioma: 13 years of experience. Neurosurgery 1992;31:171–178

43. Osborn AG. Diagnostic Neuroradiology. St. Louis: Mosby, 1994

44. Dougherty MJ, Santi M, Brose MS, et al. Activating mutations in BRAF characterize a spectrum of pediatric low-grade gliomas. Neuro-oncol 2010;12:621–630

45. Compton JJ, Laack NN, Eckel LJ, Schomas DA, Giannini C, Meyer FB. Long-term outcomes for low-grade intracranial ganglioglioma: 30-year experience from the Mayo Clinic. J Neurosurg 2012;117:825–830

46. Matsumoto K, Tamiya T, Ono Y, Furuta T, Asari S, Ohmoto T. Cerebral gangliogliomas: clinical characteristics, CT and MRI. Acta Neurochir (Wien) 1999;141:135–141

47. Pilcher WH, Silbergeld DL, Berger MS, Ojemann GA. Intraoperative electrocorticography during tumor resection: impact on seizure outcome in patients with gangliogliomas. J Neurosurg 1993;78:891–902

48. Prayson RA, Khajavi K, Comair YG. Cortical architectural abnormalities and MIB1 immunoreactivity in gangliogliomas: a study of 60 patients with intracranial tumors. J Neuropathol Exp Neurol 1995;54:513–520

49. Hummel TR, Miles L, Mangano FT, Jones BV, Geller JI. Clinical heterogeneity of desmoplastic infantile ganglioglioma: a case series and literature review. J Pediatr Hematol Oncol 2012;34:e232–e236

50. Gelabert-Gonzalez M, Serramito-García R, Arcos-Algaba A. Desmoplastic infantile and non-infantile ganglioglioma. Review of the literature. Neurosurg Rev 2010;34:151–158

51. Trehan G, Bruge H, Vinchon M, et al. MR imaging in the diagnosis of desmoplastic infantile tumor: retrospective study of six cases. AJNR Am J Neuroradiol 2004;25:1028–1033

52. Sugiyama K, Arita K, Shima T, et al. Good clinical course in infants with desmoplastic cerebral neuroepithelial tumor treated by surgery alone. J Neurooncol 2002;59:63–69

53. Mallucci C, Lellouch Tubiana A, Salazar C, et al. The management of desmoplastic neuroepithelial tumours in childhood. Childs Nerv Syst 2000;16:8–14

54. Duffner PK, Burger PC, Cohen ME, et al. Desmoplastic infantile gangliogliomas: an approach to therapy. Neurosurgery 1994;34:583–589, discussion 589

55. Bächli H, Avoledo P, Gratzl O, Tolnay M. Therapeutic strategies and management of desmoplastic infantile ganglioglioma: two case reports and literature overview. Childs Nerv Syst 2003;19:359–366

56. Tamburrini G, Colosimo C Jr, Giangaspero F, Riccardi R, Di Rocco C. Desmoplastic infantile ganglioglioma. Childs Nerv Syst 2003;19:292–297

57. De Munnynck K, Van Gool S, Van Calenbergh F, et al. Desmoplastic infantile ganglioglioma: a potentially malignant tumor? Am J Surg Pathol 2002;26:1515–1522

58. Chan CH, Bittar RG, Davis GA, Kalnins RM, Fabinyi GC. Long-term seizure outcome following surgery for dysembryoplastic neuroepithelial tumor. J Neurosurg 2006;104:62–69

59. Thom M, Toma A, An S, et al. One hundred and one dysembryoplastic neuroepithelial tumors: an adult epilepsy series with immunohistochemical, molecular genetic, and clinical correlations and a review of the literature. J Neuropathol Exp Neurol 2011;70:859–878

60. O'Brien DF, Farrell M, Delanty N, et al; Children's Cancer and Leukaemia Group. The Children's Cancer and Leukaemia Group guidelines for the diagnosis and management of dysembryoplastic neuroepithelial tumours. Br J Neurosurg 2007;21:539–549

61. Daumas-Duport C, Varlet P, Bacha S, Beuvon F, Cervera-Pierot P, Chodkiewicz JP. Dysembryoplastic neuroepithelial tumors: nonspecific histological forms—a study of 40 cases. J Neurooncol 1999;41:267–280

62. Sakuta R, Otsubo H, Nolan MA, et al. Recurrent intractable seizures in children with cortical dysplasia adjacent to dysembryoplastic neuroepithelial tumor. J Child Neurol 2005;20:377–384

63. Taratuto AL, Pomata H, Sevlever G, Gallo G, Monges J. Dysembryoplastic neuroepithelial tumor: morphological, immunocytochemical, and deoxyribonucleic acid analyses in a pediatric series. Neurosurgery 1995; 36:474–481

64. Nolan MA, Sakuta R, Chuang N, et al. Dysembryoplastic neuroepithelial tumors in childhood: long-term outcome and prognostic features. Neurology 2004;62:2270–2276

65. Suh YL, Koo H, Kim TS, et al; Neuropathology Study Group of the Korean Society of Pathologists. Tumors of the central nervous system in Korea: a multicenter study of 3221 cases. J Neurooncol 2002;56: 251–259

66. Myung JK, Byeon SJ, Kim B, et al. Papillary glioneuronal tumors: a review of clinicopathologic and molecular genetic studies. Am J Surg Pathol 2011;35:1794–1805

67. Eng C, Murday V, Seal S, et al. Cowden syndrome and Lhermitte-Duclos disease in a family: a single genetic syndrome with pleiotropy? J Med Genet 1994;31:458–461

68. Zhou XP, Marsh DJ, Morrison CD, et al. Germline inactivation of PTEN and dysregulation of the phosphoinositol-3-kinase/Akt pathway cause human Lhermitte-Duclos disease in adults. Am J Hum Genet 2003; 73:1191–1198

69. Nowak DA, Trost HA. Lhermitte-Duclos disease (dysplastic cerebellar gangliocytoma): a malformation, hamartoma or neoplasm? Acta Neurol Scand 2002;105:137–145

70. Kumar R, Vaid VK, Kalra SK. Lhermitte-Duclos disease. Childs Nerv Syst 2007;23:729–732

71. Ragel BT, Osborn AG, Whang K, Townsend JJ, Jensen RL, Couldwell WT. Subependymomas: an analysis of clinical and imaging features. Neurosurgery 2006;58:881–890, discussion 881–890

72. Ryken TC, Robinson RA, VanGilder JC. Familial occurrence of subependymoma. Report of two cases. J Neurosurg 1994;80:1108–1111

73. Zhang J, Babu R, McLendon RE, Friedman AH, Adamson C. A comprehensive analysis of 41 patients with rosette-forming glioneuronal tumors of the fourth ventricle. J Clin Neurosci 2013;20:335–341

27 Brainstem Tumors

Sarah T. Garber and John Kestle

■ Epidemiology and Classification

Brainstem tumors (BSTs) are predominantly found in the pediatric population, with a mean age at presentation of between 7 and 9 years.[1–3] Overall, BSTs represent 10 to 15% of pediatric brain tumors.[4–6] The incidence in the United States is estimated to be between 5 and 10 cases per 10 million people per year,[1,7–15] and BSTs do not appear to have a predilection based on sex, race, or geographic location.

Historically, BSTs were considered as a uniform group of inoperable tumors. It was not until the advent of neuroimaging in recent decades that classifications began to emerge to describe the heterogeneity of this group of neoplasms.[9,10,16] Although minor variations exist between the various classification systems, they all aim to classify BSTs according to biological behavior and location and are the basis for selecting patients for surgery. For example, BSTs have been classified as diffuse or focal, and the focal tumors were further subdivided into midbrain, pontine, dorsally exophytic, and medullary.[17] A simplified classification into diffuse, focal, and exophytic has also been proposed.[18] This system has been found to be very valuable in selecting patients for surgery and discussing prognosis with families (see text box).

Several large series have now reported the distribution and prognosis of BSTs among the various subgroups. It has been estimated that between 58% and 75%[9,10,16] of BSTs are diffuse, and approximately 25% are focal. Diffuse tumors originate from the pons and are now often referred to as diffuse intrinsic pontine gliomas (DIPGs). These lesions have a dismal prognosis and were previously thought not to be amenable to surgical therapy. Focal tumors can be found in any part of the

brainstem and may be completely surrounded by brainstem tissue or may reach the surface. Focal tumors that grow out of the brainstem are referred to as exophytic. The exophytic portion may be dorsally, laterally, or ventrally located. In general, the focal and exophytic tumors are lower grade, present with a longer history, are sometimes surgically resectable, and have a much better prognosis than the diffuse tumors.

The dorsally exophytic tumors, a special subtype of the focal tumors, were first described about 25 years ago.[12] They are unique in several respects. They are almost completely extramedullary, filling the fourth ventricle and mimicking other fourth ventricle tumors. The exophytic component often enhances. They are usually pilocytic,[15] and, as a result of these favorable features, they are considered by many to be a surgically curable subtype with favorable long-term outcomes.

A second type of focal BST is the tectal glioma. This lesion usually presents with hydrocephalus secondary to obstruction of the aqueduct. Typically, these tumors do not enhance and have a very indolent course such that management of the hydrocephalus is the main issue.

Once exophytic and focal BSTs were described, surgical approaches to these lesions were introduced. As experience in the surgical treatment of BSTs increased, a variety of pathological diagnoses were encountered, including pilocytic and fibrillary astrocytomas, gangliogliomas (low-grade and anaplastic), gangliocytomas, primitive neuroectodermal tumors (medulloepitheliomas), and ependymomas.[19] Nevertheless, gliomas, especially low-grade gliomas, are the most common histology for the focal and exophytic tumor groups, and surgery should be considered for these lesions.

Clinical Presentation

The clinical presentation of BSTs provides essential information for their diagnosis and management. The congruence of clinical presentation and magnetic resonance imaging (MRI) strongly predicts the BST type and is the basis for management decisions. Children with diffuse BSTs typically present with a triad of cerebellar dysfunction (87%), cranial neuropathies (77%), and long-tract signs (53%). Cerebellar dysfunction is often in the form of gait instability, whereas paresis is a common manifestation of long-tract compromise. The cranial nerves most frequently affected are V, VI, and VII. Hydrocephalus is a relatively uncommon finding at presentation (< 20%). Leptomeningeal dissemination has been reported in 4 to 39% of cases during relapse.[20] Although not all children present with the triad, the multiplicity of symptoms is strongly predictive of a poor outcome. In one report the presence of symptoms from at least two of the three categories in the triad predicted death within 18 months, with a 97% positive predictive value in 33 children.[21]

Rapid evolution of symptoms is another hallmark of diffuse BSTs. Among children with diffuse BSTs, the interval from onset of symptoms to diagnosis was less than 1 month in 55% of patients, less than 3 months in 80%, and within 6 months in 94%.[13] Similar to symptom multiplicity, the duration of symptoms prior to diagnosis also correlates with survival. A median survival of 12.9 months was reported with an interval of 1 to 4 weeks, compared with 19.5 months with a longer duration prior to diagnosis.[22] Other studies have also reported similar findings, with decreased survival for patients with symptoms of less than 1 month's duration compared with those with symptoms lasting 6 months or longer.[7,8,17,21]

In contrast to the diffuse BSTs, the presentation of focal BSTs is much more indolent and is usually measured in months to years. In our series of 28 children with focal pilocytic tumors of the brainstem, the most common presentation (86%) was a focal neurologic deficit of cranial nerves with or without motor or sensory long-tract findings. Of those patients, 25% also presented with hydrocephalus and one of them suffered from seizures. Two patients presented with hydrocephalus only, and two others presented with headaches alone. As expected, the nature of the cranial nerve deficits and the presence of hydrocephalus corresponded to the anatomical location of the tumor. Midbrain tumors, most commonly tectal gliomas, usually present with signs and symptoms of progressive hydrocephalus. Parinaud syndrome, oculomotor palsies, and long-tract findings are less common except for tumors that involve the tegmentum. Patients with intrinsic focal pontine tumors may present with diplopia, facial weakness or numbness, hearing loss, and paresis, whereas the dorsally exophytic variant, which typically arises from the medulla, presents more often with hydrocephalus from fourth ventricular obstruction. Additionally, patients with medullary tumors can present with dysphagia, hoarseness, nausea and vomiting, ataxia, and paresis, often in the context of recurrent upper respiratory tract infections and pneumonia as a result of silent aspiration. The

prolonged history, often with gastrointestinal or respiratory investigations, is a hallmark of the medullary tumors.

Molecular Genetics

Studies have shown that diffuse BSTs share similar genetic alterations with pediatric high-grade gliomas but have molecular characteristics that distinguish them from adult gliomas. The role of epidermal growth factor and downstream signaling pathways in high-grade gliomas has been well established.[23] In diffuse BSTs, both p53 mutation (a tumor suppressor gene mutation associated with secondary glioblastomas) and epidermal growth factor receptor amplification (associated with primary glioblastomas) have been identified.[24] This may explain their similarities with glioblastomas in terms of their aggressive biological behavior. Studies have also shown molecular alterations leading to overexpression of the platelet-derived growth factor receptor (PDGFR) in diffuse pediatric pontine gliomas.[25,26] This may serve as a useful target for treatment of these therapeutically challenging tumors. Furthermore, the association with secondary glioblastomas raises the possibility of malignant transformation in these diffuse BSTs, which could explain the long-standing problem of the poor predictive value of biopsies of these tumors.

Neurofibromatosis Type 1 and Brainstem Tumors

Patients with neurofibromatosis type 1 (NF1) who have brainstem tumors appear to have a more favorable prognosis than those without NF1. With a median follow-up of 3.75 years, none of the nine NF1 patients with diffuse BSTs progressed and required intervention in one report.[27] In another study (in which 14 of 17 patients had primary focal medullary lesions), a 5-year progression-free survival (PFS) of 82% was reported with a median follow-up of 52 months.[28] This is in contrast to the 51% 5-year PFS in our series of non-NF1 patients with predominantly focal medullary tumors.[14]

In NF1 patients, it is particularly important not to confuse the diagnosis of BSTs with the commonly identified T2 signal abnormalities in the brainstem, which exhibit few, if any, symptoms and little growth.[29–31] Another clue to the diagnosis of NF1 is T2 signal abnormality in the globus pallidus. Because of the more indolent nature of these NF1 BSTs, the current recommendation is a conservative one with observation, and intervention should be reserved only for lesions that exhibit clinical or imaging changes.

■ Imaging Studies

Although computed tomography (CT) may aid the diagnosis in a few selected cases (the presence of calcium may suggest oligodendroglioma or an occult vascular malformation[32]), smaller focal tumors are often missed on routine CT imaging. At present, MRI is the imaging modality of choice in the evaluation of BSTs. The neuroimaging features of diffuse BSTs can be misleading and often do not correlate with clinical features.[33] For example, MRI is not specific for distinguishing lower from higher grade neoplasms unless focal enhancement or diffusion restriction (implying a higher-grade lesion) is present. The most striking feature is an enlarged ("fat") pons (**Fig. 27.1a**). On T1-weighted images (T1WIs), the lesion appears hypointense with ill-defined margins blurring into the adjacent parenchyma. On T2-weighted images (T2WIs), the lesion is hyperintense, and the extent of tumor infiltration is much better appreciated because signal intensities extend cranially into the midbrain or caudally into the medulla usually beyond the margin of the T1 abnormality (**Fig. 27.1b**). With gadolinium, about a third of diffuse BSTs enhance, usually heterogeneously (**Fig. 27.1c**). The role of biopsy in these tumors remains controversial. Biopsy is considered when the presentation (clinical or imaging) is atypical (**Fig. 27.2**). Recent advances in the molecular genetics of diffuse BSTs may lead to a paradigm shift favoring biopsy to better understand tumor biology and to identify new therapeutic targets.[33]

In contrast, focal BSTs are usually smaller and are well demarcated on MRI (**Fig. 27.3**). They have homogeneous en-

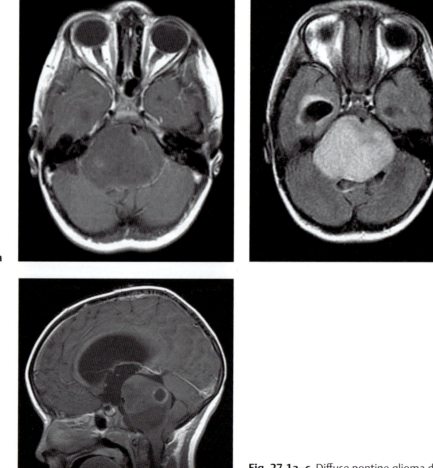

a

b

c

Fig. 27.1a–c Diffuse pontine glioma demonstrating a diffusely enlarged "fat" pons that (**a**) is hypointense on T1-weighted magnetic resonance imaging (MRI), (**b**) is bright on T2-weighted MRI, and (**c**) shows enhancement around a small cystic component.

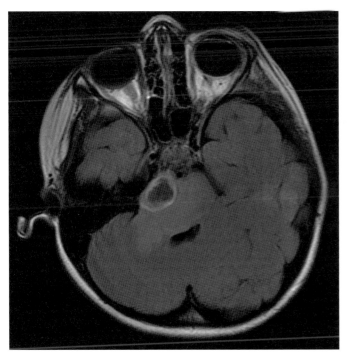

Fig. 27.2 Axial T2-weighted fluid-attenuated inversion recovery (FLAIR) image of an atypical biopsy-proven pontine glioblastoma,

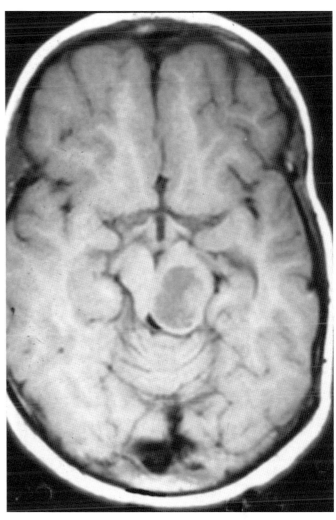

hancement, especially when they are pilocytic in origin, and they may have a cystic component. Unlike their diffuse counterparts, these lesions are typically noninfiltrative with their T1WIs and T2WIs superimposable (**Fig. 27.4**). Focal BSTs may present on the surface of the brainstem and may have an exophytic component.

The dorsally exophytic tumors typically present as a fourth ventricular mass with variable brainstem involvement. They

Fig. 27.3 Noncontrast, T1-weighted MRI of a focal tumor of the midbrain tegmentum enlarging the left cerebral peduncle.

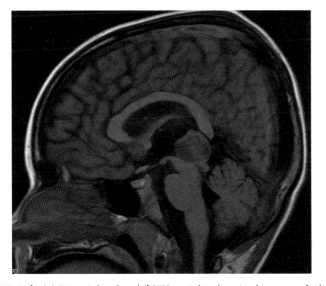

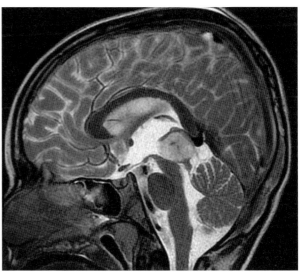

a

b

Fig. 27.4a,b (**a**) T1-weighted and (**b**) T2-weighted sagittal images of a biopsy-proven pilocytic astrocytoma of the tectum.

are hypointense on T1WI and bright on T2WI and enhance with gadolinium, similar to the focal BSTs. Unlike the diffuse and other focal intrinsic BSTs, the differential diagnosis of the dorsally exophytic variant is broader and should include other fourth ventricular tumors such as ependymomas or medulloblastomas (**Fig. 27.5**).

Tumor classification (focal/exophytic versus diffuse) and location (midbrain, pons, or medulla) correlate well with survival. A 5-year survival of 75% was reported for patients with midbrain tumors, 65% for those with medullary tumors, but only 18% of those with pontine tumors (**Fig. 27.2**).[10] The same study reported a 5-year survival of 70% for those with focal tumors compared with 22% for those with diffuse lesions.

In the future, other diagnostic tools may play an important role as adjuncts to conventional MRI in the diagnosis of BSTs. At present, both thallium single photon emission CT (SPECT) and magnetic resonance spectroscopy (MRS) appear particularly promising. Compared with thallium studies, longitudinal MRS offers the additional possibility of monitoring early response to radiation or other therapies through detecting levels of different glial and neuronal metabolites. Typically, an elevated ratio of choline to *N*-acetyl aspartate implies a more

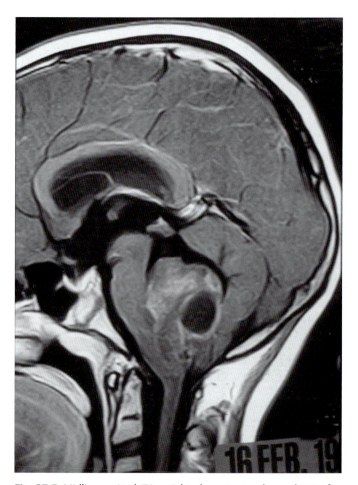

Fig. 27.5 Midline sagittal, T1-weighted, contrast-enhanced MRI of a dorsally exophytic brainstem tumor.

Pearls

- Diffuse BSTs can be confidently diagnosed solely on the basis of MRI, negating the need for a biopsy. The most striking finding is a fat pons.
- Focal BSTs have T1WIs and T2WIs that are almost superimposable.

aggressive tumor pathology. Use of MRS alone or in combination with apparent diffusion coefficient maps may help to differentiate progressive tumor from postradiation effects in malignant brainstem gliomas.[33]

■ Treatment

Surgery

Indications

Surgical decision making for patients with brainstem tumors is based on the focal/exophytic/diffuse classification system described earlier. For this reason, particular attention should be paid to the history and physical examination. A slowly progressive focal abnormality in association with focal imaging suggests low-grade pathology and should prompt a consideration of surgical resection. Patients with rapidly progressive symptoms and an MRI that is characteristic of a diffuse pontine glioma should be treated with prompt radiation therapy, as this is the only therapeutic modality that has consistently shown clinical and imaging improvement in children with diffuse BSTs, although the effects are often short-lived.[33] If the clinical course or imaging are not characteristic of a diffuse pontine glioma, a stereotactic biopsy may be considered.[34]

In patients with nonenhancing tectal gliomas who present with hydrocephalus (**Fig. 27.6**), endoscopic third ventriculostomy usually relieves the hydrocephalus. The underlying tumor is usually very indolent and should be monitored by serial imaging with contrast. Enhancement is a worrisome finding in these lesions, but biopsy is reserved for those with clear signs of progression on imaging. Occasionally, large midbrain lesions with significant mass effect, well-defined borders, and a large exophytic component can be considered for surgical resection.

Focal intrinsic pontine tumors are rare lesions that are usually best observed unless they come to a pial or ependymal surface, allowing surgical access. They can be biopsied stereotactically through a coronal transpeduncular approach or resected if the lesion is located superficially. In contrast, the dorsally exophytic variant usually has a large extramedullary component that is very amenable to resection.

Regarding focal medullary tumors, certain accessible lesions that present to the surface can be resected or debulked

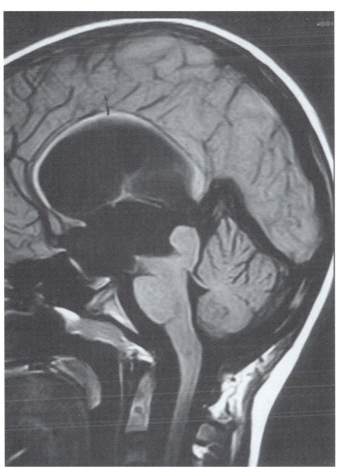

Fig. 27.6 T1-weighted, noncontrast MRI of a tectal tumor with obstructive hydrocephalus.

(**Fig. 27.7**). In the medulla, there is a separate distinct entity called a cervicomedullary tumor. These lesions typically present with a very long history of upper cervical/lower medulla dysfunction characterized by recurrent aspiration pneumonia, change in voice, or long tract problems. They can be quite large at diagnosis (**Fig. 27.8**). They are often pilocytic and therefore should be considered for surgery. The potential morbidity of tumor removal in this location must be openly discussed with the child's parents, and subtotal resection may be preferable to a permanent tracheostomy and gastrostomy. In summary, surgical resection should only be considered in BSTs that are focal, enhancing, and accessible because these tumors tend to be low grade or pilocytic and PFS can be improved significantly with resection. With documented progression, repeat resections of focal accessible low-grade lesions has been our preference.[14]

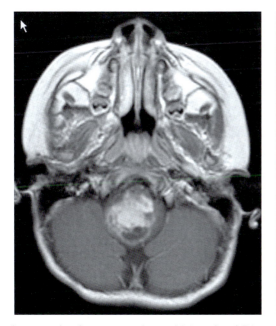
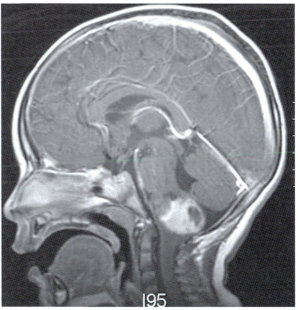

a   b

Fig. 27.7a–d T1-weighted, contrast-enhanced (**a**) axial and (**b**) sagittal preoperative images of a focal tumor of the medulla. (*continued on next page*)

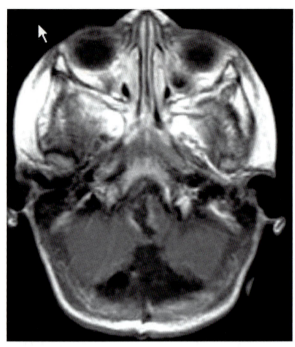
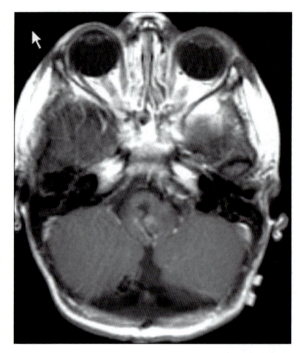

c

d

Fig. 27.7a–d (*continued*) (**c,d**) Postoperative images.

Surgical Technique

The surgical approach to tumors of the brainstem is individualized to the specific location and tumor anatomy, but there are several helpful principles: (1) Choose the shortest route through the tissue. (2) If there is an accessible tumor cyst, use it as a corridor to approach the tumor. (3) The brainstem should be entered through regions of distorted anatomy where the tumor bulges toward the surface and causes discoloration (**Fig. 27.9**). (4) When approaching intrinsic tumors in the medulla, the route is through the midline, and the superior limit of the midline incision is kept below the obex to reduce the risk to the lower cranial nerves. (5) Exophytic tumors are approached so that the exophytic portion is encountered first. (6) For dorsally exophytic lesions, resection is carried down to the floor of the fourth ventricle, and great care is taken not to enter the brainstem. (7) Tumor resection is performed by entering the center of the lesion and gradually working toward the margins. Because these tumors do not have a surrounding gliotic zone, do not attempt to dissect outside the tumor at the tumor–brainstem interface. Resection is terminated when the tissue color and texture begin to look normal. Bipolar elec-trocautery and laser change the tissue characteristics and make the transition between tumor and normal tissue more difficult to identify and should thus be used as little as possible. (8) Neurophysiological monitoring, including brainstem auditory evoked responses, somatosensory evoked potentials, motor nuclei mapping, electromyography, and motor evoked potentials, is very helpful in selected cases.

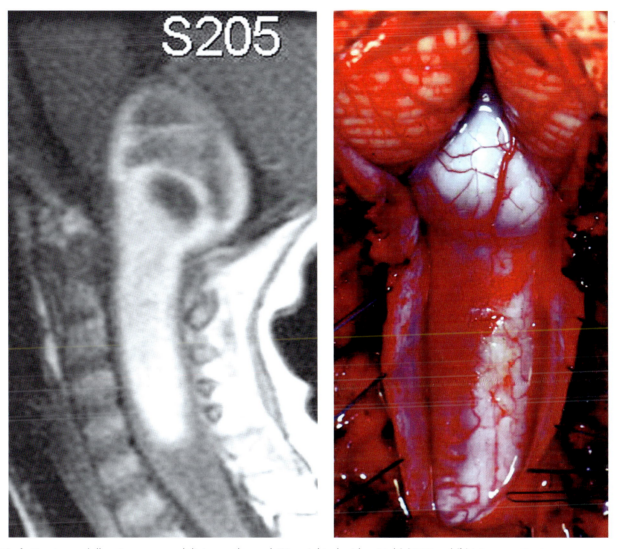

Fig. 27.8a,b Cervicomedullary tumor on gadolinium-enhanced, T1-weighted midsagittal (**a**) MRI and (**b**) intraoperative image.

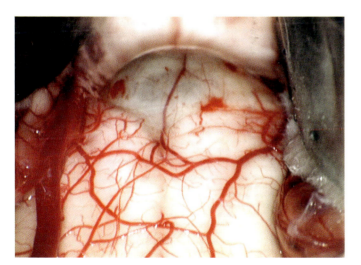

Fig. 27.9 Intraoperative image of the obex and the floor of the fourth ventricle demonstrating discoloration and distortion of the floor of the fourth ventricle over an intrinsic tumor of the medulla.

Complications

Specific surgical complications are related to the anatomic location of the tumor. Surgery of the medulla carries risks of postoperative swallowing and airway difficulties, occasionally requiring a feeding gastrostomy and tracheostomy. At the level of the pons, surgery can result in diplopia and facial weakness due to injuries of cranial nerve VI and VII nuclei and the medial longitudinal fasciculus. In addition, cerebellar mutism can occur with the dorsally exophytic variant, especially with large tumors that require extensive vermian splitting. Similarly, surgery at the level of the midbrain can also result in diplopia through oculomotor palsies.

In our series of 28 children who underwent surgical resection for focal brainstem pilocytic astrocytomas, immediate surgery-related complications were present in 20 of 28 patients (71%).[14] These complications resolved often, and persistent deficits remained in six patients at the last follow-up. The deficits were observed in two of the 12 patients with gross total resection (GTR) or near GTR, in three of 13 patients with residual tumor, and in one of three patients in whom a biopsy was performed (**Table 27.1**).

Outcomes

The prognosis for patients with brainstem tumors varies greatly among the categories outlined in **Table 27.1**. The diffuse pontine glioma, which in the past was thought to represent all BSTs, has a dismal prognosis. Survival is measured in months to a year or two despite adjuvant therapy. Nonenhancing tectal tumors usually have a very indolent course for years, with the only issue being management of hydrocephalus. Dorsally exophytic lesions are usually pilocytic and have an excellent prognosis after resection. In our series of focal brainstem pilocytic astrocytomas, 25 of the 28 patients underwent resection as initial treatment.[14] Twelve patients demonstrated GTR or residual linear enhancement (RLE) in the tumor bed. Seven of 12 received no further treatment, and, in one patient, local tumor progression occurred 1.1 years later. In none of the remaining six was there evidence of progression at last follow-up. Four of the 12 received radiotherapy, and progression was observed in one patient at 0.63 years. One of the 12 patients was treated with adjuvant chemotherapy only, but tumor progression occurred at 0.42 years.

In 13 of 25 patients with residual solid tumor, 10 of the 13 received no adjuvant therapy and 5 of the 10 progressed. Four of the 10 tumors were stable and one actually regressed, a phenomenon documented in some supratentorial pilocytic astrocytomas[35] (**Fig. 27.10**). Two of the 13 underwent radiotherapy and both progressed. One had undergone a biopsy, radiation, and chemotherapy prior but was stable after resection with no further adjuvant therapy.

All patients were alive at the last follow-up (mean 5.8 years). In the entire study population, PFS was 51% at 5 years and 44% at 10 years. The rates were higher (74% at 5 years, 62% at 10 years) with GTR or RLE rather than residual solid tumor (19% at 5 years and 10 years).

Recurrence or progression occurred in 11 of the 28 patients (39%). At that time repeat resection was performed in 10 patients and one patient underwent radiotherapy. GTR or

Table 27.1 Summary of Neurologic Status After Surgery of a Juvenile Pilocytic Astrocytoma of the Brainstem

Postoperative Deficit	Number of Cases		
	Gross Total Resection or Residual Linear Enhancement	Solid Residual Lesion	Biopsy Sampling
Immediate	8 of 12	10 of 13	2 of 3
Last follow-up	2 of 12*	3 of 13[†]	1 of 3[‡]

*Dysfunction involved (1) a seventh cranial nerve palsy requiring reanimation (medullary tumor) and (2) ambulatory paraparesis treated with the baclofen pump.
[†]Dysfunction involved (1) a seventh cranial nerve palsy (pontine tumor); (2) mild hemiparesis (midbrain peduncle tumor; the patient can write and walk); and (3) nonambulatory quadriparesis (medullary tumor) in a patient presenting with spastic triplegia.
[‡]Dysfunction involved a third cranial nerve palsy (midbrain tumor).

RLE was achieved in 7 of the 10 patients, with stable tumor in six and progression in one (subsequently treated with chemotherapy). The other three with residual solid tumor underwent adjuvant radiotherapy.

Based on our cohort, excision (GTR or RLE) appeared to give the best chance of PFS at initial surgery or at the time of recurrence. The use of adjuvant therapy was not associated with increased PFS, regardless of the extent of surgical resection.

Radiotherapy

Children diagnosed with diffuse BSTs are treated with fractionated radiation therapy. Corticosteroids are often given in addition for symptomatic relief. Although the clinical response rate is approximately 70% for patients undergoing radiation, the median time to progression of diffuse BSTs is about 6 months, with a median survival of slightly less than 1 year.[11] In a series of 119 cases, 1-, 2-, and 3-year survival rates of 37%, 20%, and 13%, respectively, were reported.[13] Conventional radiotherapy consists of a 54-Gy total dose delivered in 30 fractions over 6 weeks. Radiation-related morbidity follows a typical dose–response pattern, and at 78 Gy, steroid dependency, hearing loss, ischemic events, hormone deficits, and late seizures were reported. Several studies using higher doses of radiation (75.6–78 Gy) have not shown a benefit in terms of improved survival rate.[36,37]

Hyperfractionated radiation therapy, which involves a more frequent delivery of a smaller radiation dose, can achieve a higher total dose and offers the theoretical advantage of being more selective for tumor cells. Nevertheless, the results from several clinical trials have been disappointing, and hyperfractionated radiotherapy did not appear to improve the outcome or prolong survival. At present, the role of stereotactic radiosurgery in the treatment of focal BSTs is still under investiga-

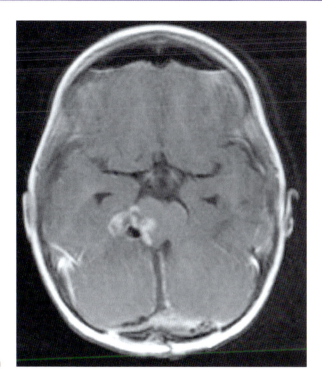
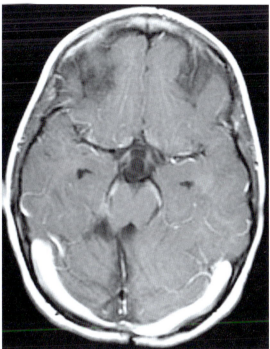

Fig. 27.10a,b Postoperative axial, T1-weighted, gadolinium-enhanced images of a pilocytic astrocytoma taken (**a**) immediately postoperatively and (**b**) 2.5 years later with no intervening therapy.

tion. In a study of five patients harboring focal pilocytic BSTs, a significant decrease in tumor size was noted in four patients with a mean follow-up of 19 months. The remaining patient demonstrated stable disease, and none of the patients suffered neurologic dysfunction related to radiosurgery.[38]

Chemotherapy

Chemotherapy as a single agent or in combination has been explored in both an adjuvant and neoadjuvant role for diffuse BSTs. A randomized trial evaluating the efficacy of adjuvant chemotherapy was performed in 74 patients who received vincristine, lomustine, and prednisone after radiation treatment versus no therapy after radiation treatment. The 5-year survival rate was 17% in the radiation-alone group versus 23% in the group receiving adjuvant chemotherapy, although there was no statistical difference between the groups.[39] Pre-radiation chemotherapy with 1,3-bis(2-chloroethyl)-1-nitro-soureacisplatin and high-dose methotrexate led to an increase in overall survival in one study to 17 months[40]; however, there was significant myelotoxicity associated with this regimen. To date, no single chemotherapeutic agent alone or in combination, adjuvant or neoadjuvant, has been proven to alter the overall survival in children with diffuse BSTs. Additionally, the eloquent location of these tumors and the limited ability of chemotherapeutic agents to traverse the blood–brain barrier has impaired therapeutic advances. The dearth of successful therapeutic options for diffuse BSTs may be due in part to the practice of not obtaining tissue diagnosis prior to treatment. This again raises the question of a paradigm shift where performing a biopsy of these tumors to better understand their molecular biology may become standard management.

■ Conclusion

Brainstem tumors are a group of diverse lesions largely confined to the pediatric population. Diffuse BSTs remain a leading cause of therapeutic failure among pediatric brain tumors; however, the advent of neuroimaging, surgical techniques, and intraoperative monitoring has allowed many of the low-grade focal and dorsally exophytic BSTs to be approached surgically with acceptable mortalities and morbidities. In this small subgroup of BSTs, resection either at initial surgery or at the time of recurrence can result in long-term PFS. For diffuse BSTs, tissue diagnosis via biopsy prior to starting adjuvant treatment modalities may become the new standard of care as the molecular characteristics and behavior of these lethal tumors have yet to be fully elucidated.

Editor's Note

Brainstem tumors are a daunting challenge for the neuro-oncology team. Neurosurgeons are usually the first members of the team to see these patients, and surgery may play a minimal role, although specific indications for surgery (including resection of exophytic portions, biopsy, and cerebrospinal fluid diversion) do arise, especially in children. Care is mostly in the hands of the radiation oncologist and neuro-oncologist. The diffuse pontine gliomas carry a death sentence, whereas the other tumors in this group have more favorable prognoses. In adults, treatment usually consists of conformal radiation without the requirement for tissue diagnosis, as the risk–benefit analysis favors not subjecting the patient to the risk of biopsy, although it is always better to have tissue diagnosis if possible. As in other areas of neuro-oncology, developments in molecular diagnostics may provide improved prognostic information, and new options for therapeutic intervention include a trend toward more tumor- and patient-specific therapy. (Bernstein)

References

1. Berger MS, Edwards MS, LaMasters D, Davis RL, Wilson CB. Pediatric brain stem tumors: radiographic, pathological, and clinical correlations. Neurosurgery 1983;12:298–302

2. Littman P, Jarrett P, Bilaniuk LT, et al. Pediatric brain stem gliomas. Cancer 1980;45:2787–2792

3. Pierre-Kahn A, Hirsch JF, Vinchon M, et al. Surgical management of brain-stem tumors in children: results and statistical analysis of 75 cases. J Neurosurg 1993;79:845–852

4. Lee BC, Kneeland JB, Walker RW, Posner JB, Cahill PT, Deck MD. MR imaging of brainstem tumors. AJNR Am J Neuroradiol 1985;6:159–163

5. Schoenberg BS, Schoenberg DG, Christine BW, Gomez MR. The epidemiology of primary intracranial neoplasms of childhood. A population study. Mayo Clin Proc 1976;51:51–56

6. Yates AJ, Becker LE, Sachs LA. Brain tumors in childhood. Childs Brain 1979;5:31–39

7. Cohen ME, Duffner PK, Heffner RR, Lacey DJ, Brecher M. Prognostic factors in brainstem gliomas. Neurology 1986;36:602–605

8. Epstein F, McCleary EL. Intrinsic brain-stem tumors of childhood: surgical indications. J Neurosurg 1986;64:11–15

9. Epstein F, Wisoff JH. Intrinsic brainstem tumors in childhood: surgical indications. J Neurooncol 1988;6:309–317

10. Fischbein NJ, Prados MD, Wara W, Russo C, Edwards MS, Barkovich AJ. Radiologic classification of brain stem tumors: correlation of magnetic resonance imaging appearance with clinical outcome. Pediatr Neurosurg 1996;24:9–23

11. Freeman CR, Suissa S. Brain stem tumors in children: results of a survey of 62 patients treated with radiotherapy. Int J Radiat Oncol Biol Phys 1986;12:1823–1828

12. Hoffman HJ, Becker L, Craven MA. A clinically and pathologically distinct group of benign brain stem gliomas. Neurosurgery 1980;7:243–248

13. Kaplan AM, Albright AL, Zimmerman RA, et al. Brainstem gliomas in children. A Children's Cancer Group review of 119 cases. Pediatr Neurosurg 1996;24:185–192

14. Kestle J, Townsend JJ, Brockmeyer DL, Walker ML. Juvenile pilocytic astrocytoma of the brainstem in children. J Neurosurg 2004;101(1, Suppl):1–6

15. Khatib ZA, Heideman RL, Kovnar EH, et al. Predominance of pilocytic histology in dorsally exophytic brain stem tumors. Pediatr Neurosurg 1994;20:2–10

16. Nishio S, Fukui M, Tateishi J. Brain stem gliomas: a clinicopathological analysis of 23 histologically proven cases. J Neurooncol 1988;6:245–250

17. Albright AL, Guthkelch AN, Packer RJ, Price RA, Rourke LB. Prognostic factors in pediatric brain-stem gliomas. J Neurosurg 1986;65:751–755

18. Abbott R. Brain stem gliomas. In: McLone DG, ed. Pediatric Neurosurery: Surgery of the Developing Nervous System, 4th ed. Philadelphia: WB Saunders, 2001:859–867

19. Molloy PT, Yachnis AT, Rorke LB, et al. Central nervous system medulloepithelioma: a series of eight cases including two arising in the pons. J Neurosurg 1996;84:430–436

20. Sethi R, Allen J, Donahue B, et al. Prospective neuraxis MRI surveillance reveals a high risk of leptomeningeal dissemination in diffuse intrinsic pontine glioma. J Neurooncol 2011;102:121–127

21. Sanford RA, Freeman CR, Burger P, Cohen ME. Prognostic criteria for experimental protocols in pediatric brainstem gliomas. Surg Neurol 1988;30:276–280

22. Shuper A, Kornreich L, Loven D, Michowitz S, Schwartz M, Cohen IJ. Diffuse brain stem gliomas. Are we improving outcome? Childs Nerv Syst 1998;14:578–581

23. Bredel M, Pollack IF, Hamilton RL, James CD. Epidermal growth factor receptor expression and gene amplification in high-grade non-brainstem gliomas of childhood. Clin Cancer Res 1999;5:1786–1792

24. Raffel C. Molecular biology of pediatric gliomas. J Neurooncol 1996; 28:121–128

25. Thorarinsdottir HK, Santi M, McCarter R, et al. Protein expression of platelet-derived growth factor receptor correlates with malignant histology and PTEN with survival in childhood gliomas. Clin Cancer Res 2008;14:3386–3394

26. Wakabayashi T, Natsume A, Hatano H, et al. p16 promoter methylation in the serum as a basis for the molecular diagnosis of gliomas. Neurosurgery 2009;64:455–461, discussion 461–462

27. Pollack IF, Shultz B, Mulvihill JJ. The management of brainstem gliomas in patients with neurofibromatosis 1. Neurology 1996;46:1652–1660

28. Molloy PT, Bilaniuk LT, Vaughan SN, et al. Brainstem tumors in patients with neurofibromatosis type 1: a distinct clinical entity. Neurology 1995;45:1897–1902

29. Milstein JM, Geyer JR, Berger MS, Bleyer WA. Favorable prognosis for brainstem gliomas in neurofibromatosis. J Neurooncol 1989;7:367–371

30. Packer RJ, Nicholson HS, Johnson DL, Vezina LG. Dilemmas in the management of childhood brain tumors: brainstem gliomas. Pediatr Neurosurg 1991-1992;17:37–43

31. Raffel C, McComb JG, Bodner S, Gilles FE. Benign brain stem lesions in pediatric patients with neurofibromatosis: case reports. Neurosurgery 1989;25:959–964

32. Zimmerman RA. Neuroimaging of primary brainstem gliomas: diagnosis and course. Pediatr Neurosurg 1996;25:45–53

33. Khatua S, Moore KR, Vats TS, Kestle JR. Diffuse intrinsic pontine glioma-current status and future strategies. Childs Nerv Syst 2011;27:1391–1397

34. Pincus DW, Richter EO, Yachnis AT, Bennett J, Bhatti MT, Smith A. Brainstem stereotactic biopsy sampling in children. J Neurosurg 2006; 104(2, Suppl):108–114

35. Balkhoyor KB, Bernstein M. Involution of diencephalic pilocytic astrocytoma after partial resection. Report of two cases in adults. J Neurosurg 2000;93:484–486

36. Freeman CR, Krischer JP, Sanford RA, et al. Final results of a study of escalating doses of hyperfractionated radiotherapy in brain stem tumors in children: a Pediatric Oncology Group study. Int J Radiat Oncol Biol Phys 1993;27:197–206

37. Prados MD, Wara WM, Edwards MS, Larson DA, Lamborn K, Levin VA. The treatment of brain stem and thalamic gliomas with 78 Gy of hyper-fractionated radiation therapy. Int J Radiat Oncol Biol Phys 1995;32: 85–91

38. Somaza SC, Kondziolka D, Lunsford LD, Flickinger JC, Bissonette DJ, Albright AL. Early outcomes after stereotactic radiosurgery for growing pilocytic astrocytomas in children. Pediatr Neurosurg 1996;25: 109–115

39. Jenkin RD, Boesel C, Ertel I, et al. Brain-stem tumors in childhood: a prospective randomized trial of irradiation with and without adjuvant CCNU, VCR, and prednisone. A report of the Children's Cancer Study Group. J Neurosurg 1987;66:227–233

40. Frappaz D, Schell M, Thiesse P, et al. Preradiation chemotherapy may improve survival in pediatric diffuse intrinsic brainstem gliomas: final results of BSG 98 prospective trial. Neuro-oncol 2008;10:599–607

28 Pediatric Posterior Fossa Tumors

Marc Remke, Vijay Ramaswamy, and Michael D. Taylor

More than half of pediatric brain tumors are located in the posterior fossa. These neoplasms encompass some of the most favorable, and some of the worst, primary brain tumors seen in children. Complete surgical removal of a cerebellar astrocytoma virtually guarantees a cure. In contrast, a medulloblastoma patient can go on to expire after gross total resection, craniospinal irradiation, and chemotherapy. The four most common lesions seen in the posterior fossa of children are medulloblastoma, ependymoma, cerebellar astrocytoma, and less commonly brainstem glioma; the first three are discussed in this chapter, and the fourth was discussed in Chapter 27.

> **Pearl**
>
> - Fewer than 5% of medulloblastoma patients present due to symptomatic metastases. Presentation due to involvement of the cauda equina by "drop mets" is very unusual, but children who present de novo with multiple intradural lesions compressing the spinal cord or cauda equina should have posterior fossa imaging to rule out a cerebellar neoplasm.

Medulloblastoma

Medulloblastoma is the most common malignant brain tumor of childhood and comprises up to 18% of all pediatric brain tumors.[1] Although it used to be regarded as a single heterogeneous entity, current consensus recognizes four biologically distinct subgroups—WNT, SHH, Group 3, and Group 4—with distinct genomic, clinical, and prognostic features (**Table 28.1**).[2–4] Across subgroups, the mean age of medulloblastoma patients is between 5 and 7 years; more than half of medulloblastomas occur in the first 10 years of life but are uncommon under the age of 1 year. There is a male preponderance in most reported series (M/F ratio 1.8:1). Most cases have no known cause, but rare examples do arise in the setting of familial syndromes such as Turcot's syndrome (polyposis of the colon and primary brain tumors), Gorlin's syndrome (multiple cutaneous basal cell carcinomas, congenital anomalies, and medulloblastoma), and Li-Fraumeni syndrome.[5] Isochromosome 17q is seen commonly in Group 3 and Group 4 and *MYC* amplifications in Group 3 medulloblastomas.[2,6] Thus, these somatic copy number alterations are useful to identify subsets of patients with poor prognosis.[7–10] In contrast, WNT tumors are associated with a good prognosis and frequently display monosomy 6, and *CTNNB1* mutations/nuclear positivity.[2,11]

Clinical Presentation

Most patients present with a short history; in the Toronto Hospital for Sick Children (HSC) experience, symptoms had been present for less than 1.5 months in 51% of patients and less than 3 months in 76%.[12] Early symptoms of a posterior fossa medulloblastoma include behavioral changes such as lethargy, irritability, and loss of appetite. These nonspecific symptoms are often not initially diagnosed as secondary to a posterior fossa tumor, and children often have extensive investigations before the correct diagnosis is finally made. Most patients present with symptoms due to increased intracranial pressure or compression of surrounding neural structures. The most common presentation is the "midline triad" of headache, lethargy, and vomiting.[13] Headache is often present on awakening in the morning due to hypoventilation during sleep and a consequent rise in carbon dioxide levels, causing increased intracranial pressure. Vomiting often relieves the headache due to accompanying hyperventilation and reduction in intracranial pressure.

Cerebellar signs such as truncal ataxia (62%), limb ataxia/dysmetria (44%), and nystagmus may be present. Many children have papilledema at the time of diagnosis. Sixth nerve palsies may be seen and are usually due to hydrocephalus and increased intracranial pressure rather than direct brainstem invasion. Facial or bulbar palsies, when present, do suggest brainstem invasion. Head tilt secondary to impaction of the cerebellar tonsils into the foramen magnum with compression of the C1 and C2 nerve roots is commonly seen in patients with cerebellar neoplasms. Infants with open sutures may have atypical presentations and can present with asymptomatic head enlargement.

There is no pathognomonic symptom or sign in patients with medulloblastoma that differentiates them from children with other types of cerebellar neoplasms. However, neck stiffness, intense neck pain, and vomiting in the absence of headache are more typical of ependymoma; lateral cerebellar signs are more common in patients with cerebellar astrocytoma. Clinically evident spontaneous tumor hemorrhage can be seen in both primary and recurrent tumors (5.6% of patients in the HSC series).[12]

Table 28.1 Clinicopathological and Molecular Characteristics of Medulloblastoma Subgroups

	WNT	SHH	Group 3	Group 4
Gender distribution	M = F	M = F	M > F	M > F
Peak age	Pediatric	Infant/adult	Pediatric	Pediatric
Histology	Classic, rarely LCA	Desmoplastic / MBEN, classic, LCA	Classic, LCA	Classic, LCA
Metastatic propensity	Low	Extremely low	High	Intermediate
Prognosis	Very good	Infants good, others intermediate	Poor	Intermediate
Characteristic SCNA	Monosomy 6	3q gain, 9p deletion	*MYC* amplification	*SNCAIP* duplication

Abbreviations: WNT, wingless pathway; SHH, sonic hedgehog pathway; M, male; F, female; LCA, large-cell, anaplastic histology; MBEN, medulloblastomas with extensive nodularity; SCNA, somatic copy number alterations.

Medulloblastoma can spread along cerebrospinal fluid (CSF) pathways and also rarely to systemic sites (bone, lung). Any child with a known medulloblastoma who presents with bone pain must have a metastatic lesion ruled out.

Imaging Studies

Classic features of a medulloblastoma on computed tomographic (CT) scan are increased density on the noncontrast scan, midline location, well-defined margins, and dense, homogeneous enhancement with injection of contrast[14] (**Fig. 28.1**). The hyperdensity on plain CT scan, seen in medulloblastoma and in some ependymomas, is secondary to the high cellularity of these tumors that have scanty cytoplasm and areas of desmoplasia.[5] The tumor is usually in the cerebellar vermis (85%) but can be found in the cerebellar hemisphere

Special Consideration

- Any patient with a posterior fossa tumor that might be medulloblastoma or ependymoma should undergo preoperative imaging of the spinal axis to rule out leptomeningeal spread. In addition to prognostication, the absence or presence of metastatic disease may prompt the surgeon to be more, or less, aggressive, respectively, at the time of resection. Patients who do not undergo preoperative spinal imaging need to wait at least 2 weeks postoperatively to facilitate optimum interpretation of imaging.

(more commonly the SHH subgroup), or, rarely, in the cerebellopontine angle. Calcification is seen in 7 to 10% of cases,

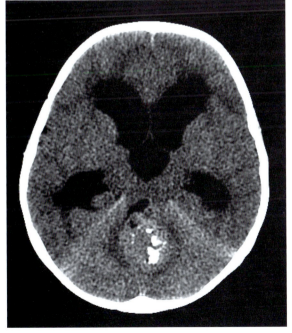
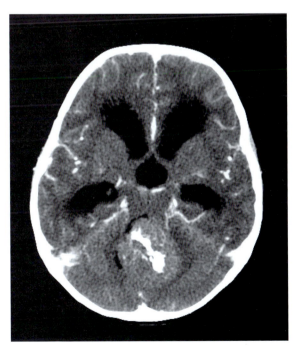

a   b

Fig. 28.1a,b (**a**) Non–contrast-enhanced computed tomography (CT) of a medulloblastoma showing a hyperdense mass occupying and obstructing the fourth ventricle. Note the extreme enlargement of the lateral ventricles consistent with noncommunicating hydrocephalus. (**b**) Contrast-enhanced CT showing diffuse enhancement of the lesion with administration of contrast.

and true macrocysts are uncommon. Almost all medulloblastomas enhance in children, but, on occasion, adult medulloblastomas will not take up contrast. Heterogeneity of enhancement within the tumor is due to regions of necrosis.

Obstructive hydrocephalus with enlargement of the lateral, third, and rostral fourth ventricles is extremely common on preoperative imaging. Tumor signal on T1-weighted magnetic resonance imaging (MRI) shows low or intermediate signal compared with adjacent white matter. T2-weighted MRI is

Controversial Point

- Intermittent surveillance imaging is frequently performed but is of no proven benefit.

varied and can be hypo-, iso-, or hyperintense to surrounding white matter (**Fig. 28.2**). Medulloblastomas display heterogeneous enhancement with infusion of gadolinium with lower

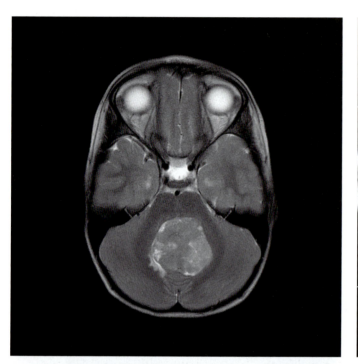

a

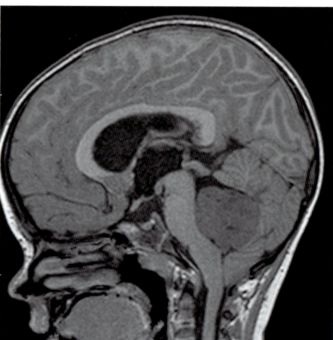

b

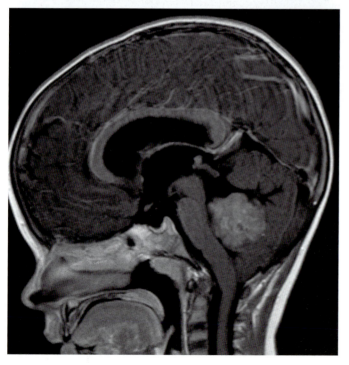

c

Fig. 28.2a–f (**a**) Axial T2-weighted magnetic resonance imaging (MRI) showing a midline hyperintense solid mass occupying the fourth ventricle. (**b**) Sagittal T1-weighted MRI without contrast showing a hypointense mass occupying the fourth ventricle and compressing the brainstem, and (**c**) with gadolinium enhancement showing homogeneous enhancement upon administration of gadolinium. (**d**) Apparent diffusion coefficient map and (**e**) diffusion-weighted B1000 MRI showing restricted diffusion of medulloblastoma. (**f**) Axial T2-weighted MRI of a lateral desmoplastic medulloblastoma.

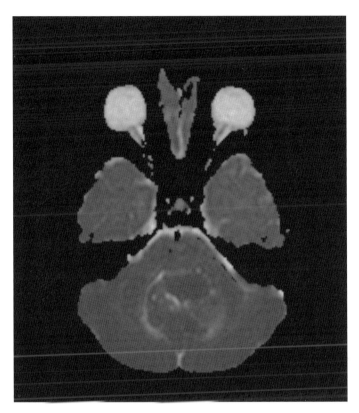

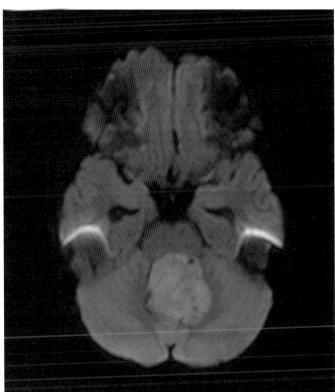

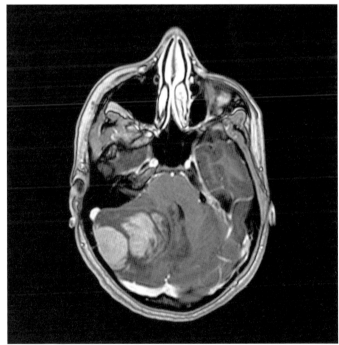

Fig. 28.2a–f (*continued*) (**d**) Apparent diffusion coefficient map and (**e**) diffusion-weighted B1000 MRI showing restricted diffusion of medulloblastoma. (**f**) Axial T2-weighted MRI of a lateral desmoplastic medulloblastoma.

apparent diffusion coefficient values compared with ependymomas due to relatively higher cellularity in medulloblastomas. MRI demonstrates the extent of the tumor; medulloblastoma is less likely than ependymoma to extend through the exit foramina of the fourth ventricle into the subarachnoid space of the upper cervical spinal cord or into the cerebellopontine angle. Intratumoral hemorrhage in young children should alert neurosurgeons to a possible diagnosis of atypical teratoid/rhabdoid tumor (AT/RT). Leptomeningeal dissemination is evident in 25 to 35% of cases at diagnosis. Gadolinium-enhanced MRI is more sensitive than CT in detecting small cortical and basal metastases (**Fig. 28.3**).

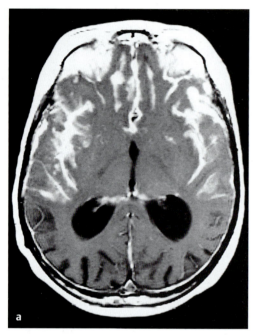
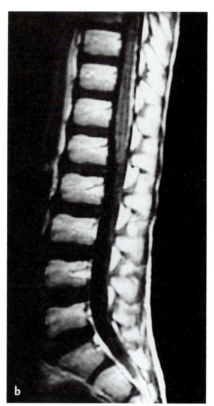
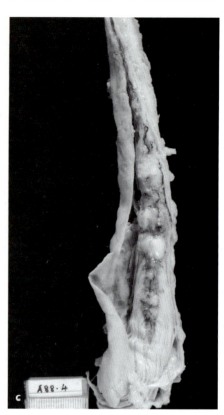

Fig. 28.3a–c (**a**) Axial T1-weighted MRI with contrast shows enhancement in the subarachnoid spaces over the hemispheres and in the sylvian fissures bilaterally. This is indicative of diffuse cerebrospinal fluid dissemination in a medulloblastoma patient. (**b**) Midsagittal T1-weighted MRI of the spine showing drop metastases from medulloblastoma as enhancement along the posterior aspect of the spinal cord and conus medullaris. (**c**) Postmortem specimen of the thecal sac, spinal cord, and cauda equina with extensive metastases from a medulloblastoma.

Surgical assessment of the extent of resection is often poor. Postoperative imaging should be performed within 48 hours of surgery when imaging artifacts due to postsurgical change are at a minimum.[15]

The most common site of intracranial recurrence is the primary site in the posterior fossa. Other common sites include the infundibular stalk, ventricular system, surface of the spinal cord, and the subfrontal subarachnoid space.

Pathology

Grossly, the surgeon finds a pinkish, gray mass that fills the fourth ventricle and often has tiny vessels around the periphery.[1] The tumor typically arises from the medullary velum. CSF dissemination has occurred in 20 to 50% of cases at the time of operation, and on occasion can be seen as a whitish layer or "sugar coating" over the exposed cerebellum. Histopathological examination reveals an extremely cellular tumor with round cells, basophilic nuclei, a high nuclear to cytoplasmic ratio, and frequent mitoses.

Five histological variants are recognized by the 2007 World Health Organization (WHO) classification[16]: (1) Classic medulloblastomas (70 to 80% of cases) have densely packed and primarily undifferentiated cells with highly hyperchromatic nuclei surrounded by scanty cytoplasm and numerous Homer-Wright rosettes (tumor cell nuclei arranged in a circle around tangled cytoplasmic processes) (**Fig. 28.4**). (2) Desmoplastic tumors (15% of cases) occasionally show maturation to more differentiated ganglion cell tumors, and a biphasic pattern with distinctive lucent areas referred to as "pale islands" and areas with abundant internodular reticulin. The desmo-

Controversial Point

- Some authorities liken medulloblastoma to pineoblastoma and supratentorial primitive neuroectodermal tumor (PNET), all of which have similar histopathological appearance. These authorities group all of these tumors together under the rubric of PNET. More recent biological studies show that these tumors are in fact distinct entities with different clinical and biological profiles, and that they should not be lumped together.

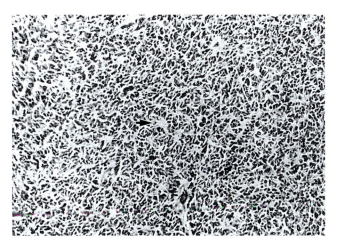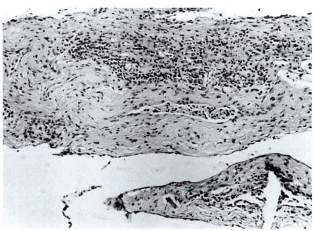

Fig. 28.4a,b (**a**) Histological section of medulloblastoma showing a cellular tumor with pleomorphic nuclei, a high nuclear to cytoplasmic ratio, and the presence of a Homer-Wright rosette (*arrowhead*)

(hematoxylin and eosin [H&E] stain.) (**b**) Histological section showing medulloblastoma cells invading the leptomeninges (H&E stain).

plastic variant is more likely than the classic medulloblastoma to occur laterally in the cerebellar hemisphere and may have a better prognosis. Immunohistochemistry of medulloblastoma may show glial, neuronal, and ependymal differentiation. (3) Medulloblastomas with extensive nodularity (MBEN) consist almost entirely of nodules with large areas of neuropil and little or no desmoplastic internodular tissue. This variant is rare and shows extensive neuronal differentiation, has a very good prognosis, and occurs in very young children.[17,18] (4) Anaplastic tumors have pleomorphic, enlarged nuclei and an increased cytoplasm-to-nucleus ratio and brisk mitotic activity. The nuclei display angulation and molding. (5) Large-cell medulloblastomas are composed of large cells with round nuclei and prominent nucleoli. Characteristic features include high mitotic rate, extensive apoptosis, and wrapping of tumor cells over each other.

Atypical teratoid/rhabdoid tumor can also occur in the posterior fossa, and under the microscope some areas may contain only sheets of small blue cells, making it difficult to differentiate from medulloblastoma. The diagnosis of AT/RT is made by the presence of rhabdoid cells, which are medium-sized cells with an eccentric nucleus and a pink cytoplasmic inclusion body.[19] The great majority of AT/RTs have mutations of the *hSNF5/INI1* gene on chromosome 22, encoding for a protein that facilitates the transcriptional activation of genes by altering the structure of chromatin.[20] Indeed, because histological identification of an AT/RT can be difficult, current Children's Oncology Group (COG) protocols that include infants with AT/RT require that the *hSNF5/INI1* gene be analyzed, as well as looking for deletions on chromosome 22. In addition, loss of *INI1* expression is a very sensitive and specific molecular characteristic of AT/RTs.[16] Patients with AT/RTs have a much worse prognosis than patients with medulloblastoma, despite recent improvements in treatment success with intensive multimodality treatment.[21]

Cerebrospinal Fluid Diversion

Many, if not most, children with medulloblastoma present with hydrocephalus. In the past many surgeons placed preoperative shunts or external ventricular drains in these patients. This was thought to immediately decrease the intracranial pressure; to enable the child to recover emotionally, physically, and nutritionally before the resection; to give the parents time to adjust to the diagnosis; and to allow resective surgery to be done on an elective basis by the best neurosurgical operating team. More recently, some groups are treating all children with posterior fossa tumors with a pre-resection endoscopic third ventriculostomy.[22] Currently preoperative CSF diversion surgery is not recommended; most patients can be managed with corticosteroids followed by semiurgent tumor resection. Not all patients require a CSF diversionary procedure once the tumor is removed, and preoperative shunting or third ventriculostomy may expose these children to unnecessary risks.

About 25% of patients with medulloblastoma ultimately develop postoperative hydrocephalus requiring definitive treatment. The clinical presentation of postoperative hydrocephalus is that of increased intracranial pressure, or it may take the form of a pseudomeningocele at the site of the surgical incision. Many pseudomeningoceles resolve with serial lumbar

---

Controversial Point

- In most patients with medulloblastoma, a preoperative ventriculoperitoneal (VP) shunt, third ventriculostomy, or external ventricular drain is unnecessary and undesirable because symptomatic patients can usually be managed with corticosteroids alone until posterior fossa surgery is performed.

punctures, but others may require VP shunting or cyst-peritoneal shunting. The risk of subsequent hydrocephalus and the need for a shunt is typically higher in younger patients and in the setting of metastatic disease, aseptic meningitis, and incomplete resection.

Treatment

Surgery

Surgical goals in the treatment of posterior fossa medulloblastoma include establishing a tissue diagnosis, reconstitution of CSF pathways, and removal of as much of the tumor as can be done safely. The tumor is approached through a midline suboccipital incision and can often be seen as a mass hanging down between the tonsils after the dura is opened. The surgeon should inspect the surface of the exposed cerebellum and spinal cord for evidence of leptomeningeal spread of disease. Gross total resection of disease is the surgeon's aim; however, in about one third of cases the tumor will have invaded the brainstem. The tumor should not be "chased" into the brainstem because this will lead to serious neurologic morbidity.

The mortality rate for posterior fossa tumor surgery is low, but there is considerable morbidity secondary to damage to nearby structures such as the cerebellum, brainstem, and cranial nerves. Mutism is observed in over 20% of patients,[23] and has been pathophysiologically linked with splaying of the middle cerebellar peduncles.[24] The patient's speech usually recovers in a few weeks to months after a brief period of dysarthria, but may not recover completely in some cases.[25]

Radiotherapy

Following the introduction of craniospinal radiotherapy (CSRT), the survival rate for this malignant tumor rose from 0 to 50%.[26] Total neuraxis radiation is standard treatment for patients with medulloblastoma with the exception of children under the age of 3 years.[27–29] Standard treatment for children > 36 months is craniospinal irradiation with a boost to the posterior fossa up to 55 to 59 Gy followed by adjuvant chemotherapy. The dose of craniospinal irradiation is risk-adapted, where patients with average-risk disease receive 23.4 Gy and patients with high-risk disease receive 36 Gy.[30,31] Reduced-dose craniospinal irradiation followed by adjuvant cisplatin-based chemotherapy results in 5-year survival of up to 85% for average-risk medulloblastoma.[30] An additional boost of radiation is given to areas with metastases so that they receive the same dose as the primary tumor. The immature nervous system of children younger than 36 months of age is particularly sensitive to radiation, and complications of radiation treatment in that group are extremely high, including severe cognitive impairment, endocrinopathy, moyamoya disease, and radiation-induced tumors. Children without evidence of dissemination may be treated with a lower craniospinal dose. Future trials will evaluate reduction of radiotherapy for WNT tumors to minimize radiation-induced side effects in this patient population with good prognosis.

Side effects of radiation are seen in at least 56% of long-term survivors. Prospective studies have shown that patients with medulloblastoma who receive radiation develop cognitive deficits, which is not observed in children with cerebellar astrocytomas who do not receive radiation.[15] In the Toronto experience, the only fatal complication of radiotherapy for medulloblastoma was the induction of secondary tumors at an incidence of 10%. Other side effects of radiation include growth retardation, hypopituitarism, severe sensorineural hearing loss, and leukoencephalopathy.

Chemotherapy

Patients with medulloblastoma can be divided into high-risk and low-risk groups for assessment of prognosis and perhaps the need for chemotherapy. Standard-risk patients are 3 years of age or older, have no residual tumor on postoperative imaging, and have no distant metastases identified. High-risk patients are younger than 3 years of age, have residual tumor on postoperative MRI, or have evidence of metastatic disease. Historically, all children with medulloblastoma have been treated with standard-dose craniospinal irradiation, but only achieved a 5-year survival rate of up to 60%. However, several studies over the past 15 years have shown that children with average-risk medulloblastoma can be treated with reduced-dose craniospinal irradiation with adjuvant cisplatin-based chemotherapy, with several studies showing 5-year survivals of up to 85%.[30,31] Children with high-risk disease are treated with standard-dose craniospinal irradiation followed by adjuvant chemotherapy regimens, with 5-year survivals ranging from 40 to 70%.[31–33]

In infants, chemotherapy is used to delay or even avoid radiotherapy to minimize neurotoxicity.[34] Several studies have shown that infants can be successfully treated with only chemotherapy by using several approaches including systemic induction followed by high-dose chemotherapy with autologous stem cell support (Headstart, COG, SFOP), systemic chemotherapy with conformal local irradiation (UK, COG), and intraventricular methotrexate (HIT2000). All these approaches have shown that infants with desmoplastic disease can achieve 5-year survivals of up to 90%, and 5-year survivals across all patients of 50 to 70%. The intraventricular methotrexate approach, however, is associated with a dose-dependent leukoencephalopathy of varying severity, and these patients are at risk of radiation necrosis if subsequently salvaged with radiation. High-dose chemotherapy has also been used at the time of relapse with leptomeningeal dissemination in combination with autologous bone marrow transplant; this has resulted in the longest reported event-free survival in the relapse setting, but it remains an investigational protocol.[35]

Prognostic Factors

Current stratification of treatment intensity is based primarily on clinical parameters, with high-risk patients identified as being younger than 3 years of age and having metastatic dissemination at diagnosis or an incomplete surgical resection.[31] The size of the tumor at the time of diagnosis and brainstem invasion are not used to stratify patients. Increasing evidence suggests that molecular markers may help to refine patient stratification. The next generation of clinical trials will include MYC/MYCN amplification and isochromosome 17q to identify high-risk patients, whereas WNT subgroup markers (nuclear accumulation of CTNNB1, CTNNB1 mutations, monosomy 6) stratify low-risk patients.

In light of the classification of the four subgroups of medulloblastoma, it is important now to develop subgroup-specific treatment protocols. The first subgroup-specific treatment protocol employs SHH inhibitors in relapsed medulloblastomas with SHH activation.[36] More recently, molecular markers have been shown to be prognostic in children with medulloblastoma. Elevated expression of beta-catenin and TrkC are associated with a good prognosis, whereas high levels of ERB-B2 expression are associated with a poor prognosis.[37] High FSTL5 expression identified high-risk tumors across and within medulloblastoma subgroups, suggesting additional heterogeneity within subgroups.[38] Dissemination is found at the time of

> **Pearl**
>
> - Long-term survivors often have significant learning disabilities, and patients should have neuropsychiatric assessments for several years after the cessation of therapy to maximize their level of functioning.

presentation in 20 to 30% of patients overall but in 50% of younger children. Patients with dissemination at the time of diagnosis are less likely to respond to initial therapy and are more likely to relapse early in the course of treatment. Extent of resection is certainly a prognostic factor but it is controversial in the literature whether there is a difference to the patient between a 90% and a 100% resection.

Leptomeningeal dissemination constitutes the most common pattern of recurrence for Group 3 and Group 4 patients, and usually leads to a quick progressive clinical decline despite therapy. Isolated recurrence to the posterior fossa may permit the patient to live for some time after repeat surgical resection and possibly further adjuvant treatments. Five-year survivals for standard-risk medulloblastoma are about 80%, and, for high risk patients, 60%. Aggressive therapy may improve the outlook for these patients. Even among children who are cured of their disease, the cost can be high in terms of focal and global neurologic deficits.

■ Ependymoma

Ependymomas represent 2 to 8% of all central nervous system (CNS) neoplasms, and, in childhood, are the third most common CNS neoplasm, accounting for 6 to 12% of intracranial tumors.[39] They are highly prevalent in young children, representing 30% of brain tumors in children younger than 3 years of age. Ependymomas can occur throughout the CNS but are infratentorial in two thirds of cases.[40] The mean age in the HSC series was 3.7 years; there is no gender predilection. There are no clear etiologic associations for posterior fossa ependymoma.

Clinical Presentation

Children with ependymoma present with a median 3-month history of symptoms prior to diagnosis. The most common presentation is increased intracranial pressure secondary to hydrocephalus. The predominant symptoms at diagnosis are headache, nausea, and vomiting. Vomiting may be secondary to hydrocephalus causing increased intracranial pressure, or it may be from tumor infiltration of the area postrema in the floor of the fourth ventricle. Extension of tumor into the cervical subarachnoid space is more common in ependymoma than other posterior fossa tumors (30 to 50% of cases) and, as such, these patients are more likely to present with nuchal rigidity, neck pain, torticollis, and head tilt. Children younger than 2 years of age usually present with irritability, lethargy, cranial neuropathies, and vomiting due to the presence of open cranial sutures. The most common signs at presentation in children are papilledema, ataxia, nystagmus, and gaze palsies. Fewer than 5% of children with ependymoma have disseminated disease at the time of diagnosis, and therefore it is very uncommon for a patient with an ependymoma to present with symptoms from a leptomeningeal metastasis.

Imaging Studies

On unenhanced CT images, ependymomas can be isodense, hyperdense, or of mixed density. They have calcifications in 50% of cases and are more heterogeneous than medulloblastoma. Most tumors enhance intensely with contrast. On MRI these tumors are seen to arise in the region of the fourth ventricle and often track along the lateral recesses into the cerebellopontine angle and the cerebellomedullary cistern. MRI shows marked heterogeneity of the tumor due to small cysts as well as areas of old hemorrhage. Extension of the tumor through the foramen of Magendie into the upper cervical subarachnoid space and compression of the upper cervical spinal cord is characteristic of ependymomas, whereas medulloblastomas are more likely to extend up into the tentorial incisura.

> **Pearl**
>
> • Ependymomas enhance inhomogeneously and therefore may have nonenhancing portions. If these are not appreciated on the preoperative MRI, these portions may be missed at surgery.

Postoperative imaging should be obtained in all patients within 48 hours of surgery to determine the extent of resection (**Fig. 28.5**). Imaging of the spine should also be done to look for leptomeningeal dissemination of tumor.

Pathology

Ependymomas are glial neoplasms that histologically resemble the cells lining the ventricles. Grossly, the tumor is usually solid, well circumscribed, gray in color, soft in consistency, and has occasional flecks of calcification. The tumor may arise from the roof of the fourth ventricle, the floor of the fourth ventricle, or laterally in the cerebellopontine angle. The three classic histological findings are monomorphic round-to-oval nuclei with "salt and pepper" speckling of the chromatin, true ependymal rosettes, and perivascular pseudorosettes (glial tumor cells radially arranged around blood vessels) (**Fig. 28.6**).

> **Controversy**
>
> • There is great controversy in the literature as to whether the grading of infratentorial ependymoma has any prognostic significance.

True ependymal rosettes are present in only a minority of cases (28%).[41]

Although many institutions use the two-tiered WHO classification of ependymoma (ependymoma and anaplastic ependymoma), it is unclear how reliable the histological assessment of anaplasia is in the clinical setting, and the degree to which it reflects a poor prognosis. The histological differences between ependymoma and anaplastic ependymoma include the presence of nuclear atypia, marked mitotic activity, and high cellularity in the anaplastic tumors.[16] Although ependymomas from the supratentorial space, posterior fossa, and spinal cord have very similar histology, they are biologically distinct diseases with their own transcriptional profiles and distinct sets of (epi)genetic abnormalities.[42–44]

Treatment

Surgery

The surgical approach to a fourth ventricular ependymoma is removal through a midline suboccipital approach. Hydrocephalus is dealt with as outlined earlier for medulloblastomas. As with other lesions in this location, surgical goals include tissue diagnosis, total tumor removal, and reconstitution of CSF pathways.

In patients with ependymoma, the extent of tumor resection is the single most significant prognostic factor, and as such there is a definite advantage for gross total resection. Surgery alone can probably cure a small percentage of patients with supratentorial ependymoma if the tumor is completely removed. The surgeon's impression of the extent of resection is poor, and postoperative imaging is essential.[39] In patients for whom postoperative imaging shows residual disease that is surgically accessible, there may be a role for early second-look surgery or perhaps delayed surgery for resection of residual disease after chemotherapy and radiation.[40] Tumors arising

> **Pearl**
>
> • A midsagittal MRI defines the lower limit of the tumor and thus the minimum number of cervical lamina that should be removed to achieve total removal. Unnecessary removal of lamina in the pediatric upper cervical spine is undesirable because it may lead to the delayed occurrence of a swan-neck deformity.

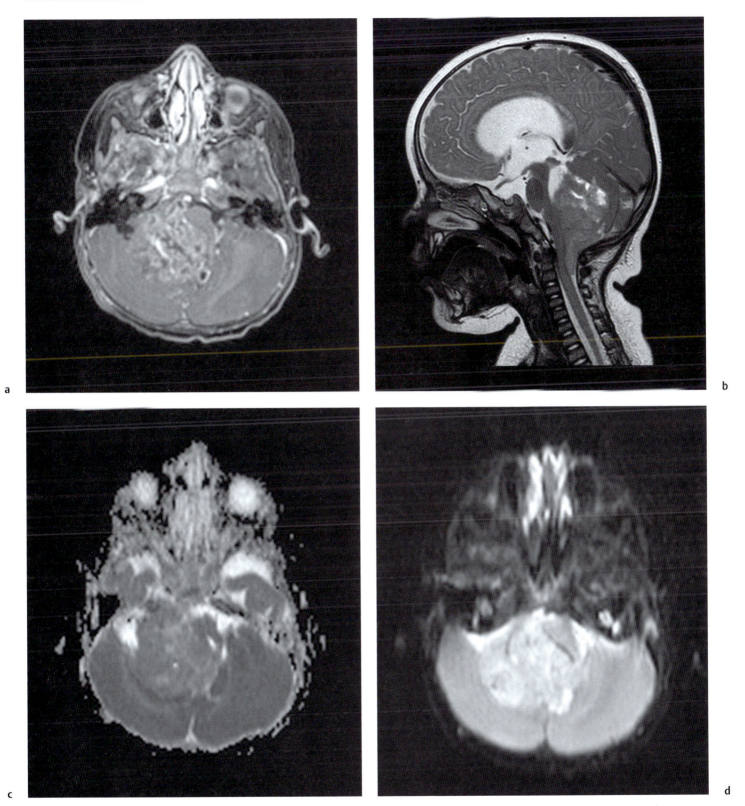

Fig. 28.5a–d (**a**) Axial T1-weighted MRI with gadolinium enhancement of a fourth ventricular ependymoma showing patchy enhancement throughout the lesion. (**b**) Sagittal T2-weighted MRI through the midline showing infiltration of the fourth ventricular ependy- moma caudally through the foramen of Magendie. (**c**) Axial apparent diffusion coefficient (ADC) map and (**d**) axial B1000 at the same level showing lack of diffusion restriction of the solid fourth ventricular mass.

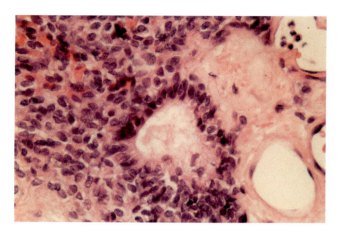

Fig. 28.6 Histological section of an ependymoma showing a true ependymal rosette (H&E stain).

from the roof of the fourth ventricle are the easiest to totally remove. Lateral tumors with a large cerebellopontine angle component are the most difficult to totally remove because they are often adherent to cranial nerves and vascular structures.[45] In highly specialized centers, surgical mortality is under 1%; however, morbidity remains high (10 to 30%) secondary to brainstem and cranial nerve injury.

Radiotherapy

Most children with ependymoma are treated postoperatively with conformal irradiation to the tumor bed. Although disseminated disease is seen in about 30% of patients at autopsy, it is seen in far fewer patients at presentation. Ependymoma recurrences are usually at the primary site in the posterior fossa. Most incidences of spinal metastases follow failure in the posterior fossa and it is very unusual to see isolated recurrence in the spine. Craniospinal irradiation is therefore unnecessary in the absence of documented leptomeningeal dissemination. Recently, conformal radiation treatment of the tumor bed alone, rather than the entire posterior fossa, has been shown to be a safe and effective technique.[46] Indeed, with conformal therapy it is probably safe to treat infants with localized radiotherapy.

At present there is little evidence to support the beneficial role of adjuvant chemotherapy in the routine treatment of infratentorial ependymoma of childhood as it has not been shown to increase progression-free survival in patients who have received radiotherapy. Reirradiation has shown some therapeutic effect in recurrent ependymomas.[47]

Prognostic Factors

Poor prognostic factors include age younger than 24 months, incomplete resection, infratentorial location, duration of symptoms less than 1 month, and perhaps anaplastic histology.[39] Good prognostic factors include adult age, supratentorial lo-

cation, benign pathology, and total surgical resection. The most important variable is probably the presence or absence of total resection confirmed with postoperative imaging. Malignant histology may be a risk factor for CSF dissemination. The majority of fourth ventricular ependymomas that recur remain low grade on repeat resection, and recurrence is usually at or immediately adjacent to the original tumor site.[46] The median time to progression after a total resection is 22 to 24 months, although late recurrences more than 5 years after therapy have been reported. Virtually all patients with a subtotal resection have a recurrence in 12 to 14 months. In cases with gross total resection, no dissemination, and adequate radiotherapy, 5-year survival rates as high as 85% have been reported. Recent evidence suggests two posterior fossa subgroups, called A and B, with distinct biological, clinical, and prognostic features. Group A patients are younger, display lateral tumor location with balanced genome, and with a higher proportion of recurrent disease, metastasis, and tumor-related death compared with Group B patients.[43]

■ Cerebellar Astrocytoma

Cerebellar astrocytoma (CA) constitutes 20% of pediatric brain tumors, making it the most common brain tumor in the pediatric age group. More than half of pediatric astrocytomas are located in the posterior fossa, and more than 70% of cerebellar astrocytomas occur in children.[48] The peak incidence of CA is in the middle of the first decade (mean age in the HSC series was 7.3 years), and these tumors are rarely found in children under 1 year of age or in adults over the age of 40.[49] There is no gender predilection for CA. Virtually all CA display *BRAF*-mediated activation of the mitogen-activated protein kinase (MAPK) pathway, which may comprise an attractive target for molecular-based therapy.[50–52]

Clinical Presentation

The median duration of symptoms before diagnosis is decreasing due to the availability of modern imaging; current symptomatic periods range from 5 to 9 months.[49] Because of the slow growth pattern, the length of symptomatic time before diagnosis is often longer in patients with CA than in patients with posterior fossa medulloblastoma or ependymoma. The clinical presentation of CA varies widely with the age of the child, depending on the stage of development and the status of the cranial sutures. Most children present with symptoms due to increased intracranial pressure or cerebellar dysfunction; common symptoms at diagnosis include headache (84%), nausea and vomiting (74%), altered gait (70%), increasing head size (14%), and, rarely, blindness or coma.[48] Signs at diagnosis include papilledema (84%), truncal ataxia (75%), and appendicular ataxia (39%). Hydrocephalus is present in 85% of patients and may be more common with vermian rather than hemispheric lesions.[53] Location in the brainstem is associated with cranial nerve palsies including eye muscle paralysis, facial nerve palsy, and swallowing difficulties.

Imaging Studies

On an unenhanced CT scan, a CA is hypodense or isodense compared with surrounding white matter (as opposed to medulloblastoma, which is hyperdense). There may be foci of hyperdensity within the tumor in 10 to 20% of cases due to areas of calcification.[53] These tumors enhance significantly and diffusely with contrast. Tumors may be wholly solid, wholly cystic, or mixed solid-cystic in appearance (**Fig. 28.7**). In a true cystic astrocytoma, the wall will not enhance, and there will be an enhancing mural nodule. The cyst wall may enhance with contrast and in such cases will contain tumor. Thus CA may be broken into three groups: solid (32%), cystic (cyst wall does not enhance and contains no tumor, 26%), and mixed solid-cystic (42%). Cyst fluid is slightly more hyperdense than CSF on CT scan. MRI is superior to CT in the definition of anatomy and the extent of the tumor. T1-weighted images show the tumor to have decreased or similar signal to surrounding white matter, whereas T2-weighted images show it to be of increased signal. With gadolinium enhancement, an enhancing mural nodule is commonly observed. All patients should have postoperative imaging, with and without contrast,

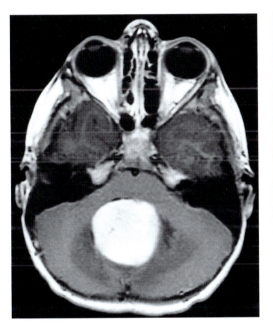

a

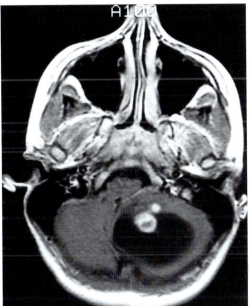

b

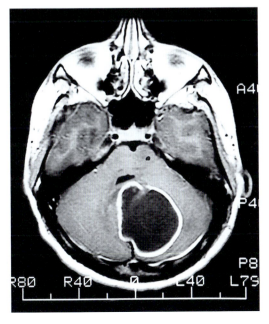

c

Fig. 28.7a–c T1-weighted MRI with gadolinium showing (**a**) wholly solid cerebellar astrocytoma (CA), (**b**) wholly cystic CA with an enhancing mural nodule, and (**c**) mixed solid/cystic CA with enhancing cyst walls.

within 48 hours of surgery. Early postoperative scans avoid the difficulty of distinguishing between postoperative changes and residual tumor; postoperative imaging is a much more reliable indicator of the extent of resection than the impression of the operating surgeon.[54]

Pathology

These tumors most commonly arise from the vermis but have been documented to grow in every part of the cerebellum. There is a tendency to invade the subarachnoid space and grow along the surface of the cerebellum, but this is not ominous and does not usually portend a negative prognosis. Most CAs are low-grade neoplasms, especially in children. In the HSC series, 88% of CAs were pilocytic astrocytomas, which virtually never show malignant progression to high-grade astrocytoma. Histological features include Rosenthal fibers, microcysts, areas of mineralization, and endothelial proliferation. In the setting of a pilocytic astrocytoma, the presence of endothelial proliferation does not imply the same negative prognosis as it does in adult fibrillary astrocytomas. Some low-grade fibrillary astrocytomas are seen in the cerebellum of children. Malignant or anaplastic CAs are exceedingly rare in children, and when they are seen, there is often a history of prior radiation treatment to the area.[55]

Controversy

- Distinctions in the subtype of astrocytoma of the cerebellum (e.g., pilocytic vs fibrillary) have not been useful in predicting prognosis.

Treatment

Surgery

Gross total resection is almost always curative. Surgical goals include making a tissue diagnosis, reestablishing CSF pathways, and accomplishing complete surgical removal of the tumor. Preoperative CSF diversion is unnecessary because most patients can be temporized with corticosteroids as out-

---

Pearl

- It is not uncommon to observe small, contrast-enhancing foci on postoperative imaging of patients with CA. These foci may represent residual or recurrent tumor. However, because the growth potential of these neoplasms is low, the neurosurgeon can safely follow these patients with serial imaging studies.

Pitfall

- Rarely, CA invades the brainstem (about 10% of cases), necessitating an incomplete removal. Due to the indolent nature of this disease, surgeons should not chase this tumor into the brainstem, where it can cause significant morbidity.

Special Consideration

- Although radiotherapy and chemotherapy for CA are of no clear benefit, it may be considered in cases with brainstem invasion or clearly documented progression on postoperative imaging. Radiotherapy should be omitted in neurofibromatosis type 1–associated astrocytomas.

---

lined in the section on medulloblastoma. The tumor is removed through a posterior fossa craniotomy. Total removal is essential because recurrent tumor arises from residual tumor. Watchful waiting is the management of choice for incompletely resected CAs with serial neuroimaging.

Low-grade glioma protocols or involved field radiation should be considered only for incompletely resected CA that is not amenable to additional surgery, and that is observed to increase in size over time on serial imaging. In addition, vinblastine- or temozolomide-based protocols constitute another therapeutic option.[56–58]

Cases where gross total resection is impossible or ill advised should still undergo as much resection as the surgeon deems safe. In the treatment of cystic tumors it is important not to let the cyst fluid escape into the CSF pathways because it may cause chemical meningitis and increase the risk of developing long-term hydrocephalus. Approximately 10% of children with a CA will eventually require a VP shunt, the percentage being even higher among children under the age of 3 years. If surgically accessible disease is seen on the postoperative imaging, early second-look surgery and resection of tumor may be considered in some cases. There is no role for adjuvant radiation or chemotherapy once a CA has been completely removed, with confirmation by postoperative imaging.

Prognostic Factors

Long-term prognosis is dependent on the extent of resection, the presence of brainstem invasion, and the histological features of malignancy. Long-term, event-free survival after total removal of a CA of childhood approaches 90%. However, when resection is subtotal, recurrence is common and was seen in all five patients with incomplete resection at 1 to 8 years after surgery at our institution. Some authors have documented disease progression after an apparently complete resection, but the majority of recurrences are amenable to a repeat resection. Prognosis is poorest at the extremes of life. Many late recurrences have been reported because CA does not follow Collins's law (indicating that tumor relapse should occur within a period equal to the patient's age at diagnosis plus 9 months), and it is uncertain at what point in time a patient can be considered cured of a CA.

Conclusion

Great success and even greater challenges typify pediatric posterior fossa tumors. Many patients have excellent outcomes through the selective use of surgery, radiotherapy, and chemotherapy. Although current techniques have greatly improved the prognosis of patients with posterior fossa tumors, many challenges persist. Some patients go on to progressive disease despite modern, aggressive therapy; among the long-term survivors there is a great deal of iatrogenic morbidity. The imminent arrival of molecularly based systems of tumor classification, and the development of future therapies based

on tumor molecular biology should continue to improve the outlook for these patients.

Editor's Note

Posterior fossa tumors in children represent a huge challenge for neurosurgeons, radiation oncologists, neuro-oncologists, and patients and their families. It appears that for some tumors in this group, especially medulloblastoma, the extent of resection may be an important prognostic factor, although, as with supratentorial gliomas in adults, no randomized class I evidence exists to show us this, and such a study most certainly never will be done.[59] Like other groups of tumors that affect the nervous system, the real hope for the future may lie in learning more about the molecular profile of the tumor, and the recent discovery of four subgroups of medulloblastoma based on molecular analysis should be seen as a very exciting development for all those caring for and studying brain tumor patients. (Bernstein)

References

1. Rutka JT. Medulloblastoma. Clin Neurosurg 1997;44:571–585
2. Taylor MD, Northcott PA, Korshunov A, et al. Molecular subgroups of medulloblastoma: the current consensus. Acta Neuropathol 2012; 123:465–472
3. Northcott PA, Korshunov A, Pfister SM, Taylor MD. The clinical implications of medulloblastoma subgroups. Nat Rev Neurol 2012;8:340–351
4. Northcott PA, Korshunov A, Witt H, et al. Medulloblastoma comprises four distinct molecular variants. J Clin Oncol 2011;29:1408–1414
5. Taylor MD, Mainprize TG, Rutka JT. Molecular insight into medulloblastoma and central nervous system primitive neuroectodermal tumor biology from hereditary syndromes: a review. Neurosurgery 2000;47: 888–901
6. Northcott PA, Shih DJ, Peacock J, et al. Subgroup-specific structural variation across 1,000 medulloblastoma genomes. Nature 2012;488: 49–56
7. Korshunov A, Remke M, Werft W, et al. Adult and pediatric medulloblastomas are genetically distinct and require different algorithms for molecular risk stratification. J Clin Oncol 2010;28:3054–3060
8. Pfister S, Remke M, Benner A, et al. Outcome prediction in pediatric medulloblastoma based on DNA copy-number aberrations of chromosomes 6q and 17q and the MYC and MYCN loci. J Clin Oncol 2009; 27:1627–1636
9. Traenka C, Remke M, Korshunov A, et al. Role of LIM and SH3 protein 1 (LASP1) in the metastatic dissemination of medulloblastoma. Cancer Res 2010;70:8003–8014
10. Ramaswamy V, Northcott PA, Taylor MD. FISH and chips: the recipe for improved prognostication and outcomes for children with medulloblastoma. Cancer Genet 2011;204:577–588
11. Kool M, Korshunov A, Remke M, et al. Molecular subgroups of medulloblastoma: an international meta-analysis of transcriptome, genetic aberrations, and clinical data of WNT, SHH, Group 3, and Group 4 medulloblastomas. Acta Neuropathol 2012;123:473–484
12. Park TS, Hoffman HJ, Hendrick EB, Humphreys RP, Becker LE. Medulloblastoma: clinical presentation and management. Experience at the

Hospital for Sick Children, Toronto, 1950–1980. J Neurosurg 1983;58: 543–552
13. Sutton LN, Phillips PC, Molloy PT. Surgical management of medulloblastoma. J Neurooncol 1996;29:9–21
14. Blaser SI, Harwood-Nash DC. Neuroradiology of pediatric posterior fossa medulloblastoma. J Neurooncol 1996;29:23–34
15. Albright AL, Wisoff JH, Zeltzer PM, Boyett JM, Rorke LB, Stanley P. Effects of medulloblastoma resections on outcome in children: a report from the Children's Cancer Group. Neurosurgery 1996;38:265–271
16. Louis DN, Ohgaki H, Wiestler OD, et al. The 2007 WHO classification of tumours of the central nervous system. Acta Neuropathol 2007;114: 97–109
17. Giangaspero F, Perilongo G, Fondelli MP, et al. Medulloblastoma with extensive nodularity: a variant with favorable prognosis. J Neurosurg 1999;91:971–977
18. Rutkowski S, von Hoff K, Emser A, et al. Survival and prognostic factors of early childhood medulloblastoma: an international meta-analysis. J Clin Oncol 2010;28:4961–4968
19. Rorke LB, Packer RJ, Biegel JA. Central nervous system atypical teratoid/rhabdoid tumors of infancy and childhood: definition of an entity. J Neurosurg 1996;85:56–65
20. Versteege I, Sévenet N, Lange J, et al. Truncating mutations of hSNF5/INI1 in aggressive paediatric cancer. Nature 1998;394:203–206
21. Chi SN, Zimmerman MA, Yao X, et al. Intensive multimodality treatment for children with newly diagnosed CNS atypical teratoid rhabdoid tumor. J Clin Oncol 2009;27:385–389
22. Sainte-Rose C, Cinalli G, Roux FE, et al. Management of hydrocephalus in pediatric patients with posterior fossa tumors: the role of endoscopic third ventriculostomy. J Neurosurg 2001;95:791–797
23. Robertson PL, Muraszko KM, Holmes EJ, et al; Children's Oncology Group. Incidence and severity of postoperative cerebellar mutism syndrome in children with medulloblastoma: a prospective study by the Children's Oncology Group. J Neurosurg 2006;105(6, Suppl):444–451

24. Morris EB, Phillips NS, Laningham FH, et al. Proximal dentatothalamo-cortical tract involvement in posterior fossa syndrome. Brain 2009; 132(Pt 11):3087–3095

25. Steinbok P, Cochrane DD, Perrin R, Price A. Mutism after posterior fossa tumour resection in children: incomplete recovery on long-term follow-up. Pediatr Neurosurg 2003;39:179–183

26. Jenkin D. The radiation treatment of medulloblastoma. J Neurooncol 1996;29:45–54

27. Geyer JR, Sposto R, Jennings M, et al; Children's Cancer Group. Multiagent chemotherapy and deferred radiotherapy in infants with malignant brain tumors: a report from the Children's Cancer Group. J Clin Oncol 2005;23:7621–7631

28. Grill J, Sainte-Rose C, Jouvet A, et al; French Society of Paediatric Oncology. Treatment of medulloblastoma with postoperative chemotherapy alone: an SFOP prospective trial in young children. Lancet Oncol 2005;6:573–580

29. Rutkowski S, Bode U, Deinlein F, et al. Treatment of early childhood medulloblastoma by postoperative chemotherapy alone. N Engl J Med 2005;352:978–986

30. Packer RJ, Gajjar A, Vezina G, et al. Phase III study of craniospinal radiation therapy followed by adjuvant chemotherapy for newly diagnosed average-risk medulloblastoma. J Clin Oncol 2006;24:4202–4208

31. Gajjar A, Chintagumpala M, Ashley D, et al. Risk-adapted craniospinal radiotherapy followed by high-dose chemotherapy and stem-cell rescue in children with newly diagnosed medulloblastoma (St. Jude Medulloblastoma-96): long-term results from a prospective, multicentre trial. Lancet Oncol 2006;7:813–820

32. Gandola L, Massimino M, Cefalo G, et al. Hyperfractionated accelerated radiotherapy in the Milan strategy for metastatic medulloblastoma. J Clin Oncol 2009;27:566–571

33. Jakacki RI, Burger PC, Zhou T, et al. Outcome of children with metastatic medulloblastoma treated with carboplatin during craniospinal radiotherapy: a Children's Oncology Group Phase I/II study. J Clin Oncol 2012;30:2648–2653

34. Duffner PK, Horowitz ME, Krischer JP, et al. Postoperative chemotherapy and delayed radiation in children less than three years of age with malignant brain tumors. N Engl J Med 1993;328:1725–1731

35. Cohen BH, Packer RJ. Chemotherapy for medulloblastomas and primitive neuroectodermal tumors. J Neurooncol 1996;29:55–68

36. Rudin CM, Hann CL, Laterra J, et al. Treatment of medulloblastoma with hedgehog pathway inhibitor GDC-0449. N Engl J Med 2009;361:1173–1178

37. Gajjar A, Hernan R, Kocak M, et al. Clinical, histopathologic, and molecular markers of prognosis: toward a new disease risk stratification system for medulloblastoma. J Clin Oncol 2004;22:984–993

38. Remke M, Hielscher T, Korshunov A, et al. FSTL5 is a marker of poor prognosis in non-WNT/non-SHH medulloblastoma. J Clin Oncol 2011; 29:3852–3861

39. Sanford RA, Gajjar A. Ependymomas. Clin Neurosurg 1997;44:559–570

40. Pollack IF, Gerszten PC, Martinez AJ, et al. Intracranial ependymomas of childhood: long-term outcome and prognostic factors. Neurosurgery 1995;37:655–666, discussion 666–667

41. Healey EA, Barnes PD, Kupsky WJ, et al. The prognostic significance of postoperative residual tumor in ependymoma. Neurosurgery 1991;28:666–671, discussion 671–672

42. Taylor MD, Poppleton H, Fuller C, et al. Radial glia cells are candidate stem cells of ependymoma. Cancer Cell 2005;8:323–335

43. Witt H, Mack SC, Ryzhova M, et al. Delineation of two clinically and molecularly distinct subgroups of posterior fossa ependymoma. Cancer Cell 2011;20:143–157

44. Mack SC, Witt H, Wang X, et al. Emerging insights into the ependymoma epigenome. Brain Pathol 2013;23:206–209

45. Sanford RA, Kun LE, Heideman RL, Gajjar A. Cerebellar pontine angle ependymoma in infants. Pediatr Neurosurg 1997;27:84–91

46. Merchant TE, Mulhern RK, Krasin MJ, et al. Preliminary results from a phase II trial of conformal radiation therapy and evaluation of radiation-related CNS effects for pediatric patients with localized ependymoma. J Clin Oncol 2004;22:3156–3162

47. Bouffet E, Hawkins CE, Ballourah W, et al. Survival benefit for pediatric patients with recurrent ependymoma treated with reirradiation. Int J Radiat Oncol Biol Phys 2012;83:1541–1548

48. Ilgren EB, Stiller CA. Cerebellar astrocytomas. Clinical characteristics and prognostic indices. J Neurooncol 1987;4:293–308

49. Abdollahzadeh M, Hoffman HJ, Blazer SI, et al. Benign cerebellar astrocytoma in childhood: experience at the Hospital for Sick Children 1980–1992. Childs Nerv Syst 1994;10:380–383

50. Pfister S, Janzarik WG, Remke M, et al. BRAF gene duplication constitutes a mechanism of MAPK pathway activation in low-grade astrocytomas. J Clin Invest 2008;118:1739–1749

51. Jones DT, Gronych J, Lichter P, Witt O, Pfister SM. MAPK pathway activation in pilocytic astrocytoma. Cell Mol Life Sci 2012;69:1799–1811

52. Jones DT, Kocialkowski S, Liu L, et al. Tandem duplication producing a novel oncogenic BRAF fusion gene defines the majority of pilocytic astrocytomas. Cancer Res 2008;68:8673–8677

53. Campbell JW, Pollack IF. Cerebellar astrocytomas in children. J Neurooncol 1996;28:223–231

54. Morreale VM, Ebersold MJ, Quast LM, Parisi JE. Cerebellar astrocytoma: experience with 54 cases surgically treated at the Mayo Clinic, Rochester, Minnesota, from 1978 to 1990. J Neurosurg 1997;87:257–261

55. Kulkarni AV, Becker LE, Jay V, Armstrong DC, Drake JM. Primary cerebellar glioblastomas multiforme in children. Report of four cases. J Neurosurg 1999;90:546–550

56. Ater JL, Zhou T, Holmes E, et al. Randomized study of two chemotherapy regimens for treatment of low-grade glioma in young children: a report from the Children's Oncology Group. J Clin Oncol 2012;30:2641–2647

57. Bouffet E, Jakacki R, Goldman S, et al. Phase II study of weekly vinblastine in recurrent or refractory pediatric low-grade glioma. J Clin Oncol 2012;30:1358–1363

58. Gururangan S, Fisher MJ, Allen JC, et al. Temozolomide in children with progressive low-grade glioma. Neuro-oncol 2007;9:161–168

59. De Braganca KC, Packer RJ. Treatment options for medulloblastoma and CNS primitive neuroectodermal tumor (PNET). Curr Treat Options Neurol 2013;15:593–606

29 Pediatric Supratentorial Tumors

Michael DeCuypere and Frederick A. Boop

Tumors of the central nervous system (CNS), as a group, make up approximately 25% of all childhood cancers and represent the most common solid tumors in children. Supratentorial and infratentorial tumors occur with almost equal incidence in the pediatric population. However, the relative frequency by location varies according to the age of the patient, with supratentorial tumors predominating in children up to age 3 and older than age 10.[1] Glial-based tumors make up 60% of neoplasms within the supratentorial compartment, and 80% of these are of low-grade histology.[2] This chapter reviews several supratentorial neoplasms in children. Some important supratentorial pediatric tumors, such as craniopharyngiomas and pineal region tumors, are discussed in other chapters.

Clinical Presentation in Childhood

Early diagnosis of CNS tumors in the pediatric population is a primary determinant of treatment and outcome. The symptoms of initial presentation generally relate to the tumor location and the rate of growth. For instance, tumors within the frontal lobe may lead to personality changes, seizures, or headaches. A tumor located in the temporal lobe may cause seizures or speech alterations. Tumors of the suprasellar region typically present with endocrinopathies or visual changes. Those within the thalamus usually result in motor and sensory deficits. Tumors of the tectal plate and pineal region may lead to obstructive hydrocephalus, as do tumors invading or emanating from the lateral and third ventricles. However, some symptoms may be nonlocalizing, such as vomiting. Often misdiagnosed as a gastrointestinal disease or migraine variant, it

is one of the most common presentations of childhood CNS tumors.

The confirmation of a suspected brain tumor ultimately relies on some type of neuroimaging. The decision of whether to obtain a computed tomography (CT) or magnetic resonance imaging (MRI) examination of the brain with an acute presentation in the emergency room is usually relatively straightforward. In contrast, primary care pediatricians may be following more subtle signs on a chronic basis and face a more challenging decision about whether imaging is justified.

High-Grade Tumors

High-Grade Astrocytomas

Anaplastic astrocytomas are classified as World Health Organization (WHO) grade III lesions and are characterized by rapid and infiltrative growth. They tend to occur at about the same frequency in children as lower grade diffuse astrocytomas.[3] When supratentorial, these tumors predominantly occur in the cerebral hemispheres, but may also be found in deep midline structures. Microscopically, anaplastic astrocytomas are diffusely infiltrating, with increased cellularity, nuclear pleomorphism, and high mitotic activity. Chromosomal gains of 5q and losses of 6q, 9q, 12q, and 22q are characteristic aberrations in anaplastic astrocytomas in children. Furthermore, significantly shorter survival has been noted in patients whose tumors display gain of material at chromosome arm 1q.[4]

Glioblastoma multiforme (WHO grade IV) occurs approximately 1.5 times more often than anaplastic astrocytoma, but is about 100 times less common in children than in adults. Combined frontotemporal location is typical, but parietal and occipital lobes may also be affected. Glioblastomas are diffusely infiltrating tumors defined by the presence of prominent microvascular proliferation or necrosis. These highly malignant tumors typically demonstrate high cellularity with marked nuclear atypia and brisk mitotic activity.

Genomic amplification of the *EGFR* gene, the most frequent genetic change in adult primary glioblastoma, is rarely observed in pediatric tumors.[5,6] The *TP53* mutations, rarely found in primary glioblastomas in adults, frequently occur in de novo pediatric tumors. Similarly, whereas pediatric glioblastomas rarely harbor mutations of the *PTEN* tumor suppressor gene at 10q23, they are found quite commonly in adult primary glioblastomas.[7,8] However, if mutations of *PTEN* are observed, they are generally associated with poor prognosis in the pediatric population.[9,10]

Surgery remains the primary treatment modality of most supratentorial high-grade astrocytomas in children.[11] However, the higher the grade of the tumor, the more locally infiltrative it becomes. This makes complete surgical resection practically impossible without significant damage to surrounding normal tissue. Nevertheless, radical surgical resection has been shown to improve outcome, and high-dose postoperative radiation plays a critical role in prolonging survival.[7,8] Craniospinal radiation is typically unnecessary, as these tumors do not usually spread via cerebrospinal fluid (CSF) pathways. Although chemotherapy has not played a major treatment role historically, recent studies utilizing temozolomide, an alkylating agent with relatively good CNS penetration, have shown some promise.[12]

High-grade astrocytomas generally carry a very poor prognosis. Despite aggressive treatment with surgery and radiation, fewer than 50% of patients are alive 2 years after diagnosis, and long-term survival rates are low.[13] Generally speaking, patients with anaplastic astrocytoma do tend to survive longer than patients with glioblastoma. After initial therapy, children should be carefully monitored with follow-up MRI exams.

Ependymomas

Predominantly an infratentorial lesion, ependymomas are well-circumscribed tumors that arise in children with an incidence peak at 6 years of age. However, approximately 30% of ependymomas arise supratentorially, most commonly from the lateral or third ventricle (60%) or from the cerebral hemisphere (40%). They account for 10% of all pediatric tumors and approximately 30% of tumors in children younger than 3 years of age. Histologically, ependymomas (WHO grade II) classically exhibit perivascular pseudorosettes of tumor cells radially arranged around blood vessels and true ependymal rosettes that form a central lumen. Anaplastic ependymomas (WHO grade III) demonstrate increased cellularity and brisk mitotic

activity. Perivascular pseudorosettes are frequently encountered with microvascular proliferation and necrosis. Histopathological distinction between grades II and III is often difficult and entails frequent disagreement among neuropathologists.[14] As a result, an impact of tumor histology on clinical outcome remains controversial.

Genetic aberrations are frequent in ependymomas and range from 61 to 79% of the studied populations.[15] Oncogene amplifications are infrequent in ependymomas, and only single cases harbor the homozygous deletion of the *CDKN2A/B* gene.[16] Importantly, the gain of chromosome 1q is a common finding in several studies associated with poor prognosis.[15,17] In contrast, a better prognosis has been associated with the loss of 6q25.3 in patients with anaplastic ependymomas.[18] One study has demonstrated frequent gains and even amplification of the *EGFR* locus and has confirmed that overexpression was an independent marker for poor survival in patients with grade II tumors.[17] Interestingly, there is a correlation between anatomic location and type of genomic alteration, suggesting distinct genetic pathways in ependymoma. Gene expression profiling has identified specific expression signatures, demonstrating the involvement of both Notch and Hedgehog signaling pathways in intracranial ependymomas and suggests that radial glial cells are the origin for tumor formation.[19]

The benefit of complete surgical resection has been clearly demonstrated for pediatric ependymomas, and gross total resection should be the first-line therapy when possible. Additional resection is justified when the postoperative imaging suggests residual disease.[20] Postoperative radiation to the resection cavity has been shown to improve survival for children with ependymoma.[21] In general, ependymomas are not chemoresponsive tumors. Current clinical trials are investigating the role of postradiation chemotherapy in preventing recurrence.

Children with ependymoma who have undergone gross total resection followed by focal radiation generally have a good prognosis, with approximately an 80% 5-year survival. If gross total resection is not achieved, 5-year survival dramatically worsens, with most studies reporting a drop to approximately 20 to 30%. Due to the possibility of late disease recurrence, children with ependymoma require follow-up for many years.

Choroid Plexus Tumors

Tumors of the choroid plexus are rare, comprising only about 1% to 2% of pediatric brain tumors. Although the histological

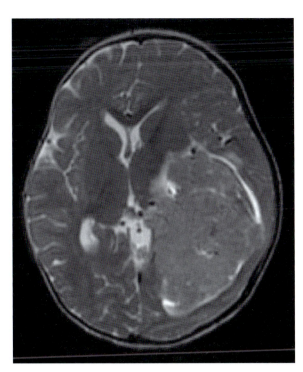

Fig. 29.1 Axial T2-weighted image of a large left parietal mass involving the atrium of the lateral ventricle consistent with a choroid plexus carcinoma. Aggressive lesions may show invasion through the ependyma into hemispheric parenchyma.

classification can be ambiguous, two types of choroid plexus tumors are distinguished, the choroid plexus carcinoma (WHO grade III; **Fig. 29.1**) and choroid plexus papilloma (WHO grade I). Microscopically, papillomas may resemble normal choroid plexus, but may demonstrate a higher degree of columnar epithelium, nuclear pleomorphism, hyperchromasia, and sparse mitotic figures. In contrast, carcinomas are characterized by marked cytological and architectural atypia. They may be invasive, with high mitotic index and areas of necrosis. Germline mutations of the tumor suppressor gene *TP53* are frequently observed, and genetic testing for Li-Fraumeni syndrome should be considered.[22]

The presenting signs of a choroid plexus tumor can include a bulging fontanel with accelerated head circumference, irritability, seizures, vomiting, and lethargy. Due to open fontanels in infants, these tumors can be exceptionally large at presentation. For the lower grade papillomas, surgical resection may be the only treatment required. In the more aggressive carcinomas, gross total resection with adjuvant chemotherapy or radiation will offer the best opportunity for cure. However, the decision to deliver craniospinal radiation therapy to a population with a median age of 2 years is daunting due to long-term side effects. Postoperative chemotherapy for carcinoma does improve survival rates, and intensive chemotherapy is often used with the aim of delaying or avoiding radiation.[23]

Although both tumors have been shown to metastasize, the survival rate of patients with papilloma is significantly higher. However, progression from papilloma to carcinoma has been reported.[24] Nevertheless, the rarity of choroid plexus tumors makes it difficult to establish exact rates of recurrence and cure. Follow-up recommendations for carcinoma survivors are similar to those for other pediatric brain tumors, with routine MRI at 3- or 4-month intervals in the first year. Neuropsychological assessments are essential for following cognitive development in this young group of patients.

Supratentorial Primitive Neuroectodermal Tumors

Supratentorial primitive neuroectodermal tumors (PNETs) (**Fig. 29.2**) are the most common group of malignant childhood brain tumors. They are embryonal tumors with divergent degrees of differentiation along neuronal, astrocytic, muscular, or melanocytic lines. For example, cerebral neuroblastomas (neuronal differentiation) and ganglioneuroblastomas (ganglion and neuronal differentiation) are histologically unique. Additionally, infrequent tumor types such as medulloepithelioma, ependymoblastoma, and embryonal tumor with abundant neuropil and true rosettes are delineated in the current WHO classification. These tumors are solely en-

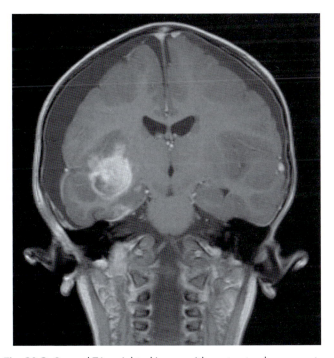

Fig. 29.2 Coronal T1-weighted image with contrast enhancement showing a right temporal primitive neuroectodermal tumor (PNET). Supratentorial PNET tends to present as a heterogeneous mass centered in deep white matter. Solid portions of the tumor tend to show isodensity to gray matter on T2-weighted images. Enhancement after contrast administration is typically heterogeneous in appearance.

- Primitive neuroectodermal tumors are typically composed of sheets of small round blue cells, and during the 1980s and 1990s there was a major controversy over whether the "small round blue cell tumors" involved distinct, location-specific entities (e.g., medulloblastomas) or whether these were different manifestations of a common underlying molecular pathway. Genome-wide profiling has since revealed specific DNA copy number alterations and messenger RNA expression signatures in supratentorial PNETs as compared with medulloblastomas. For instance, the loss of chromosome 17p, which comprises a cytogenetic hallmark of medulloblastoma, is rarely found in supratentorial PNET.

countered in the cerebrum and occasionally in the suprasellar region.

In the pediatric population, aggressive clinical behavior and the high risk of leptomeningeal dissemination are encountered in supratentorial PNETs to an extent similar to that in medulloblastomas. Thus, current treatment strategies for supratentorial PNETs are essentially based on those for medulloblastomas. However, the long-term prognosis is considerably worse than for medulloblastomas. As such, surgery plays a vital role in the treatment of all embryonal tumors, with gross total resection as the goal. The role of chemotherapy is uncertain and has not been tested in a randomized setting. Craniospinal irradiation followed by a boost to the primary tumor site is typically a requirement for an optimal outcome.

Atypical Teratoid/Rhabdoid Tumor

A relatively rare rhabdoid tumor occurring within the central nervous system, atypical teratoid/rhabdoid tumor (AT/RT)

comprises only 1 to 2% of all pediatric brain tumors. These neoplasms typically present in children younger than 3 years of age, with approximately equal supratentorial and infratentorial distribution. Supratentorial tumors are typically located in the cerebral hemispheres (**Fig. 29.3**) and the sellar region. Dissemination of AT/RT via CSF is relatively common and found in 25% of patients at presentation.[25] Microscopically, AT/RTs are heterogeneous lesions composed of rhabdoid cells with eccentrically placed nuclei and abundant cytoplasm with eosinophilic inclusions. Tumors may contain variable tissue components with primitive neuroectodermal, epithelial, and mesenchymal features.

Immunohistochemical staining with integrase interactor 1 (INI1) antibody shows a very sensitive and specific pattern in AT/RT. AT/RTs typically show a loss of nuclear expression, often in association with mutation or deletion of the genomic locus of the encoding gene, *SMARCB1*. Loss of INI1 protein is detected in almost all AT/RTs, and most tumors (75%) have detectable deletions and mutations of the *INI* locus. The localization of mutations within the *INI1* gene appears to vary between tumors from different sites of origin, and exons 5 and 9 are considered hot spots for AT/RTs located within the CNS.[26] Thus, rapid identification of these tumors is possible using immunohistochemical staining for *INI1* expression supplemented with mutation analysis.[27,28]

Patients with AT/RT have significantly shorter survival than patients with PNET undergoing comparable therapy (mean survival less than 12 months) and often exhibit rapid progression. No difference in outcome has been observed in patients with various types of *INI1* alterations, including mutations in specific *INI1* exons. However, patients who are older than 3 years of age at presentation appear to have a longer survival. Current treatment protocols for AT/RT are evaluating alternative high-intensity chemotherapy and the early utilization of radiation therapy. This approach is based on the observation that long-term survivors in previous studies have often re-

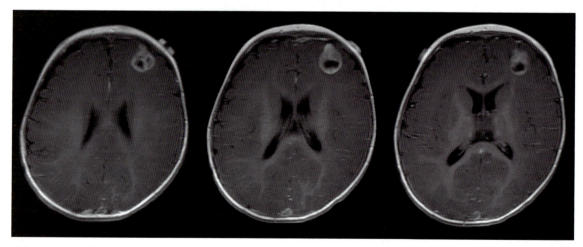

Fig. 29.3 Serial axial T1-weighted images with contrast enhancement showing a left frontal atypical teratoid/rhabdoid tumor (AT/RT). The imaging appearance of AT/RT is similar to that of PNET, with solid portions showing signal intensity similar to that of gray matter, as well as marked heterogeneity resulting from frequent necrosis and hemorrhage.

ceived multiagent chemotherapy, early radiation therapy, or a combination of the two.[29,30]

Low-Grade Tumors

Low-Grade Astrocytomas

Pilocytic astrocytomas are the most common primary brain tumor of childhood, comprising about 20% of all tumors in children up to 14 years of age, and 15% of tumors in teenagers aged 15 to 18 years.[31] Pilocytic astrocytomas are noninfiltrating lesions with a morphologically benign appearance (WHO grade I). Cyst formation is common and often used as a diagnostic feature on neuroimaging. These tumors usually have a low-to-moderate cellularity with pleomorphic nuclei and rare mitotic figures. Rosenthal fibers and eosinophilic granular bodies are frequently observed. Supratentorially, these tumors are typically observed within the hypothalamic/optic pathways, thalamic region, and cerebral hemispheres. Circumscribed and noninfiltrative growth patterns are typical histological features of these tumors, although optic pathway gliomas (**Fig. 29.4**) and diencephalic pilomyxoid astrocytomas may infiltrate surrounding brain. The pilomyxoid variant demonstrates a prominent mucoid matrix with tumor cells arranged concentrically around vessels. Pilomyxoid astrocytomas are prone to rapid recurrence and are therefore considered WHO grade II lesions.

Diffuse astrocytomas (WHO grade II) are about six times less common in children than are pilocytic astrocytomas. These tumors are considered biologically distinct from pilocytic astrocytomas and may progress to higher grade lesions in approximately 10% of cases.[32] Diffuse astrocytomas may be located in any region of the CNS, with the most frequent location being the frontal and temporal lobes. Diffuse astrocytomas display moderate cellularity composed of differentiated

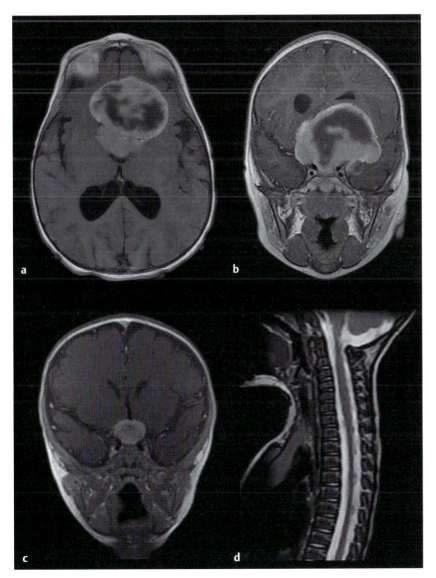

Fig. 29.4a–d (**a**) Axial and (**b**) coronal T1-weighted images after gadolinium contrast showing a large heterogeneously enhancing tumor arising from the suprasellar region in a child consistent with optic pathway glioma. (**c**) A coronal T1-weighted image with contrast enhancement showing a small homogeneously enhancing suprasellar optic glioma associated with (**d**) metastatic nodules along the dorsum of the thoracic spine. Heterogeneous enhancement of solid components is identified in most tumors. In addition, fusiform expansion of the optic nerves is a common appearance.

fibrillary or gemistocytic cells with a general absence of mitotic figures.

Conventional comparative genomic hybridization studies have revealed a balanced karyotype in most pilocytic astrocytomas. However, the most frequent aberrations noted are gains of chromosomes 5 and 7, with tandem duplications of 7q34 found in more than 50% of low-grade astrocytomas in children.[33–35] Several other studies have demonstrated that the *BRAF* proto-oncogene is duplicated in 55% of pilocytic tumors.[33–35] Interestingly, subsequent studies have shown that tandem duplication at 7q34 results in an in-frame fusion gene incorporating the kinase domain of the *BRAF* oncogene, fused to *KIAA1549,* a previously uncharacterized gene located approximately 2 megabase (Mb) from *BRAF.*[35] This frequent tumor specific aberration has great potential as a novel therapeutic target.

Neurofibromatosis type 1 (NF1) has been linked to pilocytic astrocytoma formation in several locations (optic nerve, hypothalamus, and cerebellum). This syndrome is caused by mutations of the *NF1* gene on chromosome 17q. This gene encodes neurofibromin, a guanosine triphosphatase (GTPase)-activating protein that controls astrocytic proliferation and neuronal differentiation by silencing mitogen-activated protein kinase (MAPK) signaling. Inactivating mutations of the *NF1* gene leads to increased Ras activity and astrocyte proliferation. Aberrant activation of Ras signaling may thus be responsible for the formation of low-grade astrocytomas in 15 to 20% of NF1 patients. Activating mutations of *KRAS* also result in the activation of MAPK signaling and have been reported in a small fraction of sporadic pilocytic astrocytomas.[36] Interestingly, genome-wide RNA profiling demonstrates that MAPK pathway target genes are induced in sporadic as well as NF1-associated pilocytic astrocytomas. Finally, some sporadic pilocytic astrocytomas that do not show a loss of the *NF1* gene demonstrate activation of the mammalian target of rapamycin (mTOR) pathway, albeit through different mechanisms.

Low-grade astrocytomas generally occur in a single location and do not tend to spread via CSF pathways. Low-grade astrocytomas typically are well circumscribed, and gross total resection can be curative (90% overall survival at 5 years).[31,37] In contrast, optic pathway gliomas are generally not surgically resectable without severely compromising vision. For most children, every attempt should be made to delay radiation as long as possible.

In older patients, radiation is generally well tolerated and can be effective in treating growing lesions in unforgiving locations. However, with the desire to avoid radiation therapy in young patients, several trials have demonstrated a role for chemotherapy in stabilizing or attenuating lesions.[38,39]

Oligodendrogliomas

Oligodendrogliomas are rare tumors that account for approximately 2% of all primary brain tumors, approximately 6% of gliomas, and approximately 1% of all pediatric brain tumors.[40] In children, the majority of oligodendrogliomas are supratentorial (**Fig. 29.5**), commonly found in frontal, temporal, parietal, hypothalamic, and intraventricular locations. Seizures are the typical presentation of grade II lesions, whereas manifestations of mass effect are typical of the faster-growing, anaplastic variant (WHO grade III).

Histologically, low-grade oligodendroglioma (grade II) is characterized by uniformly round to oval cells with round nuclei and bland chromatin. The morphology of these cells is often referred to as the "fried-egg" appearance, largely due to a perinuclear halo. A network of branching blood vessels in a "chicken-wire" pattern is also indicative. Over time, low-grade oligodendrogliomas tend to gradually become more anaplastic, demonstrating high cell density, mitoses, nuclear atypia, microvascular proliferation, and necrosis (grade III). However, anaplastic tumors may occasionally present in children without a low-grade precursor lesion.

The most frequently reported chromosomal aberrations in oligodendroglioma are the allelic loss of 1p and 19q loci.[41] The incidence of either 1p or 19q chromosomal deletions in oligodendroglioma is approximately 75%, whereas the combined loss of 1p and 19q is observed in 60 to 70% of all oligodendrogliomas.[42] Anaplastic tumors usually have additional chromosomal deletions, in particular loss of heterozygosity for 9p and deletion of the *CDKN2A* gene. This occurs in 33 to 42% of anaplastic oligodendrogliomas, and deletions on chromosome 10 occur in 19 to 25% of cases.[43] Combined morphological and genetic analyses suggest that oligodendroglial tumors with classic histological appearance show 1p/19q co-deletions, whereas in tumors with an atypical appearance other chromosomal abnormalities are found (e.g., *TP53* mutations).[44] Furthermore, isocitrate dehydrogenase (IDH) mutations have been detected in up to 80% of grade II and III oligodendrogliomas.[45] Interestingly, it has been shown that virtually all 1p/19q co-deleted lesions harbor IDH mutation, suggesting a potential link between both alterations.[46] More recently, recurrent point mutations of CIC (*Drosophila capicua*) and FUBP1 (far upstream element binding protein 1) have been identified in oligodendrogliomas and particularly in 1p/19q co-deleted tumors using high-throughput sequencing.[47,48]

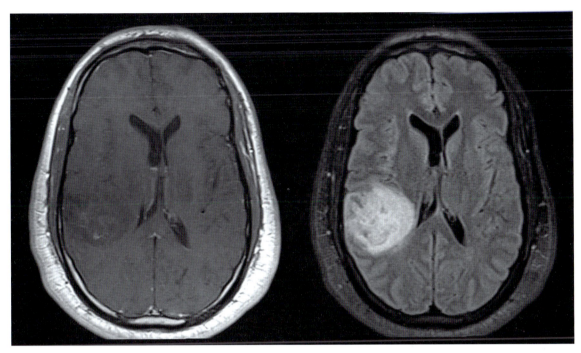

Fig. 29.5 T1-weighted axial image with contrast and an axial fluid-attenuated inversion recovery (FLAIR) image showing an intrinsic right parietal oligodendroglioma with effacement of the overlying gyri. Solid components tend to show homogeneous T2 prolongation. Prominent cortical thickening may distinguish these tumors from other astrocytic neoplasms.

Pitfall

- The clinical behavior of oligodendroglioma is heterogeneous, even within the same pathological grade, with a median overall survival of patients varying from 3.5 to 15 years and from 2 to 5 years in grade II and grade III tumors, respectively.

Oligodendrogliomas are managed with a combination of surgery, radiation, and chemotherapy. In children, low-grade tumors may behave in a more benign fashion, with no additional therapy required postoperatively. Unfortunately, no histology-based subgroup analysis of radiotherapy in children with oligodendroglioma is available. Until randomized controlled studies are conducted, a prudent approach for treating young patients with low-grade oligodendroglioma that have undergone a complete or near-complete resection may be to observe the patient and withhold radiotherapy until progression. In contrast, patients with large unresectable or incompletely resected tumors, or those with anaplastic histology, should receive radiotherapy without delay.

In 1994, Cairncross and Macdonald[49] first observed very favorable responses in recurrent anaplastic oligodendroglioma treated with PCV chemotherapy (consisting of procarbazine, chloroethylcyclohexylnitrosourea [CCNU], and vincristine). Further studies demonstrated that approximately two thirds of patients with recurrent lesions have either a complete or partial response to PCV. This has made PCV the standard treatment for patients with recurrent oligodendroglioma following radiotherapy, regardless of the grade of the tumor. More recent publications focus on first-line temozolomide in recurrent anaplastic oligodendroglioma after prior radiotherapy. Response rates vary between 46% and 55%, with 12-month progression-free survival between 40% and 50% and a median progression-free survival of 10 to 12 months.[50,51]

Glioneuronal Tumors

The classification of glioneuronal tumors has grown over time, and the recently updated WHO Classification of Tumors of the Central Nervous System expands the classification of tumors of mixed glioneuronal type.[52] This is largely due to the availability of new histological techniques, which have enabled improved identification of neuronal differentiation in tumors that morphologically resemble glial neoplasms.

Ganglioglioma represents approximately 4 to 8% of primary brain tumors in children. This tumor is marked by the presence of both an atypical ganglion cell component combined with a glioma component. The astrocytic element often resembles a low-grade fibrillary astrocytoma, pilocytic astrocytoma, or occasionally oligodendroglioma. Gangliogliomas are designated as WHO grade I lesions with an excellent prognosis. Rare examples of more aggressive behaving tumors, marked by increased mitotic activity and areas of necrosis, have been recognized with a designation of anaplastic ganglioglioma (grade III).[53] Approximately 90% of gangliogliomas are supratentorial (**Fig. 29.6**), with the temporal lobe being the most common location followed by the frontal, occipital, and parietal lobes, and the diencephalon.[54,55] Imaging may reveal cystic, well-circumscribed components with gyral expansion. Most patients with ganglioglioma typically present with a long history of medically intractable epilepsy, and frequently there is cortical dysplasia of adjacent cortex. The desmoplastic infantile ganglioglioma is marked by superficial location, early age of presentation, and a morphology demonstrating a collagenous matrix supporting a mixture of spindled astrocytic and ganglionic cells.[56] These tumors generally behave in a benign fashion as well and are designated as grade I neoplasms.

The dysembryoplastic neuroepithelial tumor (DNET) is a mixed glioneuronal neoplasm that may arise during embryogenesis. These grade I lesions often present in children and teenagers, typically during the first or second decade of life, as an incidental finding or with seizures. On imaging studies, it usually presents as a multinodular, focally cystic lesion in the temporal or frontal cortex (**Fig. 29.7**). It carries a good prognosis after surgical excision, with only rare recurrence. Histologically, cells resemble mature oligodendrocytes intermixed with normal-appearing neurons that appear to float within mucinous pools. As with gangliogliomas, adjacent areas of cortical dysplasia may be found in association. A specific genetic basis for DNET has not been identified, although it has been proposed that DNET arises from the secondary germinal matrix.

The treatment of ganglioglioma and DNET involves gross total surgical resection and is aimed primarily at seizure control and prevention of recurrence. Many authors utilize electrocorticography to ensure removal of abnormal peritumoral cortex and report increased rates of seizure cure.[57,58] Some support the addition of anterior temporal lobectomy and amygdalohippocampectomy into the surgical plan to ensure better long-term seizure control.[57] For lesions outside the temporal lobe, lesionectomy alone will provide good seizure control.

Central neurocytoma often arises from the fornix, the subependymal cell layer of the lateral ventricle near the foramen of Monro, or the septum pellucidum, and extends into the lateral or third ventricle. It represents only 0.1 to 0.5% of all intracranial tumors.[59] Central neurocytoma presents in young

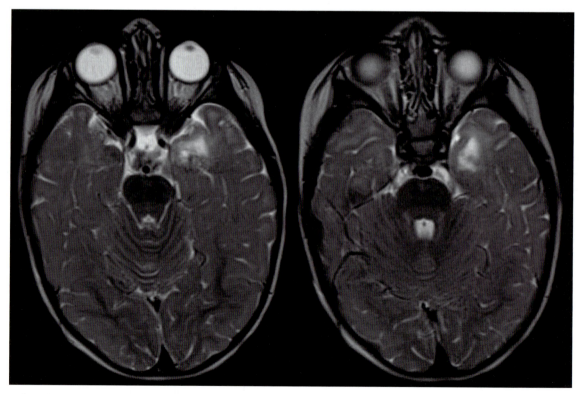

Fig. 29.6 Serial axial T2-weighted images consistent with an anterior left temporal ganglioglioma. These tumors may be completely solid or partly cystic in appearance. Solid components of these tumors show T1 and T2 prolongation relative to gray matter. Contrast enhancement is a variable finding.

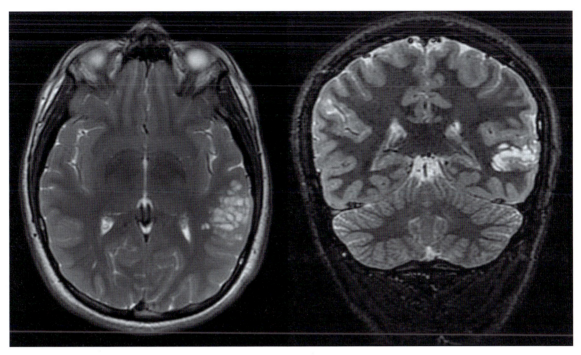

Fig. 29.7 Axial T2-weighted and coronal FLAIR images showing the "soap bubble" appearance of a tumor of the left superior temporal gyrus consistent with dysembryoplastic neuroepithelial tumor (DNET). Cystic components are common, and contrast enhancement, if present, tends to be nodular.

adults as a well-demarcated, often calcified lesion. Patients typically present with signs and symptoms of CSF outflow obstruction at the foramen of Monro (progressive headache, nausea, vomiting, diplopia, etc.). The neuronal component of this tumor is composed of a monotonous proliferation of cells, which can sometimes exhibit a "salt-and-pepper" chromatin staining pattern. Central neurocytomas sometimes show Homer Wright rosettes with occasional perivascular rosettes. Central neurocytoma is considered a benign lesion, and surgical resection is necessary in most cases for diagnosis and relief of CSF outflow obstruction. Most patients experience good long-term tumor control, with gross total resection providing cure.

■ Benign Tumors

Pediatric Meningiomas

Supratentorial meningiomas are relatively uncommon in children, accounting for approximately 4% of pediatric brain tumors and approximately 1.5% of all meningiomas. As in adult meningiomas, these tumors arise from arachnoid cap cells of the dura but tend to have a propensity for more aggressive histology.[60] Children typically present with larger tumors than adults (**Fig. 29.8**), with an average diameter of 5 to 6 cm.[61] Common locations in the pediatric population include the skull base and tentorium, as well as intraventricular and even

intraparenchymal sites with no proximity to the dural surface.[62] Intraventricular tumors may present with obstructive hydrocephalus or seizures, whereas skull base lesions may present with visual loss or proptosis.[63] The pathognomonic whorls and psammoma bodies of adult meningiomas are rarely seen in pediatric tumors. Childhood lesions are typically composed of uniform cells with oval nuclei that may resemble normal arachnoid cap cells.[52]

Neurofibromatosis type 2 (NF2) and Gorlin syndrome are both associated with an increased incidence of meningiomas in pediatric patients.[64] NF2 is caused by mutation of the gene responsible for production of the merlin protein, located on chromosome 22. This disorder is inherited in autosomal dominant fashion, and 50 to 75% of NF2 patients may develop meningiomas in several locations.[64] Gorlin syndrome (multiple basal cell nevus syndrome) is an autosomal dominant disorder caused by mutations in the *PTCH* gene (patched) found on chromosome 9q and is associated with a constellation of neoplasms, notably medulloblastomas and meningiomas. In addition, children who have been radiated early in life (patients with medulloblastoma, leukemia, etc.) may develop

Pearl

- Neurofibromatosis type 2 (NF2) and Gorlin syndrome are both associated with an increased incidence of meningiomas in pediatric patients.

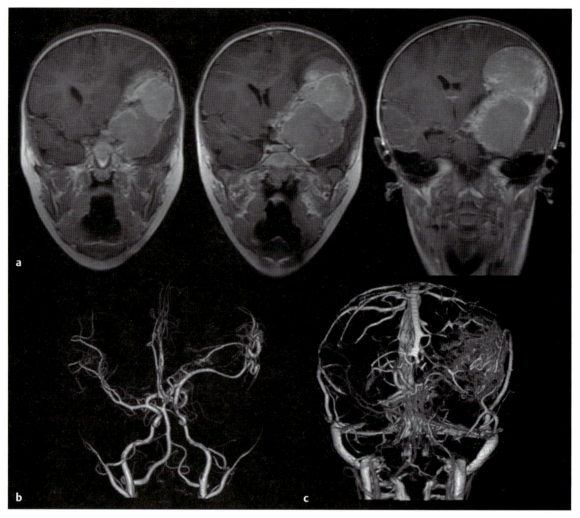

Fig. 29.8a–c (**a**) Serial coronal T1-weighted images with contrast showing a large anterior left skull base meningioma in a child with extension into the frontal and temporal lobes. (**b**) Arterial and (**c**) venous computed tomography (CT) angiographic imaging shows significant vascularity. In children, these tumors tend to show CT density and magnetic resonance signal intensity similar to that of gray matter with intense, homogeneous contrast enhancement.

radiation-induced meningiomas as early as 2 years after therapy. Thus, surveillance MRI scans well into adulthood are recommended in all children receiving cranial radiation.

As with most benign tumors, definitive treatment for meningiomas is complete surgical resection. As in adults, endovascular embolization of the arterial blood supply can aid in resection by drastically decreasing intraoperative blood loss, which may be especially important in smaller children. Although complete surgical resection remains the preferred treatment modality, radiation is effective adjuvant therapy, especially for unresectable, recurrent, or high-grade tumors.[65] Moderate success with interferon-α_{2B} and hydroxyurea chemotherapy has been noted in refractory meningiomas.[66,67]

In general, overall prognosis in children with meningioma is worse than in adults. This has been attributed largely to more aggressive pathology in combination with greater tumor volume at presentation. In a large series of pediatric tumors,

5-year survival for grade I, II, and III lesions are 84%, 44%, and 35%, respectively.[65] Confounding associations such as NF2 and Gorlin syndrome generally worsen the prognosis. Thus, serial imaging and lifelong follow-up are needed in children with meningioma.

■ Conclusion

A diverse array of tumors arises within the supratentorial compartment of children, representing both glial and nonglial neoplasms. Presenting symptoms may vary extensively, largely dependent on tumor location and rate of growth. Diagnosis of these lesions remains paramount in affecting survival and may be difficult based on neuroimaging alone. At present, the extent of surgical resection is the most important determinant of survival for the majority of patients with these neoplasms. Optimal patient care and treatment of these tumors is obtained at centers staffed by experienced practitioners of pediatric neurosurgery, neuroradiology, neuropathology, and neuro-oncology. Such multidisciplinary centers should be sought out soon after identification of brain tumors in children.

Editor's Note

Not much has changed over the past decade in this area of pediatric neuro-oncology in terms of classification and management. These tumors are various types of low-grade lesions that are cortically based or within the ventricle, although high-grade tumors can and do occur in this age group. Our understanding of the molecular genetics of these different lesions has improved significantly, allowing us to better understand how to predict the clinical course of these diseases. These lesions need to be aggressively resected, and in virtually every setting, whether they are high- or low-grade tumors, these children do better when a radical resection is done before any therapeutic regime is started. The goal has always been to do this with the least amount of morbidity, and, fortunately, with improvements in microsurgical technique as well as intraoperative navigation and intraoperative MRI scanning, the extent of surgery has continued to improve without increasing morbidity. These are very rare lesions and are best managed by pediatric neurosurgeons who are well versed in operating on very young children. The overarching goal is to present to the pediatric neuro-oncologist a child that is neurologically intact with the least amount of residual disease prior to any further therapy. In certain cases, such as low-grade gliomas, many of these children do not need to be treated once a radical resection has been completed, thus avoiding the potential problems associated with radiation and chemotherapy. (Berger)

References

1. Panigrahy A, Blüml S. Neuroimaging of pediatric brain tumors: from basic to advanced magnetic resonance imaging (MRI). J Child Neurol 2009;24:1343–1365
2. Pollack IF. Brain tumors in children. N Engl J Med 1994;331:1500–1507
3. Kaatsch P, Rickert CH, Kühl J, Schüz J, Michaelis J. Population-based epidemiologic data on brain tumors in German children. Cancer 2001;92:3155–3164
4. Rickert CH, Sträter R, Kaatsch P, et al. Pediatric high-grade astrocytomas show chromosomal imbalances distinct from adult cases. Am J Pathol 2001;158:1525–1532
5. Bredel M, Pollack IF, Hamilton RL, James CD. Epidermal growth factor receptor expression and gene amplification in high-grade non-brain-stem gliomas of childhood. Clin Cancer Res 1999;5:1786–1792
6. Sung T, Miller DC, Hayes RL, Alonso M, Yee H, Newcomb EW. Preferential inactivation of the p53 tumor suppressor pathway and lack of EGFR amplification distinguish de novo high grade pediatric astrocytomas from de novo adult astrocytomas. Brain Pathol 2000;10:249–259
7. Wisoff JH, Boyett JM, Berger MS, et al. Current neurosurgical management and the impact of the extent of resection in the treatment of malignant gliomas of childhood: a report of the Children's Cancer Group trial no. CCG-945. J Neurosurg 1998;89:52–59
8. Cohen KJ, Broniscer A, Glod J. Pediatric glial tumors. Curr Treat Options Oncol 2001;2:529–536
9. Raffel C, Frederick L, O'Fallon JR, et al. Analysis of oncogene and tumor suppressor gene alterations in pediatric malignant astrocytomas reveals reduced survival for patients with PTEN mutations. Clin Cancer Res 1999;5:4085–4090
10. Cheng Y, Ng HK, Zhang SF, et al. Genetic alterations in pediatric high-grade astrocytomas. Hum Pathol 1999;30:1284–1290
11. Pollack IF. The role of surgery in pediatric gliomas. J Neurooncol 1999;42:271–288
12. Cohen KJ, Pollack IF, Zhou T, et al. Temozolomide in the treatment of high-grade gliomas in children: a report from the Children's Oncology Group. Neuro-oncol 2011;13:317–323
13. Qaddoumi I, Sultan I, Gajjar A. Outcome and prognostic features in pediatric gliomas: a review of 6212 cases from the Surveillance, Epidemiology, and End Results database. Cancer 2009;115:5761–5770
14. Godfraind C. Classification and controversies in pathology of ependymomas. Childs Nerv Syst 2009;25:1185–1193
15. Dyer S, Prebble E, Davison V, et al. Genomic imbalances in pediatric intracranial ependymomas define clinically relevant groups. Am J Pathol 2002;161:2133–2141
16. Milde T, Pfister S, Korshunov A, et al. Stepwise accumulation of distinct genomic aberrations in a patient with progressively metastasizing ependymoma. Genes Chromosomes Cancer 2009;48:229–238
17. Mendrzyk F, Korshunov A, Benner A, et al. Identification of gains on 1q and epidermal growth factor receptor overexpression as independent prognostic markers in intracranial ependymoma. Clin Cancer Res 2006;12(7 Pt 1):2070–2079
18. Monoranu CM, Huang B, Zangen IL, et al. Correlation between 6q25.3 deletion status and survival in pediatric intracranial ependymomas. Cancer Genet Cytogenet 2008;182:18–26
19. Taylor MD, Poppleton H, Fuller C, et al. Radial glia cells are candidate stem cells of ependymoma. Cancer Cell 2005;8:323–335
20. Ridley L, Rahman R, Brundler MA, et al; Children's Cancer and Leukaemia Group Biological Studies Committee. Multifactorial analysis of predictors of outcome in pediatric intracranial ependymoma. Neuro-oncol 2008;10:675–689
21. Merchant TE, Li C, Xiong X, Kun LE, Boop FA, Sanford RA. Conformal radiotherapy after surgery for paediatric ependymoma: a prospective study. Lancet Oncol 2009;10:258–266
22. Krutilkova V, Trkova M, Fleitz J, et al. Identification of five new families strengthens the link between childhood choroid plexus carcinoma and germline TP53 mutations. Eur J Cancer 2005;41:1597–1603

23. Wrede B, Liu P, Wolff JE. Chemotherapy improves the survival of patients with choroid plexus carcinoma: a meta-analysis of individual cases with choroid plexus tumors. J Neurooncol 2007;85:345–351

24. Wolff JE, Sajedi M, Brant R, Coppes MJ, Egeler RM. Choroid plexus tumours. Br J Cancer 2002;87:1086–1091

25. Hilden JM, Meerbaum S, Burger P, et al. Central nervous system atypical teratoid/rhabdoid tumor: results of therapy in children enrolled in a registry. J Clin Oncol 2004;22:2877–2884

26. Zhang F, Tan L, Wainwright LM, Bartolomei MS, Biegel JA. No evidence for hypermethylation of the hSNF5/INI1 promoter in pediatric rhabdoid tumors. Genes Chromosomes Cancer 2002;34:398–405

27. Eaton KW, Tooke LS, Wainwright LM, Judkins AR, Biegel JA. Spectrum of SMARCB1/INI1 mutations in familial and sporadic rhabdoid tumors. Pediatr Blood Cancer 2011;56:7–15

28. Judkins AR, Burger PC, Hamilton RL, et al. INI1 protein expression distinguishes atypical teratoid/rhabdoid tumor from choroid plexus carcinoma. J Neuropathol Exp Neurol 2005;64:391–397

29. Finkelstein-Shechter T, Gassas A, Mabbott D, et al. Atypical teratoid or rhabdoid tumors: improved outcome with high-dose chemotherapy. J Pediatr Hematol Oncol 2010;32:e182–e186

30. Tekautz TM, Fuller CE, Blaney S, et al. Atypical teratoid/rhabdoid tumors (ATRT): improved survival in children 3 years of age and older with radiation therapy and high-dose alkylator-based chemotherapy. J Clin Oncol 2005;23:1491–1499

31. Burkhard C, Di Patre PL, Schüler D, et al. A population-based study of the incidence and survival rates in patients with pilocytic astrocytoma. J Neurosurg 2003;98:1170–1174

32. Broniscer A, Baker SJ, West AN, et al. Clinical and molecular characteristics of malignant transformation of low-grade glioma in children. J Clin Oncol 2007;25:682–689

33. Pfister S, Janzarik WG, Remke M, et al. BRAF gene duplication constitutes a mechanism of MAPK pathway activation in low-grade astrocytomas. J Clin Invest 2008;118:1739–1749

34. Bar EE, Lin A, Tihan T, Burger PC, Eberhart CG. Frequent gains at chromosome 7q34 involving BRAF in pilocytic astrocytoma. J Neuropathol Exp Neurol 2008;67:878–887

35. Jones DT, Kocialkowski S, Liu L, et al. Tandem duplication producing a novel oncogenic BRAF fusion gene defines the majority of pilocytic astrocytomas. Cancer Res 2008;68:8673–8677

36. Sharma MK, Zehnbauer BA, Watson MA, Gutmann DH. RAS pathway activation and an oncogenic RAS mutation in sporadic pilocytic astrocytoma. Neurology 2005;65:1335–1336

37. Sievert AJ, Fisher MJ. Pediatric low-grade gliomas. J Child Neurol 2009;24:1397–1408

38. Packer RJ, Ater J, Allen J, et al. Carboplatin and vincristine chemotherapy for children with newly diagnosed progressive low-grade gliomas. J Neurosurg 1997;86:747–754

39. Gururangan S, Fisher MJ, Allen JC, et al. Temozolomide in children with progressive low-grade glioma. Neuro-oncol 2007;9:161–168

40. Creach KM, Rubin JB, Leonard JR, et al. Oligodendrogliomas in children. J Neurooncol 2012;106:377–382

41. Reifenberger J, Reifenberger G, Liu L, James CD, Wechsler W, Collins VP. Molecular genetic analysis of oligodendroglial tumors shows preferential allelic deletions on 19q and 1p. Am J Pathol 1994;145:1175–1190

42. Smith JS, Alderete B, Minn Y, et al. Localization of common deletion regions on 1p and 19q in human gliomas and their association with histological subtype. Oncogene 1999;18:4144–4152

43. Bigner SH, Matthews MR, Rasheed BK, et al. Molecular genetic aspects of oligodendrogliomas including analysis by comparative genomic hybridization. Am J Pathol 1999;155:375–386

44. van den Bent MJ, Looijenga LH, Langenberg K, et al. Chromosomal anomalies in oligodendroglial tumors are correlated with clinical features. Cancer 2003;97:1276–1284

45. Yan H, Parsons DW, Jin G, et al. IDH1 and IDH2 mutations in gliomas. N Engl J Med 2009;360:765–773

46. Labussière M, Idbaih A, Wang XW, et al. All the 1p19q codeleted gliomas are mutated on IDH1 or IDH2. Neurology 2010;74:1886–1890

47. Bettegowda C, Agrawal N, Jiao Y, et al. Mutations in CIC and FUBP1 contribute to human oligodendroglioma. Science 2011;333:1453–1455

48. Yip S, Butterfield YS, Morozova O, et al. Concurrent CIC mutations, IDH mutations, and 1p/19q loss distinguish oligodendrogliomas from other cancers. J Pathol 2012;226:7–16

49. Cairncross G, Macdonald D, Ludwin S, Lee D, Cascino T, Buckner J, et al. Chemotherapy for anaplastic oligodendroglioma. J Clin Oncol 1994;12(10):2013–2021

50. Brandes AA, Tosoni A, Cavallo G, et al; GICNO. Correlations between O6-methylguanine DNA methyltransferase promoter methylation status, 1p and 19q deletions, and response to temozolomide in anaplastic and recurrent oligodendroglioma: a prospective GICNO study. J Clin Oncol 2006;24:4746–4753

51. van den Bent MJ, Taphoorn MJ, Brandes AA, et al; European Organization for Research and Treatment of Cancer Brain Tumor Group. Phase II study of first-line chemotherapy with temozolomide in recurrent oligodendroglial tumors: the European Organization for Research and Treatment of Cancer Brain Tumor Group Study 26971. J Clin Oncol 2003;21:2525–2528

52. Louis DN, Ohgaki H, Wiestler OD, et al. The 2007 WHO classification of tumours of the central nervous system. Acta Neuropathol 2007;114:97–109

53. Luyken C, Blümcke I, Fimmers R, Urbach H, Wiestler OD, Schramm J. Supratentorial gangliogliomas: histopathologic grading and tumor recurrence in 184 patients with a median follow-up of 8 years. Cancer 2004;101:146–155

54. Blümcke I, Wiestler OD. Gangliogliomas: an intriguing tumor entity associated with focal epilepsies. J Neuropathol Exp Neurol 2002;61:575–584

55. Zentner J, Wolf HK, Ostertun B, et al. Gangliogliomas: clinical, radiological, and histopathological findings in 51 patients. J Neurol Neurosurg Psychiatry 1994;57:1497–1502

56. VandenBerg SR, May EE, Rubinstein LJ, et al. Desmoplastic supratentorial neuroepithelial tumors of infancy with divergent differentiation potential ("desmoplastic infantile gangliogliomas"). Report on 11 cases of a distinctive embryonal tumor with favorable prognosis. J Neurosurg 1987;66:58–71

57. Morioka T, Hashiguchi K, Nagata S, et al. Additional hippocampectomy in the surgical management of intractable temporal lobe epilepsy associated with glioneuronal tumor. Neurol Res 2007;29:807–815

58. Pilcher WH, Silbergeld DL, Berger MS, Ojemann GA. Intraoperative electrocorticography during tumor resection: impact on seizure outcome in patients with gangliogliomas. J Neurosurg 1993;78:891–902

59. Schmidt MH, Gottfried ON, von Koch CS, Chang SM, McDermott MW. Central neurocytoma: a review. J Neurooncol 2004;66:377–384

60. Gao X, Zhang R, Mao Y, Wang Y. Childhood and juvenile meningiomas. Childs Nerv Syst 2009;25:1571–1580

61. Lakhdar F, Arkha Y, El Ouahabi A, et al. Intracranial meningioma in children: different from adult forms? A series of 21 cases. Neurochirurgie 2010;56:309–314

62. Liu Y, Li F, Zhu S, Liu M, Wu C. Clinical features and treatment of meningiomas in children: report of 12 cases and literature review. Pediatr Neurosurg 2008;44:112–117

63. Rohringer M, Sutherland GR, Louw DF, Sima AA. Incidence and clinicopathological features of meningioma. J Neurosurg 1989;71(5 Pt 1):665–672

64. Goutagny S, Kalamarides M. Meningiomas and neurofibromatosis. J Neurooncol 2010;99:341–347

65. Glaholm J, Bloom HJ, Crow JH. The role of radiotherapy in the management of intracranial meningiomas: the Royal Marsden Hospital experience with 186 patients. Int J Radiat Oncol Biol Phys 1990;18:755–761
66. Kaba SE, DeMonte F, Bruner JM, et al. The treatment of recurrent unresectable and malignant meningiomas with interferon alpha-2B. Neurosurgery 1997;40:271–275
67. Schrell UM, Rittig MG, Anders M, et al. Hydroxyurea for treatment of unresectable and recurrent meningiomas. II. Decrease in the size of meningiomas in patients treated with hydroxyurea. J Neurosurg 1997; 86:840–844

30 Pineal Region Tumors

Adam M. Sonabend, Alfred T. Ogden, and Jeffrey N. Bruce

Despite sharing a common anatomic location and often displaying similar imaging characteristics, pineal region tumors are extremely heterogeneous with respect to histopathology, natural history, and response to therapy. Moreover, due to their relatively uncommon nature (only 1.2% of all primary central nervous system [CNS] tumors),[1] the study of their behavior and outcomes is compromised by limited clinical information. Historically, these tumors were considered unresectable, and the first strides in treatment were made with conventional radiotherapy, often pursued without a tissue diagnosis. At the time, this approach was justified because some previously untreatable pineal region tumors could be cured with radiotherapy.

Under current standards, conventional radiation is only appropriate for certain histologically verified malignant tumors. Approximately 30% of pineal tumors are benign and can be cured with gross total resection, which, in the contemporary microsurgery era, can be achieved with low rates of morbidity. Stereotactic radiosurgery is a potential alternative, particularly in patients with medical contraindications to open surgery.

Determining the most effective treatment strategies for malignant lesions is an ongoing process. The roles of all modalities, including surgery, radiation, radiosurgery, and chemotherapy, are being defined by outcomes from clinical trials and databases. As a result of these efforts, the prognoses of certain types of malignant tumors have already greatly improved. Advances in diagnosis and treatment of these rare and heterogeneous tumors are predicated on accurately establishing tumor cell type and grade. Although, in rare cases, a diagnosis can be made on the basis of circulating tumor-specific markers, the vast majority of pineal tumors can only be accurately diagnosed with ample tissue sampling.

Historical Background

In the first half of the 20th century, small surgical series from some of the early giants in neurosurgery, including Cushing, Dandy, and van Wagnenen, illustrated the futility of safe pineal region surgery using the rudimentary surgical equipment of the time. In the words of Dandy, this experience was "disastrous ... almost to indicate the futility of other efforts."[2] When radiotherapy was introduced in the middle of the 20th cen-

> **Controversial Point**
>
> - Tissue diagnosis for a pineal region tumor can be made via a diagnostic biopsy or an open surgical approach. The decision should be made after a thorough discussion of the risks and benefits of each option between the physician and patient.

tury, pineal region surgery had advanced little, and surgical approaches were still considered too dangerous, even for the limited goal of obtaining diagnostic tissue. Contemporary opinion was reflected through Poppen, a pioneer in surgical approaches to the pineal region, who, as recently as 1968, favored "X-ray therapy unless unusually critical conditions necessitate immediate surgical intervention."[3]

Radiotherapy without tissue diagnosis, along with shunting for hydrocephalus, became the standard of care. This strategy resulted in acceptable 5-year survival rates ranging from 58 to 70%, reflecting the prevalence and exquisite radiosensitivity of germinomas and the overall slow growth rates of many tumors found in the pineal region.[4–6]

By the early 1970s, routine use of the operating microscope, the development of microneurosurgical techniques, advances in neuroanesthesia, and the advent of neurologic critical care as a subspecialty helped to usher in the modern era of neurosurgery, in which many operative goals that were considered too dangerous or impossible were now attainable.

The demonstration of safe, effective pineal region surgery by Stein[7] using the infratentorial supracerebellar approach adapted from Krause, and by Jamieson[8] using the occipital transtentorial approach adapted from Poppen, required that the role of radical surgery be reexamined. Since these seminal papers were published in 1971, numerous surgical series have demonstrated safe effective surgical approaches to the pineal region over a large number of patients (**Table 30.1**). Similarly, the introduction and refinement of stereotaxy have improved the safety and efficacy of biopsies in the pineal region. Thus surgical management of pineal region tumors has advanced to the point where a tissue diagnosis to direct therapy is mandatory for patients with negative serum tumor markers, and open surgical resection is a viable tool whose relative merits depend on tumor histology.

Table 30.1 Results of Large Microsurgical Series of Pineal Region Tumors

Authors	Year	No. of Cases	Approach	Patient Population	Pathology	GTR (%)	Mortality (%)	Major Morbidity (%)	Permanent Minor Morbidity (%)
Hoffman et al[68]	1994	61	TCIH ITSC	Pediatric	All	NA	20	NA	NA
Neuwelt et al[69]	1985	13	OTT	Adult/pediatric	All	60	0	0	20
Lapras et al[70]	1987	86	TCIH OTT	Adult/pediatric	All	65	5.8	5.8	28
Edwards et al[57]	1988	36	TT OTT ITSC	Pediatric	All	?	0	3.3	3.3
Pluchino et al[71]	1989	40	ITSC	Adult/pediatric	All	25	5	NA	NA
Luo et al[72]	1989	64	OTT	Adult/pediatric	All	21	10		NA
Vaquero et al[73]	1992	29	TCIH ITSC OTT	Adult/pediatric	All	NA	11	NA	NA
Herrmann et al[74]	1992	49	TCIH ITSC	Adult/pediatric	All	NA	8	NA	NA
Bruce and Stein[21]	1995	160	ITSC TCIH OTT	Adult/pediatric	All	45	4	3	19
Chandy and Damaraju[29]	1998	48	ITSC OTT	Adult/pediatric	"Benign lesions"	55	0	NA	NA
Kang et al[75]	1998	16	OTT ITSC TCIH	Adult/pediatric	All	37.5	0	0	19
Shin et al[76]	1998	21	OTT	Pediatric/adult	All	54.5	0	0	5
Konovalov et al[23]	2003	201	OTT ITSC	Adult/pediatric	All	58	10	NA	> 20
Bruce[13]	2011	128	ITSC TCIH OTT	Adult/pediatric	All	49	2	1	NA
Hernesniemi et al[12]	2008	119	ITSC OTT	Adult/pediatric	All	88	0	1	4.9

Abbreviations: TCIH, transcallosal interhemispheric; ITSC, infratentorial supracerebellar; OTT, occipital transtentorial; TT, transcortical transventricular; NA, not available.

Clinical Presentation and Preoperative Evaluation

The vast majority of patients with pineal region tumors present with symptoms of obstructive hydrocephalus: headache, nausea/vomiting, lethargy, and midbrain compression resulting in Parinaud's phenomena: impaired up-gaze, near-light dissociation, and convergence nystagmus.

Initial evaluation of a pineal region mass entails a directed medical history, a careful neurologic exam, serum assays for germ cell tumor markers, and a contrast-enhanced magnetic resonance imaging (MRI) study. Determination of the degree of hydrocephalus is critical to optimize immediate and subsequent management decisions. Elevated serum β-human chorionic gonadotrophin (β-hCG) is consistent with choriocarcinoma,

Pitfalls

- The standard workup for a pineal mass includes assays for germ cell markers. If they are present, radiation treatment can proceed without the need for a tissue diagnosis. Failure to order marker studies can result in an unindicated surgical procedure.
- Pineal cysts are simple cysts that are isointense to CSF and may show some rim enhancement on MRI. They should not be confused with pineal region tumors that are hyperintense to CSF and more densely enhancing. Pineal cysts can be followed with serial imaging and rarely require treatment.

although slight elevations can be found in germinomas with syncytiotrophoblastic elements. Elevated α-fetoprotein (AFP) is consistent with yolk sac and some embryonal carcinomas. Cerebrospinal fluid (CSF) is only marginally more sensitive for tumor markers than serum and, as such, carries little additional diagnostic potential. Whether detected in the serum or the CSF, positive germ markers are diagnostic for malignant germ cell tumors and obviate the need for a tissue diagnosis.

Cerebrospinal Fluid Sampling and Diversion

Hydrocephalus, usually from obstruction of the sylvian aqueduct, can be treated with ventriculoperitoneal shunting or endoscopic third ventriculostomy. In rare cases of mild hydrocephalus, a CSF-diverting procedure can be deferred if an open tumor resection is planned that will likely relieve the obstruction. In general, third ventriculostomy is preferred because it achieves CSF diversion without exposing patients to shunt-related complications, such as shunt malfunction, shunt infection, and abdominal seeding of a malignancy. Either procedure offers an opportunity to assay CSF for tumor markers and cytology. In rare cases, when hydrocephalus is not present, CSF sampling by lumbar puncture may be desirable prior to surgery, especially if CSF dissemination is apparent on preoperative imaging studies. After CSF diversion, if cytology and markers are negative, a procedure to obtain tissue is indicated, via a stereotactic, an endoscopic, or an open approach.

Pearls

- Endoscopic third ventriculostomy offers many advantages over ventriculoperitoneal shunting in cases of obstructive hydrocephalus from a pineal region mass.
- Mild asymptomatic hydrocephalus might resolve following resection of a pineal mass, obviating the need for CSF diversion.

Pitfall

- In the absence of positive tumor markers, treatment of pineal region tumors requires a histological diagnosis. Upfront radiation can result in an ineffective and unnecessary radiation exposure.

Diagnostic Biopsy

Stereotactic Biopsy

Stereotactic biopsy of tumors in the pineal region carries an increased risk of hemorrhage compared with biopsies in other regions of the brain, although the clinical impact of this risk may be small. Proximity to numerous vascular structures and CSF spaces raises the likelihood of bleeding during tissue sampling and the possibility that even minor bleeding will fail to tamponade. Additionally, biopsy trajectories typically pass adjacent to the lateral ventricle, risking penetration of pial surfaces en route to the stereotactic target. Biopsy series in which hemorrhage rates were calculated from systematic postoperative computed tomography (CT) scans found only a mildly increased incidence of biopsy-associated hemorrhages, the majority of which carried little, if any, clinical relevance.[9,10]

Some series have found a higher morbidity associated with pineal region biopsies compared with routine biopsies, whereas others have not. One retrospective multicenter study of 370 patients reported a mortality rate of 1.3%.[11] Overall, reported complications seen after stereotactic biopsy of pineal region tumors are almost always transient exacerbations of existing symptoms.

Although safe in experienced hands, stereotactic biopsy in the pineal region does require foresight and an appreciation of the complex anatomy surrounding the pineal region. An anterolateral-superior approach originating anterior to the coronal suture and lateral to the midpupillary line is usually preferred. Often a point just behind the hairline, at the superior temporal line, is convenient and cosmetic. This trajectory traverses the frontal lobe and internal capsule, staying lateral to the lateral ventricle (**Fig. 30.1**). Alternatively, a posterolateral-superior approach through an entry point at the parieto-occipital junction can be utilized but is most appropriate for tumors with lateral extension. In either case, multiple biopsies can be performed along the trajectory path to increase the diversity of tissue sampled.

Endoscopic Biopsy

Tissue can also be obtained endoscopically in the same sitting as a third ventriculostomy. Although a potentially elegant, "minimally invasive" surgical solution to CSF diversion and tissue diagnosis, it is only truly less invasive than separate diversion and biopsy procedures if performed through a single bur hole. With the vast majority of pineal region tumors, this requires the use of a flexible endoscope. Endoscopic biopsies carry a potentially higher risk of bleeding because the biopsy is taken through a ventricular surface where even minor and delayed bleeding can be difficult to control.

Drawbacks to Diagnostic Biopsy

The major drawback to diagnostic biopsies in the pineal region is limited tissue sampling. Pineal region tumors are incredibly varied, are sometimes of mixed histology, and require different treatment paradigms depending on histological differences that are subtle and difficult to recognize even in experienced hands. Thus whether tissue obtained through a

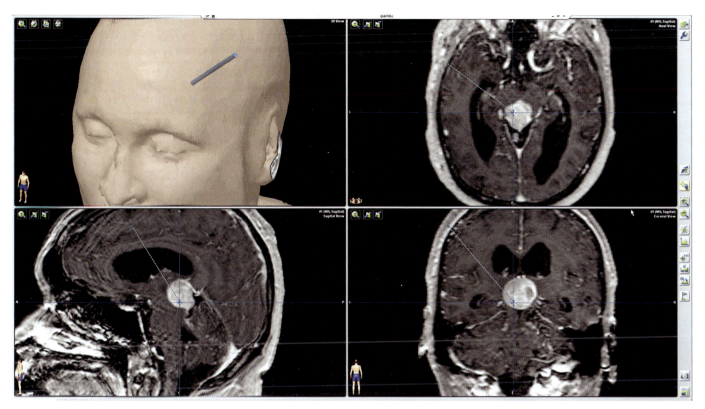

Fig. 30.1 Illustrative example of the trajectory employed for a stereotaxic needle biopsy of a pineal lesion. The trajectory has a precoronal and slightly lateral entry point to avoid the ventricular system, minimizing the traversing of pial boundaries and eloquent cortical territory.

diagnostic procedure is truly representative of the entire tumor is always debatable (**Fig. 30.2**).

have a complete contrast-enhanced MRI of the spine to look for metastases.

■ Staging

Once a histological diagnosis has been made, a management strategy should be developed in collaboration with radiation and oncology specialists. Patients with ependymomas, malignant germ cell tumors, or malignant pineal cell tumors should

Special Considerations

- Tumor types such as ependymoma, pineoblastoma, and germinoma that are known to spread along CSF spaces require contrast-enhanced total spine imaging after diagnosis to rule out drop metastases (**Fig. 30.3**).
- Pineal parenchymal tumors are notoriously difficult to grade accurately. Pathological diagnoses should be performed with as much representative tissue as possible, and confirmed by a neuropathologist with specific expertise in pineal tumors.

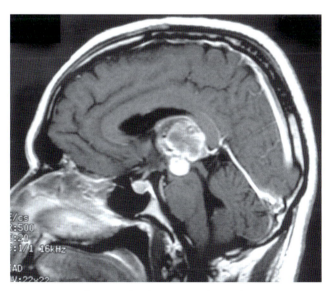

Fig. 30.2 Sagittal T1-weighted contrast-enhanced magnetic resonance imaging (MRI) shows a pineal region tumor with a heterogeneous pattern of enhancement. Tissue obtained after craniotomy demonstrated a mixed germ cell tumor.

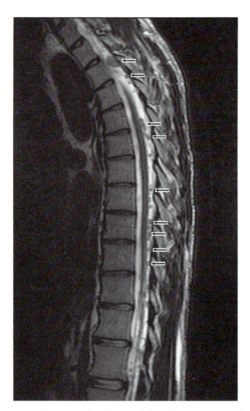

Fig. 30.3 Sagittal T2-weighted MRI of the thoracic spine of a patient with a history of a pineoblastoma shows nodular metastatic disease throughout the spinal axis (*arrows*).

◼ Open Surgery

Overview

Although a diagnostic biopsy is a reasonable first option in selected cases, an open approach is preferable in the majority of cases. Open surgery offers the potential to provide generous tissue sampling, to obviate a shunt by relieving obstructive hydrocephalus, and to proceed with a radical resection if indicated. Once tissue is obtained via an open approach, the decision to proceed with radical resection depends on an accurate histopathological diagnosis and the extent to which a particular diagnosis dictates a benefit from radical resection with an accepted rate of surgical morbidity.

Complications from open surgery range from transient exacerbations of existing symptoms to potentially devastating neurologic injury. Serious morbidity typically results from postoperative hematoma, venous infarction from vein sacri-

Pearl

• In some cases, gross total resection of a pineal region mass can obviate the need for a CSF diversion procedure.

fice, thalamic injury, air embolism in the setting of a sitting-position craniotomy, and visual deficits from occipital lobe retraction. Pineal region surgery is certainly not trivial, but within the last 25 years major morbidity and mortality from published surgical series have improved dramatically and have dropped to 0 to 2% in published surgical series (**Table 30.1**).[12,13]

Approaches

Several operative approaches to the pineal region have been described. The most effective and the most utilized are the supracerebellar-infratentorial approach, the interhemispheric transcallosal approach, and the occipital transtentorial approach.[7,13,14] The optimal approach for a specific patient depends, to a degree, on the anatomic features of the tumor but is also influenced by the surgeon's level of experience and comfort.

The supracerebellar-infratentorial approach is the most widely used and has the benefit of providing a direct midline approach through a natural corridor between the dorsal cerebellum and the tentorium (**Fig. 30.4**). This approach facilitates the dissection of the tumor from its attachment along the velum interpositum and deep venous system, which often represents the most difficult aspect of surgical removal.

The supratentorial approaches, including the occipital-transtentorial and the transcallosal-interhemispheric approaches, provide wider exposure than the infratentorial alternative but have the disadvantage of forcing the surgeon to work around and in between components of the deep venous

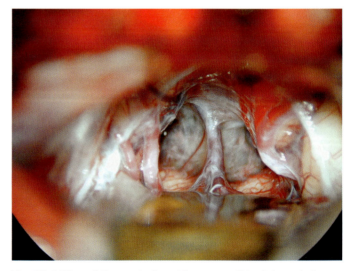

Fig. 30.4 View of the surgical corridor accomplished through the supracerebellar-infratentorial approach to the pineal region. Note the metal blade retracting the superior surface of the cerebellum on the floor of the corridor as well as the tentorium on the superior aspect of the corridor. Note the precentral cerebellar vein in the center of the field. This vein can be sacrificed to gain direct access the pineal gland and lesion (*center,* behind the vein).

Pearl

- Craniotomy as opposed to craniectomy for open pineal approaches results in better wound healing and more rapid postoperative recovery.

Controversy

- The incidence of spinal seeding is relatively low, and there is no compelling evidence supporting spinal radiation to prevent metastasis to the spine when no tumor is present on postoperative staging. Thus, the use of prophylactic spinal radiation for pineal region tumors is at best controversial, and has been largely abandoned.

system during tumor resection. The occipital-transtentorial approach requires occipital lobe retraction, which can result in visual field deficits, but once the tentorium is divided, excellent exposure to the pineal region from the quadrigeminal plate into the third ventricle is achievable. The transcallosal-interhemispheric approach requires retraction of the parietal lobe and often the sacrifice of bridging cortical veins to access the interhemispheric corridor.

Positioning

Several patient positions have been described and are somewhat interchangeable for the various approaches.[13,15] The sitting position is preferred for the supracerebellar-infratentorial approach because gravity aids tumor dissection while drawing venous blood away from the operative field.[15,16] Air embolus can be avoided with careful hemostatic technique, but the risk is increased in the sitting position. Still, the anesthesia team must be equipped to detect embolus early on, using a precordial Doppler and measuring end-tidal carbon dioxide. Other complications associated with the sitting position such as cortical collapse and subdural hematoma occur rarely.

The three-quarter-prone/lateral decubitus position is useful with the occipital transtentorial approach because gravity helps the dependent hemisphere to fall away from the falx. This position is relatively comfortable for the surgeon, although it does not avoid venous pooling. The prone position is suitable for parietal interhemispheric approaches; however, it often results in awkward lines of vision when used with an infratentorial approach. The Concorde position is supposed to combine elements of prone and sitting positions.[16] This position can be cumbersome, however, especially in adults, where the shoulder can be a vexing impediment to a comfortable arm position. The advantages of the Concorde position are perhaps best realized in pediatric patients whose small shoulders are easier for the surgeon to work around.

■ Radiation Therapy and Chemotherapy

Fractionated radiotherapy is indicated for patients with malignant glial, pineal, and germ cell tumors, and is usually withheld for patients with benign tumor histology who undergo gross total resection. The recommended radiation dose is 5,500 cGy given in 180-cGy daily fractions, with 4,000 cGy to the ventricular system and an additional 1,500 cGy to the tumor bed.[17,18]

Spinal radiation consisting of 3,500 cGy is given to all patients with pineoblastomas or any patient with documented CSF seeding (**Fig. 30.3**).

Chemotherapy is reserved for patients with nongerminomatous malignant germ cell tumors and children who are too young to receive radiation. There is no clear mandate on the role of adjuvant therapy for mixed pineal parenchymal neoplasms.

■ Stereotactic Radiosurgery

Studies of stereotactic radiosurgery demonstrate mixed results over small numbers of patients with tumors of a variety of histologies. Overall, the results reflect the natural history of the histology of the tumors treated, with good outcomes for benign lesions[18–20] and poor outcomes for malignant lesions.[17–19,21,22] The promising outcomes achieved with gross total resection of pineocytomas have set a high bar for efficacy of novel treatments for these low-grade tumors.[12,22,23] Outcomes following radiosurgical treatment of pineocytoma have been favorable as well,[17–19] although the few reported adult cases had only had a short follow-up[18] and included at least one adult treatment failure resulting in death from CNS metastasis.[17] One pediatric pineocytoma radiosurgical series reported four of seven treatment failures resulting in death during a follow-up of 3 months to 4 years,[24] although more recently, more favorable results have been reported.[25] The few published cases of stereotactic radiosurgery for pineoblastomas report poor results, with one report showing local tumor control of 30% at 2 years from diagnosis,[17–19,24,26] reflecting these tumors' malignant nature and potential to spread through CSF.

Stereotactic radiosurgery has an undefined role for nongerminomatous germ cell tumors (NGGCTs). One report of four patients who received radiosurgery along with fractionated radiation and chemotherapy showed tumor regression in three patients after a follow-up of 2 years.[20]

The relative utility of radiosurgery cannot be ascertained based on a few published cases except to say that radiosurgery is not a "magic bullet" for these lesions and does not address the metastatic potential of these tumors. Thus, it seems difficult to justify radiosurgical treatment without tissue diagnosis when such a course will result in ineffectual treatment and a delay to appropriate therapy in a larger percentage of patients. The relative merits of radiosurgery versus open surgery for tissue-diagnosed tumors will only be defined by further study.

■ Treatment Outcomes According to Histologic Type

Benign Pineal Region Tumors

Benign tumors account for about one third of the masses found in the pineal region. This group includes well-differentiated ependymomas, meningiomas, teratomas, pineocytomas, and rare pilocytic astrocytomas. In each case, gross total resection is the standard of care as long as it can be performed within a reasonable degree of safety. Surgical series demonstrate good outcomes over a range of pathologies, although there is a need in the literature for surgical outcomes to be analyzed according to specific histologies, with longer follow-up that includes data regarding adjuvant therapy. To date, there are only a few small surgical series, case reports, or systematic reviews that have been dedicated to benign pineal lesions of a single histological type.[27–32]

Glial Tumors

Pineal region tumors of glial differentiation are of four recognizable types: "true" pineal astrocytomas, brainstem astrocytomas, oligodendrogliomas, and ependymomas.[27,28,30,33,34] "True" pineal astrocytomas arise from the supporting astrocytes of the pineal gland itself. These tumors are cystic, encapsulated, and resemble pilocytic astrocytomas on histology.[28,35] They can be completely resected and have excellent long-term results. Brainstem astrocytomas arising from the tectum can extend rostrally into the pineal region. These lesions can manifest with obstructive hydrocephalus. Often, resection of lesions in the tectum is associated with auditory deficits. These tumors are solid, and, although they may be "low grade," are generally invasive. Therefore, some authors recommend irradiation after biopsy.[14,36–40] Ependymomas can arise anywhere along the third ventricle and can grow posteriorly in the pineal region.[41] Surgical outcomes from ependymomas are binary, depending on the degree of anaplasia. Pineal region ependymomas with low cellularity and few mitoses have excellent long-term outcomes, although they may recur more readily than ependymomas associated with the lateral ventricles.[41]

Papillary Tumor of the Pineal Region

Papillary tumor of the pineal region (PTPR) was first described in 2003,[42] and introduced as a distinct pathological tumor entity in the 2007 WHO classification of CNS tumors.[43] The cell of origin for these lesions is presumed to be specialized ependyma of the subcommissural organ.[42,44,45] Due to their recent identification as a separate entity, and their rarity, not much is known about their clinical behavior. A retrospective study of 31 patients by Fèvre-Montange et al,[46] the largest published series of these tumors, reported an age range from 5 to 66 years (median age, 29 years) and slight female predominance. Gross total resection was performed on 21 of 31 patients, and in 15, adjuvant radiotherapy was given. Despite aggressive treatment, the majority of patients had recurrences. The 5-year overall survival was 73%, with progression-free survival of 27%.[46] Details on these tumors' histological and immunohistochemical profile, as well as reliable methods for distinguishing papillary tumors from a differential diagnosis list that includes choroid plexus papillomas and metastatic carcinomas, have been reported.[44,46]

Pineal Parenchymal Tumors

Arising from the melatonin-producing cells of the pineal gland, pineal parenchymal tumors exist along a histopathological continuum from benign and indolent pineocytomas to malignant and aggressive pineoblastomas. Tumors of intermediate grade are referred to as mixed pineal parenchymal tumors or pineal parenchymal tumors of intermediate differentiation (PPTID) and various classification schemes tied to prognosis have been proposed.[22,47] Because making an accurate pathological diagnosis is difficult even with generous tissue sampling, grading along the parenchymal pineal tumor spectrum is especially challenging in the setting of an incisional biopsy. The value of an extensive specimen for pathological assessment is also supported by a series of markers that have been shown to bear prognostic implications independent of the tumor grade. For instance, a series of 33 pineal parenchymal tumors included six pineocytomas and 16 pineoblastomas, and all the pineocytomas and three of the pineoblastomas expressed neurofilament (NF) protein, a finding that proved to be a favorable prognostic factor independent of tumor grade. The median disease-free survival in NF-negative pineoblastomas was 5 months, compared to 32 months in NF-positive pinealoblastomas.[48] Ki-67 labeling index, a marker of proliferation, also differed among tumors of different grades, with mean labeling of 1.58% for pineocytomas, 16.1% for PPTID, and 23.52% for pineoblastomas.[48]

Pearl

- Pineocytomas should be managed with radical resection. Radiation therapy for residual disease does not seem to offer any benefit over observation.

The goal for all true pineocytomas should be a cure, at least in adults. The standard of care for pineocytoma has been validated by clinical experience of low recurrence rates with gross total resection as suggested by series where radical resection led to 100% survival at 40 months median follow-up.[12,22,23] In general, no adjuvant therapy is indicated for these tumors. Indeed, in the setting of subtotal resection, radiation does not seem to offer a significant benefit over observation, although these conclusions are based on retrospective data.[32] Gross total resection of pineocytomas may be unrealistic in children, in whom these tumors tend to behave more aggressively.[49]

Pineoblastomas often appear identical to pineocytomas on MRI. They are histologically indistinguishable from medulloblastomas and behave in a similar clinical fashion. Like medulloblastomas they tend to be more aggressive in children than in adults.[50] Moreover, within the pediatric population greater aggressivity correlates with decreasing age of presentation.[4,5,51] Although the data are not conclusive, there is some indication of increased survival in both adults[52] and children[53] undergoing open surgery. Given the similarities in histology and natural history between pineoblastomas and medulloblastomas, it is reasonable to apply to pineoblastoma the standard of care for medulloblastoma, for which significant survival benefits are apparent after surgical reduction of a tumor mass less than 1.5 cm.[3,54] As with medulloblastomas, whole neuraxis imaging for detection of metastatic disease is crucial following diagnosis of pineoblastoma. Similar to medulloblastomas, the major prognostic factors for pineoblastoma include age at presentation and metastatic dissemination at the time of diagnosis.

Pineal parenchymal tumors of intermediate differentiation behave in an unpredictable fashion, and there is little agreement on their optimal clinical management.[47,52,55] This is attributed to the fact that these intermediate-grade tumors can contain areas characteristic of a pineocytoma, whereas other areas may have a component representative of a pineoblastoma.[48] Although patients with subtotally resected intermediate-grade pineal parenchymal tumors are routinely irradiated after surgery, it is unclear whether this is universally required in cases with gross total resection of encapsulated tumors. A retrospective analysis of 101 adult patients with malignant pineal parenchymal tumors whose treatment included radiation therapy was reported.[52] The median follow-up period was 38 months, and the median overall survival was 100 months. In this study, disseminated disease,

grade (PPTID versus pineoblastoma), and > 50% of residual disease following resection were independent negative prognostic factors influencing overall survival following radiation on a multivariate analysis. The median survival in patients with local or spinal failure was 15 months; 20% of the treatment failures presented more than 5 years after diagnosis, stressing the need for prolonged follow-up in future studies of these tumors.

Germ Cell Tumors

Germ cell tumors are considered and studied in two separate groups—germinomas and NGGCTs—consisting of endodermal sinus tumors, choriocarcinomas, embryonal carcinomas, mature teratomas, and immature teratomas. The role of open surgery, radiation, and chemotherapy is perhaps as well defined for these lesions as for any pineal region tumors.

Germinomas are the most common pineal region tumors, especially in adolescent boys and young men. Because they do not secrete a specific tumor marker and they cannot be distinguished radiographically from other types of tumors that call for different treatment paradigms, diagnosis should be made with tissue confirmation regardless of age of presentation. Cytoreduction has not been shown to improve the excellent outcomes with radiation alone,[56] and thus the overwhelming majority of germinomas are diagnosed by open or stereotactic biopsy and treated with radiation. Long-term control of these tumors has been reported in up to 90% of the patients. Five-year survival greater than 75% and 10-year survival of 69% have been reported with radiation doses of 5,000 cGy, but lower radiation doses have shown a higher incidence of local failure.[57–60] A small percentage of patients fail radiation and suffer CSF dissemination that is ultimately fatal. Treatment failure is much more likely when syncytiotrophoblastic giant cells are mixed in the usual histological features, and failure rates in this histological subtype have been reported as high as 40%.[61–63] Because many patients with intracranial germinoma are cured, the long-term sequelae of whole-brain radiation, particularly in the pediatric population, are another major concern. Strides in chemotherapy have been made in trials with children too young to receive full doses of whole-brain radiation.[64,65] Stereotaxic radiotherapy for germinomas has also been evaluated, with local tumor control rates at 3 and 5 years of 82% and 72%, respectively, although germinomas with syncytiotrophoblastic giant cells had 5-year control rate of 62%.[26]

Nongerminomatous germ cell tumors have historically had a much worse prognosis that germinomas. Because the individual types are so rare and they are frequently of mixed histology, they have been lumped together in retrospective analyses and clinical trials. These are the only pineal region tumors that should be treated without a tissue diagnosis because elevated levels of markers in the serum or CSF are pathognomonic for specific histopathologies. Although open surgery in a preadjuvant-therapy cytoreductive role has been examined with variable results, the best results seem to occur when radiation or chemotherapy is followed by "second-look" surgery when a persistent radiographic lesion exists.[64–67] Using this approach, only residual teratomatous elements or scar tissue has been removed, and 5-year survival rates have improved dramatically to > 90%.

◼ Conclusion

Pineal region tumors present a formidable clinical challenge. Because of the variety of tumor types that occur in the pineal region, tissue diagnosis is mandatory to direct appropriate therapy. The only exceptions to this rule are marker-positive, malignant germ cell tumors. Tissue is usually best obtained via an open surgical approach so that gross total resection can be pursued if indicated by intraoperative pathological consultation. Prognoses for most pineal region tumors are excellent after appropriate histologically directed therapy.

Editor's Note

The management of pineal region tumors has come full circle. There was a period of time in the 1960s and 1970s when open surgical procedures were in vogue. However, as stereotactic frames with CT and MRI became more readily available, there were a considerable number of biopsies done during the 1970s and 1980s. Then, with improvements in the microscope and with navigation, there was a reawakening of interest in open surgical procedures especially with microsurgical techniques. Then the endoscope came into play and we found more examples of biopsies conducted via endoscopic imaging and less open surgery.

At the present time most pineal region tumors are approached with open microsurgical techniques, with the goal of surgical resection. However, the exception to this is in the classic case of a germ cell tumor where a biopsy can be done endoscopically along with a third ventriculostomy. I suspect these two modalities are going to continue to be critical for the management of patients with these tumors, thus producing better outcomes with lower morbidity. In almost every circumstance it is imperative to obtain serum markers to decide whether or not the diagnostic accuracy can be improved along with obtaining tissue when absolutely essential. That said, for most pineal region tumors other than the pure germ cell tumors, the treatment of choice is an open radical resection with the goal of complete removal. (Berger)

References

1. Dolecek TA, Propp JM, Stroup NE, Kruchko C. CBTRUS statistical report: primary brain and central nervous system tumors diagnosed in the United States in 2005-2009. Neuro-oncol 2012;14(Suppl 5):v1–v49
2. Dandy W. An operation for the removal of pineal tumors. Surg Gynecol Obstet 1921;33:113–119
3. Poppen JL, Marino R Jr. Pinealomas and tumors of the posterior portion of the third ventricle. J Neurosurg 1968;28:357–364
4. Abay EO II, Laws ER Jr, Grado GL, et al. Pineal tumors in children and adolescents. Treatment by CSF shunting and radiotherapy. J Neurosurg 1981;55:889–895
5. Jenkin RD, Simpson WJ, Keen CW. Pineal and suprasellar germinomas. Results of radiation treatment. J Neurosurg 1978;48:99–107
6. Marsh WR, Laws ER Jr. Shunting and irradiation of pineal tumors. Clin Neurosurg 1985;32:384–396
7. Stein BM. The infratentorial supracerebellar approach to pineal lesions. J Neurosurg 1971;35:197–202
8. Jamieson KG. Excision of pineal tumors. J Neurosurg 1971;35:550–553
9. Field M, Witham TF, Flickinger JC, Kondziolka D, Lunsford LD. Comprehensive assessment of hemorrhage risks and outcomes after stereotactic brain biopsy. J Neurosurg 2001;94:545–551
10. Sawin PD, Hitchon PW, Follett KA, Torner JC. Computed imaging-assisted stereotactic brain biopsy: a risk analysis of 225 consecutive cases. Surg Neurol 1998;49:640–649
11. Regis J, Bouillot P, Rouby-Volot F, Figarella-Branger D, Dufour H, Peragut JC. Pineal region tumors and the role of stereotactic biopsy: review of the mortality, morbidity, and diagnostic rates in 370 cases. Neurosurgery 1996;39:907–912, discussion 912–914
12. Hernesniemi J, Romani R, Albayrak BS, et al. Microsurgical management of pineal region lesions: personal experience with 119 patients. Surg Neurol 2008;70:576–583
13. Bruce J. Youman's Neurological Surgery: Pineal Tumors. Philadelphia: WB Saunders, 2011:1011–1029
14. Stein BM, Bruce JN. Surgical management of pineal region tumors (honored guest lecture). Clin Neurosurg 1992;39:509–532
15. Bruce JN. Sitting position for the removal of pineal region lesions. World Neurosurg 2012;77:657–658
16. Kobayashi S, Sugita K, Tanaka Y, Kyoshima K. Infratentorial approach to the pineal region in the prone position: Concorde position. Technical note. J Neurosurg 1983;58:141–143
17. Hasegawa T, Kondziolka D, Hadjipanayis CG, Flickinger JC, Lunsford LD. The role of radiosurgery for the treatment of pineal parenchymal tumors. Neurosurgery 2002;51:880–889
18. Manera L, Régis J, Chinot O, et al. Pineal region tumors: the role of stereotactic radiosurgery. Stereotact Funct Neurosurg 1996;66(Suppl 1):164–173
19. Kobayashi T, Kida Y, Mori Y. Stereotactic gamma radiosurgery for pineal and related tumors. J Neurooncol 2001;54:301–309

20. Hasegawa T, Kondziolka D, Hadjipanayis CG, Flickinger JC, Lunsford LD. Stereotactic radiosurgery for CNS nongerminomatous germ cell tumors. Report of four cases. Pediatr Neurosurg 2003;38:329–333

21. Bruce JN, Stein BM. Surgical management of pineal region tumors. Acta Neurochir (Wien) 1995;134:130–135

22. Vaquero J, Ramiro J, Martínez R, Coca S, Bravo G. Clinicopathological experience with pineocytomas: report of five surgically treated cases. Neurosurgery 1990;27:612–618, discussion 618–619

23. Konovalov AN, Pitskhelauri DI. Principles of treatment of the pineal region tumors. Surg Neurol 2003;59:250–268

24. Raco A, Raimondi AJ, D'Alonzo A, Esposito V, Valentino V. Radiosurgery in the management of pediatric brain tumors. Childs Nerv Syst 2000; 16:287–295

25. Yianni J, Rowe J, Khandanpour N, et al. Stereotactic radiosurgery for pineal tumours. Br J Neurosurg 2012;26:361–366

26. Mori Y, Kobayashi T, Hasegawa T, Yoshida K, Kida Y. Stereotactic radiosurgery for pineal and related tumors. Prog Neurol Surg 2009;23: 106–118

27. Barnett DW, Olson JJ, Thomas WG, Hunter SB. Low-grade astrocytomas arising from the pineal gland. Surg Neurol 1995;43:70–75, discussion 75–76

28. DeGirolami U, Armbrustmacher VW. Juvenile pilocytic astrocytoma of the pineal region: report of a case. Cancer 1982;50:1185–1188

29. Chandy MJ, Damaraju SC. Benign tumours of the pineal region: a prospective study from 1983 to 1997. Br J Neurosurg 1998;12:228–233

30. Levidou G, Korkolopoulou P, Agrogiannis G, Paidakakos N, Bouramas D, Patsouris E. Low-grade oligodendroglioma of the pineal gland: a case report and review of the literature. Diagn Pathol 2010;5:59

31. Clark AJ, Ivan ME, Sughrue ME, et al. Tumor control after surgery and radiotherapy for pineocytoma. J Neurosurg 2010;113:319–324

32. Clark AJ, Sughrue ME, Ivan ME, et al. Factors influencing overall survival rates for patients with pineocytoma. J Neurooncol 2010;100:255–260

33. Baehring J, Vives K, Duncan C, Piepmeier J, Bannykyh S. Tumors of the posterior third ventricle and pineal region: ependymoma and germinoma. J Neurooncol 2004;70:273–274

34. Dashti SR, Robinson S, Rodgers M, Cohen AR. Pineal region giant cell astrocytoma associated with tuberous sclerosis: case report. J Neurosurg 2005;102(3, Suppl):322–325

35. Epstein FJ, Farmer JP, Freed D. Adult intramedullary astrocytomas of the spinal cord. J Neurosurg 1992;77:355–359

36. Bognar L, Fischer C, Turjman F, et al. Tectal plate gliomas. Part III. Apparent lack of auditory consequences of unilateral inferior collicular lesion due to localized glioma surgery. Acta Neurochir (Wien) 1994; 127:161–165

37. Matsuno A, Nagashima H, Ishii H, Iwamuro H, Nagashima T. Aggressive and invasive growth of tectal glioma after surgical intervention and chemoradiotherapy. Br J Neurosurg 2006;20:246–249

38. Meyer B, Kral T, Zentner J. Pure word deafness after resection of a tectal plate glioma with preservation of wave V of brain stem auditory evoked potentials. J Neurol Neurosurg Psychiatry 1996;61:423–424

39. Rees J. Tectal plate glioma presenting as generalised myasthenia in an adult. J Neurol 2001;248:630–631

40. Stark AM, Fritsch MJ, Claviez A, Dörner L, Mehdorn HM. Management of tectal glioma in childhood. Pediatr Neurol 2005;33:33–38

41. Schwartz TH, Kim S, Glick RS, et al. Supratentorial ependymomas in adult patients. Neurosurgery 1999;44:721–731

42. Jouvet A, Fauchon F, Liberski P, et al. Papillary tumor of the pineal region. Am J Surg Pathol 2003;27:505–512

43. Brat DJ, Scheithauer BW, Fuller GN, Tihan T. Newly codified glial neoplasms of the 2007 WHO Classification of Tumours of the Central Nervous System: angiocentric glioma, pilomyxoid astrocytoma and pituicytoma. Brain Pathol 2007;17:319–324

44. Hasselblatt M, Blümcke I, Jeibmann A, et al. Immunohistochemical profile and chromosomal imbalances in papillary tumours of the pineal region. Neuropathol Appl Neurobiol 2006;32:278–283

45. Shibahara J, Todo T, Morita A, Mori H, Aoki S, Fukayama M. Papillary neuroepithelial tumor of the pineal region. A case report. Acta Neuropathol 2004;108:337–340

46. Fèvre-Montange M, Hasselblatt M, Figarella-Branger D, et al. Prognosis and histopathologic features in papillary tumors of the pineal region: a retrospective multicenter study of 31 cases. J Neuropathol Exp Neurol 2006;65:1004–1011

47. Fauchon F, Jouvet A, Paquis P, et al. Parenchymal pineal tumors: a clinicopathological study of 76 cases. Int J Radiat Oncol Biol Phys 2000; 46:959–968

48. Arivazhagan A, Anandh B, Santosh V, Chandramouli BA. Pineal parenchymal tumors—utility of immunohistochemical markers in prognostication. Clin Neuropathol 2008;27:325–333

49. D'Andrea AD, Packer RJ, Rorke LB, et al. Pineocytomas of childhood. A reappraisal of natural history and response to therapy. Cancer 1987; 59:1353–1357

50. Chang SM, Lillis-Hearne PK, Larson DA, Wara WM, Bollen AW, Prados MD. Pineoblastoma in adults. Neurosurgery 1995;37:383–390, discussion 390–391

51. Jakacki RI, Zeltzer PM, Boyett JM, et al. Survival and prognostic factors following radiation and/or chemotherapy for primitive neuroectodermal tumors of the pineal region in infants and children: a report of the Childrens Cancer Group. J Clin Oncol 1995;13:1377–1383

52. Lutterbach J, Fauchon F, Schild SE, et al. Malignant pineal parenchymal tumors in adult patients: patterns of care and prognostic factors. Neurosurgery 2002;51:44–55, discussion 55–56

53. Reddy AT, Janss AJ, Phillips PC, Weiss HL, Packer RJ. Outcome for children with supratentorial primitive neuroectodermal tumors treated with surgery, radiation, and chemotherapy. Cancer 2000;88:2189–2193

54. Zeltzer PM, Boyett JM, Finlay JL, et al. Metastasis stage, adjuvant treatment, and residual tumor are prognostic factors for medulloblastoma in children: conclusions from the Children's Cancer Group 921 randomized phase III study. J Clin Oncol 1999;17:832–845

55. Jouvet A, Saint-Pierre G, Fauchon F, et al. Pineal parenchymal tumors: a correlation of histological features with prognosis in 66 cases. Brain Pathol 2000;10:49–60

56. Wara WM, Fellows CF, Sheline GE, Wilson CB, Townsend JJ. Radiation therapy for pineal tumors and suprasellar germinomas. Radiology 1977;124:221–223

57. Edwards MS, Hudgins RJ, Wilson CB, Levin VA, Wara WM. Pineal region tumors in children. J Neurosurg 1988;68:689–697

58. Sano K, Matsutani M. Pinealoma (Germinoma) treated by direct surgery and postoperative irradiation. A long-term follow-up. Childs Brain 1981;8:81–97

59. Sung DI, Harisiadis L, Chang CH. Midline pineal tumors and suprasellar germinomas: highly curable by irradiation. Radiology 1978;128:745–751

60. Kersh CR, Constable WC, Eisert DR, et al. Primary central nervous system germ cell tumors. Effect of histologic confirmation on radiotherapy. Cancer 1988;61:2148–2152

61. Uematsu Y, Tsuura Y, Miyamoto K, Itakura T, Hayashi S, Komai N. The recurrence of primary intracranial germinomas. Special reference to germinoma with STGC (syncytiotrophoblastic giant cell). J Neurooncol 1992;13:247–256

62. Utsuki S, Kawano N, Oka H, Tanaka T, Suwa T, Fujii K. Cerebral germinoma with syncytiotrophoblastic giant cells: feasibility of predicting prognosis using the serum hCG level. Acta Neurochir (Wien) 1999;141: 975–977, discussion 977–978

63. Utsuki S, Oka H, Tanaka S, Tanizaki Y, Fujii K. Long-term outcome of intracranial germinoma with hCG elevation in cerebrospinal fluid but not in serum. Acta Neurochir (Wien) 2002;144:1151–1154, discussion 1154–1155

64. Balmaceda C, Heller G, Rosenblum M, et al. Chemotherapy without irradiation—a novel approach for newly diagnosed CNS germ cell tumors: results of an international cooperative trial. The First International Central Nervous System Germ Cell Tumor Study. J Clin Oncol 1996;14:2908–2915

65. Kochi M, Itoyama Y, Shiraishi S, Kitamura I, Marubayashi T, Ushio Y. Successful treatment of intracranial nongerminomatous malignant germ cell tumors by administering neoadjuvant chemotherapy and radiotherapy before excision of residual tumors. J Neurosurg 2003; 99:106–114

66. Weiner HL, Lichtenbaum RA, Wisoff JH, et al. Delayed surgical resection of central nervous system germ cell tumors. Neurosurgery 2002; 50:727–733, discussion 733–734

67. Friedman JA, Lynch JJ, Buckner JC, Scheithauer BW, Raffel C. Management of malignant pineal germ cell tumors with residual mature teratoma. Neurosurgery 2001;48:518–522, discussion 522–523

68. Hoffman HJ, Yoshida M, Becker LE, Hendrick EB, Humphreys RP. Pineal region tumors in childhood. Experience at the Hospital for Sick Children. 1983. Pediatr Neurosurg 1994;21:91–103, discussion 104

69. Neuwelt EA. An update on the surgical treatment of malignant pineal region tumors. Clin Neurosurg 1985;32:397–428

70. Lapras C, Patet JD, Mottolese C, Lapras C Jr. Direct surgery for pineal tumors: occipital-transtentorial approach. Prog Exp Tumor Res 1987; 30:268–280

71. Pluchino F, Broggi G, Fornari M, Franzini A, Solero CL, Allegranza A. Surgical approach to pineal tumours. Acta Neurochir (Wien) 1989; 96:26–31

72. Luo SQ, Li DZ, Zhang MZ, Wang ZC. Occipital transtentorial approach for removal of pineal region tumors: report of 64 consecutive cases. Surg Neurol 1989;32:36–39

73. Vaquero J, Ramiro J, Martínez R, Bravo G. Neurosurgical experience with tumours of the pineal region at Clinica Puerta de Hierro. Acta Neurochir (Wien) 1992;116:23–32

74. Herrmann HD, Winkler D, Westphal M. Treatment of tumours of the pineal region and posterior part of the third ventricle. Acta Neurochir (Wien) 1992;116:137–146

75. Kang JK, Jeun SS, Hong YK, et al. Experience with pineal region tumors. Childs Nerv Syst 1998;14:63–68

76. Shin HJ, Cho BK, Jung HW, Wang KC. Pediatric pineal tumors: need for a direct surgical approach and complications of the occipital transtentorial approach. Childs Nerv Syst 1998;14:174–178

31 Intraventricular Tumors

Jason L. Schroeder and Gene H. Barnett

Intraventricular (IV) tumors are a relatively rare subset of all intracranial tumors[1] (**Fig. 31.1**). They represent a diverse group of histopathologies spanning from low-grade or benign lesions to highly malignant primary or metastatic lesions. These lesions are located within the fluid-filled spaces of the ventricular system. As such, they represent a challenging group of tumors to treat, not only because of the wide variety of pathologies but also because they are deep-seated lesions and they are in close proximity to a variety of critical neurologic and vascular structures, leading to the potential for significant morbidity as a side effect of treatment. Tumors are considered primarily IV if they arise completely within the ventricular system or secondarily IV due to exophytic growth of a parenchymal tumor directly adjacent to the ventricular system. This chapter provides a general overview of the types and distribution of IV tumors, describes commonly used surgical approaches to these tumors, and offers representative examples.

Special Consideration

- Intraventricular tumors are deep-seated lesions whose morbidity and potential mortality arise due to their close anatomic proximity to important neurovascular structures such as the genu of the internal capsule, the internal cerebral veins, and the thalamic perforators. This is due to the structures that must be sacrificed or transgressed to reach the lesions such as cortical bridging veins, the functional cortex, and deep white matter tracts.

Epidemiology

The differential diagnosis for any given IV tumor depends on its location, patient characteristics (e.g., age), and the radiographic characteristics of the lesion on multiple imaging platforms [typically magnetic resonance imaging (MRI), but potentially computed tomography (CT) and angiography][2,3] (**Fig. 31.2** and **Table 31.1**). A simple list of the potential pathologies to be considered for any intraventricular lesion includes at least choroid plexus papilloma (CPP), choroid plexus carcinoma, ependymoma, anaplastic ependymoma, subependymoma, meningioma, subependymal giant cell astrocytoma

Pearl

- Using a combination of tumor location in the ventricular system, imaging characteristics of the tumor, specific patient demographics, and history can often help to significantly narrow the differential diagnosis for a given IV tumor.

(SEGA), central neurocytoma, oligodendroglioma, glioblastoma, and metastasis.[2–5] Beyond this already lengthy list of primarily solid tumors, there are other diagnostic possibilities including cysts (e.g., colloid and ependymal cysts); other less common tumors, including perineurinomas, hemangiopericytomas, and solitary fibrous tumors; and potentially even some inflammatory or infectious lesions, such as neurocysticercosis.[2,4]

Some diagnostic possibilities can be narrowed down based on patient demographics and the location of the tumor. For example, CPP in childhood is more likely to be within the lateral ventricles, whereas CPP in adulthood is most commonly seen in the fourth ventricle.[4] Some tumors may be seen preferentially in patients who have specific tumor syndromes, such as subependymal giant cell astrocytoma in tuberous sclerosis or intraventricular meningioma in neurofibromatosis.[3–5] Finally, for IV metastases, many different primary pathologies have been reported: renal, pulmonary, breast, colon, gastric, bladder, lymphoma, thyroid, and melanoma; however, although breast and lung cancer are by far the most common systemic cancers to produce intracranial metastases, the risk of having a CNS metastasis in an intraventricular location may be highest in renal cell carcinoma.[6]

Intraventricular tumors are also varied with regard to their histological and imaging properties. Some tumors show well-differentiated histological patterns including the papillary structures with fibrovascular cords seen in CPP or the perivascular pseudorosettes that can be seen in well-differentiated ependymoma. Calcification may be found in many types of IV tumors including meningioma, CPP, ependymoma, subependymoma, central neurocytoma, and SEGA, and as a result may not by itself be as useful for narrowing the differential diagnosis. On imaging, some of these tumors may show relatively uniform enhancement, such as meningioma and CPP, or no enhancement in central neurocytoma, whereas others have more heterogeneous imaging characteristics, such as nonuniform enhancement in ependymoma, subependymoma,

Fig. 31.1a,b Two pie graphs showing (**a**) the relative distribution of primary versus metastatic tumors in all intracranial locations and (**b**) the distribution of primary intracranial tumors by location. Note the small percentage of tumors located within the ventricular system (1.2%). (Reproduced with permission of the Cleveland Clinic Center for Medical Art and Photography. Copyright 2013. All rights reserved.)

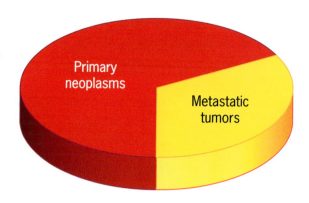

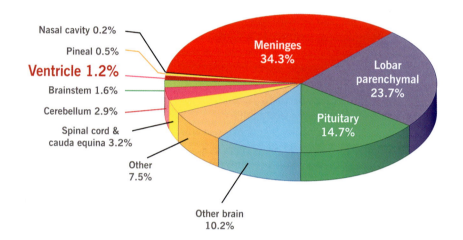

- Many IV lesions have either low-grade or benign histologies. Enthusiasm for resection must be appropriately balanced with the potential for complications in order to tailor treatment and maximize the outcome for each patient.

and atypical teratoid/rhabdoid tumor, or heterogeneous intrinsic T1 or T2 signal from hemorrhage or areas of necrosis in higher grade ependymoma or glioblastoma.[2,3,5] Finally, some IV tumors appear to be well demarcated from the surrounding structures, such as subependymoma (often attached to the ventricular wall via a stalk) or meningioma, as well as metastases, which tend to be attached to the choroid plexus, in contrast to other tumors that are growing into the ventricle as an exophytic component of an intraparenchymal tumor, such as glioblastoma or brainstem glioma.

■ Clinical Presentation

Patients with IV tumors seem to preferentially present with signs or symptoms of increased intracranial pressure (ICP) as opposed to clear focal neurologic deficits. Several authors have documented the presenting symptoms in their specific case series,[7,8] with the more common presenting symptoms of an IV tumor being nonlocalizing neurologic problems such as headache, nausea and vomiting, visual disturbance, gait problems, and memory difficulties.[7–10] Also, acute obstruction from a third or fourth ventricular tumor or cyst may result in spastic paraparesis and altered level of consciousness, including coma. This is in contrast to the focal deficits like focal motor or sensory deficit, aphasia, or agnosia that may more commonly be seen in patients with parenchymal tumors or cranial nerve deficits that may be seen in skull base tumors. Although potentially less common with IV tumors, seizures can still be a part of the constellation of presenting symptoms with a reported incidence of 5.6% in a series of IV metastases.[11]

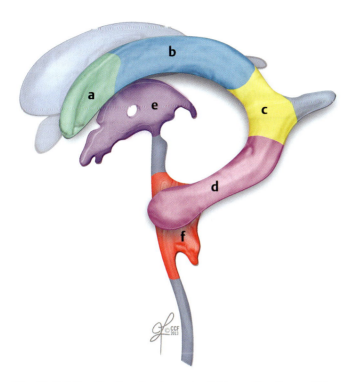

Fig. 31.2 A line drawing showing potential tumor locations within the ventricular system; *a*, frontal horn (*green*); *b*, body (*cyan*); *c*, trigone (*yellow*); *d*, temporal horn (*magenta*); *e*, third ventricle (*deep purple*); *f*, fourth ventricle (*red*). (Reproduced with permission of the Cleveland Clinic Center for Medical Art and Photography. Copyright 2013. All rights reserved.)

Surgical Management

The surgical treatment of IV tumors can be categorized based on the approach used. The modern neurosurgical literature describes in detail the traditional open approaches to IV tumors[7,8,10,12–14] and the more recent endoscopic approaches for some of the same lesions.[15,16] Chapter 13 discusses endo-scopic treatment approaches, so those approaches to IV tumors are not discussed here.

The surgical approach for any particular tumor is largely determined by its location (e.g., temporal horn versus adjacent to the foramen of Monro), the surrounding neurovascular anatomy, the proposed differential diagnosis, and the overall goals of the surgery. The goals for surgery are similar to those for any other cranial tumors. These include the specific goals of obtaining a histological diagnosis and debulking or completely resecting the lesion, typically described as maximal safe resection, to relieve mass effect. An additional goal that may be present for IV or periventricular tumors is that of reestablishing patency of the cerebrospinal fluid (CSF) pathways. Given that many IV tumors present with hydrocephalus and signs and symptoms of increased ICP, often one of the main goals is to reestablish normal CSF flow and to relieve the "mass effect" caused by excess CSF trapped within the ventricular system "upstream" of the tumor.

General Surgical Principles

Each patient should provide a full history and be given a physical examination not only to describe and document their neurologic disabilities but also to evaluate and compensate for any systemic derangements that may affect perisurgical and intraoperative care, such as diabetes, heart disease, and chronic steroid dependence. Once the decision has been made to pursue surgical intervention, preoperative planning includes selection of appropriate antibiotic and thromboembolism prophylaxis as well as imaging to define the lesion and for neuronavigation. Other important perioperative considerations include potential CSF diversion with external ventricular drainage and preoperative estimation of the potential for blood loss so that appropriate provisions are available for blood loss/volume replacement as needed. Finally, careful consideration needs to be given to the proposed positioning for

Table 31.1 Representative Intraventricular Tumors Arranged by Location Within the Ventricular System

Frontal Horn	Anterior Third	Fourth Ventricle
Astrocytoma	Colloid cyst	Ependymoma
Oligodendroglioma	Subependymoma	Subependymoma
Central neurocytoma	Gliomas	Medulloblastoma
Subependymoma	Craniopharyngioma	Choroid plexus papilloma
Metastasis	Central neurocytoma	
Atrium	**Posterior Third**	**Temporal Horn**
Meningioma	Astrocytoma	Metastasis
Metastasis	Pineal tumor	Meningioma
Choroid plexus papilloma	Metastasis	

surgery to protect the patient during a potentially long period of immobility, to maximize exposure of the lesion, and to reduce surgeon fatigue during the course of the operation.

Important general postoperative considerations include (1) duration of anticonvulsant therapy, if used, and antibiotics; (2) prevention of common postoperative complications, including infection, via meticulous wound and ventriculostomy care, and thromboembolism, via early mobilization; and (3) early imaging or laboratory evaluation if there are concerns about the potential for retained tumor, continued hydrocephalus. or other complications.

■ Surgical Approaches to Intraventricular Tumors

The following subsections describe some of the common approaches to intraventricular tumors based on lesion location.

These descriptions are illustrated with imaging from representative cases.

Anterior Portion of the Lateral Ventricle/ Anterior Third Ventricle

The classic open approaches to this location include the frontal transcortical approach and the interhemispheric transcallosal approach. More detailed descriptions of both of these approaches can be found elsewhere.[8,12,14] Here we outline the interhemispheric transcallosal and frontal transcortical approaches, and discuss how they differ.

Interhemispheric Approach

Typically, the patient is positioned supine on the operating table with the head in pin fixation and the neck flexed approximately 10 to 15 degrees. The incision is planned to expose the proposed craniotomy, which should have its medial border at the midline and be created about two thirds anterior and one third posterior to the coronal suture (**Fig. 31.3a**). The dura is opened based on the midline superior sagittal sinus (SSS), and when the dura is tacked up to maintain exposure, care must be taken not to occlude the sinus at the bony edges of the cranial opening. Careful review of preoperative imaging and the use of neuronavigation may help tailor the craniotomy to decrease the likelihood of having to sacrifice midline bridging veins. Once the falx has been identified in the midline, the plane between the ipsilateral frontal lobe and

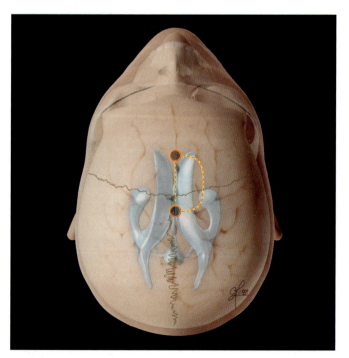

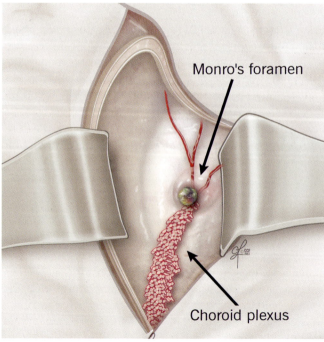

a

b

Fig. 31.3a–d (a) The planned cranial opening and **(b)** the deep exposure for a patient with a third ventricular colloid cyst undergoing the transcallosal approach.

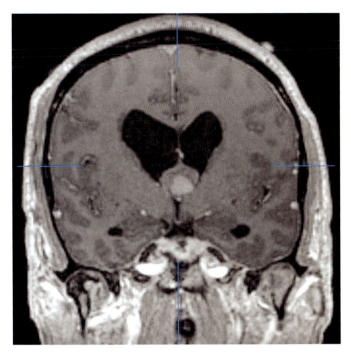
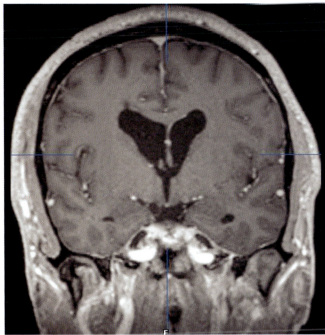

c

d

Fig. 31.3a–d (*continued*) (**c**) Pre- and (**d**) postoperative magnetic resonance imaging (MRI) scans for this patient. (Reproduced with permission of the Cleveland Clinic Center for Medical Art and Photography. Copyright 2013. All rights reserved.).

the falx is developed with microdissection and maintained with a self-retaining retractor. At the depth of the dissection, the arachnoidal adhesions between the paired cingulate gyri are divided sharply, the pericallosal arteries are separated, and the corpus callosum is identified.

The callosotomy is created longitudinally between the pericallosal arteries over a distance of 2 to 3 cm to allow access to the frontal horn of the lateral ventricle (**Fig. 31.3b**). If the tumor is situated in the frontal horn or body of the lateral ventricle, then the tumor capsule can be evaluated, and devascularization and internal debulking of the lesion can begin. For tumors of the third ventricle, further exposure needs to be accomplished prior to tumor resection (**Fig. 31.3c,d**). There are three potential routes of access to the third ventricle from the lateral ventricle: transforaminal, transchoroidal, and interforniceal (**Fig. 31.4a**). All of them are well described in the literature.[8,14,17] Because the access corridor to the tumor is deep and relatively small, once the third ventricle has been entered and the tumor is identified, the lesion is opened and internal debulking is completed prior to final detachment of the tumor from its point of origin to complete the resection. Meticulous hemostasis must be obtained while removing the retractors from the deep exposure, and copious irrigation can help to clear blood and other surgical debris from the ventricular system, which may otherwise contribute to postoperative hydrocephalus. An external ventricular drain (EVD) may be kept in place to provide CSF diversion and to allow for invasive ICP monitoring in case of impaired neurologic functioning.

Frontal Transcortical Approach

Typically the patient is positioned supine with the head fixed in pins and rotated approximately 30 degrees to the side opposite the tumor. The incision is designed to accommodate an adequate bone flap exposing the middle frontal gyrus. The size of the corticotomy/corticectomy is determined by the tumor extension and its vascular attachments. Neuronavigation can be helpful to plan the entry trajectory, and subcortical dissection is carried down through the white matter to the frontal horn of the lateral ventricle. Once the tumor is visible, the sites of vascular attachment are identified and coagulated to decrease bleeding during resection.

For extensive IV tumors, the septum pellucidum may need to be opened to enable resection of the portion of the tumor that crosses the midline, and the corticotomy/corticectomy may need to be expanded to enable more posterior access to the trigone area (**Fig. 31.4b,c**). Also, as described above, adjunctive maneuvers may be needed if any portion of the tumor extends into the third ventricle (transchoroidal or trans-

---

Pitfall

- Careful attention must be paid to the delicate perforating vessels that may arise from the anterior or posterior choroidal vessels, which are the feeding vessels for the majority of IV tumors.

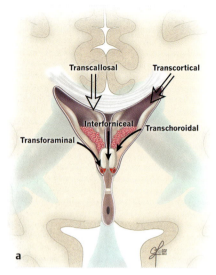
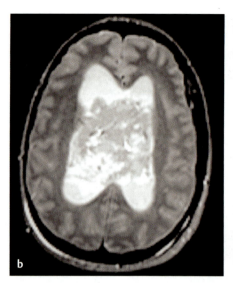
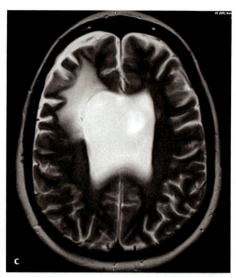

Fig. 31.4a–c (**a**) Illustration of the potential corridors to access the anterior third ventricle from the frontal horn of the lateral ventricle. (**b**) Pre- and (**c**) postoperative axial MRI from a central neurocytoma involving the bilateral frontal horns, third ventricle, and right trigone

removed via the frontal transcortical approach. (Reproduced with permission of the Cleveland Clinic Center for Medical Art and Photography. Copyright 2013. All rights reserved.)

foraminal exposure). Most lesions require sequential devascularization and debulking in pieces from the deep IV space. Final hemostasis after tumor resection needs to be precise, and CSF diversion may be needed during the postoperative period.

Potential advantages for the interhemispheric transcallosal approach over the frontal transcortical approach include good access in the setting of small ventricles, exposure in the midline and to both foramina of Monro, and a shorter trajectory to the third ventricle.[8] Disadvantages include the risk of injury to bridging veins, retraction injury, and the potential consequences of hemispheric "disconnection." There are conflicting data both supporting and refuting the possibility of a lower incidence of seizures when utilizing the interhemispheric transcallosal approach compared with a transcortical route for accessing the lateral ventricle.[8,9] Transcortical approaches may impact numerous white matter fasciculi[18] (**Fig. 31.5**), and the neuropsychological consequences of this potential fiber disruption are poorly defined.

If the frontal transcortical approach is used to provide initial access to the lateral ventricle, the subsequent routes of access to the third ventricle are limited to the transforaminal

approach and the transchoroidal approach, because the angle of approach is too lateral to allow midline exposure between the fornices for the interforniceal approach (**Fig. 31.4a**). For pathologies that enlarge the foramen of Monro, typically a transforaminal approach suffices to expose the lesion and enable internal decompression and then resection. An adjunct procedure that is often completed in conjunction with resection of obstructing lesions at the anterior third ventricle is fenestration of the septum pellucidum in an effort to create one communicating lateral ventricular system that can drain into the third ventricle via either foramen of Monro to circumvent any postoperative scarring that may occur at the site of tumor resection. Some of the potential complications associated with accessing the anterior part of the lateral ventricle or the third ventricle for tumor resection include alteration of consciousness, seizures, hemiparesis, and memory loss.[8]

Atrium of the Lateral Ventricle

For trigone area IV tumors, the most commonly described approaches include the superior parietal lobule approach, parieto-occipital approach, middle temporal gyrus approach, and transoccipital approach, which is used only for patients with a preoperative fixed homonymous hemianopsia.

For the parietal transcortical approach, the patient is placed either in the supine position with an ipsilateral shoulder roll or in the park bench position with the tumor side up. The head is in pin fixation and positioned with the parietal area as the highest point in the field, and the head of the bed is elevated about 15 degrees. The skin incision and craniotomy are tailored to the needs for the individual exposure with the aid

Controversy

- There is disagreement in the literature regarding whether the risk of postoperative seizure is higher after the frontal transcortical approach or the interhemispheric transcallosal approach.

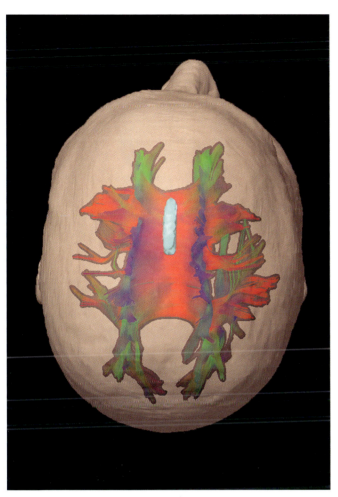
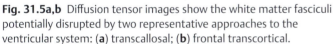
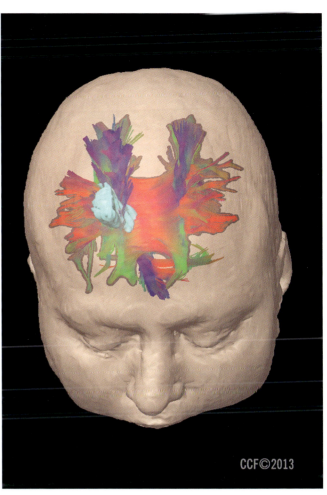

Fig. 31.5a,b Diffusion tensor images show the white matter fasciculi potentially disrupted by two representative approaches to the ventricular system: (**a**) transcallosal; (**b**) frontal transcortical.

(Reproduced with permission of the Cleveland Clinic Center for Medical Art and Photography. Copyright 2013. All rights reserved.)

of image guidance (**Fig. 31.6a**). Preoperative functional MRI and diffusion tensor imaging can aid the selection of a trajectory that avoids the major white matter bundles traversing the parietal area. After completing the craniotomy, the corticotomy and deep dissection proceed through either the gyrus or an adjacent sulcus, and self-retaining retractors maintain the exposure during tumor removal (**Fig. 31.6b**). The cortical opening should provide adequate access to the lesion and should decrease the tension on the adjacent cortex and white matter during retraction. Once the IV tumor is identified, every effort is made to devascularize it prior to debulking and resection in order to decrease bleeding within the ventricles, which can be difficult to control, can obstruct vision, and can contribute to postoperative hydrocephalus (**Fig. 31.6c,d**).

In addition to the typical complications that can occur after any cranial surgery, such as hematoma, infection, and incomplete resection, other potential neurologic complications for approaches to the trigone area of the lateral ventricle include motor or sensory deficits if the approach is too anterior, visual deficits if the approach traverses the occipital cortex or the optic radiations, language deficits if the approach is too lateral on the dominant side, disconnection syndrome, and parietal syndromes including apraxia, acalculia, and alexia without agraphia from cortical transgression.[7,8]

Temporal Horn of the Lateral Ventricle

Tumors in the temporal horn of the lateral ventricle are typically approached through a transcortical approach in either the middle or inferior temporal gyrus (**Fig. 31.7**). The head is fixed in pins and rotated 30 to 60 degrees contralateral to the exposure. The skin incision and craniotomy are low enough to identify the floor of the temporal fossa. The superior temporal gyrus is typically avoided because of its proximity to the vessels in the sylvian fissure and because of the potential for language deficits in the dominant hemisphere. The dura is

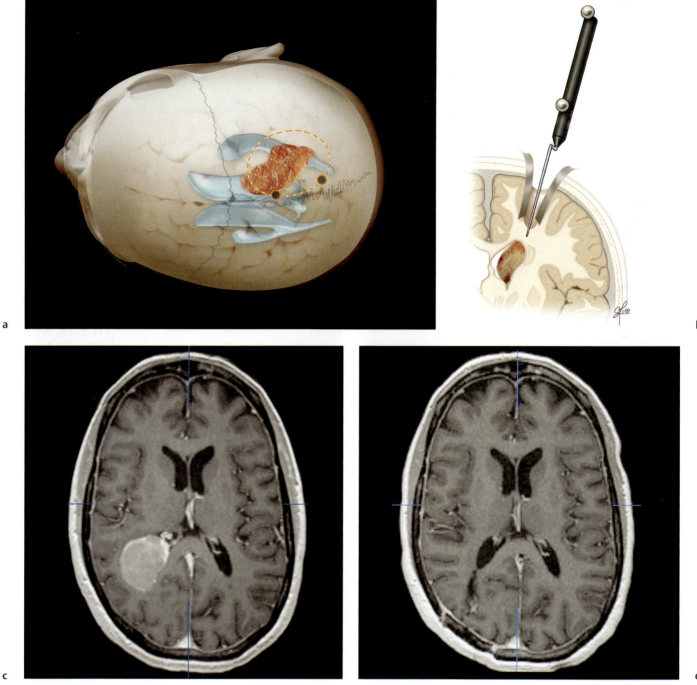

Fig. 31.6a–d (**a**) Tumor location and (**b**) parietal transcortical approach with the aid of neuronavigation for resection of a meningioma. (**c**) Pre- and (**d**) postoperative axial MRI. (Reproduced with permission of the Cleveland Clinic Center for Medical Art and Photography. Copyright 2013. All rights reserved.)

opened carefully to protect against injuring the vein of Labbé posteriorly. The corticotomy is made horizontally into the middle temporal gyrus, keeping in mind that the optic radiations pass superior and lateral to the temporal horn. Neuronavigation may be helpful for maintaining an appropriate trajectory to the IV tumor. A retractor is used to maintain the deeper exposure so that the tumor feeding vessels can be identified and coagulated. The hippocampus and other medial structures must be protected to help prevent postoperative cognitive impairment, and the extent of the corticotomy and retraction in the dominant hemisphere must be minimized to help prevent language impairment.

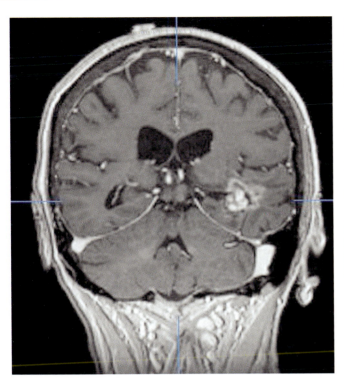
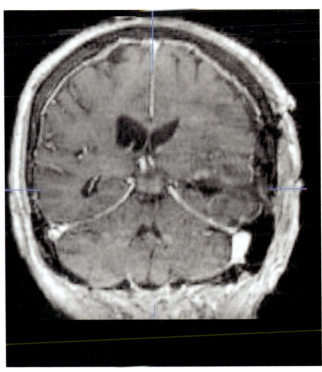

a   b

Fig. 31.7a,b (**a**) Pre- and (**b**) postoperative coronal MRI of a thyroid cancer metastasis removed through the middle temporal gyrus approach. (Reproduced with permission of the Cleveland Clinic Center for Medical Art and Photography. Copyright 2013. All rights reserved.)

Midline of the Fourth Ventricle

Midline tumors of the fourth ventricle are most commonly approached through a midline suboccipital craniotomy or craniectomy and splitting of the vermis (**Fig. 31.8**). Typically the patient is placed in the prone or the three-quarter prone position with the head fixed in pins. The head should be maintained neutral without rotation, and the neck may be flexed to increase access to the suboccipital region. Sufficient time and attention must be given to positioning the remainder of the patient's body to decrease the risk of pressure ulcers and thromboembolism. For tumors causing significant obstructive hydrocephalus, an EVD may be placed at the beginning of the procedure to relieve pressure and prevent downward herniation during the suboccipital exposure. A linear incision is created from just above the inion to approximately the spinous process of C2.

The dissection continues in the relatively avascular midline down to the bone of the suboccipital area and the posterior elements of the upper cervical spine. As the dissection is carried laterally, care must be taken to identify and protect the vertebral arteries during their extradural course along the upper margin of C1. The exposure is maintained with retractors, and cranially the muscles should be detached just below the superior nuchal line, leaving a cuff of muscle for reattachment at the end of the procedure (**Fig. 31.8c**). The suboccipital bone is then removed with a high-speed drill either as a craniectomy or as a craniotomy depending on the surgeon's preference.

Depending on the exposure required, the bone can be removed from the level of the transverse sinus bilaterally down to and including the posterior aspect of the foramen magnum. If there is tonsillar herniation from mass effect or hydrocephalus, then the posterior ring of C1 and possibly C2 needs to be removed as well. The dura is opened in the midline over the upper cervical cord, and then the opening is angled outward in a Y shape over each cerebellar hemisphere. The dura is tacked back with suture to the adjacent muscle to maximize exposure. The initial plane for microdissection is identified between and beneath the cerebellar tonsils while protecting the arachnoid over the spinal cord and lower brainstem. Ribbon retractor blades from a self-retaining system can be used to elevate and laterally displace the cerebellar tonsils once the arachnoid has been sharply opened (**Fig. 31.8d**). As the dissection proceeds cranially, the plane around the tumor is developed with a combination of sharp and blunt dissection and maintained by gently introducing paddies into the spaces that have been opened. Depending on the type of tumor, the site of attachment may be primarily in the superior medullary velum or on the floor of the fourth ventricle. It is possible that some tumor tissue may need to be left in place to avoid injury to the brainstem parenchyma, long tracts, and cranial nerve nuclei. Once the tumor resection is completed and hemostasis is satisfactory, the dura may or may not be closed. If closed, it should be done in a watertight fashion, often using some type of patch material. The cranial bone or a titanium cranioplasty can be replaced followed by layered closure of the muscle and skin.

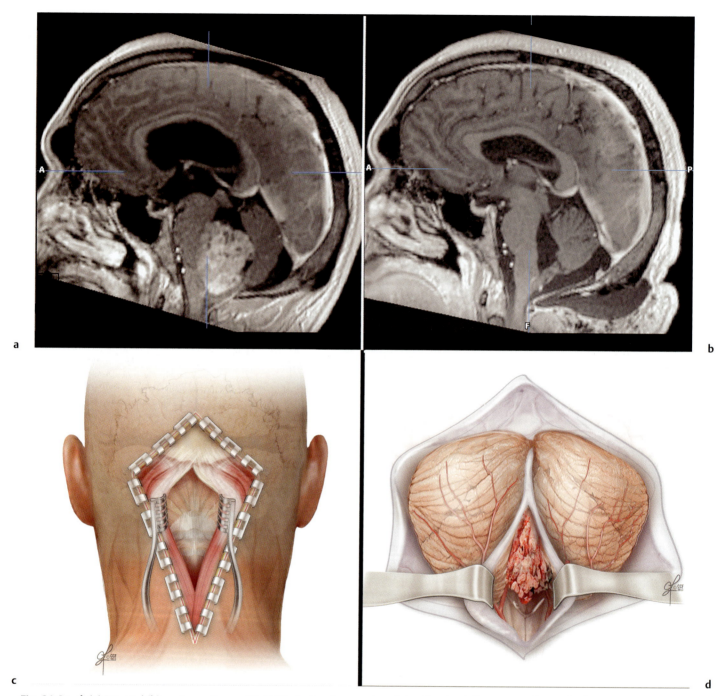

Fig. 31.8a–d (**a**) Pre- and (**b**) postoperative sagittal MRI of a fourth ventricular ependymoma removed via (**c**) a midline suboccipital approach with (**d**) splitting of the vermis. (Reproduced with permis-sion of the Cleveland Clinic Center for Medical Art and Photography. Copyright 2013. All rights reserved.)

Potential Complications

Tumors of the cranial ventricular system are deep lesions that are in close proximity to important neurologic and vascular structures. All of the trajectories for removing these tumors require trespassing through normal tissue,[8] and as a result the potential complications from removing these tumors encom-pass a wide variety of neurologic problems. Seizures, altered mental status, language deficits, and motor and sensory defi-cits can result from the transcortical resection of intraven-tricular tumors. However, there is at least one report of the risk for seizure being higher from the interhemispheric tran-scallosal approach to the frontal horn than from the frontal transcortical approach (25% for transcallosal versus 8% for

Pearl

- The fundamental principles that determine the success of IV tumor surgery include minimal retraction for adequate exposure, early control of the blood supply, piecemeal removal of large masses, and an understanding of the function of the surrounding anatomic structures.

transcortical in that series).[9] Language deficits can result from ischemia, retraction-related edema, and manipulation of the cortex or the deeper white matter connection fibers when resections are completed in the dominant hemisphere.

Motor deficits including hemiparesis may be seen in up to 30% of patients after intraventricular tumor removal.[7] The cause of the motor deficit may be direct invasion or attenuation of motor control or relay structures by tumor that is subsequently perturbed by the operation, a change in regional blood flow from arterial or venous manipulation during retraction or tumor resection, or inadvertent direct violation of the motor cortex or deeper motor structures due to their proximity to the approach corridor or tumor resection bed. Sensory deficits may occur due to transgression of the sensory cortex in a parietal transcortical approach or the primary visual sensory cortex in an occipital transcortical approach, or due to interruption of deep sensory circuits (e.g., a sensory language deficit with injury to the arcuate fasciculus in the dominant hemisphere, a visual deficit with injury to the optic radiations in the posterior temporal or parietal lobe, or a disconnection syndrome with injury to the posterior corpus callosum in some approaches). In addition, other complications that can be seen after transcallosal tumor resection include memory deficits, apraxia, and mutism. The most common cognitive complication in one series was transient recent memory loss in 30% of the patients.[8]

Some deficits may result from sectioning a portion of the corpus callosum itself and others may be related to retraction injury or mechanical trauma to surrounding structures, including cortical bridging veins, perforating arteries, components of Papez circuit, the cingulate gyrus itself, the fornices in the interforniceal approach to the third ventricle, or deep anterior thalamic nuclei. For tumors of the deep anterior third ventricle, postoperative disturbances in memory function may result from trauma to the mammillary bodies, and endocrine dysfunction may result from traction on the hypothalamus or infundibulum.[19]

Other more common postoperative complications from cranial surgery, though not specific to IV tumor surgery, are still important to note. They include new or persistent hydrocephalus, metabolic derangements, infectious or aseptic meningitis, and intracranial bleeding—epidural, subdural, intraparenchymal, or intraventricular. Pseudomeningocele may occur as a result of creating a corridor from the wound to the ventricular system; some authors suggest closure of the transparenchymal corridor with biological "glue" or other methods. For any patient undergoing neurosurgery for intracranial pathology, general postoperative care includes careful clinical, laboratory, and targeted imaging evaluations to prevent further sequelae from these types of potential complications. Ultimately, patient outcomes are maximized when surgeons painstakingly use the appropriate resources at their disposal to provide care before, during, and after the operation.

■ Conclusion

Patients with intraventricular tumors pose significant challenges for the treating neurosurgeon, but with deliberate attention to detail in all phases of the patient's care appropriate outcomes can often be achieved. Because many IV tumors are low-grade or benign lesions, the potential for long-term survival or cure exists when complete resection is feasible; however, the potential morbidity from iatrogenic injury to the adjacent neural and vascular structures during surgery also produces the possibility of long survival with substantial disability after treatment. In some cases a staged approach combining subtotal resection with subsequent stereotactic radiosurgery may achieve tumor control at less risk than that associated with complete surgical resection alone. In-depth neuroanatomical knowledge, careful planning, precise surgical technique, and dedication to overall patient care provide the best opportunity for good outcomes in these patients.

Editor's Note

Intraventricular tumors often present challenges primarily for neurosurgeons, although radiation oncologists may be involved in the care of gliomas and occasional neurocytomas that recur after surgery. The results of these operations tend to be acceptable for both the patient and the surgeon, but one of the main judgment calls to be made is whether such a tumor requires surgery at all. For example, meningiomas arising in the lateral ventricle, subependymomas, and small colloid cysts are often asymptomatic and diagnosed incidentally on brain imaging done for nonspecific headaches or other symptoms unrelated to the tumor. In these cases, these tumors can be safely watched with regular MRI and often do not grow and may never require treatment. If they grow and require intervention, the risk of surgery has been deferred. Several neurosurgical approaches exist depending mainly on the location of the tumor and the size of the ventricles, which give rise to interesting surgical planning for the surgeon. (Bernstein)

References

1. Central Brain Tumor Registry of the United States (CBTRUS). CBTRUS Statistical Report: Primary Brain and Central Nervous System Tumors Diagnosed in the United States in 2004–2008 (March 23, 2012 revision). Hinsdale, IL: CBTRUS, 2012. www.cbtrus.org

2. Osborn AG. Diagnostic Neuroradiology. Philadelphia: Mosby, 1994

3. Smith AB, Smirniotopoulos JG, Horkanyne-Szakaly I. From the radiologic pathology archives: intraventricular neoplasms: radiologic-pathologic correlation. Radiographics 2013;33:21–43

4. Waldron JS, Tihan T. Epidemiology and pathology of intraventricular tumors. Neurosurg Clin N Am 2003;14:469–482

5. Fenchel M, Beschorner R, Naegele T, Korn A, Ernemann U, Horger M. Primarily solid intraventricular brain tumors. Eur J Radiol 2012;81: e688–e696

6. Hassaneen W, Suki D, Salaskar AL, et al. Surgical management of lateral-ventricle metastases: report of 29 cases in a single-institution experience. J Neurosurg 2010;112:1046–1055

7. Piepmeier JM, Spencer DD, Sass KJ, George TM. Lateral ventricular masses. In: Brain Surgery: Complication Avoidance and Management. New York: Churchill Livingstone, 1993:581–599

8. Amar AP, Ghosh S, Apuzzo MLJ. Ventricular tumors. In: Winn HR, ed. Youmans' Neurological Surgery, 5th ed. Philadelphia: Saunders, 2003: 1237–1263

9. Milligan BD, Meyer FB. Morbidity of transcallosal and transcortical approaches to lesions in and around the lateral and third ventricles: a single-institution experience. Neurosurgery 2010;67:1483–1496, discussion 1496

10. Anderson RCE, Ghatan S, Feldstein NA. Surgical approaches to tumors of the lateral ventricle. Neurosurg Clin N Am 2003;14:509–525

11. Vecil GG, Lang FF. Surgical resection of metastatic intraventricular tumors. Neurosurg Clin N Am 2003;14:593–606

12. Ocal E, Baehring JM, Piepmeier J. Surgical approaches to intraventricular tumors (lateral ventricles). In: Badie B, ed. Neurosurgical Operative Atlas: Neuro-Oncology, 2nd ed. New York: Thieme, 2007:54–57

13. Nayar VV, DeMonte F, Yoshor D, Blacklock JB, Sawaya R. Surgical approaches to meningiomas of the lateral ventricles. Clin Neurol Neurosurg 2010;112:400–405

14. Yao KC, Lang FF. Surgical approaches to tumors of the third ventricle. In: Badie B, ed. Neurosurgical Operative Atlas: Neuro-Oncology, 2nd ed. New York: Thieme, 2007:42–53

15. Souweidane MM. Endoscopic approaches for intraventricular brain tumors. In: Badie B, ed. Neurosurgical Operative Atlas: Neuro-Oncology, 2nd ed. New York: Thieme, 2007:33–41

16. Schroeder HWS. Intraventricular tumors. World Neurosurg 2013;79(2, Suppl):e15–e19

17. Tew JM, van Loveren HR, Keller JT. Atlas of Operative Microneurosurgery, Volume 2: Brain Tumors. Philadelphia: Saunders, 2001

18. Park ES, Cho YH, Kim JH, Kim SJ, Khang SK, Kim CJ. Frontal transcortical approach in 12 central neurocytomas. Acta Neurochir (Wien) 2012; 154:1961–1971, discussion 1972

19. Chamoun R, Couldwell WT. Transcortical-transforaminal microscopic approach for purely intraventricular craniopharyngioma. Neurosurg Focus 2013;34(1, Suppl):4

32 Meningiomas

Corinna C. Zygourakis, Roxanna M. Garcia, and Michael W. McDermott

It is fair to say that few procedures in surgery may be more immediately formidable than an attack upon a large tumor of the [meningioma type], and that the ultimate prognosis hinges more on the surgeon's wide experience with the problem in all its many aspects than is true of almost any other operation that can be named.[1]

Much of what was written about meningiomas by Harvey Cushing and Louise Eisenhardt in 1938 still applies today. However, there have been many recent advances in the understanding of the biology and molecular genetics of these tumors. New developments in imaging, endovascular treatments, and surgical and radiotherapy techniques have significantly improved treatment outcomes for meningioma patients. Although more technically sophisticated, our surgical approaches have become less aggressive over recent years for all meningiomas, given recent findings of no significant difference in recurrence-free survival in patients undergoing less versus more aggressive resections, as determined by the Simpson grading system.[2] This is particularly true for tumors in certain high-risk locations, such as the cavernous sinus[3] or those involving major venous sinuses,[4] for which we now favor combined approaches of surgery and adjuvant radiotherapy, providing good tumor control with excellent functional outcomes.

Epidemiology

The recent report of the Central Brain Tumor Registry of the United States, reviewing primary brain tumor statistics from 49 population-based cancer registries, indicates that the most frequently reported histology is meningioma, accounting for 35.5% of all tumors, followed by glioblastoma (15.8%).[5] By comparison with other benign histologics, meningiomas appear to be the predominant tissue type, with pituitary tumors accounting for only 14.1% and benign nerve sheath tumors 8.3% of all primary brain tumors. Benign intracranial meningiomas are more prevalent in women, but atypical and anaplastic forms appear more commonly in men. Meningiomas account for about 38% of all intracranial tumors in women and 20% in men. Generally their incidence increases with age, ranging from a low of 0.3 per 100,000 in childhood to a high of 8.4 per 100,000 in the elderly population.[6] In childhood, meningiomas account for only 1 to 4% of all brain tumors and there is no female predominance. In most surgical series, the predominant tumor locations are convexity, falx/parasagittal, sphenoid wing, and skull base locations (**Table 32.1**).

Classification

In 1922, Harvey Cushing coined the term *meningioma* to describe a benign globoid tumor arising from the leptomeninges. Since that time, various pathological classification systems have used different morphological features, proliferation indices, and pathological grading systems. The current World Health Organization (WHO) system groups meningiomas by likelihood of recurrence into three grades (**Table 32.2**).[7,8] Meningiomas with a low risk of recurrence and nonaggressive growth are classified as grade I, whereas those with a higher likelihood of recurrence and more aggressive behavior are classified as either grade II or grade III meningiomas. Generally, grade I meningiomas are referred to as benign, grade II as atypical, and grade III as malignant.

Beyond the histology classification, the degree of meningioma resection is characterized by the system described by Simpson in 1957 (**Table 32.3**).[9] This system takes into account the extent of tumor resection and removal of involved dura, bone, and venous sinuses. Traditionally, many studies have found that higher Simpson grade resections, when tumor is residing within dura or bone, are associated with increased risk of tumor recurrence.[10,11] More recent studies, however, suggest that recurrence-free survival is not statistically different between patients undergoing Simpson grade I, II, III, or IV resections.[2] Despite this, the Simpson grade of surgical resection should be part of the routine reporting of surgical results, as it reflects more subtle involvement of the dura, arachnoid, arteries, veins, and nerves that only the surgeon can observe at open operation and that is not always obvious on routine postoperative magnetic resonance imaging (MRI).

Pearl

- Adding the Simpson grade of resection and labeling index to pathological grading improves the comparability of results for different methods of treatment of meningioma.

Table 32.1 Meningioma Locations: UCSF Surgical Series 1992–2005

Location	Number	Percent
Convexity	246	30
Falx/parasagittal	227	27
Sphenoid wing	126	15
Tentorium	53	6
Cerebellopontine angle	50	6
Olfactory groove	44	5
Multifocal	30	4
Suprasellar	22	3
Intraventricular	15	2
Foramen magnum	13	2
Pineal	3	<1
Total	829	100

Table 32.2 World Health Organization Classification of Meningiomas

Meningiomas with Low Risk of Recurrence/Aggressive Behavior	
Meningothelial meningioma	WHO grade I
Fibrous (fibroblastic) meningioma	WHO grade I
Transitional (mixed) meningioma	WHO grade I
Psammomatous meningioma	WHO grade I
Angiomatous meningioma	WHO grade I
Microcystic meningioma	WHO grade I
Secretory meningioma	WHO grade I
Lymphoplasmacyte-rich meningioma	WHO grade I
Metaplastic meningioma	WHO grade I
Meningiomas with Higher Risk of Growth/Aggressive Behavior	
Atypical meningioma	WHO grade II
Clear cell meningioma	WHO grade II
Chordoid meningioma	WHO grade II
Brain invasive meningioma	WHO grade II
Rhabdoid meningioma	WHO grade III
Papillary meningioma	WHO grade III
Anaplastic (malignant) meningioma	WHO grade III

Immunohistochemical markers of proliferation potential such as Ki-67, MIB-1, and proliferating cell nuclear antigen (PCNA) indices have also been correlated with risk of recurrence.[12–17] Ideally, pathological grade and histology, Simpson surgical grade, and a marker of proliferation index should be included in the reporting/analysis of operative meningioma specimens (**Table 32.4**).

■ Molecular Biology

Chromosomal and Genetic Abnormalities

It has long been recognized that the arachnoid cap cell is the cell of origin of meningiomas. Early karyotypic analysis of meningioma cells revealed abnormalities of the long arm of chromosome 22 as a characteristic feature. However, over the years, much more has been learned about the chromosomal and genetic aberrations underlying meningiomas. Progression from benign to atypical meningioma is associated with losses on chromosome 1p, 6q, 10, 14q, and 18q, and gains on 1p, 9q, 12q, 15q, and 20.[18–20] The progression from an atypical to a malignant meningioma has been associated with losses

on 9p and 17q.[18] More recent gene expression array studies identified nine genes that are overexpressed (*TPX2, RRM2, TOP2A, PI3, BIRC5, CDC2, NUSAP1, DLG7, SOX11*) and two that are underexpressed (*TIMP3, KCNMA1*) in grade III versus grade I meningiomas.[21]

The loss of the long arm of chromosome 22 occurs in 40 to 70% of meningiomas and is associated with loss of the tumor suppressor gene for neurofibromatosis type 2 (NF2), located at 22q12.[22–25] The product of this gene, merlin, is thought to be critical for meningioma tumorigenesis. Merlin belongs to the family of structural proteins that link the cytoskeleton to several proteins of the cytoplasmic membrane, and some authors have suggested that merlin may act as a tumor suppressor via its interactions with the cellular cytoskeleton.[26] Recent genomic analysis of non-*NF2* meningiomas reveals mutations in *TRAF7* (a proapoptotic E3 ubiquitin ligase), *KL4* (a transcription factor involved in inducing pluripotency), *AKT1* (a phosphatidylinositol 3-kinase [PI3K] activator), and *SMO* (a

Table 32.3 Simpson Classification of Surgical Resection

Grade	Tumor Removal			Dural Attachment		Bone/Sinus Excised
	Complete	Partial	Biopsy	Excised	Coagulated	
I	X			X		X
II	X				X	
III	X					
IV		X				
V			X			

Source: From Simpson D. The recurrence of intracranial meningiomas after surgical treatment. J Neurol Neurosurg Psychiatry 1957;20:22–39. Reproduced with permission from BMJ Publishing Group Ltd.

Table 32.4 Recommended Reporting of Surgical Cases

Index	Option
Pathological grade	WHO (2007)
Extent of surgical resection	Simpson grade
Marker of proliferation potential	MIB-1, PCNA, K_i-67

Hedgehog signaling activator).[27] These non-*NF2* meningiomas with their unique genomic profile are also clinically distinctive. They are nearly always benign, have chromosomal stability, and originate from the medial skull base. In contrast, *NF2* meningiomas are more likely to be atypical, have genomic instability, and arise from the cerebral or cerebellar hemispheres.[27]

Cell Surface Receptors

Meningiomas express a variety of nuclear and cell surface receptors.[6] Somatostatin, dopamine, epidermal growth factor (EGF), platelet-derived growth factor (PDGF), vascular endothelial growth factor (VEGF), insulin-like growth factor (IGF), transforming growth factor (TGF), basic fibroblast growth factor (bFGF), and endothelin-1 have all been found in meningiomas, although their role as therapeutic targets is still under investigation. Bevacizumab, an anti-VEGF antibody, demonstrated only modest activity against meningiomas in two recent reports.[28,29] Several other PDGF-receptor inhibitors (tandutinib, dasatinib, nilotinib, sunitinib, pazopanib, and CHIR 265) are currently being studied as potential therapeutic targets for meningiomas.[30]

Sex steroid hormone receptors such as progesterone, androgens, and estrogen, have long been linked to meningiomas, although their significance in relation to tumor development and growth remains unclear.[6,31] Most clinical studies demonstrate the female predominance for intracranial meningiomas (2:1), yet the majority of meningiomas are estrogen receptor negative. There are many reports of meningiomas changing in size with menstrual cycle phase, menopausal status, and pregnancy.[31,32] Women on hormone replacement therapy, which is primarily estrogen-based, are frequently taken off their medication if a meningioma is incidentally discovered. However, there is no convincing evidence of a causal relationship between hormone replacement therapy and meningioma development or growth.[33] The progesterone receptor is

Controversy

- The role of estrogen and progesterone in the development and growth of meningiomas remains to be clarified. Until then, the use of oral contraceptives and hormone replacement therapy in patients with a known meningioma should be considered on a case-by-case basis.

active in normal meninges but is also strongly expressed in benign meningiomas, suggesting a role in tumorigenesis. However, it is significantly reduced or absent in higher grade tumors, and prior attempts to control tumor growth of recurrent benign and malignant meningiomas with antiprogesterone agents have been unsuccessful.

▪ Imaging Studies

Meningiomas are often discovered incidentally when patients are worked up for headaches. Most meningiomas are isodense to surrounding brain but may have microcalcifications that are seen much more clearly on computed tomography (CT) than on MRI (**Fig. 32.1**). Psammomatous meningiomas can have particularly striking calcifications. CT imaging also provides better definition of bony involvement such as hyperostosis, which contains meningothelial cells within haversian canals at the histological level. The extent of bony involvement on pre- and postoperative CT imaging is important for determining the extent of surgical removal and the risk of recurrence. CT can also be used with image-guided surgical systems particularly for the excision of hyperostotic skull base meningiomas. Following the administration of intravenous contrast agents, these tumors show intense enhancement on CT. Their margins are usually smooth, and the enhancement pattern homogeneous. Surrounding vasogenic edema is often not well visualized on CT and can be better seen on MRI sequences.

Magnetic resonance imaging is the current gold standard for imaging of intracranial meningiomas. These tumors are usually isointense on T1-weighted images and have variable signal characteristics on T2-weighted images. Following the administration of gadolinium contrast, there is intense enhancement, which may persist for several hours after the imaging studies. Many globular meningiomas show a characteristic dural tail, which is thought to represent a hypervascularity in the dura immediately adjacent to the tumor base.[34] Features such as heterogeneous enhancement in the absence of embolization, irregular borders, mushrooming, regional multifocality, and abundant surrounding vasogenic edema may be imaging signs of aggressive histopathological meningioma types and clinical behavior (**Fig. 32.2**). The presence of edema usually also indicates for the surgeon that the arachnoid plane will be obliterated by the pial blood supply, making the dissection more tedious and less discrete.

Metabolic information related to in vivo imaging studies is currently evolving, whereas magnetic resonance (MR) spectroscopy has not yet been widely applied for meningiomas. However, MR perfusion studies may help distinguish between meningiomas and durally based hemangiopericytomas or schwannomas.[35,36] A recent application of MR perfusion imaging involves intra-arterial injection of dilute contrast media into selective intracranial vessels by interventional radiolo-

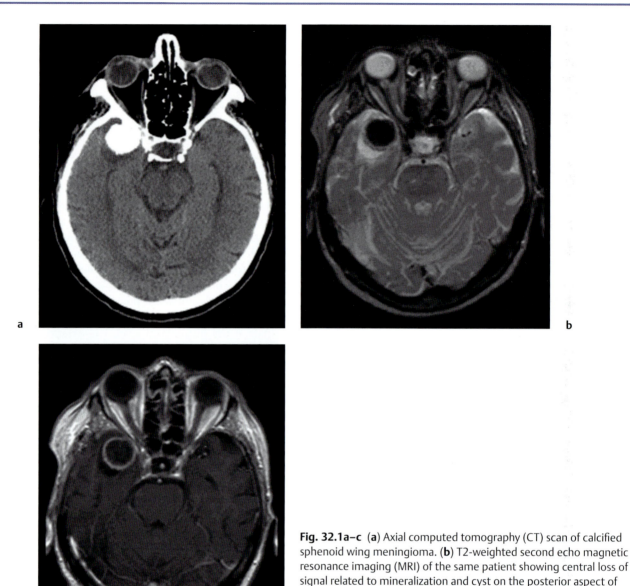

a

b

c

Fig. 32.1a–c (**a**) Axial computed tomography (CT) scan of calcified sphenoid wing meningioma. (**b**) T2-weighted second echo magnetic resonance imaging (MRI) of the same patient showing central loss of signal related to mineralization and cyst on the posterior aspect of tumor but no associated edema. (**c**) T1-weighted postcontrast image showing peripheral enhancement of the noncalcified portion of tumor. This patient was reassured and recommended to have annual follow-up scans.

gists, followed by perfusion-weighted dynamic-susceptibility contrast MRI. This enables good assessment of tissue fed by specific vessels before and after embolization treatment, which is often used as a preoperative adjuvant therapy to mitigate surgical blood loss.[37]

Cerebral angiography is sometimes used to assess the arterial supply of larger meningiomas, the status of major blood vessels displaced or narrowed by basal meningiomas, and the patency of large venous sinuses in the case of convexity, parasagittal, peritorcular, or tentorial meningiomas. For large convexity meningiomas, preoperative embolization can lead to reduced blood loss, shorter hospital stays, and decreased operating times.[38] Studies have also shown that angiography complication rates are low, approximately 2.5%.[39] However,

some surgeons have questioned whether preoperative embolization for certain tumor locations offers any advantage. The decision to embolize preoperatively should therefore be made on a case-by-case basis.

Pitfall

- For large meningiomas and those with surrounding edema, there may not be a clear arachnoid plane that separates tumor from brain. The resulting operative dissection may be subpial and associated with new transient or permanent neurologic deficits.

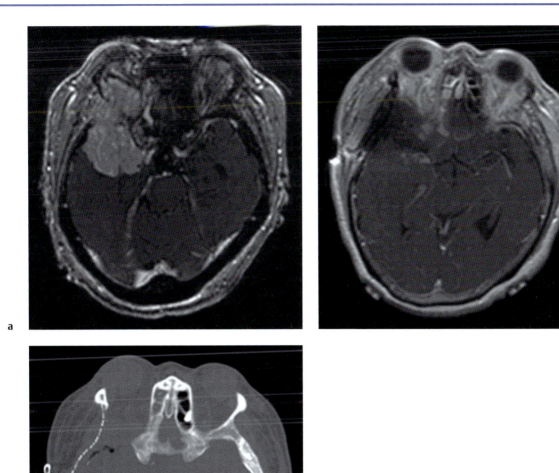

a

b

c

Fig. 32.2a–c (**a**) T1-weighted postcontrast image of atypical meningioma invading the posterolateral wall of the orbit and the bone of the pterion, causing headaches, seizures, and proptosis. (**b**) Postoperative T1-weighted MRI with contrast showing what appears to be complete resection. Intraoperative observations make this a Simpson grade III resection due to residual disease at the carotid ring, cavernous sinus wall, and posterolateral orbit. (**c**) CT scan showing the extent of bone resection and reconstruction with titanium mesh to achieve an acceptable cosmetic result.

▦ Treatment

Selection of Treatment Method

Not all patients with intracranial meningiomas require surgery. The decision to operate should take into account both patient- and tumor-specific factors, as well as surgical risk/benefit ratios. The surgeon should decide whether the meningioma seen on imaging studies correlates with the patient's symptoms and signs. If the patient has no symptoms or signs consistent with the meningioma seen on imaging, then a period of observation is recommended. In patients with no underlying medical conditions, interval 6-month MRI scans for 1 year are reasonable. If there is more than 2 mm of growth

in one dimension in 1 year, then a decision regarding treatment is warranted. If there is no documented growth by 1 year, then annual interval scans should be used to help determine the biological behavior.

The neurosurgeon should consider a patient's age, expected survival based on life table analyses, performance status, and

---

Special Consideration

- Incidental, asymptomatic meningiomas can be safely monitored with regular imaging, thus deferring or avoiding surgery.

> **Pitfall**
>
> - T1-weighted post–gadolinium contrast imaging should not be used with perfusion sequences to visualize meningiomas, as both tumor and arteries will appear white.

> **Pitfall**
>
> - Preservation of the cerebral venous system is a key to successful outcome from meningioma surgery. Interruption of transosseous and diploic venous drainage of the frontal lobes can lead to unexpected venous infarction.

neurologic condition when deciding to operate. The surgical risks are affected by associated medical conditions such as hypertension, diabetes, coronary artery disease, and prior cerebral vascular disease. Tumor factors such as size, location, vascularity, and involvement of sinuses must also be considered in determining the extent of resection that is possible. In the past 20 years, refined skull base techniques were developed for approaching tumors within the cavernous sinus; but over time, experience has indicated that many of these tumors can be treated with less aggressive surgery and adjuvant therapies to preserve good quality of life. In those patients who are symptomatic from their meningioma or in whom tumor growth is documented, surgery remains the primary form of treatment, but stereotactic radiation or radiosurgery is also an excellent option for smaller tumors.

Surgical patients require preoperative evaluation of medical conditions and often need preoperative steroids to optimize surgical conditions. Many surgeons also prescribe perioperative antiepileptics for these patients. To date, there are no class 1 data to indicate that seizure prophylaxis provides long-term reduction in seizures. However, surgery for meningiomas is frequently associated with perioperative seizures, particularly in certain locations, so perioperative antiepileptics may be helpful in reducing them. Frontal, temporal, and parietal locations have a higher incidence of associated seizures than occipital locations, and parasagittal/falx locations are at greater risk for seizures than basal or convexity locations.

Currently most surgical approaches are undertaken with the assistance of intraoperative image guidance, often with magnetic resonance angiography (MRA) and magnetic resonance venography (MRV) superimposed on T1-weighted MRI. The use of surgical navigation has become routine for confirming the localization of meningiomas before skin incisions and then before the actual bone work of the craniotomy, especially for parasagittal and convexity meningiomas.[40] For large skull base meningiomas that are not subject to shift during surgical resection, these intraoperative systems are of great help.

Surgical Treatment by Tumor Site

When the patient is deemed a suitable candidate for surgical intervention, the risks of surgery should be discussed frankly with the patient. Complications include those related to general anesthesia such as pneumonia, urinary tract infection, deep venous thrombosis, and compression neuropathy. Those specific to the surgery include wound infection, postoperative hematoma, perioperative seizures, postoperative cerebrospinal fluid (CSF) leakage, arterial or venous infarction, stroke, and death.

The most common meningioma locations in surgical series are convexity, parasagittal, falx, and sphenoid wing. In adults, 90% of meningiomas occur in the supratentorial compartment, 8% occur within the posterior fossa, and 1.3% are intraventricular.[6,41] Most intraventricular tumors occur in the lateral ventricle, usually in the atrium, 15% occur within the third ventricle, and 5% within the fourth ventricle. Intraventricular meningiomas are more common on the left than the right. The clinical presentation is similar to that of other intracranial mass lesions, including headaches, seizures, progressive focal neurologic deficit, or change in personality and behavior. However, given their dural attachments adjacent to cranial nerves, many meningiomas have symptom complexes specific to their tumor location.

Olfactory Groove Meningiomas

Meningiomas of the olfactory groove usually present with slow onset of mood changes, headaches, or visual disturbance.[1,6,42] Given their location and slow growth, these meningiomas often grow to large sizes before they present with clinical symptoms. Smaller tumors, less than 3 cm, can usually be removed by unilateral subfrontal, pterional, or cranio-orbital approaches. For larger tumors, bifrontal or extended frontal craniotomies are preferred (**Fig. 32.3**).

The general principle of surgical treatment of meningiomas includes intracapsular debulking followed by peripheral dissection of the arachnoid plane and sequential excision of the dissected meningioma. The aim is to remove all of the gross tumor, as well as to excise the involved dura and bone. Infrequently, larger olfactory groove meningiomas extend into the ethmoid sinuses, and transbasal approaches are necessary to completely remove these tumors. However, in older patients, it may be appropriate to aim for subtotal removal, leaving the intranasal portion behind for observation. Documented growth in this location can later be controlled with adjuvant therapy such as three-dimensional conformal radiotherapy (3DCRT), intensity-modulated radiotherapy (IMRT), stereotactic radiotherapy (SRT), or stereotactic radiosurgery (SRS), depending on the tumor size, location, and proximity to the optic apparatus or brainstem.[43] Nasal sinus invasion and anterior cerebral artery (ACA) encasement are

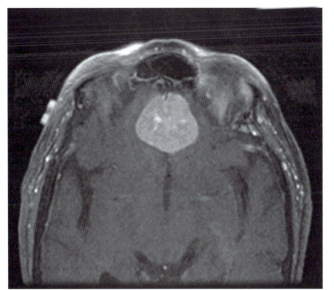
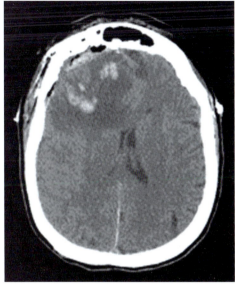

a   b

Fig. 32.3a,b (**a**) T1-weighted postcontrast MRI showing a medium-sized olfactory groove meningioma. The patient, an elderly woman, presented with headaches, and the meningioma was observed to grow before surgery. The patient was operated via a right frontal cranio-orbital approach. Simpson grade II resection was achieved. (**b**) CT scan on postoperative day 3 after a sudden unexpected decline, showing features of venous infarction. Review of the MRI suggested that frontal lobe venous outflow was mostly transdiploic. The patient had an excellent outcome after management of swelling without removal of infarcted tissue.

associated with higher risk profiles when surgery becomes necessary.[44]

Tuberculum Sellae Meningiomas

Tuberculum sellae meningiomas account for less than 10% of meningiomas in most surgical series. Patients often present with insidious, progressive visual loss, which is usually asymmetric.[45,46] Frequently these tumors are mistaken for pituitary adenomas, but they are centered on the chiasmatic sulcus of the tuberculum and grow down the front face of the sella as well as over the planum. Characteristically, on imaging studies, there is involvement of the proximal medial portion of one or both optic canals. Small to medium-sized tumors may be successfully removed with unilateral approaches such as pterional, cranio-orbital, or unilateral subfrontal approaches. Larger tumors are best treated with a bilateral approach such as a bifrontal extended frontal craniotomy. The bilateral approach provides a greater degree of flexibility because the surgeon can approach the tumor from the left, right, or down the middle. In addition, the bone in the region of the tuberculum can be drilled down to access that component of tumor extending down into the sella. The roofs of both optic canals can be drilled to expose medial extensions of meningioma down the optic canal. With bifrontal extended frontal approaches, both olfactory nerves need to be dissected back to just above the optic nerves to try to preserve function. Once dissected, the nerves should be covered with a rubber dam to avoid dehydration during the procedure. Recently, the extended transsphenoidal approach has been used to remove these tumors with endoscopic assistance.[47,48]

Optic Nerve Sheath Meningiomas

Optic nerve sheath tumors are a rare form of meningioma that no longer should be approached surgically unless the entire tumor is confined to the orbit and the patient has no useful vision. Most often these tumors are diagnosed by imaging studies and treated with fractionated external beam radiotherapy.[49,50] Surgical approaches to the orbit include a combined neurosurgical and ophthalmologic approach with a frontotemporal orbitozygomatic craniotomy.

Sphenoid Wing Meningiomas

Sphenoid wing meningiomas account for 12 to 23% of all meningiomas in larger surgical series.[51,52] Clinoid meningiomas

> **Pitfall**
>
> - When dissecting meningiomas near the optic apparatus, the blood supply to the optic nerves and chiasm from the superior hypophyseal vessels must be identified, dissected, and preserved. Postoperatively, hydration, and blood pressure should be maintained slightly above normal for 48 hours.

usually present with unilateral visual loss or retro-orbital headaches. Middle third meningiomas present with headaches, seizures, and altered mental status, and pterional meningiomas can reach large sizes before becoming symptomatic.

Clinoidal meningiomas are usually approached with a cranio-orbital or orbitozygomatic craniotomy, which allows the extradural removal of the clinoid and exposure of the optic canal to facilitate the identification of the optic nerve later in the resection. Middle third sphenoid wing meningiomas can be operated with a standard pterional approach for small tumors and frontotemporal orbitozygomatic approach for larger tumors. Lateral third or pterional meningiomas are usually approached with the standard pterional craniotomy. The unusual hyperostosing en plaque sphenoid wing meningioma, which typically involves the bone of the sphenoid wing and presents with painless proptosis, is usually best approached with an orbitozygomatic craniotomy, enabling removal of the involved bone of the greater sphenoid wing and posterolateral orbit. With such removals, the surgeon should be careful to reconstruct the posterolateral wall of the orbit to prevent enophthalmos. Symptomatic pulsating exophthalmos is a rare complication in long-term follow-up. For sphenoid wing meningiomas in general, a recent study found a 19% rate of new or worsened neurologic deficits after surgical resection.[53]

Cavernous Sinus Meningiomas

Cavernous sinus meningiomas present with double vision, facial numbness, headache, and reduced visual acuity. In the past, these were aggressively treated with skull base approaches. However, pathological postmortem specimens demonstrate infiltration of the epineurium of cranial nerves in the lateral wall of the cavernous sinus, and now these tumors are frequently treated surgically only for their exophytic middle fossa component, leaving the treatment of the truly intracavernous part to radiotherapy techniques.[54,55] Recent studies have shown improved rates of tumor control with adjuvant radiotherapy, regardless of initial extent of resection.[3]

Parasagittal Meningiomas

Parasagittal meningiomas are classified by their location in the anterior, middle, and posterior thirds of the superior sagittal sinus.[56] The symptom complex on presentation depends on the tumor location along with the sinus. Anterior third sagittal sinus tumors present with headaches, seizures, and changes in mental status. Middle third meningiomas located in the pericentral region are frequently associated with seizures and progressive focal weakness. Tumors of the posterior third of the superior sagittal sinus cause headaches, visual symptoms, and, later, seizures.

Anterior third parasagittal meningiomas can usually be approached by a frontal craniotomy that clearly exposes the midline, providing the surgeon better exposure of the lateral wall of the superior sagittal sinus to dissect the parasagittal draining veins, reducing tension on veins with retraction of the medial hemisphere. Middle third parasagittal meningiomas are approached by a parietal craniotomy and posterior one-third parasagittal meningiomas by an occipital craniotomy, again clearly exposing the midline. It is generally not advisable to attempt to excise the lateral wall of the superior sagittal sinus in cases where the sinus is still patent on MRV or formal angiography. One can try to separate the inner and outer layer of the dura on the lateral wall to help achieve a Simpson II resection while avoiding the need of a reconstruction (**Fig. 32.4**). For patients with complete occlusion of the sinus on angiography, care must be taken to identify the anterior and posterior extent of venous sinus occlusion with intraoperative adjuncts such as ultrasound, Doppler, or image guidance. Involved convexity dura is usually excised as close as possible to the lateral margin of the sinus. A recent report

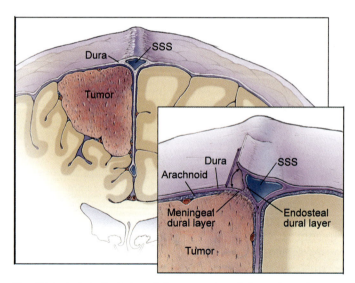

Fig. 32.4 Artist's depiction of the separation of the endosteal and meningeal layers of the dura in the lateral wall of the superior sagittal sinus (SSS) that can be dissected to improve the extent of resection.

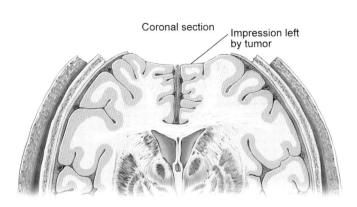
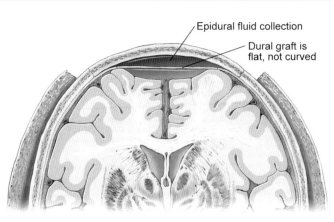

Fig. 32.5a,b (**a**) Coronal image of a dural defect and brain impression after resection of an occluded midline superior sagittal sinus and parasagittal meningioma. (**b**) The effect of not re-creating the convex shape of the dura with closure results in epidural collection. The dural graft is too short and results in a flat surface.

found a complication rate of 19% and good tumor control rates regardless of subtotal versus gross total resection.[4]

In cases where the superior sagittal sinus is occluded and a decision is made to resect a parasagittal tumor with the sinus, care should be taken to reconstruct the proper convex shape of the dura so as to avoid epidural collections on postoperative scans that may confuse the clinical picture (**Figs. 32.5** and **32.6**).

Falcine Meningiomas

Falcine meningiomas present with symptoms similar to those of parasagittal meningiomas. By definition, falcine meningiomas are covered at their surface by a cap of cerebral cortex. Only parasagittal meningiomas present in the angle between the falx, lateral wall superior sagittal sinus, and convexity dura. For the larger tumors, because the anterior falx artery cannot

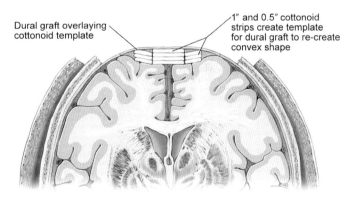
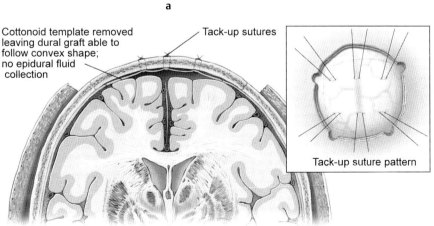

Fig. 32.6a,b (**a**) Convexity shape can be re-created using a template of cottonoids over which the dural graft can be cut to the proper size and shape. (**b**) After the cottonoid template is removed, the dural graft is sutured in and tacked up on both sides as well as in the midline. The epidural potential space is eliminated.

be embolized from its origin off the ethmoid and ophthalmic arteries, it is frequently advantageous to identify the falx anterior to the tumor and then to open it just below the superior sagittal sinus, working down the falx to coagulate and incise the falx to its inferior edge. The tumor is usually debulked to a minor degree immediately and the attachments along with the blood supply to the falx are taken down as a first step. Then internal debulking is done, followed by peripheral dissection.

Tentorial Meningiomas

Tentorial meningiomas account for less than 5% of all intracranial meningiomas but approximately 30% of posterior fossa meningiomas. Surgeons have previously divided them into medial, lateral, and falcotentorial regions, with the medial and lateral groups further subdivided into anterior, middle, and posterior locations. These tumors frequently present with headache, ataxia, nausea, and vomiting. Approaches to tentorial meningiomas can be complex and may involve ligation of affected and occluded transverse, straight, and superior sagittal sinuses. For lateral and falcotentorial meningiomas, the status of the major venous sinuses should be determined preoperatively with angiography.[57] For the most part, U-shaped inferiorly based flaps are used, with the flap centered over the direct line of approach to the tumor.

Petroclival Meningiomas

Petroclival meningiomas are thought to arise near the spheno-occipital synchondrosis and generally occupy the upper two thirds of the clivus medial to the fifth nerve. Common clinical symptoms are headache, gait disturbance, vertigo, and double vision. Today, many smaller tumors that are symptomatic or have documented growth are managed with radiosurgery. The larger tumors are still a surgical disease and can be managed with single- or two-stage approaches. A single-stage operation is best handled with a temporal craniotomy combined with a retrolabirinthine posterior fossa craniectomy, the so-called petrosal approach.[58] Alternatively, staged retrosigmoid and extended middle fossa approaches can be used for this tumor. Morbidity for the surgical treatment of these tumors remains significant, although, fortunately, cranial nerve deficits such as those that derive from dissection of cranial nerves IV, V, VI, and VII, frequently recover. Monitoring of auditory evoked brainstem potentials is necessary in those patients with useful hearing preoperatively.

Cerebellopontine Angle Meningiomas

Cerebellopontine angle meningiomas are attached to the dura medial to the sigmoid sinus below the superior petrosal sinus and above the jugular bulb. They can have attachments entirely posterior or both anterior (anterior petrous face) and posterior (posterior petrous face) to the internal auditory canal.

Clinical symptoms usually have insidious onset and include dysfunction of cranial nerves V, VII, and VIII. With large posterior lesions, cerebellar signs predominate. Most of these tumors can be operated on using standard retrosigmoid craniotomy, or a modified far lateral approach can be used to increase the exposure and allow for release of CSF from the upper cervical region after opening the foramen magnum and performing a C1 hemilaminectomy. Routine placement of a lumbar subarachnoid drain with intraoperative drainage of CSF can assist with the dural opening and with postoperative wound healing, decreasing the rate of postoperative CSF leakage.

Cerebellar Convexity Meningiomas

Cerebellar convexity meningiomas are infrequent and usually present with signs of increased intracranial pressure. These tumors can frequently be approached via a suboccipital craniotomy using a linear incision centered over the tumor. Image-guided systems are particularly useful for identifying the position of the transverse sinuses, and medial and lateral margins of the tumors. Suboccipital craniotomy may be preferable to craniectomy in an attempt to minimize the ingrowth of suboccipital musculature into the dura, which may be associated with prolonged postoperative headaches.

Foramen Magnum Meningiomas

Foramen magnum meningiomas present with variable symptoms. Most patients have a history of neck or suboccipital pain, and motor sensory symptoms develop, usually in one arm, and then in the contralateral leg. Because of the lower cranial nerve morbidity associated with surgical resection of these tumors, incidentally discovered tumors in this location can initially be followed. The standard approach for these tumors is the far lateral suboccipital approach with the patient in the three-quarter prone position.[59] The posterior one third of the occipital condyle is removed to improve access to the ventral dura. Once the dura is opened, the vertebral artery can be identified and is usually not directly invaded by meningioma. Sharp dissection of the arachnoid plane is key to preserving the rootlets of cranial nerves IX, X, XI, and XII. The patient should be warned that for the larger tumors such dissections could result in transient and possibly permanent problems with dysphasia and dysphonia.

Intraventricular Meningiomas

Intraventricular meningiomas account for less than 5% of all intracranial meningiomas.[60] The most common location is the atrium of the lateral ventricle. A patient usually presents with symptoms related to obstructive hydrocephalus such as headaches, nausea, and vomiting. Seizures can occur with large tumors in either hemisphere, and speech disturbance can occur for left-sided lesions. For nondominant tumors of

Special Consideration

- To assist with safe intraventricular meningioma resection, diffusion tensor imaging (DTI) can be used to display visual and somatosensory fiber pathways on image-guided system displays.

Pearl

- Using modern-day delivery systems for meningiomas, radiotherapy complication rates are low, and tumor control rates high.

the trigone, a temporal parietal craniotomy is used, with a middle temporal gyrus approach for access to the anterior choroidal supply early on in the operation. For giant nondominant lesions, a parieto-occipital craniotomy and a superior parietal lobule approach is also an option. For lesions of the dominant hemisphere, a superior parietal lobule approach is standard.

Postoperative Care

For all postoperative meningioma patients, intravenous fluids are run at maintenance levels, or slightly above maintenance levels. Normal hydration has not created any increased problems with hyponatremia and may serve to protect patients from the consequences of venous infarction, which typically becomes manifest on the second to fifth day postoperatively. Low molecular weight heparin may be given at a dose of 40 mg subcutaneously beginning the second day after surgery and continued for 7 days postoperatively.[61] Early mobilization is also key to preventing thromboembolic complications.

Radiotherapy

Approximately one in three meningiomas are not fully resectable, and this percentage may be higher for skull base tumors.[49] Although subtotal resection of a globular mass is an important goal when decompression is expected to result in improvement of symptoms, it is inadequate as a sole modality, with 5-, 10-, and 15-year progression-free survival rates of 50%, 40%, and 30%.[62] It is now clear that in many cases adjuvant radiotherapy techniques can prolong periods of tumor control and provide for excellent functional outcomes with low morbidity.

A variety of radiotherapy techniques using photon energy can be employed, and include fractionated radiotherapy with 3DCRT planning, IMRT, hypofractionated SRT, and single-session or multisession radiosurgery. Irrespective of the delivery system, modern-day imaging and planning systems provide excellent outcomes.

Fractionated radiotherapy techniques (3DCRT, IMRT, SRT) can be performed for well-circumscribed or diffuse tumors of all sizes in all locations.[43] Tumors adjacent to the optic apparatus require special consideration of dose limitations to these structures to preserve function, but tumor control rates with complete tumor coverage are excellent. Optimal therapy requires MRI, and when there is bony involvement, composite CT-MR volumes are helpful. Modern results for radiotherapy techniques with extensive follow-up indicate that 5- and 10-year progression free survivals range from 91 to 100%, and complication rates are acceptably low (**Table 32.5**).[63–65]

Patients who have Simpson grade I and grade II resections of benign meningiomas can be followed with interval scans and observed for occurrence. Patients with grade III or less extensive resection are candidates for adjuvant radiotherapy. Current evidence indicates that patients with known residual tumor who are followed have a shorter time to tumor recurrence than those who are treated with radiotherapy in the adjuvant setting. Atypical meningiomas have a higher recurrence rate and are frequently recommended for adjuvant radiotherapy irrespective of the extent of resection, although in some cases close interval follow-up may be appropriate. All malignant meningiomas should be irradiated to the maximum tolerated dose of 60 Gray (Gy).

In skull base meningiomas treated with fractionated radiotherapy after subtotal resection, comparable rates of long-term freedom from tumor recurrence were achieved with or without prior surgery.[66] In 14 patients with optic nerve

Table 32.5 Results of External Irradiation from Selected Series in the Modern Era

Author	Era	Dose (Gy) (Median)	5-/10-year PFS (%)	Complication Rate (%)
Metellus et al[63]	1990–2002	52.9[a]	98/96	<1
Litré et al[64]	1995–2006	45	94/NA	0
Milker-Zabel et al[65]	1985–2001	57.6	91/89	2.5
Mendenhall et al[66]	1984–2001	54	95/92	6
Narayan et al[67b]	1986–2001	54	100/NA	0 grade 3

[a] Mean Gy delivered.
[b] Fourteen patients with optic nerve sheath meningiomas.
Abbreviations: Gy, gray; NA, not applicable; PFS, progression-free survival.

sheath meningiomas treated to a median dose of 54 Gy and followed for a period of 4 years, visual acuity improved, was stable, or worsened in 36%, 50%, and 14% of patients, respectively.[67] There was no imaging evidence of tumor progression or recurrence.

Radiosurgery

For small to medium-size tumors less than 30 mm, or less than 8 cc, at sites not associated with critical structures such as optic nerves, chiasm, or brainstem, radiosurgery is a powerful technique as either a primary form of therapy, for residual

disease, or for treatment of recurrence (**Fig. 32.7**). A variety of delivery systems are used both with and without stereotactic head frames. To date, tumor control seems to be independent

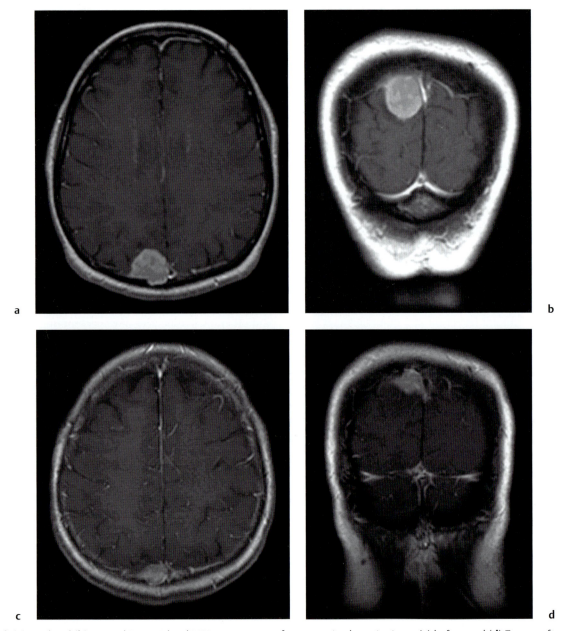

Fig. 32.7a–d (**a**) Axial and (**b**) coronal T1-weighted MRI postcontrast of a parasagittal meningioma (**c**) before and (**d**) 7 years after radiosurgery as the primary form of treatment.

Table 32.6 Results of Stereotactic Radiosurgery for Meningiomas: Selected Series since 2001

Authors	Year	No. Patients	Median Dose (Gy)	5-Year PFS (%)
Santacroce et al[69]	2012	4565	14	95
Pollock et al[70]	2012	416	16	96
dos Santos et al[71]	2011	88	14	93
Kondziolka et al[76]	2008	482	14[a]	97
Iwai et al[68]	2008	108	12	93
Malik et al[75]	2005	309	20	87
Kreil et al[74]	2005	200	12	98
DiBiase et al[73]	2004	162	14	86
Lee et al[72]	2002	159	13	93

[a] Mean Gy delivered.

Abbreviations: Gy, gray; PFS, progression-free survival.

of the delivery method, with 5-year progression-free survival between 86% and 98% in modern series (**Table 32.6**).[68–76]

In general, doses of 14 Gy or more are associated with the best tumor control rates. There is controversy about whether the dural tail needs to be included in the target volume, but the general consensus is that inclusion of the first several millimeters of the adjacent dura within the dural tail may be sufficient. The results of primary radiosurgery and resection for patients with Simpson grade I or II surgical resection were compared and, after a mean follow-up of 7 years, the progression-free survival with radiosurgery was equivalent to that achieved by Simpson grade I excision.[77] A study of a minimum of 10 years' follow-up for 85 meningiomas has confirmed that the long-term tumor control with progression-free survival is greater than 90% and tumor volume decreases in 53% of patients.[78] Complication rates were low, and no patient developed a radiation-induced tumor. One of the concerns regarding use of radiotherapy for benign tumors is the risk of malignancy generation or secondary tumor induction. However, data suggest that this risk is acceptably low, perhaps 1 to 2% at 10 to 20 years after treatment.[79]

Chemotherapy

Although there have been several early reports of the success of individual agents in small clinical series, there has been no collective experience with a single drug agent that indicates consistent responses for recurrent, benign, atypical, or malignant meningiomas. Agents such as CPT-11, temozolomide, hydroxyurea, tamoxifen, RU46, cyclophosphamide, Adriamycin, vincristine, and hydroxyprogesterone have been disappointing.[80] Newer agents such as tyrosine kinase receptor antagonists are under investigation. Alpha-interferon has been used for patients with malignant meningiomas, and there are experimental studies indicating potential for other small molecule inhibitors. Future investigations require a focus on newer agents that can help us deal with recurrent, atypical, and malignant meningiomas.

■ Conclusion

The successful management of a meningioma requires thorough knowledge of the many aspects of this tumor in all its parts, as mentioned by Cushing and Eisenhardt back in the 1930s.[1] Decisions regarding treatment must be made on a case-by-case basis, understanding that these tumors are, for the most part, benign, and that all therapy carries some risk of side effects. One algorithm for management is suggested in **Fig. 32.8**. Considering all options for treatment, a successful outcome for the patient can be achieved in the majority of cases. For those patients who require surgery, there is no substitute for the surgeon's keen knowledge of anatomy and delicate surgical technique, although recent surgical adjuncts have improved our efficiency and results in the past 20 years. For those patients in whom we cannot achieve a surgical cure, modern-day radiotherapy techniques can provide long-term tumor control with few side effects. Continued research is needed to find effective strategies for recurrent atypical and malignant meningiomas.

Editor's Note

Although non–skull base meningiomas are among the "bread and butter" operations in the practice of neurosurgery, and primarily a neurosurgical disease, they still pose substantial challenges to the whole neuro-oncology team. Advances in imaging, instrumentation, and radiation oncology tools such as stereotactic radiosurgery have transformed the care of these patients, but treatment dilemmas remain. Not as much scientific energy has been focused on meningiomas as on gliomas, because of their relatively benign nature, but we need greater understanding so that we can apply new molecular and chemotherapeutic treatments to the ones that are not completely resectable and to recurrent ones and those of WHO grade II and III.

As patients with meningioma generally have a different perioperative experience compared with patients with malignant tumors, and as they have excellent survival, increased focus on quality-of-life studies often using qualitative research methodologies is also important.[81,82] Another interesting facet of meningiomas relates to the common finding of incidental asymptomatic ones and the role of conservative management for these and even for some minimally symptomatic meningiomas.[82] (Bernstein)

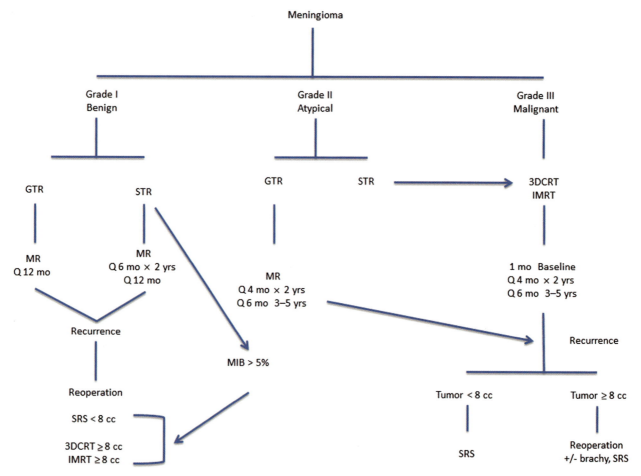

Fig. 32.8 Treatment algorithm for management of meningioma. GTR, gross total resection; MR, magnetic resonance; STR, subtotal resection; 3DCRT, three-dimensional conformal radiotherapy; IMRT, intensity-modulated radiotherapy; SRS, stereotactic radiosurgery; brachy, brachytherapy.

References

1. Cushing H, Eisenhardt L. Meningiomas. Their Classification, Regional Behaviour, Life History, and Surgical End Results. Springfield, IL: Charles C. Thomas, 1938

2. Sughrue ME, Kane AJ, Shangari G, et al. The relevance of Simpson Grade I and II resection in modern neurosurgical treatment of World Health Organization Grade I meningiomas. J Neurosurg 2010;113: 1029–1035

3. Sughrue ME, Rutkowski MJ, Aranda D, Barani IJ, McDermott MW, Parsa AT. Factors affecting outcome following treatment of patients with cavernous sinus meningiomas. J Neurosurg 2010;113:1087–1092

4. Sughrue ME, Rutkowski MJ, Shangari G, Parsa AT, Berger MS, McDermott MW. Results with judicious modern neurosurgical management of parasagittal and falcine meningiomas. Clinical article. J Neurosurg 2011;114:731–737

5. Dolecek TA, Propp JM, Stroup NE, Kruchko C. CBTRUS statistical report: primary brain and central nervous system tumors diagnosed in the United States in 2005–2009. Neuro-oncol 2012;14(Suppl 5): v1–v49

6. McDermott M, Wilson C. Meningiomas. In: Youmans J, ed. Neurological Surgery, 4th ed. Philadelphia: WB Saunders, 1996:2782–2825

7. Perry A, Louis DN, Scheithauer BW. Meningiomas. In: Louis DN, Ohgaki H, Wiestler OD, Cavenee WK, eds. WHO Classification of Tumours of the Central Nervous System, Lyon, France: IARC Press, 2007

8. Mawrin C, Perry A. Pathological classification and molecular genetics of meningiomas. J Neurooncol 2010;99:379–391

9. Simpson D. The recurrence of intracranial meningiomas after surgical treatment. J Neurol Neurosurg Psychiatry 1957;20:22–39

10. Jääskeläinen J, Haltia M, Servo A. Atypical and anaplastic meningiomas: radiology, surgery, radiotherapy, and outcome. Surg Neurol 1986; 25:233–242

11. Stafford SL, Perry A, Suman VJ, et al. Primarily resected meningiomas: outcome and prognostic factors in 581 Mayo Clinic patients, 1978 through 1988. Mayo Clin Proc 1998;73:936–942

12. Abramovich CM, Prayson RA. MIB-1 labeling indices in benign, aggressive, and malignant meningiomas: a study of 90 tumors. Hum Pathol 1998;29:1420–1427

13. Ho DM-T, Hsu C-Y, Ting L-T, Chiang H. Histopathology and MIB-1 labeling index predicted recurrence of meningiomas: a proposal of diagnostic criteria for patients with atypical meningioma. Cancer 2002;94: 1538–1547

14. Kayaselçuk F, Zorludemir S, Gümürdühü D, Zeren H, Erman T. PCNA and Ki-67 in central nervous system tumors: correlation with the histological type and grade. J Neurooncol 2002;57:115–121

15. Kunishio K, Ohmoto T, Matsuhisa T, Maeshiro T, Furuta T, Matsumoto K. The significance of nucleolar organizer region (AgNOR) score in predicting meningioma recurrence. Cancer 1994;73:2200–2205

16. Nakasu S, Li DH, Okabe H, Nakajima M, Matsuda M. Significance of MIB-1 staining indices in meningiomas: comparison of two counting methods. Am J Surg Pathol 2001;25:472–478

17. Striepecke E, Handt S, Weis J, et al. Correlation of histology, cytogenetics and proliferation fraction (Ki-67 and PCNA) quantitated by image analysis in meningiomas. Pathol Res Pract 1996;192:816–824

18. Louis DN, Scheithauer BW, Budka H, von Deimling A, Kepes JJ. Meningiomas. In: Kleihues P, Cavenee WK, eds. Pathology and Genetics of Tumours of the Nervous System. Lyon, France: IARC, 2000

19. Weber RG, Boström J, Wolter M, et al. Analysis of genomic alterations in benign, atypical, and anaplastic meningiomas: toward a genetic model of meningioma progression. Proc Natl Acad Sci U S A 1997;94:14719–14724

20. Cuevas IC, Slocum AL, Jun P, et al. Meningioma transcript profiles reveal deregulated Notch signaling pathway. Cancer Res 2005;65:5070–5075

21. Stuart JE, Lusis EA, Scheck AC, et al. Identification of gene markers associated with aggressive meningioma by filtering across multiple sets of gene expression arrays. J Neuropathol Exp Neurol 2011;70:1–12

22. Al-Mefty O, Kadri PAS, Pravdenkova S, Sawyer JR, Stangeby C, Husain M. Malignant progression in meningioma: documentation of a series and analysis of cytogenetic findings. J Neurosurg 2004;101:210–218

23. Ruttledge MH, Sarrazin J, Rangaratnam S, et al. Evidence for the complete inactivation of the NF2 gene in the majority of sporadic meningiomas. Nat Genet 1994;6:180–184

24. Ruttledge MH, Xie YG, Han FY, et al. Physical mapping of the NF2/meningioma region on human chromosome 22q12. Genomics 1994;19:52–59

25. Dumanski JP, Rouleau GA, Nordenskjöld M, Collins VP. Molecular genetic analysis of chromosome 22 in 81 cases of meningioma. Cancer Res 1990;50:5863–5867

26. Rouleau GA, Merel P, Lutchman M, et al. Alteration in a new gene encoding a putative membrane-organizing protein causes neuro-fibromatosis type 2. Nature 1993;363:515–521

27. Clark VE, Erson-Omay EZ, Serin A, et al. Genomic analysis of non-NF2 meningiomas reveals mutations in TRAF7, KLF4, AKT1, and SMO. Science 2013;339:1077–1080

28. Goutagny S, Raymond E, Sterkers O, Colombani JM, Kalamarides M. Radiographic regression of cranial meningioma in a NF2 patient treated by bevacizumab. Ann Oncol 2011;22:990–991

29. Puchner MJA, Hans VH, Harati A, Lohmann F, Glas M, Herrlinger U. Bevacizumab-induced regression of anaplastic meningioma. Ann Oncol 2010;21:2445–2446

30. Yew A, Trang A, Nagasawa DT, et al. Chromosomal alterations, prognostic factors, and targeted molecular therapies for malignant meningiomas. J Clin Neurosci 2013;20:17–22

31. Smith JS, Quiñones-Hinojosa A, Harmon-Smith M, Bollen AW, McDermott MW. Sex steroid and growth factor profile of a meningioma associated with pregnancy. Can J Neurol Sci 2005;32:122–127

32. McDermott MW. Current treatment of meningiomas. Curr Opin Neurol 1996;9:409–413

33. Claus EB, Black PM, Bondy ML, et al. Exogenous hormone use and meningioma risk: what do we tell our patients? Cancer 2007;110:471–476

34. Kawahara Y, Niiro M, Yokoyama S, Kuratsu J. Dural congestion accompanying meningioma invasion into vessels: the dural tail sign. Neuroradiology 2001;43:462–465

35. Cha S, Yang L, Johnson G, et al. Comparison of microvascular permeability measurements, K(trans), determined with conventional steady-state T1-weighted and first-pass T2*-weighted MR imaging methods in gliomas and meningiomas. AJNR Am J Neuroradiol 2006;27:409–417

36. Jun P, Garcia J, Tihan T, McDermott MW, Cha S. Perfusion MR imaging of an intracranial collision tumor confirmed by image-guided biopsy. AJNR Am J Neuroradiol 2006;27:94–97

37. Martin AJ, Cha S, Higashida RT, et al. Assessment of vasculature of meningiomas and the effects of embolization with intra-arterial MR perfusion imaging: a feasibility study. AJNR Am J Neuroradiol 2007;28:1771–1777

38. Chun JY, McDermott MW, Lamborn KR, Wilson CB, Higashida R, Berger MS. Delayed surgical resection reduces intraoperative blood loss for embolized meningiomas. Neurosurgery 2002;50:1231–1235, discussion 1235–1237

39. Waldron JS, Sughrue ME, Hetts SW, et al. Embolization of skull base meningiomas and feeding vessels arising from the internal carotid circulation. Neurosurgery 2011;68:162–169, discussion 169

40. Wadley J, Dorward N, Kitchen N, Thomas D. Pre-operative planning and intra-operative guidance in modern neurosurgery: a review of 300 cases. Ann R Coll Surg Engl 1999;81:217–225

41. McDermott MW. Intraventricular meningiomas. Neurosurg Clin N Am 2003;14:559–569

42. Turazzi S, Cristofori L, Gambin R, Bricolo A. The pterional approach for the microsurgical removal of olfactory groove meningiomas. Neurosurgery 1999;45:821–825, discussion 825–826

43. Bauman G, Wong E, McDermott M. Fractionated radiotherapy techniques. Neurosurg Clin N Am 2006;17:99–110, v v

44. Zygourakis C, Sughrue ME, Parsa AT, Berger MS, McDermott MW. Modern Treatment of Planum/Olfactory Meningiomas. Unpublished. 2013

45. Chi JH, McDermott MW. Tuberculum sellae meningiomas. Neurosurg Focus 2003;14:e6

46. Fahlbusch R, Schott W. Pterional surgery of meningiomas of the tuberculum sellae and planum sphenoidale: surgical results with special consideration of ophthalmological and endocrinological outcomes. J Neurosurg 2002;96:235–243

47. Laufer I, Anand VK, Schwartz TH. Endoscopic, endonasal extended transsphenoidal, transplanum transtuberculum approach for resection of suprasellar lesions. J Neurosurg 2007;106:400–406

48. Ogawa Y, Tominaga T. Extended transsphenoidal approach for tuberculum sellae meningioma—what are the optimum and critical indications? Acta Neurochir (Wien) 2012;154:621–626

49. Goldsmith B, McDermott MW. Meningioma. Neurosurg Clin N Am 2006;17:111–120, vi vi

50. Goldsmith BJ, Wara WM, Wilson CB, Larson DA. Postoperative irradiation for subtotally resected meningiomas. A retrospective analysis of 140 patients treated from 1967 to 1990. J Neurosurg 1994;80:195–201

51. McDermott MW, Durity FA, Rootman J, Woodhurst WB. Combined frontotemporal-orbitozygomatic approach for tumors of the sphenoid wing and orbit. Neurosurgery 1990;26:107–116

52. DeMonte F. Surgical treatment of anterior basal meningiomas. J Neurooncol 1996;29:239–248

53. Sughrue ME, Rutkowski MJ, Chen CJ, et al. Modern surgical outcomes following surgery for sphenoid wing meningiomas. J Neurosurg 2013;119:86–93

54. Metellus P, Regis J, Muracciole X, et al. Evaluation of fractionated radiotherapy and gamma knife radiosurgery in cavernous sinus meningiomas: treatment strategy. Neurosurgery 2005;57:873–886, discussion 873–886

55. Al-Mefty O, Smith RR. Surgery of tumors invading the cavernous sinus. Surg Neurol 1988;30:370–381

56. Ransohoff J. Removal of convexity, parasagittal, and falcine meningiomas. Neurosurg Clin N Am 1994;5:293–297
57. Quinones-Hinojosa A, Chang EF, McDermott MW. Falcotentorial meningiomas: clinical, neuroimaging, and surgical features in six patients. Neurosurg Focus 2003;14:e11
58. Couldwell WT, Fukushima T, Giannotta SL, Weiss MH. Petroclival meningiomas: surgical experience in 109 cases. J Neurosurg 1996;84:20–28
59. Sekhar LN, Wright DC, Richardson R, Monacci W. Petroclival and foramen magnum meningiomas: surgical approaches and pitfalls. J Neurooncol 1996;29:249–259
60. Criscuolo GR, Symon L. Intraventricular meningioma. A review of 10 cases of the National Hospital, Queen Square (1974–1985) with reference to the literature. Acta Neurochir (Wien) 1986;83:83–91
61. Agnelli G, Piovella F, Buoncristiani P, et al. Enoxaparin plus compression stockings compared with compression stockings alone in the prevention of venous thromboembolism after elective neurosurgery. N Engl J Med 1998;339:80–85
62. Condra KS, Buatti JM, Mendenhall WM, Friedman WA, Marcus RB Jr, Rhoton AL. Benign meningiomas: primary treatment selection affects survival. Int J Radiat Oncol Biol Phys 1997;39:427–436
63. Metellus P, Batra S, Karkar S, et al. Fractionated conformal radiotherapy in the management of cavernous sinus meningiomas: long-term functional outcome and tumor control at a single institution. Int J Radiat Oncol Biol Phys 2010;78:836–843
64. Litré CF, Colin P, Noudel R, et al. Fractionated stereotactic radiotherapy treatment of cavernous sinus meningiomas: a study of 100 cases. Int J Radiat Oncol Biol Phys 2009;74:1012–1017
65. Milker-Zabel S, Zabel A, Schulz-Ertner D, Schlegel W, Wannenmacher M, Debus J. Fractionated stereotactic radiotherapy in patients with benign or atypical intracranial meningioma: long-term experience and prognostic factors. Int J Radiat Oncol Biol Phys 2005;61:809–816
66. Mendenhall WM, Morris CG, Amdur RJ, Foote KD, Friedman WA. Radiotherapy alone or after subtotal resection for benign skull base meningiomas. Cancer 2003;98:1473–1482
67. Narayan S, Cornblath WT, Sandler HM, Elner V, Hayman JA. Preliminary visual outcomes after three-dimensional conformal radiation therapy for optic nerve sheath meningioma. Int J Radiat Oncol Biol Phys 2003;56:537–543
68. Iwai Y, Yamanaka K, Ikeda H. Gamma Knife radiosurgery for skull base meningioma: long-term results of low-dose treatment. J Neurosurg 2008;109:804–810
69. Santacroce A, Walier M, Régis J, et al. Long-term tumor control of benign intracranial meningiomas after radiosurgery in a series of 4565 patients. Neurosurgery 2012;70:32–39, discussion 39
70. Pollock BE, Stafford SL, Link MJ, Brown PD, Garces YI, Foote RL. Single-fraction radiosurgery of benign intracranial meningiomas. Neurosurgery 2012;71:604–612, discussion 613
71. dos Santos MA, de Salcedo JBP, Gutiérrez Diaz JA, et al. Long-term outcomes of stereotactic radiosurgery for treatment of cavernous sinus meningiomas. Int J Radiat Oncol Biol Phys 2011;81:1436–1441
72. Lee JYK, Niranjan A, McInerney J, Kondziolka D, Flickinger JC, Lunsford LD. Stereotactic radiosurgery providing long-term tumor control of cavernous sinus meningiomas. J Neurosurg 2002;97:65–72
73. DiBiase SJ, Kwok Y, Yovino S, et al. Factors predicting local tumor control after gamma knife stereotactic radiosurgery for benign intracranial meningiomas. Int J Radiat Oncol Biol Phys 2004;60:1515–1519
74. Kreil W, Luggin J, Fuchs I, Weigl V, Eustacchio S, Papaefthymiou G. Long term experience of gamma knife radiosurgery for benign skull base meningiomas. J Neurol Neurosurg Psychiatry 2005;76:1425–1430
75. Malik I, Rowe JG, Walton L, Radatz MWR, Kemeny AA. The use of stereotactic radiosurgery in the management of meningiomas. Br J Neurosurg 2005;19:13–20
76. Kondziolka D, Mathieu D, Lunsford LD, et al. Radiosurgery as definitive management of intracranial meningiomas. Neurosurgery 2008;62:53–58, discussion 58–60
77. Pollock BE, Stafford SL, Utter A, Giannini C, Schreiner SA. Stereotactic radiosurgery provides equivalent tumor control to Simpson Grade 1 resection for patients with small- to medium-size meningiomas. Int J Radiat Oncol Biol Phys 2003;55:1000–1005
78. Kondziolka D, Nathoo N, Flickinger JC, Niranjan A, Maitz AH, Lunsford LD. Long-term results after radiosurgery for benign intracranial tumors. Neurosurgery 2003;53:815–821, discussion 821–822
79. Rowe J. Late neoplastic complications after radiation treatments for benign intracranial tumors. Neurosurg Clin N Am 2006;17:181–185, vii vii
80. Schrell UM, Rittig MG, Koch U, Marschalek R, Anders M. Hydroxyurea for treatment of unresectable meningiomas. Lancet 1996;348:888–889
81. Wong J, Mendelsohn D, Nyhof-Young J, Bernstein M. A qualitative assessment of the supportive care and resource needs of patients undergoing craniotomy for benign brain tumours. Support Care Cancer 2011;19:1841–1848
82. Jagadeesh H, Bernstein M. Patients' anxiety around incidental brain tumors: a qualitative study. Acta Neurochir (Wien) 2014;156:375–381

Skull Base Meningiomas and Other Tumors

Kaith K. Almefty, Kadir Erkmen, and Ossama Al-Mefty

A wide range of tumor pathologies occur at the skull base. They are often slow-growing, benign, extra-axial tumors that cause symptoms by involvement of the cranial nerves or a mass effect on the brainstem and cerebellum. They are frequently located in critical areas with brainstem compression and involvement of delicate neurovascular structures that are especially hard to reach with routine surgical techniques. The introduction of microsurgical techniques heralded an era of technical advances that ultimately translated into decreased patient morbidity and mortality.

The 1980s witnessed the popularization of skull base techniques. The combination of microsurgical and skull base surgery techniques has allowed access to areas of the brain once considered inaccessible. The addition of neuromonitoring, neuronavigation, improved optics, and surgeon experience has advanced the field to its current state. Most benign skull base lesions once considered inoperable are now curable with excellent rates of morbidity and mortality. The addition of stereotactic radiosurgery has further supplemented the field, providing tumor control in lesions not dissectible from essential structures and in poor surgical candidates.

◼ Skull Base Meningioma

Meningiomas occur frequently, constituting 20% or more of all intracranial tumors. Their incidence in community-based series and clinical series varies from 1 to 6 cases per 100,000 persons per year and on average is estimated to be around 2.6 cases per 100,000 persons per year.[1] However, in autopsy-based studies, meningiomas are present in 2.3% of people,[2] suggesting that many people harbor undiagnosed asymptomatic meningiomas.

The modern widespread use of magnetic resonance imaging (MRI) has resulted in a large number of these meningiomas being discovered incidentally. The asymptomatic incidentally discovered meningioma is a management challenge. Tumor progression in conservatively managed meningiomas is reported to range from 22 to 90% in natural history studies,[3–8] with higher rates reported in studies using volumetric rather than linear growth analysis. Significant factors associated with a higher likelihood of progression are age < 60, large tumor size (> 25 mm), lack of calcification, associated edema, and hyperintensity on T2-weighted MRI sequences.[4,6,9] Close follow-up is necessary, particularly of skull base tumors. In a study of the natural history of petroclival meningiomas, growth was noted in 76% of cases, with 63% of the growing tumors causing a functional decline.[10] Prudent surgeons should have an understanding of this natural history, allowing them to avoid the potential morbidities of surgery in the patient who is likely to receive little benefit from intervention, while not withholding a potential surgical cure from the patient who would otherwise be devastated by the disease.

Forty percent of meningiomas occur at the skull base. The sphenoid ridge is the most commonly involved location at the skull base[11] (**Fig. 33.1a**). Other locations include the olfactory groove, planum sphenoidale, tuberculum sella, anterior clinoid, cavernous sinus, cerebellopontine angle, clivus and petroclival area, and foramen magnum.

Imaging Studies

Computed tomography (CT) scan of meningiomas typically reveals a hyperdense extra-axial lesion relative to the adjacent brain. In up to 25% of cases, tumoral calcification may be present. In particular, bone sclerosis and hyperostosis may be seen at the site of origin of meningiomas of the skull base, which is believed to be tumor invasion. An MRI examination of these tumors typically demonstrates marked enhancement of the tumor with a dural tail. Mushrooming of the tumor is a concerning sign and has been associated with higher grade meningiomas and higher likelihood of recurrence.[12,13] Imaging should be carefully reviewed for multiple lesions, particularly at the skull base. On T1-weighted images most of these tumors are isointense as compared with gray matter. On T2-weighted sequences, these lesions typically demonstrate similar or increased intensity relative to the gray matter. The T2 sequence is also useful in identifying a hyperintense band between the tumor and the brain. Absence of this band is a concerning sign and often represents an inability to dissect the tumor safely from the brain (**Fig. 33.1b**). Brainstem edema seen on T2 sequences is a troublesome sign and may be associated with poor outcome (**Fig. 33.1b**). MRI and magnetic res-

---

Special Consideration

- The recurrence rate of meningiomas is directly related to the extent of resection.

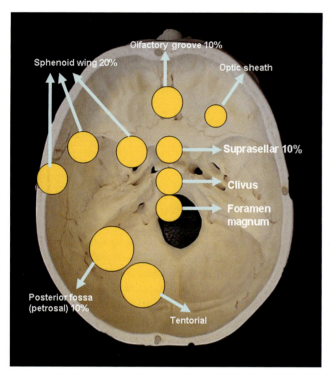

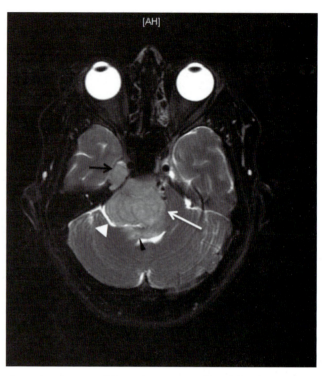

Fig. 33.1a,b (a) The distribution of meningiomas along the skull base. **(b)** Axial T2-weighted magnetic resonance imaging (MRI) of a petroclival meningioma demonstrating a hyperintense T2 band (*white arrowhead*), which indicates the presence of a dissectible arachnoid plane; the absence of the T2 hyperintense band (*black arrowhead*), indicating a lack of this plane; hyperintensity in the brainstem (*white arrow*), which is associated with worse outcomes; and extension into the cavernous sinus (*black arrow*).

onance venography (MRV) can examine the extent of dural sinus involvement and sinus patency. Angiography may be indicated for preoperative embolization of feeding vessels supplying vascular tumors. Angiography also helps in the preoperative evaluation of the venous complex of the vein of Labbé, especially when the petrosal approach is indicated or when the tentorium needs to be cut. This venous anatomy can adequately be evaluated with MRV or computed tomography venography (CTV), but angiography may still be utilized in special cases.

Surgical Management

The mainstay of meningioma management regardless of location is surgical resection. The steps involved in resection of basal meningiomas include tumor devascularization via coagulation of the tumor base followed by internal debulking and finally removal of the tumor capsule from the surrounding vital neurovascular structures while respecting the arachnoid plane (**Fig. 33.2**). Clinical features that affect the extent of resection include tumor location, size, consistency, and vascular/neural involvement. It is important to excise not only the neoplasm but also the involved dura, soft tissue, and bone to decrease the risk of recurrence. The extent of meningioma resection is directly associated with the risk of tumor recur-

rence. The extent of meningioma resection has been graded based on the Simpson classification. Grade I or II is radical tumor removal with resection of the involved dura and bone at the tumor origin (grade I) or coagulation of the tumor origin (grade II).[14] The skull base approaches facilitate tumor resection along with the involved bone and dura while placing minimal retraction on the brain and providing a flat wide surgical corridor to promote safe dissection of the vital neurovascular structures. A selection of these approaches along with the meningiomas for which they are well suited are described below.

■ Tuberculum Sellae, Olfactory Groove Meningiomas, and the Supraorbital Approach

Tuberculum sella meningiomas comprise 5 to 10% of intracranial meningiomas (**Fig. 33.3a**). They typically present with progressive asymmetrical visual loss, incongruous visual field defects, and rarely panhypopituitarism. Visual field defects are identified in 84% of patients. Seizures are present in 10%, and pituitary dysfunction in 9%. These meningiomas originate from the tuberculum sella, chiasmatic sulcus, limbus sphe-

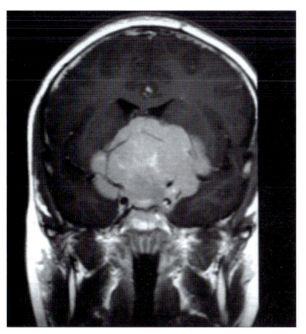
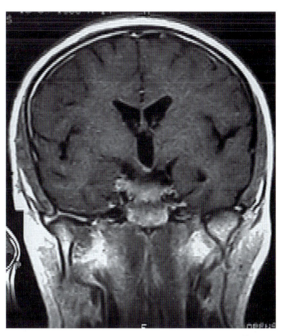

a

b

Fig. 33.2a,b (**a**) Preoperative coronal T1-weighted MRI with contrast demonstrating a giant suprasellar meningioma encasing the circle of Willis. (**b**) Postoperative coronal T1-weighted MRI with contrast demonstrating a gross total removal. Resection is facilitated by the presence of an arachnoid plane between the tumor and the neuro-vascular structures.

noidale, and diaphragma sella, and have a small dural attachment. The bone may be involved with exostosis at the anterior margin of the sella. The optic nerves are usually elevated and displaced laterally. Tumor invasion into the optic canals was present in 67% of tuberculum sellae meningiomas. Unroofing of the optic canal is typically necessary for safe tumor resection and decompression of the nerve. The carotid arteries are displaced laterally. The pituitary stalk and basilar artery are usually displaced posteriorly and separated by the membrane of Liliequist, which often provides an excellent dissection plane. Outcomes are generally good, as in most cases a Simpson grade I resection is achievable (86% in the senior author's [OA] experience). Also visual outcomes are typically excellent, with visual improvement reported in 70 to 80% of patients, and these improvements are often dramatic.[15] A small subset of anterior cranial fossa meningiomas arises directly from the diaphragma sella. These tumors typically grow retrochiasmatically, compress the hypothalamus, and are challenging.[16]

Patients with olfactory groove meningiomas may present with symptoms and signs of frontal lobe dysfunction, including changes in mental status, particularly mood and motivation. They may have anosmia. The Foster Kennedy syndrome of anosmia, optic atrophy in the ipsilateral eye associated with papilledema in the contralateral eye, is uncommon but associated with olfactory meningiomas. These meningiomas are typically discovered late and may become very large prior to correct diagnosis. The tumor arises in the midline of the anterior fossa over the cribriform plate of the ethmoid bone and the planum sphenoidale. The tumor's blood supply is

Controversy

- Expanded endonasal transsphenoidal approaches are applied in selected cases of anterior cranial fossa meningiomas.

from the anterior ethmoidal artery. The tumors may extend into the ethmoids and nasal cavity.[17]

The supraorbital approach (**Fig. 33.3b**), which includes the orbital rim with a frontal flap, is the authors' preferred approach for tuberculum sellae and olfactory groove meningiomas. It provides a basal approach, eliminating the need for brain retraction, and affords the advantage of unroofing the optic canals bilaterally. The endonasal, endoscopic, and extended endonasal transsphenoidal approaches have been reported to remove smaller tuberculum sellae meningiomas (< 3.5 cm).[18–28] To use this approach effectively, these tumors should have no vascular or neural encasement and present no extension into the optic canal.[18,23] Several studies discussing the endonasal endoscopic approaches have shown relatively higher recurrence rates, in the range of 33%, as well as a greater proportion of patients with residual tumor (15 to 57%).[20,21,25,27] Visual improvements ranged from 0 to 60% in patients with tuberculum sellae meningiomas treated via this approach.[23,28] Worsening of vision was seen in up to 33% of patients.[21] Series that limit the endonasal approach to carefully selected small

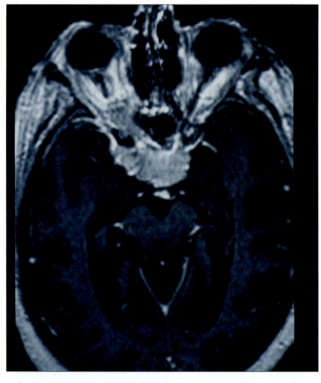

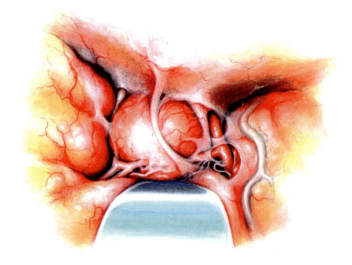

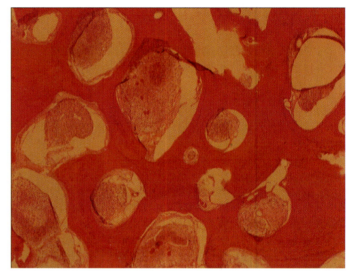

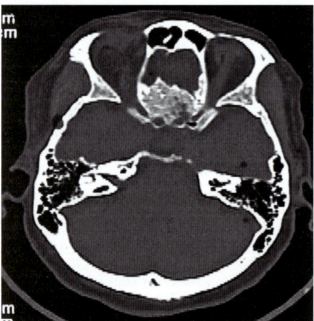

Fig. 33.3a–d (**a**) T1-weighted axial enhanced MRI demonstrating extension into the optic canals. Complete resection and improved visual outcomes are achieved with opening the optic canal. (**b**) Operative illustration of the supraorbital approach used for resection. (**c**) Computed tomography (CT) scan with hyperostosis of the bone caused by tumor invasion. (**d**) Histological section demonstrating the infiltration of tumor into the haversian canals of the bone. (From Al-Mefty O. Operative Atlas of Meningiomas. Philadelphia: Lippincott Williams & Wilkins, 1998:40. Reproduced with permission from Lippincott Williams & Wilkins.)

midline lesions without major vessel encasement have demonstrated good results.[21,26]

The patient is placed in the supine position and the trunk is elevated 20 degrees, with the head moderately hyperextended and fixed in a Mayfield headrest to allow the frontal lobes to fall backward. The head is kept straight to facilitate orientation. The scalp incision is started 1 cm anterior to the tragus and continued behind the hairline to the level of the superior temporal line on the opposite side. In this manner, the superficial temporal artery course is posterior to the incision, whereas the branches of the facial nerve are anterior. The scalp behind the incision is elevated and freed from the pericranium, leaving the thick areolar tissue with the pericranium. A large pericranial flap based on the supraorbital and frontal vessels is then incised as far posteriorly as possible, dissected forward, and reflected over the scalp flap. Both layers of the temporalis fascia are incised posterior to and along the course of the upper branches of the facial nerve until muscle fibers are seen. The deep fascia, the fat pad, and the superficial fascia are then retracted anteriorly. The upper portion of the temporal muscle is detached from its insertion anteriorly and is retracted posteriorly, exposing the junction of the zygomatic, sphenoidal, and frontal bones.

The bone flap used depends on the size and location of the tumor. After the bone flap is removed, the dura is tacked up and opened under the microscope. Elevation of the frontal lobe should be minimal. The olfactory nerve is located and preserved by dissecting it for some distance from the base of the frontal lobe. Tumor feeders are encountered early; they are coagulated and severed on the basal aspect of the tumor. Devascularization is restricted to midline to avoid injury to the optic nerve on either side. Midline orientation is maintained by observing the position of the falx. The tumor is debulked with suction, ultrasonic aspirator, or a bipolar coagulator and microscissors.

Once the dissection approaches the neurovascular structures, only bipolar cautery and microdissection should be used. After the tumor is debulked, the optic nerves, which are displaced laterally, are identified. The tumor is slowly stripped from the flattened or engulfed nerve. Despite apparent encasement of or severe adherence to the nerve, a plane of dissection can be obtained under high magnification. To preserve any remaining vision, dissection of the optic nerve and its blood supply must be meticulous. Dissection may need to begin at the chiasm so that the surgeon can locate and dissect an obscured optic nerve on the opposite side.

Arterial structures should be preserved through the same method of sharp microdissection into an arachnoidal plane. The carotid artery is dissected free from the tumor with an array of microinstruments, including bipolar forceps, microdissectors, and scissors. Carotid dissection continues to free the ophthalmic artery, the posterior communicating artery, the anterior thalamic perforators, and the choroidal artery. Further dissection of the tumor progresses to the bifurcation of the internal carotid artery (ICA) and into the sylvian fissure. Dissection is then continued to free the middle and anterior cerebral arteries. In most cases, the tumor has simply displaced each vessel and their perforators, and rarely actually engulfs them. The A1 segments in particular are usually severely stretched or adherent and tend to tear. Although arterial twigs of the anterior cerebral arteries may supply the tumor, the surgeon must first be certain that these vessels are, indeed, tumor feeders and not hypothalamic perforators or the optic tract blood supply. Thus, each arterial branch should be dissected and followed to ascertain its eventual course. Particular precision is needed to spare the artery of Heubner and the vital branches to the striatum. As dissection continues, both A1 arteries and the anterior communicating artery are freed from the tumor.

The membrane of Liliequist is intact, making tumor removal from the posteriorly displaced basilar artery easy. The

pituitary stalk can be recognized by its distinctive color and vascular network. A tumor extending backward under the hypothalamus usually displaces the pituitary stalk backward and to one side. Some tumors actually engulf the pituitary stalk and require meticulous and tedious dissection. The blood supply to the pituitary gland should be preserved. The tumor impinging on the hypothalamus can be removed gently if the surgeon maintains a plane of cleavage. Excessive downward retraction of the tumor, however, should be avoided. The arachnoid membrane of Liliequist provides an excellent plane of dissection for tumor removal. Often this membrane comes away with the tumor, leaving the rostral pons, midbrain, oculomotor nerves, and basilar artery and its branches in full view.

When the tumor extends into the optic canal, the anterior clinoid process, the roof of the optic canal, and the roof of the superior orbital fissure are drilled away with the diamond bit of the high-speed air drill. The dura is then opened along the optic nerve. Tumor tissue around the optic nerve is removed with bipolar forceps and microdissectors, and the surgeon must pay particular attention to preserving the hypothalamic and central retinal arteries. This bony drilling exposes the superior aspect of the cavernous sinus, and the ICA emerges through the superior wall and is surrounded and firmly anchored to the dura by a ring. Beginning at this emergence, an incision is made in the exposed dura and extended posteriorly toward the posterior clinoid process. The ICA is then followed in retrograde fashion into the cavernous sinus where it is dissected.

Following the removal of the tumor, its dural attachment should be resected or coagulated. Involved bone (**Fig. 33.3c,d**) should be removed with a diamond bit of a high-speed drill. Any opening into a paranasal sinus requires thorough repair of the dural defect. If the sphenoid sinus was entered, its mucosa is exenterated, and the sinus is packed with fat taken from the patient's thigh. A large piece of fascia lata is laid intradurally and secured with sutures along the lesser sphenoid wing. The graft is then spread to cover the frontal fossa and then sutured to the frontal dura. The preserved pericranial flap in the frontal region is turned over the frontal sinus and extended over any defect in the floor of the frontal fossa. Titanium microplates are used here to reattach the bone flap to the cranial vault. The temporal muscle is sutured to the fascia at the lateral orbital rim, and the skin is closed in two layers.

■ Clinoidal, Cavernous Sinus, and Meckel's Cave Meningiomas, and the Cranio-Orbital Zygomatic Approach

Clinoidal meningiomas originate from the anterior clinoid and present with visual loss in 84% of cases.[29] They are divided into three groups based on their point of origin—thus the arachnoid relationship of the carotid artery and optic nerve with the tumor. Group I tumors originate proximal to the carotid cistern from the inferior aspect of the anterior clinoidal process. The carotid artery has a 1- to 2-mm course in the subdural space prior to entering the carotid cistern where it lacks an arachnoid membrane, and thus group I tumors adhere directly to the adventitia of the carotid artery, which makes it impossible to dissect the tumor from the carotid artery.[30] Group II tumors originate from the superior or lateral aspect of the anterior clinoid process. This is distal to the arachnoidal investment of the carotid artery. The arachnoid investment of the carotid and sylvian cisterns enables these tumors to be dissected from the cerebral arteries. Additionally, for group I and II tumors, the optic chiasm and nerve are wrapped in the arachnoidal membrane of the chiasmatic cistern, and these tumors can be dissected safely from the optic apparatus.[30]

Group III tumors originate at the optic foramen and extend into the optic canal. They are typically small and cause early visual symptoms. The tumors occur proximal to the chiasmatic cistern, and therefore there may be no arachnoidal plane between the tumor and the optic nerve. The arachnoidal plane investing the carotid artery is usually present.[30]

Cavernous sinus meningiomas are usually of two general types: those that originate in and may be confined to the cavernous sinus, and those that invade the cavernous sinus but originate in an adjacent area. Meningiomas originating from the cavernous sinus and confined to it, present with extraocular movement disorders and facial paresthesias. Their management is controversial, with options including surgery, radiosurgery, or observation alone. Cavernous sinus meningiomas with a significant extracavernous component resulting in neural compression should be considered for microsurgical resection. Also, tumors compressing the optic apparatus should be considered for surgical resection to prevent radiation-induced optic neuropathy.[31] A 4-mm margin should separate the tumor from the optic apparatus to avoid this complication.[32] Patients with tumors larger than 3 cm are not ideal candidates for radiosurgery.[33] Radiosurgery series with acceptable long-term follow-up report 5- and 10-year progression-free survival rates of 87 to 95% and 69 to 73%, respectively. New cranial neuropathies occurred in 10%.[34,35]

In the senior author's (OA) experience, gross total resection was obtained in 44% of patients (71 of 163),[36] with recurrence in 7% following gross total resection. Others have reported tumor-free survival following complete resection of 87% at 3 years and 62% at 5 years.[37] Cranial nerve morbidity is an important consideration for cavernous sinus meningiomas. Improvement in cranial nerve function occurs in 14% and new cranial nerve neuropathy occurred in 18%; however, this is often transient.[38]

Meckel's cave meningiomas originate within the cave itself and are rarely confined to it. Patients with these kinds of tumors usually present with a petrous apex syndrome consisting of facial numbness or pain and diplopia secondary to a

sixth nerve palsy. In rare cases, these tumors due not extend beyond the cave and they can be removed through an extended middle fossa approach. More commonly these meningiomas grow and extend anteriorly into the middle fossa and the cavernous sinus, proceed into the upper clivus and petroclival area, and are approached through the cranio-orbital zygomatic approach.[17]

The cranio-orbital zygomatic approach provides the optimal approach for these parasellar meningiomas. The skin incision originates 1 cm in front of the tragus, going behind the hairline up to the superior temporal line on the contralateral side. The cutaneous flap is elevated while preserving the pericranium and the thick areolar tissue. As a subfacial dissection of the temporal muscle is performed to preserve the branches of the facial nerve, an osteotomy of the zygoma is performed using an oscillating saw, and the bone flap is elevated in one piece containing the orbital rim. The orbital roof and the lateral wall of the orbit are then removed in one piece for later reconstruction. The rest of the sphenoid wing is resected, and the anterior clinoid is then drilled using a diamond bit under microscopic magnification and abundant irrigation to avoid thermal injury to the optic nerve.

The dura is then opened and the sylvian fissure is opened widely, and branches of the middle cerebral artery are identified and followed proximally to the carotid bifurcation that is typically either pushed laterally and superiorly by the tumor or engulfed by it, often in cases of clinoidal meningiomas. The tumor is then debulked using ultrasonic aspirator, microscissor, and suction.

The optic apparatus is identified and preserved, and the optic sheath of the optic nerve is opened and the tumor followed into the optic canal. The carotid rings are opened proximally and distally to permit mobilization of the carotid artery. For tumors involving the cavernous sinus, entering into this area may be through either the medial or the lateral triangles. Dissection of the tumor progresses in a stepwise fashion, beginning by opening the optic nerve sheath longitudinally along the length of the optic canal. The distal dural ring is opened next with the opening extending posteriorly to the ocular motor trigone and thereby also freeing the proximal dural ring and allowing a wide entry into the anterior and superior cavernous sinus space.

The carotid artery can be mobilized laterally by releasing it from its proximal and distal dural rings, which then allows entry to the medial cavernous sinus space. Lateral entry into the cavernous sinus begins by an incision beneath the projected course of the third nerve, enabling elevation of the outer dural layer of the lateral wall of the cavernous sinus that is peeled away. The ICA can be located in Parkinson's triangle by dissection between the third and fourth nerves and the first division of the trigeminal nerve. The course of the sixth nerve, running lateral to the ICA and directly opposed to it, is usually parallel but deep to V1. The tumor is removed from the cavernous sinus space using suction bipolar coagulation and microdissection. A plane of cleavage along the carotid artery can usually be developed. Venous bleeding is typically not a problem when the tumor fills the sinus. It may occur as the venous plexus is decompressed during tumor removal. In that event, hemostasis can be obtained by packing the cavernous sinus space with oxidized cellulose or similar hemostatic agent. Reconstruction is performed with the vascularized pericranial flap and standard closure technique.

Petroclival Meningiomas and the Petrosal Approaches

Petroclival and sphenopetroclival meningiomas are the most formidable meningiomas (**Fig. 33.4**). They usually present with signs and symptoms of brainstem compression as well as facial numbness, diplopia, hearing loss, and facial weakness. Petroclival meningiomas arise in the upper two thirds of the clivus at the petroclival junction medial to the fifth nerve. The brainstem and basilar artery is typically displaced laterally. Though challenging, total removal of petroclival meningiomas is achievable in 71% of cases in the senior author's (OA) experience and achieves excellent recurrence-free survival.[39] Sphenopetroclival meningiomas are more extensive lesions. They invade the posterior cavernous sinus and grow into the middle and posterior fossa. The bony clivus and the petrous apex are involved, and the sphenoid sinus is invaded. They frequently require an extended petrosal approach or a combination of the petrosal cranio-orbital zygomatic approaches. Preoperative understanding of the venous system, particularly the vein of Labbé at its insertion to the sigmoid sinus, is essential to safe resection.

Selection of the approach is based on tumor extension, venous anatomy, and preoperative hearing status. Small tumors above the internal auditory meatus (IAM) may be resected through an anterior petrosal approach. Large tumors extending below the IAM require a posterior petrosal approach. If these tumors extend beyond the midline of the clivus or involve the cavernous sinus, they will require the addition of an anterior petrosectomy (combined petrosal approach). Patients who do not have hearing and have large tumors below the IAM benefit from a total petrosectomy.[40] In the event that the vein of Labbé drains into the superior petrosal vein rather than the sigmoid sinus, the approach is modified.

For petroclival meningiomas, the patient is placed in the supine position with the shoulder elevated and the head turned 45 degrees away from the side of the tumor. The head is lowered and tilted toward the opposite side to bring the base of the petrous bone to the highest point of the operative field. The bone flap is elevated, exposing the transverse and sigmoid sinuses. A mastoidectomy is performed, exposing the sigmoid sinus and the dura anterior to it, the jugular bulb, the lateral and posterior semicircular canals, and the facial nerve in the fallopian canal. The bone overlying the sinodural angle is removed, exposing the superior petrosal sinus. If hearing is absent, a total labyrinthectomy can be performed at this point, thereby increasing the anterior lateral exposure of the tumor.

The dura is opened along the anterior border of the sigmoid sinus and along the floor of the temporal fossa. The vein of Labbé is identified and protected. The superior petrosal sinus is coagulated and divided, and this division is carried medially through the tentorium, avoiding injury to the trochlear nerve and the superior petrosal vein. Sectioning of the tentorium allows the sigmoid sinus and the cerebellar hemisphere to fall away and diminishes the need for retraction. This exposure will provide visualization of the entire vertebral basilar system and the fourth through twelfth cranial nerves. The basilar artery may be displaced posteriorly or to the opposite side, or it may be encased. The posterior cerebellar artery, superior cerebellar artery, anterior inferior cerebellar artery (AICA), and posterior inferior cerebellar artery (PICA) are usually posterior and medial to the tumor, but they too may be encased by it.

Tumor removal begins with progressive devascularization of the tumor by coagulating and dividing its vascular supply from the tentorium and from its insertion on the petrous pyramid and clivus. The arachnoid over the tumor is opened to allow entry through the capsule and debulking. The neurovascular structures may be embedded in the meningioma, requiring that great care be taken during debulking. The tumor capsule is then dissected free from the surrounding structures. The need to preserve the small perforating arteries of the brainstem and cranial nerves cannot be overemphasized. The point of dural attachment is coagulated and resected, and hyperostotic bone is drilled. The dura is closed in a watertight manner, the drilled petrous bone is covered with autologous fat, and the soft tissues are closed in multiple layers.

When the patient has lost hearing preoperatively, a total petrosectomy (**Fig. 33.4e**) is done to take advantage of the additional exposure for meningiomas of the clivus, petroclival area, and sphenopetroclival area. This technique simply adds a translabyrinthine and transcochlear resection to the petrosal approach. In patients with a tumor that extends into the middle fossa or anterior cavernous sinus or where the temporal lobe's venous anatomy forbids elevation of the posterior temporal lobe, the petrosal approach is extended with the addition of an anterior petrosectomy.

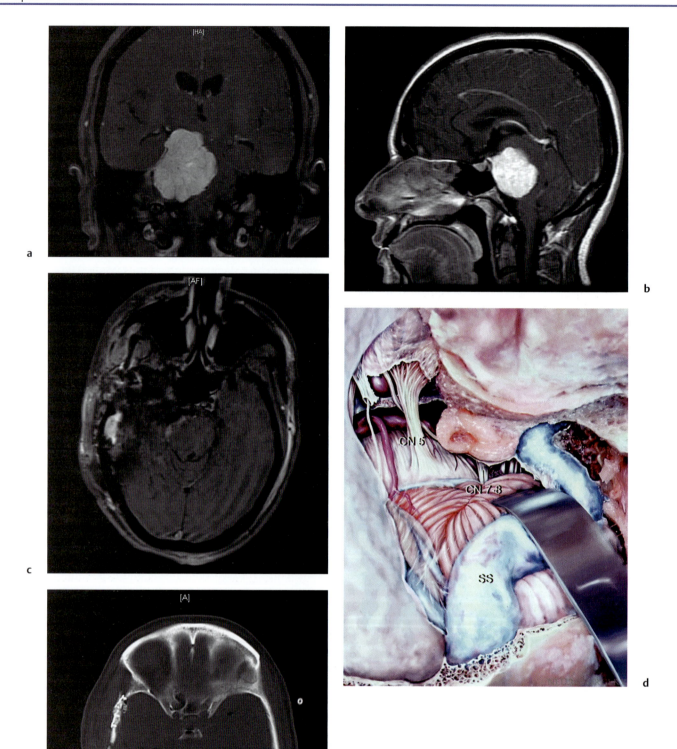

Fig. 33.4a–e (**a**) Coronal and (**b**) sagittal T1-weighted postcontrast MRI of the petroclival meningioma show in **Fig. 33.1b.** (**c**) Postoperative axial T1-weighted postcontrast MRI demonstrating gross total resection achieved with (**d**) a combined petrosal approach. CN, cranial nerve; SS, sigmoid sinus. (**e**) Postoperative CT scan shows the bone cuts of the craniotomy with preservation of the labyrinth and cochlea. (From Cho CW, Al-Mefty O. Combined petrosal approach to petroclival meningiomas. Neurosurgery 2002;51(3):708-718. Reproduced with permission from Lippincott Williams & Wilkins.)

Foramen Magnum Meningiomas and the Transcondylar Approach

Foramen magnum meningiomas arise from the dura at the craniocervical junction between the lower third of the clivus and the upper edge of the axis (**Fig. 33.5**). These lesions represent 3% of all meningiomas. Presentation is typically secondary to lower cranial nerve palsies. Ventral foramen magnum meningiomas are challenging lesions to treat due to the association of vital neurovascular, particularly the lower cranial nerves, in the region. Gross total resection is achievable with low morbidity, and was obtained in 75% of ventral foramen magnum meningiomas in the senior author's (OA) experience.[41]

The transcondylar approach (**Fig. 33.5e**) is utilized for ventral lesions in the foramen magnum. The patient is placed in the supine position with the ipsilateral shoulder and back elevated 30 to 45 degrees. A C-shaped incision begins above the ear and is extended along the edge of the sternocleidomastoid muscle. The scalp flap is elevated to the level of the external auditory canal. The sternocleidomastoid muscle is detached from the mastoid and reflected inferiorly, taking care not to injure the accessory nerve. The muscles are dissected from the lamina of C1 and C2. The C2 root is followed to the vertebral artery, which may be transposed medially by opening the transverse foramen of C1. A lateral suboccipital craniotomy and C1 and C2 laminectomies are performed, and the sigmoid sinus may be skeletonized to the jugular bulb. The occipital condyle and the lateral mass of C1 are drilled.

A lateral dural incision is made posterior to the sigmoid sinus and extends caudally to circumscribe the vertebral artery, enabling its further mobilization. The accessory nerve is identified between the dentate ligament and the spinal nerve root. The hypoglossal nerve may be either anterior or posterior to the tumor. The dentate ligament is divided and the C2 nerve root may also be divided if necessary. The tumor capsule is opened and debulking is performed. The clival dural attachment is coagulated and detached, enabling devascularization of the tumor. The tumor is dissected in the arachnoid plane from the medulla, cervical spinal cord, cranial nerves and vertebral artery. Dural attachments are removed and hyperostotic bone is drilled. The dura is closed in a watertight fashion. If tumor removal requires drilling of the entire occipital condyle, then an occipitocervical fusion should be performed.

Paragangliomas

Glomus tumors or paragangliomas originate from paraganglionic tissue of the extra-adrenal chromaffin cell system and have a close relationship to the arterial and venous structures in the neck and skull base. These tumors are named according to the site of origin: *carotid body* (from the carotid bifurcation), *glomus jugulare* (from the superior vagal ganglion), *glo-mus tympanicum* (from the auricular branch of the vagus), and *glomus intravagale* (from the inferior vagal ganglion). This discussion focuses on glomus jugulare tumors because of their involvement in the skull base and multiple lower cranial nerves.

Glomus jugulare tumors arise from glomus bodies surrounding the jugular bulb and tend to be highly vascular tumors that are usually slowly growing and benign (**Fig. 33.6**). They usually invade locally through destruction of the temporal bone. Often they invade through the skull base and have an intracranial intradural extension. The intracranial portions can involve the petrous bone, foramen magnum, and clivus.

Epidemiology and Clinical Presentation

The incidence of paragangliomas is 1 per 1.3 million people per year and they are the second most common tumor of the temporal bone after vestibular schwannomas. They often present in the fourth decade of life and are significantly more common in females. Multiple paragangliomas are reported in more than 10% of the cases, with the most common association being an ipsilateral carotid body tumor. Bilateral glomus tumors are present in 2%.[11]

The average time from symptom onset to diagnosis is 3 to 6 years. The presenting symptoms depend on the extent of tumor and compression of the surrounding neural structures. Most patients present with tinnitus, hearing loss, dizziness, and lower cranial nerve dysfunction. Cranial nerve paresis is noted in up to 35% of patients. Cranial nerve X is invaded most commonly (61%), followed by VII (54%), XI (52%), IX (48%), and least commonly XII. Facial weakness may present in large tumors. On otologic examination, a pulsatile red mass is often seen behind the tympanic membrane within the middle ear cavity.[11]

Glomus tumors can secrete low levels of catecholamines; however, only 1 to 3% of paragangliomas present with clinical symptoms of catecholamine secretion because detectable symptoms, such as hypertension, excessive perspiration, tachycardia, and headache, require high levels of secretion. Surgical manipulation of these tumors can result in the release of neuropeptides and blood pressure changes during surgery. Measurement of catecholamine levels in the serum and urine should be a part of the preoperative workup in anyone suspected of having a paraganglioma. Patients with secreting glomus tumors require pre- and intraoperative α- and β-adrenergic blocking medications.[11]

Pitfall

- Patients with hormonally active tumors require preparation with α- and β-catecholamine blockade prior to interventions.

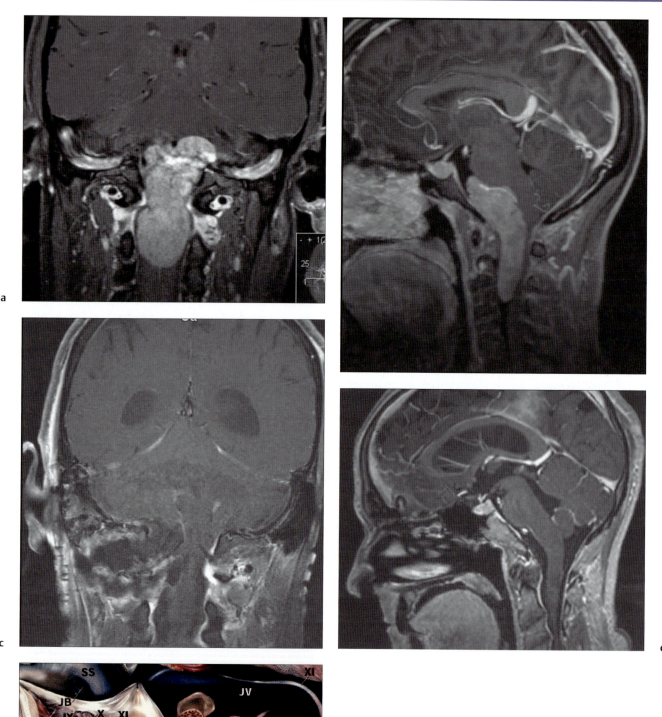

Fig. 33.5a–e (a) Coronal and (b) sagittal T1-weighted postcontrast MRI of a ventral foramen magnum meningioma. (c) Postoperative coronal and (d) sagittal T1-weighted postcontrast MRI with gross total resection of the tumor achieved with (e) the transcondylar approach. DR, Dural Ring; JB, jugular bulb; JV, jugular vein; PICA, posterior inferior cerebellar artery; SS, sigmoid sinus; VA, Vertebral artery; VA with VAVP, vertebral artery with vertebral artery with venous plexus. (From Arnautovic KI, Al-Mefty O, Husain M. Ventral foramen magnum meningiomas. J Neurosurg 2000;92:71–80. Reproduced with permission from the *Journal of Neurosurgery.*)

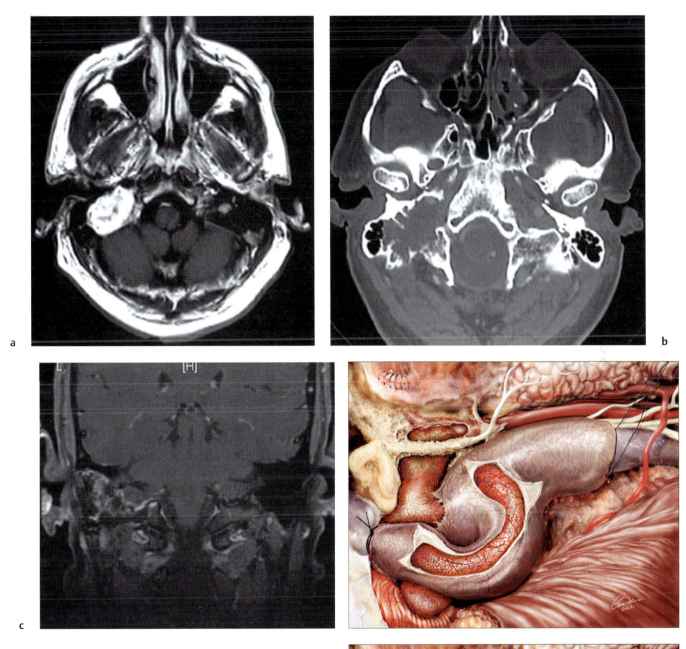

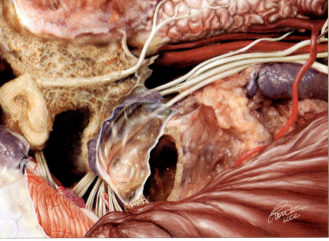

Fig. 33.6a–e (**a**) Preoperative axial contrast-enhanced T1-weighted MRI and (**b**) axial CT scan of glomus jugulare tumor. (**c**) Postoperative coronal MRI demonstrating gross total resection. (**d**) Artist's illustration of total tumor isolation prior to resection. The tumor is exposed and dissected from the carotid artery, lower cranial nerves, and facial nerve. The sigmoid sinus and the jugular vein are then ligated and the sinus and jugular bulb are opened. The external ear canal is closed and the middle ear ossicle is removed. (**e**) Illustration demonstrating the intrabulbar dissection performed by preserving the anterior and medial walls of the jugular bulb minimizing the manipulation of the lower cranial nerves. (From Al-Mefty O, Teixeira A. Complex tumors of the glomus jugulare: criteria, treatment, and outcome. J Neurosurg 2002;97:1356–1366. Reproduced with permission from the *Journal of Neurosurgery*.)

Serotonin-secreting tumors produce the carcinoid syndrome of bronchoconstriction, abdominal pain, violent headaches, diarrhea, cutaneous flushing, and electrolyte abnormalities. The presence of the carcinoid syndrome is evident by clinical symptomatology; specific laboratory testing is not required in the absence of symptoms. Octreotide can be used in the preoperative phase for symptomatic relief.[11]

Diagnostic Studies

The initial evaluation includes neurologic, neuro-ophthalmological, neuro-otologic, and endocrinologic testing. A measurement of the catecholamines in the serum and vanillylmandelic acid and metanephrines in the 24-urine collection is routine. Each patient with a glomus tumor should be studied to detect tumor multiplicity, and patients with multiple tumors should undergo genetic testing. High-resolution CT scan of the temporal bone demonstrates destruction of the jugular foramen. CT scan of the abdomen may identify associated adrenal lesions (carcinomas, sarcomas, etc.). MRI illustrates the relationship of the tumor to the important neighboring neural structures. Jugular foramen tumors have the characteristic "salt-and-pepper" appearance on MRI (**Fig. 33.6**). MRA and MRV evaluate the anatomy of the arteries and venous sinuses, which is paramount for surgical planning. Conventional angiography is used to delineate vascular anatomy in more detail, confirm the diagnosis, detect other associated paragangliomas, and provide a chance for selective embolization of very vascular tumors in expectation of surgical resection. The majority of the feeders for these tumors come from the ascending pharyngeal artery and occipital artery. However, tumors with intracranial extension may recruit blood supply from the ICA or vertebral arteries.

Histology

Histologically, these tumors show clusters (Zellballen) of epithelioid (chief) cells invested with highly vascular stroma containing capillary-size blood vessels. The pathological evaluation is uniform for paragangliomas. There are few pathological criteria that can distinguish between benign and malignant tumors. The designation of malignant or benign is based on the clinical course as opposed to histological features of the tumors. Malignant tumors result in rapid recurrence, metastasis, and death within a short time. Low levels of neuropeptides have been reported in highly undifferentiated paragangliomas.[42] These tumors may secrete a variety of other neuropeptide hormones, including adrenocorticotropic hormone (ACTH), serotonin, catecholamine, and dopamine.[43]

Treatment

Treatment planning must be tailored for each patient based on the location, extension, and invasion from the tumor. The

high morbidity of a lower cranial nerve palsies makes the management challenging. Advances in endovascular embolization have been an important addition to the surgical treatment of these tumors. Glomus tumors have been considered radioresistant in the past, but newer studies using radiosurgery for these lesions have reported good control with limited follow-up.[44,45] Treatment planning is essential for patients with multiple tumors, especially in patients with bilateral tumors. These patients present a particular management challenge, as bilateral lower cranial nerve deficits are associated with high morbidity.

Complete surgical resection can produce a cure from this disease. The specific surgical approach is tailored for each patient depending on the location of the tumor, extent of bony invasion, the patient's clinical condition, and preexisting neurologic deficits (**Fig. 33.6e**). The intracranial and extracranial aspects of the tumor are exposed together, allowing single-stage resection of the entire tumor. Preservation of the lower cranial nerves can be accomplished with intrabulbar dissection, but this technique is not effective in cases of tumor invasion through the outer venous wall. Preservation of the internal carotid artery is achieved by careful dissection under microscopic visualization. A cleavage plane is usually discovered between the tumor and arterial adventitia.

Gross total resection was achieved in 86% of the senior author's (OA) series of "complex" glomus tumors with even higher rates achieved in typical series. In small tumors, cranial nerve preservation is achieved in 85 to 90%. Preservation is more challenging in large or complex tumors but is achievable with an intrabulbar dissection technique if the tumor does not invade beyond the outer venous wall or the actual cranial nerves.[46]

Treatment of glomus jugulare tumors with stereotactic radiosurgery has gained significant popularity. Recent studies have shown promising results with glomus tumors that are within the treatment size limit for radiosurgery.[44] Treatment of these tumors with radiosurgery is safe, with an 8.5% rate of cranial neuropathy and a 2.1% rate of permanent morbidity. Tumor growth was controlled in 98% of patients, although only 36% had a decrease in the size of the tumor. Results such as these have led some authors to recommend radiosurgical treatment of glomus tumors as a primary treatment. Longer term follow-up is required to assess growth rates over time with radiosurgery, as most studies have limited follow-up and these tumors are slow growing. The advantages of surgery include complete removal of tumor and alleviation of mass effect.

Surgical resection is also able to treat tumors that are larger than the size limits of radiosurgery. Thus, surgical resection remains the treatment of choice for patients who desire complete removal and immediate cure of tumor, for large and giant tumors, for tumors with brainstem compression or significant intracranial extension, and for tumors with severe vascular encasement. Radiosurgery may have indications for residual tumors after surgical resection, for elderly patients, and bilateral tumors.

Chordoma

Chordoma is a rare neoplasm believed to arise from remnants of the notochord. About 32% of cases occur in the skull base, 33% in the spine, and 29% in the sacrum. The tumors are locally aggressive, infiltrative, and resistant to therapy. Additionally, they can be difficult to distinguish radiographically and pathologically from chondrosarcoma. Skull base chordomas occur most commonly in adults in the third and fourth decades with a small pediatric subpopulation. The most common clinical symptoms of clival chordomas are headache and diplopia. Other symptoms commonly reported include hoarseness, dysphagia, facial numbness, facial pain, ptosis, vertigo, hearing loss, visual loss, and facial paresis. Due to the slow-growing nature of chordomas, the presentation is typically insidious with the average time between onset of symptoms and presentation for diagnostic workup being 3.44 years.

Radiological Presentation

The typical radiological presentation of skull base chordoma is a midline clival lesion that is hypo- or isointense on T1-weighted MRI, hyperintense on T2-weighted MRI, and variably enhanced with contrast (**Fig. 33.7a,b**). Tumor extension into the sella, nasopharynx, or cavernous sinus is not unusual, and critical structures are frequently involved, including the brainstem and the circle of Willis vessels. Sagittal images are valuable in distinguishing the posterior extension of the tumor and intradural involvement. Coronal images are useful in depicting tumor relationship with the optic chiasm and cavernous sinus.

Computed tomography imaging is an important tool in the evaluation of chordomas due to the usual lytic bone destruction of the clivus (**Fig. 33.7c,d**). Additionally, evaluation of the odontoid process is important in planning the need for postoperative spinal stabilization. Chordomas and chondrosarcomas have similar radiographic appearances and cannot reliably be differentiated. However, chordomas typically are more midline lesions with symmetric expansion, whereas chondrosarcomas are more commonly a lateral lesion primarily involving the petrous bone; this can give some clue into the proper diagnosis.

Pathology

Chordomas are classified into three pathological categories: conventional, chondroid, and dedifferentiated.

Conventional chordomas form a well-demarcated mass within a pseudocapsule formed by overlying periosteum and dura. This results from erosion of bony structures with further expansion and displacement of overlying structures. Skull base chordomas typically present as much smaller masses than their sacral counterparts. They are grossly lobulated, nodular, gray-tan, soft masses. Microscopic examination shows the tumors pseudoencapsulated by fibrous strands forming thick hyalinized septa or thin septa creating lobules. The lobules appear as a sheet of vacuolated physaliferous cells with pools of mucin. The sheets of cells contain varying amounts of intracytoplasmic mucin ranging from hardly visible to quantities causing the cells to rupture (**Fig. 33.7f**). Mitotic figures are typically limited. Immunohistochemistry is an important tool in the diagnoses of chordomas. Chordomas are positive for cytokeratin and epithelial membrane antigen (EMA). They also stain with brachyury with a sensitivity and specificity of > 90%.[47,48]

The chondroid chordoma variant contains areas of conventional chordoma with areas of hyalin cartilage resembling low-grade hyalin-type chondrosarcoma. The tumors range from mostly chordoma with small, scattered foci of cartilaginous differentiation to mostly cartilaginous tumors with small areas of chordoma. These tumors can be potentially difficult to classify, and are frequently confused with chondrosarcomas. Immunohistochemistry can assist in this distinction, with chondroid chordomas staining positive for cytokeratin and EMA whereas chondrosarcoma is negative for both.[49]

Dedifferentiated chordoma is a rare variant with a more aggressive clinical course and poor response to treatment. It is much more common in the sacral region. It contains areas of conventional chordoma with components that appear similar to high-grade malignant fibrous histiocytoma, fibrosarcoma, or osteosarcoma.

Treatment

The appropriate management of chordoma requires a multidisciplinary team approach. Radical surgery followed by high-dose radiation therapy is the treatment of choice for skull base chordomas. Due to the involvement of critical structures, debulking procedures have commonly been employed in order to make radiation therapy possible. However, improved disease-free survival rates have been demonstrated when no residual tumor is seen on postoperative MRI.[50] Maximal surgical resection with removal of soft tissue mass and drilling into adjacent bone is recommended and should be attempted. Although radical surgical resection often requires multiple approaches, it is achievable with acceptable morbidity and mortality rates.

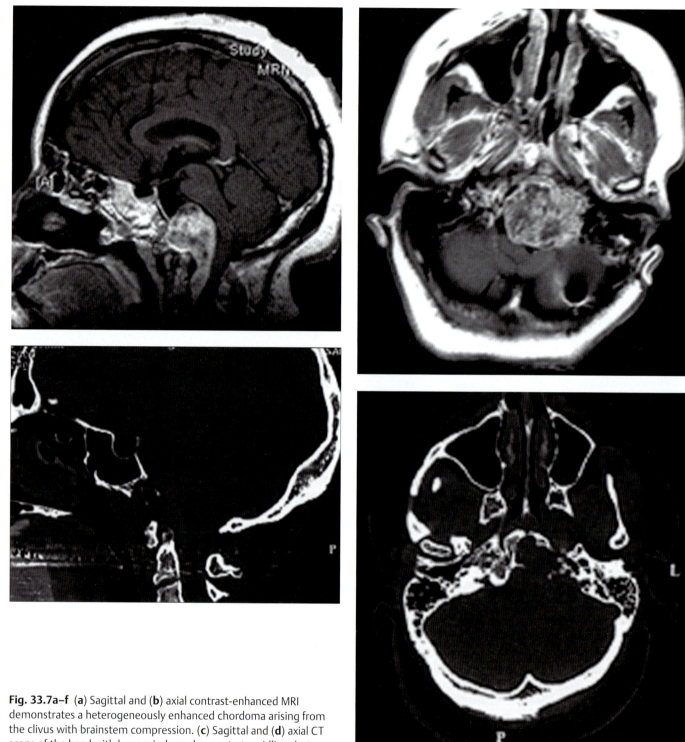

Fig. 33.7a–f (**a**) Sagittal and (**b**) axial contrast-enhanced MRI demonstrates a heterogeneously enhanced chordoma arising from the clivus with brainstem compression. (**c**) Sagittal and (**d**) axial CT scans of the head with bone windows demonstrate midline destruction of the clivus by the tumor.

Prognosis

Chordomas have an aggressive clinical course marked by a high propensity for local recurrence despite optimal treatment regimens. Improved outcomes are seen in patients with gross total removal at initial presentation.[50] High-dose local radiation, such as proton beam therapy, has been shown to improve survival.[51] Progression is local and aggressive, with short recurrence periods following second resection and an accumulation of cytogenetic abnormalities following recur-

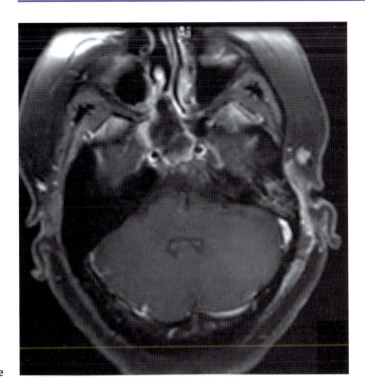

e

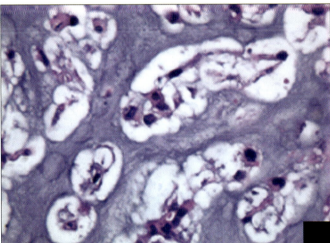

f

Fig. 33.7a–f (*continued*) (**e**) Axial postoperative MRI with contrast demonstrates gross total resection of the tumor. (**f**) Microscopic examination of the resected specimen shows vacuolated physaliferous cells containing cytoplasmic mucin with cords of eosinophilic syncytial cells.

rence.[52] The histological variant chondroid chordoma follows a similar clinical course despite prior reports of an improved prognosis.[50]

Distinction from Chondrosarcomas

Frequently, chondrosarcomas have been erroneously included with chordomas in clinical series due to their similar location, clinical presentation, and radiographic appearance. Additionally, the histological appearance of chondroid chordomas and chondrosarcomas is similar. The tumors are distinguishable with immunohistochemical staining. Chordomas are positive for cytokeratin and epithelial membrane antigen, whereas chondrosarcomas are negative for both. It is important to make this distinction, as the clinical course is markedly different. Chondrosarcomas have 5-year recurrence-free survival between 95% and 100%. Also, postoperative radiation does not appear to be necessary for chondrosarcomas as it is for chordomas.[50]

▪ Epidermoid and Dermoid Tumors

Epidermoid tumors are benign, slow-growing lesions accounting for 1.2% of all brain tumors. They may arise from misplaced cell rests during the early weeks of embryonic development. They are considered the result of inclusion of ectodermal elements at the time of closure of the neural groove between the third and fifth week of embryonic life. Epidermoid tumors should be differentiated from dermoid tumors. Dermoid tumors contain other dermal elements such as hair follicles, sebaceous glands, and sweat glands. Dermoid lesions are also more commonly located along the midline and may be accompanied by a dermal sinus. Dermoid tumors present earlier in life because of their abundant production of oily secretions and hair.

Clinical Presentation

Clinical presentation depends on the location and size of the lesion. Epidermoid tumors tend to grow as epithelial tumor cells desquamate with resultant formation of keratin and cholesterol crystals. Although the most common location for epidermoid tumors is the cerebellopontine angle followed by the parasellar and suprasellar regions, these tumors may occur anywhere within the cranial cavity, including the middle fossa, intraventricular space, or intraparenchyma.[53–55] Patients typically present with cranial nerve deficits along with headache and ataxia.

Imaging Studies

Epidermoid tumors are hypodense relative to brain parenchyma on CT scans. MRI demonstrates lesions that are hypointense on T1-weighted images and hyperintense on T2-weighted sequences with minimal or no enhancement (**Fig. 33.8a–d**). Slight enhancement in the periphery of the tumor most likely represents chemical inflammation and irritation by cyst contents or compressed vessels around the tumor. Radiological follow-up evaluation after surgery may be difficult because these tumors have signal characteristics similar to cerebrospinal fluid (CSF) on MRI. The diffusion MRI sequence provides the most reliable tool to identify tumor recurrence on follow-up postoperative imaging. Epidermoid tumors are hyperintense on diffusion images, unlike CSF, which is hypointense. Dermoid tumors are hyperintense on T1-weighted MRI sequences due to their fat content.

Histology

Histologically, epidermoid tumors contain stratified squamous epithelium with a whitish fibrous capsule containing cellular debris, including keratin and occasionally some lipid material (cholesterin) from cell membrane breakdown. Dermoid tumors contain a tough wall, composed of stratified squamous epithelium. Dermoid tumors also contain hair follicles, glands, and yellowish-white, grumous, greasy, foul-smelling material that can cause intense meningitis if the tumor ruptures.

Surgical Treatment

Surgical excision using microsurgical techniques is the only treatment with proven efficacy. Epidermoid tumors have a white, shiny, pearly appearance (**Fig. 33.8f**). Surgical removal should aim at complete resection of the tumor and its capsule during the first attempt. In most cases, the tumor may be re-moved from its capsule using a suction apparatus without significant difficulty. Removal of the tumor capsule is advocated if the capsule is not intimately attached to the vital surrounding neurovascular structures. Occasionally, dense adhesions between the capsule and surrounding arachnoid structures make surgical removal of the capsule difficult, resulting in some authors advising against removal of the tumor capsule.[56] One study, however, advocated radical excision to decrease the chance of recurrence.[57] Excision of the capsule is essential to preventing recurrence, and leaving residual capsule will entail subjecting the patient to multiple surgical procedures. For this reason capsule resection must be attempted as it is the source of growth (**Fig. 33.8g**). Resection of dermoid tumors follows similar principles, but tumor contents should not be released to prevent an intense inflammatory response.

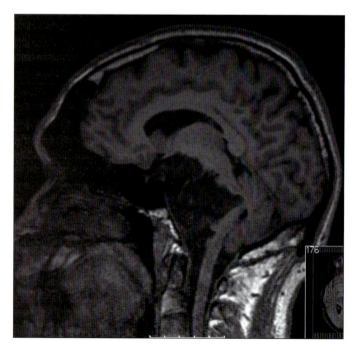

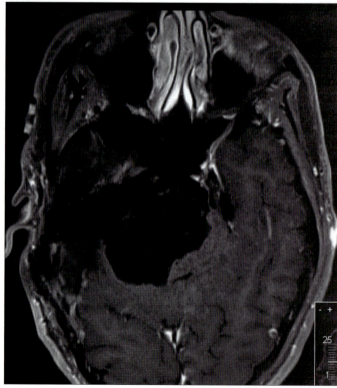

Fig. 33.8a–g (**a**) Sagittal and (**b**) axial MRI of the brain demonstrates a nonenhancing hypointense lesion compressing the brainstem.

a

b

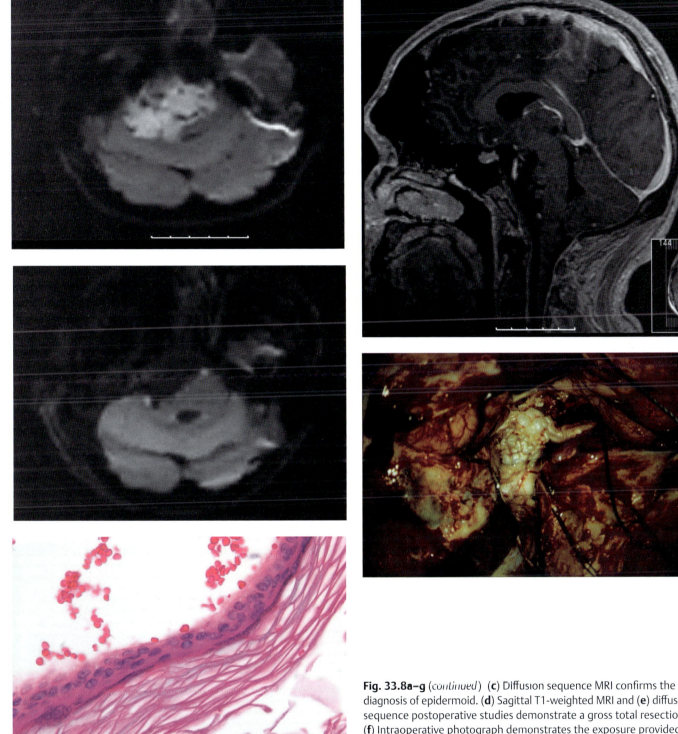

Fig. 33.8a–g (continued) (**c**) Diffusion sequence MRI confirms the diagnosis of epidermoid. (**d**) Sagittal T1-weighted MRI and (**e**) diffusion sequence postoperative studies demonstrate a gross total resection. (**f**) Intraoperative photograph demonstrates the exposure provided by the petrosal approach used for resection. (**g**) Histological section of the epidermoid illustrating the displaced cutaneous epithelium arising from the capsule. Resection of the capsule is necessary to prevent recurrence.

Conclusion

Skull base tumors are challenging lesions due to their relationship with vital neural and vascular structures. Advancements in skull base surgery have made the treatment of these lesions with low morbidity and mortality rates possible. The prognosis for most tumors at the skull base is now good; however, there remains a subset of tumors that have a malignant course.

Editor's Note

Historically, many skull base tumors were too complex or situated within regions at the base of the brain that were not amenable to safe surgical resection. Then came the era of microdissection, with advanced microscopes and superb preoperative anatomic imaging, which allowed neurosurgeons to create innovative skull base approaches and make significant inroads into an area that had always been difficult to traverse. Although skull base surgery remains one of the most difficult disciplines within neurosurgery, the techniques and methods continue to evolve. The use of endoscopes, for example, may enhance resection of the more formidable lesions.

Through genomic analysis, our understanding of the biology of these complex tumors has also evolved, providing molecular markers that may be therapeutically targeted, thus contributing to the overall success of radical surgery, especially for the malignant tumor varieties. At present, and certainly well into the future, surgery will be the mainstay of treating these complex lesions, especially since the morbidity and mortality rates remain low in experienced hands and centers. (Berger)

References

1. Porter KR, McCarthy BJ, Freels S, Kim Y, Davis FG. Prevalence estimates for primary brain tumors in the United States by age, gender, behavior, and histology. Neuro-oncol 2010;12:520–527 10.1093/neuonc/nop066
2. Nakasu S, Hirano A, Shimura T, Llena JF. Incidental meningiomas in autopsy study. Surg Neurol 1987;27:319–322
3. Hashiba T, Hashimoto N, Izumoto S, et al. Serial volumetric assessment of the natural history and growth pattern of incidentally discovered meningiomas. J Neurosurg 2009;110:675–684 10.3171/2008.8.JNS08481
4. Nakamura M, Roser F, Michel J, Jacobs C, Samii M. The natural history of incidental meningiomas. Neurosurgery 2003;53:62–70, discussion 70–71
5. Yoneoka Y, Fujii Y, Tanaka R. Growth of incidental meningiomas. Acta Neurochir (Wien) 2000;142:507–511
6. Niiro M, Yatsushiro K, Nakamura K, Kawahara Y, Kuratsu J. Natural history of elderly patients with asymptomatic meningiomas. J Neurol Neurosurg Psychiatry 2000;68:25–28
7. Olivero WC, Lister JR, Elwood PW. The natural history and growth rate of asymptomatic meningiomas: a review of 60 patients. J Neurosurg 1995;83:222–224 10.3171/jns.1995.83.2.0222
8. Yano S, Kuratsu J-I; Kumamoto Brain Tumor Research Group. Indications for surgery in patients with asymptomatic meningiomas based on an extensive experience. J Neurosurg 2006;105:538–543 10.3171/jns.2006.105.4.538
9. Oya S, Kim S-H, Sade B, Lee JH. The natural history of intracranial meningiomas. J Neurosurg 2011;114:1250–1256 10.3171/2010.12.JNS101623
10. Van Havenbergh T, Carvalho G, Tatagiba M, Plets C, Samii M. Natural history of petroclival meningiomas. Neurosurgery 2003;52:55–62, discussion 62–64
11. Erkmen K, Al-Mefty O, Adada B. Tumors of the skull base. In: Oncology of CNS Tumors. Berlin, Heidelberg: Springer Berlin Heidelberg, 2010: 279–307. doi:10.1007/978-3-642-02874-8_17
12. New PF, Hesselink JR, O'Carroll CP, Kleinman GM. Malignant meningiomas: CT and histologic criteria, including a new CT sign. AJNR Am J Neuroradiol 1982;3:267–276
13. Nakasu S, Nakasu Y, Nakajima M, Matsuda M, Handa J. Preoperative identification of meningiomas that are highly likely to recur. J Neurosurg 1999;90:455–462 10.3171/jns.1999.90.3.0455
14. Simpson D. The recurrence of intracranial meningiomas after surgical treatment. J Neurol Neurosurg Psychiatry 1957;20:22–39
15. Mahmoud M, Nader R, Al-Mefty O. Optic canal involvement in tuberculum sellae meningiomas: influence on approach, recurrence, and visual recovery. Neurosurgery 2010;67(3, Suppl Operative):ons108–ons118, discussion ons118–ons119
16. Kinjo T, al-Mefty O, Ciric I. Diaphragma sellae meningiomas. Neurosurgery 1995;36:1082–1092
17. Al-Mefty O. Operative Atlas of Meningiomas. Philadelphia: Lippincott Williams & Wilkins, 1998
18. Cook SW, Smith Z, Kelly DF. Endonasal transsphenoidal removal of tuberculum sellae meningiomas: technical note. Neurosurgery 2004;55: 239–244, discussion 244–246
19. Fatemi N, Dusick JR, de Paiva Neto MA, Malkasian D, Kelly DF. Endonasal versus supraorbital keyhole removal of craniopharyngiomas and tuberculum sellae meningiomas. Neurosurgery 2009;64(5, Suppl 2): 269–284, discussion 284–286
20. Wang Q, Lu X-J, Li B, Ji W-Y, Chen K-L. Extended endoscopic endonasal transsphenoidal removal of tuberculum sellae meningiomas: a preliminary report. J Clin Neurosci 2009;16:889–893 10.1016/j.jocn.2008.10.003
21. de Divitiis E, Cavallo LM, Esposito F, Stella L, Messina A. Extended endoscopic transsphenoidal approach for tuberculum sellae meningiomas. Neurosurgery 2007;61(5, Suppl 2):229–237, discussion 237–238
22. de Divitiis E, Esposito F, Cappabianca P, Cavallo LM, de Divitiis O. Tuberculum sellae meningiomas: high route or low route? A series of 51 consecutive cases. Neurosurgery 2008;62:556–563, discussion 556–563
23. Kaptain GJ, Vincent DA, Sheehan JP, Laws ER Jr. Transsphenoidal approaches for the extracapsular resection of midline suprasellar and anterior cranial base lesions. Neurosurgery 2001;49:94–100, discussion 100–101
24. Couldwell WT, Weiss MH, Rabb C, Liu JK, Apfelbaum RI, Fukushima T. Variations on the standard transsphenoidal approach to the sellar re-

gion, with emphasis on the extended approaches and parasellar approaches: surgical experience in 105 cases. Neurosurgery 2004;55: 539–547, discussion 547–550

25. Ceylan S, Koc K, Anik I. Endoscopic endonasal transsphenoidal approach for pituitary adenomas invading the cavernous sinus. J Neurosurg 2010;112:99–107 10.3171/2009.4.JNS09182

26. Gardner PA, Kassam AB, Thomas A, et al. Endoscopic endonasal resection of anterior cranial base meningiomas. Neurosurgery 2008;63:36–52, discussion 52–54

27. Dusick JR, Esposito F, Kelly DF, et al. The extended direct endonasal transsphenoidal approach for nonadenomatous suprasellar tumors. J Neurosurg 2005;102:832–841 10.3171/jns.2005.102.5.0832

28. Kitano M, Taneda M, Nakao Y. Postoperative improvement in visual function in patients with tuberculum sellae meningiomas: results of the extended transsphenoidal and transcranial approaches. J Neurosurg 2007;107:337–346 10.3171/JNS-07/08/0337

29. Taha ANMA, Erkmen KK, Dunn IFI, Pravdenkova SS, Al-Mefty OO. Meningiomas involving the optic canal: pattern of involvement and implications for surgical technique. Neurosurg Focus 2011;30:E12–E12 10.3171/2011.2.FOCUS1118

30. Ossama Al-Mefty. Clinoidal meningiomas. 1990. http://dxdoiorg/103171/jns19907360840

31. Pendl G, Schröttner O, Eustacchio S, Ganz JC, Feichtinger K. Cavernous sinus meningiomas—what is the strategy: upfront or adjuvant gamma knife surgery? Stereotact Funct Neurosurg 1998;70(Suppl 1):33–40

32. Nicolato A, Foroni R, Alessandrini F, Maluta S, Bricolo A, Gerosa M. The role of gamma knife radiosurgery in the management of cavernous sinus meningiomas. Int J Radiat Oncol Biol Phys 2002;53:992–1000

33. Lee JYK, Niranjan A, McInerney J, Kondziolka D, Flickinger JC, Lunsford LD. Stereotactic radiosurgery providing long-term tumor control of cavernous sinus meningiomas. J Neurosurg 2002;97:65–72 10.3171/jns.2002.97.1.0065

34. Hasegawa T, Kida Y, Yoshimoto M, Koike J, Iizuka H, Ishii D. Long-term outcomes of gamma knife surgery for cavernous sinus meningioma. J Neurosurg 2007;107:745–751 10.3171/JNS-07/10/0745

35. Williams BJ, Yen CP, Starke RM, et al. Gamma knife surgery for parasellar meningiomas: long-term results including complications, predictive factors, and progression-free survival. J Neurosurg 2011;114: 1571–1577 10.3171/2011.1.JNS091939

36. Heth JA, Al-Mefty O. Cavernous sinus meningiomas. Neurosurg Focus 2003;14:e3

37. De Jesús O, Sekhar LN, Parikh HK, Wright DC, Wagner DP. Long-term follow-up of patients with meningiomas involving the cavernous sinus: recurrence, progression, and quality of life. Neurosurgery 1996; 39:915–919, discussion 919–920

38. DeMonte F, Smith HK, al-Mefty O. Outcome of aggressive removal of cavernous sinus meningiomas. J Neurosurg 1994;81:245–251 10.3171/jns.1994.81.2.0245

39. Almefty R, Dunn IF, Pravdenkova S, Abolfotoh M, Al-Mefty O. True petroclival meningiomas: results of surgical management. J Neurosurg 2013

40. Erkmen K, Pravdenkova S, Al-Mefty O. Surgical management of petroclival meningiomas: factors determining the choice of approach. Neurosurg Focus 2005;19:E7

41. Kenan I, Arnautović KI, Al-Mefty O, Husain M. Ventral foramen magnum meningiomas. 2000. http://dxdoiorg/103171/spi20009210071

42. Linnoila RI, Lack EE, Steinberg SM, Keiser HR. Decreased expression of neuropeptides in malignant paragangliomas: an immunohistochemical study. Hum Pathol 1988;19:41–50 10.1016/S0046-8177(88) 80314-9

43. Brown JS. Glomus jugulare tumors revisited: a ten-year statistical follow-up of 231 cases. Laryngoscope 1985;95:284–288

44. Gottfried ON, Liu JK, Couldwell WT. Comparison of radiosurgery and conventional surgery for the treatment of glomus jugulare tumors. Neurosurg Focus 2004;17:E4

45. Jordan JA, Roland PS, McManus C, Weiner RL, Giller CA. Stereotactic radiosurgery for glomus jugulare tumors. Laryngoscope 2009;110: 35–38

46. Al-Mefty O, Teixeira A. Complex tumors of the glomus jugulare: criteria, treatment, and outcome. J Neurosurg 2002;97:1356–1366 10.3171/jns.2002.97.6.1356

47. Oakley GJ, Fuhrer K, Seethala RR. Brachyury, SOX-9, and podoplanin, new markers in the skull base chordoma vs chondrosarcoma differential: a tissue microarray-based comparative analysis. Mod Pathol 2008; 21:1461–1469 10.1038/modpathol.2008.144

48. Jambhekar NA, Rekhi B, Thorat K, Dikshit R, Agrawal M, Puri A. Revisiting chordoma with brachyury, a "new age" marker: analysis of a validation study on 51 cases. Arch Pathol Lab Med 2010;134.1181–1187 10.1043/2009-0476-OA.1

49. Heffelfinger MJ, Dahlin DC, MacCarty CS, Beabout JW. Chordomas and cartilaginous tumors at the skull base. Cancer 1973;32:410–420

50. Almefty K, Pravdenkova S, Colli BO, Al-Mefty O, Gokden M. Chordoma and chondrosarcoma: similar, but quite different, skull base tumors. Cancer 2007;110:2457–2467 10.1002/cncr.23073

51. Hug EB. Review of skull base chordomas: prognostic factors and long-term results of proton-beam radiotherapy. Neurosurg Focus 2001;10:E11

52. Almefty KK, Pravdenkova S, Sawyer J, Al-Mefty O. Impact of cytogenetic abnormalities on the management of skull base chordomas. J Neurosurg 2009;110:715–724 10.3171/2008.9.JNS08285

53. Dufour H, Fuentes S, Metellus P, Grisoli F. [Intracavernous epidermoid cyst. Case report and review of the literature]. Neurochirurgie 2001; 47:55–59

54. Bougeard R, Mahla K, Roche PH, Hallacq P, Vallée B, Fischer G. [Epidermoid cyst of the lateral ventricles]. Neurochirurgie 1999;45:316–320

55. Iaconetta G, Carvalho GA, Vorkapic P, Samii M. Intracerebral epidermoid tumor: a case report and review of the literature. Surg Neurol 2001;55:218–222

56. Berger MS, Wilson CB. Epidermoid cysts of the posterior fossa. J Neurosurg 1985;62:214–219 10.3171/jns.1985.62.2.0214

57. Yaşargil MG, Abernathey CD, Sarioglu AC. Microneurosurgical treatment of intracranial dermoid and epidermoid tumors. Neurosurgery 1989;24:561–567

34 Pituitary Tumors

Osaama H. Khan and Gelareh Zadeh

Pituitary adenomas account for 25% of all intracranial tumors and are the most common lesion arising in the sellar region.[1] They are present in approximately 16.9% of the general population.[2] Although men and women are equally affected, certain tumor subtypes do show a sex preference. Pituitary tumors are classified according to their morphological and functional characteristics. Such neoplasms are identified as secreting or functioning when they produce hormones in sufficient amounts to lead to clinical manifestations, including, from high to low prevalence, lactotrophic tumors (prolactinomas), somatotropinomas (acromegaly, gigantism), corticotropinomas (Cushing's disease), and, rarely, tumors secreting the glucoproteic hormones thyroid-stimulating hormone (TSH) (thyrotropinomas), luteinizing hormone (LH), and follicle-stimulating hormone (FSH) (gonadotropinomas). Pituitary adenomas can also secrete two or more hormones, with growth hormone (GH) and prolactin (PRL) co-secretion being the most prevalent of them. Pituitary neoplasms that do not produce circulating measurable amounts of intact hormones are called nonsecreting or nonfunctioning (NF) tumors.[3] Regarding their morphology, pituitary tumors are classified as microadenomas, which are less than 10 mm in diameter, generally enclosed, and less frequently invasive, and macroadenomas, which expand the sellar boundaries and are invasive.[4]

Clinical Presentation

The clinical presentation can be broadly categorized based on (1) the tumor being incidentally found; (2) headaches due to compression or stretching of the dura lining of the sella or of the diaphragm, which is innervated by the branches of the trigeminal nerve; (3) mass effect on adjacent structures, such as the optic nerve and chiasm, or occasionally cranial nerves located in the cavernous sinus; and (4) endocrinologic dysfunction. A rare emergent presentation, pituitary apoplexy, usually occurs with sudden-onset headache, meningismus, and oculomotor abnormalities, with a change in vision and disruption of the hypothalamic-pituitary-axis due to tumor hemorrhage or necrosis. However, pituitary hemorrhage occurs in up to 27% of cases of pituitary adenomas, and many of these have no clinical features of pituitary apoplexy.[5]

Optimal management of pituitary tumors requires a team approach. The unique location of the pituitary gland coupled with its complex role as the epicenter of control for hormone regulation can present unique obstacles for ideal treatment. For this reason, a series of examinations and investigations are recommended prior to surgery. These include neurologic, neuroendocrinologic, neuro-ophthalmologic, and neuroradiological assessments.

Pearl

- To obtain the optimal outcome, a team-based approach involving neurosurgery, ophthalmology, and endocrinology should be used for patient management.

Endocrine Evaluation

The endocrinologic screening is aimed at finding any hormonal deficits or hypersecretion. Pre- and postoperative endocrinologic screening includes evaluation of free cortisol, adrenocorticotropic hormone (ACTH), free thyroxine, TSH, PRL, GH, insulin-like growth factor-I (IGF-I), testosterone, estradiol, LH, and FSH to look for endocrinologic derangements. The diagnosis of a prolactinoma can be made based on serum PRL levels of > 150 ng/mL in combination with typical clinical symptoms.[6] In patients with a prolactinoma, endocrinologic remission is defined as postoperative PRL levels of < 20 ng/mL in females or < 15 ng/mL in males. The diagnosis of Cushing's disease is based on either abnormal 24-hour urinary free cortisol or abnormal results on low-dose dexamethasone suppression tests, defined as failure of 1 mg of dexamethasone to reduce plasma cortisol levels to < 1.8 mg/mL the next morning.[7,8] The diagnosis of acromegaly is based on abnormal basal fasting levels of GH and IGF-I.[9]

Pearl

- A thorough history and physical examination should include questions about genetic syndromes such as multiple endocrine neoplasia (MEN) type 1. These individuals also have neoplasms of the parathyroid gland and the pancreas.

Ophthalmologic Examination

A formal neuro ophthalmologic examination is essential in all patients. The examination includes visual field testing, both with confrontation and with Goldmann perimetry or semi-automatic perimetry. The classic bitemporal field loss is found in chiasmatic compression. Early compression may lead to upper quadrantic defects. This results from inferior chiasmal fiber compression. Evaluation of visual acuity with a Snellen chart without and with correction is essential. Funduscopy must be undertaken to evaluate the presence of optic nerve atrophy. Extraocular movements should be documented, especially in tumors extending into the surrounding cavernous sinus.

Neuroimaging

Currently, magnetic resonance imaging (MRI) is the modality of choice for the diagnosis and characterization of a pituitary lesion. The standard protocol for MRI of the pituitary and parasellar region consists of sagittal T1- and T2-weighted images performed with and without intravenous contrast.[10] Contrast enhancement may differentiate the adenoma from the displaced pituitary gland, may detect cavernous sinus invasion and demonstrate narrowing of the intracavernous internal carotid artery (ICA), and is helpful in the differential diagnosis of sellar and parasellar lesions. Thin coronal T2-weighted images provide good visualization of compression of the optic chiasm. Computed tomography (CT) is an alternative for patients with contraindications for MRI, and, in cases of bone invasiveness, CT bony window can be helpful in demonstrating the sellar floor and pneumatization of the sphenoid sinus.

A preoperative diagnosis of invasion is critical for planning surgical and adjuvant treatment strategies. Clinical signs of cavernous sinus invasion are evaluated on MRI. The Knosp-Steiner classification system uses this approach to preoperatively evaluate growth into the cavernous sinus (CS). Using mid-sella MRI in the coronal plane and the intra- and supracavernous segments of the carotid artery as reference points, a series of lines are drawn medially, through, and laterally to the ICA segments. The amount of tumor crossing these lines is divided into five grades (0 to 4). Grade 0 represents the normal condition with no invasion (the medial line is not crossed by tumor) and grade 4 represents total encasement of the ICA. Using 25 pituitary adenoma cases (functioning and nonfunctioning), Knosp et al[11] correlated the preoperative classification with surgical confirmation of CS invasion, and it was determined that all grade 3 and 4 tumors exhibited CS invasion, most of those in the grade 2 category had surgically proven invasion, and the grade 0 and 1 had no invasion. The authors suggest that once the tumor crosses the intercarotid line (grade 2), CS invasion becomes very likely.

Pitfall

- Cavernous sinus invasion has classically been considered a feature of aggressive tumor behavior, and given the anatomic location, it is difficult to achieve gross total resection of tumors with CS invasion.

A number of authors have confirmed the usefulness of the Knosp classification in their own studies. In one study, it was used to show that none of the adenomas with parasellar extension grade 0 had CS invasion, and all adenomas with grade 4 had CS invasion when correlated with surgical outcome.[12] There is also a correlation with Knosp criteria of CS invasion with surgical findings and MRI is also able to predict CS invasion with a sensitivity of 60% and a specificity of 85%.[13]

Surgical Management

After appropriate medical workup and management, surgery usually provides the final diagnosis and indicates the appropriate treatment. Goals of surgery are (1) total tumor removal, (2) decompression of the optic chiasm and nerve, (3) tumor debulking for cytoreduction, (4) preservation or restoration of endocrine function, and (5) histological confirmation. The last few decades have been marked by advances in diagnostic and surgical instruments and technology. They provide the neurosurgeon with a large armamentarium to help achieve surgical goals while reducing complications. They include, but are not limited to, intraoperative imaging (intraoperative CT or MRI[14]), neuronavigation, handheld Doppler ultrasound for carotid artery identification, use of indocyanine green to differentiate tumor margins,[15] and endoscopic endonasal instrumentation (two- and three-dimensional endoscopes). Controversies over ideal surgical approach (craniotomy versus microscopic endonasal versus endoscopic endonasal) have declined as larger surgical series have been reported with longer follow-up. Neurosurgeons in training and in practice are becoming more comfortable with the evolving technology (**Fig. 34.1**).

The advantages of an endonasal method over a craniotomy include a less invasive approach, a more direct anatomic route, no craniotomy or facial incisions, less trauma to the brain and neurovascular structures, early devascularization of the tumor blood supply, improved visualization of relevant anatomy, a better cosmetic result, and shorter recovery times. The endoscope also provides a wider field of view compared with the microscope. With advances of sellar floor reconstruction, for example with a vascularized nasoseptal flap,[16] the problem of greater cerebrospinal fluid leaks has become less prominent for surgery on adenomas isolated to the sella.

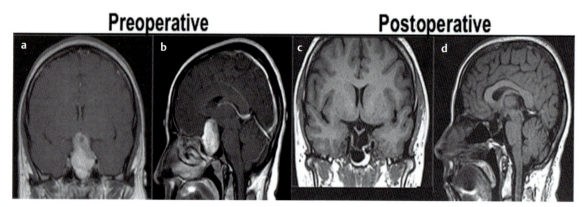

Fig. 34.1a–d Coronal (**a**) and sagittal (**b**) T1-weighted magnetic resonance imaging (MRI) of a 36-year-old woman with amenorrhea presenting with new-onset headaches and visual changes. The MRI demonstrates a giant pituitary macroadenoma measuring 4 cm in maximum diameter with suprasellar extension and heterogeneity, representing blood products or proteinaceous material. The patient underwent endoscopic endonasal surgery. (**c,d**) Postoperative imaging shows complete resection of the tumor with the optic chiasm and the pituitary stalk (**c**) now clearly visible. Pathology determined this to be a hormone-negative gonadotroph adenoma.

◼ Individual Pituitary Tumor Types

Prolactinomas

Hyperprolactinemia is among the most common of pituitary disorders, and prolactinomas account for 30 to 60% of pituitary tumors.[17] Physiological hyperprolactinemia is seen with physical and emotional stress, pregnancy, nipple stimulation, and after sexual orgasm. Iatrogenic elevation occurs by antagonizing dopamine action with such medications such as antiemetics, antidepressants, antipsychotics, and narcotics. The clinical findings, regardless of the patient's sex, can be associated with anxiety, depression, fatigue, emotional instability, and hostility.[18,19] Symptoms in women of reproductive age include amenorrhea, galactorrhea, infertility, seborrhea, and hirsutism. Low estrogen can result in a loss of libido, and long-lasting effects include osteopenia. In men, the most common presentation is a loss of libido and impotency, and less commonly oligospermia and hypogonadism. Galactorrhea or gynecomastia is present in 15 to 30% of male patients.[20]

Treatment goals are dependent on acuity and cause of presentation, with the ultimate goal being normalization of prolactin levels. Patients presenting with noniatrogenic hyperprolactinemia are usually treated medically with dopamine agonists to normalize serum levels but also to control tumor size and growth. A systematic review of the use of cabergoline and bromocriptine for prolactinomas found that cabergoline was more effective at normalization of hyperprolactinemia and associated with significantly less adverse events.[21] Patients requiring surgery have either failed medical treatment or are experiencing major adverse effects induced by all of the dopaminergic agonists. There is still some controversy as to the use of cabergoline, given the long-term adverse effects when a number of surgical series report remission rates of 85 to 89%[22–24] with recurrence rates of 18.7%.[25]

Acromegaly

Acromegaly is a disease of chronic overproduction of GH. The consequences of GH oversecretion are numerous and include, but are not limited to, facial changes (large lips, tongue, skin changes), laryngeal hypertrophy (low voice), bony hypertrophy (prognathism, thick skull, jaw, hands, cervical spine stenosis), hypertension, cardiomyopathy, barrel chest, high adrenocorticoid output, and chronic renal volume increase. Acromegaly is diagnosed by clinical features, an elevated serum IGF-I level, and a serum GH level that does not decline to < 1 ng/mL after oral glucose (75 or 100 g). The definitive test for acromegaly is the GH response to an oral glucose challenge (oral glucose tolerance test [OGTT]). The test must be performed correctly to interpret the results. Baseline serum glucose and GH are measured, then the patient drinks a glucose solution (75 or 100 g), and the serum glucose and GH levels are measured every 30 minutes for 2 hours. The current guideline for a normal response is a serum GH level of < 1 ng/mL. Cardiac disease is the most important cause of morbidity and mortality in acromegalic patients.[26,27] This is followed by respiratory disease where upper airway obstruction (obstructive sleep apnea) affects up to 70% patients.[28]

Surgery remains the first-line therapy.[9] Whether microscopic or endoscopic, the surgical techniques are the same as with other adenomas. Remission rates vary between 46% and 85%: for microadenomas, 75 to 100%; for macroadenomas, 50 to 80%.[29–32] Intraoperative biochemical testing to determine remission during resection has been employed in some cen-

---

Pitfall

- In giant prolactinomas the "hook effect" is described as a low serum prolactin level, when in reality if the samples are diluted (10-fold dilution) there is a substantially high level.

ters, with successful measurement of intraoperative GH levels as a guide to remission.[33]

Cushing's Disease

Cushing's disease specifically results from the unregulated hypersecretion of ACTH by a pituitary adenoma and consequent hypercortisolism. Excess cortisol secretion was first described by Harvey Cushing[34] in 1912. Systemic hypertension is among the most common manifestations of Cushing's disease. As many as 80% of patients with Cushing's disease have systemic hypertension and 50% of untreated patients have severe hypertension with a diastolic blood pressure > 100 mmHg. Weight gain, centripetal obesity, and fat deposits over the cheeks and temporal regions, giving rise to the rounded moon facies, are commonly observed in Cushing's disease. Glucose intolerance occurs in at least 60% of patients with Cushing's disease, with overt diabetes mellitus present in up to one third of all patients.[35] Many patients with Cushing's disease report depression, memory loss, generalized weakness, and a myopathy of the proximal muscles of the lower limb and the shoulder girdle.

Consistent overproduction of cortisol is demonstrated by three types of screening tests: elevated 24-hour urine free cortisol (preferably measured by tandem mass spectrometry), loss of circadian rhythm with elevated nighttime salivary cortisol levels, and failure of the serum cortisol to decline to <1.8 µg/dL at 8 AM after ingestion of dexamethasone at 11 PM the previous night.[7] Because 50% of patients with a pituitary adenoma causing Cushing's disease have no visible lesion on MRI, it is occasionally inappropriate to recommend pituitary surgery. An inferior petrosal sinus sampling (IPSS) study is the most precise method to determine if the source of ACTH is the pituitary gland and to exclude ectopic ACTH syndrome. This test involves comparing the central (petrosal sinus, left and right) and peripheral (inferior vena cava) ACTH levels be-

fore and after the administration of corticotropin-releasing hormone (CRH). A ratio of the basal central to the peripheral ACTH level of > 2 or a CRH-stimulated ratio of > 3 indicates a pituitary etiology.

Definitive management with surgery remains the first-line therapy.[36] Remission rates from combined microscopic and endoscopic series range from 56 to 86%.[22–24,37–40]

Nonfunctioning Adenomas

Approximately 25% of pituitary adenomas are clinically nonfunctioning. Although their presentation is usually visual, they may present with panhypopituitarism or apoplexy. The absence of biochemical criteria for remission requires an imaging estimate of the degree of resection and introduces a degree of subjectivity. Gross total resection ranges from 66 to 93%.[22,24,38,41]

■ Radiotherapy

Tumors that are refractory to medical and surgical treatment may be treated with either fractionated radiation or stereotactic radiosurgery (SRS). Fractionated radiation has the benefit of limiting radiation damage to nearby radiation-sensitive structures such as the optic apparatus, whereas radiosurgery can be conveniently performed in a single session and results in more rapid biochemical remission.[42] The long-term results of fractionated radiation for pituitary tumors have been well defined; therefore, most current research has been focused on outcomes following SRS.[43] Although radiotherapy can have a significant effect on preventing recurrences,[44,45] radiotherapy carries risks of new endocrinopathy, cognitive impairment, and induction of new neoplasms after about 10 years.[46–50]

The goal of pituitary adenoma radiosurgery is to permanently control tumor growth, to maintain pituitary function, to normalize hormonal secretion in case of functional adenomas, and to preserve neurologic function, especially vision.[51] The largest current series of SRS for pituitary adenomas reported on 418 patients.[52] Tumor control via gamma knife radiosurgery was achieved in 90.3% of patients. Biochemical remission was achieved in 53% of patients with acromegaly and 54% of patients with Cushing's disease, and the median time to remission overall was 48.9 months. Tumor control was related to margin dose, which was frequently limited by the risk of radiation to nearby structures. New pituitary hormone deficiency was present in 24.4% of patients. Thirteen patients experienced new cranial neuropathies, including eight with visual acuity or field deficits. This study has helped to better characterize the effectiveness of SRS for pituitary tumors as well as its risks. Tumor control was reported as 83% over an 80.5-month median follow-up.

Typically, acromegaly patients respond best with normalization of GH hypersecretion in over 70% of patients and in approximately half of those with Cushing's disease.[53] It was found that all patients with microadenomas and 97% of patients with macroadenomas had tumor control after radiosurgery. Gamma knife radiosurgery was essentially equally effective for control of adenomas with cavernous sinus invasion and suprasellar extension. Endocrine deficits are less common after radiosurgery, although some recent reports with detailed testing show some hormone deficiencies over time.

■ Advances in Tumor Biology

The molecular and genetic abnormalities in pituitary adenomas and the definitive mutational events that explain pituitary adenoma tumor genesis remain elusive. By investigating familial and sporadic variants of adenomas, a variety of intrinsic and extrinsic pathways have been suggested.[54] These may be genetic or epigenetic and may result in cell-cycle dysregulation, signaling defects, or loss of tumor suppressor factors.[55] Further studies of stem cells, micro-RNAs (miRNAs), and cell-cycle regulators should facilitate our understanding of these unique tumors as well as their diagnosis and treatment.

Mechanisms of adenoma invasiveness also remain poorly understood. The molecular regulators that drive one adenoma to invade the neighboring structures, such as the cavernous sinus in particular, versus another histologically identical adenoma is not known. Invasion into the cavernous sinus is of critical importance, given the difficulty of removing tumor without causing injury to the carotid and the delicate cranial nerves. Therefore, there is a need to investigate histological or molecular markers that predict pituitary tumor behavior. Although the best prognosticator in pituitary adenomas remains accurate detailed subtyping of adenomas, there is a need to identify novel protein targets for which drugs would provide adjuvant treatment.

The fibroblast growth factors (FGFs) and their receptors (FGFRs) are frequently expressed in pituitary tumors and may represent a biomarker of cavernous sinus invasion. In GH-secreting pituitary adenomas, examination of ptd-FGFR4 mRNA levels through reverse-transcriptase polymerase chain reaction (RT-PCR) determined that ptd-FGFR4–positive adenomas invaded the cavernous sinus more frequently than did ptd-FGFR4–negative adenomas.[56] With respect to FGFR4 protein expression in both functioning and nonfunctioning adeno-

mas, high levels of FGFR4 was found in invasive tumors as compared to noninvasive tumors.[57]

The matrix metalloproteinases (MMPs) are another biomarker that may contribute to invasion. They are classified as type IV collagenases, and these proteins are able to degrade type IV collagen, which composes the basement membrane of the extracellular matrix. A number of studies have provided evidence for increased protein and mRNA expression of MMP-9 and -2 in both functioning and nonfunctioning adenomas invading the cavernous sinus.[58] Furthermore, increased MMP-9 protein expression may be related to increased angiogenesis as measured through microvessel density (MVD).[13]

Angiogenesis, the process of forming new blood vessels from a preexisting vascular network, is often assessed through MVD and vascular endothelial growth factor (VEGF) expression. MVD, as assessed through the expression of F8–factor VIII–related antigen, has been shown to be increased in invasive adenomas. Expression of VEGF has also been demonstrated to have an association with CS invasion. Furthermore, VEGF is correlated with the Ki-67 labeling index, a measure of cell proliferation.[13]

Ki-67 is a nuclear protein often used to assess proliferative activity of tumor cells. Ki-67 is recognized by the MIB-1 monoclonal antibody, and it is expressed throughout the cell cycle in G_1, S, G_2, and M phases, but not in the G_0 phase. The percentage of cells immunostained for this protein (Ki-67/MIB-1) represents a reliable marker of proliferative activity. The Ki-67 proliferative index may be a useful prognostic marker for determining CS invasion. One study defined the biological significance of the MIB-1 in 159 surgically excised pituitary adenomas and found that MIB-1 correlated with adenomas invading the CS. Furthermore, bilateral CS invasion had a significantly higher MIB-1 than did unilateral extension.[54] Another study determined that expression of Ki-67 in the pituitary has associations with adenoma growth into the cavernous sinus.

■ Adenoma Recurrence

Pituitary adenomas can recur even after an initial gross total removal, and recurrence is not rare. Surgery for the removal of a lesion recurring from a residual is burdened by an increased risk of mortality and morbidity, and more often it results in incomplete resections compared with the primary surgery.[59] Attempts to identify prognostic biomarkers that may indicate possible tumor recurrence are ongoing. One study determined that in nonfunctioning adenomas, residual tumors that progressed had a significantly higher MIB-1 relative to the residuals that did not progress.[60] In GH-secreting adenomas, Ki-67 was found to be significantly lower in tumors that were cured after surgery versus those that were not.[61] The relationship between Ki-67 and the growth rate of recurrent tumor has also been examined in a few studies. These studies have used tumor volume doubling time (TVDT) as an estimate of residual growth. Ki-67 has been shown to be inversely correlated to TVDT, where short TVDT was associated with higher MIB-1.[62]

There is a paucity of data regarding the identification of other possible biomarkers that may predict tumor recurrence. The phosphatidylinositol 3-kinase (PI3K)/Akt/mammalian target of rapamycin (mTOR) pathway is involved in regulating protein translation, cell growth and motility, apoptosis, and metabolism, and has been demonstrated to be overactivated in a variety of human cancers[63] and upregulated at both the mRNA and protein level in pituitary adenomas.[64] Recently, it has been demonstrated that high levels of phosphor-Akt may predict early recurrence in nonfunctioning pituitary adenoma.[65]

Current medical treatment for pituitary adenomas includes somatostatin analogues such as octreotide or dopamine agonists such as cabergoline and bromocriptine. However, a large percent of these tumors are unresponsive to these agents. Therefore, it is necessary to investigate how to overcome the resistance to existing treatments and to identify new cytostatic agents.

Everolimus (RAD001) has been shown to inhibit mTOR signal transduction in a variety of tumor cell lines and tumors both in vitro and in vivo[66] and in leukemias.[67]

Recently, it has been demonstrated that various elements of the PI3K/Akt/mTOR pathway are upregulated in both functioning and nonfunctioning pituitary adenomas. This finding has prompted a number of studies to begin investigating the functional role of this signaling pathway in in vitro systems on both tumor cell lines and primary culture. Cell viability has also been shown to be reduced in GH,[68] PRL secretion,[69] and ACTH secretion[70] in rat pituitary adenoma cell lines following treatment with RAD001 in a dose- and time-dependent manner. Furthermore, administration of RAD001 has been shown to promote apoptosis (via increases in caspase levels) and to have cytostatic effects by inhibiting cyclin-dependent kinases, such as cyclin D1, and increasing the levels of cyclin-dependent kinase inhibitors such as p27 in nonfunctioning pituitary adenomas in primary culture.

Temozolomide (TMZ) is an effective therapy for malignant neuroendocrine tumors.[71] There is recent evidence that TMZ has efficacy in the treatment of pituitary adenomas that are resistant to other treatment options. TMZ methylates DNA and thereby exhibits an antitumor effect. The DNA repair enzyme O6-methylguanine-DNA methyltransferase (MGMT) removes methyl groups induced by TMZ, thereby counteracting its effects. Thus, MGMT is inversely correlated to TMZ efficacy. A recent meta-analysis determining the value of analyzing the MGMT status of pituitary adenoma reported that MGMT immunohistochemistry, but not methylation status, is a useful predictive tool.[72] TMZ has been shown to be effective at reducing cell proliferation and promoting apoptosis in the GH3, MMQ, and AtT20 cell lines.[51] Furthermore, TMZ also suppresses cell proliferation and induces apoptosis in the aT3 gonadotroph cell line.[73] Further clinical studies are needed to recognize TMZ's clinical indications, predictors of success, and outcomes.

Conclusion

Pituitary adenomas are relatively common tumors within the sellar and parasellar region. Surgical resection represents an important part of the treatment paradigm for patients with hypersecretory adenomas and nonsecretory adenomas exerting mass effect. Imaging and endocrine results after pituitary adenoma surgery are favorable. Long-term follow-up of these patients is required to detect recurrence. Reoperation generally affords less favorable results than the initial surgery. Radiosurgery is proving to be a viable option for selected cases where reoperation is not ideal. A team-based approach for optimum diagnosis and medical/surgical management is crucial in order to obtain the best outcomes in these complex pathologies.

Editor's Note

Pituitary tumors have also seen a transformation in care, first with the advent of transsphenoidal surgery, and then with a series of drugs that essentially converted many pituitary tumors into nonsurgical disease. Recently the use of the endoscope to replace the microscope for illumination and magnification has been embraced by many, and may well become the standard approach for many surgeons in the not too distant future. Scientific advances also have been made but, as with meningioma, not as many human or fiscal resources have been spent on the molecular biological study of these conditions. For many refractory cases, radiation modalities such as conventional fractionated conformal fractionation and stereotactic radiosurgery still play an important role.[74] As with meningioma patients, pituitary tumor patients have a unique surgical experience and long survival, so quality of life/qualitative research studies are important.[75] (Bernstein)

References

1. Asa S. Tumors of the pituitary gland. In: Atlas of Tumor Pathology. Washington, DC: Armed Forces Institute of Pathology, 1998,

2. Ezzat S, Asa SL, Couldwell WT, et al. The prevalence of pituitary adenomas: a systematic review. Cancer 2004;101:613–619

3. Al-Brahim NY, Asa SL. My approach to pathology of the pituitary gland. J Clin Pathol 2006;59:1245–1253

4. Hardy J. Transsphenoidal surgery of hypersecreting pituitary tumors. In: Kohler PO, Ross GT, eds. Diagnosis and Treatment of Pituitary Tumors. New York: Elsevier, 1973:179–194

5. Lenthall RK, Dean JR, Bartlett JR, Jeffree MA. Intrapituitary fluid levels following haemorrhage: MRI appearances in 13 cases. Neuroradiology 1999;41:167–170

6. Casanueva FF, Molitch ME, Schlechte JA, et al. Guidelines of the Pituitary Society for the diagnosis and management of prolactinomas. Clin Endocrinol (Oxf) 2006;65:265–273

7. Arnaldi G, Angeli A, Atkinson AB, et al. Diagnosis and complications of Cushing's syndrome: a consensus statement. J Clin Endocrinol Metab 2003;88:5593–5602

8. Nieman LK, Biller BM, Findling JW, et al. The diagnosis of Cushing's syndrome: an Endocrine Society Clinical Practice Guideline. J Clin Endocrinol Metab 2008;93:1526–1540

9. Giustina A, Chanson P, Bronstein MD, et al; Acromegaly Consensus Group. A consensus on criteria for cure of acromegaly. J Clin Endocrinol Metab 2010;95:3141–3148

10. Kucharczyk W, Bishop JE, Plewes DB, Keller MA, George S. Detection of pituitary microadenomas: comparison of dynamic keyhole fast spin-echo, unenhanced, and conventional contrast-enhanced MR imaging. AJR Am J Roentgenol 1994;163:671–679

11. Knosp E, Steiner E, Kitz K, Matula C. Pituitary adenomas with invasion of the cavernous sinus space: a magnetic resonance imaging classification compared with surgical findings. Neurosurgery 1993;33:610–617, discussion 617–618

12. Vieira JO Jr, Cukiert A, Liberman B. Evaluation of magnetic resonance imaging criteria for cavernous sinus invasion in patients with pituitary adenomas: logistic regression analysis and correlation with surgical findings. Surg Neurol 2006;65:130–135, discussion 135

13. Pan LX, Chen ZP, Liu YS, Zhao JH. Magnetic resonance imaging and biological markers in pituitary adenomas with invasion of the cavernous sinus space. J Neurooncol 2005;74:71–76

14. Berkmann S, Fandino J, Zosso S, Killer HE, Remonda L, Landolt H. Intraoperative magnetic resonance imaging and early prognosis for vision after transsphenoidal surgery for sellar lesions. J Neurosurg 2011;115:518–527

15. Litvack ZN, Zada G, Laws ER Jr. Indocyanine green fluorescence endoscopy for visual differentiation of pituitary tumor from surrounding structures. J Neurosurg 2012;116:935–941

16. Hadad G, Bassagasteguy L, Carrau RL, et al. A novel reconstructive technique after endoscopic expanded endonasal approaches: vascular pedicle nasoseptal flap. Laryngoscope 2006;116:1882–1886

17. Colao A, Di Sarno A, Cappabianca P, Di Somma C, Pivonello R, Lombardi G. Withdrawal of long-term cabergoline therapy for tumoral and nontumoral hyperprolactinemia. N Engl J Med 2003;349:2023–2033

18. Reavley A, Fisher AD, Owen D, Creed FH, Davis JR. Psychological distress in patients with hyperprolactinaemia. Clin Endocrinol (Oxf) 1997;47:343–348

19. Sobrinho LG. The psychogenic effects of prolactin. Acta Endocrinol (Copenh) 1993;129(Suppl 1):38–40

20. Carter JN, Tyson JE, Tolis G, Van Vliet S, Faiman C, Friesen HG. Prolactin-screening tumors and hypogonadism in 22 men. N Engl J Med 1978;299:847–852

21. dos Santos Nunes V, El Dib R, Boguszewski CL, Nogueira CR. Cabergoline versus bromocriptine in the treatment of hyperprolactinemia: a systematic review of randomized controlled trials and meta-analysis. Pituitary 2011;14:259–265

22. Kabil MS, Eby JB, Shahinian HK. Fully endoscopic endonasal vs. transseptal transsphenoidal pituitary surgery. Minim Invasive Neurosurg 2005;48:348–354

23. Dehdashti AR, Ganna A, Karabatsou K, Gentili F. Pure endoscopic endonasal approach for pituitary adenomas: early surgical results in 200 patients and comparison with previous microsurgical series. Neurosurgery 2008;62:1006–1015, discussion 1015–1017

24. Gondim JA, Schops M, de Almeida JP, et al. Endoscopic endonasal transsphenoidal surgery: surgical results of 228 pituitary adenomas treated in a pituitary center. Pituitary 2010;13:68–77

25. Kreutzer J, Buslei R, Wallaschofski H, et al. Operative treatment of prolactinomas: indications and results in a current consecutive series of 212 patients. Eur J Endocrinol 2008;158:11–18

26. Matta MP, Caron P. Acromegalic cardiomyopathy: a review of the literature. Pituitary 2003;6:203–207

27. Colao A, Marzullo P, Di Somma C, Lombardi G. Growth hormone and the heart. Clin Endocrinol (Oxf) 2001;54:137–154

28. Guilleminault C, van den Hoed J. Acromegaly and narcolepsy. Lancet 1979;2:750–751

29. Campbell PG, Kenning E, Andrews DW, Yadla S, Rosen M, Evans JJ. Outcomes after a purely endoscopic transsphenoidal resection of growth hormone-secreting pituitary adenomas. Neurosurg Focus 2010;29:E5

30. Hofstetter CP, Mannaa RH, Mubita L, et al. Endoscopic endonasal transsphenoidal surgery for growth hormone-secreting pituitary adenomas. Neurosurg Focus 2010;29:E6

31. Jane JA Jr, Starke RM, Elzoghby MA, et al. Endoscopic transsphenoidal surgery for acromegaly: remission using modern criteria, complications, and predictors of outcome. J Clin Endocrinol Metab 2011;96:2732–2740

32. Wagenmakers MA, Netea-Maier RT, van Lindert EJ, Pieters GF, Grotenhuis AJ, Hermus AR. Results of endoscopic transsphenoidal pituitary surgery in 40 patients with a growth hormone-secreting macroadenoma. Acta Neurochir (Wien) 2011;153:1391–1399

33. Ludecke DK, Abe T. Transsphenoidal microsurgery for newly diagnosed acromegaly: a personal view after more than 1,000 operations. Neuroendocrinology 2006;83:230–239

34. Cushing H. Medical classic. The functions of the pituitary body: Harvey Cushing. Am J Med Sci 1981;281:70–78

35. Smith M, Hirsch NP. Pituitary disease and anaesthesia. Br J Anaesth 2000;85:3–14

36. Biller BM, Grossman AB, Stewart PM, et al. Treatment of adrenocorticotropin-dependent Cushing's syndrome: a consensus statement. J Clin Endocrinol Metab 2008;93:2454–2462

37. Jho HD. Endoscopic transsphenoidal surgery. J Neurooncol 2001;54:187–195

38. Cappabianca P, Cavallo LM, Colao A, de Divitiis E. Surgical complications associated with the endoscopic endonasal transsphenoidal approach for pituitary adenomas. J Neurosurg 2002;97:293–298

39. D'Haens J, Van Rompaey K, Stadnik T, Haentjens P, Poppe K, Velkeniers B. Fully endoscopic transsphenoidal surgery for functioning pituitary adenomas: a retrospective comparison with traditional transsphenoidal microsurgery in the same institution. Surg Neurol 2009;72:336–340

40. Yano S, Kawano T, Kudo M, et al. Endoscopic endonasal transsphenoidal approach through the bilateral nostrils for pituitary adenomas. Neurol Med Chir (Tokyo) 2009;49:1–7

41. Cusimano MD, Kan P, Nassiri F, et al. Outcomes of surgically treated giant pituitary tumours. Can J Neurol Sci 2012;39:446–457

42. Loeffler JS, Shih HA. Radiation therapy in the management of pituitary adenomas. J Clin Endocrinol Metab 2011;96:1992–2003

43. Snead FE, Amdur RJ, Morris CG, Mendenhall WM. Long-term outcomes of radiotherapy for pituitary adenomas. Int J Radiat Oncol Biol Phys 2008;71:994–998

44. Kong DS, Lee JI, Lim H, et al. The efficacy of fractionated radiotherapy and stereotactic radiosurgery for pituitary adenomas: long-term results of 125 consecutive patients treated in a single institution. Cancer 2007;110:854–860

45. Selch MT, Gorgulho A, Lee SP, et al. Stereotactic radiotherapy for the treatment of pituitary adenomas. Minim Invasive Neurosurg 2006;49:150–155

46. Tsang RW, Brierley JD, Panzarella T, Gospodarowicz MK, Sutcliffe SB, Simpson WJ. Role of radiation therapy in clinical hormonally-active pituitary adenomas. Radiother Oncol 1996;41:45–53

47. Tsang RW, Brierley JD, Panzarella T, Gospodarowicz MK, Sutcliffe SB, Simpson WJ. Radiation therapy for pituitary adenoma: treatment outcome and prognostic factors. Int J Radiat Oncol Biol Phys 1994;30:557–565

48. Fisher BJ, Gaspar LE, Noone B. Radiation therapy of pituitary adenoma: delayed sequelae. Radiology 1993;187:843–846

49. Littley MD, Shalet SM, Beardwell CG, Robinson EL, Sutton ML. Radiation-induced hypopituitarism is dose-dependent. Clin Endocrinol (Oxf) 1989;31:363–373

50. Chang EF, Zada G, Kim S, et al. Long-term recurrence and mortality after surgery and adjuvant radiotherapy for nonfunctional pituitary adenomas. J Neurosurg 2008;108:736–745

51. Sheehan JP, Niranjan A, Sheehan JM, et al. Stereotactic radiosurgery for pituitary adenomas: an intermediate review of its safety, efficacy, and role in the neurosurgical treatment armamentarium. J Neurosurg 2005;102:678–691

52. Starke RM, Nguyen JH, Rainey J, et al. Gamma Knife surgery of meningiomas located in the posterior fossa: factors predictive of outcome and remission. J Neurosurg 2011;114:1399–1409

53. Niranjan A, Szeifert GT, Kondziolka D. Gamma Knife radiosurgery for growth hormone-secreting pituitary adenomas. Radiosurgery 2002;4:93–101

54. Chacko G, Chacko AG, Kovacs K, et al. The clinical significance of MIB-1 labeling index in pituitary adenomas. Pituitary 2010;13:337–344

55. Melmed S. Pathogenesis of pituitary tumors. Nat Rev Endocrinol 2011;7:257–266

56. Morita K, Takano K, Yasufuku-Takano J, et al. Expression of pituitary tumour-derived, N-terminally truncated isoform of fibroblast growth factor receptor 4 (ptd-FGFR4) correlates with tumour invasiveness but not with G-protein alpha subunit (gsp) mutation in human GH-secreting pituitary adenomas. Clin Endocrinol (Oxf) 2008;68:435–441

57. Qian ZR, Sano T, Asa SL, et al. Cytoplasmic expression of fibroblast growth factor receptor-4 in human pituitary adenomas: relation to tumor type, size, proliferation, and invasiveness. J Clin Endocrinol Metab 2004;89:1904–1911

58. Liu W, Matsumoto Y, Okada M, et al. Matrix metalloproteinase 2 and 9 expression correlated with cavernous sinus invasion of pituitary adenomas. J Med Invest 2005;52:151–158

59. Benveniste RJ, King WA, Walsh J, Lee JS, Delman BN, Post KD. Repeated transsphenoidal surgery to treat recurrent or residual pituitary adenoma. J Neurosurg 2005;102:1004–1012

60. Widhalm G, Wolfsberger S, Preusser M, et al. Residual nonfunctioning pituitary adenomas: prognostic value of MIB-1 labeling index for tumor progression. J Neurosurg 2009;111:563–571

61. Fusco A, Zatelli MC, Bianchi A, et al. Prognostic significance of the Ki-67 labeling index in growth hormone-secreting pituitary adenomas. J Clin Endocrinol Metab 2008;93:2746–2750

62. Ekramullah SM, Saitoh Y, Arita N, Ohnishi T, Hayakawa T. The correlation of Ki-67 staining indices with tumour doubling times in regrowing non-functioning pituitary adenomas. Acta Neurochir (Wien) 1996;138:1449–1455

63. Advani SH. Targeting mTOR pathway: a new concept in cancer therapy. Indian J Med Paediatr Oncol 2010;31:132–136

64. Musat M, Korbonits M, Kola B, et al. Enhanced protein kinase B/Akt signalling in pituitary tumours. Endocr Relat Cancer 2005;12:423–433

65. Noh TW, Jeong HJ, Lee MK, Kim TS, Kim SH, Lee EJ. Predicting recurrence of nonfunctioning pituitary adenomas. J Clin Endocrinol Metab 2009;94:4406–4413

66. Figlin RA, Brown E, Armstrong AJ, et al. NCCN Task Force Report: mTOR inhibition in solid tumors. J Natl Compr Canc Netw 2008;6(Suppl 5):S1–S20, quiz S21–S22

67. Böhm A, Aichberger KJ, Mayerhofer M, et al. Targeting of mTOR is associated with decreased growth and decreased VEGF expression in acute myeloid leukaemia cells. Eur J Clin Invest 2009;39:395–405

68. Gorshtein A, Rubinfeld H, Kendler E, et al. Mammalian target of rapamycin inhibitors rapamycin and RAD001 (everolimus) induce antiproliferative effects in GH-secreting pituitary tumor cells in vitro. Endocr Relat Cancer 2009;16:1017–1027

69. Sukumari-Ramesh S, Singh N, Dhandapani KM, Vender JR. mTOR inhibition reduces cellular proliferation and sensitizes pituitary adenoma cells to ionizing radiation. Surg Neurol Int 2011;2:22

70. Lee M, Theodoropoulou M, Graw J, Roncaroli F, Zatelli MC, Pellegata NS. Levels of p27 sensitize to dual PI3K/mTOR inhibition. Mol Cancer Ther 2011;10:1450–1459

71. Ekeblad S, Sundin A, Janson ET, et al. Temozolomide as monotherapy is effective in treatment of advanced malignant neuroendocrine tumors. Clin Cancer Res 2007;13:2986–2991

72. McCormack AI, Wass JA, Grossman AB. Aggressive pituitary tumours: the role of temozolomide and the assessment of MGMT status. Eur J Clin Invest 2011;41:1133–1148

73. Ma S, Liu X, Yao Y, et al. Effect of temozolomide on cell viability in gonadotroph adenoma cell lines. Oncol Rep 2011;26:543–550

74. Sheehan JP, Xu Z, Salvetti DJ, Schmitt PJ, Vance ML. Results of gamma knife surgery for Cushing's disease. J Neurosurg 2013;119:1486–1492

75. Lwu S, Edem I, Banton B, et al. Quality of life after transsphenoidal pituitary surgery: a qualitative study. Acta Neurochir (Wien) 2012;154:1917–1922

35 Craniopharyngiomas

Khaled M. Krisht, Oren N. Gottfried, and William T. Couldwell

Craniopharyngiomas are benign epithelial neoplasms of the sellar region that arise from embryonic squamous cells of the hypophysiopharyngeal duct (Rathke's pouch). Although Erdheim originally described these lesions in 1904, Cushing introduced the term *craniopharyngioma* in 1932 to describe these epithelial neoplasms and to denote their origin from the embryological remnant. These tumors are characterized by slow growth that may involve important neurovascular structures. Clinical presentation may be associated with endocrine, visual, and mental disturbances; these are secondary to involvement of the hypothalamus–pituitary axis, optic pathways, thalamus, and frontal lobes. Although advances in microsurgical and skull base techniques, radiotherapy, chemotherapy, and hormonal replacement have provided better long-term survival and longer recurrence-free intervals, controversies remain as to the optimal treatment of these tumors.

Typically, craniopharyngiomas are located in the parasellar region. Approximately 5 to 15% manifest within the confines of the sella.[1,2] Another 20% present as a suprasellar mass.[2] Their pattern of growth and location largely depend on where they arise from the pituitary stalk. Lesions arising from the distal portion of the stalk may grow within the sella turcica. They usually adhere to a midline location and may extend into the suprasellar compartment and third ventricle. Lesions arising from the more proximal end of the stalk may grow predominantly within the third ventricle.[3] Thirty percent of craniopharyngiomas may extend anteriorly to involve the frontal lobes; 25% grow laterally to involve the temporal lobe and structures of the middle cranial fossa; another 20% may grow posterior and inferior to encroach on the brainstem and may extend into the cerebellopontine angle or foramen magnum.[2] Papillary craniopharyngiomas more often are located in the third ventricle.[4]

Incidence

Craniopharyngiomas have an annual incidence of 0.5 to 2.0 cases/million population per year and are seen in both adults and children.[5,6] These tumors account for 1.2 to 4% of adult intracranial tumors and 6 to 10% of intracranial neoplasms in the pediatric population.[7,8]

Craniopharyngiomas exhibit a bimodal age distribution, with the first peak at age 5 to 10 years and second peak between ages 50 and 60 years. They occur equally between sexes.[7]

The classic adamantinomatous subtype occurs 10 times as often as the papillary subtype and mainly in children.[4] In contrast, the papillary subtype only occurs in adults.[4]

Embryology: Derivation from Rathke's Pouch

At approximately the fourth week of gestation, Rathke's pouch forms as a diverticulum of the embryonic stomodeum (roof of the oral cavity). Rathke's pouch migrates upward to meet with the infundibulum, which is a down-growth from the floor of the diencephalon. The migratory path of Rathke's pouch corresponds with the primitive craniopharyngeal duct. At approximately the second month of fetal life, Rathke's pouch separates to form Rathke's vesicle, which surrounds the infundibulum. The cells that compose Rathke's vesicle eventually form the pars distalis, pars tuberalis, and pars intermedia, which compose the adenohypophysis. Craniopharyngiomas were originally believed to originate from squamous cell rests found along the path of the primitive craniopharyngeal duct and adenohypophysis at the surface of the pituitary stalk,[4] but now it is thought that those cells are not remnants of the craniopharyngeal duct, but actually result from metaplasia of adenohypophyseal cells of the pituitary stalk.[9] These cells have an increased frequency with age and thus cannot be responsible for the largely juvenile onset of craniopharyngiomas.[4]

Craniopharyngiomas of both subtypes are thought to derive from Rathke's cleft/pouch as evidenced by the occasional ability of some tumor cells to express one or more pituitary hormones.[4] It has also been suggested that the adamantinomatous craniopharyngioma may arise from embryonic rests with enamel organ potential.[4,10] Papillary craniopharyngiomas may share a similar origin or represent a spectrum of a similar disease process with Rathke's cleft cysts as evidenced by the fact that these two disease entities are occasionally of very similar pathology.[4] Papillary craniopharyngiomas may have focal ciliation of epithelium or goblet cells, whereas some Rathke's cleft cysts have extensive squamous metaplasia of their cyst wall, resulting in a solid component, and these cysts may have an associated higher rate of recurrence more similar to papillary craniopharyngiomas.[4,10]

■ Genetics

Typically, craniopharyngiomas occur sporadically and do not follow a direct pattern of familial inheritance; rare cases of craniopharyngioma occurring in siblings, cousins, and children of an affected parent have been reported. Studies have shown that a subset of adamantinomatous craniopharyngiomas are of a monoclonal origin and, thus, are due to somatic genetic defects at specific chromosomal loci.[11] No consistent genetic abnormalities have been observed, and the precise molecular mechanisms involved in craniopharyngioma development are unknown[11]; however, several genetic abnormalities have been reported. Beta-catenin gene mutations have been described in adamantinomatous craniopharyngiomas but not in the papillary type.[12,13] All adamantinomatous craniopharyngiomas demonstrate expression of beta-catenin and some have beta-catenin mutations, which activate the Wnt signaling pathway, causing mitogenic stimulation and mis-specification of cells to form distinct structures, including increased expression of enamel proteins.[12,13] Adamantinomatous craniopharyngiomas have shown other gene changes. One study found that six of nine tumors displayed at least one genomic alteration and three had six or more alterations; the most common abnormality was chromosomal gains.[11] Loss of the Y chromosome has also been observed in some craniopharyngiomas. In contrast, no tumors demonstrated chromosomal imbalances or changes in DNA copy number in 20 adamantinomatous and nine papillary craniopharyngiomas evaluated in another study.[14]

■ Pathology

Adamantinomatous Type

The adamantinomatous or "childhood" type of craniopharyngioma resembles a neoplasm of tooth-forming tissues[10] and is grossly cystic with a smaller solid component with calcifica-

tion. The cystic fluid contains cholesterol and necrotic debris that impart a dark brown to black "motor oil" appearance to the fluid. The cystic fluid is believed to be secondary to desquamation of the cyst epithelium. A well-described pathological feature of the adamantinomatous type is its propensity to adhere to blood vessels and adjacent neural structures, especially the hypothalamus.[4] It commonly has a ragged interface with the surrounding anatomy.[4] This adherence promotes a glial reaction at the tissue–tumor interface characterized by an intensive gliosis with Rosenthal fiber formation.[4] This localized process provides a plane for dissection during surgical removal.

Microscopically, the epithelium is arranged in a distinctive adamantinomatous-like pattern. This pattern is characterized by a basal layer containing cells with darkly staining nuclei associated with an intermediate layer of stellate cells surrounded by a layer of columnar epithelium (**Fig. 35.1**). Histological examination of the cyst wall reveals a keratinized squamous epithelium with discrete areas of stacked clusters of desquamated cells, giving the appearance of nodules of keratin ("wet keratin"). It is the mineralization and deposition of calcium salts to this keratin-rich epithelium that accounts for the calcification seen in this neoplasm.

Papillary Type

In contrast to the adamantinomatous variety, which may occur in children and adults, the squamous papillary type occurs almost exclusively in adulthood, with only rare isolated cases reported in children. It has a distinct propensity to involve the third ventricle.[4] Upon gross examination, the squamous papillary type is mostly solid but may possess a cystic component.[4] Microscopically, the squamous papillary variant exhibits nests of well-differentiated keratinized stratified squamous epithelium forming papillae. These tumors are well circumscribed, rarely calcify, and lack the "wet keratin" and motor oil content seen in the adamantinomatous form.[4] In addition, they do not adhere to surrounding structures; however, gliosis and Rosenthal fiber formation may be present. Unlike the epithelium found in the classic craniopharyngioma, the papillary form does not resemble the tissues of enamel organs.

■ Molecular Markers

The identification of molecular markers for craniopharyngiomas has begun, but their clinical use has not been identified. A subset of craniopharyngiomas have increased insulin-like growth factor I receptor (IGF-IR) expression and display growth arrest with IGF-IR inhibitors.[15] In craniopharyngiomas that express estrogen and progesterone receptors (~30%), the incidence of regrowth after surgery is higher in patients negative for these receptors because of loss of differentiation.[16] An elevated β-human chorionic gonadotrophin level has been

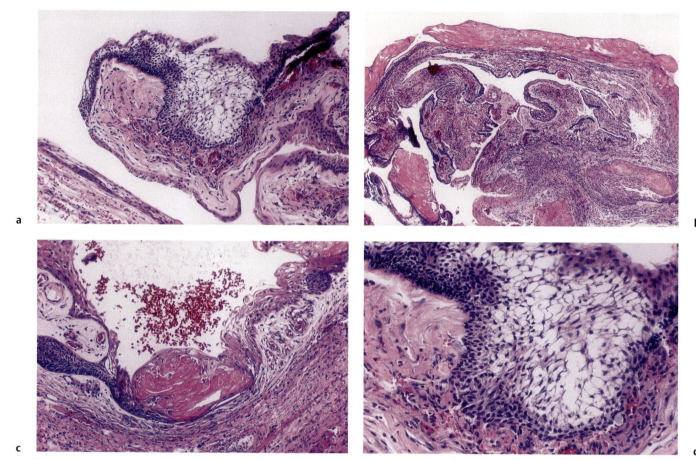

Fig. 35.1a–d (**a**) Adamantinomatous craniopharyngioma with a highly distinctive pattern of epithelial maturation. (**b**) On low-power view, the tumor consists of both solid and cystic epithelial components associated with chronically inflamed fibrous stroma. (**c**) Another characteristic feature of adamantinomatous craniophar- yngioma is the presence of nodules of plump eosinophilic keratinized cells with ghosted nuclei. (**d**) On higher power view, tumor cells abutting the stroma are palisaded, whereas centrally they readily dehisce to create a loose "stellate reticulum."

reported in the cerebrospinal fluid (CSF) of patients with craniopharyngioma, and the tumor has been found to stain positive for this hormone. Finally, a high MIB-1 staining (Ki-67 index) suggests a high possibility of tumor regrowth and was significantly higher in patients who progressed to have a recurrence compared with patients without regrowth.[16]

■ Clinical Features

Presentation

Clinical manifestations of craniopharyngiomas depend on the origin, direction of growth, degree of tumor extension, and involvement of surrounding neural structures. Patients may present with symptoms related to increased intracranial pressure from mass effect or hydrocephalus, or from compression of the optic apparatus, pituitary-hypothalamus axis, or cerebrum. Headache is encountered in more than 50% of patients and is one of the most common complaints prompting medical attention in all age groups. Children often tolerate a significant degree of visual loss; it is the headaches, vomiting, and behavioral changes that usually bring them to initial medical attention. Adults more often than children present with visual disturbance, usually in a delayed fashion because of macular sparing and because they may erroneously relate it to external causes.[17]

Pearl

- Patients with craniopharyngioma typically present with symptoms related to increased intracranial pressure from mass effect or hydrocephalus, or from compression of the optic apparatus, pituitary-hypothalamus axis, or cerebrum. Headache is one of the most common complaints prompting medical attention in all age groups.

Visual Symptoms

Although approximately 20% of children have papilledema at presentation,[1] adults appear to be more sensitive to visual deficits than children. Eighty percent of adults demonstrate visual disturbance as a presenting symptom.[1] Visual disturbance may manifest as a decrease in visual acuity,[5] diplopia, blurred vision, bitemporal hemianopia, homonymous hemianopia, various quadrantanopsias, or seesaw nystagmus.[17] Rare cases of unilateral or even bilateral blindness have been reported.

Endocrine Abnormalities

Endocrine abnormality is found in 80 to 90% of individuals at presentation.[1,7,18] Children commonly present with short stature and delayed linear growth, whereas adolescents may present with delayed or arrested puberty. Men may observe a loss of libido; women may present with secondary amenorrhea.

The most common hormonal deficiencies include growth hormone (75%), followed by luteinizing hormone or follicle-stimulating hormone (40%), adrenocorticotropic hormone (25%), and thyroid-stimulating hormone (25%). The presence of hyperprolactinemia in 20% of patients indicates impingement of areas within the hypothalamus or the pituitary stalk that normally exert an inhibitory influence on prolactin release ("stalk section" effect). Hypothalamic compression may occasionally lead to precocious puberty owing to loss of hypothalamic inhibition exerted on the gonadotropin-releasing hormones in the preadolescent phase. Precocious puberty, however, may be offset by panhypopituitarism secondary to compression of the pituitary gland. Diabetes insipidus (DI) is infrequent at presentation, occurring in 9 to 17% of patients before surgery.[18]

> **Pearl**
>
> - Diabetes insipidus is a common feature in patients postoperatively; however, fewer than 20% of patients manifest DI at presentation.

Behavioral Changes

Some patients come to medical attention as a result of changes in mental status or behavior. Although unusual in children, about 25% of adults present with mental disturbance.[17]

Psychological or intellectual manifestations are largely due to the direction of tumor expansion. Tumor growth involving the frontal lobes may cause dementia, apathy, abulia, or psychomotor slowing.[1] Three of 12 patients presenting with mental status change demonstrated characteristics of Korsakoff syndrome in one report.[19] Complex psychomotor seizures and amnesia have been documented with tumor extension into the temporal lobe and hippocampus.[1]

Imaging Studies

Plain radiographs of the skull have largely been replaced by computed tomography (CT) or magnetic resonance imaging (MRI) as the initial imaging study for diagnosis of craniopharyngioma. Approximately 66% of adults and more than 90% of children, however, exhibit some abnormality on plain skull X-ray, such as enlargement of the sella, erosion of the clinoids and dorsum sella, or suprasellar calcification. More than 80% of children and 40% of adults show calcification on plain skull radiographs.[1]

Computed tomography demonstrates calcification (**Fig. 35.2**) and the secondary skull base bone changes.[20] Calcifications are seen in 93% of childhood craniopharyngiomas.[20] The cyst fluid is iso- or hypodense on CT but may appear hyperdense if sufficient calcification is present. CT with intravenous contrast results in enhancement of the solid portion of the tumor as well as the cyst capsule.

Magnetic resonance imaging is the neuroimaging modality of choice, precisely demonstrating the extent and location of the tumor as well as the tumor's relationship to important surrounding neurovascular structures. Cystic components (**Fig. 35.3**) are identified in 54 to 94% of all craniopharyngiomas,[21] but they are found in 99% of pediatric craniopharyngiomas.[20] On MRI, the cyst exhibits a hyperintense signal on T1-weighted images. The solid component is isointense but enhances on administration of intravenous gadolinium. Mag-

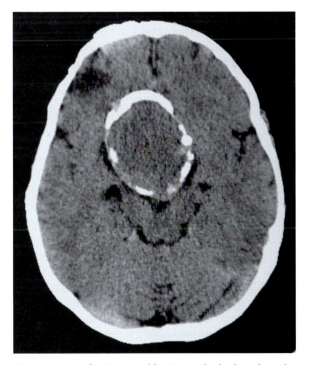

Fig. 35.2 Imaging of a 48-year-old patient who had a subtotal resection of a craniopharyngioma at age 5 and 43 years later experienced increasing headaches and decline in vision. Computed tomography demonstrated a suprasellar lesion with a calcified rim.

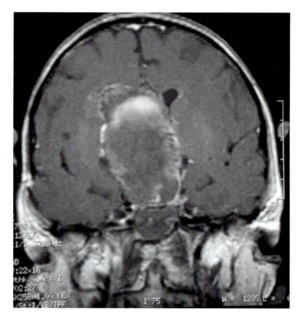 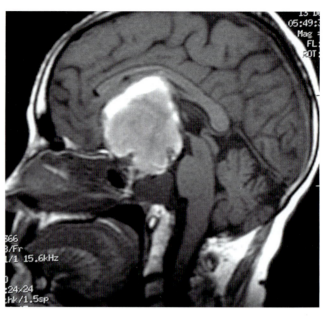

Fig. 35.3a,b (**a**) Coronal and (**b**) sagittal magnetic resonance imaging (MRI) of the same patient shown in **Fig. 35.2**. MRI demonstrated a 5 × 2 × 4 cm suprasellar mass with sellar extension and a largely cystic component. The patient underwent a right fronto- temporal orbitozygomatic craniotomy for resection of tumor. A total resection was achieved, and the patient showed no signs of clinical or imaging recurrence 30 months later.

netic resonance (MR) or CT angiography provides anatomic detail of the cerebral vasculature in relation to the tumor, which is important in surgical planning.

On imaging, craniopharyngiomas may be described in relation to the optic chiasm; craniopharyngiomas are characterized as prechiasmatic, retrochiasmatic, and subchiasmatic. Prechiasmatic tumors grow forward between the optic nerves, displacing the optic chiasm upward and backward as well as displacing the A-1 segment of the anterior cerebral artery.[2] In contrast, retrochiasmatic craniopharyngiomas displace the chiasm forward and have a propensity to fill the third ventricle, resulting in obstructive hydrocephalus. With posterior and inferior extension, retrochiasmatic tumors may displace the basilar artery.[2]

With the introduction of intraoperative imaging modalities such as intraoperative MRI, the rate of gross total resection of difficult cases has been improved. Intraoperative MRI was used during surgery in 25 selected patients in whom tumor resection was anticipated to be difficult according to preoperative findings[22]; the rate of total tumor extirpation was increased by 16% (four additional patients) after reintervention based on preoperative MRI findings of residual tumor, leading to an 80% rate of gross total resection in the entire series. The rate of new ophthalmologic and endocrine deficits was acceptable compared with previously reported rates.[22] With the further development and evolution of intraoperative MRI, we can anticipate continued improvement in the extent of safe, radical resection of challenging craniopharyngioma cases.

■ Management

Preoperative Considerations

Craniopharyngioma is a complex clinicopathological condition that requires a multidisciplinary approach to treatment involving specialists in neurosurgery, endocrinology, neuro-ophthalmology, neuropsychology, and radiation oncology. Because visual disturbance is present in many cases, full visual acuity and visual field examinations are imperative before surgery. One important aspect of initial management pertains to the evaluation and correction of underlying endocrinologic abnormalities. DI, hypocortisolism, and hypothyroidism have been shown to increase the intraoperative and postoperative morbidity when present. Therefore, all patients require extensive preoperative endocrinologic evaluation at presentation and should receive stress doses of glucocorticoids before surgery. If hypothyroidism is present, initiation of replacement therapy should be prompt because several days are required for correction; adrenocortical insufficiency may be precipitated

Controversy

• Patients presenting with hydrocephalus do not always require permanent CSF diversion. Hydrocephalus often resolves after the tumor is removed.

if thyroid replacement is initiated before steroid administration.[23] Accurate assessment and correction of electrolyte deficits must also be done before surgery.

The presence of preoperative hydrocephalus has been shown to have a negative impact on postoperative outcome. Preoperative external ventricular decompression should be performed if the patient presents with significant symptoms as a result of obstructive hydrocephalus. Because the hydrocephalus frequently resolves following tumor removal, many authors suggest that external ventricular drainage at the time of surgery, followed by weaning of the drain postoperatively, is a more effective way to manage hydrocephalus.[1] If serial CT scans demonstrate increasing ventricular size, a shunting procedure should be performed postoperatively.

Surgical Treatment

Advances in surgical technique, radiotherapy, and chemotherapy have led to a better long-term outcome for patients harboring craniopharyngiomas; however, the role of aggressive surgical removal of these tumors is still somewhat controversial. Some authors contend that total resection offers the best chance for tumor-free survival.[24,25] With advances in microsurgical and skull base techniques, safe gross total or near-total excision of these tumors has become possible in the majority of cases with low rates of morbidity and mortality.

In other series, the percent of patients with complete resections has increased from 69 to 90%, but it is well established that tumors can recur even after a radical resection.[24] Radical resection was achieved in over 70% of 112 consecutive patients treated between 1990 and 2008 in one series[26]; recurrence, however, was noted in 25% of cases, necessitating further treatment with radiotherapy, repeat surgery, or a combination of both. In another report, total resection was attempted but subtotal or partial resection was performed if intraoperative findings suggested significant risk of injuring critical neurovascular structures with radical resection.[25] Complete microsurgical removal, when safe, is arguably the treatment of choice to offer the best chance of long-term control.

Other authors support a more conservative approach consisting of subtotal resection combined with postoperative radiation. The argument is supported by the fact that a radical resection in certain cases may be associated with an increased risk of hypothalamic, pituitary, and visual complications. For primarily cystic tumors, drainage and injection of radioactive isotopes or a chemotherapeutic agent may be an alternative to surgical resection.[27]

Controversy

- Either total resection or subtotal resection followed by radiotherapy is a good treatment option in individual patients.

Pitfall

- A radical resection in certain cases may be associated with an increased risk of hypothalamic, pituitary, and visual complications. The goal of surgery is decompression of the optic and ventricular pathways regardless of whether a total or subtotal resection is undertaken.

Surgical Approaches

Choosing the appropriate surgical approach depends primarily on the location and extent of the tumor. The approach must provide exposure that is close to the lesion, adequate visualization, control of critical neurovascular structures, and minimal brain retraction. The goal of surgery is decompression of the optic and ventricular pathways regardless of whether a total or subtotal resection is undertaken. Some commonly used approaches are the subfrontal, pterional, orbitozygomatic, and transsphenoidal approaches. Transcallosal and subtemporal approaches have been described but their use is limited.

Subfrontal Approach

The subfrontal approach is a versatile approach for removing craniopharyngiomas that are midline with extension along the anterior skull base and suprasellar cistern. This approach has the advantage of a straight frontal trajectory with good visualization of both optic nerves and internal carotid arteries. It also has the advantage of accessing the anterior third ventricle via the lamina terminalis if there is intraventricular extension of the tumor. This approach is commonly used for resection of prechiasmatic craniopharyngiomas and for some retrochiasmatic tumors that extend anteriorly and fill the third ventricle. It may not be suitable for patients with a prefixed chiasm.

Pterional (Frontotemporal)

The pterional (frontotemporal) approach may be used for large retrochiasmatic craniopharyngiomas with significant anterior and posterior extension. It is the best route to craniopharyngiomas involving primarily the suprasellar cistern because it provides the shortest distance to the suprasellar region via a transcranial approach. This is the preferred method in patients with a prefixed chiasm because the tumor can be resected beneath the chiasm. A combined pterional and subfrontal approach provides access to both anterior and posterior portions of the tumor.

For craniopharyngiomas with significant suprasellar extension or superior extension into the third ventricle, the orbitozygomatic variation may be useful because it offers an improved inferior-to-superior ("looking-up") view to the hypothalamic and suprasellar regions. Because the orbital rim and lateral sphenoid region are removed, the bony obstruction that typically limits adequate superior exposure is circumvented. In essence, the angle of exposure, based on the fulcrum of the inferior frontal lobe, is significantly improved. Removal of the zygomatic arch allows more inferior mobilization of the temporalis muscle and reduces the muscle bulk that may otherwise obstruct visualization.

Transsphenoidal Approach

Transsphenoidal resection is favorable for craniopharyngiomas that occupy both sellar and suprasellar regions, primarily if the sella is enlarged. The transsphenoidal approach may be a suitable choice for cystic tumors confined to the sella, but even in mostly suprasellar cases an extended transsphenoidal approach can afford a complete resection. In one series, 90% of 68 craniopharyngiomas were totally resected via a transsphenoidal approach.[28] This approach is associated with a lower surgical morbidity and a lower incidence of postoperative DI than is conventional craniotomy.[29]

Intrasellar craniopharyngiomas frequently lack the intimate adherence to vital neurovascular structures such as the hypothalamus,[1,29] but the surgeon must be aware of the nearby cavernous sinus, which contains the internal carotid artery and cranial nerves. Although rare, intraoperative hemorrhage has been reported. In addition, the transsphenoidal approach has a potential for CSF leaks. This approach is contraindicated for large calcified craniopharyngiomas with significant suprasellar or lateral extension as well as tumors demonstrating adherence to the optic nerves or hypothalamus.[1] The transsphenoidal approach may be more difficult in young children who do not have a pneumatized sphenoid sinus. In these cases, access to the sella requires additional drilling of the sphenoid bone with the aid of stereotactic CT guidance.

Transcallosal Approach

The transcallosal approach is advocated primarily for craniopharyngiomas arising from within the third ventricle[3] or with marked superior extension within the third ventricle. The transcallosal route may also be applied for the planned staged resection of the superior component of a large tumor extending superiorly into the third or lateral ventricles in conjunction with a pterional or subfrontal approach. In the aforementioned scenario, it is advisable to start with the pterional approach to help achieve brain relaxation by opening the basal cisterns and rendering the inferior portion of the tumor mobile after dissecting it from the optic apparatus and anterior cerebral artery complex and then resort to the transcallosal approach to complete the resection.

Endoscopic Endonasal Approach

As discussed earlier, the microscope-assisted transsphenoidal approach with its various extensions and variations has demonstrated good resection results with no brain retraction. One of its limitations, however, is its inability to tackle lesions permeating the third ventricle or extending posterior to the optic chiasm through this approach. This restriction can be overcome with the use of the endoscope, making the endonasal route a viable option for more involved cases with superior extension while avoiding brain retraction. Indeed, over the past several years, the scientific and technical refinements made in endoscopic surgery, with the advent of new high-definition optics have enabled minimally invasive resection of large sellar and suprasellar craniopharyngiomas.[29] In another series, 16 patients underwent an expanded endoscopic endonasal approach (EEA) for craniopharyngioma between 1999 and 2006.[30] In these patients, 73% (8 of 11) had a gross total resection without recurrence during a mean follow-up time of 34 months. None of the patients experienced worsening vision. The postoperative rate of DI was 8%. These results were comparable with those obtained with the more conventional methods of resection via the pterional and microscopic transsphenoidal approaches. There was, however, a large discrepancy in the rate of CSF leak (58% with EEA vs. 1 to 5% with microscopic transcranial and transsphenoidal methods).

A CSF leak is more commonly encountered with craniopharyngiomas than with pituitary adenomas because of the extensive cisternal and arachnoid dissection that is undertaken throughout the tumor resection and the resulting direct communication with the third ventricle in cases where there is intraventricular involvement. Several reconstruction strategies, including nasoseptal flaps, multilayered planes of reconstruction material such as fat and fascia lata, and the use of a Foley catheter balloon to hold the reconstruction material in place, have been attempted with varying success rates. With the continued evolution of endoscopy and its growing role in addressing craniopharyngiomas, improvements in the reconstruction strategy are likely to reduce the postoperative CSF leak rate to that of transsphenoidal pituitary surgery.

Surgical Complications

Since the availability of hormone replacement therapy, the surgical mortality rate has dropped from 41% to less than 2% in some series.[24,25] Surgical complications may involve visual, hormonal, behavioral, or vascular sequelae. DI is the most frequently encountered complication seen postoperatively.[24]

Pitfall

- The gliotic reaction around some craniopharyngiomas provides an excellent plane for dissection; however, adherence at the tissue–tumor interface may be tenacious, and neurologic sequelae can result if an aggressive attempt at removal is undertaken, especially in the area of the hypothalamus.

The incidence of postoperative DI ranges from 76 to 94%, but in almost 75% of patients the DI is transient. Other complications include panhypopituitarism, memory deficits, and psychological abnormalities. These complications can be attributed to manipulation of the pituitary stalk and hypothalamus at surgery. Vascular complications resulting from attempts at radical resection have also been reported; although rare, intraoperative laceration or delayed formation of a fusiform dilation of the internal carotid artery may occur from dissection of the tumor. As mentioned earlier, CSF leak is a potential complication after transnasal transsphenoidal approaches whether microscopically or endoscopically assisted. Those cases can be treated with a lumbar drain for CSF diversion with or without repacking of the nasal cavity.

Radiotherapy

Radiation following subtotal resection is associated with a better long-term, recurrence-free survival than is subtotal resection alone. A 20-year survival of 60% was reported for patients treated with adjuvant radiotherapy following subtotal removal.[31] Radiation modalities used in the treatment of craniopharyngiomas have included external fractionated field treatments, stereotactic radiosurgery (SRS; via gamma knife or linear accelerator), fractionated stereotactic radiotherapy (SRT), and stereotactic intracavitary implantation of radionuclides.

Generally, radiation is reserved for the treatment of children older than 3 years but is preferred for children older than 5 years.[32] Radiotherapy in children may negatively impact neurocognitive development and the IQ. Decline is typically associated with several risk factors, including younger age at time of treatment, radiotherapy dose, and the volume of the brain that received treatment. Technical advances in radiotherapy hold promise for lowering the frequency of neurocognitive sequelae.[33]

A fractionated approach with conventional external beam treatment or with SRT results in fewer and less severe adverse radiation-related sequelae, and a higher overall total radiation dose can be more safely delivered. Normal brain tissue tolerates multiple small doses of radiation much better than it does a single large dose. Thus, fractionation enables the delivery of large doses of radiation while sparing normal tissue. Optimum response occurs with radiation doses ranging from 50 to 65 Gy in fractionated doses of 180 to 200 cGy/d.[31,34] Although notable long-term survival rates exist, complications following radiotherapy include radiation necrosis, optic neuritis, dementia, calcification of the basal ganglia, radiation-induced

---

Pearl

- Radiation following subtotal removal is associated with better long-term survival than subtotal resection alone.

Special Consideration

- Stereotactic radiosurgery is a viable treatment alternative for recurrent disease but should be reserved for solid craniopharyngiomas less than 3 cm in size and preferably a safe distance (> 5 mm) away from the optic pathway.

---

vasculopathy, hypothalamic-pituitary dysfunction, and a decrease in intellectual performance in the very young. This latter complication has led to the avoidance of fractionated field radiotherapy by most practitioners for tumors in early childhood. Additionally, neoplasms, including meningiomas, sarcomas, and gliomas, have all been reported at varying latencies following radiotherapy. In one study with a median follow-up of 17 years after treatment, there were radiation-related complications in 58% of children and 46% of adults.[35] Two new pediatric cases (4-year-old boy and 6-year-old girl) were reported in addition to three previously reported cases of malignant transformation of craniopharyngioma 7 to 8 years after external beam radiation therapy.[36] Six similar cases of malignant transformation following radiotherapy have been reported in the adult literature.[37–39]

Stereotactic Radiosurgery

Stereotactic radiosurgery enables accurate and precise application of multiple convergent beams of ionizing radiation to a focally distinct volume of tissue with a single dose. The use of multiple beams results in a sharp dose fall-off beyond the target area, which spares normal adjacent tissue. Typically, SRS has been used as treatment for recurrent disease. In one study, stereotactic gamma knife radiosurgery (GKRS) was employed in 10 cases of craniopharyngioma with a median follow-up of 14 months; seven patients had considerable shrinkage of the tumor and the remaining three patients had no overall change in tumor size, but on follow-up MRI showed central low-intensity signal changes consistent with central necrosis. In another series of 10 patients treated with GKRS, four patients had complete regression and another four had tumor shrinkage at last follow-up at a median of 63 months.[40] Between these two series, three patients experienced visual deterioration. Whereas the mean marginal tumor dose was 16.4 and 14.3 Gy in these series, respectively, the 13 patients in another series were treated with only 6 Gy, and 11 suffered tumor progression at a mean of 17 years follow-up.[41]

In another study, 23 patients with recurrent craniopharyngioma were treated with GKRS with a mean of 10.8 Gy, and 61% of patients had tumor reduction at a mean of 22.6 months, but local control was achieved in another 13% after a second radiosurgical intervention.[42] Currently, SRS is generally contraindicated in craniopharyngiomas with solid components larger than 2.5 to 3 cm, primarily cystic tumors, tumors involving the hypothalamus and brainstem, as well as tumors less than 3 to 5 mm in distance from the optic apparatus,[34] although a single fractionated dose less than 8 to 10 Gy to the optic apparatus is considered to be safe.

Stereotactic radiotherapy uses fractionated irradiation under stereotactic guidance. It enables delivering multiple doses of fractionated radiation to focal areas and offers the advantage of treating tumors more than 3 cm in size as well as tumors adjacent to critical neural structures, which normally limit the application of SRS.[43] Excellent relapse-free survival without any evidence of radiation-induced optic neuropathy has been reported.[43]

Intracavitary irradiation has been primarily recommended for solitary cystic craniopharyngioma. It is also possible to treat the cystic component of a mixed tumor with intracavitary irradiation while the solid component is treated with another modality. Intracavitary irradiation employs placement of β-emitting isotopes (^{32}P or ^{90}Y) into the cyst cavity following stereotactic aspiration of the cyst contents. Currently, it is possible to aspirate the cyst and instill the isotope through a minimally invasive approach with image guidance. Results have demonstrated stabilization or a decrease in the size of the cyst in greater than 75% of patients treated for primary cystic craniopharyngiomas[21,44]; however, in one series, 33% of patients required additional surgery and 10% died.[44] Although many patients have improved vision, side effects can include decreased visual acuity or decrease in visual fields, which typically occur in approximately one third of patients.[44] Yttrium-90 is associated with a higher incidence of visual dysfunction because of its higher maximum energy and greater depth of tissue penetration.[44] Unlike these β-emitting isotopes, interstitial irradiation with iodine-125 may be useful in patients with solid tumors.[45] Iodine-125 was used in a patient with a solid craniopharyngioma and one with a mixed solid and cystic tumor, with resolution of the tumors at 12 and 24 months and without recurrence or toxicity.[45]

Chemotherapy

The role of chemotherapy in the treatment of craniopharyngioma has yet to be clearly defined, and most articles are case reports. There has been interest in the use of intracavitary bleomycin injection into cystic craniopharyngiomas. In one series of 11 patients with cystic craniopharyngiomas with follow-up of 3 to 16 years. The cyst resolved completely in

Special Consideration

- Although the role of chemotherapy for the treatment of craniopharyngioma is unclear at this time, some success has been achieved with intracavitary injection of chemotherapy into cystic lesions.

three patients and decreased in size by 80 to 90% in four patients who were monitored with serial imaging. In three patients there was a reduction of size of 60 to 70% and these patients were also treated with radiosurgery. One patient died of hormone insufficiency.[46] In another study, 24 craniopharyngiomas were treated with only bleomycin; nine tumors completely resolved and 15 cysts decreased in size by 50 to 70%. At a median of 5 years, there were no recurrences.[47] The most serious problem associated with intralesional injection of bleomycin relates to the neurotoxic effects of drug leakage on normal neural tissue, particularly the hypothalamus.

Intralesional injection of bleomycin into solid or mixed craniopharyngiomas has demonstrated minimal or no effect.[27] A substitute for bleomycin might be interferon-α (IFN-α), which has low neurotoxicity.[48] Its intralesional use was described in nine patients with cystic craniopharyngiomas and resulted in disappearance of the tumor in seven and partial tumor reduction in the other two at a mean of 20 months of follow-up.[48] More recently, the use of pegylated interferon-α-2b (PI), a well-known antitumor protein that affects cell growth and differentiation, was reported for treating children with recurrent craniopharyngioma.[49] Five children were treated for up to 2 years with subcutaneous injections of PI at a dose of 1 to 3 μg/kg/week. Tumor response was assessed with MRI. All patients had stable disease or improvement in tumor burden in response to PI.[49] Intralesional administration of nonpegylated interferon has also shown efficacy against craniopharyngioma.

■ Recurrence

Although craniopharyngiomas are histologically benign, they are characterized by a high incidence of tumor recurrence. The pathogenesis of recurrence is unclear. One hypothesis contends that "brain invasion" is the most likely nidus for tumor regrowth. This invasion, seen in some specimens of craniopharyngioma, is in fact islets of tumor cells surrounded by neural tissue and does not represent true invasion.[1]

Overall recurrence rates approach 28%,[1] with the average time interval to recurrence of 2 to 5 years.[15] Adults show a lower recurrence rate (20%) than children (30%),[1] possibly because of the difference in the histopathological variants seen in the pediatric versus the adult population, although some series suggest that recurrence rates do not differ between papillary and adamantinomatous tumors.[8] Overall, the extent of surgical resection is the most significant factor associated with recurrence.[8]

In the most extensive single surgical experience encompassing 144 patients over 22 years, a 90% gross total resection was reported with a recurrence rate of 7%.[24] Others have noted a recurrence rate of up to 33% following gross total resection. In contrast, 63 to 90% of the tumors subtotally removed increase in size.[1] This figure was reduced to 30% when subtotal removal was combined with adjuvant radiotherapy.[1] Complete resection without recurrence with tumors less than 2 cm has been reported, supporting the finding that smaller tumors are more likely to be completely resected and are therefore associated with a decreased rate of recurrence.[8]

Many authors agree that an attempt at gross total resection offers the best possible long-term outcome. Radical surgery is not without risk, however, especially in those patients with tumor adherent to vital visual pathway structures or the hypothalamus, damage to which may have disastrous consequences. On the other hand, radiotherapy has its own inherent risks that are compounded in the developing nervous system.

Various modalities exist for the treatment of recurrent tumor. Most authors still advocate surgery for accessible recurrent disease, with radiation reserved for those tumors deemed not amenable to surgery.[1] Reoperation for tumor regrowth carries a higher morbidity, and the possibility of total removal is decreased.[1,24] Patient age and location of tumor are important factors for consideration in the surgical treatment for recurrent disease. The deleterious effects of irradiation on the developing nervous system warrant an attempt at radical resection in young children. Similarly, patients harboring residual tumor in accessible areas are good candidates for reoperation.

Outcome

In a review of the literature, the 5- and 10-year survival rates were 58 to 100% and 24 to 100% for total resection, 37 to 71% and 31 to 52% for subtotal excision, and 69 to 95% and 62 to 84% for subtotal resection and postoperative radiotherapy.[50] No significant difference in overall survival was observed in a study of 75 patients, when comparing patients treated with surgery alone versus subtotal resection plus radiotherapy.[32] Also, the timing of radiotherapy (immediately after surgery with a subtotal resection or after a relapse) was not significant, and the two groups had comparable tumor control rates.[32]

Craniopharyngioma is one of the main causes of hypothalamic-pituitary dysfunction in childhood; this dysfunction may arise from the tumor itself or as a result of the treatment. The incidence of endocrine dysfunction is arguably greater after total resection than after subtotal resection.[7,18] It is also possible that radiotherapy after partial resection results in less endocrine dysfunction than a total resection, and that radiotherapy may not be as harmful on the pituitary-hypothalamic axis.[7] Other studies have not noted a difference between the extent of resection and endocrine dysfunction, with the exception of an increased incidence of DI after a radical dissection.[24]

Multiple endocrinopathies occur in 84 to 97% of patients after treatment.[32,33] The most common hypothalamic dysfunctions after treatment include growth hormone deficiency, gonadotropin deficiency, thyroid deficiency, adrenal insufficiency, DI, hypothyroidism, and hyperprolactinemia. Most patients require long-term hormone replacement after treatment.

Morbidity can be significant even when the tumor can be resected completely. Patients with a childhood craniopharyngioma often suffer from severe obesity, which significantly affects the quality of life and is typically refractory to conventional treatments. Hypothalamic damage can also result in defective short-term memory, limited concentration span, defective thirst sensation, and sleep disturbance.

Poor functional outcomes are associated with large tumors infiltrating or displacing the hypothalamus, the occurrence of hydrocephalus, young age at diagnosis, and multiple surgeries because of tumor recurrence.[33] Cognitive dysfunction and disability occur frequently in patients with craniopharyngiomas. Neurocognitive dysfunction, including difficulties with concentration, learning, and memory, is a well-known complication of radical craniopharyngioma surgery.[33] Epilepsy and visual complications, including decreased visual acuity or constriction of the visual field, have also been reported.[24,33]

Conclusion

Advances in neurosurgical technique, radiotherapy, and adjuvant endocrine treatment have provided a better prognosis; however, craniopharyngiomas still present a difficult management problem. The surgeon must bear in mind the goals of therapy as well as the possible sequelae of the treatment. Therapy should be individualized for each patient to achieve the best overall management while maintaining quality of life, with a solid understanding of limitations and risks of treatment.

Editor's Note

Craniopharyngiomas are uncommon, and, because of their adhesion to and intimate relationship with extremely important structures such as the chiasm and hypothalamus, are very challenging lesions for most neurosurgeons. Original thought was that radical resection was necessary, and although this is still the desired goal in many cases, the overzealous manipulation of the hypothalamus can produce devastating results for the patient, especially children. The lesion's location and various combinations of cystic and solid components and directions of growth result in numerous possible approaches that further confuse decision making. In one report, one craniopharyngioma case e-consulted on by 40 neurosurgeons yielded 10 different surgical approaches, indicating the wide variety and lack of standardization of surgical approaches for this tumor.[51] The expanded endoscopic approach may be the most important recent surgical innovation, and when complete surgical resection is not possible, adjuvant radiotherapy is effective in delaying or preventing recurrence. (Bernstein)

References

1. Samii MT, Tatagiba M. Craniopharyngioma. In: Kaye A, Laws EJ, eds. Brain Tumors. New York: Churchill Livingstone, 1995:873–894
2. Harwood-Nash DC. Neuroimaging of childhood craniopharyngioma. Pediatr Neurosurg 1994;21(Suppl 1):2–10
3. Fukushima T, Hirakawa K, Kimura M, Tomonaga M. Intraventricular craniopharyngioma: its characteristics in magnetic resonance imaging and successful total removal. Surg Neurol 1990;33:22–27
4. Burger PC, Scheithauer BW, Vogel FS. Surgical Pathology of the Nervous System and Its Coverings, 4th ed. New York: Churchill Livingstone, 2002:475–483
5. Adamson TE, Wiestler OD, Kleihues P, Yaşargil MG. Correlation of clinical and pathological features in surgically treated craniopharyngiomas. J Neurosurg 1990;73:12–17
6. Bunin GR, Surawicz TS, Witman PA, Preston-Martin S, Davis F, Bruner JM. The descriptive epidemiology of craniopharyngioma. J Neurosurg 1998;89:547–551
7. Thomsett MJ, Conte FA, Kaplan SL, Grumbach MM. Endocrine and neurologic outcome in childhood craniopharyngioma: Review of effect of treatment in 42 patients. J Pediatr 1980;97:728–735
8. Weiner HL, Wisoff JH, Rosenberg ME, et al. Craniopharyngiomas: a clinicopathological analysis of factors predictive of recurrence and functional outcome. Neurosurgery 1994;35:1001–1010, discussion 1010–1011
9. Asa SL, Kovacs K, Bilbao JM. The pars tuberalis of the human pituitary. A histologic, immunohistochemical, ultrastructural and immunoelectron microscopic analysis. Virchows Arch A Pathol Anat Histopathol 1983;399:49–59
10. Bernstein ML, Buchino JJ. The histologic similarity between craniopharyngioma and odontogenic lesions: a reappraisal. Oral Surg Oral Med Oral Pathol 1983;56:502–511
11. Rienstein S, Adams EF, Pilzer D, Goldring AA, Goldman B, Friedman E. Comparative genomic hybridization analysis of craniopharyngiomas. J Neurosurg 2003;98:162–164
12. Kato K, Nakatani Y, Kanno H, et al. Possible linkage between specific histological structures and aberrant reactivation of the Wnt pathway in adamantinomatous craniopharyngioma. J Pathol 2004;203:814–821
13. Sekine S, Shibata T, Kokubu A, et al. Craniopharyngiomas of adamantinomatous type harbor beta-catenin gene mutations. Am J Pathol 2002;161:1997–2001
14. Rickert CH, Paulus W. Lack of chromosomal imbalances in adamantinomatous and papillary craniopharyngiomas. J Neurol Neurosurg Psychiatry 2003;74:260–261
15. Ulfarsson E, Karström A, Yin S, et al. Expression and growth dependency of the insulin-like growth factor I receptor in craniopharyngioma cells: a novel therapeutic approach. Clin Cancer Res 2005;11:4674–4680
16. Izumoto S, Suzuki T, Kinoshita M, et al. Immunohistochemical detection of female sex hormone receptors in craniopharyngiomas: correlation with clinical and histologic features. Surg Neurol 2005;63:520–525, discussion 525
17. Cohen ME, Duffner PK. Brain Tumors in Children: Principles of Diagnosis and Treatment. New York: Raven Press, 1994:285–301
18. Sklar CA. Craniopharyngioma: endocrine sequelae of treatment. Pediatr Neurosurg 1994;21(Suppl 1):120–123
19. Kahn EA, Gosch HH, Seeger JF, Hicks SP. Forty-five years' experience with the craniopharyngiomas. Surg Neurol 1973;1:5–12
20. Zhang YQ, Wang CC, Ma ZY. Pediatric craniopharyngiomas: clinicomorphological study of 189 cases. Pediatr Neurosurg 2002;36:80–84
21. Voges J, Sturm V, Lehrke R, Treuer H, Gauss C, Berthold F. Cystic craniopharyngioma: long-term results after intracavitary irradiation with stereotactically applied colloidal beta-emitting radioactive sources. Neurosurgery 1997;40:263–269, discussion 269–270
22. Hofmann BM, Nimsky C, Fahlbusch R. Benefit of 1.5-T intraoperative MR imaging in the surgical treatment of craniopharyngiomas. Acta Neurochir (Wien) 2011;153:1377–1390, discussion 1390
23. Ingbar SH. Disease of the thyroid. In: Harrison's Principles of Internal Medicine, Vol 2, 11th ed. New York: McGraw-Hill, 1987:1732–1752
24. Yaşargil MG, Curcic M, Kis M, Siegenthaler G, Teddy PJ, Roth P. Total removal of craniopharyngiomas. Approaches and long-term results in 144 patients. J Neurosurg 1990;73:3–11
25. Fahlbusch R, Honegger J, Paulus W, Huk W, Buchfelder M. Surgical treatment of craniopharyngiomas: experience with 168 patients. J Neurosurg 1999;90:237–250
26. Mortini P, Losa M, Pozzobon G, et al. Neurosurgical treatment of craniopharyngioma in adults and children: early and long-term results in a large case series. J Neurosurg 2011;114:1350–1359
27. Takahashi H, Nakazawa S, Shimura T. Evaluation of postoperative intratumoral injection of bleomycin for craniopharyngioma in children. J Neurosurg 1985;62:120–127
28. Chakrabarti I, Amar AP, Couldwell W, Weiss MH. Long-term neurological, visual, and endocrine outcomes following transnasal resection of craniopharyngioma. J Neurosurg 2005;102:650–657
29. Coppens JR, Couldwell WT. Staged use of the transsphenoidal approach to resect superior third ventricular craniopharyngiomas. Minim Invasive Neurosurg 2010;53:40–43
30. Gardner PA, Kassam AB, Snyderman CH, et al. Outcomes following endoscopic, expanded endonasal resection of suprasellar craniopharyngiomas: a case series. J Neurosurg 2008;109:6–16

31. Regine WF, Kramer S. Pediatric craniopharyngiomas: long term results of combined treatment with surgery and radiation. Int J Radiat Oncol Biol Phys 1992;24:611–617

32. Stripp DC, Maity A, Janss AJ, et al. Surgery with or without radiation therapy in the management of craniopharyngiomas in children and young adults. Int J Radiat Oncol Biol Phys 2004;58:714–720

33. Poretti A, Grotzer MA, Ribi K, Schönle E, Boltshauser E. Outcome of craniopharyngioma in children: long-term complications and quality of life. Dev Med Child Neurol 2004;46:220–229

34. Tarbell NJ, Barnes P, Scott RM, et al. Advances in radiation therapy for craniopharyngiomas. Pediatr Neurosurg 1994;21(Suppl 1):101–107

35. Regine WF, Mohiuddin M, Kramer S. Long-term results of pediatric and adult craniopharyngiomas treated with combined surgery and radiation. Radiother Oncol 1993;27:13–21

36. Aquilina K, Merchant TE, Rodriguez-Galindo C, Ellison DW, Sanford RA, Boop FA. Malignant transformation of irradiated craniopharyngioma in children: report of 2 cases. J Neurosurg Pediatr 2010;5:155–161

37. Akachi K, Takahashi H, Ishijima B, et al. [Malignant changes in a craniopharyngioma]. No Shinkei Geka 1987;15:843–848

38. Kristopaitis T, Thomas C, Petruzzelli GJ, Lee JM. Malignant craniopharyngioma. Arch Pathol Lab Med 2000;124:1356–1360

39. Suzuki F, Konuma I, Matsumoto M, Aoki M, Hayakawa I. [Craniopharyngioma with malignant transformation—a report of two cases]. Gan No Rinsho 1989;35:723–728

40. Chiou SM, Lunsford LD, Niranjan A, Kondziolka D, Flickinger JC. Stereotactic radiosurgery of residual or recurrent craniopharyngioma, after surgery, with or without radiation therapy. Neuro-oncol 2001;3:159–166

41. Ulfarsson E, Lindquist C, Roberts M, et al. Gamma knife radiosurgery for craniopharyngiomas: long-term results in the first Swedish patients. J Neurosurg 2002;97(5, Suppl):613–622

42. Mokry M. Craniopharyngiomas: a six year experience with gamma knife radiosurgery. Stereotact Funct Neurosurg 1999;72(Suppl 1):140–149

43. Kalapurakal JA, Goldman S, Hsieh YC, Tomita T, Marymont MH. Clinical outcome in children with recurrent craniopharyngioma after primary surgery. Cancer J 2000;6:388–393

44. Pollock BE, Lunsford LD, Kondziolka D, Levine G, Flickinger JC. Phosphorus-32 intracavitary irradiation of cystic craniopharyngiomas: current technique and long-term results. Int J Radiat Oncol Biol Phys 1995;33:437–446

45. Barlas O, Bayindir C, Can M. Interstitial irradiation for craniopharyngioma. Acta Neurochir (Wien) 2000;142:389–395

46. Takahashi H, Yamaguchi F, Teramoto A. Long-term outcome and reconsideration of intracystic chemotherapy with bleomycin for craniopharyngioma in children. Childs Nerv Syst 2005;21:701–704

47. Mottolese C, Stan H, Hermier M, et al. Intracystic chemotherapy with bleomycin in the treatment of craniopharyngiomas. Childs Nerv Syst 2001;17:724–730

48. Cavalheiro S, Dastoli PA, Silva NS, Toledo S, Lederman H, da Silva MC. Use of interferon alpha in intratumoral chemotherapy for cystic craniopharyngioma. Childs Nerv Syst 2005;21:719–724

49. Yeung JT, Pollack IF, Panigrahy A, Jakacki RI. Pegylated interferon-α-2b for children with recurrent craniopharyngioma. J Neurosurg Pediatr 2012;10:498–503

50. Heideman RL, Packer RJ, Albright LA, Freeman CR, Rorke LB. Tumors of the central nervous system. In: Pizzo PA, Poplak DG, eds. Principles and Practice of Paediatric Oncology. Philadelphia: Lippincott-Raven, 1997: 633–697

51. Bernstein M, Khu KJ. Is there too much variability in technical neurosurgery decision-making? Virtual Tumour Board of a challenging case. Acta Neurochir (Wien) 2009;151:411–412, discussion 412–413

36 Vestibular Schwannomas

Martin J. Rutkowski, Taemin Oh, and Andrew T. Parsa

Over the past three decades, a shift has occurred in the treatment of sporadic vestibular schwannoma (sVS). Rather than relying solely on surgical resection, noninvasive therapies such as external beam radiotherapy and gamma knife radiosurgery (GKR) have been widely studied and employed as sole and adjuvant management strategies.[1–3] The literature has seen a surge in publications addressing the relative merits of less morbid interventions, including rates of tumor control, hearing preservation, and complication profiles. Importantly, developments in our understanding of the pathological characteristics and natural history of untreated sVS have allowed practitioners to more confidently select the most appropriate modality of treatment for their patients.

In the evaluation of sVS patients, it is paramount that the needs and preferences of each patient be taken into consideration. sVS is a benign brain tumor, and as such, treatment decisions should center on the tumor's impact on the patient's quality of life. Treatment selection must take into account audiometric studies, interval growth rate, and anatomic parameters such as intracanalicular extension and overall size. Such considerations may influence the decision to employ radiation-based treatment versus open surgery, surgical approach selection, and goals for the extent of resection. Weighing the pros and cons of each option with the preferences of the individual patient offers the best chance of achieving a mutually satisfactory treatment result.

In the evaluation of patients with familial schwannomas, similar due diligence must be applied to ensure optimal quality of life and tumor control. However, given the association of familial tumors with neurofibromatosis type 2 (NF2) and bilateral involvement, such patients can present with additional challenges in management.[4,5]

◼ Management of Sporadic Vestibular Schwannomas

Observation

As a benign brain tumor, sVS can be conservatively managed without compromising the overall survival of a patient. Since the introduction and widespread adoption of MRI, incidentally detected sVS has become more commonplace, with recent evidence indicating an incidence of 0.2% across all imaging scans among asymptomatic patients.[6] Because many sVS pa-

tients present without symptoms or are unwilling to accept the risks of intervention, observation is an important first-line management strategy. Even for patients who are minimally symptomatic, an initial MRI scan provides an important baseline for future treatment decisions; growth can be documented over time with interval imaging, and, at each stage, a provider can discuss management options should the clinical condition deteriorate.

Despite a rich literature on sVS, there remains an incomplete understanding of the manner in which these tumors actually cause symptoms. Beyond the obvious impact of mass effect on adjacent structures, including cranial nerves such as the trigeminal nerve, it has been observed that tumor size does not always correlate with vestibulocochlear symptoms; more specifically, larger tumors do not always cause hearing loss, whereas patients with smaller tumors may present with hearing loss. Thus, in the absence of intolerable presenting symptoms, tumor size on initial MRI may not be the most reliable metric on which to base treatment planning. Size does not always correlate with symptomatology, nor does it predict tumor growth, potentially leaving patients better served by interval brain scans to document tumor growth.

To better document the relationship of tumor growth with patient outcomes, two populations of conservatively treated sVS patients were studied to determine growth rates and their effect on the development of hearing loss.[7] These patients included those presenting with serviceable hearing (American Academy of Otolaryngology–Head and Neck Surgery [AAO-HNS] grade A or B) and tumors less than 25 mm in initial diameter. Using a data set of 982 patients observed with interval scans, it was found that patients who experienced growth of greater than 2.5 mm per year were more than twice as likely to suffer hearing loss, whereas initial size had no bearing on the development of hearing loss during the observation period (**Fig. 36.1**). These results were corroborated by a second study analyzing 59 conservatively managed patients over a 22-year period.[8] In this prospectively collected database, patients were at greater risk for hearing loss if their tumors grew

Pearl
• Tumor size does not always correlate with symptomatology or predict growth rate.

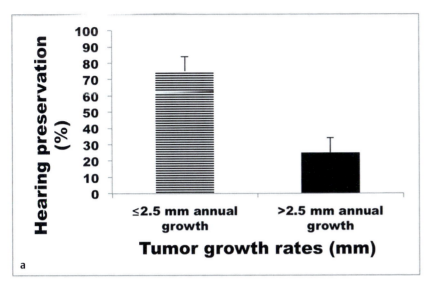

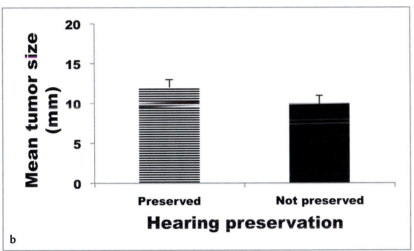

Fig. 36.1a,b Results of hearing outcomes from the literature review. (**a**) Differences in hearing preservation rates based on tumor growth rates ($p < 0.0001$). (**b**) Differences in hearing preservation based on initial tumor size (mm; $p < 0.001$). (Adapted from Suqhrue ME, Yang I, Aranda D, et al. The natural history of untreated sporadic vestibular schwannomas: a comprehensive review of hearing outcomes. J Neurosurg 2010;112:165.)

more than 2.5 mm per year (**Fig. 36.2**), with a median time to hearing loss of 7 years (versus almost 15 years in the patients with slower growing tumors). Thus, in the absence of intolerable presenting symptoms, watchful waiting can serve as a viable initial strategy, with the caveat that documented growth rates greater than 2.5 mm per year pose greater risk for hearing loss during the observation period.

Hearing loss has been observed in sVS patients followed for more than a decade without evidence of tumor growth on imaging. In these patients, it is possible that pathological characteristics such as microhemorrhage or fibrosis may be responsible for vestibulocochlear damage and hearing loss,

potentially prognostic features that are intriguing due to the ability of high-resolution MRI to detect them.[9] Further study into the clinicopathological characteristics of sVS will undoubtedly improve understanding to aid the practitioner in counseling patients on conservative versus interventional management.

Radiotherapy

In a select subset of patients, noninvasive treatment with stereotactic GKR provides an attractive management strategy. Treatment with this modality does not typically require hospitalization and avoids the risks attendant to open surgery. However, radiosurgery is not without its risks, which limits its applicability. Radiation exposure to adjacent neurologic structures can cause tissue toxicity such as cranial neuropathies, whereas other complications such as cerebral edema and hydrocephalus have also been reported. Furthermore, tumors greater than 30 mm in diameter are not currently candidates for single fraction GKR.

Special Consideration

- Observation is an important first-line treatment strategy, but patients whose tumors grow at a rate greater than 2.5 mm per year are at increased risk for hearing loss.

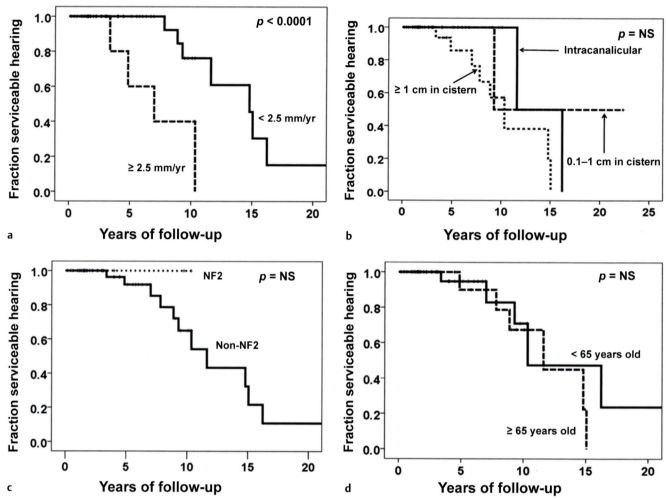

Fig. 36.2a–d (**a**) Kaplan-Meier analysis comparing the rate of hearing loss between patients with tumors growing < 2.5 mm/year versus those growing ≥ 2.5 mm/year, (**b**) patients with small, medium, and large initial tumor sizes, (**c**) patients with and without a known history of neurofibromatosis type 2 (NF2), and (**d**) patients < 65 years of age versus those ≥ 65 years of age.(From Sughrue ME, Kane AJ, Kaur R, et al. A prospective study of hearing preservation in untreated vestibular schwannomas. J Neurosurg 2011;114:384. Reproduced with permission.)

As the role of GKR has become better established for benign skull base tumors such as sVS, there has been an effort to identify factors that predict postinterventional hearing preservation, including tumor size, patient age, and radiation dose given. GKR would appear to have excellent tumor control rates largely in excess of 90%, and acceptable overall hearing preservation rates, with numerous studies reporting rates over 50%. More specifically, radiation dose less than 13 Gy is predictive of increased hearing preservation, whereas age and tumor volume have little effect (**Fig. 36.3**).[10,11]

Any discussion of radiosurgical intervention with patients must also include a consideration of complication rates, especially those involving adjacent cranial nerves. Facial nerve preservation has been reported as high as 96% following GKR, with lower radiation dose (less than 13 Gy), smaller tumor size (less than 15mm³), and younger age (less than 60 years) acting as positive predictors of outcome (**Fig. 36.4**).[1] Radiation dose greater than 13 Gy was also significantly associated with higher rates of cranial nerve V dysfunction.[12]

Surgery

Long a mainstay in therapeutic intervention for sVS, open surgical resection offers an important option to patients with documented rapid tumor growth, tumors that are too large

Pearls

- Tumors greater than 30 mm in diameter are not currently candidates for single-fraction GKR.
- Radiation doses less than 13 Gy are associated with better hearing and facial nerve preservation.

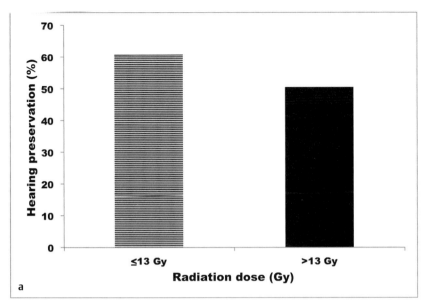

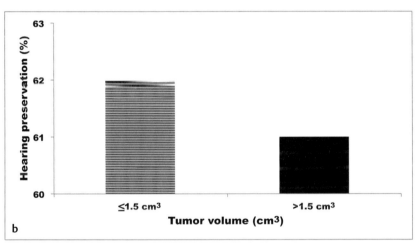

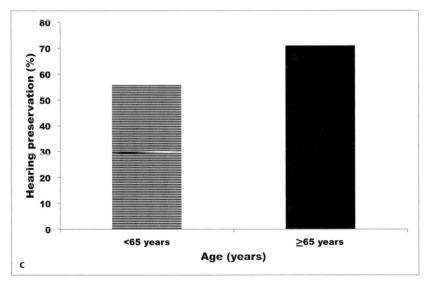

Fig. 36.3a–c (**a**) Differences in hearing preservation based on high versus low radiation dose (>13 vs ≤ 13 Gy), $p = 0.0005$. (**b**) Differences in hearing preservation based on tumor volume (≤ 1.5 cm^3 vs > 1.5 cm^3), $p = 0.8968$. (**c**) Differences in hearing preservation based on patient age (< 65 vs ≥ 65 years), $p = 0.1134$. (Adapted from Yang I, Sughrue ME, Han SJ, et al. A comprehensive analysis of hearing preservation after radiosurgery for vestibular schwannoma: clinical article. J Neurosurg 2010;112:855–856.)

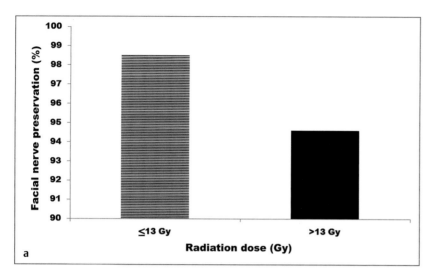

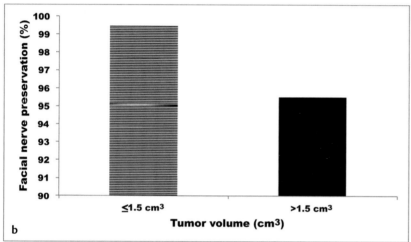

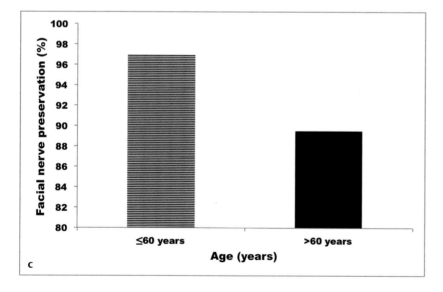

Fig. 36.4 (a) Differences in facial nerve preservation based on high versus low radiation dose (>13 vs ≤13 Gy), $p < 0.0001$. (**b**) Differences in facial nerve preservation based on tumor volume (≤ 1.5 cm³ vs > 1.5 cm³), $p < 0.0001$. (**c**) Differences in hearing preservation based on patient age (≤ 60 vs > 60 years), $p < 0.0001$. (Adapted from Yang I, Sughrue ME, Han SJ, et al. Facial nerve preservation after vestibular schwannoma gamma knife radiosurgery. J Neuro-Oncol 2009;93:43–44.)

for GKR, and for patients who require immediate, durable, and long-term freedom from tumor mass effect. Similar to observation or treatment with GKR, the relative advantages and disadvantages of surgical resection must be considered, in addition to the inherent risks and benefits of approach selection. The middle cranial fossa, translabyrinthine, and retrosigmoid approaches are selected on the basis of tumor size, intracanalicular extension, and level of preoperative hearing loss, in an effort to better achieve more complete resection while minimizing comorbid complications including cerebrospinal fluid (CSF) leaks and vascular infarction (**Fig. 36.5**). Each patient requires a customized approach based on the anatomic features of their tumor.

Ample evidence supports the long-term durability of open surgical resection. For example, in a study of 772 surgically treated sVS patients, there was no significant relationship between extent of resection and tumor recurrence (**Fig. 36.6**).[13] These results suggest that subtotal resections performed with the intent of avoiding manipulation and damage to adjacent neurovascular structures, such as cranial nerves VII and VIII, may minimize comorbidity while achieving similar rates of tumor control. In particular, facial nerve dysfunction can have devastating functional and cosmetic effects on patients.[14] When considering that there may be an association between larger tumor size and postoperative facial nerve dysfunction, a less aggressive resection may be better tolerated while providing equivalent durability. Furthermore, when controlling for extent of resection, surgical approach did not affect rates of tumor control, which implies that a wide repertoire of surgical strategies can be employed and still lead to favorable outcomes.[15]

Preservation of hearing function (cranial nerve VIII) is also an important factor in the patient's quality of life. Although the role of age as a predictive variable for hearing preservation remains somewhat equivocal, surgical resection holds promise in the achievement of long-term tumor control in patients who present with sVS at less than 40 years of age. In a series of patients followed for 15 years, 89% showed no evidence of recurrence or progression, whereas hearing preservation was 68% in patients presenting with tumors less than 30 mm.[16]

Fortunately, advances in microsurgery have made it possible to minimize the risk of complications. In a systematic review of over 30,000 patients treated operatively, the overall mortality rate was only 0.2%, whereas postoperative cranial neuropathies manifested in 15%. Rates of nonaudiofacial complications such as CSF leak, infection, and vascular ischemia/infarction were 8.5%, 3.8%, and 1%, respectively.[17] Reports such as these could prove informative when counseling patients who may be conflicted between choosing microsurgical removal and less invasive approaches such as GKR.

Management Decision Making

The importance of respecting a patient's wishes cannot be understated, and ultimately the management strategy must be determined through open dialogue between patient and provider. Patients' expectations must be carefully guided, as they are presented with the advantages and disadvantages of each course of treatment available to them. In an artificially constructed scenario in which patients and otolaryngologists were asked to consider how specific outcomes might affect their treatment decision making, based on likelihoods of deafness, temporary facial weakness, incurable cancer, and recovery time, there were several interesting results. First, patients preferred GKR, despite the risk of missing the potential diagnosis of malignancy with a surgical biopsy; second, age had no bearing on treatment selection, implying that all patients should be presented with all options; third, surgeons were less likely to choose approaches that favored hearing sparing, likely due to the prioritization of facial nerve preservation over hearing preservation.[18] Although not universally applicable, this study highlights both patient and provider biases, and underscores the need to objectively present treatment options in order to reach a mutually satisfactory assessment and plan.

Special Consideration

- It is critical to take into account a patient's preferences and disposition. The management strategy must be determined through open dialogue between patient and provider.

Special Consideration

- Hearing preservation and cranial nerve preservation are important factors for quality of life and patients need to be appropriately counseled on the risks and benefits of surgery versus radiotherapy.

■ Management of Neurofibromatosis Type 2

Neurofibromatosis type 2 is a genetic disorder inherited in an autosomal dominant fashion that predisposes patients to the development of various intracranial tumors, including vestibular schwannoma (VS). Patients presenting with bilateral schwannomas or early-age unilateral schwannomas raise clinical suspicion for NF2.[4,5] Pursuant with the management strategy for sVS, nonsporadic schwannomas can be treated much in the same manner, although patients do not fare as well.[3] Overall, the majority of issues attendant to the management of sVS apply to NF2 schwannomas. However, innovations in treatment paradigms unique to NF2 schwannomas

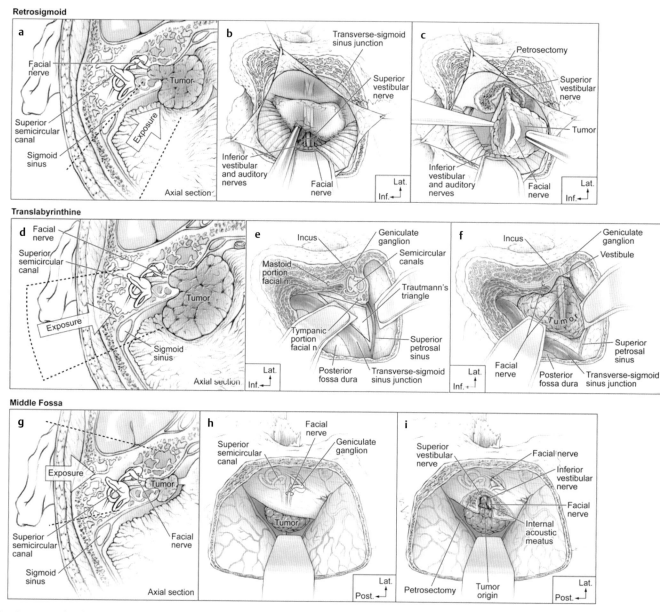

Fig. 36.5a–i The three surgical approaches for VS resection are the retrosigmoid (**a–c**), the translabyrinthine (**d–f**), and the middle fossa (**g–i**). The middle fossa approach is typically used for small tumors to preserve hearing but requires temporal lobe retraction and results in poor exposure of the posterior fossa. The translabyrinthine approach is often used for tumors with internal auditory canal (IAC) extension with no serviceable hearing. The retrosigmoid approach is used primarily for cisternal tumor, but can be used for different sizes of tumors. It is also the most familiar approach for many neurosurgeons. The retrosigmoid approach is performed posterior to the sigmoid sinus and provides access to the cerebellopontine angle (CPA) without sacrificing the labyrinth. The IAC is exposed by drilling its posterior wall. The translabyrinthine approach enables lateral access to the IAC and the CPA lesions with no cerebellar retraction. This approach, however, sacrifices the labyrinth, and thus hearing. (**e,f**) The Trautmann's triangle is entered via this approach. It is demarcated by the bony labyrinth, sigmoid sinus, and superior petrosal sinus or dura. The middle fossa approach enables complete exposure of the IAC from the porus to the fundus with a limited exposure of the CPA through the superior surface of the temporal bone; thus, this approach enables hearing preservation. (**h,i**) The approach to Kawase's triangle can be seen, and is demarcated by the greater petrosal nerve, trigeminal nerve (V₃), the arcuate eminence, and the medial edge of the petrous ridge (or superior petrosal sinus). Lat., lateral; n., nerve; Post., posterior. (From Sun MZ, Oh MC, Safaee M, et al. Neuroanatomical correlation of the House-Brackmann grading system in the microsurgical treatment of vestibular schwannoma. Neurosurg Focus 2012;33:E7. Reproduced with permission.)

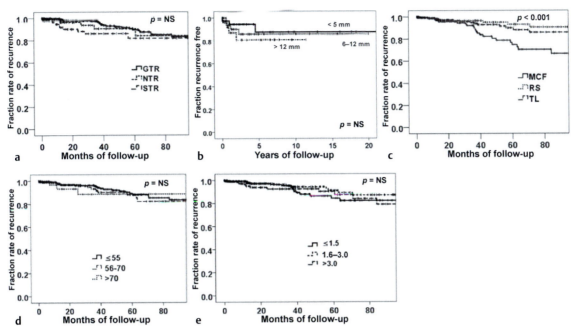

Fig. 36.6a–d (**a**) Kaplan-Meier analysis comparing the rate of tumor recurrence between extent of resection (gross total resection [GTR] vs Intentional nonresection of a thin layer of tumor in order to preserve audiofacial function [NTR] vs subtotal resection [STR]), (**b**) a subgroup analysis of STR patients divided by size of the lesion on postoperative imaging, (**c**) surgical approaches (middle cranial fossa [MCF] vs retrosigmoid craniotomy [RS] vs translabyrinthine craniotomy [TL]), (**d**) patient age (≤ 55 years vs those 56–70 years vs those > 70 years of age), (**e**) and preoperative tumor size (≤ 1.5 cm vs 1.6–3.0 cm vs > 3.0 cm) . NS, not significant. (From Sughrue ME, Kaur R, Rutkowski MJ, et al. Extent of resection and the long-term durability of vestibular schwannoma surgery. J Neurosurg 2011;114: 1221. Reproduced with permission.)

> **Pearl**
>
> - Nonsporadic vestibular schwannoma associated with NF2 can be treated in the same manner as sVS, but patients with NF2 tend to have worse outcomes.

are on the horizon. In particular, pharmaceutical treatment with the antiangiogenic agent bevacizumab has demonstrated great promise as primary treatment in place of more traditional treatment modalities, with associated reductions in tumor burden and improvements in functional outcomes.[19,20]

▪ Conclusion

Inherent in any discussion of treatment decision making for patients with sVS is the realization that patient customization is a critical component. Any assessment of options must take into consideration a provider's strengths as well as a patient's preferences and ability to accept risk. With very few exceptions, such as a young patient whose tumor shows brainstem compression requiring urgent decompression, management options for sVS are complex. Provider and patient bias can negatively impact objectivity, and must be acknowledged openly and honestly. Each individual patient has a different

tolerance for potential complications, and only in fully discussing the pros and cons of observation, radiation, and surgery can a well-informed decision be reached. In doing so, both the physician and patient will contribute equally to the strength of the therapeutic alliance while balancing expectations with treatment goals.

Editor's Note

There are numerous issues to consider when deciding how best to manage the patient, including the extent of hearing loss as well as whether this tumor is a component of neurofibromatosis. The other controversial issue for the single lesion has to do with whether the tumor should be removed or whether it could be treated with radiosurgery. Certainly patients under the age of 60 or 70 will demonstrate growth of these lesions in nearly all circumstances. However, patients of ages 70 and older often have a very indolent clinical course, with the lesion not growing to any significant degree; thus, watchful waiting is reasonable unless there is mass effect from the tumor. There is no doubt that patients with NF2 have worse outcomes due to the bilateral nature of these lesions. The overarching theme with this type of lesion is that there must be extensive discussion with the patient and family regarding the risk/benefit ratio of surgery versus radiosurgery. The good news is that with surgery or radiosurgery for a single lesion, the likelihood of long-term control is excellent, and therefore it is important to make a decision soon after the tumor is diagnosed and to come up with a treatment plan that is acceptable for the patient and family, weighing all of the benefits and risks of surgery versus radiotherapy. (Berger)

References

1. Yang I, Sughrue ME, Han SJ, et al. Facial nerve preservation after vestibular schwannoma gamma knife radiosurgery. J Neurooncol 2009;93: 41–48

2. Timmer FC, Hanssens PE, van Haren AE, et al. Gamma knife radiosurgery for vestibular schwannomas: results of hearing preservation in relation to the cochlear radiation dose. Laryngoscope 2009;119:1076–1081

3. Combs SE, Volk S, Schulz-Ertner D, Huber PE, Thilmann C, Debus J. Management of acoustic neuromas with fractionated stereotactic radiotherapy (FSRT): long-term results in 106 patients treated in a single institution. Int J Radiat Oncol Biol Phys 2005;63:75–81

4. Gutmann DH, Aylsworth A, Carey JC, et al. The diagnostic evaluation and multidisciplinary management of neurofibromatosis 1 and neurofibromatosis 2. JAMA 1997;278:51–57

5. Sughrue ME, Yeung AH, Rutkowski MJ, Cheung SW, Parsa AT. Molecular biology of familial and sporadic vestibular schwannomas: implications for novel therapeutics. J Neurosurg 2011;114:359–366

6. Vernooij MW, Ikram MA, Tanghe HL, et al. Incidental findings on brain MRI in the general population. N Engl J Med 2007;357:1821–1828

7. Sughrue ME, Yang I, Aranda D, et al. The natural history of untreated sporadic vestibular schwannomas: a comprehensive review of hearing outcomes. J Neurosurg 2010;112:163–167

8. Sughrue ME, Kane AJ, Kaur R, et al. A prospective study of hearing preservation in untreated vestibular schwannomas. J Neurosurg 2011; 114:381–385

9. Sughrue ME, Kaur R, Kane AJ, et al. Intratumoral hemorrhage and fibrosis in vestibular schwannoma: a possible mechanism for hearing loss. J Neurosurg 2011;114:386–393

10. Yang I, Aranda D, Han SJ, et al. Hearing preservation after stereotactic radiosurgery for vestibular schwannoma: a systematic review. J Clin Neurosci 2009;16:742–747

11. Yang I, Sughrue ME, Han SJ, et al. A comprehensive analysis of hearing preservation after radiosurgery for vestibular schwannoma. J Neurosurg 2010;112:851–859

12. Sughrue ME, Yang I, Han SJ, et al. Non-audiofacial morbidity after gamma knife surgery for vestibular schwannoma. Neurosurg Focus 2009;27:E4

13. Sughrue ME, Kaur R, Rutkowski MJ, et al. Extent of resection and the long-term durability of vestibular schwannoma surgery. J Neurosurg 2011;114:1218–1223

14. Sun MZ, Oh MC, Safaee M, Kaur G, Parsa AT. Neuroanatomical correlation of the House-Brackmann grading system in the microsurgical treatment of vestibular schwannoma. Neurosurg Focus 2012;33:E7

15. Bloch O, Sughrue ME, Kaur R, et al. Factors associated with preservation of facial nerve function after surgical resection of vestibular schwannoma. J Neurooncol 2011;102:281–286

16. Sughrue ME, Kaur R, Rutkowski MJ, et al. A critical evaluation of vestibular schwannoma surgery for patients younger than 40 years of age. Neurosurgery 2010;67:1646–1653, discussion 1653–1654

17. Sughrue ME, Yang I, Aranda D, et al. Beyond audiofacial morbidity after vestibular schwannoma surgery. J Neurosurg 2011;114:367–374

18. Cheung SW, Aranda D, Driscoll CL, Parsa AT. Mapping clinical outcomes expectations to treatment decisions: an application to vestibular schwannoma management. Otol Neurotol 2010;31:284–293

19. Plotkin SR, Merker VL, Halpin C, et al. Bevacizumab for progressive vestibular schwannoma in neurofibromatosis type 2: a retrospective review of 31 patients. Otol Neurotol 2012;33:1046–1052

20. Plotkin SR, Stemmer-Rachamimov AO, Barker FG II, et al. Hearing improvement after bevacizumab in patients with neurofibromatosis type 2. N Engl J Med 2009;361:358–367

Primary Central Nervous System Lymphoma

Elina Tsyvkin and Lisa M. DeAngelis

Primary central nervous system lymphoma (PCNSL) is a rare aggressive non-Hodgkin lymphoma (NHL) confined to the craniospinal axis including the brain parenchyma, leptomeninges, eyes, or spinal cord. It is recognized as a discrete entity in the 2008 World Health Organization classification.[1] It represents about 1% of all NHLs and 2 to 5% of all primary intracranial tumors. Men and women are equally affected, with an annual incidence rate of 0.47 per 100,000 person-years and a median age of 60.[2] PCNSL is associated with congenital or acquired immunodeficiency, particularly with human immunodeficiency virus (HIV), but the incidence in immunocompetent patients has risen over the past three to four decades.[3]

Biology and Pathogenesis

Primary central nervous system lymphoma is restricted to the central nervous system (CNS), despite there being no lymphoid tissue in the nervous system. About 90% of PCNSLs are diffuse large B-cell lymphomas (DLBCLs). Only a small proportion have Burkitt (5%), lymphoblastic (5%), marginal zone (3%), or T-cell lymphoma histotype (2–3%). PCNSL typically has an angiocentric growth pattern and phenotypically expresses pan–B-cell markers (CD20, CD19, CD22, CD79a). Approximately 80% represent nongerminal center lymphomas, and only about 20% have a germinal center phenotype; all are negative for Epstein-Barr virus (EBV), unlike PCNSL in immunocompromised patients, which is characteristically EBV-driven. The proliferating index is usually 50 to 90%.[4]

Clinical Presentation

At presentation, cerebral symptoms are the most common, followed by ocular, leptomeningeal, and spinal cord symptoms (**Table 37.1**).

Seizures occur less frequently (10%) in PCNSL than in gliomas or metastatic lesions (25–35%). Symptom duration prior to definitive diagnosis averages 1 to 3 months, reflecting its rapid growth rate.

Ocular involvement is seen in approximately 20% of PCNSL patients and may be unilateral or bilateral. Ocular symptoms typically include floaters and blurred or diminished vision, but many patients have no visual symptoms, and ocular in-

Table 37.1 Symptoms of Primary Central Nervous System Lymphoma

Cranial
Personality/cognitive changes
Lateralized: e.g., hemiparesis, aphasia
Seizures
Headache
Cranial neuropathy
Ocular
Floaters
Blurred or cloudy vision
Diminished visual acuity
Spinal
Back pain
Radiculopathy
Limb weakness
Sensory level or paresthesias
Bowel or bladder dysfunction

volvement is detected only on slit-lamp examination. About 15% of patients have a positive cerebrospinal fluid (CSF) cytology, although focal leptomeningeal involvement can be identified in almost all patients at autopsy.

> **Pearl**
>
> - When systemic NHL metastasizes to the CNS, it usually involves the leptomeninges and only rarely the brain parenchyma, whereas PCNSL primarily involves the brain.

Diagnostic Procedures

Imaging

Magnetic resonance imaging (MRI) is the preferred imaging modality, unless contraindicated, to identify brain or spinal cord PCNSL, which is typically hypointense to isointense on T1-weighted images, with intense homogeneous contrast enhancement (**Fig. 37.1**). Nonenhancing lesions can occur, and peritumoral edema is often less than expected. Acquired immunodeficiency syndrome (AIDS)-related PCNSL lesions are often ring-enhancing on T1-weighted images and may be

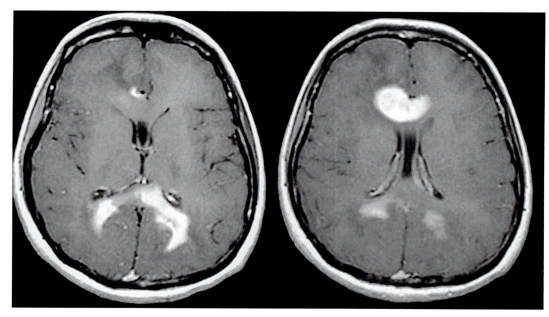

Fig. 37.1 Gadolinium-enhanced T1-weighted magnetic resonance imaging showing intense contrast enhancement and multifocality in a patient with primary central nervous system lymphoma.

Pitfall

- Steroid response should not be used intentionally as a diagnostic test for PCNSL because other CNS processes, such as multiple sclerosis or sarcoidosis, can have a similar imaging appearance and response to steroids.

associated with hemorrhage or necrosis. PCNSL lesions are typically supratentorial, periventricular, and involve deep structures such as the basal ganglia. They are single in approximately 60% of patients and multiple in 40% (**Fig. 37.1**); more than 90% of AIDS patients have multiple lesions. Unlike other primary brain tumors, PCNSL is usually bright on diffusion sequences with corresponding hypointensity on apparent diffusion coefficient (ADC) sequences. Single photon emission computed tomography (SPECT) scanning using gallium 67 and thallium 201, positron emission tomography (PET), and methionine PET all show increased uptake in PCNSL tumors.

Biomarkers

In a multicenter retrospective series, CXC chemokine ligand (CXCL)13 and interleukin-10 (IL-10) in the CSF were identified as a complementary biomarker pair that yields diagnostic information in most PCNSL cases, with sensitivity significantly greater than with standard CSF tests, cytology, and flow cytometry, and equivalent to the sensitivity of results obtained from brain biopsy.[5] More recently, CXCL13 alone was found to discriminate greater than 70% of PCNSL cases with 94.9%

specificity; diagnostic sensitivity can be improved to 84% by parallel evaluation of IL-10, which also provides prognostic information while maintaining greater than 90% specificity.[6] Although the precision of the cutoff points for maximal diagnostic accuracy need to be defined prospectively, CXCL13 and IL-10 may be used to guide the workup of potential PCNSL in patients for whom brain biopsy may be of heightened risk or low diagnostic yield.

■ Staging and Pretreatment Investigations

Primary central nervous system lymphoma is classified as a stage I_E NHL because it is restricted to a single extranodal site.

Systemic workup identifies extraneural disease in approximately 6% of patients, and all sites can be identified by abdominal and pelvic computed tomography (CT) scan or bone marrow biopsy, suggesting that, if performed, systemic staging can be limited to these tests.[7] In all patients, outcome is determined by the CNS disease and not by the systemic lymphoma. More importantly, staging of the nervous system must be thorough (**Table 37.2**).

■ Prognosis

Two main prognostic scoring systems have been developed. In the International Extranodal Lymphoma Study Group (IELSG),

Table 37.2 Essential Studies for Staging Disease in Patients with Primary Central Nervous System Lymphoma

Contrast-enhanced imaging of the brain, preferably MRI
Ophthalmologic evaluation (including slit-lamp examination)
Lumbar puncture
Human immunodeficiency virus test
Body CT scan ± body PET
Contrast-enhanced MRI of the spine (if clinically indicated)

age older than 60 years, Eastern Cooperative Oncology Group (ECOG) performance status greater than 1, elevated serum lactate dehydrogenase, high CSF protein concentration, and involvement of deep brain regions were all independently associated with worse survival.[8] The Memorial Sloan-Kettering Cancer Center group established and validated a simpler and widely applicable model with three risk groups: age ≤ 50 years (low); age > 50 years and Karnofsky Performance Scale (KPS) score ≥ 70 (intermediate); and age > 50 years and KPS < 70 (high).[9]

There are likely pathological prognostic factors in PCNSL similar to what has been identified in systemic DLBCL.[10] In systemic NHL, germinal center phenotype, defined by either gene expression profiling or a pattern of cell surface marker expression by immunohistochemistry (IHC), is associated with better survival. Most such reports on PCNSL also suggest that germinal center phenotype predicts better outcome, but this is not universal and needs verification in larger cohorts.

Imaging may help predict the clinical course of patients. Early complete response (CR) assessed by MRI indicated long-term survival in a cohort of 88 patients treated with a polychemotherapy regimen. A significantly longer survival was observed for those patients who achieved complete remission after two treatment cycles compared with those who reached CR after six cycles.[11]

■ Treatment

Primary central nervous system lymphoma is sensitive to chemotherapy and radiotherapy, so that durable complete remissions are possible. However, the outcome is still unsatisfactory when compared to other NHLs. There is consensus that high-dose methotrexate (HD-MTX) is the single most important chemotherapeutic agent, but there is no standardized combination regimen.

Current therapeutic knowledge in PCNSL is based primarily on single-arm phase 2 studies; only one randomized phase 2 trial[12] and one phase 3 trial[13] have been reported. Besides the rarity of the disease, the success of clinical trials is limited by the fact that many patients present with severe symptoms and various comorbidities, compromising enrollment. Thus, the level of evidence for therapeutic choices in PCNSL remains low.

Surgery

Gross total resection is often not possible due to the deep location and multifocality of most PCNSL lesions. Most reports suggest there is no survival advantage to gross total resection, but a recent report suggests that debulking may improve outcome.[14,15] Furthermore, tumor debulking may be indicated for urgent decompression in a patient with neurologic deterioration because of mass effect. However, in most patients, image-guided/stereotactic biopsy is the preferred method for obtaining a tissue diagnosis in patients suspected of having PCNSL.

Pitfall

- Administration of glucocorticoids prior to performing a biopsy may lead to a nondiagnostic specimen and hinder establishing the correct diagnosis. Corticosteroids are oncolytic in PCNSL, identical to their activity against systemic NHL. The initial approach to patients with lesions consistent with PCNSL is to withhold steroids prior to biopsy unless the patient is decompensating clinically. The lympholytic effect of steroids can be seen in CSF and vitreal specimens as well.

Radiotherapy

Primary central nervous system lymphoma is a radiosensitive tumor, and radiotherapy (RT) was the first treatment modality to prolong median survival to between 12 and 18 months,[16] a marked increase from the 2- to 3-month survival of untreated patients. Whole-brain radiotherapy (WBRT) is recommended because of the diffuse, infiltrative, and often multifocal nature of PCNSL. Doses in the range of 40 to 50 Gy are used, with single fractions of 2 Gy or less. Higher doses or the addition of a boost does not enhance disease control, but is associated with increased neurotoxicity.[17]

Radiotherapy in Combination with Chemotherapy

To increase remission rates and prolong overall survival (OS), the first structured efforts to use systemic chemotherapy combined it with WBRT. Better response rates and improved survival were reported in clinical trials using HD-MTX–based chemotherapy followed by WBRT. Complete response rates ranged between 69% and 87% using combined chemo-radiotherapy, with a median progression-free survival (PFS) of 24 to 40 months.[18,19] This resulted in widespread use of combined modality treatment in the primary management of PCNSL. Unfortunately, with longer follow-up, severe neurologic impairment developed after combined treatment particularly in older patients.[20] This led to the investigation of RT dose reduction and RT omission in patients with a CR after chemotherapy alone. Neurotoxicity risks are age-related and the risk rises with increasing age.

The only randomized control trial (G-PCNSL-SG) completed in PCNSL examined the role of WBRT in combination with MTX-based therapy.[13] All patients received six cycles of single-agent MTX, 4 g/m^2, ± ifosfamide (1.5 g/m^2) in 14-day cycles. Patients who achieved a CR were randomized to be followed or to receive 45 Gy WBRT. A total of 551 patients were enrolled, but only 58% completed the study as per the protocol. In all patients, WBRT prolonged PFS from 12 to 18 months ($p = 0.041$ in the intent to treat [ITT] population), but OS was similar at 37 versus 34 months (0.94, ITT population). The CR rate following chemotherapy was 35% overall and was similar in patients younger and older than 60 years of age. However, the overall response rate (CR + partial remission) was better in younger patients (63% vs 49%). Although remarkable for its size, the study was limited by high dropout rates, variable chemotherapy, underpowered noninferiority design, and insufficient neurotoxicity evaluation. These data suggest that WBRT does not prolong survival and, therefore, can be eliminated to reduce neurotoxicity. However, the G-PCNSL-SG trial did not really study neurotoxicity, and the potentially negative impact of early relapse and salvage therapy on cognitive function has never been evaluated.

As an alternative strategy, reduced-dose WBRT has been examined in a series of studies that suggest that it retains efficacy in patients with a response to chemotherapy, and there are various reports on its risk of neurotoxicity. In an early study,[21] reducing the dose of WBRT to 30.6 Gy compromised survival in patients younger than but not older than 60 years. In Radiation Therapy Oncology Group (RTOG) trial 9310, decreasing WBRT from 45 to 36 Gy in patients achieving a CR to chemotherapy did not compromise survival but also did not reduce the frequency of neurotoxicity, although onset was delayed. More recently, in a phase 2 trial, patients achieving a CR after R-MVP (rituximab, MTX 3.5 g/m^2, vincristine, procarbazine) received dose-reduced WBRT (23.4 Gy), whereas others received standard WBRT (45 Gy). Initial results reported a 2-year OS and PFS of 67% and 57%, respectively, and no treatment-related neurotoxicity was observed.[22,23] These results suggest that reduced-dose WBRT achieves disease control comparable to that of full-dose WBRT; neurotoxicity, which was assessed with prospective neuropsychiatric testing, was not observed. A randomized phase 2 study is currently underway comparing R-MPV followed by reduced-dose RT (23.4 Gy), with chemotherapy only (RTOG trial 1114, NCT01399372).

Although microscopic CSF dissemination is common, craniospinal irradiation does not confer additional survival benefit and is associated with significant morbidity.[24] No data presently exist to support a role for stereotactic radiosurgery (SRS) for PCNSL. Given the highly infiltrative nature of PCNSL, focal treatments such as SRS would be expected to treat only a small volume of tumor. As a result, SRS is not recommended as a routine treatment for PCNSL.

Chemotherapy

Primary central nervous system lymphoma is a typical NHL histologically, so there have been efforts to treat this tumor in the same manner as its systemic counterpart using cyclophosphamide, hydroxydaunomycin (doxorubicin), Oncovin (vincristine), and prednisone (CHOP). CHOP, or comparable regimens in combination with WBRT, did not improve survival over WBRT alone in PCNSL, and these regimens have been abandoned.

High-dose Methotrexate

High-dose MTX constitutes the backbone of chemotherapy for PCNSL (**Fig. 37.2**), with efficacy established in prospective phase 2 trials. Unfortunately, the great variability in patient characteristics and regimens used in these studies makes comparisons difficult. MTX doses from 1 to 8 g/m^2 intravenously every 10 to 21 days are used in PCNSL (**Table 37.3**). Total dose and infusion rate are important to achieve concentrations of MTX that cross the blood–brain barrier (BBB) sufficiently. Patients treated with ≥ 3 g/m^2 reliably achieve sufficient CSF levels of MTX with a rapid (3-hour) infusion, but even doses as low as 1 g/m^2 can achieve therapeutic CSF levels.[25] Dose reduction due to impaired creatinine clearance was needed in 45% of patients in trials using MTX 8 g/m^2, whereas in the 3.5-g/m^2 trials, few patients needed reduction in MTX dose. Thus, the MTX dose target is variably achieved depending on the normalized dose outlined in a given study.[26]

Pearl

- High-dose methotrexate constitutes the backbone of chemotherapy for PCNSL.

High-Dose Methotrexate Monotherapy

Two studies examined single-agent MTX at 8 g/m^2 given every 2 weeks during induction and monthly for 12 cycles.[27–29] In both studies, PFS was approximately 12 months, meaning 50% of patients were relapsing while on induction or maintenance. One study was closed before accrual was complete.[27,28] Although OS was prolonged in these studies, this could be attributed to effective salvage regimens, so single-agent therapy has largely been abandoned. The only effort to directly compare single-agent MTX with combination therapy was a randomized phase 2 trial of MTX alone or MTX with cytarabine followed by WBRT in both arms.[12] The addition of cytarabine significantly improved outcome, with CR rates increased

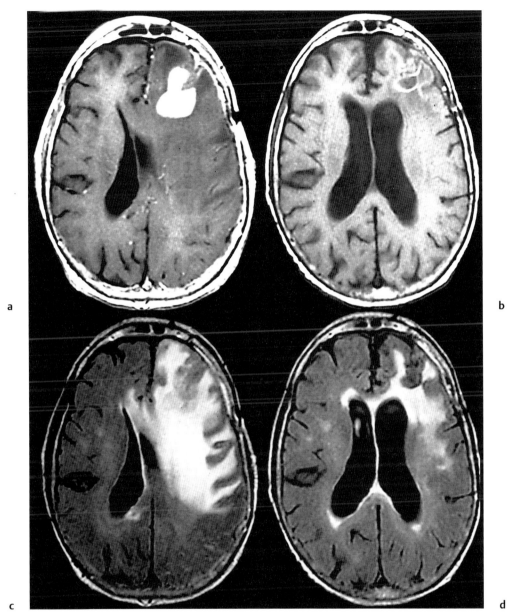

a

b

c

d

Fig. 37.2a–d Enhanced T1-weighted (**a,b**) and fluid-attenuated inversion recovery (FLAIR) T2-weighted (**c,d**) magnetic resonance imaging of an elderly patient with primary central nervous system lymphoma before (**a,c**) and after (**b,d**) treatment with four cycles of high-dose methotrexate, procarbazine, and vincristine.

from 18% to 46% (*p* = 0.006) and 3-year OS from 32% to 46% (*p* = 0.07). The combination was clearly superior, but not necessarily optimal as both response rate and survival in both arms were lower than in other PCNSL trials, likely reflecting its multicenter conduct and the low-intensity MTX schedule (every 3 weeks).

Methotrexate-Based Multidrug Regimens

There is a great heterogeneity of both combination chemotherapy regimens employed in newly diagnosed PCNSL. MTX

has been combined with one or more of the following chemotherapy drugs: cytarabine, vincristine, procarbazine, dexamethasone, carmustine, lomustine, etoposide, ifosfamide and methylprednisolone (**Table 37.3**). The goal of adding chemotherapeutic agents to HD-MTX is to improve the outcomes of HD-MTX monotherapy and to achieve a balance between long-term relapse control and neurotoxicity.

A recently published phase 2 trial (CALGB 50202) demonstrated that dose-intensive consolidation for PCNSL yields rates of PFS and OS at least comparable to those involving WBRT.[30] Forty-four patients with newly diagnosed PCNSL were treated

Table 37.3 Selected Studies of First-Line Therapy in Immunocompetent Patients with Primary Central Nervous System Lymphoma

First Author	Design	N	Chemotherapy Regimen	WBRT	ORR (%)	OS
Chemotherapy + WBRT						
DeAngelis[56]	Phase 2	31	M (1 g/m^2), IT M, AraC	40 Gy (14.4 Gy boost)	94	mOS 43 mo
Shah[22]	Phase 2	30	M (3.5 g/m^2), R, P, V, AraC	23.4 Gy if CR 45 Gy if no CR	93	2-yr 67%
Ferreri[12]	Phase 2	40 39	M (3.5 g/m^2) M (3.5 g/m^2), AraC	30–49 Gy (both groups)	40 69	3 yr 32% ; 5 yr 26% 3 yr 46%; 5 yr 46%
Thiel[13]	Phase 3	154 164	M (4 g/m^2) ± ifosfamide (both groups)	45 Gy None	54 54	mOS 32 mo mOS 37 mo 2 yr 63% (in both arms)
Chemotherapy Alone						
Batchelor[29]	Phase 2	25	M (8 g/m^2)	None	74	2 yr 70%
Chamberlain[37]	Phase 2	40	M (8 g/m^2), R	None	70	2 yr 60%
Fritsch[35]	Phase 2	28 (> 65 years)	M (3g/m^2), R, P, CCNU	None	82	mOS 29 mo in < 80 yo (1yr 82%) mOS 4.3 mo in > 80 yo (1 yr 17%) In both groups 3 yr 31%
Rubenstein[30]	Phase 2	44	M (98 g/m^2), TMZ, R; if CR: E + AraC	None	77	mOS NR; 2 yr PFS 0.57
HDC and ASCT ± WBRT						
Illerhaus[44]	Phase 2	30	M (8 g/m^2), AraC, T + ASCT (HD: BCNU, T)	25/30 pts 45 Gy	70 after induction; 100 after ASCT	2 yr 83%; 5 yr 69%
Colombat[45]	Phase 2	25 (< 65 years)	M, E, BCNU, Methylpred (HD: BEAM)	30 Gy	84 after induction; 94 after ASCT	2 yr 70%
Alimohamed[47]	Retrospective	21	T, B, C + ASCT	None	85	5 yr 52%

Abbreviations: WBRT, whole-brain radiation therapy; ORR, overall response rate (partial response and complete response); OS, overall survival; CR, complete response; mOS, median overall survival; M, methotrexate; IT, intrathecal; AraC, cytarabine; I, ifosfamide; R, rituximab; P, procarbazine; Methylpred, methylprednisolone; V, vincristine; TMZ, temozolomide; BEAM, bischloroethylnitrosourea (BCNU), etoposide, cytarabine, melphalan; C, cyclophosphamide; E, etoposide; HDC, high-dose chemotherapy; ASCT, autologous stem cell transplant; B, busulfan; T, thiotepa; PFS, progression-free survival; NR, not reached.

with induction MT-R (MTX 8 g/m^2 IV every 2 weeks for seven doses, rituximab 375 mg/m^2 weekly for six doses, temozolomide 150 mg/m^2 on days 7 to 11 of the first 5 months); patients who achieved CR received EA consolidation (etoposide 5 mg/kg IV every 12 hours for eight doses, cytarabine 2 g/m^2 IV every 12 hours for eight doses). The CR rate for MT-R was 66%. The overall 2-year PFS was 57%, which exceeds that of other chemotherapy-alone studies (**Table 37.3**), and is at least comparable to combined-modality approaches with reduced-dose WBRT.[22] The median time to progression of the 44 patients of 4 years was double that achieved with combined-modality therapy in multicenter trials using standard-dose WBRT.[13,31] Survival for the cohort of patients who completed EA dose-intensive consolidation is promising, confirming prior single-institution data.[32] The survival curves show encourag-

ing evidence of a stable plateau, and the median OS has not yet been reached, with a median follow-up of 4.9 years.

Immunotherapy

The monoclonal CD-20 antibody rituximab has excellent efficacy against a variety of systemic B-cell NHLs, but rituximab penetrates the BBB poorly, with CSF levels of 3% or usually much less of the serum concentration.[22] However, the BBB is disrupted in parenchymal PCNSL lesions, which is indicated by the pronounced contrast-enhancement on brain MRI. Using radiolabeled tositumomab,[33] it is clear that an anti–CD-20 monoclonal antibody can penetrate into a bulky PCNSL lesion with clinical response, but there is rapid progression likely due to disease residing behind an intact BBB that the antibody could not reach. Supporting these considerations,[34] an imaging response to rituximab monotherapy was observed in four of 11 patients with recurrent PCNSL. Thus, rituximab might be mostly efficacious before chemotherapy or glucocorticoids are given and during the early treatment cycles.

A German pilot trial ($n = 28$) evaluating rituximab, MTX (3 g/m^2), lomustine and procarbazine (R-MCP) in elderly PCNSL patients (i.e., > 65 years) observed a CR of 64% (relative risk [RR] 82%).[35] In a previous study using the identical regimen without rituximab ($n = 30$), the same group reported a CR of 44% (RR 70%).[36] In a separate phase 2 study ($n = 40$), the CR rate was 60% after four to six cycles of rituximab and MTX.[37] Previous studies using MTX monotherapy without rituximab have reported a CR of 30 to 58%.[28,38]

To evaluate the effect of rituximab on the CR rate after chemotherapy with MTX and ifosfamide of patients with newly diagnosed PCNSL, a retrospective trial compared 19 patients who were treated with six cycles of MTX (4 g/m^2) and ifosfamide (1.5 g/m^2 on days 3 to 5) with 17 patients who were treated with the same regimen plus rituximab (375 mg/m^2 on day 0 during the first three cycles). The addition of rituximab to MTX and ifosfamide was correlated with a significant increase in the CR rate (100.0 vs. 68.4%, $p = 0.02$). Furthermore, 6-month PFS was significantly higher for the rituximab group (94.1 vs. 63.2%, $p = 0.04$).[39]

A recent retrospective study examining the impact of rituximab in the context of concurrent therapies, including MTX, cytarabine, and radiotherapy, in 100 patients aged 21 to 81 years demonstrated that the addition of rituximab was associated with improved OS (5-year OS 46%).[40] Intrathecal administration of rituximab has also been investigated and has demonstrated some benefit.[41] All of these studies suffer from small patient numbers and are retrospective, but the weight of the evidence suggests that adding rituximab to HD-MTX–based regimens is helpful.

Other Drugs in First-Line Therapy

Other alkylating agents with good CNS penetration, such as temozolomide, thiotepa, ifosfamide, nitrosoureas, and procarbazine, have been included in chemotherapy combinations for PCNSL. Temozolomide is an oral alkylating agent that can penetrate the BBB and has a good safety profile. As upfront monotherapy in elderly patients, temozolomide was associ-

ated with a CR of 47%, and median OS of 21 months. This drug can be combined safely with MTX in elderly patients, and the combination of HD-MTX, rituximab, and temozolomide is associated with a 63% CR, and a 3-year PFS of 50%.[42]

Ifosfamide, another alkylating agent, improved the CR of HD-MTX from 32% to 42% and reduced the primary progression rate from 26% to 15% in the G-PCNSL-SG1 trial; however, it has a higher toxicity profile, particularly in elderly patients.[13]

Thiotepa is a lipophilic alkylator that has been combined with HD-MTX, HD-cytarabine, idarubicin, and WBRT. This regimen resulted in an overall response rate of 83%, a median PFS of 13 months, and a 5-year OS of 41% in a phase 2 trial with a plateau in the survival curve; however, the regimen had a 10% toxicity-related mortality.[19] Thiotepa was also included as part of induction and conditioning regimens in programs of high-dose chemotherapy (HDCT) supported by autologous stem cell transplantation (ASCT).

Carmustine has been used in patients with PCNSL both as part of primary chemotherapy or in conditioning regimens before ASCT.

Use of osmotic BBB disruption prior to intra-arterial infusion of MTX-based chemotherapy to increase drug delivery to the tumor has been assessed. In the most recent multiinstitutional analysis of this approach, results comparable to those achieved with conventional treatments were reported, with a 5-year PFS of 31% and 7-year PFS of 25%. The procedure, however, can be associated with acute toxicity and is currently available only at specialized centers.[43]

High-Dose Chemotherapy with Autologous Stem Cell Transplantation

High-dose chemotherapy (HDC) followed by ASCT has been evaluated in PCNSL patients with newly diagnosed and recurrent disease, based on the promising experiences in other hematologic malignancies. HDC followed by ASCT may allow for higher drug availability in the CNS and may help to overcome resistance to conventional chemotherapy. HD-MTX–based chemotherapy is mainly used for induction treatment followed by various conditioning regimens. Studies of HD–ASCT vary considerably regarding regimens and outcomes.

Upfront HDC-ASCT has been assessed in several studies. A phase 2 study treated 30 patients aged < 65 years with HD-MTX (8 g/m^2), HD cytarabine (two doses of 3 g/m^2), and thiotepa (40 mg/m^2), followed by a conditioning regimen involving carmustine and thiotepa, ASCT, and WBRT (45 Gy). With a median follow-up of 63 months, the 5-year OS was 69% for all patients.[44] A prospective trial of 25 patients with newly diagnosed PCNSL assessed HD-MTX–based polychemotherapy followed by HDC and ASCT. WBRT at a dose of 30 Gy was delivered after ASCT. This regimen yielded a promising response rate of 84%.[45] However, neither of the studies examined neurotoxicity in their survivors.

Long-term neurotoxicity appears to be significantly less frequent when WBRT can be deferred after ASCT, as shown in a trial comprising 23 patients treated with HD-MDX followed by high-dose busulfan/thiotepa and ASCT.[46] A combination of high-dose thiotepa, busulfan, and cyclophosphamide with subsequent ASCT also showed promising results without significant neurotoxicity.[47] However, acute treatment-related toxicity causing therapy-associated deaths was observed in patients older than 60 years.

A recent analysis of 43 patients from two prospective single-arm studies of HD–ASCT revealed encouraging results, with median OS of 104 months and 2-year and 5-year OS of 81% and 70%.[48] However, 30 of these patients also received WBRT post-ASCT. Moreover, late relapses still occurred, and neurotoxicity, which was evaluated only clinically and was, therefore, probably underestimated, was observed in 20% of patients despite a median age of only 54 years. The role of HD–ASCT in initial treatment of PCNSL, therefore, remains undefined, and is currently being explored in a multicenter randomized phase 2 trial in the United States. A randomized trial in Europe comparing HDC-ASCT with WBRT (NCT01011920) continues.

Recurrent or Refractory Tumor

A large proportion of PCNSL patients suffer progression or relapse, the overwhelming majority of which occur in the brain, but may not be at the original site; relapse is seen in 25 to 55% usually within the first few years of diagnosis.[36,49] The prognosis of relapsed PCNSL is poor, with reported median survival of only 2 months if left untreated; with treatment, the median survival is 14 months (**Table 37.4**). There is no standard treatment for patients with recurrent or refractory PCNSL, and treatment is often based on the location of relapse

(brain, CSF, eye), the type of initial therapy, and the time interval since last treatment.

Whole-brain RT is useful as a salvage strategy, with a response rate of 60 to 79% and an OS of 11 to 16 months. Response rates and survival after WBRT were similar between primary refractory and recurrent patients.[50]

High-dose MTX–based regimens remain the most effective salvage therapy for patients with PCNSL who previously responded to HD-MTX, with reported response rates of 71 to 91% and OS of 23 to 61 months.[51] Alkylating agents such as temozolomide or nitrosoureas, with or without rituximab, are commonly used in the relapse setting. A phase 2 trial of temozolomide monotherapy showed a response rate of 31% (25% CR and 6% partial response [PR]) and a 1-year OS of 31% in a group of 36 patients.[52] Pemetrexed, an antifolate agent similar to MTX, has activity in recurrent and refractory PCNSL.[53] Eleven patients, 10 of whom had prior HD-MTX treatment, were treated with Pemetrexed for a mean of five cycles and had a response rate of 55% and disease control in 91%. The 6-month mean PFS was 5.7 months, and the OS was 10.1 months.[53]

Topotecan, a topoisomerase I inhibitor, has limited activity in relapsed and refractory PCNSL, and hematologic toxicity remains a major concern especially in elderly patients. In a phase 2 study of 15 refractory or relapsed PCNSL patients with a median age of 56 years, three patients achieved CR with a median PFS of 2 months.[54] Eleven of the 15 patients had grade 3/4 neutropenia and three patients had grade 3 thrombocytopenia.

Promising results were reported for HDC-ASCT in patients at relapse. Utilizing an induction chemotherapy regimen of cytarabine and etoposide followed by HDC with stem-cell rescue,[55] the median PFS was 12 months in the ITT population, and 41.1 months in those who were transplanted; the median OS was 18.3 and 58.6 months, respectively. However, the in-

Table 37.4 Selected Studies of Salvage Treatment in Immunocompetent Patients with Relapsed/Refractory Primary Central Nervous System Lymphoma

First Author	N	Chemotherapy Regimen	WBRT	ORR%	OS
Pels[67]	65	M (5 g/m^2), V, ifosfamide, C, Vindesine, Dex +IT M, AraC, Prednisone	None	68	mOS 54 mo 2 yr 69%; 5 yr 43%
Voloschin[54]	15	Topotecan	None	40	32.7 mo
Raizer[53]	11	Pemetrexed	None	55	10.1 mo; 1 yr 45%
Reni[52]	36	Temozolomide	None	31	mOS 3.9 mo; 1 yr 31%
Hottinger[50]	48	None	40 Gy	79	mOS 16 mo 1 yr 54%
Soussain[55]	43(< 65 years)	AraC, E + ASCT (HD: B, T, C)	2/43 pts 30–40 Gy	47 after induction; 96 after ASCT	mOS 18.3 mo ITT mOS 58.6 mo transplanted 1 yr 60% whole group
Batchelor[34]	12	Rituximab	None	47	1 yr OS 60%

Abbreviations: WBRT, whole-brain radiation therapy; ORR, overall response rate (partial response and complete response); OS, overall survival; M, methotrexate; V, vincristine; C, cyclophosphamide; Dex, dexamethasone; IT, intrathecal; AraC, cytarabine; I, ifosfamide; E, etoposide; ASCT, autologous stem cell transplant; B, busulfan; T, Thiotepa; mOS, median overall survival; ITT, intent to treat.

duction chemotherapy was highly toxic, and this approach was restricted to high-performing patients, all younger than 65 years. Because the optimal salvage approach is unclear, patients with relapsed disease should be treated in a clinical trial if available.

Treatment-Related Neurotoxicity

Leukoencephalopathy is a serious complication of effective PCNSL treatment but is apparent only when the patient is in a durable remission.[56] Therefore, it is rarely observed in patients treated with WBRT alone but has been seen in patients treated with combined modality therapy, especially HD-MTX–based regimens, and in those treated with MTX-based chemotherapy alone. There is additive toxicity when MTX is combined with WBRT, but most regimens administer the MTX prior to RT to reduce neurotoxicity. In a small study of patients who received WBRT for salvage, if the time interval between MTX and WBRT was more than 6 months, then the risk of neurotoxicity was substantially reduced, demonstrating that close timing of the two modalities affects risk.[50] In addition, treatment-related leukoencephalopathy occurs primarily in patients who are older than 60 at the time therapy is initiated. Neurotoxicity presents with a syndrome similar to normal pressure hydrocephalus with cognitive impairment, gait ataxia, and incontinence; some patients improve with ventriculoperitoneal shunting.[57] In a retrospective analysis of 183 patients for the development of long-term treatment-related toxicity, only administration of RT was identified as an independent risk factor.[58]

Neurotoxicity also remains a concern with chemotherapy alone, especially in older patients. In the G-PCNSL-SG1 trial, clinically determined neurotoxicity was seen in 26% of long-term survivors in the chemotherapy alone arm, which was less than the 49% incidence seen in patients who received chemotherapy and WBRT.[13] Thus, omitting WBRT substantially reduces but does not eliminate the risk of treatment-related cognitive impairment following successful treatment of PCNSL.

Most reports do not include long-term follow-up of patients to assess the true risk of neurotoxicity associated with a regimen. Recently, a panel of neuropsychological tests to assess, quantify, and follow treatment-related neurologic deterioration in patients with PCNSL was established in an effort to standardize this assessment.[59]

Primary Central Nervous System Lymphoma and AIDS

Acquired immunodeficiency syndrome–related PCNSL is more aggressive than PCNSL in the immunocompetent patient. Median survival for AIDS-related PCNSL was found to be 27 days without treatment. However, WBRT produced both clinical and imaging responses in 76% and 69% of AIDS patients, respectively, and a median survival of 119 days for those com-

pleting the RT protocol.[60] In patients treated with RT, the cause of death was opportunistic infection in 87%, whereas progressive PCNSL caused death in 77% when untreated.

Of 15 AIDS patients treated with MTX (3 g/m^2), 47% achieved a complete remission with a median survival of 19 months.[61] Combined chemotherapy with intravenous MTX (3 g/m^2) and intrathecal MTX, procarbazine, thiotepa, and WBRT was used in 10 patients with AIDS.[62] Eight patients completed both chemotherapy and RT; six had a complete remission with a median survival of 7 months, but two patients survived more than 1 year. Although the sample was small, it appeared that patients with a CD4 count > 50 cells/mm^3, KPS > 50, and a single cerebral lesion fared better. A recent study endorsed the use of rituximab even in patients with a CD4 count < 100 cells/mm^3 at the time of lymphoma diagnosis.[63] These studies suggest a role for combined modality therapy or possibly chemotherapy alone in AIDS-related PCNSL, but it should be reserved for those patients with good KPS score, high CD4 counts, and no concomitant opportunistic infections.

The addition of highly active antiretroviral therapy (HAART) in the treatment of AIDS has reduced the incidence of PCNSL and improved survival in patients with PCNSL. Skiest and Crosby[64] studied HAART therapy in 25 patients diagnosed with AIDS and PCNSL. Median survival for patients treated with HAART was not reached versus 52 days for those not receiving HAART. Six of seven patients treated with HAART were alive at a median of 667 days, compared with 0 of 18 patients not treated with HAART. Improved survival has been reported when HAART is combined with WBRT (median survival 92 days vs 38 days).[65] Long-term remission has been described in HIV-associated PCNSL patients who demonstrate rapid immune recovery and prolonged lymphoma regression with potent HAART alone.[66] These studies suggest an important role for HAART therapy in the treatment of AIDS patients with PCNSL.

◼ Conclusion

Primary central nervous system lymphoma is a rare but highly treatable brain tumor. Its characteristic diffuse enhancement on MRI should raise the diagnostic consideration of PCNSL and enable the physician to withhold corticosteroids until histologic confirmation is obtained. Treatment should begin with chemotherapy in virtually all patients and an HD-MTX–based regimen is most appropriate. Full-dose cranial irradiation should be avoided in all older patients and probably in patients of all ages. The role of low-dose WBRT and HDC-ASCT remains to be defined. However, effective therapy can produce durable remissions and improved function in many patients.

Editor's Note

Primary central nervous system lymphoma was often confused with brain metastasis or glioblastoma, particularly in the pre-MRI era when it was less clear on CT and when it was a much less commonly recognized entity. When surgeons operated thinking it was one of the two former diagnoses, aggressive resections were often done, which is not necessary or indicated. Nowadays this disease is cared for primarily with chemotherapy by neuro-oncologists and sometimes radiation, and the role of the surgeon is to provide a tissue diagnosis by biopsy. It is important to note that the disappearance of the tumor with steroid administration, although classic, is not sufficient evidence for definitive diagnosis, as this phenomenon can rarely be seen with gliomas, and occasionally with certain inflammatory diagnoses that can mimic tumors. (Bernstein)

References

1. Swerdlow S, Campo E, Harris N, et al. WHO Classification of Tumour of Haematopoietic and Lymphoid Tissues, 4th ed. Geneva: WHO press, 2008

2. Dolecek TA, Propp JM, Stroup NE, Kruchko C. CBTRUS statistical report: primary brain and central nervous system tumors diagnosed in the United States in 2005-2009. Neuro-oncol 2012;14(Suppl 5):v1–v49

3. Bayraktar S, Bayraktar UD, Ramos JC, Stefanovic A, Lossos IS. Primary CNS lymphoma in HIV positive and negative patients: comparison of clinical characteristics, outcome and prognostic factors. J Neurooncol 2011;101:257–265

4. Camilleri-Broët S, Crinière E, Broët P, et al. A uniform activated B-cell-like immunophenotype might explain the poor prognosis of primary central nervous system lymphomas: analysis of 83 cases. Blood 2006; 107:190–196

5. Josephson SA, Papanastassiou AM, Berger MS, et al. The diagnostic utility of brain biopsy procedures in patients with rapidly deteriorating neurological conditions or dementia. J Neurosurg 2007;106:72–75

6. Rubenstein JL, Wong VS, Kadoch C, et al. CXCL13 plus interleukin 10 is highly specific for the diagnosis of CNS lymphoma. Blood 2013;121: 4740–4748 Epub ahead of print

7. Abrey LE, Batchelor TT, Ferreri AJ, et al; International Primary CNS Lymphoma Collaborative Group. Report of an international workshop to standardize baseline evaluation and response criteria for primary CNS lymphoma. J Clin Oncol 2005;23:5034–5043

8. Ferreri AJ, Blay JY, Reni M, et al. Prognostic scoring system for primary CNS lymphomas: the International Extranodal Lymphoma Study Group experience. J Clin Oncol 2003;21:266–272

9. Abrey LE, Ben-Porat L, Panageas KS, et al. Primary central nervous system lymphoma: the Memorial Sloan-Kettering Cancer Center prognostic model. J Clin Oncol 2006;24:5711–5715

10. Lenz G, Staudt LM. Aggressive lymphomas. N Engl J Med 2010;362: 1417–1429

11. Pels H, Juergens A, Schirgens I, et al. Early complete response during chemotherapy predicts favorable outcome in patients with primary CNS lymphoma. Neuro-oncol 2010;12:720–724

12. Ferreri AJ, Reni M, Foppoli M, et al; International Extranodal Lymphoma Study Group (IELSG). High-dose cytarabine plus high-dose methotrexate versus high-dose methotrexate alone in patients with primary CNS lymphoma: a randomised phase 2 trial. Lancet 2009; 374:1512–1520

13. Thiel E, Korfel A, Martus P, et al. High-dose methotrexate with or without whole brain radiotherapy for primary CNS lymphoma (G-PCNSL-SG-1): a phase 3, randomised, non-inferiority trial. Lancet Oncol 2010;11:1036–1047

14. Weller M, Martus P, Roth P, Thiel E, Korfel A; German PCNSL Study Group. Surgery for primary CNS lymphoma? Challenging a paradigm. Neuro-oncol 2012;14:1481–1484

15. Bellinzona M, Roser F, Ostertag H, Gaab RM, Saini M. Surgical removal of primary central nervous system lymphomas (PCNSL) presenting as space occupying lesions: a series of 33 cases. Eur J Surg Oncol 2005; 31:100–105

16. Deangelis LM. Current management of primary central nervous system lymphoma. Oncology (Williston Park) 1995;9:63–71, discussion 71, 75–76, 78

17. Schultz CJ, Bovi J. Current management of primary central nervous system lymphoma. Int J Radiat Oncol Biol Phys 2010;76:666–678

18. Abrey LE, Yahalom J, DeAngelis LM. Treatment for primary CNS lymphoma: the next step. J Clin Oncol 2000;18:3144–3150

19. Ferreri AJ, Dell'Oro S, Foppoli M, et al. MATILDE regimen followed by radiotherapy is an active strategy against primary CNS lymphomas. Neurology 2006;66:1435–1438

20. Feugier P, Virion JM, Tilly H, et al. Incidence and risk factors for central nervous system occurrence in elderly patients with diffuse large-B-cell lymphoma: influence of rituximab. Ann Oncol 2004;15:129–133

21. Bessell EM, López-Guillermo A, Villá S, et al. Importance of radiotherapy in the outcome of patients with primary CNS lymphoma: an analysis of the CHOD/BVAM regimen followed by two different radiotherapy treatments. J Clin Oncol 2002;20:231–236

22. Shah GD, Yahalom J, Correa DD, et al. Combined immunochemotherapy with reduced whole-brain radiotherapy for newly diagnosed primary CNS lymphoma. J Clin Oncol 2007;25:4730–4735

23. Correa DD, Rocco-Donovan M, DeAngelis LM, et al. Prospective cognitive follow-up in primary CNS lymphoma patients treated with chemotherapy and reduced-dose radiotherapy. J Neurooncol 2009;91: 315–321

24. Ferreri AJ, DeAngelis L, Illerhaus G, et al. Whole-brain radiotherapy in primary CNS lymphoma. Lancet Oncol 2011;12:118–119, author reply 119–120

25. Shapiro WR, Young DF, Mehta BM. Methotrexate: distribution in cerebrospinal fluid after intravenous, ventricular and lumbar injections. N Engl J Med 1975;293:161–166

26. Joerger M, Huitema AD, Illerhaus G, et al. Rational administration schedule for high-dose methotrexate in patients with primary CNS lymphoma. Leuk Lymphoma 2012;53:1867–1875

27. Herrlinger U, Schabet M, Brugger W, et al. German Cancer Society Neuro-Oncology Working Group NOA-03 multicenter trial of single-agent high-dose methotrexate for primary central nervous system lymphoma. Ann Neurol 2002;51:247–252

28. Herrlinger U, Küker W, Uhl M, et al; Neuro-Oncology Working Group of the German Society. NOA-03 trial of high-dose methotrexate in primary central nervous system lymphoma: final report. Ann Neurol 2005;57:843–847

29. Batchelor T, Carson K, O'Neill A, et al. Treatment of primary CNS lymphoma with methotrexate and deferred radiotherapy: a report of NABTT 96-07. J Clin Oncol 2003;21:1044–1049

30. Rubenstein JL, Hsi ED, Johnson JL, et al. Intensive chemotherapy and immunotherapy in patients with newly diagnosed primary CNS lymphoma: CALGB 50202 (Alliance 50202). J Clin Oncol 2013;31:3061–3068

31. DeAngelis LM, Seiferheld W, Schold SC, Fisher B, Schultz CJ; Radiation Therapy Oncology Group Study 93-10. Combination chemotherapy and radiotherapy for primary central nervous system lymphoma: Radiation Therapy Oncology Group Study 93-10. J Clin Oncol 2002;20: 4643–4648

32. Zhu JJ, Gerstner ER, Engler DA, et al. High-dose methotrexate for elderly patients with primary CNS lymphoma. Neuro-oncol 2009;11: 211–215

33. Iwamoto FM, Schwartz J, Pandit-Taskar N, et al. Study of radiolabeled indium-111 and yttrium-90 ibritumomab tiuxetan in primary central nervous system lymphoma. Cancer 2007;110:2528–2534

34. Batchelor TT, Grossman SA, Mikkelsen T, Ye X, Desideri S, Lesser GJ. Rituximab monotherapy for patients with recurrent primary CNS lymphoma. Neurology 2011;76:929–930

35. Fritsch K, Kasenda B, Hader C, et al. Immunochemotherapy with rituximab, methotrexate, procarbazine, and lomustine for primary CNS lymphoma (PCNSL) in the elderly. Ann Oncol 2011;22:2080–2085

36. Illerhaus G, Marks R, Müller F, et al. High-dose methotrexate combined with procarbazine and CCNU for primary CNS lymphoma in the elderly: results of a prospective pilot and phase II study. Ann Oncol 2009;20:319–325

37. Chamberlain MC, Johnston SK. High-dose methotrexate and rituximab with deferred radiotherapy for newly diagnosed primary B-cell CNS lymphoma. Neuro-oncol 2010;12:736–744

38. Cobert J, Hochberg E, Woldenberg N, Hochberg F. Monotherapy with methotrexate for primary central nervous lymphoma has single agent activity in the absence of radiotherapy: a single institution cohort. J Neurooncol 2010;98:385–393

39. Birnbaum T, Stadler EA, von Baumgarten L, Straube A. Rituximab significantly improves complete response rate in patients with primary CNS lymphoma. J Neurooncol 2012;109:285–291

40. Gregory G, Arumugaswamy A, Leung T, et al. Rituximab is associated with improved survival for aggressive B cell CNS lymphoma. Neuro-oncol 2013;15:1068–1073

41. Rubenstein JL, Li J, Chen L, et al. Multicenter phase 1 trial of intraventricular immunochemotherapy in recurrent CNS lymphoma. Blood 2013;121:745–751

42. Omuro AM, Taillandier L, Chinot O, Carnin C, Barrie M, Hoang-Xuan K. Temozolomide and methotrexate for primary central nervous system lymphoma in the elderly. J Neurooncol 2007;85:207–211

43. Angelov L, Doolittle ND, Kraemer DF, et al. Blood-brain barrier disruption and intra-arterial methotrexate-based therapy for newly diagnosed primary CNS lymphoma: a multi-institutional experience. J Clin Oncol 2009;27:3503–3509

44. Illerhaus G, Marks R, Ihorst G, et al. High-dose chemotherapy with autologous stem-cell transplantation and hyperfractionated radiotherapy as first-line treatment of primary CNS lymphoma. J Clin Oncol 2006;24:3865–3870

45. Colombat P, Lemevel A, Bertrand P, et al. High-dose chemotherapy with autologous stem cell transplantation as first-line therapy for primary CNS lymphoma in patients younger than 60 years: a multicenter phase II study of the GOELAMS group. Bone Marrow Transplant 2006; 38:417–420

46. Kiefer T, Hirt C, Späth C, et al; Ostdeutsche Studiengruppe Hämatologie und Onkologie. Long-term follow-up of high-dose chemotherapy with autologous stem-cell transplantation and response-adapted whole-brain radiotherapy for newly diagnosed primary CNS lymphoma: results of the multicenter Ostdeutsche Studiengruppe Hamatologie und Onkologie OSHO-53 phase II study. Ann Oncol 2012;23: 1809–1812

47. Alimohamed N, Daly A, Owen C, Duggan P, Stewart DA. Upfront thiotepa, busulfan, cyclophosphamide, and autologous stem cell transplantation for primary CNS lymphoma: a single centre experience. Leuk Lymphoma 2012;53:862–867

48. Kasenda B, Schorb E, Fritsch K, Finke J, Illerhaus G. Prognosis after high-dose chemotherapy followed by autologous stem-cell transplantation as first-line treatment in primary CNS lymphoma—a long-term follow-up study. Ann Oncol 2012;23:2670–2675

49. Ferreri AJ, Verona C, Politi L, et al. Consolidation radiotherapy in primary CNS lymphomas: impact on outcome of different fields and doses in patients in complete remission after upfront chemotherapy. Int J Radiat Oncol Biol Phys 2011;80:169–175

50. Hottinger AF, DeAngelis LM, Yahalom J, Abrey LE. Salvage whole brain radiotherapy for recurrent or refractory primary CNS lymphoma. Neurology 2007;69:1178–1182

51. Pentsova E, DeAngelis LM, Omuro A. Methotrexate re-challenge for recurrent primary central nervous system lymphoma. J Neurooncol 2014;117:161–165

52. Reni M, Zaja F, Mason W, et al. Temozolomide as salvage treatment in primary brain lymphomas. Br J Cancer 2007;96:864–867

53. Raizer JJ, Rademaker A, Evens AM, et al. Pemetrexed in the treatment of relapsed/refractory primary central nervous system lymphoma. Cancer 2012;118:3743–3748

54. Voloschin AD, Betensky R, Wen PY, Hochberg F, Batchelor T. Topotecan as salvage therapy for relapsed or refractory primary central nervous system lymphoma. J Neurooncol 2008;86:211–215

55. Soussain C, Hoang-Xuan K, Taillandier L, et al; Société Française de Greffe de Moëlle Osseuse-Thérapie Cellulaire. Intensive chemotherapy followed by hematopoietic stem-cell rescue for refractory and recurrent primary CNS and intraocular lymphoma: Société Française de Greffe de Moëlle Osseuse-Thérapie Cellulaire. J Clin Oncol 2008;26: 2512–2518

56. DeAngelis LM, Yahalom J, Thaler HT, Kher U. Combined modality therapy for primary CNS lymphoma. J Clin Oncol 1992;10:635–643

57. Thiessen B, DeAngelis LM. Hydrocephalus in radiation leukoencephalopathy: results of ventriculoperitoneal shunting. Arch Neurol 1998; 55:705–710

58. Omuro AM, Ben-Porat LS, Panageas KS, et al. Delayed neurotoxicity in primary central nervous system lymphoma. Arch Neurol 2005;62: 1595–1600

59. Correa DD, Maron L, Harder H, et al. Cognitive functions in primary central nervous system lymphoma: literature review and assessment guidelines. Ann Oncol 2007;18:1145–1151

60. Baumgartner JE, Rachlin JR, Beckstead JH, et al. Primary central nervous system lymphomas: natural history and response to radiation therapy in 55 patients with acquired immunodeficiency syndrome. J Neurosurg 1990;73:206–211

61. Jacomet C, Girard PM, Lebrette MG, Farese VL, Monfort L, Rozenbaum W. Intravenous methotrexate for primary central nervous system non-Hodgkin's lymphoma in AIDS. AIDS 1997;11:1725–1730

62. Forsyth PA, Yahalom J, DeAngelis LM. Combined-modality therapy in the treatment of primary central nervous system lymphoma in AIDS. Neurology 1994;44:1473–1479

63. Wyen C, Jensen B, Hentrich M, et al. Treatment of AIDS-related lymphomas: rituximab is beneficial even in severely immunosuppressed patients. AIDS 2012;26:457–464

64. Skiest DJ, Crosby C. Survival is prolonged by highly active antiretroviral therapy in AIDS patients with primary central nervous system lymphoma. AIDS 2003;17:1787–1793

65. Newell ME, Hoy JF, Cooper SG, et al. Human immunodeficiency virus-related primary central nervous system lymphoma: factors influencing survival in 111 patients. Cancer 2004;100:2627–2636

66. Travi G, Ferreri AJ, Cinque P, et al. Long-term remission of HIV-associated primary CNS lymphoma achieved with highly active antiretroviral therapy alone. J Clin Oncol 2012;30:e119–e121

67. Pels H, Juergens A, Glasmacher A, et al. Early relapses in primary CNS lymphoma after response to polychemotherapy without intraventricular treatment: results of a phase II study. J Neurooncol 2009;91:299–305

Metastatic Brain Tumors

Akash J. Patel, Frederick Lang, and Raymond Sawaya

Brain metastases, aside from being the most common brain tumors, are one of the most feared consequences of systemic cancer because of their poor prognosis if left untreated. Although 10 to 30% of cancer patients ultimately develop brain metastases, the incidence is increasing due to increased cancer survival.[1] Treatment of brain metastasis consists of surgical resection, radiation therapy, or a combination of the two. With advances in surgery and stereotactic radiosurgery (SRS), therapeutic options have increased, and long-term survival has become a reasonable goal. When to use the available treatments has been the source of considerable debate. This chapter reviews the therapeutic options and provides a rational basis for their appropriate application.

Epidemiology

The incidence of brain metastasis is estimated to range from 21,000 to over 100,000 new cases per year[2] in the United States and is thought to be increasing with improved cancer survival, an aging population, increased awareness of the disease, and better diagnostic tests.[1]

Overall, lung cancer is the most common source of brain metastasis, and is responsible for over half of all cases, followed by breast cancer, melanoma, renal cell cancer, and colorectal cancer.[1] Whereas the lung is the most common primary cancer source in men, breast cancer predominates in women. However, the percentage of patients with brain metastases is highest in patients having melanoma, with 40 to 60% developing brain metastases,[3] and 60% percent of brain metastases occur in patients who are 50 to 70 years old.[4]

Based on magnetic resonance imaging (MRI) studies, 50 to 80% of brain metastases are multiple, whereas autopsy studies report that 60 to 85% of brain metastases are multiple. The relative frequency of multiple metastases varies with the type of primary tumor. Melanoma has the highest tendency to produce multiple lesions,[5] whereas renal cancer metastases are more often single lesions.[1]

Pathology

Although on gross examination most metastases are spheroid and well demarcated from surrounding brain tissue, on microscopic examination these tumors may have an infiltrative appearance.[1] Histologically, they appear similar to those of the primary lesion or to the systemic metastases that arise from the primary. Metastases are most often located at the junction of the gray and white matter of the brain, where tumor emboli are trapped in the cerebral vasculature. The cerebrum is the site of localization of 80 to 85% of brain metastases, the cerebellum 10 to 15%, and the brainstem, 3 to 5%.[4]

Special Consideration

- Although metastases are infiltrative much less often than gliomas, this quality may account for tumor recurrences and may justify the use of postoperative irradiation.

Clinical and Imaging Features

Up to two thirds of all brain metastases are symptomatic at some time during a cancer patient's life. The signs and symptoms of metastatic tumors are the same as the signs and symptoms of other expanding intracranial mass lesions.[6] In patients with known systemic cancer, the appearance of neurologic symptoms and a lesion evident on imaging consistent with brain metastasis are virtually diagnostic. Of patients with a history of cancer, 89 to 93% who present with a single supratentorial lesion have a brain metastasis.[7] In patients without a diagnosis of systemic cancer who have a single brain lesion with the imaging features of a metastasis, the probability is less than 15% that the mass is a metastasis.

Contrast-enhanced MRI is the single best tool for imaging evaluation of patients with suspected brain metastasis. MRI is more sensitive and specific than computed tomography (CT) in determining presence or absence, location, and number of metastases. On T1 MRI, metastases appear as loci of increased

---

Pearl

- Any primary cancer can metastasize to the brain, and there are multiple reports in the literature of brain metastases from rare or unusual systemic tumors. Consequently, metastasis should always be considered in the differential diagnosis of a brain lesion in a cancer patient.

signal intensity. Larger tumors often appear to have peripheral enhancement with a nonenhancing core, representing central necrosis. Peritumoral edema appears on a T1 image as a region of decreased signal intensity. In T2 images, tumors often have decreased intensity, whereas edema appears as increased intensity. The presence and extent of edema are far better appreciated on T2 than on T1 imaging.

■ Treatment

Patients with symptomatic brain metastases receive corticosteroid therapy initially, which decreases edema and often alleviates neurologic symptoms. Treatment of brain metastasis consists of surgical resection, radiation therapy, or a combination of the two. Determining which of these modalities is best for a particular patient depends on the number, size, and location of the lesion(s), the status of the systemic disease, the general health and neurologic condition of the patient, and the radiosensitivity or chemosensitivity of the lesion. The status of the systemic disease, both the primary tumor and noncerebral metastases, is a particularly important determinant of outcome in patients with cerebral metastases. In general, patients with controlled primary tumors who have few or no noncerebral metastases are expected to have the best outcome and should be treated with the goal of local cure. More palliative approaches with limited risk for immediate morbidity should be considered for patients who have advanced primary tumors and multiple systemic metastases.

Whole-Brain Radiation Therapy

The use of whole-brain radiation therapy (WBRT) for the treatment of brain metastasis was first reported in 1954.[8] Since then, numerous studies have analyzed the role of WBRT in the treatment of brain metastases.[1] The advantage of WBRT is that it is a simple, noninvasive method of treating the entire brain. Unlike local treatments such as surgery or SRS, WBRT can control metastatic deposits throughout the brain, particularly small or microscopic ones. Consequently, WBRT is best suited for patients with multiple brain metastases. The effectiveness of WBRT depends at least in part on the histology of the lesion. Although breast and lung cancers may respond favorably, tumors such as melanoma and renal cancer are more radioresistant.

The major disadvantage of WBRT is that the normal brain is exposed to the effects of ionizing radiation, which may result in untoward side effects depending on the total dose, fraction size, and dosing interval. Acute side effects include dry desquamation, hair loss, headaches, nausea, lethargy, otitis media, and brain edema. A "somnolence syndrome" of increased fatigue can appear 1 to 4 months after treatment. Late effects can be more serious and include radiation necrosis, atrophy, leukoencephalopathy, and dementia.[1] Large daily radiotherapy fraction sizes have been shown to increase the risk of neurocognitive deficits.[9] In patients with the potential to survive for longer than 1 year, radiation injury to the central nervous system can be a significant problem, and more attention to the potential cognitive effects of WBRT is warranted.[10]

Many series have shown that a median survival time of 3 to 6 months can be expected after WBRT depending on the number of lesions, their radiosensitivity, and the status of any extracranial lesions present. The Radiation Therapy Oncology Group (RTOG) has analyzed the effectiveness of various treatment schedules.[1] These studies indicated that 30 Gy delivered in 10 fractions over 2 weeks results in a rate and length of palliation equivalent to more protracted and higher dose schedules. Yet the risk of radiation-induced leukoencephalopathy, as a consequence of damage to microvessels, increases with radiotherapy fraction sizes > 2 Gy.[11] Consequently, at The University of Texas M.D. Anderson Cancer Center, patients with favorable prognostic factors are frequently treated with 15 fractions of 2 Gy to a total dose of 30 Gy instead of the more customary 10 fractions of 3 Gy.

Whole-brain radiation therapy may be used as primary therapy or as adjuvant treatment after surgical resection or SRS. As primary therapy, WBRT should be considered for all patients with multiple brain metastases and for all patients whose tumors are highly radiosensitive. For patients with single brain metastases, surgery or SRS are probably better options, except in patients with highly radiosensitive tumors such as small-cell lung cancer or germ-cell tumor metastases, in whom WBRT is the best option. In fact, in a randomized trial, prophylactic cranial irradiation has been shown to reduce the incidence of symptomatic brain metastasis and to improve disease-free and overall survival for patients with small-cell lung cancer.[12]

Whole-brain radiation therapy may be a better option than surgery or SRS in patients whose condition makes them a high risk for surgery or SRS. As an adjunctive treatment, patients undergoing surgery or SRS are often given WBRT afterward in an attempt to reduce the possibility of recurrence.

- Whole-brain radiation therapy is generally recommended for patients with multiple brain metastases. For patients with single brain metastases, WBRT may be used as the primary therapy when the tumor is radiosensitive, when the patient has advanced uncontrolled systemic disease, or for patients who cannot tolerate other treatments.

Surgical Resection

Although surgical resection was initially viewed with much nihilism, in the modern era, surgery has become an important treatment option. Surgical resection has several advantages over WBRT or SRS: (1) Surgery is the only modality that establishes a histological diagnosis. This is important because 5 to 11% of patients with single brain lesions and known systemic cancer have lesions that are not metastases.[7] (2) Surgery rapidly relieves symptoms by reducing intracranial pressure, relieving local compression, and eliminating the source of edema. This reduces the need for prolonged steroid administration and lessens the incidence of associated complications that may occur with WBRT or SRS. (3) Unlike SRS, conventional surgery is effective against large tumors (> 3 cm in maximal diameter). The disadvantages of surgery are that it is invasive and has inherent morbidity.

Surgical resection of single brain metastases is associated with a median survival time of 8 to 16 months and local recurrence rates of 7 to 15%.[13,14] Modern techniques of microsurgery, computer-assisted stereotaxy, intraoperative ultrasonography, cortical mapping, and a better understanding of surgical approaches have made most lesions amenable to surgery, including those in deep locations (**Fig. 38.1**).[13] These techniques have reduced the surgical morbidity to about 10% and mortality to less than 5%.

Nevertheless, the limited survival time of patients with systemic cancer demands that patients have short postoperative recovery times and incur no neurologic deficits that necessitate extensive rehabilitation. Therefore, metastases in the basal ganglia, thalamus, and brainstem are not usually resected. When reviewing our experience in patients who underwent surgery alone without WBRT, for a single, previously untreated brain metastasis, we identified two factors that independently affected local recurrence: tumor volume and method of resection.[14] En bloc resection decreases the risk

- Until the 1990s, the role of surgical resection versus WBRT for treatment of single brain metastases was an area of considerable debate, but now surgical resection is often the preferred initial option.

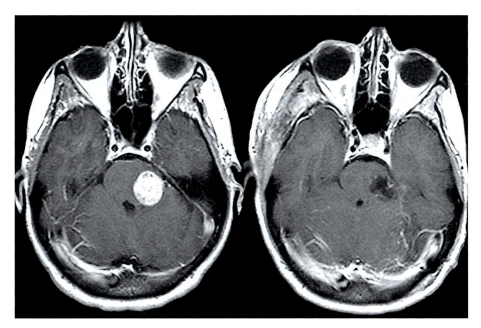

a   b

Fig. 38.1a,b (**a**) Preoperative and (**b**) postoperative contrast-enhanced, T1-weighted magnetic resonance imaging (MRI) scans of a 35-year-old woman with breast cancer metastatic to the pons. The patient was discharged on the fourth postoperative day, fully capable of independent living. (From Sawaya R. Surgical treatment of brain metastases. Clin Neurosurg 1999;45:41–47. Reproduced with permission.)

of leptomeningeal dissemination and local recurrence relative to piecemeal resection, particularly in tumors with a volume < 9.71 cm[3,14-16] without incurring increased risk of neurologic deficit, even in eloquent areas.

In general, surgery is most appropriate for patients with a single brain metastasis, limited systemic disease, and a favorable Karnofsky Performance Scale (KPS) score (typically ≥ 70). Unless they are highly radiosensitive, most single lesions that are ≥ 3 cm in maximal diameter should be resected, as both SRS and WBRT have limited effectiveness against large tumors.

Although many retrospective studies suggest that surgery offers longer survival than WBRT, proponents of WBRT argue that surgical candidates are a select group whose long-term outcome depends on their good functional status rather than treatment with surgery. In 1996, a prospective randomized trial reported that surgery followed by WBRT did not show a survival advantage over WBRT alone in patients with single brain metastasis[17] (**Table 38.1**), but 73% of their patients had advanced extracranial systemic cancer. In contrast, two other prospective randomized trials[7,18] (**Table 38.1**) in the 1990s demonstrated that surgery plus WBRT was superior to WBRT alone. In both studies, patients with single brain metastases, KPS scores ≥ 70, and limited systemic disease, who were treated with surgery, lived significantly longer, had fewer recurrences, and had a better quality of life than the patients treated with WBRT alone.

Surgery has traditionally been contraindicated once multiple lesions are identified.[19] However, a retrospective review of patients harboring multiple brain metastases, comparing patients who had three lesions or less and underwent resection of either all lesions or just some of the lesions showed that patients with multiple metastases that were all resected survived significantly longer (median 14 months) than patients in whom at least one lesion was left unresected (median 6 months).[20] These two groups were compared with a control group of patients undergoing resection of a single brain metastasis. Moreover, patients with resected multiple metastases survived just as long as patients in the control group, with a single metastasis that was resected. Other retrospective studies have subsequently corroborated these findings.[21,22]

Table 38.1 Summary of all Class I Studies Evaluating Treatment of Brain Metastasis

Year	Study	Groups	Local Control	Distant Control	Median Survival (Months)
1990	Patchell et al[7]	WBRT (n = 23)	48%[1]	87%[1]	3.5[1]
		Surgery + WBRT (n = 25)	80%[1]	80%[1]	9.2[1]
1993	Vecht et al[18]	WBRT (n = 31)	N/A	N/A	6[1]
		Surgery + WBRT (n = 32)	N/A	N/A	10[1]
1996	Mintz et al[17]	WBRT (n = 43)	N/A	N/A	6.3
		Surgery + WBRT (n = 41)	N/A	N/A	5.6
1998	Patchell et al[28]	Surgery (n = 46)	54%[1]	30%[1]	9.9
		Surgery + WBRT (n = 49)	90%[1]	82%[1]	11.1
1999	Kondziolka et al[55]	WBRT (n = 14)	0%[1]	N/A	9.9
		SRS + WBRT (n = 13)	92%[1]	N/A	11.1
2004	Andrews et al[38]	WBRT (n = 164)	71%[1]	N/A	4.9[2]
		WBRT + SRS boost (n = 167)	82%[1]	N/A	6.5[2]
2006	Aoyama et al[39]	SRS (n = 67)	73%	36%	8
		SRS + WBRT (n = 65)	89%	58%	7.5
2008	Muacevic et al[53]	SRS (n = 31)	97%	74%	10.3
		Surgery + WBRT (n = 33)	82%	97%	9.5

Abbreviations: N/A, data not available; SRS, stereotactic radiosurgery; WBRT, whole-brain radiation therapy.
[1] Difference is statistically significant.
[2] Mean, not median.

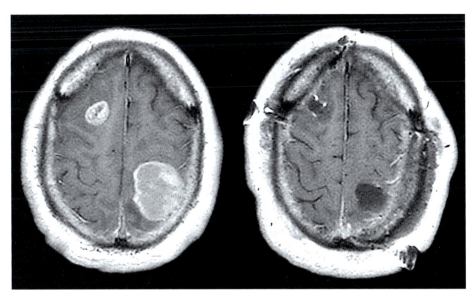

a   b

Fig. 38.2a,b Example of resectable multiple cerebral metastases. (**a**) Preoperative and (**b**) postoperative gadolinium-enhanced T1-weighted axial MRI scans of bilateral brain metastases. The lesions were resected via two separate craniotomies performed at the same sitting. (From Lang FF, Sawaya R. Surgical treatment of metastatic brain tumors. Semin Surg Oncol 1998;14:53–63. Reproduced with permission.)

Nevertheless, based on current retrospective studies, not all patients with multiple brain metastases are candidates for surgery. Only patients with two or three resectable metastases should be considered for surgery (**Fig. 38.2**). Moreover, candidates should have limited or controlled systemic disease. Surgery is most often considered when the lesions are relatively resistant to radiation, such as in the case of renal cancer. Patients expected to survive for less than 3 months based on their systemic disease status are generally not surgical candidates, and patients with radiosensitive primaries such as small-cell lung cancer should be treated with WBRT alone.

Other patients with multiple metastases who may benefit from surgical resection are those with one symptomatic lesion, especially if it is large and immediately life threatening, and one or two smaller asymptomatic lesions. Resection of the symptomatic lesion allows time for treatment of the smaller lesions with WBRT or SRS (**Fig. 38.3**). Only prospective trials will determine the extent to which surgery influences the outcome of patients with multiple brain metastases.

Several reports have retrospectively compared surgery alone with surgery plus WBRT.[23–26] Studies have concluded that postoperative WBRT could reduce the rate of recurrence but that overall survival might not be influenced and that the toxicity at high, daily hypofractionated radiation doses can be significant.[25–27] The study authors recommended that for patients with no evidence of disease after surgery for single metastases, better control could be achieved by using "curative" total doses of 4000 to 4500 cGy, rather than the usual 3000 cGy palliative dose, and that toxicity could be reduced by limiting the daily fractions to 180 to 200 cGy.[25,26]

Controversies

- The role of surgery in treating multiple brain metastases will remain controversial until a prospective trial is undertaken, but retrospective analysis suggests that in patients with two or three lesions, resection of all lesions followed by WBRT may improve survival.
- The role of adjunctive WBRT after surgery and SRS has become increasingly controversial. In randomized trials comparing surgery with WBRT, the patients in the surgical groups received adjuvant WBRT. Advocates of adjuvant WBRT argue that it eradicates microscopic residual disease at the resection site and microscopic deposits at distant sites, thereby delaying both local and distant recurrences. Critics of WBRT cite the potential risk of dementia and other irreversible neurotoxicities in long-term survivors and emphasize that these problems are often compounded by systemic chemotherapy.

A phase III prospective, randomized trial evaluated the benefit of postoperative WBRT in patients with single brain metastases.[28] After surgical resection, patients were randomly assigned to either observation or treatment with 50.4 Gy over 5.5 weeks. Patients were stratified according to the extent of their systemic disease and the primary tumor type. Tumor recurrence anywhere in the brain was drastically lower in the WBRT group than in the observation group (18% vs 70%, respectively), and local recurrence at the surgical site was also less frequent.

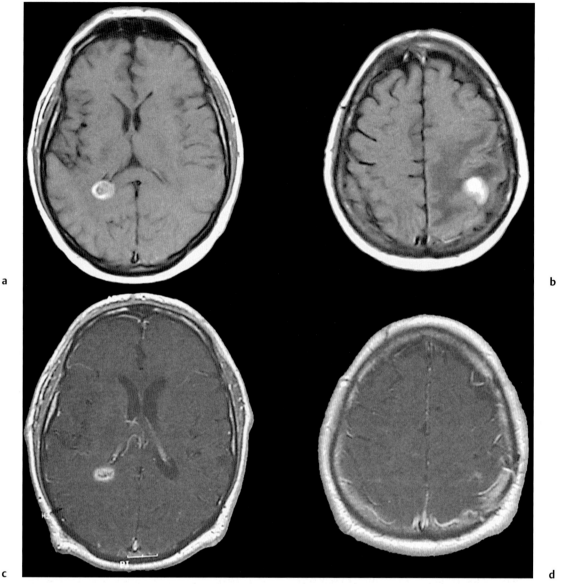

a

b

c

d

Fig. 38.3a–d (**a,b**) Preoperative and (**c,d**) postoperative gadolinium-enhanced, T1-weighted MRI scans of two brain metastases from lung cancer presenting synchronously in a 50-year-old man. (**b**) Edema surrounds the larger lesion, which was symptomatic (producing right hemiparesis) and (**d**) was surgically excised. (**a,c**) The second, smaller lesion was asymptomatic and deeply located and was treated radiosurgically.

The European Organization for Research and Treatment of Cancer (EORTC) conducted a larger randomized phase III trial and found that adjuvant WBRT after surgery or SRS reduced both local (from 59% to 27%) and distant (from 42% to 23%) intracranial tumor recurrences and neurologic deaths but did not improve overall survival or functional independence in patients with one to three brain metastases.[29]

Yet, despite the observation of a reduced rate of local and distant tumor recurrence in these studies, many neuro-oncologists still withhold WBRT after surgical resection. This approach may reflect the findings that the KPS scores of pa-tients treated with WBRT declined at the same rate as for the group receiving surgery alone, suggesting that the toxicity of WBRT offsets its beneficial effects.[28] Furthermore, adjunctive WBRT did not improve the overall survival time of patients. Moreover, when the EORTC analyzed the health-related quality of life (HRQOL) results in patients who received adjuvant WBRT, they found that WBRT resulted in worse HRQOL scores.[30]

Given this controversy, the question arises as to how to treat patients with relatively radioresistant brain metastases, such as those from melanoma and renal cell carcinoma. The aforementioned prospective studies did not address this subset of patients, but a retrospective study did find that even in patients with radioresistant tumors, withholding WBRT did result in a higher rate of distant recurrence.[31]

Stereotactic Radiosurgery

The technique of SRS (now known as gamma knife) was first developed in Sweden in 1951.[32] Since then, other radiosurgical systems have been developed by modification of standard linear accelerators (LINACS).

Stereotactic radiosurgery uses small, well-collimated beams of ionizing radiation to ablate intracranial lesions in three-dimensional space, and the radiation dose rapidly falls off away from the target in a ratio dependent on the size of the target. With a small target, surrounding normal brain tissue receives a smaller radiation dose than with a larger target, which is the main advantage of SRS relative to WBRT. Its advantage relative to surgery lies primarily in its ability to treat small, deep lesions that are not amenable to resection. In addition, SRS is minimally invasive, has fewer immediate risks, requires no overnight hospital stay, and is probably less expensive than surgery. Rapid treatment of multiple lesions is possible with SRS, although as the number of lesions increases, the inability to avoid overlapping of fields results in excessive irradiation of normal brain.

A disadvantage of SRS is that it does not provide histological verification that a lesion is truly a metastasis. Also important, it is necessary to reduce the radiation dose as the lesion size increases to avoid damage to normal tissue. A dramatic decrease has been shown in complete response with increasing tumor size, such that although tumors smaller than 2 cm^3 in volume (maximal diameter of 1.5 cm) showed a total response rate of 78%, the response rate of tumors of 10 cm^3 or larger was less than 50%.[33] Another study analyzed 153 intracranial melanoma metastases treated with SRS.[34] Local control in smaller tumors with a volume of 2 cm^3 or less (75.2%) surpassed that in larger lesions (42.3%) ($p < 0.05$). In addition, in a study of brain metastases of different histological types treated with SRS,[35] the 1- and 2-year actuarial local control rates for tumors no more than 1 cm (0.5 cm^3) in maximal diameter were 86% and 78%, respectively, and were significantly higher than the corresponding rates of 56% and 24% for lesions

larger than 1 cm in maximal diameter ($p = 0.0016$). Moreover, lesions treated with SRS that were > 1 cm^3 had a higher rate of local recurrence than smaller ones; this was statistically significant in a multivariate analysis.[36] The factors that predict response of larger brain lesions to SRS have been identified; tumors of > 16 cm^3 had a statistically significantly lower response rate than smaller lesions.[37] These data suggest that the size of the lesion is important and that the use of SRS to treat brain metastases of ≥ 3 cm in maximal diameter may not be as appropriate or effective as for lesions that are ≤ 1.5 cm in maximal diameter.

Although surgery removes the tumor in one procedure, the beneficial effects of SRS are delayed, and thus symptoms are not as quickly reversed. Because metastases often induce significant amounts of edema, patients treated with SRS may require higher doses of steroids for a longer time than those undergoing surgery, thereby increasing the rate of steroid-related complications.

The RTOG employed recursive partitioning analysis (RPA) in a large multi-institutional randomized trial comparing treatment of brain metastases using WBRT alone (164 patients) with WBRT plus an SRS boost (167 patients).[38] As determined by univariate analysis, patients with single brain metastases who underwent SRS survived significantly longer (mean survival time, 6.5 months) than those who did not (median survival time, 4.9 months) ($p - 0.039$).

A randomized controlled trial of 132 patients with one to four brain metastases, who were treated with SRS alone or SRS plus WBRT, found no survival benefit by adding WBRT (7.5 months vs 8 months), but the 1-year recurrence rate for patients treated with SRS alone was 76.4% versus 46.8% in the SRS plus WBRT group ($p < 0.001$).[39] Retrospective clinical series of brain metastases treated by SRS have demonstrated median survival times as high as 11 months.[40–47] These results are comparable with surgical results, but patients in SRS series usually have smaller tumors than patients in surgical series. Because of the many reports describing favorable results obtained with SRS, several authors have suggested that SRS should replace surgery whenever a metastatic lesion is amenable to this treatment.[48]

The complications associated with SRS are distinct from those associated with surgery. Whereas surgical complications are usually evident immediately, complications from SRS are frequently delayed, like other radiation effects, which may cause them to go unrecorded. SRS carries the potential for injury to the surrounding brain. Increases in posttreatment MRI

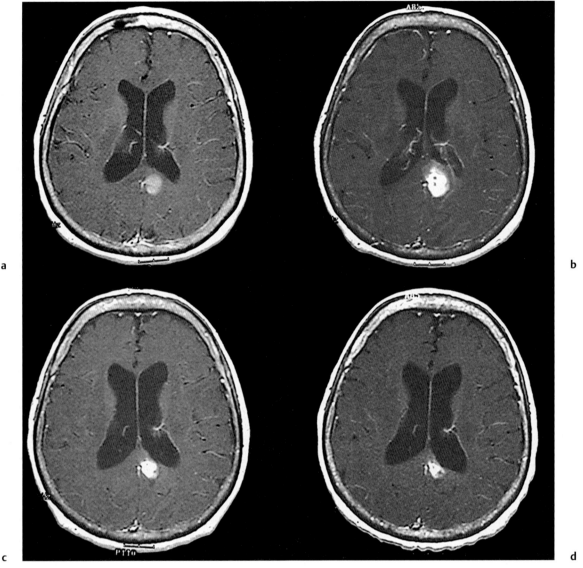

Fig. 38.4a–d Gadolinium-enhanced, T1-weighted MRI scans of a single brain metastasis from non–small-cell lung carcinoma in a 54-year-old woman. (**a**) The lesion was treated with SRS and (**b**) had increased in size after 1 month relative to its pretreatment state. (**c**) At 2 months after treatment, the lesion had returned to approximately its original size, and (**d**) at 4 months posttreatment, it showed some shrinkage.

contrast enhancement and edema (**Fig. 38.4**) are not uncommon after SRS and, although usually transient, may require surgical intervention.[49]

One series of patients with brain metastases treated with SRS alone found a complication rate of only 8%,[46] but 70% of the complications were acute and included increases in seizures and worsening of preexisting neurologic symptoms. Studies reviewing patients treated at M.D. Anderson[50] have reported a 3.8% rate of significant peritumoral edema and a 6.4% rate of hemorrhage within 2.5 months of treatment with SRS, half of which required surgical intervention. A review of 273 patients found that complications occurred in 40% of the treated lesions, with new neurologic symptoms occurring in 32%.[51]

Radiation-induced necrosis is a later complication that can be difficult to differentiate from recurrent disease. Magnetic resonance spectroscopy can be useful in differentiating between the two. Radiation-induced neoplasia is another long-term complication of radiation therapy, but owing to the limited survival of patients with metastatic disease, this is not commonly an issue.

The common notion that SRS is safer to use than conventional surgery for lesions within or near eloquent brain areas may not be warranted. At M.D. Anderson, a retrospective study of neurologic complications in patients treated with SRS for brain metastases[51,52] found that complications (e.g., radiation necrosis, seizures, and neurologic symptom development or worsening) were highest for tumors in eloquent brain and reached 25% for complications severe enough (RTOG grade 3 or higher) to require medical management, typically by administration of steroids or antiepileptic drugs.

There are three categories of patients with single brain metastases: (1) Those with large (≥ 3 cm in maximal diameter) tumors that can only be treated surgically; SRS is ineffective here because to prevent injuring normal brain, the radiation dose must be decreased as tumor size increases, causing tumor control rates to become unfavorable. (2) Those with small (< 3 cm in maximal diameter) surgically inaccessible tumors deep within the brain, for which WBRT was previously the only treatment; SRS is effective and most indicated for these small deep lesions. (3) Those with a surgically accessible single metastasis that is also < 3 cm in maximum diameter; such lesions can be treated with either SRS or surgery, depending on which treatment affords better tumor control.

Surgery Versus Stereotactic Radiosurgery

Although there is no question that surgery or SRS in addition to WBRT reduces local recurrence compared with WBRT alone, whether surgery or SRS is the optimal treatment for lesions < 3 cm in maximal diameter remains controversial.

In patients who underwent surgery and WBRT compared with those who received SRS alone, it was found that the respective mean times to recurrence were 25 months and 7.2 months.[36] The results of a prematurely terminated (due to poor patient accrual) randomized trial comparing surgery plus WBRT with SRS alone found no difference in local tumor control between these two groups.[53] However, each of these studies had only about 30 patients in each arm and did not directly compare surgery and SRS, because the SRS group did not receive WBRT. A prospective study at M.D. Anderson with both randomized and nonrandomized arms compared patients receiving surgery or SRS for single brain metastases. The randomized arm included 30 patients in the surgical

group and 29 in the SRS group; the nonrandomized arm had 89 and 66 patients, respectively. A multivariate analysis to eliminate confounding covariables demonstrated that both SRS groups had significantly more local recurrences than those undergoing surgical excision. As expected, distant recurrence rates were the same in the surgery and the SRS groups.[54]

It is difficult to compare surgery and SRS because of differences in the way recurrence is defined. Published values of local control after SRS permit an increase in tumor size of up to 25%. This must be considered when comparing these two treatment modalities, as it can overstate the level of local control in patients receiving SRS. Nevertheless, most of the retrospective and prospective studies in the literature report a better local control rate with surgery than SRS, particularly as lesion size increases.

Although much debate exists over the relative advantages and disadvantages of surgery and SRS, a rational recommendation can be made to most patients based on tumor size and location, and clinical presentation. Patients with tumors > 3 cm in maximal diameter are almost always treated with surgery, whereas those with small lesions (< 1.5 cm in maximal diameter) that are deeply located are treated with SRS. The treatment for lesions amenable to either therapy (1.5 to 3 cm in maximal diameter) is determined by the patient's symptoms. Patients who are asymptomatic can be treated with SRS, whereas those with symptomatic lesions are more frequently treated surgically. This approach may be modified depending on the patient's medical condition or systemic disease status. For example, patients with conditions that increase surgical risk may undergo SRS, or patients who are to receive chemotherapeutic agents for systemic disease that are likely to cause a bleeding diathesis may be treated surgically to remove the lesion prior to commencing such therapies and to thereby decrease the risk of tumoral hemorrhage.

■ Conclusion

Brain metastases are common in patients with systemic cancer. The vast number of available treatment options has greatly increased the complexity of decision making. The approaches presented here are general guidelines. The surgeon must tailor therapy to the needs of the individual patient.

Editor's Note

Metastatic brain tumors were, until about 20 years ago, viewed as a palliative situation much as glioblastoma was, but even worse. Then randomized studies demonstrated the benefit of surgery for single metastases prior to whole-brain radiation, and a trend that was already beginning blossomed, and single and even multiple brain metastases were aggressively and routinely resected by neurosurgeons everywhere. The efficacy and safety of surgery for many cases was enhanced by the increasingly widespread availability of surgical navigation, and the resurgence of awake craniotomy with cortical mapping. Then came radiosurgery, which not only can replace surgery for small metas-

tases that are also resectable with similar control rates and less morbidity, but also can be used to boost or treat primarily metastases in impossible locations, such as the brainstem, with superb results, and fairly easily re-treat a patient several times as new lesions arise. The result is that many cases of brain metastases nowadays no longer carry a death sentence but actually are a potentially curative situation, such that the patient has an excellent overall survival or at least is spared a neurologic death. (Bernstein)

Acknowledgment

We thank David M. Wildrick, PhD, for reviewing and editing the mansucript.

References

1. Sawaya R, Bindal RK, Lang FF, Suki D. Metastatic brain tumors. In: Kaye AH, Laws ER, eds. Brain Tumors: An Encyclopedic Approach, 3rd ed. Edinburgh: Saunders/Elsevier, 2012:866–894
2. Stelzer KJ. Epidemiology and prognosis of brain metastases. Surg Neurol Int 2013;4(Suppl 4):S192–S202
3. Barnholtz-Sloan JS, Sloan AE, Davis FG, Vigneau FD, Lai P, Sawaya RE. Incidence proportions of brain metastases in patients diagnosed (1973 to 2001) in the Metropolitan Detroit Cancer Surveillance System. J Clin Oncol 2004;22:2865–2872
4. Hojo S, Hirano A. Pathology of metastases affecting the central nervous system. In: Takakura K, Sano K, Hojo S, Hirano A, eds. Metastatic tumors of the nervous system. Tokyo: Igaku-Shoin, 1982:5–111
5. Fox BD, Cheung VJ, Patel AJ, Suki D, Rao G. Epidemiology of metastatic brain tumors. Neurosurg Clin N Am 2011;22:1–6, v
6. Hirsch FR, Paulson OB, Hansen HH, Vraa-Jensen J. Intracranial metastases in small cell carcinoma of the lung: correlation of clinical and autopsy findings. Cancer 1982;50:2433–2437
7. Patchell RA, Tibbs PA, Walsh JW, et al. A randomized trial of surgery in the treatment of single metastases to the brain. N Engl J Med 1990; 322:494–500
8. Chao JH, Phillips R, Nickson JJ. Roentgen-ray therapy of cerebral metastases. Cancer 1954;7:682–689
9. Klein M, Taphoorn MJ, Heimans JJ, et al. Neurobehavioral status and health-related quality of life in newly diagnosed high-grade glioma patients. J Clin Oncol 2001;19:4037–4047
10. Laack NN, Brown PD. Cognitive sequelae of brain radiation in adults. Semin Oncol 2004;31:702–713
11. Soffietti R, Rudā R, Mutani R. Management of brain metastases. J Neurol 2002;249:1357–1369
12. Slotman B, Faivre-Finn C, Kramer G, et al; EORTC Radiation Oncology Group and Lung Cancer Group. Prophylactic cranial irradiation in extensive small-cell lung cancer. N Engl J Med 2007;357:664–672
13. Lang FF, Sawaya R. Surgical management of cerebral metastases. Neurosurg Clin N Am 1996;7:459–484
14. Patel AJ, Suki D, Hatiboglu MA, et al. Factors influencing the risk of local recurrence after resection of a single brain metastasis. J Neurosurg 2010;113:181–189
15. Suki D, Abouassi H, Patel AJ, Sawaya R, Weinberg JS, Groves MD. Comparative risk of leptomeningeal disease after resection or stereotactic

radiosurgery for solid tumor metastasis to the posterior fossa. J Neurosurg 2008;108:248–257
16. Suki D, Hatiboglu MA, Patel AJ, et al. Comparative risk of leptomeningeal dissemination of cancer after surgery or stereotactic radiosurgery for a single supratentorial solid tumor metastasis. Neurosurgery 2009; 64:664–674, discussion 674–676
17. Mintz AH, Kestle J, Rathbone MP, et al. A randomized trial to assess the efficacy of surgery in addition to radiotherapy in patients with a single cerebral metastasis. Cancer 1996;78:1470–1476
18. Vecht CJ, Haaxma-Reiche H, Noordijk EM, et al. Treatment of single brain metastasis: radiotherapy alone or combined with neurosurgery? Ann Neurol 1993;33:583–590
19. Patchell RA. Metastatic brain tumors. Neurol Clin 1995;13:915–925
20. Bindal RK, Sawaya R, Leavens ME, Lee JJ. Surgical treatment of multiple brain metastases. J Neurosurg 1993;79:210–216
21. Paek SH, Audu PB, Sperling MR, Cho J, Andrews DW. Reevaluation of surgery for the treatment of brain metastases: review of 208 patients with single or multiple brain metastases treated at one institution with modern neurosurgical techniques. Neurosurgery 2005;56:1021–1034, discussion 1033–1034
22. Iwadate Y, Namba H, Yamaura A. Significance of surgical resection for the treatment of multiple brain metastases. Anticancer Res 2000;20:573–577
23. Smalley SR, Schray MF, Laws ER Jr, O'Fallon JR. Adjuvant radiation therapy after surgical resection of solitary brain metastasis: association with pattern of failure and survival. Int J Radiat Oncol Biol Phys 1987;13:1611–1616
24. Dosoretz DE, Blitzer PH, Russell AH, Wang CC. Management of solitary metastasis to the brain: the role of elective brain irradiation following complete surgical resection. Int J Radiat Oncol Biol Phys 1980;6:1727–1730
25. DeAngelis LM, Mandell LR, Thaler HT, et al. The role of postoperative radiotherapy after resection of single brain metastases. Neurosurgery 1989;24:798–805
26. Hagen NA, Cirrincione C, Thaler HT, DeAngelis LM. The role of radiation therapy following resection of single brain metastasis from melanoma. Neurology 1990;40:158–160
27. Choi KN, Withers HR, Rotman M. Metastatic melanoma in brain. Rapid treatment or large dose fractions. Cancer 1985;56:10–15

28. Patchell RA, Tibbs PA, Regine WF, et al. Postoperative radiotherapy in the treatment of single metastases to the brain: a randomized trial. JAMA 1998;280:1485–1489

29. Kocher M, Soffietti R, Abacioglu U, et al. Adjuvant whole-brain radiotherapy versus observation after radiosurgery or surgical resection of one to three cerebral metastases: results of the EORTC 22952-26001 study. J Clin Oncol 2011;29:134–141

30. Soffietti R, Kocher M, Abacioglu UM, et al. A European Organisation for Research and Treatment of Cancer phase III trial of adjuvant whole-brain radiotherapy versus observation in patients with one to three brain metastases from solid tumors after surgical resection or radiosurgery: quality-of-life results. J Clin Oncol 2013;31:65–72

31. McPherson CM, Suki D, Feiz-Erfan I, et al. Adjuvant whole-brain radiation therapy after surgical resection of single brain metastases. Neuro Oncol 2010;12:711–719

32. Leksell L. The stereotaxic method and radiosurgery of the brain. Acta Chir Scand 1951;102:316–319

33. Mehta MP, Rozental JM, Levin AB, et al. Defining the role of radiosurgery in the management of brain metastases. Int J Radiat Oncol Biol Phys 1992;24:619–625

34. Selek U, Chang EL, Hassenbusch SJ III, et al. Stereotactic radiosurgical treatment in 103 patients for 153 cerebral melanoma metastases. Int J Radiat Oncol Biol Phys 2004;59:1097–1106

35. Chang EL, Hassenbusch SJ III, Shiu AS, et al. The role of tumor size in the radiosurgical management of patients with ambiguous brain metastases. Neurosurgery 2003;53:272–280, discussion 280–281

36. Shinoura N, Yamada R, Okamoto K, Nakamura O, Shitara N. Local recurrence of metastatic brain tumor after stereotactic radiosurgery or surgery plus radiation. J Neurooncol 2002;60:71–77

37. Yang HC, Kano H, Lunsford LD, Niranjan A, Flickinger JC, Kondziolka D. What factors predict the response of larger brain metastases to radiosurgery? Neurosurgery 2011;68:682–690, discussion 690

38. Andrews DW, Scott CB, Sperduto PW, et al. Whole brain radiation therapy with or without stereotactic radiosurgery boost for patients with one to three brain metastases: phase III results of the RTOG 9508 randomised trial. Lancet 2004;363:1665–1672

39. Aoyama H, Shirato H, Tago M, et al. Stereotactic radiosurgery plus whole-brain radiation therapy vs stereotactic radiosurgery alone for treatment of brain metastases: a randomized controlled trial. JAMA 2006;295:2483–2491

40. Adler JR, Cox RS, Kaplan I, Martin DP. Stereotactic radiosurgical treatment of brain metastases. J Neurosurg 1992;76:444–449

41. Coffey RJ, Flickinger JC, Lunsford LD, Bissonette DJ. Solitary brain metastasis: radiosurgery in lieu of microsurgery in 32 patients. Acta Neurochir Suppl (Wien) 1991;52:90–92

42. Sturm V, Kimmig B, Engenhardt R, et al. Radiosurgical treatment of cerebral metastases. Method, indications and results. Stereotact Funct Neurosurg 1991;57:7–10

43. Auchter RM, Lamond JP, Alexander E, et al. A multiinstitutional outcome and prognostic factor analysis of radiosurgery for resectable single brain metastasis. Int J Radiat Oncol Biol Phys 1996;35:27–35

44. Flickinger JC, Kondziolka D. Radiosurgery instead of resection for solitary brain metastasis: the gold standard redefined. [editorial] [see comments] Int J Radiat Oncol Biol Phys 1996;35:185–186

45. Hasegawa T, Kondziolka D, Flickinger JC, Germanwala A, Lunsford LD. Brain metastases treated with radiosurgery alone: an alternative to whole brain radiotherapy? Neurosurgery 2003;52:1318–1326, discussion 1326

46. Lutterbach J, Cyron D, Henne K, Ostertag CB. Radiosurgery followed by planned observation in patients with one to three brain metastases. Neurosurgery 2003;52:1066–1073, discussion 1073–1074

47. Sneed PK, Suh JH, Goetsch SJ, et al. A multi-institutional review of radiosurgery alone vs. radiosurgery with whole brain radiotherapy as the initial management of brain metastases. Int J Radiat Oncol Biol Phys 2002;53:519–526

48. Mehta MP, Tsao MN, Whelan TJ, et al. The American Society for Therapeutic Radiology and Oncology (ASTRO) evidence-based review of the role of radiosurgery for brain metastases. Int J Radiat Oncol Biol Phys 2005;63:37–46

49. Vecil GG, Suki D, Maldaun MV, Lang FF, Sawaya R. Resection of brain metastases previously treated with stereotactic radiosurgery. J Neurosurg 2005;102:209–215

50. Chang EL, Wefel JS, Maor MH, et al. A pilot study of neurocognitive function in patients with one to three new brain metastases initially treated with stereotactic radiosurgery alone. Neurosurgery 2007;60:277–283, discussion 283–284

51. Williams BJ, Suki D, Fox BD, et al. Stereotactic radiosurgery for metastatic brain tumors: a comprehensive review of complications. J Neurosurg 2009;111:439–448

52. Dare AO, Sawaya R, Part II. Surgery versus radiosurgery for brain metastasis: surgical advantages and radiosurgical myths. Clin Neurosurg 2004;51:255–263

53. Muacevic A, Wowra B, Siefert A, Tonn JC, Steiger HJ, Kreth FW. Microsurgery plus whole brain irradiation versus Gamma Knife surgery alone for treatment of single metastases to the brain: a randomized controlled multicentre phase III trial. J Neurooncol 2008;87:299–307

54. Lang FF, Suki D, Maor M, et al. Conventional surgery versus stereotactic radiosurgery in the treatment of single brain metastases: a prospective study with both randomized and nonrandomized arms. American Association of Neurological Surgeons Meeting [abstract]. Article ID: 48938, 2008

55. Kondziolka D, Lunsford LD, Flickinger JC. The radiobiology of radiosurgery. Neurosurg Clin N Am 1999;10:157–166

39 Intradural Spinal Tumors

Alfred T. Ogden and Paul C. McCormick

Spinal tumors encompass a range of histologies that reflect the diversity of cell types within the spinal cord and nerve roots as well as supporting structures inside the thecal sac. They most frequently present with pain, often in the absence of discrete neurologic findings early in the course of the illness. Most spinal cord tumors are best treated and often cured with complete surgical resection. Because functional outcomes after surgery are closely linked to the preoperative neurologic condition, systematic inclusion of spinal cord tumors in the differential diagnosis for back or limb pain can result in a timely diagnosis that can profoundly impact patient outcomes. Adjuvant radiation has a variable role for malignant tumors depending on histology, and remains the subject of some controversy. Radiosurgery for the spine is now widely available, but its role in the management of these heterogeneous, predominantly benign neoplasms is still being assessed.

■ Histology and Epidemiology

Although there is significant crossover, intradural spinal tumors are divided into two main anatomic categories: intramedullary and extramedullary. Intramedullary tumors arise within spinal cord parenchyma and are primarily of glial origin (astrocytomas, ependymomas, gangliogliomas) or vascular origin (hemangioblastomas). Extramedullary tumors grow within the subarachnoid space and arise mostly from cells within the nerve roots (neurofibromas, schwannomas) or the meninges (meningiomas). Other, rarer tumors stem from ectopic tissues found in association with these structures. Some of these are a result of embryological errors (dermoids, epidermoids, teratomas, lipomas) and others a result of systemic malignancy (intramedullary or extramedullary intradural spinal cord metastases).

Intramedullary tumors occur throughout the spinal cord. Age of presentation is bimodal, with the first peak occurring in children 5 to 10 years of age and the second occurring in adults in their mid-30s. To a degree, the patient's age can anticipate the histology of spinal cord tumors. Ependymomas are the most common intramedullary lesions in adults,[1] whereas in children, astrocytomas are much more prevalent.[2] In adults, 35 to 40 years as a mean age of presentation is remarkably constant over series of patients with the three most common adult intramedullary tumors: ependymomas,[3,4] astrocytomas,[5] and hemangioblastomas.[6] High-grade astrocytomas have been found most commonly in adolescents.[7] Adult extramedullary lesions tend to present later in life, with large series showing peak ages of presentation between 45 and 50 years of age for schwannomas[8] and between 50 and 65 years of age for meningiomas.[9,10] The incidence of lesions resulting from embryological errors increases significantly with decreasing age, reaching 31% of spinal tumors in children under 15 years of age[11] and 65% of spinal tumors in children under 1 year of age.[12]

■ Clinical Presentation

Although patients can present with a range of symptoms, the most common complaint in adults with spinal tumors is pain.[3] The development of motor deficits, in particular gait disturbances, may ultimately be the symptom most likely to attract medical attention in young children because of their inability to verbalize effectively complaints of pain. The pain generated by an intramedullary tumor is typically axial, dull, and aching; of gradual onset; and not easily explained by pathological changes to known sensory pathways. Because this symptom is somewhat vague and is often not associated with any neurologic deficit early on, the lapse between symptom onset and diagnosis is often prolonged. Pain from extramedullary lesions may be radicular, mimicking a herniated disk, or axial depending on histology and cord involvement. Sensory changes, including paresthesias and sensory loss, are approximately as common as weakness as a second presenting symptom.

> **Pitfall**
>
> - The classic syndrome of an intramedullary tumor is a central, dull, aching pain of gradual onset, not easily explained by pathological changes to known sensory pathways. Because this symptom is somewhat vague and is often not associated with any neurologic deficit early in the course of the illness, the lapse between symptom onset and diagnosis is often prolonged.

■ Differential Diagnosis

The signs and symptoms of spinal tumors can resemble many other disorders affecting the spinal axis, including musculo-skeletal pain syndromes (fibromyalgia), autoimmune disorders (transverse myelitis, multiple sclerosis), degenerative disease (ruptured intervertebral disks, spinal stenosis, synovial cysts), vascular lesions (cavernous malformations, arteriovenous malformations), infectious processes (epidural abscess, viral radiculitis, syphilis), traumatic lesions (syringomyelia, chronic dens fracture), congenital malformations of the spine and skull base (Klippel-Feil), motor neuron disease (amyotrophic lateral sclerosis [ALS]), and other miscellaneous disorders (arachnoiditis, hypertrophic arthritis, B_{12} deficiency). Information gathered from a careful medical history and a detailed neurologic examination can help to navigate through this extensive differential diagnosis. For example, a relapsing, remitting course compared with a slow, steady decline is much more typical of multiple sclerosis than of a spinal tumor. A patient with motor findings in the absence of any sensory disturbances hints at a motor neuron disease. As a practical matter, however, there are two critical branch points in the clinician's decision analysis: (1) when to order spinal imaging; and (2) how to distinguish between spinal tumors and other, nonoperative lesions that can resemble them on imaging studies.

As a general rule, any patient with a new neurologic complaint localizing to the spine requires spinal imaging. The same applies to patients whose pain falls in a radicular pattern. Patients with vague complaints of back pain in the absence of neurologic symptoms may present a bit of a dilemma; however, a patient with gradual onset of constant, dull midback pain over weeks to months should pique enough suspicion to merit an imaging study.

■ Imaging Studies

When imaging is deemed appropriate, magnetic resonance imaging (MRI) is the modality of choice. Often, a noncontrast MRI specific to the spinal level to which signs and symptoms localize is the initial study to detect a lesion. If such a study is suggestive of a spinal tumor or of an associated abnormality such as a syrinx, a full spinal axis gadolinium-enhanced MRI is indicated. Lesions that can resemble spinal cord tumors on MRI include inflammatory processes, such as transverse

---

Pitfall

- Any syrinx needs contrast-enhanced imaging of the entire spine.

Pearl

- Spinal cord tumors can usually be distinguished from inflammatory lesions because they are more likely to be enhancing and they expand the cord significantly.

---

myelitis, multiple sclerosis, and sarcoidosis; degenerative processes, such as synovial cysts; and traumatic lesions, such as cord edema and syringes. Spinal tumors enhance with contrast in a fashion that is specific enough to remove ambiguity in most cases; however, the enhancing tumor may be sufficiently remote from the sentinel lesion discovered on initial imaging studies that it can be missed if the entire spinal axis is not imaged. Spinal cord tumors can also be distinguished from other nonneoplastic lesions because they produce a redundancy of tissue that dramatically enlarges cord diameter.

When imaging studies are consistent with a spinal tumor, additional specialized MRI modalities can point to specific diagnoses. Nonenhancing congenital lesions with high lipid content are suggested when fat-suppressed MRI sequences decrease signal intensity in all or part of the lesion. Gradient echo is useful in identifying blood products or finding tiny hemorrhagic lesions that cannot be resolved by conventional MRI modalities. Although MRI is usually sufficient to identify the relative positions of key vascular structures, such as the vertebral artery, to tumor, an angiogram is sometimes useful and will also provide the surgeon with a blueprint of a tumor's blood supply.

■ Treatment

Surgery: Operative Planning and Techniques

Most intramedullary glial tumors (e.g., ependymomas, astrocytomas) are approached via a midline incision and a joint-sparing laminectomy that extends about one level above and below the tumor. Intramedullary tumors are usually accessed through a midline myelotomy; however, a myelotomy through the dorsal root entry zone can be used for tumors lateral in the cord or if the cord is rotated. In either case, the myelotomy should be extended just beyond the rostral and caudal poles of the tumor if more than a biopsy is anticipated.

Establishment of a plane between tumor and cord parenchyma is the paramount early goal because the ability to maintain and develop this plane will dictate the aggressiveness and safety of resection. An intraoperative pathological consultation should be obtained early in the procedure and may inform the operative process; however, frozen sections are not reliable enough to distinguish between tumors for which aggressive surgical resection is indicated and tumors for which surgical goals are more limited. In practice, as long as a clear plane exists between tumor and spinal cord, gross total resection should remain the operative objective. When possible, the tumor should be removed en bloc, although this is often not practical for larger tumors for which an en bloc technique can obscure visualization of the dissection plane of the anterior portion of the tumor. Intraoperative monitoring is advocated by most surgeons, and may provide useful information regarding spinal cord function. More recently, anterior approaches have been utilized to access ventrally situated intramedullary tumors.[13,14]

Intradural extramedullary tumors are usually encapsulated and noninvasive. The goal of surgery is almost always gross total resection. A posterior midline approach is sufficient for the vast majority of tumors, even those with anterior extension. The lateral extracavitary approach or a costotransversectomy may be useful for small ventrally located tumors. Some authors have advocated anterolateral approaches for dumbbell lesions with anterior extradural extension, and good results have been achieved in experienced hands; however, these approaches have the disadvantage of leaving decompression of neural elements until the final stages of the tumor resection. In recent years, ventral and minimally invasive techniques have been described for ventrally located extramedullary tumors.[14,15]

Following laminectomy, the first priority is decompression of the spinal cord. For tumors with both intradural and extradural components, this may require durotomy and intradural resection as a first step if the tumor is located anteriorly or anterolaterally, or extradural debulking to permit sufficient exposure to the intradural portion of the tumor if the tumor is located posteriorly. Once the tumor is exposed, cauterization of tumor capsule both shrinks and devascularizes the mass. Small tumors can be carefully dissected from neural elements and rolled away from the cord as the dissection plane develops. Large tumors often require internal debulking with a sonic aspirator. For nerve sheath tumors it is usually impossible to save the affected nerve root; however, one should

always stimulate it to confirm nonfunctionality prior to cauterization and ligation. For meningiomas, excision of part of the dura mater is sometimes required for complete tumor removal. After tumor removal and hemostasis, the dura is closed primarily with patching of any dural defect with dural substitute.

Adjuvant Therapy

The overwhelming majority of clinical experience regarding adjuvant therapy is with conventional radiotherapy for intramedullary tumors. Although the benefits of radiotherapy remain controversial, many clinicians advocate a local cumulative dose of 5,040 cGy for low-grade ependymomas and astrocytomas with radiographic residual disease following surgery. High-grade lesions receive slightly higher doses, and disseminated disease requires complete craniospinal irradiation.[16] Various chemotherapy strategies have been reported, but nothing approaching a consensus exists for any particular histology.[17] Radiosurgery remains an investigational modality for most spinal tumors, although recent reports appear to support an expanding role of radiosurgery in the treatment of both benign and malignant intradural neoplasms.[18,19]

◼ Intradural Intramedullary Tumors

Ependymomas

Ependymomas are usually slow-growing, benign lesions that are nonencapsulated but noninvasive. They are estimated to account for 37 to 60% of all intramedullary tumors in adults and 30% of those in children.[12] They most commonly present with axial pain, roughly arising from the level of the tumor or dysesthesias that are referred to limbs or dermatomes.[4,20] Sensory changes and motor deficits are common as well. Ependymomas tend to be hypointense to isointense to neural tissue on T1-weighted MRI and uniformly enhancing[21] (**Fig. 39.1**). They can be associated with a syrinx, exhibiting polar "capping" phenomenon, or may contain intratumoral cysts. Although the typical ependymoma is centrally located within the cord, the myxopapillary subtype arises in association with the cauda equina, and subependymomas appear eccentrically

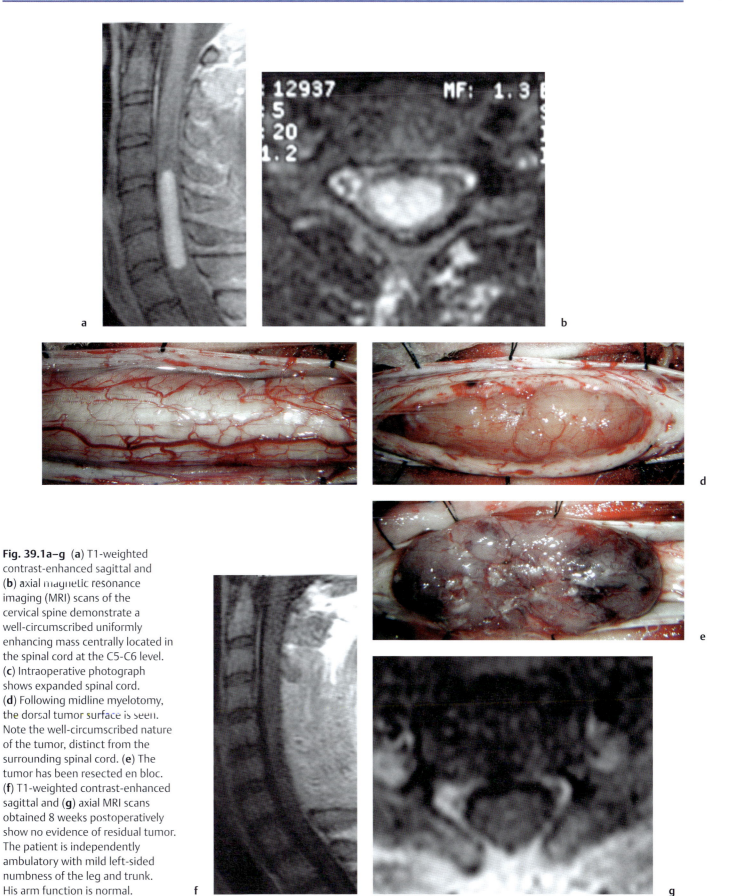

Fig. 39.1a–g (**a**) T1-weighted contrast-enhanced sagittal and (**b**) axial magnetic resonance imaging (MRI) scans of the cervical spine demonstrate a well-circumscribed uniformly enhancing mass centrally located in the spinal cord at the C5-C6 level. (**c**) Intraoperative photograph shows expanded spinal cord. (**d**) Following midline myelotomy, the dorsal tumor surface is seen. Note the well-circumscribed nature of the tumor, distinct from the surrounding spinal cord. (**e**) The tumor has been resected en bloc. (**f**) T1-weighted contrast-enhanced sagittal and (**g**) axial MRI scans obtained 8 weeks postoperatively show no evidence of residual tumor. The patient is independently ambulatory with mild left-sided numbness of the leg and trunk. His arm function is normal.

within the cord. Overall, histology varies from benign subtypes, such as cellular, papillary, and myxopapillary, that carry excellent prognoses, to anaplastic varieties that may portend a more aggressive course. Metastatic spread occurs infrequently.

Identification of possible risk factors for recurrence following gross total microscopic resection (GTMR) is difficult because surgical series often fail to report specific information regarding histology and anatomic location. In adults, recurrence rates in most surgical series after GTMR without adjuvant therapy of any kind have been very low, ranging from 0 to 4% to as high as 9% with a follow-up period of 2 to > 10 years.[4,20,22] Similar numbers have been generated for pediatric cases of ependymoma.[23] Many patients who were cured by surgery in these series had previously failed radiotherapy, and most of the radiation oncology literature shows a correlation between the extent of resection and survival, as well as a relatively high rate of progression after irradiation of tumors that were either subtotally resected or biopsied.[24,25]

Published series of spinal ependymomas treated with radiotherapy claim a benefit, reporting long-term rates of local failure at 0 to 33% and survival at 60 to 100% over 5 years[16,24,25]; however, a dose–response relationship across a range of 4,000 to 5,400 Gy has not been demonstrated.[16] Whether these data demonstrate a therapeutic impact or merely reflect the natural history of the disease can only be answered by randomized, prospective studies. Given the indolent nature of most spinal ependymomas, some clinicians choose to follow small recurrences or residuals radiographically without adjuvant therapy. If a lesion progresses, reoperation is always an option, as is delayed radiotherapy.

The majority of experience regarding chemotherapy for ependymomas comes from the pediatric literature and involves intracranial disease.[17] There is a curious disparity between long-term survival in intracranial as opposed to spinal ependymomas. Although ependymomas in both locations respond poorly to chemotherapy and radiation, and disease progression for both is closely tied to the extent of resection, spinal ependymomas are usually cured with GTMR, whereas intracranial ependymomas usually recur.[25,26] This inconsistency is poorly understood but suggests significant pathophysiological differences between spinal and intracranial ependymoma that preclude extrapolations vis-á-vis chemotherapy. A few individual successes using etoposide for spinal ependymoma have been reported.[27,28]

Ependymomas of the filum terminale, so-called myxopapillary ependymomas, warrant special consideration because their lack of a well-defined tumor capsule and apposition to the subarachnoid space render them susceptible to either preoperative or postoperative cerebrospinal fluid (CSF) dissemination, despite the histologically benign nature of these neoplasms. Early surgical intervention with en bloc resection is usually recommended for midline cauda equina tumors, even for small asymptomatic lesions, to prevent this potentially devastating occurrence.

Astrocytomas

Astrocytomas are estimated to account for 36 to 45%[1,29] of all intramedullary tumors in adults and 60% of those in children.[2] They most commonly present with pain and other sensory symptoms, with motor deficits occurring after disease progression. Like ependymomas, astrocytomas are hypointense to isointense on MRI, but, unlike ependymomas, they tend to enhance more heterogeneously and to lack defined margins. They are often eccentric within the cord and are more likely than ependymomas to be cystic[21] (**Fig. 39.2**). Histologically they are classified by the same World Health Organization (WHO) grading system governing intracranial lesions: grade I, pilocytic astrocytoma; grade II, fibrillary; grade III, anaplastic; and grade IV, glioblastoma. The vast majority of spinal astrocytomas in adults are fibrillary, indolent, and invasive. There is more histological variability in children, where low-grade astrocytomas are usually fibrillary but can contain neural elements (gangliogliomas) or pilocytic features. Gangliogliomas and pilocytic astrocytomas tend to be more circumscribed and may carry a better prognosis.

Unlike their intracranial counterparts, grade III and IV lesions are rare, but when diagnosed carry a similarly dismal prognosis, with life expectancy ranging from a few months to 2 years after diagnosis.[30] High-grade spinal gliomas metastasize along CSF spaces in about half of reported cases, and extraneural metastases have been reported as well.[7,30] Surgical intervention is indicated for all astrocytomas if only for the limited goal of obtaining tissue. For high-grade lesions there is no recognized benefit from aggressive surgery, and these are routinely irradiated after biopsy.

For low-grade lesions, controversy exists regarding the roles of both radical resection and radiation. Some authors have found both a survival and a symptomatic benefit from aggressive surgical resection,[5] whereas others have not, neither in adults[22,31] nor in children.[27,32] Some studies quote an 88% 5-year survival rate with maximal resection alone and see no advantage of adjuvant radiation.[5] Others point toward a modest benefit to radiation, with 5-year survival rates of 50 to 91%, and recommend adjuvant radiation in cases of residual radiographic disease.[16,33,34] Various chemotherapy regimens, described in a few published reports, have been attempted for spinal gliomas; lomustine (chloroethylcyclohexylnitrosourea [CCNU]) and vincristine; and carboplatin and vincristine.[17,35] Still, no standard of care exists regarding chemotherapy.

Hemangioblastomas

Hemangioblastomas are benign, vascular tumors thought to arise from erythrocyte precursors. They can occur anywhere in the body but, for unknown reasons, occur most frequently in the posterior fossa and the spinal cord. In the spinal cord they account for 3 to 6% of all intramedullary tumors.[6,36] They

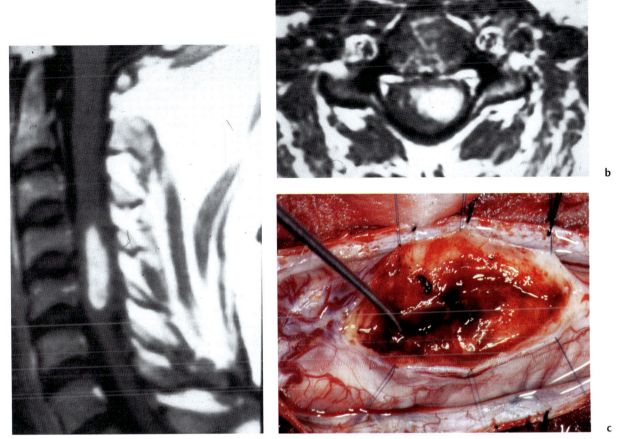

Fig. 39.2a–c (**a**) T1-weighted contrast-enhanced sagittal and (**b**) axial MRI scans of the cervical spine demonstrate a uniformly enhancing eccentric lesion at the C4-C5 level. Note the somewhat indistinct tumor margins on the axial image. This is typical for most intramedullary astrocytomas. (**c**) Intraoperative photograph shows intramedullary tumor. The central portion of the tumor is well defined but the margins at the tumor–spinal cord interface are not.

are twice as common in men as in women and are associated with the genetic neurocutaneous disorder von Hippel–Lindau disease (VHL), with which 20 to 30% of patients with hemangioblastomas are diagnosed.[6,36] Despite a much higher risk of hemangioblastoma formation in individuals with VHL, VHL-associated and sporadic tumors are histologically identical and thought to be generated through mutations in the same tumor-suppressor gene.[37]

On MRI, the classic appearance of a hemangioblastoma is a brightly, homogeneously enhancing nidus in association with a much larger syrinx or cyst (**Fig. 39.3**). Surgical series have reported the presence of an associated cyst 50 to 100% of the time,[38,39] and in their absence even small hemangioblastomas are typically surrounded by a widened, edematous cord. Although always intradural lesions, 70% of hemangioblastomas are entirely or partially intramedullary and 30% are entirely extramedullary and may resemble other, more common extramedullar lesions such as meningiomas and schwannomas.[39] Longitudinal radiographic studies of hemangioblastomas in patients with VHL have demonstrated a stepwise progression from nidus appearance to the development of perinidal edema to syrinx formation.[40] This process may be mediated in part by vascular endothelial growth factor (VEGF), which is the target of new molecular therapies designed for patients with unresectable tumors or a diffuse manifestation of VHL called hemangioblastomatosis.[41]

Patients with hemangioblastomas present with a range of symptoms that are usually attributable to syrinx formation or peritumoral edema. In sporadic cases the most common first symptom is pain, although weakness and paresthesias are common as well.[6,36] Patients with VHL frequently harbor asymptomatic lesions that are followed for long periods of time without intervention. Surgery is generally performed when lesions become symptomatic, and, in such cases, pain is a much less common feature than numbness and weakness.

Surgical resection is the only accepted treatment for spinal hemangioblastomas. Fortunately, most hemangioblastomas arise from the dorsal or dorsolateral pia on the spinal cord surface with varying degrees of extension into the spinal cord. This superficial location often facilitates surgical resection.[6] Gross

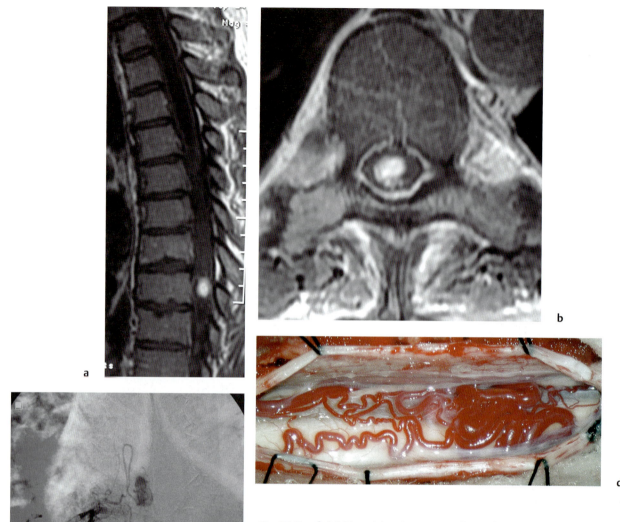

Fig. 39.3a–d (**a**) T1-weighted contrast-enhanced sagittal and (**b**) axial MRI scans of the thoracic spine demonstrate intensely enhancing well-circumscribed tumor at the T9 level. (**c**) Selective spinal angiogram shows typical hemangioblastoma tumor blush and feeding anterior spinal artery. (**d**) Intraoperative photograph shows vascular tumor mass with markedly enlarged draining veins.

total resection cures sporadic cases and results in local eradication in patients with VHL. The principal impediment to a complete surgical resection is excessive bleeding, and because of the highly vascular nature of these tumors, some authors have recommended preoperative embolization.[36] Some authors have reported improvement in symptoms after surgery,[6,36] whereas others reported mild exacerbations in symptoms that did not impair function and resolved over several days.[39] Rare neurologic deterioration after surgery appears to be related to incomplete resection, ventral location, and tumor size.[37,39]

Intramedullary Spinal Cord Metastases

Although intracranial metastases and epidural metastases from systemic cancers are common, direct metastases to the spinal cord parenchyma are rare. Intramedullary spinal cord metastases (ISCMs) follow two patterns: direct invasion of a leptomeningeal metastasis across the pia and intramedullary hematogenous spread from a pulmonary source. The latter appears to be exclusively from bronchogenic carcinomas, which are responsible for most cases of ISCM.[42] Other cancers known to metastasize to the spinal cord include breast, melanoma, and renal cell carcinoma. Although most patients develop ISCM in the setting of known metastatic disease, as many as 25% of patients present with ISCM as the initial manifestation of a systemic cancer. Some advocate surgical excision of ISCM in addition to radiation and histology-specific chemotherapy. Although life expectancy in patients with ISCM is usually less than a year, directed therapy can significantly extend this generalization.

■ Intradural Extramedullary Tumors

Nerve Sheath Tumors

Nerve sheath tumors arise from nonneural supporting cells within spinal roots and peripheral nerves. Although they can appear anywhere along the course of a nerve once it has left the spinal cord, nerve sheath tumors are commonly found in association with nerve roots or very proximal peripheral nerves and thus may affect the spinal cord and adjacent nerve roots. Symptoms are usually referable to the afflicted nerve root but may also result from cord compression. Because nerve sheath tumors typically arise from the dorsal sensory root, they most commonly present with pain, which is usually radicular but can be vague and dysesthetic.[8,43] Peak presentation is in the fourth decade of life, and there has been no consistent anatomic or gender predilection across surgical series.[8]

On MRI, nerve sheath tumors are isointense to neural tissue and enhance uniformly with contrast, although encystation frequently confers a heterogeneous appearance[21] (**Fig. 39.4**). Depending on the exact point of origin and the size of tumor, nerve sheath tumors can be entirely intradural, extradural, or have both intradural and extradural components

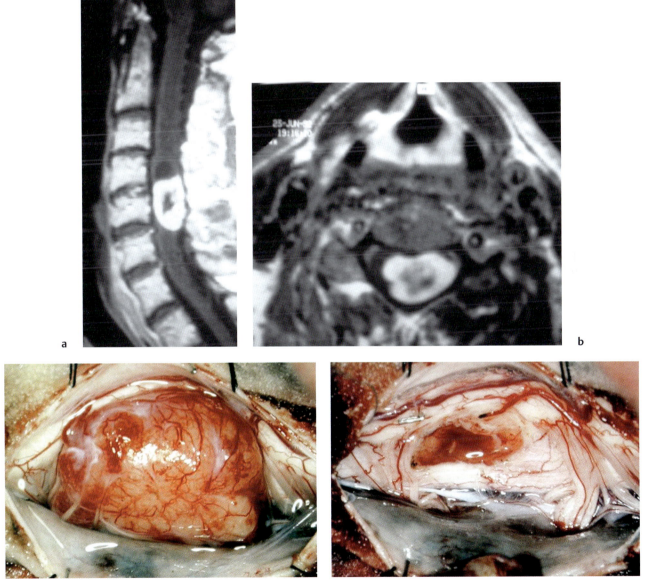

Fig. 39.4a–d (**a**) T1-weighted contrast-enhanced sagittal and (**b**) axial MRI scans of the cervical spine demonstrate a well-circumscribed, heterogeneously enhancing mass at the C5 level with severe spinal cord compression. Note the rostrally located syrinx on the sagittal image. (**c**) Operative photograph of the initial tumor exposure and (**d**) following tumor resection.

that evince a characteristic dumbbell shape. Because they often arise from the dorsal root, they typically lie dorsolateral to the cord. Lesions with a significant extradural presence will often erode bone over time and can displace important local anatomic structures, although these will always lie outside the tumor margin if the tumor is benign.

The overwhelming majority of nerve sheath tumors are benign, with schwannomas accounting for 85% and neurofibromas 15%.[8] Histologically, the salient distinguishing feature of a neurofibroma is the presence of axons admixed with tumor cells, whereas schwannomas grow tangentially to nerve fibers. Approximately 3% of these lesions are malignant nerve sheath tumors, as evidenced by a high mitotic index and spindle-shaped cells.

Neurofibromas are seen with increased frequency in association with neurofibromatosis type 1 (NF1); indeed, the presence of two or more neurofibromas or a single plexiform neurofibroma is considered pathognomonic for NF1. Schwannomas are seen in association with neurofibromatosis type 2 (NF2), and the presence of multiple schwannomas is pathognomonic for NF2. Compared with sporadic cases, patients with neurofibromatosis are much more likely to present with neurologic deficits than with pain. A diagnosis of neurofibromatosis should be considered in any patient who presents with a nerve sheath tumor, even though the majority of cases are sporadic.

Nerve sheath tumors are slow-growing lesions that can reach an impressive size before causing symptoms. When symptomatic, they should be removed surgically. For large dumbbell lesions, a surgical plan that addresses the entire tumor is required and may include surgeons from multiple disciplines. In general, spinal cord decompression should be the initial operative goal. Although an attempt to dissect the tumor from the nerve or nerve root of origin should be attempted, this is usually not possible. Fortunately, sacrifice of the nerve root of origin results in lasting functional deficits in only 2 to 4% of patients.[8,43,44] These patients potentially can be identified intraoperatively using neurostimulation.[45] Overall, surgical series report improvement in functional status in the majority of patients after 6 months, with pain as the most

reliable symptom to respond.[8,43] Accurate recurrence rates after surgery are difficult to assess because of a lack of studies with long-term follow-up. One study found 5-year recurrence rates of 10.7% in sporadic cases of spinal schwannoma and 39.2% in patients with NF2.[43] In the authors' experience, tumor recurrence for sporadic nerve sheath tumors usually occurs following subtotal resection of dumbbell tumors with paraspinal tumor extension beyond the surgical field or the inability to achieve a safe intradural marginal resection due to the proximity of the spinal cord or concern with injury to an important functional motor nerve of origin (e.g., C5-C8, L2-S1).

Meningiomas

Meningiomas are the second most common intradural, extramedullary spinal tumor after schwannomas. The female preponderance seen in intracranial meningiomas is even more pronounced in the spine, with surgical series reporting female/male ratios of 4:1[46] to as high as 9:1.[47] Spinal meningiomas are thought to arise from cells within arachnoid villi, found at highest density around nerve root exit sites. This formulation likely influences the finding that the majority of spinal meningiomas are intradural, extramedullary, lie lateral to the cord, and are most prevalent in the segment of the spine with the most nerve roots, the thoracic spine.[9,46–48] The thoracic predilection, as high as 82%,[9] and the paucity of lumbar tumors, as low as 2%,[48] is perhaps not completely explained by the density of cell of origin, and some authors have found a more even distribution of thoracic and cervical meningiomas in men.[42] Meningiomas peak in late middle age, are uncommon in young adults, and are very rare in children.

Most patients present with a slowly progressive level-appropriate myelopathy. Although the most common presenting symptom is pain, concomitant motor deficits are much more prevalent in patients with meningiomas than other kinds of tumors.[9,46,48]

On MRI, spinal meningiomas are isointense to neural tissue and homogeneously enhance with contrast administration. They are often obviously associated with the dura mater with the tumor mass compressing the spinal cord (**Fig. 39.5**). Less than 10% of the time, spinal meningiomas exhibit significant extradural extension, although they may be entirely extradural.[9,46] Rarely have intramedullary meningiomas been reported.

Histologically, the vast majority of spinal meningiomas are benign and fall into the same subtypes as seen intracranially. The psammomatous subtype, however, is far more prevalent in the spine and there is a suggestion in the literature that it is associated with less favorable neurologic outcomes after surgery. Younger patients are more likely to harbor the surgically recalcitrant angioblastic subtype, but true malignant meningiomas are exceedingly rare in the spine.[9]

The first line of therapy for spinal meningiomas is surgical resection, which usually results in a cure after GTMR. Subtotal resection is associated with en plaque morphology, malignant

---

Special Consideration

- Patients who present with multiple nerve sheath tumors should be evaluated for neurofibromatosis. Patients who present with a hemangioblastoma should be evaluated for von Hippel–Lindau disease, especially if surgery is contemplated because of the possible presence of a pheochromocytoma. The likelihood of these diagnoses dramatically increases with the presence of other associated lesions or a family history of the disease. Genetic testing is available for both disorders and should be pursued in conjunction with the consultation of a genetic counselor.

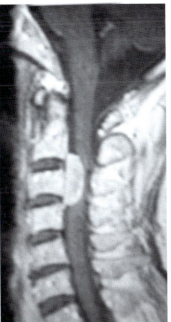

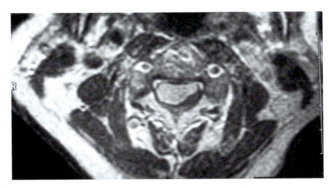

Fig. 39.5a–d (**a**) T1-weighted contrast-enhanced sagittal and (**b**) axial MRI scans demonstrate durally based tumor of the ventral spinal canal at the C3 level. (**c**) Intraoperative photograph following laminectomy and dural opening does not show the ventrally located tumor. (**d**) Following section of the dentate ligaments and gentle spinal cord rotation the tumor can now be clearly seen.

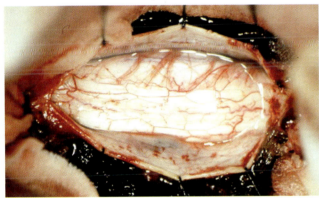

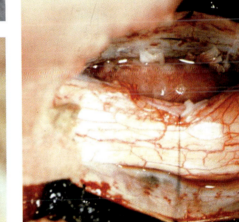

histological features, and anterior location.[9,46,48] Outcomes after resection are linked to preoperative neurologic condition, but improvements in neurologic condition are seen in the majority of patients. Surgical series report the reacquisition of ambulation in 80 to 90% of nonambulatory patients,[9,46–48] and one series reports complete neurologic recovery in 46% of paraplegic patients.[49]

Congenital Tumors

Dermoids, Epidermoids, Lipomas, and Teratomas

Congenital spinal tumors are thought to result from embryological errors during neural tube closure between the third and fifth week postconception. Either as a result of the dis-placement of cells with nonneural fates or the failure of properly positioned cells to receive the appropriate differentiation signals, these rare lesions grow slowly in association with neural tissue and usually present in early childhood, often in conjunction with spinal dysraphisms such as dermal sinus tracts. Depending on the potentiality and fate of the ectopic cells, tumors form that mimic cutaneous and subcutaneous tissues. Epidermoids are growths of keratinized squamous epithelium and some are thought to be seeded iatrogenically during lumbar puncture or surgical repair of myelomeningoceles. Dermoids contain sebaceous material and hair. Lipomas are ectopic fat deposits. Teratomas contain elements of all three embryological layers. The majority of congenital tumors occur in association with the conus and lumbar nerve roots.[12] Still, they may be entirely intramedullary and can occur throughout the neuraxis, although cervical lesions are exceedingly rare.[12] When involving the conus, leg pain and urinary incontinence are common presenting symptoms, but many are diagnosed in asymptomatic patients after the discovery of a sacral skin abnormality leads to imaging studies.

On MRI, congenital tumors are generally nonenhancing. Epidermoids are homogeneously hypointense to neural tissue on T1-weighted images and hyperintense on T2-weighted images. Dermoids and lipomas reflect lipid content, which appears hyperintense on both T1 and contemporary fast spin echo T2 sequences.[21]

When symptomatic, surgical resection is indicated, although total resection is sometimes limited by attachment of tumor capsule to neural elements. Because these are indolent lesions, disease control is often achieved, even with incomplete resection.

Conclusion

Spinal tumors reflect a range of histologies, the majority of which are benign and effectively treated with surgical excision. Pain symptoms usually precede neurologic deficits, and outcomes are optimized with an early diagnosis and timely surgical intervention. Adjuvant therapy is generally reserved for subtotally resected, recurrent, or disseminated tumors, with the majority of clinical experience involving radiotherapy.

Editor's Note

Tumors involving the spinal cord, or if located either completely intradurally or partially in the epidural space, are largely surgical problems. There are not a lot of pathological entities that occur in this location and most are primary central nervous system tumors. However, tumors involving the peripheral nervous system can also encroach upon the spinal cord via intradural or epidural compression. This is particularly true in the case of neurofibromatosis. Then again, there are numerous possibilities when these lesions are metastatic to the spinal axis with encroachment in the epidural space.

Because most of these lesions cause acute or subacute compression of the spinal cord, surgical intervention is typically necessary and for the most part these lesions can be radically, if not completely, resected with excellent surgical results, including gain of function, which can significantly affect the quality of life. Perhaps the most critical issue with these entities is that early detection takes place with good anatomic imaging and that the default mechanism is not just to treat with radiation therapy. We learn from randomized studies that have been done in the past that when neurologic deficits occur, the best action to take is to decompress the spinal cord surgically. (Berger)

References

1. Lunardi P, Missori P, Gagliardi FM, Fortuna A. Long-term results of the surgical treatment of spinal dermoid and epidermoid tumors. Neurosurgery 1989;25:860–864
2. Nadkarni TD, Rekate HL. Pediatric intramedullary spinal cord tumors. Critical review of the literature. Childs Nerv Syst 1999;15:17–28
3. Sonneland PR, Scheithauer BW, Onofrio BM. Myxopapillary ependymoma. A clinicopathologic and immunocytochemical study of 77 cases. Cancer 1985;56:883–893
4. Epstein FJ, Farmer JP, Freed D. Adult intramedullary spinal cord ependymomas: the result of surgery in 38 patients. J Neurosurg 1993;79:204–209
5. Jallo GI, Danish S, Velasquez L, Epstein F. Intramedullary low-grade astrocytomas: long-term outcome following radical surgery. J Neurooncol 2001;53:61–66
6. Mandigo C, Ogden FT, Angevine PD, McCormick PC. Intramedullary hemangioblastoma of the spinal cord. Neurosurgery 2009;65:1166–1177
7. Cohen AR, Wisoff JH, Allen JC, Epstein F. Malignant astrocytomas of the spinal cord. J Neurosurg 1989;70:50–54
8. Seppälä MT, Haltia MJ, Sankila RJ, Jääskeläinen JE, Heiskanen O. Long-term outcome after removal of spinal schwannoma: a clinicopathological study of 187 cases. J Neurosurg 1995;83:621–626
9. Solero CL, Fornari M, Giombini S, et al. Spinal meningiomas: review of 174 operated cases. Neurosurgery 1989;25:153–160
10. Roux FX, Nataf F, Pinaudeau M, Borne G, Devaux B, Meder JF. Intraspinal meningiomas: review of 54 cases with discussion of poor prognosis factors and modern therapeutic management. Surg Neurol 1996;46:458–463, discussion 463–464
11. Matson DD, Tachdjian MO. Intraspinal tumors in infants and children: review of 115 cases. Postgrad Med 1963;34:279–285
12. Takeuchi J, Ohta T, Kajikawa H. Congenital tumors of the spinal cord. In: Vinken PJ, Bruyn GW, Myrianthopoulos NC, eds. Handbook of Clinical Neurology, Vol 32. New York: North-Holland, 1978:xii, 588
13. Ogden AT, Feldstein NA, McCormick PC. Anterior approach to cervical intramedullary pilocytic astrocytoma. Case report. J Neurosurg Spine 2008;9:253–257
14. Angevine PD, Kellner C, Haque RM, McCormick PC. Surgical management of ventral intradural spinal lesions. J Neurosurg Spine 2011;15:28–37
15. Uribe JS, Dakwar E, Le TV, Christian G, Serrano S, Smith WD. Minimally invasive surgery treatment for thoracic spine tumor removal: a mini-open, lateral approach. Spine 2010;35(26, Suppl):S347–S354
16. Isaacson SR. Radiation therapy and the management of intramedullary spinal cord tumors. J Neurooncol 2000;47:231–238
17. Balmaceda C. Chemotherapy for intramedullary spinal cord tumors. J Neurooncol 2000;47:293–307
18. Veeravagu A, Lieberson RE, Mener A, et al. CyberKnife stereotactic radiosurgery for the treatment of intramedullary spinal cord metastases. J Clin Neurosci 2012;19:1273–1277
19. Sachdev S, Dodd RL, Chang SD, et al. Stereotactic radiosurgery yields long-term control for benign intradural, extramedullary spinal tumors. Neurosurgery 2011;69:533–539, discussion 539
20. Hanbali F, Fourney DR, Marmor E, et al. Spinal cord ependymoma: radical surgical resection and outcome. Neurosurgery 2002;51:1162–1172, discussion 1172–1174
21. Osborn AG. Diagnostic Neuroradiology. St. Louis: Mosby, 1994

22. Guidetti B, Mercuri S, Vagnozzi R. Long-term results of the surgical treatment of 129 intramedullary spinal gliomas. J Neurosurg 1981; 54:323–330

23. Lonjon M, Goh KY, Epstein FJ. Intramedullary spinal cord ependymomas in children: treatment, results and follow-up. Pediatr Neurosurg 1998;29:178–183

24. Shaw EG, Evans RG, Scheithauer BW, Ilstrup DM, Earle JD. Radiotherapeutic management of adult intraspinal ependymomas. Int J Radiat Oncol Biol Phys 1986;12:323–327

25. Schild SE, Nisi K, Scheithauer BW, et al. The results of radiotherapy for ependymomas: the Mayo Clinic experience. Int J Radiat Oncol Biol Phys 1998;42:953–958

26. Nazar GB, Hoffman HJ, Becker LE, Jenkin D, Humphreys RP, Hendrick EB. Infratentorial ependymomas in childhood: prognostic factors and treatment. J Neurosurg 1990;72:408–417

27. Chamberlain MC. Salvage chemotherapy for recurrent spinal cord ependymoma. Cancer 2002;95:997–1002

28. Chamberlain MC. Etoposide for recurrent spinal cord ependymoma. Neurology 2002;58:1310–1311

29. Helseth A, Mørk SJ. Primary intraspinal neoplasms in Norway, 1955 to 1986. A population-based survey of 467 patients. J Neurosurg 1989; 71:842–845

30. Santi M, Mena H, Wong K, Koeller K, Olsen C, Rushing EJ. Spinal cord malignant astrocytomas. Clinicopathologic features in 36 cases. Cancer 2003;98:554–561

31. Kim MS, Chung CK, Choe G, Kim IH, Kim HJ. Intramedullary spinal cord astrocytoma in adults: postoperative outcome. J Neurooncol 2001;52: 85–94

32. Bouffet E, Pierre-Kahn A, Marchal JC, et al. Prognostic factors in pediatric spinal cord astrocytoma. Cancer 1998;83:2391–2399

33. Shirato H, Kamada T, Hida K, et al. The role of radiotherapy in the management of spinal cord glioma. Int J Radiat Oncol Biol Phys 1995;33: 323–328

34. Linstadt DE, Wara WM, Leibel SA, Gutin PH, Wilson CB, Sheline GE. Postoperative radiotherapy of primary spinal cord tumors. Int J Radiat Oncol Biol Phys 1989;16:1397–1403

35. Allen JC, Aviner S, Yates AJ, et al; Children's Cancer Group. Treatment of high-grade spinal cord astrocytoma of childhood with "8-in-1" chemotherapy and radiotherapy: a pilot study of CCG-945. J Neurosurg 1998; 88:215–220

36. Lee DK, Choe WJ, Chung CK, Kim HJ. Spinal cord hemangioblastoma: surgical strategy and clinical outcome. J Neurooncol 2003;61:27–34

37. Lee JY, Dong SM, Park WS, et al. Loss of heterozygosity and somatic mutations of the VHL tumor suppressor gene in sporadic cerebellar hemangioblastomas. Cancer Res 1998;58:504–508

38. Xu QW, Bao WM, Mao RL, Yang GY. Magnetic resonance imaging and microsurgical treatment of intramedullary hemangioblastoma of the spinal cord. Neurosurgery 1994;35:671–675, discussion 675–676

39. Lonser RR, Weil RJ, Wanebo JE, DeVroom HL, Oldfield EH. Surgical management of spinal cord hemangioblastomas in patients with von Hippel-Lindau disease. J Neurosurg 2003;98:106–116

40. Lonser RR, Vortmeyer AO, Butman JA, et al. Edema is a precursor to central nervous system peritumoral cyst formation. Ann Neurol 2005; 58:392–399

41. Aiello LP, George DJ, Cahill MT, et al. Rapid and durable recovery of visual function in a patient with von Hippel-Lindau syndrome after systemic therapy with vascular endothelial growth factor receptor inhibitor su5416. Ophthalmology 2002;109:1745–1751

42. Schiff D, O'Neill BP. Intramedullary spinal cord metastases: clinical features and treatment outcome. Neurology 1996;47:906–912

43. Klekamp J, Samii M. Surgery of spinal nerve sheath tumors with special reference to neurofibromatosis. Neurosurgery 1998;42:279–289, discussion 289–290

44. Celli P. Treatment of relevant nerve roots involved in nerve sheath tumors: removal or preservation? Neurosurgery 2002;51:684–692, discussion 692

45. Lot G, George B. Cervical neuromas with extradural components: surgical management in a series of 57 patients. Neurosurgery 1997;41: 813–820, discussion 820–822

46. Klekamp J, Samii M. Surgical results for spinal meningiomas. Surg Neurol 1999;52:552–562

47. Levy WJ Jr, Bay J, Dohn D. Spinal cord meningioma. J Neurosurg 1982; 57:804–812

48. King AT, Sharr MM, Gullan RW, Bartlett JR. Spinal meningiomas: a 20-year review. Br J Neurosurg 1998;12:521–526

49. Haegelen C, Morandi X, Riffaud L, Amlashi SF, Leray E, Brassier G. Results of spinal meningioma surgery in patients with severe preoperative neurological deficits. Eur Spine J 2005;14:440–444

Spinal Column Tumors

Anick Nater, Frederick Vincent, and Michael G. Fehlings

Spinal tumors arise from all tissue types from which neoplastic changes could occur, including neural element, meninge, bone, cartilage, and muscle. This chapter addresses the clinical presentation, diagnosis, management, and outcomes of primary and secondary osseous neoplasms affecting the spine. Advances in evidence-based medicine and treatment options, especially with regard to surgical interventions, have initiated a paradigm shift in the management of both primary tumors, where treatment aims to cure, and secondary tumors, where surgery is now not only a palliative measure but also has increasingly been used for improving functional outcomes and quality of life.

■ Primary Tumors

Primary spinal tumors are rare, accounting for less than 5% of osseous tumors and 0.2% of all cancers.[1] They are classified as benign (**Table 40.1**) and malignant (**Table 40.2**). Both benign and malignant tumors may be associated with spinal instability and deformity (**Table 40.3**). They also typically present as persistent local back pain, often occurring at night. Age and location provide provide central clues to help physician distinguish between spinal benign and malignant tumors. While over 65% of the pediatric spinal tumors are benign, the same proportion of lesion is malignant in adults. In addition, 75% of the neoplasms located in the vertebral body are malignant, but 65% of those involving the posterior elements are benign.[2]

Benign spinal tumors can be difficult to diagnose; they may be incidental findings, and they tend to affect young adults. Although they can be associated with radiating radicular symptoms in the lower extremities, they seldom cause focal neurologic deficits as a result of spinal cord or nerve root compression.

Malignant osseous tumors commonly present with unremitting axial back pain that often does not respond well to analgesics. They normally affect older adults, tend to progress more rapidly, and recur more often. They are also associated with higher morbidity, including more risk of neurologic deficits and mortality. In fact, they have a greater propensity (1) to create pathological fractures; (2) invade and destroy adjacent structures, which can compromise the spinal cord, nerves, or blood vessels; and (3) metastasize to other organs.

Clinical evaluation of primary spinal tumors includes a thorough history and physical examination and adequate imaging [including plain X-rays, computed tomography (CT), and magnetic resonance imaging (MRI)]. CT-guided needle biopsy is often indicated to guide therapy, and bone scans may be required to search for other bone lesions. CT of the spine is the best modality to characterize bony involvement, quality, and anatomy, which can be very valuable for surgical planning.[6]

Staging

Enneking and Weinstein-Boriani-Biagini (WBB) classification systems have been used for primary spinal tumors. Boriani et al modified the original Enneking staging system to classify benign and malignant primary spinal tumors. This classification divides benign tumors into three stages (SI, SII, and SIII) and malignant spinal tumors into six stages (IA, IB, IIA, IIB, IIIA, and IIIB) based on surgical grade (G, G1, G2), local extent (T, T1, T2), and presence or absence of metastasis (M0, M1) (**Table 40.4**). The stage of the tumor dictates the extent of surgical resection and margins.[2-5]

Primary benign spinal tumors in the SI (latent/inactive) stage are either not growing or doing so extremely slowly; have a true capsule, and thus well-defined margins; and are generally asymptomatic. These tumors include incidental vertebral body hemangioma, occurring in about 10% of the population. Unless palliative intracapsular excision is required for decompression or stabilization, SI tumors are typically managed conservatively, with reassurance and observation.[2,5]

SII benign lesions (active) are bordered with a thin/pseudocapsule surrounded by a layer of host reactive tissue and confined to the vertebral osseous elements; bone scans are often positive. They are slow-growing tumors and cause mild symptoms. Benign osteoblastomas may present as such and typically appear as a radiolucent nidus (> 20 mm) surrounded by a sclerotic rim and located in the posterior elements of the

Pearls

- Osteoid osteoma/osteoblastoma presents as painful scoliosis in about 50% of children or young adults, which typically disappears after the tumor is completely surgically excised.
- Serum protein and immune electrophoresis should be done in all adult patients with pathological vertebral compression fracture with no obvious primary malignancy to rule out multiple myeloma/plasmocytoma.

Table 40.1 Benign Primary Spinal Tumors (alphabetical order)

Tumor Type	Characteristics
Aneurysmal bone cyst	Consist of blood-filled cavity; often occur in patients in 20s; slow, gradual onset of back pain; possible palpable mass; lytic and expansile lesions in thoracolumbar area often in posterior elements, in multiple continuous levels
Eosinophilic granuloma	Results from Langerhans' cell histiocytosis; usually males < 10 years old; more often in vertebral body of thoracic spine; may be associated with systemic involvement (Hand-Schüller-Christian or Letterer-Siwe disease)
Giant cell tumor	Most often in vertebral body; 20–50 years of age; progressive back pain; expansile, radiolucent, "soap-bubble" appearance; vascular; often locally aggressive with bony destruction; en bloc excision with wide margins
Hemangioma	Most common benign spinal tumor; Incidence increases with age; Multiple ~ 30% of the time; Typically incidental finding ~10% of patients; Often asymptomatic vascular intraosseous lesions in thoracolumbar area
Neurofibroma	Derived from Schwann cells; most frequent in cervical and thoracic areas; occur in isolation or associated with neurofibromatosis; dumbbell-shaped
Osteoblastoma	Similar to osteoid osteoma, but larger diameter (> 20 mm), histologically, and clinically more aggressive; surgically managed with en bloc resection
Osteochondroma	Most frequent in posterior element; often in cervical area (C2), because of osteocartilaginous proliferation at a growth plate
Osteoid osteoma	Small bone-forming tumor (15–20 mm); ~10% primary bone tumors; ~10% occur in vertebrae, primarily in posterior elements; progressive back pain, typically at night; males more affected than females; most common cause painful scoliosis in adolescent population; radiolucent nidus with sclerotic rim; typically respond to anti-inflammatory medication; surgery is curative

Table 40.2 Malignant Primary Spinal Tumors (alphabetical order)

Tumor Type	Characteristics
Chondrosarcoma	Often males in 40s; tumor divided into low, intermediate, and high grades; destructive lesion often with paraspinal calcified mass causing axial pain with neurologic deficits
Chordoma	Often slow growing, locally invasive, not likely to metastasize; > 40 years old; often cranial or sacral origin; median survival is 50 months
Ewing's sarcoma	Typically males in 20s; often lytic, sacral, poorly delineated from normal bone lesion that invades surrounding tissues; chemotherapy ± radiation
Lymphoma	"Epidural lymphoma," which is a tumor within the epidural space that can compress the spinal cord without obvious bony involvement; treatment involves chemotherapy
Malignant fibrous histiocytoma	Osteolytic destruction of vertebrae and invasion of paraspinal structures at multiple levels, can cause neurologic deficits; tends to recur and metastasize
Osteosarcoma	Peak occurrence during onset of puberty; mostly osteoblastic; when metastasis present, most often to lungs; 18% survival rate at 5 years
Plasmocytoma/multiple myeloma	Most frequent primary malignant lesion of spine; osteolytic bone lesion(s) or diffuse osteoporosis ± fractures; high serum proteins and Bence Jones proteins in urine, renal dysfunction, high erythrocyte sedimentation rate

Table 40.3 Clinical Features of Benign and Malignant Primary Spinal Tumors

Clinical Features	Benign	Malignant
Age	Young adults (20–30 years)	Middle-aged adults (40–60 years)
Axial spinal pain, often occurring at night	Common (75%)	Common (95%) Severity progresses more rapidly than with benign tumors
Neurological deficits	20%	55%
Scoliosis/Spinal deformity	May occur	May occur
Vertebral body involvement	40%	80%

Table 40.4 Enneking Staging Classification for Primary Benign and Malignant Spinal Tumors

Tumor	Stage and G; T; M[a]	Features	Management
Benign			
	SI: latent/ inactive G0; T0; M0	Not growing or very slow growing; true capsule; few if any symptoms	Observation Intracapsular excision
	SII: active G0; T0; M0	Slow growing; thin capsule; mild symptoms	Extracapsular/intralesional excision
	SIII: aggressive G0; T1/2; M0/1	Rapidly growing; invades neighboring compartments	Marginal en bloc resection ± adjuvants
Malignant			
	Low grade: IA: G1; T0; M0 IIB: G1; T1; M0	Pseudocapsule with tumor foci: Confined to the vertebra Paravertebral invasion	Wide en bloc resection with adjuvant radiation
	High grade II: IIA: G2; T1; M0 IIB: G2; T2; M0	No pseudocapsule, seeding: Intracompartmental Invasion, pathological fracture	Wide en bloc resection with effective adjuvants radiation ± chemotherapy
	High grade III IIIA/B G1/2; T0/1/2; M0/1	Metastatic intra (IIIA) / extra (IIIB): Compartmental	Typically palliation; wide en bloc resection with effective adjuvants

[a] S: stage; G: surgical grade (G0: benign lesion; G1: low-grade malignant lesion; G2: high-grade malignant lesion); T: local extent (T0: benign lesion, intracompartmental; T1: benign aggressive or malignant, intracompartmental; T2: benign aggressive or malignant, extracompartmental invasion); M: metastasis (M0: no metastasis; M1: regional or distant metastasis).

spine. They are generally managed by intralesional excision or curettage with low reported recurrence rates.[2,5]

SIII tumors (aggressive) have a very thin, incomplete, or absent capsule, often associated with a reactive and hypervascularized pseudocapsule. They are rapidly growing and invade neighboring compartments. Bone scans on this type of tumor are positive. Giant cell tumors (**Fig. 40.1**) and aneurysmal bone cysts are examples of these lesions. Management involves aggressive marginal en bloc resection. Adjuvant treatments, such as preoperative embolization, are often needed.[2,5] The benefits of adjuvant radiation in cases of incomplete resection and local recurrence or to prevent delayed local recurrence must be weighed against the risk of developing radiation-induced myelopathy, spinal deformity, and malignant conversion (sarcomatous degeneration).[6]

Low-grade malignant spinal tumors (I) are subdivided into those that are confined to the vertebra (stage IA) and those that invade paravertebral compartments (stage IB). They have no true capsule, but a thick pseudocapsule of reactive tissue containing islands of tumor tissue. Despite safe optimal wide en bloc resection, which is sometimes not feasible, residual active tumor foci might be left behind; thus, postoperative radiotherapy is recommended.[2,5]

Special Consideration

- In primary spine tumors, the Enneking and Weinstein-Boriani-Biagini staging classification systems are very useful in assisting surgical staging and operative planning.

High-grade stage IIA (intracompartmental confined) and IIB (spread beyond the vertebral compartment) have such rapid growth that there is no host-reactive tissue forming around the lesion; thus, there is no pseudocapsule forming. These tumors are constantly seeding with neoplastic nodules (satellites); they are often associated with neoplastic nodules occurring at some distance from the main tumor mass (skip metastases). When those neoplastic seedings create distant metastasis, they are stage IIIA (intracompartmental confined lesion of origin) and IIIB (extracompartmental lesion of origin). These radiolucent high-grade lesions are often associated with pathological fractures and extensive invasion of adjacent compartments, such as the epidural space, leading to important neurologic deficits. High-grade stage II tumors are managed with wide en bloc resection and adjuvant therapies, including radiation and chemotherapy based on the histological type of the tumor, for local control and prevention of distant spread.[2,5] A recent study reported that patients who underwent a surgical resection for a primary chordoma, chondrosarcoma, Ewing's sarcoma, or osteosarcoma had longer overall survival independently of patient age, extent of local spread, or location.[7] High-grade stage III tumors are typically treated palliatively.[5]

The Enneking staging system has several limitations. Because it was originally based on the natural evolution of mesenchymal musculoskeletal appendicular tumors, it is not applicable to tumors originating in the marrow or reticuloendothelial system, including lymphoma, multiple myeloma/plasmocytoma, Ewing's sarcoma, and other round cell neoplasms. Also, the Enneking classification does not take into account the dimension of the primary tumor. The size of a

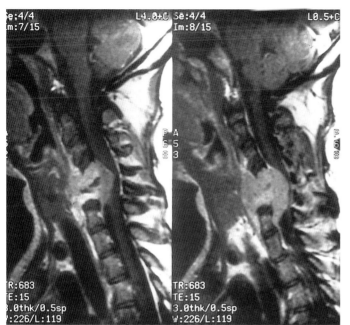

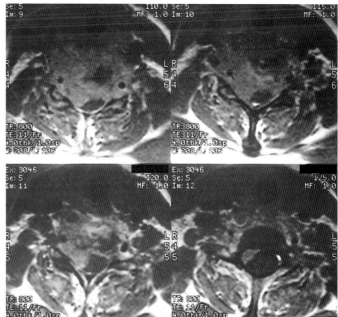

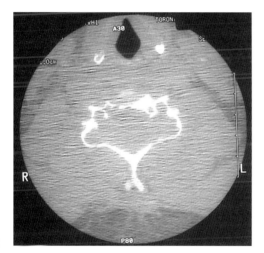

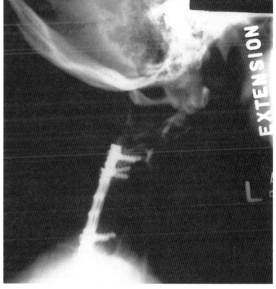

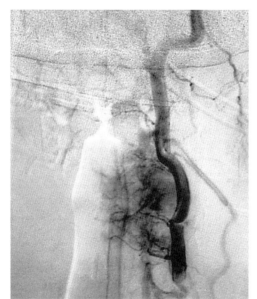

Fig. 40.1a–e This 24-year-old woman presented with severe neck pain and progressive quadriparesis. (**a**) Sagittal and (**b**) axial magnetic resonance imaging (MRI) scans show extensive involvement of C4 and C5 with severe cord compression and extension into both foramina transversaria. (**c**) The axial computed tomography (CT) scan at C4 shows the characteristic "soap bubble" involvement of the anterior and posterior elements. (**d**) A vertebral angiogram shows the highly vascular nature of the tumor. Because of the proximity of the spinal cord blood supply to the tumor feeding vessels, it was not possible to embolize the lesion. (**e**) The involvement of both pedicles and vertebral arteries precluded an en bloc resection. As an alternative, the patient underwent a combined anteroposterior resection of the lesions with anterior strut grafting and posterior lateral mass plating. At 6 months postoperatively (once fusion had been confirmed), the patient underwent adjuvant radiotherapy. The patient remained free of recurrence at 10 years postoperative follow-up.

tumor is often a significant prognostic factor, with larger lesions being more likely to metastasize. Lastly, this system does not consider (1) the presence of the epidural space as a continuous compartment, (2) the need for maintaining or restoring spinal stability, and (3) the close proximity of crucial structures, notably the spinal cord and nerve roots, which, if sacrificed, lead to important neurologic deficits; consequently, honoring Enneking surgical margins can be difficult.[3-5]

Treatment

Surgery

The WBB classification was developed to assist decision making with respect to feasible surgical margins in spinal oncological surgery. In this system, the involvement of the vertebra, neural canal, and surrounding soft tissues are determined based on the axial plane, in terms of 12 radiating zones numbered 1 to 12 in a clockwise fashion and of five concentric tissue layers identified as A to E from the paravertebral extraosseous region to the dura, which relate to the compartments

of tissue penetration involved (**Fig. 40.2**). The longitudinal extent of the tumor is identified as the number of vertebrae involved. The WBB system promotes optimal surgical tumor margins without violating the spinal cord. Therefore, it is a helpful surgical planning tool which helps determine the type of resection as well as its feasibility.[8]

In primary spinal tumors, the Enneking and WBB staging classification systems are key tools that assist with surgical staging and operative planning. Moreover, these classification systems show near-perfect intraobserver and moderate interobserver reliability.[3,5] Due to the low incidence of primary osseous spine tumors and consequently the lack of clinical experience and high-quality evidence-based research, there is no validated oncological treatment management protocol. Fisher et al[9] reported that using the surgical principles of the Enneking classification, originally introduced for the management of appendicular musculoskeletal tumors, is associated with a significant decrease in local recurrence and mortality. Indeed, the Enneking system helps avoid entering the tumor and an intralesional or piecemeal removal. Thus, it favors removing the tumor as one whole piece (en bloc) with a margin along the pseudocapsule of the tumor (marginal resection) or with a margin of normal tissue around the tumor (wide resection).[9]

Because residual tumor tissue is the single most important predictor of local recurrence, the goal of marginal or wide en bloc resection is to prevent tumor cell contamination during surgical removal of the primary tumor and ensure total tumor

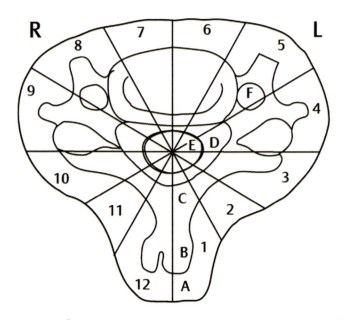

Cervical spine

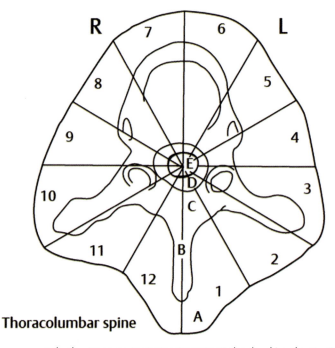

Thoracolumbar spine

Fig. 40.2 The Weinstein-Boriani-Biagini surgical staging system. On the axial plane of the cervical and thoracolumbar spine, the radiating zones numbered 1 to 12 identify the transverse extension of the vertebral lesion, and the five concentric layers A to E described the paravertebral extraosseous compartments to the dural involvement; in the cervical spine, the layer F indicates the involvement of the vertebral artery. The number of vertebral bodies involved determined the longitudinal extension of the tumor.

resection.[10] It has been suggested that better local control, prognosis, and quality of life justifies marginal or wide en bloc resection in the management of aggressive benign and low-grade malignant primary spine tumors in spite of the associated significant morbidity.[11] Indeed, spinal en bloc resections may involve sacrificing relevant structures such as the nerve roots and blood vessels, thus increasing the morbidity and compromising neurologic function.

Multiple surgical techniques have been described in the literature to achieve en bloc resection in primary osseous spinal neoplasms. A staged approach has been described as an excellent option (**Fig. 40.3**).[12] The initial stage implies placing posterior spinal instrumentation and performing laminectomies, rib head resections, corpectomies, and diskectomies in order to isolate the tumor from the spine. Then, the second stage involves the marginal or wide en bloc resection encasing the tumor using a combined anterior and posterior approach, followed by reconstruction and stabilization of the anterior spinal column.

Pitfall

- Spinal oncological en bloc resections are high-risk and demanding interventions that should be performed in properly equipped centers by experienced surgeons.

Spinal oncological en bloc resections are high-risk and demanding interventions, which should be performed in tertiary care centers by experienced surgeons. In addition, patients should be evaluated by a multidisciplinary team involving spine surgeons, radiologists, radiation and medical oncologists, and pathologists. Management decisions should include careful consideration of tumor size, histology, neurologic deficits, patient's age and medical status, as well as realistic long-term goals and expectations. Increasing age, the presence of metastasis, and more extensive tumor invasion have been identified as independent factors associated with poor survival in patients with primary malignant osseous tumors, specifically

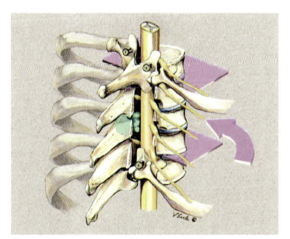
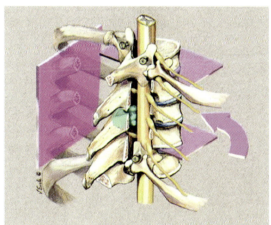
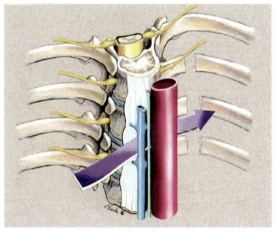
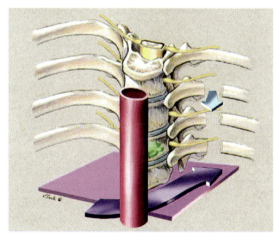

Fig. 40.3a–f Graphic depiction of the surgical technique for en bloc resection. (**a**) Posterior isolation of the tumor is initiated by performing multiple unilateral laminectomies. The upper and lower margins of the resection are defined through diskectomies. (**b**) Multiple rib head resection and ligation of roots allowed further posterior isolation of the tumor. (**c**) Anterior isolation of the tumor by dissecting the great vessels from the anterior longitudinal ligament of the vertebrae to be resected. (**d**) Simultaneous anterior and posterior dissection aimed at delivering the tumor with wide margins through the anterior surgical incision. (*continued on next page*)

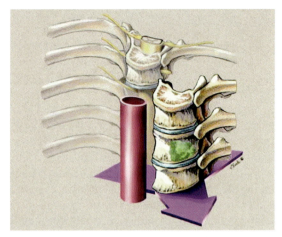
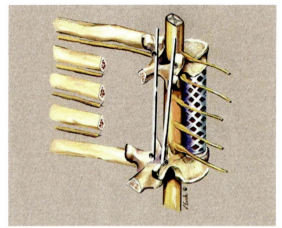

e

f

Fig. 40.3a–f (*continued*) (**e**) Anterior removal of the tumor with wide margins. (**f**) Titanium mesh cage reconstruction of the resulting defect in the spinal column after en bloc resection of the tumor.

(From Fisher CG, Keynan O, Boyd MC, Dvorak MF. The surgical management of primary tumors of the spine. Spine 2005;30: 1899–1908. Reproduced with permission.)

osteosarcomas, chondrosarcomas, and chordomas.[13] McGirt et al[13] have proposed a five-grade system in which higher scores are closely correlated with decreased survival (**Table 40.5**). Although this system is still pending validation, it could potentially assist with survival prognostication and consequently guide the aggressiveness of the treatment strategy proposed.

Stereotactic Radiosurgery

Stereotactic radiosurgery (SRS) entails radiating a highly specific target volume under image guidance with a high dose per fraction, sparing adjacent nontumor tissue. Its usage in the treatment of intracranial and extracranial tumors is blooming as an adjunct to surgery, fractioned radiotherapy, and chemotherapy, as well as being a primary treatment option, with good target localization and delineation from adjacent structures. The well-established role of SRS in the treatment of intracranial metastatic lesions is now extended to both primary and metastatic spinal osseous neoplasms, optimizing local control and pain relief.[14-16]

Although excisional surgery is the mainstay treatment of primary spinal bone tumors, open surgery can be difficult or risky to perform in some patients due to advanced age, medical comorbidities, anatomic location or multiple locations of the tumor, recurrent tumor after an open resection, or location in an area to which external beam radiation has already been applied. Therefore, patients with well-circumscribed lesions, relatively little direct compression on the spinal cord,

Patient Selection for Stereotactic Radiosurgery

- Well-circumscribed lesions
- Minimal spinal cord compromise
- Previously irradiated lesions precluding further external beam irradiation
- Recurrent surgical lesions
- Lesions requiring difficult surgical approaches
- Relatively short life expectancy as an exclusion criterion for open surgical intervention
- Significant medical comorbidities precluding open surgical intervention
- Lesions not requiring open spinal stabilization techniques

(Modified with permission from Gerszten PC, Ozhasoglu C, Burton S, et al. CyberKnife frameless stereotactic radiosurgery for spinal lesions: clinical experience in 125 cases. Neurosurgery 2004;55:89–98.)

lesions not requiring open surgery for spinal stabilization, and relatively short life expectancy might benefit from SRS.[14-16]

■ Metastatic Tumors

Metastatic osseous tumors are by far the most common tumor affecting the spinal column; they are about 25 times more frequent than primary bone cancers.[17] Aging of the popu-

Table 40.5 McGirt Cumulative Grading Score

	0 point	1 point	2 points	3 points
Age (years)		< 30	30–65	> 65
Tumor invasion	Limited to periosteum	Extends to adjacent tissue	Metastasis	

lation and advances in diagnostic and treatment options are increasing the number of primary cancer survivors; indeed, both the prevalence and the incidence of cancer are increasing.[18] Consequently, the incidence of metastatic spine cancer is also expected to rise.

Although metastatic bone disease rarely causes death directly, it is associated with shorter life expectancy and significant morbidity, such as pain, fractures, hypercalcemia, and neurologic deficits resulting from spinal cord or nerve root compression and damage.[17,19,20] Consequently, quality of life may be dramatically affected. Primary tumor type influences the patient's prognosis. The median survival in patients with bone metastases ranges from a few months for lung cancer to several years for breast or prostate cancer.[17,20] Metastatic epidural spinal cord compression (MESCC) is an oncological emergency that requires early diagnosis and expedited treatment.

Epidemiology

After the lungs and the liver, bones are the third most common site for cancer metastasis, with the spinal column being the most frequent skeletal location affected.[17,19] Not all bone metastases are clinically significant; 30 to 90% of patients who die from cancer are found to have bone metastasis at autopsy.[19,20] However, the actual incidence of bone metastasis is impossible to report. Peak incidence of cancer and spinal metastases are in patients 40 to 65 years of age and most often result from prostate, breast, kidney, lung, and thyroid primary cancers. Secondary to the high prevalence of prostate, breast, and lung cancer, they account for over 50% of all bone metastases.[19] Although the posterior aspect of the vertebral body is usually the first site of spine metastasis, changes in the pedicles are detected earliest on plain X-rays. Thus, if the pedicles are affected, the vertebral body is definitively involved.[17,20] The higher the relative bone mass and blood flow, the greater the likelihood to develop bone metastasis. Consequently, spinal metastases occur more commonly in the thoracic (60–70%), then the lumbar (20–25%), and finally the cervical (5–10%) and sacral (5–10%) segments.[19] More than 50% of patients have lesions at multiple levels, of which 10 to 38% are noncontiguous.[17]

Symptomatic spinal bone metastasis (i.e., MESCC) occurs in approximately 5 to 10% of all cancer patients, of whom 50% will need treatment.[19] Steroids, radiation therapy (RT), surgery, and chemotherapy are the principal treatment options to achieve better pain and local tumor control, obtain mechanical stability, and maintain, preserve, or improve neurologic functions as well as quality of life. A multidisciplinary team, involving a medical oncologist, radiation oncologist, radiolo-

gist, and surgeon, is required to establish the optimal treatment plan. Although RT remains the mainstay of treatment for most cancer patients with spinal metastasis, advances in surgical techniques have significantly improved surgical outcomes in this challenging population.[19,21]

Pathophysiology

Metastatic bone tumors are thought to result from three factors: metastasis pathway, tissue receptivity to tumor cells, and intrinsic features of tumor cells.[20] The first factor, metastasis pathway, implies several different routes by which a primary cancer can spread to another location, such as hematogenous (venous and arterial), direct invasion, cerebrospinal fluid, and even, perhaps, lymphatic seeding, which is not well understood. Direct arterial embolization of tumor cells with affinity for spine bone marrow is thought to be the main process of spinal metastasis.[22] In addition, the venous route is considered an important metastasis pathway. Changes in intrathoracic or intra-abdominal pressure can cause venous reflux from the caval, portal, azygous, intercostal, pulmonary, and renal venous systems to the vertebral and spinal veins, as well as to the Batson valveless venous plexus.[17,19,20] Because the azygous veins draining the breast connect to the Batson plexus of the thoracic spine and the prostatic veins communicate with the pelvic plexus in the lumbosacral region, breast and prostate cancers often metastasize to the thoracic and lumbosacral spine, respectively.[17,20] In addition, tumor cells, especially from lung cancers, can spread to the well-supplied vertebral bodies via the arterial blood system.[17,19,20] The hematogenous (venous and arterial) pathway leads to deposition of tumor cells at multiple spinal locations.[19,20]

Less frequently, direct extension of a thoracic, abdominal, or pelvic primary cancer can create symptomatic spinal metastases.[19] Tumor cells can also spread to the spine or spinal cord through cerebrospinal fluid seeding, which can notably occur after a cerebral or cerebellar primary tumor surgery.[19] Similarly to the hematogenous pathway, cerebrospinal fluid seeding often results in multicentric metastatic lesions.[19]

The second factor is tissue receptivity to tumor cells. The "seed and soil" theory hypothesizes that the bone marrow of the vertebral bodies constitutes a suitable environment to support tumor cell implantation and proliferation.[17,20]

The third factor is the intrinsic characteristics of tumor cells. These biochemical features of the primary tumor promote survival and growth of tumor cells in the spine. For example, breast cancer cells secrete prostaglandin and osteoclast-activating factors stimulating bone resorption leading to osteoblastic spinal metastasis.[17,20]

Metastatic epidural spinal cord compression occurs when (1) a vertebral body mass extends into the epidural space; or (2) a vertebral body fracture dislocates bony fragments into the epidural space. More rarely, MESCC results from a mass protruding from the vertebral foramen from the paraspinal region.[20,22]

In animal studies, MESCC is associated with white matter and axonal swelling, which can lead to white matter necrosis and gliosis. Changes in white matter depend on how fast MESCC occurs: slow development leads to venous congestion and white matter vasogenic edema, usually creating reversible neurologic deficits if the pressure on the spinal cord is relieved rapidly. However, fast development may impede arterial blood flow, resulting in ischemia and spinal cord infarction, which is associated with irreversible neurologic deficits.[20,22]

Clinical Presentation and Diagnosis

Metastatic spinal disease may present with a myriad of symptoms, including signs of systemic disease such as weight loss, anorexia, asthenia, and night sweats.[10] Early diagnosis of spinal metastasis is essential because the neurologic status at presentation is a crucial factor in predicting functional outcome after initiating treatment.[21] Back pain is the most common presenting symptom of spinal metastasis, often preceding the onset of neurologic symptoms by weeks or months, and occurs in 90% of patient with MESCC.[19,20] Any patient with a known history of cancer who presents with new onset of back pain or neurologic symptoms should be investigated to rule out spinal metastasis.[19]

Spinal metastasis is typically associated with three types of back pain: tumor related, mechanical, and radicular, arising alone or in combination.[19] Tumor-related back pain probably results from inflammatory mediators or periosteal stretching of the vertebral body due to tumor growth, which increases with the distention of the epidural venous plexus and lengthening of the spine. Therefore, this deep aching pain worsens when patients lie down and with Valsalva. It thus primarily occurs at night or early in the morning. In addition, this pain may be elicited by palpation or percussion of the spinous processes. It usually responds to anti-inflammatory drugs and low doses of corticosteroids, radiation, and surgery. Recurrence of the pain may indicate local tumor recurrence.[19,21] Structural abnormalities of the spine give rise to mechanical back pain, which is associated with movement, and thus varies with position and activities. It might be exacerbated by sitting or standing, which increase the axial loading on the spine. Corticosteroid and narcotics are often ineffective for mechanical back pain, but stabilization of the spine via bracing or surgical fixation can help.[19,20] On the other hand, radicular pain results from compression or irritation of nerve roots as they exit the spine by the tumor itself or bony elements due to pathological fracture. It is a sharp, shooting, or stabbing pain that tends to respect a dermatomal distribution.[18,20]

Neurologic symptoms often begin with radiculopathy followed by myelopathy. In MESCC, radiculopathy initially typically leads to motor dysfunction. In the 1990s, 50% of patients presenting with MESCC were not ambulatory. Nowadays, with physicians having a higher index of suspicion and better diag-

Special Consideration

- Nearly half of patient with a known history of cancer may present with clinical symptoms of MESCC caused by other etiologies, including various degenerative spinal disorders, paraneoplastic syndromes, radiation myelopathy, or complications of chemotherapy.

nostic imaging, more than 60% of patients presenting with MESCC are ambulatory. Most patients with MESCC also have sensory and autonomic disturbances, which most often involve bladder dysfunction (urinary retention). Bladder and bowel dysfunction arise relatively late and are typically associated with poor functional outcome after radiotherapy alone.[22]

Imaging Studies

Plain spinal radiographs are often the first test to evaluate patients complaining of new-onset back pain. They are useful in screening for blastic or lytic lesion, fractures, spinal deformities, and extensive masses.[19,21] Anteroposterior (AP) views may demonstrate pedicle erosion (the "winking owl" sign) or evidence of a paraspinal mass (paraspinal soft tissue shadow).[20] In addition, dynamic X-rays can be useful in assessing the stability of the spine.[21] However, plain radiographs are overall a poor screening test for metastases. In fact, most metastatic tumors are lytic in nature, infiltrating the bone marrow of the vertebral body without cortical bone involvement, and radiolucent defect becomes apparent only when about 50% of the vertebral body is destroyed.[19,21] Following surgery, plain radiographs are ideal to assess spinal alignment and integrity of instrumental construct.[21]

Although myelography has been largely supplanted by MRI, it is still sometimes used for patients with contraindication to MRI (e.g., a pacemaker).[20,22] MRI is the imaging modality with the greatest sensitivity and specificity for spinal metastasis, allowing excellent delineation of the location and extent of MESCC.[19,21,22] Although short tau inversion recovery (STIR) images may be the most sensitive screening modality for tumor, with enhanced contrast between the lipid marrow (hypointense) and tumor (hyperintense),[19,21] it provides less anatomic detail than do T1 and fast spin echo T2 sequences.[21]

In addition, the clinical and MRI features of MESCC can help distinguished from vertebral osteomyelitis.[22] In fact, infection often involves the disk space and end plate, which is atypical for tumors.[21]

Computed tomography (CT) scan provides complementary information to MRI, presenting highly detailed images of the spinal osseous anatomy, which not only delineate the extent of bone destruction and spinal instability, but also assist surgical planning of the approach and the extent of instrumentation. Moreover, CT-guided needle biopsy is an option to consider in patients with a spinal column tumor but no known primary tumor. It is important to acknowledge that this technique can yield nondiagnostic results in as many as 25% of cases. A closed, CT-guided biopsy is not indicated in patients with a known history of metastatic spinal cancer or when there is rapid neurologic deterioration.

Computed tomography angiography (CTA) or spinal angiography is beneficial in identifying the source of arterial blood supply to the cord. Determining the level of major radiculomedullary vessels, including the artery of Adamkiewicz, may be important in surgical planning for tumors in the lower thoracic and thoracolumbar spine, particularly if a far lateral extracavitary approach is used.

Another use of spinal angiography can be therapeutic. Surgical treatment of spinal metastases is often impeded by significant blood loss. Renal cell carcinoma, melanoma, and thyroid carcinoma are particularly vascular, and intraoperative bleeding from these tumors may limit the extent of surgical resection and cause significant morbidity. Preoperative embolization allows greater resection and a reduction in transfusion of blood products and its associated risks.

Bone scans (nuclear scintigraphy) rely on an osteoblastic mechanism or bone deposition to detect spinal metastases. They are relatively sensitive in early detection of pathology, but generally lack specificity. In fact, fractures, degenerative disease, and benign disorders of the spine, such as hemangioma, may be positive. Also, they are relatively insensitive to multiple myeloma and tumors confined to the bone marrow.

Classification

Based on anatomic location, metastatic spinal tumors are classically characterized as extradural, intradural-extramedullary, and intramedullary. The great majority of metastatic spinal tumors are extramedullary, which mainly extend from the vertebral body with various degrees of posterior element involvement. Intradural-extramedullary and intramedullary metastatic lesions are rare and often result from cerebrospinal fluid seeding.[19]

Management of MESCC aims to provide the least invasive treatment to maintain or restore neurologic functions and spinal stability, as well as to reduce pain and preserve or improve quality of life. Factors that influence treatment decisions for MESCC include spinal cord or nerve root compression resulting in myelopathy or motor radiculopathy; the patient's functional activity and disability status; tumor histology and radiosensitivity; spinal stability; extent of systemic disease; medical comorbidities; and patient's personal preferences.

Several scoring systems have been developed to assist treatment decision making. The Tokuhashi score, initially published in 1990 and revised in 2005, is a preoperative prediction of survival tool in patients with MESCC. It relies on six parameters generating a total score from 0 to 15 points; higher scores are associated with longer life expectancy. Overall, surgery is not indicated for patients with survival prognosis of 6 months or less (total score of 8 or less), who had poor general status or rapid progression of neurologic function and who responded well to either oral analgesic or radiotherapy (**Tables 40.6** and **40.7**).

The Tomita et al[23] classification system guides surgical strategies based on three prognostic factors: tumor grade, visceral metastases, and bone metastases. It provides a prognostic score, which determines the treatment goal and consequently the recommended surgical option. The total score may range from 2 to 10, where a score of 10 represents the worse prognosis (**Table 40.8**).

Bilsky et al[24] validated a 6-point grading system to describe epidural spinal cord compression based on axial T2-weighted MRI (**Fig. 40.4**). This classification system is particularly relevant to help identify stereotactic radiosurgery and surgical candidates. Indeed, in grade 1a and 1b, there is a distance of 1 to 2 mm between the spinal cord and the tumor, allowing for less potential cytotoxic consequences of radiation than with grade 1c, which abuts the spinal cord. Furthermore, high-grade MESCC is often regarded as an indication for surgical treatment.

Spinal instability is an important indication for a surgical intervention. The Spinal Instability in Neoplastic Score (SINS) is a new classification system that not only assists physicians identifying patients with metastatic spinal disease who require a surgical consultation, but also guides surgeons choosing the most appropriate surgical treatment. For each specific spinal metastatic lesion, points are given to six different items

Table 40.6 Tokuhashi Revised Classification System for Prognosis of Metastatic Spine Tumors

Parameters	Score
Performance status (PS)	
Poor (10–40%)	0
Moderate (50–70%)	1
Good (80–100%)	2
Primary cancer	
Lung, osteosarcoma, stomach, bladder, esophagus, pancreas	0
Liver, gallbladder, unidentified	1
Others	2
Kidney, uterus	3
Rectum	4
Thyroid, breast, prostate, carcinoid tumor	5
No. of vertebral body metastases	
≥3	0
2	1
1	2
No. of extraspinal bone metastases foci	
≥3	0
1–2	1
0	2
Metastases to major internal organs	
Unremovable	0
Removable	1
None	2
Motor deficit	
Profound (ASIA A, B)	0
Some (ASIA B, C, D)	1
None (ASIA E)	2

Abbreviation: ASIA, American Spinal Injury Association.

for a total possible score of 2 to 18 points[25] (**Table 40.9**). A near-perfect inter- and intraobserver reliability has been reported in assessing the relative stability score when the SINS was grouped into three stability categories: stable (scores 2 to 6), intermediate/possible impending instability (scores 7 to 12), and instability (scores 13 to 18).[26]

Treatment

The overall survival rate of patients with metastatic spinal cancer is poor. Palliation is a realistic treatment goal. Although the management of these patients is primarily directed toward preserving or improving their quality of life, it would be wrong to think that they are "too sick to be treated." Treatment aims to relieve morbid pain caused by the spinal lesion and resultant pathological fractures or dislocations and to preserve or improve neurologic function and ambulatory status. The principal treatment modalities are corticosteroids, radiotherapy, surgery, and chemotherapy. More specifically, the management of MESCC involves optimal surgical intervention in combination with medical treatment as dictated by tumor histology and prognosis.

Role of Steroids

Corticosteroids are known to have antioxidant activity, which may limit ischemia, lipid peroxidation, and hydrolysis. Dexamethasone is the most common corticosteroid used in MESCC. It inhibits prostaglandin E_2 and vascular endothelial growth factor (VEGF) production, decreasing vasogenic edema and inflammation, and promoting stabilization of vascular membranes, which relieves pain and helps maintain or restore functional condition.[22,27] Corticotherapy is recommended

Table 40.7 Strategy of Treatment Based on Tokuhashi Revised Classification System for Prognosis of Metastatic Spine Tumors

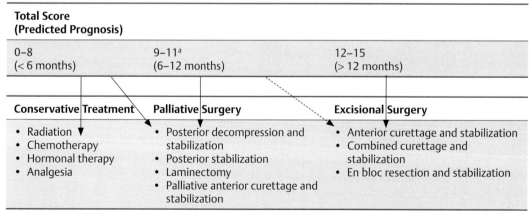

Total Score (Predicted Prognosis)		
0–8 (< 6 months)	9–11[a] (6–12 months)	12–15 (> 12 months)
Conservative Treatment	Palliative Surgery	Excisional Surgery
• Radiation • Chemotherapy • Hormonal therapy • Analgesia	• Posterior decompression and stabilization • Posterior stabilization • Laminectomy • Palliative anterior curettage and stabilization	• Anterior curettage and stabilization • Combined curettage and stabilization • En bloc resection and stabilization

[a] In patients with score 9 to 11, excisional strategies might be considered if there is a single lesion without metastases to major internal organs.

Table 40.8 Tomita's Classification System and Recommended Surgical Options

Points	Primary Tumor	Visceral Metastases	Bone Metastases Including Spinal Metastases
		Prognostic Factors	
1	Slow growth (breast, thyroid, etc.)	No point	Solitary or isolated
2	Moderate growth (kidney, uterus, etc.)	Treatable	Multiple
4	Rapid growth (lung, stomach, etc.)	Untreatable	

Total Score	2	3	4	5	6	7	8	9	10
Treatment goal	Long-term local control		Middle-term local control		Short-term palliation		Terminal care		
Surgical strategy	Wide or marginal excision		Marginal or interlesional excision		Palliative surgery		Supportive care		

for patients with suspected or confirmed MESCC showing neurologic deficits, if they have no medical contraindication to steroids. Although there is no consensus on the optimal corticosteroid dose and schedule, a general practice is to give a bolus dose of dexamethasone of 8 to 10 mg IV followed by 4 mg PO/IV every 6 hours; the duration of the therapy is dependent on the definitive treatment.[28] Corticosteroids can be used for short-term relief in painful spine metastases; how-ever, given its known side effects, long-term treatment is not recommended.[29]

Radiotherapy

Radiotherapy (RT) is the usual treatment for focal painful bone metastases not associated with pathological fractures or spinal cord compression,[29] and the combination of RT and

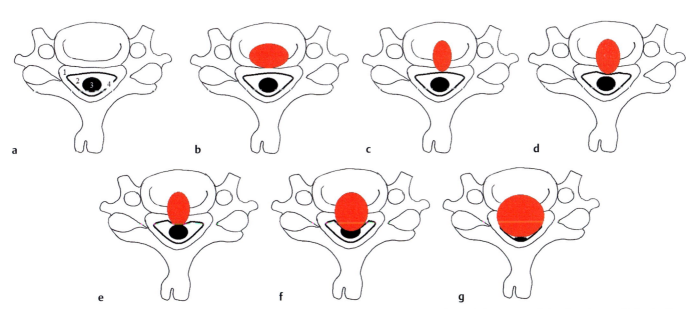

Fig. 40.4a–f Schematic representation of Bilsky 6-point grading system to describe epidural spinal cord compression based on axial T2-weighted MRI imaging. (**a**) Normal vertebral anatomy: (A.1) spinal canal space, (A.2) intradural space, where CSF is contained and surrounds the spinal cord, (A.3) spinal cord, (A.4) thecal sac; (**b**) Grade 0, bone involvement only; (**c**) Grade 1a, epidural impingement without deformation of the thecal sac; (**d**) Grade 1b, deformation of the thecal sac without spinal cord abutment; (**e**) Grade 1c, deformation of thecal sac with spinal cord abutment, but without spinal cord compression; (**f**) Grade 2, spinal cord compression with CSF visible around the cord; (**g**) Grade 3, Spinal cord compression without CSF visible around the cord.

Table 40.9 Spinal Instability in Neoplastic Score (SINS)

Characteristics	Score
Location	
Junctional (occiput-C2; C7-T2; T11-L1; L5-S1)	3
Mobile spine (C3-C6; L2-L4)	2
Semirigid (T3-T10)	1
Rigid (S2-S5)	0
Pain, which improves with recumbency and/or pain with movement/loading of spine	
Yes	3
Occasional pain but not mechanical	1
Pain-free lesion	0
Bone lesion	
Lytic	2
Mixed (lytic and blastic)	1
Blastic	0
Radiographic spinal alignment	
Subluxation/translation present	4
De novo deformity (kyphosis/scoliosis)	2
Normal alignment	0
Vertebral body collapse	
≥ 50% collapse	3
< 50% collapse	2
No collapse with ≥ 50% body involved	1
None of the above	0
Posterolateral involvement of spinal elements (facet, pedicle, or costovertebral joint fracture or replacement with tumor)	
Bilateral	3
Unilateral	1
None of the above	0

steroids has been the cornerstone of treatment for MESCC. Lymphoreticular tumors are very radiosensitive, breast and prostate carcinomas are moderately radiosensitive, and lung, renal cell, melanoma, and gastrointestinal carcinomas are relatively radioresistant. However, even these latter tumors do show some response to radiation.

Radiotherapy should be offered to all patients not having surgery as the primary treatment because it has been shown to reduce back pain and help maintain or improve ambulation.[27,28] Treatment typically involves either a single posterior field or opposed fields to encompass the metastatic lesion plus one to two normal vertebral bodies above and below. Complications related to high-dose radiotherapy delivered to the spinal cord such as radiation myelopathy represent the major limiting treatment factor.[22]

In the treatment of MESCC, optimal RT dose and regimen are still not well established. No difference in back pain relief and posttreatment maintenance, toxicities, or improvement in the ability to walk was found among five studies using di-

verse radiation courses.[27] However, others have shown better local control of spinal metastases with long-course RT.[30]

Different treatment plans are generally recommended in relation to the goal of treatment relevant to each specific patient considering the overall prognosis. For patients with poor prognosis (< 6 months survival), or as group I or II on the MESCC prognosis scale (**Table 40.10**), short-course radiotherapy, such as a single fraction of 8 Gy or 5 × 4 Gy in 1 week, is recommended.[22,31] Loblaw et al[28] define poor prognosis as either (1) poor histology tumors (melanoma or lung, sarcoma, gastrointestinal, head and neck or kidney cancers); or (2) good histology tumors associated with functional impairment or poor performance status.[28]

Patients with better prognosis (> 6 months survival after RT) should be enrolled in clinical trials to gather evidence regarding whether they would benefit from higher doses of RT. However, outside clinical trials, the most common RT treatment course for these patients involves 30 Gy in 10 fractions, especially when local control at the site of spinal cord compression is important or close follow-up is difficult.[28] In fact, longer course radiotherapy is associated with better remineralization of osteolytic bone, thus less risk of pathological fractures, and better local control than short-course regimens.[22]

Stereotactic Radiosurgery

Stereotactic radiosurgery (SRS) is reported to be a relatively safe and efficient treatment modality for spinal metastatic tumors offering various advantages. It provides a higher biologically effective dose of radiation delivered specifically to the lesion in a low number (1 to 5) of treatments. Other advantages include (1) reducing the duration of treatment, which could be consequential for patients with limited life expectancy; (2) minimizing the exposure of critical structures such as the spinal cord, thus reducing the risk of complication related to radiation toxicity; (3) avoiding radiating large segments, thus preserving bone marrow function, which is essential for continuous chemotherapy; (4) treating metastatic lesions early before they become symptomatic or create spinal instability, potentially avoiding the need for surgery; (5) providing a postoperative adjunct that may allow for less aggressive surgery, thus minimizing surgical morbidity; and (6) improving localization and control as well as preserving or improving motor function.[32-34]

However, SRS requires near-rigid body immobilization, usually longer treatment sessions (45 to 90 minutes per fraction), and, if toxicity occurs, it may be associated with more serious consequences related to permanent radiation myelopathy. Moreover, given the complexity of the technology used, the treatment cannot be given on the same day as the planning, which is not only more time consuming but also precludes SRS from being a suitable emergency procedure option.[28,35] Finally, vertebral compression fractures (VCFs) appear to occur more often following SRS. Lytic tumor and kyphotic or scoliotic

Table 40.10 Maranzano's Metastatic Epidural Spinal Cord Compression Prognosis Scale

Prognostic Factor	Category	Score
Type of tumor		
	Myeloma/lymphoma	9
	Breast cancer	8
	Prostate cancer	7
	Other tumors	4
	Lung cancer	3
Other bone metastases (at time of RT)		
	No	7
	Yes	5
Visceral metastases (at time of RT)		
	No	8
	Yes	2
Tumor diagnosis to metastatic epidural spinal cord compression		
	> 15 months	7
	≤ 15 months	4
Ambulatory status pretreatment		
	Ambulatory	7
	Nonambulatory	3
Time to develop motor deficits before treatment		
	> 14 days	8
	8–14 days	6
	1–7 days	3

Group	Score	6-Month OS	1-Year Estimated OS	Median Estimated OS (Months)
I	20–30	14%	8%	2
II	31–35	48%	26%	6
III	36–45	81%	68%	25

Abbreviations: OS, overall survival; RT, radiation therapy.

Controversy

- Although SRS is a relatively safe and efficient treatment for spinal metastases, it may increase the risk of developing VCFs.

deformity are predictors of VCF based on the SINS criteria.[25] Patients with lung and hepatocellular cancers treated SRS in a single fraction of 20 Gy are at higher risk of VCFs.[36]

Surgery

Traditionally, surgery has been often reserved for patients in whom radiotherapy has failed.[21] However, the risk of wound complications is higher when operating through irradiated tissues. Furthermore, in principle, radiotherapy will be more effective if the tumor burden is first decreased by operative means, i.e. cytoreduction. This, in part, has prompted support of de novo surgical management of spinal metastatic tumors. Proponents of radiotherapy maintain that, historically, the outcome after decompressive surgery and radiotherapy is no better than that after radiotherapy alone. However, most of these retrospective series and only one prospective study compared laminectomy as the surgical procedure combined with adjuvant radiotherapy to radiotherapy alone.[35] It has been demonstrated that laminectomy, especially in the presence of significant vertebral body disease or collapse, has a high risk of major neurologic deterioration and increased incidence of spinal instability. There is now widespread agreement that simple laminectomy is inadequate or inappropriate and is potentially harmful in most patients with spinal metastases. Simple laminectomy is indicated only if the compressing mass is localized primarily to the dorsal surface of the dural sac.

The management of patients with vertebral column metastases and spinal cord compression has been dramatically

Indications and Contraindications for Surgery for Spinal Metastases

- **Surgical indications**
  - Radiological diagnosis in an unknown primary
  - Reconstruction of an unstable spine (pathological fracture, progressive deformity) with or without neurologic compromise
  - Progression of disease or neurologic symptoms despite radiotherapy, chemotherapy, or hormonal therapy
  - Known radioresistant tumor
  - Neurologic compromise with focal accessible disease
  - Rapid neurologic deterioration, specifically from bone elements/fragments
  - Patients who reached spinal cord tolerance after prior radiation therapy
- **Relative Contraindication to Surgery**
  - Paralysis > 24 hours
  - Life expectancy < 3 months
  - Radiosensitive tumors (lymphoma, myeloma, prostate)

Special Consideration

- A randomized controlled trial has shown the superiority of combined surgical resection, stabilization, and radiotherapy for isolated spinal column metastases with spinal cord compression, over radiotherapy alone. The results of this trial have changed management algorithms for patients with vertebral column metastases.[37]

changed with the publication of randomized trial data demonstrating the superiority of combined surgical resection, stabilization, and radiotherapy over radiotherapy alone. A study compared a circumferential decompression of the spinal cord followed by 10×3 Gy radiotherapy with the same radiotherapy regimen without surgery; the primary end point was the patient's ambulatory time after treatment.[37] The trial was ended after the enrollment of 123 patients when interim analysis showed the superiority of surgical treatment with regard to neurologic recovery. In fact, 84% of patients retained the ability to walk after surgical treatment, compared with 57% after radiotherapy. In the surgical group 10 of 16 paraplegic patients regained the ability to walk, compared with three of 16 in the radiotherapy group. Narcotic analgesics and steroids were used less in the surgical group. Moreover, there was a trend for survival to be improved in the surgical group also (126 days vs 100 days). Surgery did not increase the hospital stay, and 30-day morbidity was worse in the radiotherapy group.

With recent advances in surgical approaches to the spine and stabilization techniques with instrumentation, the current indications for surgical intervention in the setting of metastatic spinal lesions have been broadened.

In essence, the surgical strategies are decompression of neural elements and the provision of spinal column stabilization with appropriate spinal reconstruction. The lack of benefit of surgery for metastatic spinal lesions reported in previous studies reflects the now-outdated use of laminectomy to treat anteriorly based pathology and the lack of instrumentations to manage spinal instability. The evolution of posterolateral and anterolateral surgical approaches to the spine, coupled with advances in spine instrumentation and knowledge re-

garding spinal biomechanics, have greatly improved results for surgery of spinal tumors.

Anterior or Anterolateral Approach

The anatomic location of the tumor is of paramount importance in selecting the operative approach for surgical management. The anterior vertebral body and pedicles account for approximately two thirds of spinal metastases. With anteriorly placed pathology, laminectomy alone does not address the site of compression and can actually further destabilize the spine. Anterior approaches to the spine typically require a thoracotomy or retroperitoneal approach, and are therefore technically more challenging. In addition, ventral access involves dealing with great vessels and mediastinal or retroperitoneal organs; they are consequently generally associated with greater surgical morbidity and mortality. Spinal reconstruction is performed with methyl methacrylate or bone graft, or both, with a metal construct. Bone graft may be used if long-term survival is anticipated. In MESCC, however, bony fusion is rarely a realistic goal (**Fig. 40.5**). Involvement of more than two adjacent vertebral bodies and the lack of bony integrity at the adjacent normal levels are important factors to consider prior to choosing an anterior approach. Although they are not absolute contraindications to an anterior approach, a posterior or posterolateral approach in those instances is preferable. Alternatively, involvement of both anterior and posterior elements of the spine may require both anterior and posterior decompressive and stabilization procedures. Furthermore, it is important to realize that the anterolateral approach enables effective decompression of the anterior dural sac and ipsilateral nerve roots. However, decompression of the contralateral roots can be challenging.

Posterior or Posterolateral Approach

Posterior and posterolateral approaches are familiar to most neurosurgeons. Whereas simple laminectomy is indicated for only a small number of patients, a wide laminectomy with resection of posterolateral elements including costotransversectomy and transpedicular decompression is often required for metastatic tumors situated dorsally and dorsolaterally. In addition, patients with medical risk factors for thoracot-

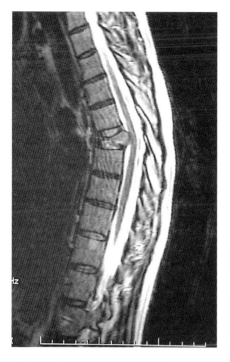
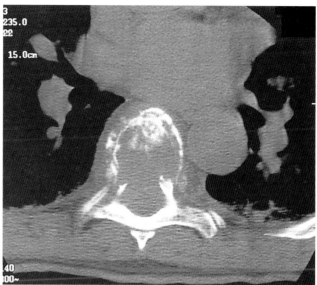

a

b

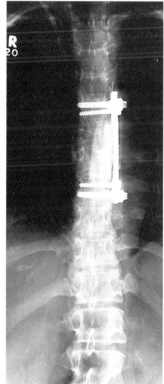
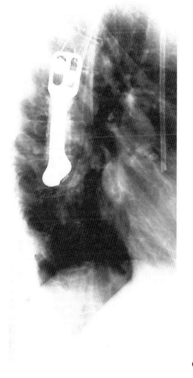

c

d

Fig. 40.5a–d A 46-year-old woman presented with back pain and rapidly progressive paraparesis. (**a**) The midsagittal MRI scan shows collapse of T7 with compression of the spinal cord by a soft tissue mass. (**b**) The axial CT scan through T7 illustrates the extent of bone destruction. (**c,d**) The patient underwent a left transthoracic resection, strut grafting (with supplemental methyl methacrylate), and plating for myeloma. At surgery, the T6 vertebral body was also diffusely involved by tumor and was resected. The patient received postoperative radiotherapy and chemotherapy and did well until succumbing to her disease 4 years later.

omy and patients with anterior compression extending more than two levels should be considered for the posterolateral approaches. With such wide exposure, decompression of tumor extending anterior to the dura is also often possible. Reconstruction with posterior instrumentation and methyl methacrylate to stabilize the spine is then performed. The posterolateral decompression has the advantage that it can be applied bilaterally, allowing a circumferential decompression of the dural sac. In addition, with a costotransversectomy or far lateral approach, access to the anterior column can be obtained, which can permit the use of a cage or other strut for vertebral reconstruction.

Percutaneous Vertebroplasty and Balloon Kyphoplasty

Nonsolid metastases, myeloma, and aggressive vertebral hemangioma are examples of neoplastic lesions that may cause pathological VCF and pain. Vertebroplasty refers to the injection of polymethylmethacrylate (PMMA) cement directly into the fractured vertebral body with intact cortex under direct fluoroscopic guidance. Percutaneous balloon kyphoplasty represents a more recent evolution in technique (**Fig. 40.6**), which applies the principles of balloon angioplasty to vertebroplasty. Balloon kyphoplasty in theory restores the vertebral body height and, thus, may correct focal kyphotic deformity.[39] The kyphoplasty technique creates an intravertebral void surrounded by impacted trabecular bone. This allows the bone cement to be injected with moderate pressure and minimizes the leakage of cement. The Cancer Patient Fracture Evaluation (CAFE) study was a randomized multicenter controlled trial involving 134 cancer patients with one to three painful VCFs, in which 70 patients received kyphoplasty and 64 had nonsurgical management. It was demonstrated that kyphoplasty reduces pain and helps improve function rapidly, effectively, and safely in cancer patients with painful VCFs. The potential disadvantages of kyphoplasty include higher cost and slightly higher radiation exposure.[40]

Both vertebroplasty and kyphoplasty are minimally invasive, percutaneous techniques that have been shown to be effective in controlling pain and improving function.[39] In patients with an osteolytic vertebral lesion, the injection of methyl methacrylate into the vertebral body by a vertebroplasty or kyphoplasty, not only restores the strength and stabilizes VCFs, but also helps to reduce pain by destroying pain receptors via (1) an exothermic reaction of the cement and

> **Pearl**
>
> - Vertebroplasty and kyphoplasty are excellent minimally invasive options to stabilize painful malignant vertebral compression fractures, particularly in patients with myeloma or lymphoma.

(2) physical compression of small nerve endings.[41] However, by increasing the stiffness of the vertebrae, it may adversely predispose the adjacent segment to new fractures.

The best candidate for vertebroplasty or kyphoplasty is a patient who has a fracture with pain and tenderness at one level. In the case of multiple lesions, the vertebrae to be treated should be chosen based on clinical criteria combined with the physical finding of worst pain location. Contraindications include active infection, uncorrectable coagulopathy, an unstable fracture with involvement of the posterior elements, a fracture that is asymptomatic, and breach of the posterior cortex by the fracture. Relative contraindications include osteoblastic metastasis, severe vertebra plana, and very old fractures.[42]

A transpedicular, parapedicular, or transvertebral body approach should be performed to avoid pleural, neurologic, or dural sac injuries. The transpedicular is the safest as long as the medial pedicle cortex is not violated. The parapedicular (i.e., approaching the spine from the lateral side of the pedicle at its junction with the vertebral body) and the costovertebral approaches (i.e., the needle enters the vertebral body at the costovertebral junction) are also safe. The major risk is related to venous embolism and epidural extrusion with neurologic compromise. However, in experienced hands, the risk of significant complications is less than 1%. Defects in the posterior vertebral cortex may increase the risk of epidural extrusion

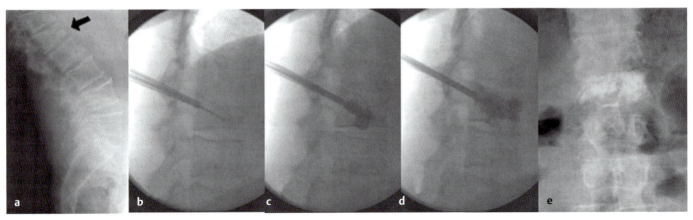

Fig. 40.6a–d (**a**) Painful L1 lytic fracture (*arrow*) from multiple myeloma treated by kyphoplasty. (**b**) Lateral view of pedicular approach to L1 under fluoroscopy. (**c**) Percutaneous balloon inflation and (**d**) injection of methyl methacrylate to fill the ventral body. (**e**) At 6-month follow-up, the patient had significantly reduced pain with excellent reconstruction of the vertebral body.

of bone cement and thus need to be assessed carefully. Both vertebroplasty and kyphoplasty are associated with excellent clinical outcomes, although kyphoplasty has the potential theoretical advantages of partially restoring body height and reducing the risk of bone cement extrusion.

Outcome and Prognosis After Treatment

Overall, the neurologic outcome of surgical decompression and stabilization using modern reconstruction techniques combined with radiotherapy is promising. In most series, 70 to 90% of patients have significant relief of pain, and 60 to 100% of patients either improve to or retain ambulatory status after surgery.

The median survival in patients with metastatic spine disease ranges from 3 to 18 months, but patients with thyroid, prostate, or breast cancer may live longer. Several studies have demonstrated that patients with preoperative and postoperative ambulatory status have significantly better survival rates than do nonambulatory patients. Finally, involvement of more than one or two vertebral sites combined with other negative prognostic indicators results in shorter life expectancy. Aggressive surgical treatment may not be warranted in such patients.

Editor's Note

Spinal column tumors include a variety of benign and malignant lesions that tax the decision-making skills of neurosurgeon/spine surgeons and oncologists, as well as the technical skills of the surgical team. There was a time when oncologists generally referred patients with suspected metastatic spinal cord compression for palliative radiation, which, combined with steroids, could certainly ameliorate the pain for some period of time. But results with surgery eventually revealed that many patients lived longer and better following surgical decompression often combined with fusion. More daring surgical approaches expanded from the original laminectomy and transpedicular body decompression to more complex lateral and anterior approaches, which have become more commonplace. More recently, SRS techniques have been adapted to treat spinal tumors, and sometimes a planned approach includes a surgical decompression to reduce the tumor burden to be followed in a staged fashion by stereotactic radiation. As with brain metastases the outlook for patients with metastatic spinal column tumors is markedly better than it was two decades ago. (Bernstein)

References

1. Nathoo N, Mendel E. The National Cancer Institute's SEER registry and primary malignant osseous spine tumors. World Neurosurg 2011;76:531–532
2. Sundaresan N, Boriani S, Rothman A, Holtzman R. Tumors of the osseous spine. J Neurooncol 2004;69:273–290
3. Chan P, Boriani S, Fourney DR, et al. An assessment of the reliability of the Enneking and Weinstein-Boriani-Biagini classifications for staging of primary spinal tumors by the Spine Oncology Study Group. Spine 2009;34:384–391
4. Jawad MU, Scully SP. In brief: classifications in brief: Enneking classification: benign and malignant tumors of the musculoskeletal system. Clin Orthop Relat Res 2010;468:2000–2002
5. Davis JH. Anatomical classification and surgical considerations: primary spinal tumours. An overview. SA Orthopaedic Journal 2011;10:26–30
6. Thakur NA, Daniels AH, Schiller J, et al. Benign tumors of the spine. J Am Acad Orthop Surg 2012;20:715–724
7. Mukherjee D, Chaichana KL, Parker SL, Gokaslan ZL, McGirt MJ. Association of surgical resection and survival in patients with malignant primary osseous spinal neoplasms from the Surveillance, Epidemiology, and End Results (SEER) database. Eur Spine J 2012
8. Boriani S, Weinstein JN, Biagini R. Primary bone tumors of the spine. Terminology and surgical staging. Spine 1997;22:1036–1044
9. Fisher CG, Saravanja DD, Dvorak MF, et al. Surgical management of primary bone tumors of the spine: validation of an approach to enhance cure and reduce local recurrence. Spine 2011;36:830–836
10. Cloyd JM, Acosta FL Jr, Polley MY, Ames CP. En bloc resection for primary and metastatic tumors of the spine: a systematic review of the literature. Neurosurgery 2010;67:435–444, discussion 444–445
11. Boriani S, Bandiera S, Donthineni R, et al. Morbidity of en bloc resections in the spine. Eur Spine J 2010;19:231–241
12. Fisher CG, Keynan O, Boyd MC, Dvorak MF. The surgical management of primary tumors of the spine: initial results of an ongoing prospective cohort study. Spine 2005;30:1899–1908
13. McGirt MJ, Gokaslan ZL, Chaichana KL. Preoperative grading scale to predict survival in patients undergoing resection of malignant primary osseous spinal neoplasms. Spine J 2011;11:190–196
14. Gerszten PC, Chen S, Quader M, Xu Y, Novotny J Jr, Flickinger JC. Radiosurgery for benign tumors of the spine using the Synergy S with cone-beam computed tomography image guidance. J Neurosurg 2012;117 (Suppl):197–202
15. Gerszten PC, Ozhasoglu C, Burton SA, et al. CyberKnife frameless stereotactic radiosurgery for spinal lesions: clinical experience in 125 cases. Neurosurgery 2004;55:89–98, discussion 98–99
16. Hsu W, Nguyen T, Kleinberg L, et al. Stereotactic radiosurgery for spine tumors: review of current literature. Stereotact Funct Neurosurg 2010;88:315–321
17. Maccauro G, Spinelli MS, Mauro S, Perisano C, Graci C, Rosa MA. Physiopathology of spine metastasis. Int J Surg Oncol 2011;2011:107969
18. Canadian Cancer Statistics, 2012
19. Sciubba DM, Petteys RJ, Dekutoski MB, et al. Diagnosis and management of metastatic spine disease. A review. J Neurosurg Spine 2010;13:94–108
20. Lee CS, Jung CH. Metastatic spinal tumor. Asian Spine J 2012;6:71–87
21. Bilsky MH, Lis E, Raizer J, Lee H, Boland P. The diagnosis and treatment of metastatic spinal tumor. Oncologist 1999;4:459–469
22. Rades D, Abrahm JL. The role of radiotherapy for metastatic epidural spinal cord compression. Nat Rev Clin Oncol 2010;7:590–598
23. Tomita K, Kawahara N, Kobayashi T, Yoshida A, Murakami H, Akamaru T. Surgical strategy for spinal metastases. Spine 2001;26:298–306

24. Bilsky MH, Laufer I, Fourney DR, et al. Reliability analysis of the epidural spinal cord compression scale. J Neurosurg Spine 2010;13:324–328

25. Fisher CG, DiPaola CP, Ryken TC, et al. A novel classification system for spinal instability in neoplastic disease: an evidence-based approach and expert consensus from the Spine Oncology Study Group. Spine 2010;35:E1221–E1229

26. Fourney DR, Frangou EM, Ryken TC, et al. Spinal instability neoplastic score: an analysis of reliability and validity from the spine oncology study group. J Clin Oncol 2011;29:3072–3077

27. L'espérance S, Vincent F, Gaudreault M, et al; Comité de l'évolution des pratiques en oncologie. Treatment of metastatic spinal cord compression: cepo review and clinical recommendations. Curr Oncol 2012;19:e478–e490

28. Loblaw DA, Mitera G, Ford M, Laperriere NJA. A 2011 updated systematic review and clinical practice guideline for the management of malignant extradural spinal cord compression. Int J Radiat Oncol Biol Phys 2012;84:312–317

29. Rades D, Schild SE, Abrahm JL. Treatment of painful bone metastases. Nat Rev Clin Oncol 2010;7:220–229

30. Rades D, Lange M, Veninga T, et al. Final results of a prospective study comparing the local control of short-course and long-course radiotherapy for metastatic spinal cord compression. Int J Radiat Oncol Biol Phys 2011;79:524–530

31. Maranzano E, Latini P, Perrucci E, Beneventi S, Lupattelli M, Corgna E. Short-course radiotherapy (8 Gy × 2) in metastatic spinal cord compression: an effective and feasible treatment. Int J Radiat Oncol Biol Phys 1997;38:1037–1044

32. Sahgal A, Bilsky M, Chang EL, et al. Stereotactic body radiotherapy for spinal metastases: current status, with a focus on its application in the postoperative patient. J Neurosurg Spine 2011;14:151–166

33. Dahele M, Fehlings MG, Sahgal A. Stereotactic radiotherapy: an emerging treatment for spinal metastases. Can J Neurol Sci 2011;38:247–250

34. Sohn S, Chung CK. The role of stereotactic radiosurgery in metastasis to the spine. J Korean Neurosurg Soc 2012;51:1–7

35. Young RF, Post EM, King GA. Treatment of spinal epidural metastases. Randomized prospective comparison of laminectomy and radiotherapy. J Neurosurg 1980;53:741–748

36. Al-Omair A, Smith R, Kiehl TR, et al. Radiation-induced vertebral compression fracture following spine stereotactic radiosurgery: clinico-pathological correlation. J Neurosurg Spine 2013;18:430–435

37. Patchell RA, Tibbs PA, Regine WF, et al. Direct decompressive surgical resection in the treatment of spinal cord compression caused by metastatic cancer: a randomised trial. Lancet 2005;366:643–648

38. Sundaresan N, Galicich JH, Lane JM, Bains MS, McCormack P. Treatment of neoplastic epidural cord compression by vertebral body resection and stabilization. J Neurosurg 1985;63:676–684

39. Hadjipavlou AG, Tzermiadianos MN, Katonis PG, Szpalski M. Percutaneous vertebroplasty and balloon kyphoplasty for the treatment of osteoporotic vertebral compression fractures and osteolytic tumours. J Bone Joint Surg Br 2005;87:1595–1604

40. Berenson J, Pflugmacher R, Jarzem P, et al; Cancer Patient Fracture Evaluation (CAFE) Investigators. Balloon kyphoplasty versus non-surgical fracture management for treatment of painful vertebral body compression fractures in patients with cancer: a multicentre, randomised controlled trial. Lancet Oncol 2011;12:225–235

41. Bhatt AD, Schuler JC, Boakye M, Woo SY. Current and emerging concepts in non-invasive and minimally invasive management of spine metastasis. Cancer Treat Rev 2013;39:142–152

42. Guglielmi G, Andreula C, Muto M, Gilula LA. Percutaneous vertebroplasty: indications, contraindications, technique, and complications. Acta Radiol 2005;46:256–268

41 Peripheral Nerve Tumors and Tumor-Like Conditions

Robert J. Spinner and B. Matthew Howe

Peripheral nerve tumors and tumor-like conditions are being increasingly well characterized and understood. There has been a particular increase in experience and expertise with imaging of peripheral nerve lesions. High-resolution magnetic resonance imaging (MRI) and ultrasound facilitate identifying tumors of peripheral nerves and often distinguish between benign and malignant disease. They also help distinguish many tumors from other tumor-like lesions that may not require biopsy for diagnosis. They can localize the safest site for biopsy with the highest yield. Clinical patterns can be correlated with radiological findings to help establish the correct diagnosis or generate a differential diagnosis, but misdiagnosis is common and leads to suboptimal treatment. Ultimately, familiarity with these clinical and radiological patterns can improve patient outcomes. This chapter discusses the role that pattern recognition plays in determining the effective treatment for these peripheral nerve lesions.

■ General Principles

Clinical Evaluation

Patterns are established with a good history and clinical examination supplemented by tests and imaging. Evaluation of the tests and imaging may be done in conjunction with a neurologist, geneticist, oncologist, or oncologic surgeon. The imaging studies and the planning and interpretation of new studies should be reviewed with a radiologist. Similar discussions should be held with a neuropathologist.

> **Pearl**
>
> - Clinical patterns can be correlated with radiological findings that can often help establish the correct diagnosis or generate a differential diagnosis. Familiarity with these patterns can improve patient outcomes.

Radiological Evaluation

Magnetic resonance imaging, ultrasound, ^{18}F-fluorodeoxy-glucose (FDG)-positron emission tomography (PET), and computed tomography (CT) are useful modalities in the evaluation of peripheral nerve tumors. The development and availability

> **Pearl**
>
> - High-resolution MRI with standard imaging sequences and the clinician's knowledge of patterns of peripheral nerve tumors and tumor-like conditions are the most valuable tools in peripheral nerve imaging.

of 3-tesla (T) MRI has led to a significant growth in peripheral nerve imaging, and MRI is the best single imaging tool available for evaluating peripheral nerve tumors and tumor-like conditions.[1,2] High-resolution MRI requires not only an MRI with increased field strength, but also knowledge of proper radiofrequency coil use and sequence selection to produce optimum images. The evaluation of peripheral nerve tumors is best performed with the use of intravenous gadolinium. Postgadolinium enhancement characteristics are a critical component in the evaluation of peripheral nerve tumors and tumor-like conditions and gadolinium should be included in the MR evaluation unless contraindicated. In the future, MRI techniques such as three-dimensional (3D) isotropic and diffusion tensor imaging may prove to be valuable sequences in the evaluation of the peripheral nerves.

The lumbosacral plexus and brachial plexus can be imaged with standardized MRI protocols. The basic components should include the key sequences of high-resolution T1-weighted, fluid sensitive, and postgadolinium fat-saturated sequences. The fluid-sensitive sequences vary depending on preference and include different methods of fat saturation, such as inversion recovery, chemical saturation, and Dixon separation techniques. Imaging planes for the brachial and lumbosacral plexus should be altered from standard anatomic planes to better visualize the oblique course of these structures. The evaluation of peripheral nerves outside of the plexus can be successfully performed with the proper knowledge, but often requires a tailored protocol for each study. Excellent multiplanar MRI studies can be performed easily in localized lesions of the extremities, but become challenging in lesions that are poorly localized clinically, and multiple coil types and patient positions may be required to evaluate a region suspected of having a nerve lesion.

Intraneural location, solitary versus fascicular, internal signal characteristics, and degree and pattern of enhancement are important features for developing a differential diagnosis. MRI can localize mass lesions as intraneural or extraneural. Once a lesion has been identified as intraneural, high-resolution imaging can differentiate a solitary intraneural mass from a plexiform process. Solitary intraneural masses can be evaluated for location within the nerve, that is, central versus eccentric, which may aid in planning for surgical resection. The internal signal characteristics are evaluated using muscle as an internal control for T1- and T2-weighted signal characteristics. Homogeneity, heterogeneity, and patterns of postgadolinium enhancement are used to determine the composition of tumors and in the identification of tumor-like conditions. This combination of imaging characteristics can often lead to a confident diagnosis without the need for biopsy.

Treatment

Performing preoperative biopsy of mass lesions remains controversial. At some institutions, image-guided biopsy of nerve tumors is routinely performed when they are not characteristic on imaging or they have features that provoke concerns about malignancy. Having a diagnosis in these cases facilitates treatment planning, as neoadjuvant therapy is indicated for some malignant tumors. Potential problems that have been described with biopsy include new neurologic deficit or pain, inadequate or faulty biopsy, and tumor seeding, but these are rare. The advantages of biopsy outweigh the potential disadvantages. The open surgical technique of targeted fascicular biopsy (**Fig. 41.1**) can be used to evaluate lesions in patients with otherwise indeterminate neuropathies who have MRI abnormalities without an overt mass-like lesion.[3] These patients often have had extensive evaluations, in many instances having had unrevealing distal cutaneous nerve biopsies or unsuccessful empiric treatment.

Symptomatic lesions should be resected whenever possible. The goal should be maintaining neurologic function. When this is not possible or not obtained, consideration should be given to reconstruction if feasible, either in the early or later stage depending on circumstances. Different options might be available ranging from nerve surgery (nerve grafting or nerve transfers) to secondary reconstruction (such as tendon transfer, free muscle transfer, or other soft tissue or bony procedures). For malignancies, chemotherapy or radiation might

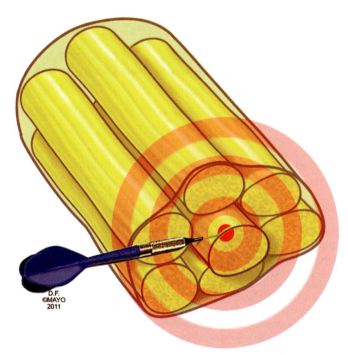

Fig. 41.1 Targeted fascicular biopsy. This drawing shows schematically how an MRI abnormality is utilized along with clinical and operative data to select the region of a nerve for open biopsy (Used with permission of the Mayo Foundation for Medical Education and Research, 2013. All rights reserved.)

well be indicated. Patients should be reevaluated in the immediate postoperative period. A baseline imaging study is often helpful to gauge complete resection. In many instances, long-term clinical and imaging follow-up is recommended.

■ Benign Nerve Sheath Tumors

Pattern

Schwannomas (neurilemommas) and neurofibromas are the most common benign nerve sheath tumors. Sporadic cases are more frequently schwannomas. Syndromic cases are often neurofibromas with neurofibromatosis type 1 (NF1) and schwannomas with neurofibromatosis type 2 (NF2), or schwannomatosis. Hybrid cases of combined schwannomas and neurofibromas (and even perineuriomas) have been described, though their incidence is not known. Benign peripheral nerve sheath tumors typically present with a mass lesion and mild to moderate paresthesias or dysesthesias. Motor examination is typically normal.

Significant overlap exists in the MRI appearance of schwannomas and neurofibromas. The classic MRI appearance of a schwannoma is an eccentrically placed round intraneural mass with well-defined smooth borders (**Fig. 41.2**). The parent nerve may be seen at the proximal and distal margins of the mass. The "split fat sign" refers to a thin rim of fat about the mass, best seen on T1-weighted images, indicating the mass is arising in an intermuscular location. T1-weighted signal ranges from isointense to skeletal muscle to slightly hyperintense and T2-weighted images classically demonstrate a "target sign" with T2-hyperintensity and relative decreased signal centrally. Conventional schwannomas demonstrate diffuse homogeneous enhancement on postgadolinium images; however, the signal characteristics are variable and range from solid and homogeneous to cystic. On PET, approximately one third of schwannomas have avid uptake. Neurofibromas are more classically fusiform lesions and less likely to be cystic, but the remainder of the MRI findings are similar to those of schwannomas. Both schwannomas and neurofibromas may produce plexiform lesions, the latter commonly involving the proximal peripheral nerve. In some cases, patients may have extensive plexiform lesions assuming a lobulated appearance; these patients may have mild or moderate neurologic deficit. The differential diagnosis of plexiform nerve sheath tumor includes other hypertrophic neuropathies such as chronic inflammatory demyelinating polyneuropathy (CIDP). Plexiform neurofibromas tend to demonstrate marked enhancement on postgadolinium images that help distinguish them from other hypertrophic neuropathies.

Treatment

Surgery is performed for several reasons. It best treats patients' symptoms, eliminates the tumor, and decreases the need or interval for follow-up examinations. Surgery tends to be easier and safer when tumors are smaller. Tumors tend to grow over a patient's lifetime, but this is not always the case. Thus, the life expectancy of a patient needs to be considered. Surgical resection provides definitive tissue diagnosis. There is also a small risk (5–10%) that neurofibromas can transform into a malignant peripheral nerve sheath tumor (MPNST); the risk of a schwannoma transforming is nearly nil.

In cases of benign peripheral nerve tumors, the aim of surgical resection is to save the nerve and preserve neural function, which can be achieved in 80 to 90% of patients. Outcomes are slightly better for patients with schwannomas than for patients with neurofibromas. Patients with larger tumors (> 5 cm) and previous surgery (or even open biopsy) have less favorable outcomes. Recurrence after gross total resection is

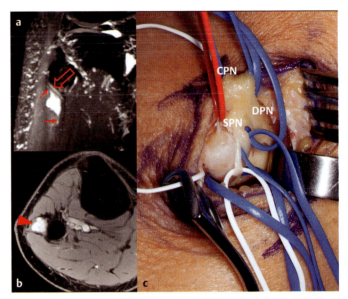

Fig. 41.2a–c Schwannoma of the superficial peroneal nerve at the fibular neck. This patient presented with focal chronic pain near the lateral knee without any neurologic deficit. (**a**) Sagittal oblique maximum intensity projection from a three-dimensional T2-weighted fat-saturated sequence demonstrates a hyperintense mass in the superficial peroneal nerve with superior and inferior "tails" (arrows). There is mass effect on the deep peroneal nerve (open arrow). (**b**) The mass demonstrates intense postgadolinium enhancement (arrowhead) on this axial postgadolinium fat-saturated image. (**c**) At operation, the schwannoma of the superficial peroneal nerve (SPN) is removed. The single entering fascicle (seen in a red vasoloop) of the SPN schwannoma has been identified, having been dissected away from the main SPN and two SPN en passant fascicles (in white vasoloops). The common peroneal nerve (CPN) and the deep peroneal nerve (DPN) have been mobilized in blue vasoloops.

low (1 to 2%). A standardized approach can be utilized to maximize good results.[4] Surgical exposure is generous enough to allow proximal and distal control of the affected nerve.

The temptation to concentrate on the tumor itself from the start should be avoided. Neighboring nerves and vessels at risk should first be identified and protected prior to attempting the tumor resection. Vasoloops help mobilize the nerve(s). The nerves and the tumor should be carefully mobilized in a 360-degree fashion. The nerve can then be rolled so that the nerve (fascicles) can be mapped on the tumor surface either with direct visualization or with a disposable stimulator. Schwannomas are typically eccentric tumors, whereas neurofibromas are often more centrally located. A bare area where the tumor is seen without intervening fascicles is identified. A longitudinal epineurotomy is performed in the tumor capsule, and the pseudocapsule around the tumor is maintained. Using blunt dissection techniques, the entering and exiting fascicle(s) can be identified. These fascicles, if tested, do not produce muscle contraction. All of the other fascicles are preserved in the outer shell of the tumor capsule and swept to the sides. The tumor can be rolled out. Resecting the entering or exiting fascicle can help mobilize the larger tumors. Sharp dissection should be delayed as long as possible (**Fig. 41.2**). Occasionally, larger tumors are removed in a piecemeal fashion or drained of cystic contents. This facilitates the dissection. Plexiform (multifascicular) lesions must be treated with caution (see Syndromes, below).[5]

◼ Syndromes

More detailed discussion of NF1, NF2, and schwannomatosis is presented in standard neurooncology textbooks. However, it is important to note that peripheral nerve tumors are often part of syndromes. The peripheral nerve tumors may be identified only as part of routine testing in patients with other central nervous system (CNS) lesions. Alternatively, the syndrome may be diagnosed only after several peripheral nerve lesions have been found.

Pattern

Specific criteria for the diagnosis of these syndromes are widely available. NF1 is the most common of these syndromes, occurring in 1/3,000 individuals. Its features include café-au-lait spots, axillary freckling, Lesch nodules, and subcutaneous neurofibromas. It is inherited as an autosomal dominant trait in 50% of patients and occurs sporadically in 50% of patients. It is associated with other CNS tumors, such as gliomas and astrocytomas. In the periphery, it is associated with conventional and plexiform neurofibromas, as well as malignant peripheral nerve sheath tumors. MRI findings can be quite extensive. NF2 and schwannomatosis occur in 1/30,000 individuals. These syndromes typically have conventional or plexiform schwannomas in the peripheral nervous system. They may be associated with other intracranial tumors, most commonly schwannomas and meningiomas. Bilateral vestibular schwannomas (acoustic neuromas) are well known to occur in patients with NF2.

Treatment

In the peripheral nerve, surgical resection is indicated for symptomatic, large, or rapidly growing lesions. Neurofibromas associated with NF1 can often be resected safely, though with slightly less favorable results than the sporadic cases of neurofibromas in patients without NF1. For plexiform lesions, surgery should be limited to carefully debulking symptomatic, large, or growing nodules; this type of surgery can often help with pain but will typically not improve neurologic function. In contrast, more aggressive attempts at surgical resection may well result in neurologic decline. Rapidly enlarging or painful plexiform neurofibromas in a patient with NF1 should be evaluated for possible malignant transformation. Long-term surveillance is necessary, and patients with these syndromes are often best followed in an interdisciplinary clinic.

◼ Miscellaneous Benign Intraneural Tumors/Lesions

In contrast to benign nerve sheath tumors that present without neurologic deficit, miscellaneous benign intraneural lesions typically present with neurologic deficit. They also have their own pathognomonic appearance on MRI, which differs from that of other benign or malignant intraneural lesions.

Intraneural Ganglia

Pattern

Mucinous cysts may develop within peripheral nerves. Intraneural ganglia present with acute or chronic features of neuropathy and are frequently found within the peroneal nerve near the knee. These patients present with a prominent deep peroneal nerve palsy with the common loss of ankle dorsiflexion. Intraneural ganglia have been described in major nerves throughout the body. They occur near joints and are most common in middle-aged men. There is evidence that they are derived from neighboring synovial joints.[6] They dissect along articular branches and propagate within the parent nerves following a path of least resistance, dependent on intra-articular pressures and pressure fluxes. The prototype peroneal nerve example originates in the superior tibiofibular joint and dissects along the articular branch into the common peroneal nerve assuming a tubular mass.

Intraneural ganglia may be discovered by MRI or ultrasound. It is critical to confirm the cystic nature of the lesion as well as a joint connection through the articular branch. Classic peroneal intraneural ganglion cysts may be easy to identify with

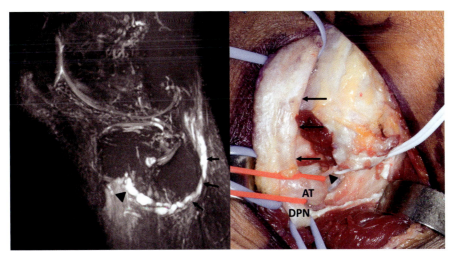

Fig. 41.3a,b Peroneal intraneural ganglion. This patient presented with the spontaneous onset of a foot drop. On examination he had severe weakness of the tibialis anterior, extensor digitorum, and extensor hallucis longus but preserved peronei. (**a**) Sagittal T2-weighted fat-saturated maximum intensity project of the left knee demonstrates an intraneural ganglion cyst arising from the superior tibiofibular joint. An intraneural cyst is well seen extending along the articular branch (*arrowhead*) and into the common peroneal nerve (*arrows*). (**b**) At operation, a peroneal intraneural cyst is seen. The cyst extends along the deep peroneal portion of the common peroneal nerve (*arrows*). The terminal branches have been identified: superficial peroneal nerve (retracted in a blue vasoloop at bottom left of the figure), deep peroneal nerve (DPN), and the cystic appearing articular trunk (AT). The white vasoloop encircles the small pathological articular branch near the superior tibiofibular joint (*arrowhead*).

knowledge of the entity and the normal anatomy (**Fig. 41.3**). On MRI, they appear homogeneous, with low signal intensity on T1 and high signal intensity on T2, and with no or minimal peripheral enhancement after intravenous administration of contrast. When an intraneural periarticular cystic lesion is identified without an identifiable joint connection, care should be taken to exclude a cystic peripheral nerve sheath tumor. Additionally, intraneural ganglion cysts may spontaneously rupture and decompress or vary in size with changes in intra-articular pressure leading to uncertain findings on MRI. Magnetic resonance arthrography of the knee after mild exercise of the joint helps confirm cases that remain unclear after high-resolution standard MRI. Three-dimensional renderings may facilitate identification of the joint connection.

Treatment

Surgery can often improve or restore useful function. Careful dissection is necessary to expose the articular branch connection, which is not always immediately obvious or known about prior to surgery. The articular branch must be explored. The articular branch may not necessarily appear enlarged. The articular branch is disconnected near the joint. The cyst itself can be decompressed but it does not need to be removed. The superior tibiofibular joint may also be resected. This combination of procedures decreases or eliminates the risk of recurrence of both intraneural and extraneural ganglia

and minimizes the risk of intraneural dissection. At other joints, the articular branch is disconnected but the joint is not resected.

Perineuriomas

Pattern

Perineuriomas have been shown to produce progressive neuropathy typically affecting teenagers or young adults. Patients present with motor weakness more so than with sensory abnormalities.[7] Most reports describe involvement of one nerve or a plexus. The origin of these hypertrophic lesions is controversial (i.e., whether or not they are a tumor). Intraneural perineuriomas are fusiform lesions on MRI that are isointense to muscle on T1-weighted images and markedly hyperintense to muscle on T2-weighted images. They demonstrate marked diffuse enhancement on postgadolinium images. A fascicular pattern can be seen on high-resolution MRI that cannot be seen on MRI at low field strength. The fascicular architecture is a key imaging feature, and, without a high-resolution technique, the MRI appearance is very similar to that of benign nerve sheath tumors.

Treatment

Confirming a diagnosis can be reassuring in many cases. Most surgeons do not recommend resection of these lesions. Focal or distal perineuriomas potentially can be resected and grafted.[8] Either the deficit is accepted or other forms of reconstruction to improve function are employed, including distal nerve transfers or tendon transfers. The long-term natural history of perineurioma is not known.

Adipocytic Lesions of Nerve

Three different types of adipocytic lesions have been described. Two are intraneural (lipomatosis of nerve and intraneural lipomas, discussed below) and one is extraneural (extraneural lipoma, discussed later in the chapter). These subtypes may also have overlapping forms.[9]

Lipomatosis of Nerve

Pattern

Lipomatosis of nerve (LN), also known as fibrolipomatous hamartoma (FLH) or lipofibromatous hamartoma (LFH), has a portion of the affected nerve interspersed with fat between fascicles. The lesion results in an enlarged nerve. Likely a congenital lesion, patients typically present with progressive neuropathy as early as a few years of life, but sometimes in their 30s or 40s. Approximately half of the patients present with or develop soft tissue (lipomas) or bony overgrowth (macrodactyly, limb length discrepancy, or osteochondromas) in the nerve territory. It most commonly occurs in the median nerve

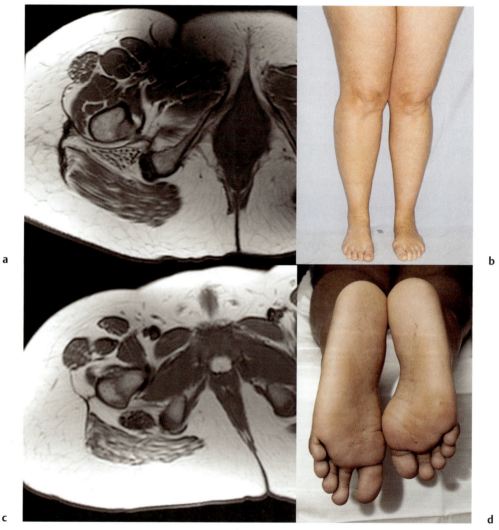

Fig. 41.4a–d (**a,b**) Lipomatosis of nerve (fibrolipomatous hamartoma) and (**c,d**) neuromuscular choristoma. Axial T1-weighted images of the proximal right thighs in two separate patients. (**a**) Sciatic nerve lipomatosis. (**c**) Neuromuscular choristoma. Note the prominent intraneural fat in lipomatosis of the nerve compared to the paucity of intraneural fat in the neuromuscular choristoma.

(**b**) The adult with lipomatosis of the sciatic nerve has longstanding overgrowth of the soft tissues in the right leg and mild-moderate sciatic neuropathy. (**d**) The teenager with neuromuscular choristoma has undergrowth of the right foot (cavovarus deformity) and mild-moderate sciatic neuropathy.

and in digital nerves in the wrist/palm, but it may occur in other nerves including the sciatic nerve (**Fig. 41.4**). LN demonstrates characteristic MRI features. The nerve is markedly enlarged with prominent fat between the individual bundles of the nerve. The intraneural fat is best appreciated on the T1-weighted transverse images of the nerves (**Fig. 41.4a**). MRI may also identify associated findings such as osseous overgrowth or adjacent soft tissue lipomatosis.

Treatment

Biopsy of the lesion is not necessary, as the appearance on MRI is pathognomonic. Although this is controversial, most surgeons perform decompression of the affected tunnel, and sometimes open the epineurium to provide more space. Resection of the fat is not recommended by most surgeons. Addressing the soft tissue or bony overgrowth may be necessary and challenging. This type of surgery is often best performed by a reconstructive surgeon.

Intraneural Lipomas

Pattern

Intraneural lipomas are the rarest form of this lesion. These intraneural masses of encapsulated fat form within the epineurium of a nerve. The most common site for their occurrence is the median nerve within the carpal tunnel. Unlike with LN, there is no association with overgrowth phenomena. The MRI in these patients also demonstrates a focal intraneural mass that follows the signal characteristics of subcutaneous fat on all MRI sequences. These masses are bright on T1-weighted images and demonstrate low signal intensity with fat-saturation techniques.

Treatment

These rare lesions can be resected safely using microsurgical technique. An opening is made in the epineurium and the mass can be separated from the fascicles and resected.

Neuromuscular Choristomas

Pattern

These nonneoplastic lesions present with progressive neuropathy and nerve-territory undergrowth (e.g., short limb, cavus foot) (**Fig. 41.4d**). Choristomas have normal elements found in abnormal locations. In neuromuscular choristomas, muscle is found within nerves, and the nerves are enlarged. Choristomas most commonly occur in the sciatic nerve in the thigh or buttock or proximal elements of the brachial plexus. They may extend longitudinally for a great distance. Given their rarity, they are often interpreted as indeterminate nerve lesions. Their imaging features are relatively characteristic on MRI. The lesions typically have marked overall enlargement

---

> **Pitfall**
>
> - Biopsy of neuromuscular choristoma has been associated with transformation to a desmoid tumor. Diagnosis should be established with imaging alone.

of the nerve. Unlike with LN, there is a paucity of intraneural fat (**Fig. 41.4c**). There is a fascicular pattern of enlargement, and the MRI signal characteristics follow muscle on all imaging sequences. They do not typically demonstrate postgadolinium enhancement. Sometimes the regional bone and soft tissue undergrowth can be identified on MRI. Over time, these lesions have been associated with the formation of desmoid (fibromatosis).[10] Biopsy of the lesion has been associated with catalyzing the transformation (see Desmoid Tumors, below). MRI of fibromatosis reveals a heterogeneous mass intimately associated with the abnormal nerve. The mass demonstrates variable areas of decreased T1- and T2-weighted signal that corresponds to the fibrotic tissue with heterogeneous enhancement on postgadolinium images.

Treatment

The best treatment for a neuromuscular choristoma is not known. Its diagnosis should be established by the MRI appearance rather than by biopsy.[11] Surgical resection is typically not an option because of the sacrifice of a (partially) functioning nerve. The best treatment for the associated fibromatosis is also not known (see Desmoid Tumors, below).

Chronic Inflammatory Demyelinating Polyneuropathy and Other Lesions

Patients with CIDP present with neurologic deficit and enlarged nerves (**Fig. 41.5**). Based on the characteristic appearance of classic forms, CIDP lesions are not biopsied. In the classic form of CIDP the nerves demonstrate marked fusiform enlargement. The involved nerves demonstrate marked T2-weighted hyperintensity, which can approach the signal intensity of adjacent vessels. CIDP may be confused with a plexiform neurofibroma on MRI without intravenous gadolinium; however, the postgadolinium characteristics are markedly different. Unlike plexiform neurofibromas that demonstrate prominent post gadolinium, little to no enhancement is seen with CIDP. A subtle thin peripheral rim of enhancement may be seen in CIDP with high-resolution MRI, but this should be easily distinguished from the prominent enhancement seen with plexiform neurofibromas.

A host of rarer lesions have been described, including granular cell tumors and amyloidomas. These lesions are too rare to be characterized. Tissue examination is necessary for their diagnosis.

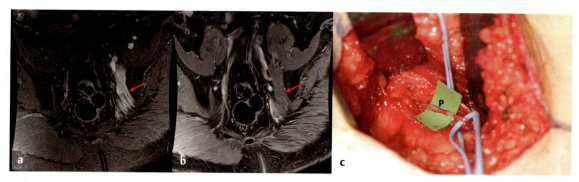

Fig. 41.5a–c Chronic inflammatory demyelinating polyneuropathy of the left lumbosacral plexus. This middle-aged patient presented with a moderately severe lumbosacral plexopathy of indeterminate etiology. (**a**) Coronal oblique fat saturated T2-weighted and (**b**) post-gadolinium images of the lumbosacral plexus. The *arrows* demon- strate the markedly enlarged and T2-hyperintense left lumbosacral plexus with no appreciable postgadolinium enhancement. (**c**) At operation, an enlarged fascicular bundle from the peroneal division (P) of the sciatic nerve is noted (in blue vasoloop).

■ Benign Extraneural Lesions

Pattern

Any soft tissue or bony lesion may secondarily affect the nerve. The differential diagnosis is broad. The most common extraneural masses are soft tissue masses, including lipomas and ganglia, or bony masses, including osteochondromas. One rare extraneural mass is cystic hygroma (**Fig. 41.6**). Benign extraneural lesions may develop and secondarily compress neighboring nerve. Patients with these lesions present with signs of nerve compression. The mass may be visible or palpable or seemingly occult and detected only at the time of imaging or surgical exploration. High-resolution imaging is recommended when nerve compression is suspected clinically at unusual locations. The nerve compression may occur at predisposed sites, such as Guyon's canal, the cubital tunnel, and the arcade of Frohse. MRI is a useful tool for preoperative planning for extraneural soft tissue masses. The goal of MRI is to describe the location of the mass in relation to the nerve and to attempt to characterize the tumor as benign, malignant, or indeterminate. The common lesions above (lipomas, ganglia, and osteochondromas) can be confidently diagnosed on MRI, precluding the need for a preoperative biopsy.

As previously discussed for intraneural lipomas, extraneural lipomas should follow the signal characteristics of the adjacent subcutaneous fat on all imaging sequences. The masses are bright on T1 and dark on fat-saturated sequences; however, fat-containing lesions that are large and internally complex, with thick septations or internal soft tissue, raise the possibility of atypical lipomatous tumors. Extraneural ganglion cysts are diagnosed on MRI by fluid signal on T1 and T2 fat saturated or inversion recovery imaging sequences with an identifiable joint connection. In the absence of an identifiable joint connection, intravenous gadolinium is recommended to exclude a soft tissue mass.

Treatment

The goal of surgical resection for these benign extraneural lesions is to identify, decompress, and protect the compressed nerve first, and then resect the mass (**Fig. 41.6**).

Desmoid Tumors (Fibromatosis)

Pattern

Desmoids are benign but locally infiltrative lesions. They may occur anywhere in the soft tissues, but they seem to have a propensity to arise near and encase neurovascular bundles.[12] They present as mass lesions or with neural symptoms. Desmoid tumors are characteristically heterogeneous masses that often demonstrate variable areas of decreased T1- and T2-weighted signal secondary to the fibrous component and heterogeneous post gadolinium enhancement (**Fig. 41.7**).

Treatment

Surgical resection is difficult. The mass may have finger-like projections that are not always seen or that may become adherent to neurovascular elements. Desmoids have a high recurrence rate following surgical resection. Wide resection is often not practical due to neurologic loss. In extreme cases, amputation has been performed. Chemotherapy and radiation may be employed.

■ Malignant Tumors

Primary Malignant Tumors of Peripheral Nerve

Pattern

Of malignant intraneural lesions, the most common are malignant peripheral nerve sheath tumors (MPNSTs). Other lesions,

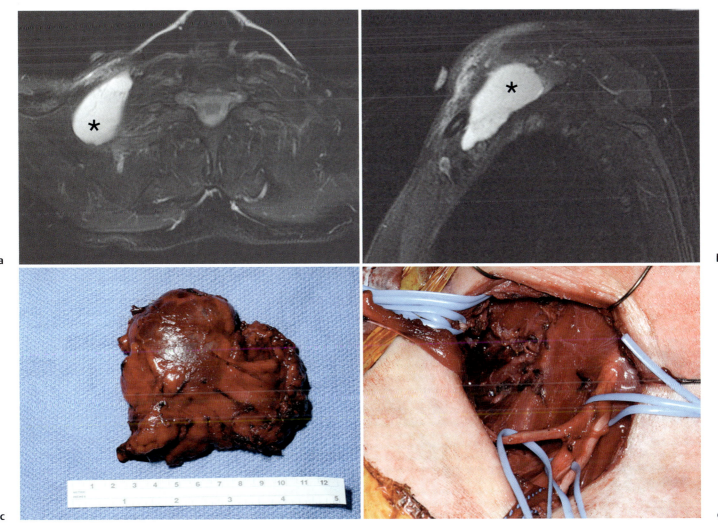

Fig. 41.6a–d Cystic hygroma. This patient presented with shoulder pain of several years' duration without deficit. T2-weighted fat-saturated (**a**) axial and (**b**) sagittal oblique images of the right brachial plexus demonstrate a large cystic mass (*asterisk*) in the region of the right supraclavicular brachial plexus. (**c**) The extraneural lesion has been resected. The underlying brachial plexus had been identified prior to mass resection and protected and decompressed. (**d**) After mass resection, the upper trunk and its divisions along with the suprascapular nerve are seen to the right of the figure, the spinal accessory nerve to the left (all in blue vasoloops). The surgical defect lies in between the two regions.

such as synovial sarcomas, may occur and appear similar on clinical and even histological examination. Patients who present with malignant intraneural lesions experience pain, which is characteristically, but not always, severe and problematic. Patients tend to have a rapidly progressive neuropathy and a rapidly growing mass. A patient presenting with a mass lesion and with the above symptoms and signs should arouse the clinician's suspicion of a malignant lesion, especially in the context of NF1 or prior radiation (on average 10 years earlier). A biopsy should be considered. MPNSTs are suspected on MRI in large intraneural masses with heterogeneous internal signal characteristics and enhancement (**Fig. 41.8**). Ill-defined margins, peritumoral edema, and an accelerated growth pat-

tern are also characteristics associated with MPNSTs. However, there is some overlap between benign nerve sheath tumors and MPNSTs, and biopsy is recommended for tumors that do not have a characteristically benign MRI appearance. PET/CT is often employed in these cases for evaluation of the meta-

> **Pitfall**
>
> • On PET/CT imaging, approximately one third of benign schwannomas have avid uptake, which may lead to false-positive diagnoses.

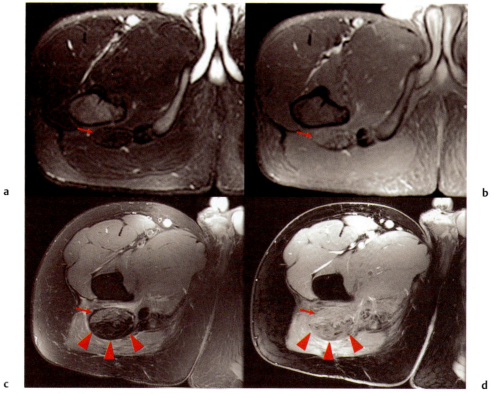

Fig. 41.7a–d Neuromuscular choristoma associated with desmoid (fibromatosis). This young adult had a neuromuscular choristoma and was found to have a new hard mass on the thigh, which was thought to be a sarcoma. (**a**) Axial T2 fat-saturated and (**b**) axial postgadolinium fat-saturated images demonstrate marked enlargement of the proximal right sciatic nerve. There is marked enlargement of the individual nerve bundles with a paucity of intraneural fat (*arrow*) consistent with neuromuscular choristoma. (**c,d**) Similar images of the right thigh in the same patient 11 years later demonstrate a new heterogeneous T2 hypointense mass (*arrowheads*) associated with the abnormal sciatic nerve, consistent with fibromatosis.

Pearl

- For patients who present with severe pain, progressive neuropathy, and rapidly growing masses, MPNST should be suspected and biopsy should be considered.

Controversy

- The benefit of chemotherapy for MPNST has not been well established.

---

bolic activity of the tumor and serves as an excellent modality for staging the disease (CT of the chest/abdomen/pelvis can also be used to stage the patient).

Treatment

Treatment is often based on surgical resection with radiation (either preoperatively or postoperatively).[13,14] Surgery consists of wide resection with negative margins. Sometimes, depending on the location of the tumor, amputation is offered. Chemotherapy may also be recommended, though its benefit is controversial. These malignant tumors are best treated by

specialized units. The 5-year survival of MPNSTs is about 50% in many large series.

Secondary Neoplasia

Pattern

In many cases, secondary neoplasia is not easy to document. It is not considered even in those individuals with neuropathic pain and a progressive neurologic deficit. Misdiagnosis is common. For example, prior radiation or chemotherapy may be presumed to be responsible for the symptoms and signs rather than recurrent cancer. Furthermore, those patients

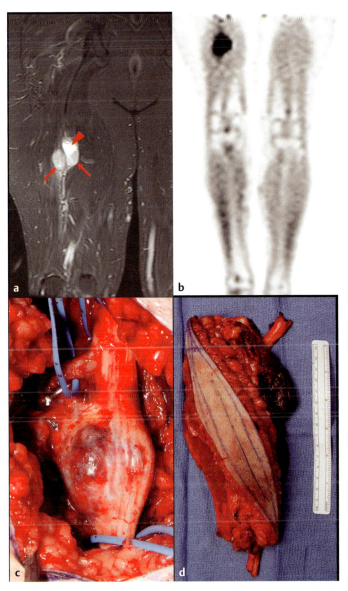

Fig. 41.8a–d Malignant peripheral nerve sheath tumor (MPNST) of the sciatic nerve. This middle-aged man presented with a several-month history of "sciatica" refractory to narcotics and a severe, progressive weakness in ankle dorsiflexion and plantarflexion and foot numbness. (**a**) Coronal T2-weighted fat-saturated MRI demonstrates a heterogeneous mass in the right sciatic nerve. The mass is heterogeneous with solid (*arrow*) and cystic (*arrowhead*) areas. (**b**) The mass demonstrates intense ^{18}F-FDG uptake on the coronal PET image of the lower extremities. (**c**) An open biopsy was performed of the lesion involving the sciatic nerve. The diagnosis of an MPNST was established, and the patient underwent a 6-week course of radiation. (**d**) A wide resection was then performed.

without a history of malignancy or who are in remission are not suspected of having recurrent malignancy. Outside of the head and neck, perineural spread of malignancy is known to occur in the brachial plexus with breast carcinoma[15] and in the lumbosacral plexus with prostate cancer[16]; there can also

be pelvic or gastrointestinal malignancies as well as hematologic disorders (such as lymphoma or leukemia). These may be challenging cases for which to distinguish neoplastic from radiation plexopathy on MRI in the setting of prior radiation. Both entities result in T2 hyperintensity of the involved nerves and this is not typically helpful as a differentiating feature unless the signal changes are sharply isolated to the radiation port. Perineural spread of malignancy typically alters the normal fascicular architecture of the nerve, but this can also be seen in the setting of radiation neuritis.

The pattern of postgadolinium enhancement is the best distinguishing feature in this clinical scenario. Radiation neuritis typically results in a thin "tram track" pattern of enhancement on postgadolinium MRI, whereas perineural spread of malignancy is a space-occupying process resulting in a thicker irregular pattern of enhancement. ^{18}F-FDG PET/CT may be a useful adjunct to MRI in these complex cases, and, in the setting of prostate carcinoma, ^{11}C choline PET/CT. Lymphoma of peripheral nerve typically demonstrates fusiform enlargement with loss of the normal fascicular architecture and mild to moderate T2-weighted hyperintensity. Postgadolinium enhancement imaging typically demonstrates diffuse contrast enhancement, but the degree of contrast enhancement is variable. The imaging findings in lymphoma are worrisome for malignancy, but are nonspecific.

Other malignant tumors may locally invade, infiltrate, metastasize to, or compress neighboring nerve(s). Malignant extraneural masses may be secondary to soft tissue masses, as seen with advanced local disease, such as apical lung carcinomas[17] (Pancoast tumors) or primary bony pathology, such as chondrosarcomas. MRI is an excellent modality for determining classically benign extraneural lesions as discussed above, or for planning for image-guided or open biopsy of extraneural masses with malignant or indeterminate imaging characteristics. For known malignant extraneural tumors, MRI is used for planning the surgical resection. T1-weighted images can be used to identify fat planes between the tumor and nerve, aiding in preoperative planning.

Treatment

A multimodality, multidisciplinary approach may be utilized to treat these aggressive lesions. This may consist of radiation, chemotherapy, and/or surgery. Specific protocols should be sought for each disease entity.

■ Conclusion

Clinicoradiological patterns facilitate the diagnosis and guide treatment of patients with peripheral nerve tumors and tumor-like conditions. More experience with rare conditions may help identify patterns that are currently unrecognized.

Editor's Note

The detection and management of peripheral nerve tumors have changed dramatically over the past decade. We now have superb imaging modalities, such as magnetic resonance neurography, to diagnosis these conditions, and we have physiological studies, such as nerve conduction tests, that can detect where along the nerve a lesion may be located. This area becomes extremely important for us when we treat patients with neurofibromatosis as these tumors can typically start out as low grade but transform to a more malignant peripheral nerve sheath tumor. Therefore, we must be vigilant when following these patients with these types of tumors. For the most part, the management of these tumors lies in surgery, and the surgical techniques have changed dramatically over the past many years. We can now better define the area of abnormality within the nerve or its fascicles using microdissection techniques as well as intraoperative physiological mapping of the nerve. We also have better techniques to achieve functional recovery with nerve grafts that have become an integral part of our surgical management of these types of lesions. However, this is a highly specialized field, and it requires referral to a surgeon or neurooncologist who has expertise in peripheral nerve tumors and their associated conditions. (Berger)

References

1. Ahlawat S, Chhabra A, Blakely J. Magnetic resonance neurography of peripheral nerve tumors and tumorlike conditions. Neuroimaging Clin N Am 2014;24:171–192

2. Amrami KK, Felmlee JP, Spinner RJ. MRI of peripheral nerves. Neurosurg Clin N Am 2008;19:559–572, vi

3. Spinner RJ, Dyck PJB, Amrami KK. Targeted fascicular biopsy: a surgeon's perspective. In: Dyck PJ, Dyck PJB, Engelstad JN, Low PA, Amrami KK, Spinner RJ, Klein CJ, eds. Companion to Peripheral Neuropathy: Illustrated Cases and New Developments. Philadelphia: Elsevier, 2010: 19–23

4. Desai KI. Primary benign brachial plexus tumors: an experience of 115 operated cases. Neurosurgery 2012;70:220–233, discussion 233

5. Hébert-Blouin MN, Amrami KK, Scheithauer BW, Spinner RJ. Multinodular/plexiform (multifascicular) schwannomas of major peripheral nerves: an underrecognized part of the spectrum of schwannomas. J Neurosurg 2010;112:372–382

6. Spinner RJ, Scheithauer BW, Amrami KK. The unifying articular (synovial) origin of intraneural ganglia: evolution-revelation-revolution. Neurosurgery 2009;65(4, Suppl):A115–A124

7. Mauermann ML, Amrami KK, Kuntz NL, et al. Longitudinal study of intraneural perineurioma—a benign, focal hypertrophic neuropathy of youth. Brain 2009;132(Pt 8):2265–2276

8. Gruen JP, Mitchell W, Kline DG. Resection and graft repair for localized hypertrophic neuropathy. Neurosurgery 1998;43:78–83

9. Spinner RJ, Scheithauer BW, Amrami KK, Wenger DE, Hébert-Blouin MN. Adipose lesions of nerve: the need for a modified classification. J Neurosurg 2012;116:418–431

10. Hébert-Blouin MN, Scheithauer BW, Amrami KK, Durham SR, Spinner RJ. Fibromatosis: a potential sequela of neuromuscular choristoma. J Neurosurg 2012;116:399–408

11. Hébert-Blouin MN, Amrami KK, Spinner RJ. Addendum: Evidence supports a "no-touch" approach to neuromuscular choristoma. J Neurosurg 2013;119:252–254

12. Dafford K, Kim D, Nelson A, Kline D. Extraabdominal desmoid tumors. Neurosurg Focus 2007;22:E21

13. Fuchs B, Spinner RJ, Rock MG. Malignant peripheral nerve sheath tumors: an update. J Surg Orthop Adv 2005;14:168–174

14. Gachiani J, Kim D, Nelson A, Kline D. Surgical management of malignant peripheral nerve sheath tumors. Neurosurg Focus 2007;22:E13

15. Hébert-Blouin MN, Amrami KK, Loukas M, Spinner RJ. A proposed anatomical explanation for perineural spread of breast adenocarcinoma to the brachial plexus. Clin Anat 2011;24:101–105

16. Hébert-Blouin MN, Amrami KK, Myers RP, Hanna AS, Spinner RJ. Adenocarcinoma of the prostate involving the lumbosacral plexus: MRI evidence to support direct perineural spread. Acta Neurochir (Wien) 2010;152:1567–1576

17. Davis GA, Knight SR. Pancoast tumors. Neurosurg Clin N Am 2008; 19:545–557, v–vi

42 Familial Tumor Syndromes

Xin Wang, Vijay Ramaswamy, and Michael D. Taylor

Although most tumors of the nervous system occur sporadically, both the central nervous system (CNS) and the peripheral nervous system are affected by a diverse and challenging collection of familial tumor syndromes.[1] Knowledge of these hereditary tumor syndromes is important from a diagnostic, therapeutic, and prognostic standpoint.

In the past many of these syndromes were known as phakomatoses because they involved both the skin and the nervous system. More recently, several genetic syndromes have been described that predispose to brain tumors but do not have cutaneous manifestations. Conversely, some of the classic phakomatoses, like Sturge-Weber, do not predispose to neoplasia. As such, the term *phakomatosis* is probably best abandoned in favor of *cancer predisposition syndrome* (CPS). Some CPSs are largely limited to the nervous system (e.g., neurofibromatosis type 2 [NF2]), whereas others predispose to cancers throughout the body (e.g., Li-Fraumeni syndrome). Targeted cancer surveillance and prevention is crucial among patients with an inherited genetic mutation conferring increased susceptibility to certain neoplasia.[2]

■ Diagnosing Cancer Predisposition Syndrome

Family History

The clinician should suspect the presence of a CPS whenever there are multiple cancers within a family, or especially multiple cancers within a single individual. Suspicion of a CPS must be tempered by the frequency of the cancer types being diagnosed. For example, two cousins in their 70s with colon cancer, a very common malignancy, are not nearly as alarming as two siblings under the age of 10 with pineoblastoma, a very rare tumor. A CPS should also be suspected when an individual also has one or more congenital anomalies or cutaneous abnormalities. The same genetic mutations that predispose to cancer often cause problems during normal development, such that mutation carriers have both developmental anomalies and cancer. When questioning a family to ascertain the presence of a CPS, the clinician should inquire about relatives with cancer, congenital abnormalities, epilepsy, frequent miscarriages, and psychiatric disorders. In the past, and today in developing countries, a brain tumor diagnosis could be missed or passed off as epilepsy or psychosis. Tumors diagnosed at a

---

Special Consideration

- Individuals and family members suspected of having a cancer predisposition syndrome should be referred to a medical geneticist so that they can better understand their own personal risks, as well as their risks of passing the disease on to their children.

---

very early age like a colon cancer in a teenager should also suggest a CPS. Individuals who present with multiple simultaneous tumors such as synchronous renal and CNS rhabdoid tumors, likely have a CPS. It is not uncommon for family members to change the reported history over time as they recollect additional details prompted by the initial questioning. Questions about family history should probably be asked of every individual, and his or her family, with a primary brain tumor.

Importance of Diagnosis

It is clinically important to make the diagnosis of a CPS. In many cases, the spectrum of neoplastic disease and the natural history is known and can therefore influence future clinical management. For example, the treatment of vestibular schwannoma in a patient with NF2 is very different from the treatment of a sporadic vestibular schwannoma. Some tumors occur only in the setting of a CPS such as subependymal giant cell astrocytoma in tuberous sclerosis, and tumors have a different prognosis when made in the setting of a CPS. For example, malignant astrocytomas in patients with Turcot's syndrome often have a comparatively mild course as compared with sporadic astrocytomas. The presence of a CPS may ultimately alter therapy for the neoplasm at hand. Sporadic optic gliomas are much more likely to be treated with radiation therapy than are optic gliomas in patients with neurofibromatosis type 1 (NF1) because NF1 patients are prone to developing malignancies after radiation. The clinical or genetic diagnosis of a CPS can profoundly affect individual and family decisions. In some cases interventions may be available to prevent neoplasia. For example, some women who carry mutations in the *BRCA* breast cancer susceptibility genes are choosing to undergo subcutaneous mastectomy to diminish their eventual chance of developing breast cancer. Similar approaches to prevent brain tumors in patients at risk are not yet available but are being developed in many centers. The ability of genetic tests to rule in or rule out a given genetic disorder can help unaffected individuals avoid a life of surveillance imaging and worry.

Some individuals may choose to alter their plans for procreation based on the presence or absence of a CPS. Excitingly, couples at risk to produce a child with a CPS can now elect to have preimplantation genetic testing, followed by transferring of only mutation-free embryos back to the mother using standard in vitro fertilization (IVF) techniques. This has been used to produce healthy children in cases of NF1, NF2, familial adenomatous polyposis coli, Li-Fraumeni syndrome, and von Hippel–Lindau disease.[3,4] Thus, it is important to make the diagnosis of a CPS because it will enable the accurate diagnosis and appropriate treatment of the neoplasm, predict and conduct appropriate surveillance for future neoplasms, in some cases provide prophylaxis against future neoplasia, as well as enable patients to plan their life course and procreation. In many cases, having prior knowledge of a CPS will allow for informed genetic counseling and family planning.

Genetic Considerations

Cancer is caused by DNA mutations that result in the gain of function of proto-oncogenes, or loss of function of tumor suppressor genes. Mutations can exist at the time of conception (germline mutation in every cell of the body), or can arise later in a single cell (somatic mutation). In almost every case, cancer predisposition syndromes are secondary to germline loss of function mutations in tumor suppressor genes. Mutations can be inherited from a parent or occur de novo in the embryo. In almost every case, inheritance of a CPS is autosomal dominant, seen in 50% of children, with variable penetrance. In many cases, the affected gene and chromosomal locus is known, and genetic testing is available. Clinicians and families seeking genetic testing in their community are encouraged to refer the family to a local medical geneticist.

■ Specific Cancer Predisposition Syndromes

More than 20 CPSs of the nervous system have been well defined, and a great deal more have been described in less detail. The following subsections outline several of the more common and well-characterized syndromes that have prominent CNS manifestations.

Li-Fraumeni Syndrome

Li-Fraumeni syndrome (LFS) was initially recognized by clinicians in the late 1960s who noticed that among their pediatric patients with sarcoma, there was a high incidence of other types of cancer in family members. Individuals with LFS are at increased risk for several malignancies, most notably soft tissue and bone sarcomas, breast cancer, adrenal cortical carcinoma, brain tumors, and leukemia.[5] The actual diagnosis of LFS is clinical, the definition is a proband under the age of 45 with a sarcoma who has a first-degree relative aged 45 or under with any cancer, and an additional first- or second-degree relative under 45 years in the same lineage with any cancer or a sarcoma. Families with a cancer spectrum similar to LFS who do not meet the criteria for a diagnosis of LFS are often said to have Li-Fraumeni–like (LFL) syndrome.[6] Criteria for LFL are a proband with any childhood tumor or sarcoma, brain tumor, or adrenocortical tumor under the age of 45 years, plus a first- or second-degree relative with a typical LFS tumor at any age, and another first- or second-degree relative with any cancer under the age of 60.

About 12% of neoplasms seen in LFS families are in the CNS. Brain tumors seen in LFS include astrocytoma, medulloblastoma, primitive neuroectodermal tumor (PNET), choroid plexus carcinoma, and ependymoma. Patients with LFS are at risk to develop multiple tumors over their life span and thus must be observed in perpetuity. The variability in age of onset and spectrum of cancer types among LFS families suggest coexisting genetic events that can modify the underlying contribution of the mutant p53. Recent integrated genomics efforts have identified mutations and polymorphisms in the p53 regulatory pathway, such as the MDM2-SNP309 polymorphism, which significantly decrease the age at onset among carriers.[7] Prospective biochemical and imaging surveillance has been shown to be feasible in detecting new cancers, and early results suggest a significant increase in survival in families undergoing a surveillance protocol.[8]

Two groups identified germline mutations of the p53 tumor suppressor gene in families with LFS.[9] About 30% of families with LFS and a higher percentage of LFL families have no detectable p53 mutation. Most germline mutations of p53, localized on chromosome 17p13.1, are located between exons 5 and 8 that encode for the DNA-binding region of the p53 protein. LFS families with a high incidence of brain tumors have been reported, but no clear phenotype–genotype relationships are evident. However, germline missense mutations of p53 result in a more severe phenotype than protein-truncating mutations because individuals with missense mutations in the DNA-binding domain have a higher incidence of cancer and an earlier age at diagnosis. This is consistent with data suggesting that missense mutations can act in a dominant negative manner by binding to and inhibiting wild-type p53 protein.

Animal studies of both *p53+/–* and *p53–/–* mice are viable, and both types are predisposed to develop a variety of tumors, especially hematological malignancies and sarcomas.[10] They only rarely develop brain tumors. Similarly, *nf1* knock-out mice do not commonly develop astrocytomas. However, *p53+/–nf1+/–* mice develop a range of astrocytic tumors with histology very reminiscent of human glial tumors.[11] The availability of mice with one mutant and one wild-type *p53* allele (*p53[R172H/+]*) has enabled the study of the dominant negative behavior of mutant *p53*.

Efforts by the International Agency for Research on Cancer (IARC) have resulted in the *TP53* Mutation Database, which includes both germline and somatic mutations reported in the literature since 1989. This important resource, which includes data on mutation prevalence and cumulative cancer risk, is invaluable for clinicians when discussing the diagnosis with LFS patients.

Neurofibromatosis Type 1

Neurofibromatosis type 1 is a common autosomal dominant CPS that afflicts one in 3,000 people. It is probably the most common CPS known. Clinical features include skin lesions such as café-au-lait spots, intertriginous freckling, subcutaneous neurofibromas, and various neoplasms such as neurofibromas, plexiform neurofibromas, pilocytic astrocytoma, leukemia,

---

NF1 Diagnostic Criteria (National Institutes of Health [NIH] Consensus Criteria)

Two or more of the following clinical features signify the presence of NF1 in a patient:

- Six or more café-au-lait macules
  - 0.5 cm at largest diameter in prepubertal individuals
  - 1.5 cm in individuals past puberty
- Axillary freckling or freckling in inguinal regions
- Two or more neurofibromas of any type or one plexiform neurofibroma
- Two or more Lisch nodules (iris hamartomas)
- A distinctive osseous lesion
  - For example, dysplasia of the sphenoid bone or dysplasia or thinning of long bone cortex
- A first-degree relative with NF1 diagnosed by using the above-listed criteria

(Adapted from Ferner et al.[14] Reproduced with permission from BMJ Publishing Group Ltd.)

Special Consideration

- Malignant gliomas seldom arise in patients with NF1 in the absence of radiation. Therefore, radiation is usually a treatment of last resort for optic glioma in patients with NF1.

---

and malignant peripheral nerve sheath tumor (**Fig. 42.1**).[12,13] Currently, the diagnosis of NF1 is made based on the presence of two of the following clinical features: café-au-lait spots, intertriginous freckling, Lisch nodules, neurofibromas, optic pathway gliomas (OPGs), distinctive bony lesions, and a first-degree family relative with NF1 (see text box).

Pilocytic astrocytoma of the optic pathway is particularly common in patients with NF1, who are also at high risk for developmental delay and cognitive disorders. With both cutaneous and neoplastic manifestations, NF1 is probably the classic phakomatosis. Due to the wide spectrum of disease phenotypes and severity, proper monitoring and thorough screening are critical. The role of genetic testing for asymptomatic patients is currently unclear in NF-1 specifically; genotype–phenotype correlations cannot currently be established.

The NF1 CPS is secondary to germline mutation of the *NF1* gene on chromosome 17. This is an extremely large gene that is prone to mutation. As such, up to 50% of cases are new mutations, with the other 50% being inherited from the parents. All patients with an *NF1* mutation will have some manifestation of the disease, but its severity is highly variable, even within families.[12,13] The *NF1* gene encodes the neurofibromin protein. Importantly, the neurofibromin protein is responsible for inactivating the *ras* oncogene, and tumors from individuals with NF1 show overactivity of the Ras pathway. This has been shown to affect downstream signaling of the Akt/mammalian target of rapamycin (mTOR) pathway. Another pathway that has been implicated in the pathogenesis of disease is neurofibromin's role in regulating cyclic adenosine monophosphate, resulting in aberrant cell growth. Inhibitors targeting the mTOR pathway and Ras activity are currently underway to study the efficacy in the treatment of NF1-related tumors.[15,16]

Curiously, even though pilocytic astrocytomas are often found in individuals with NF1, somatic mutations of the *NF1* gene are almost never found in sporadic pilocytic astrocytoma, although other somatic genetic events that activate the Ras pathway are frequently seen. OPGs are among the most common manifestations in patients with NF1, present in approximately 15% of patients. Several clinical trials have found that NF1-related OPGs respond better to chemotherapy and exhibit overall a milder progression than do sporadic OPGs.[16] Moreover, children with NF1 are at high risk for radiation-induced vasculopathies, specifically moyamoya syndrome, and as such radiation should be avoided in children with NF1 and brain tumors.[17] The molecular elucidation of NF1-related neoplasms have led the way for biological agents targeting dis-

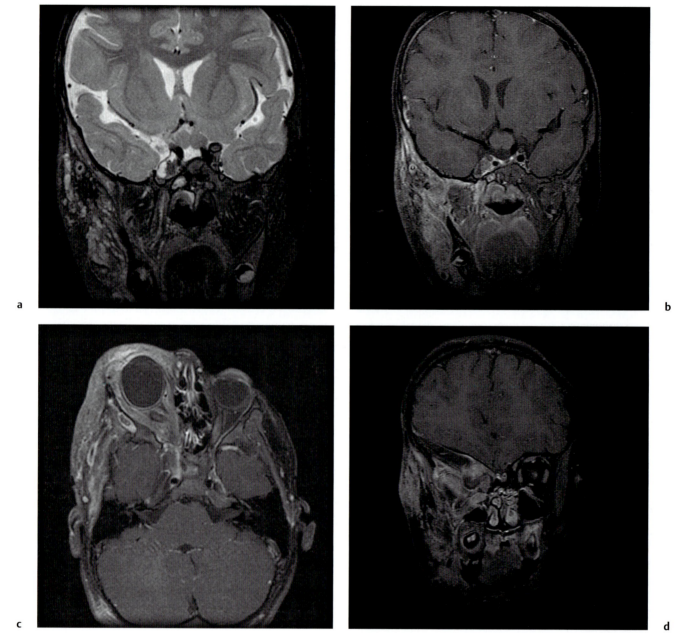

Fig. 42.1a–d Neurofibromatosis type 1. Multiple magnetic resonance imaging (MRI) scans of a patient with NF1. (**a**) Coronal T2 image of the brain shows bilateral enlargement of the optic nerves secondary to an optic glioma. (**b**) Coronal T1 image with gadolinium enhancement shows enlargement of the right cavernous sinus secondary to a cranial nerve neurofibroma. (**c**) Axial and (**d**) coronal T1 images with gadolinium enhancement show a plexiform neurofibroma of the right orbit.

ease. This emphasizes the importance of research into the biological basis of CPS.

Neurofibromatosis Type 2

Neurofibromatosis type 2 is an autosomal-dominant CPS with limited similarity to NF1. Affected individuals have limited cutaneous manifestations such as café-au-lait spots, subcutaneous schwannomas, and an increased incidence of cataracts, and are predisposed to several neoplasms, including schwan-nomas, particularly of the vestibular nerve, meningiomas, and spinal intramedullary ependymomas (**Fig. 42.2**).[18] The classic finding in NF2 is bilateral cerebellopontine angle vestibular schwannomas. Although NF2 patients can develop schwan-nomas on sensory nerves throughout the body, the predilection to develop tumors of the vestibular nerve is not well understood.

There exists some controversy regarding the diagnostic criteria for NF2, as several criteria for NF2 currently exist (National Institutes of Health [NIH], Manchester, National Neuro-

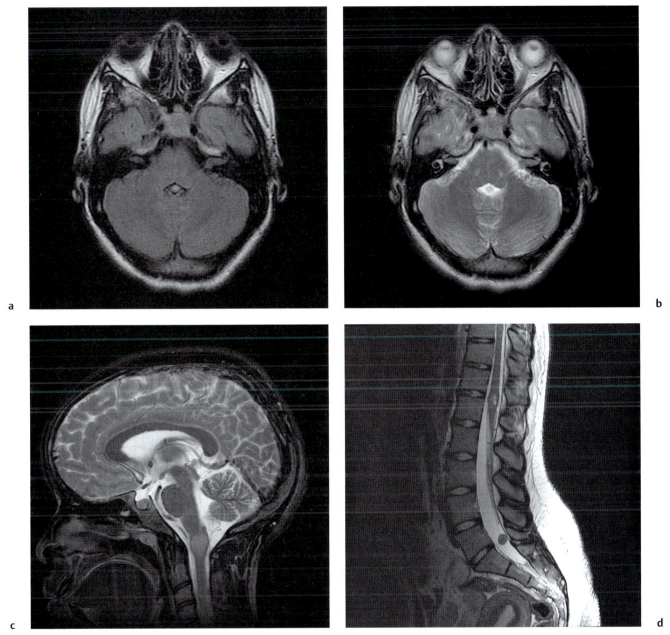

Fig. 42.2a–d Neurofibromatosis type 2 (NF2). Multiple MRI scans of a patient with NF2. (**a**) Axial T1 image shows bilateral enlargement of the internal auditory canal, with bilateral vestibular schwannomas. This is diagnostic of NF2. (**b**) Same tumors seen in **a** on T2 images. (**c**) Midsagittal T2 image of the brain and upper cervical spine shows expansion of the upper cervical spinal cord with increased T2 signal. In a patient with NF2 this is diagnostic of an intramedullary ependymoma. (**d**) T2 image of the lower spine shows multiple small tumors of the cauda equina, with one larger schwannoma seen posterior to the L5–S1 disk.

fibromatosis Foundation [NNFF]); however, all these criteria share several components, including the presence of bilateral vestibular schwannomas or a unilateral vestibular schwannoma in the setting of a first-degree relative with NF2. A recently revised set of diagnostic criteria, the Baser criteria, have been developed to assist in the complex diagnosis based on a series of clinical features.[19] NF2 mutation is about one tenth as common as NF1 (1:25,000 individuals), and is frequently a new mutation because it is much more lethal than NF1. It is important to note that the peripheral nerve tumors in NF2 are schwannomas, whereas those in NF1 are neurofibromas. Meningiomas in patients with NF2 usually belong to the fibroblastic subgroup. The role of NF2 mutation testing in asymptomatic patients is currently unclear and remains controversial.

Individuals with NF2 have germline mutations in the *NF2* gene on chromosome 22. *NF2* encodes for a protein called merlin that belongs to the protein 4.1 family of proteins that includes moesin, radixin, and ezrin.[20,21] This family of proteins is thought to be important in communication between the extracellular space and intracellular cytoskeleton. Phosphorylation of merlin leads to downstream regulation of oncogenic pathways, especially through the phosphatidylinositol-3 kinase and mitogen-activated protein kinase pathways. Sporadic schwannomas, meningiomas, and spinal intramedullary ependymomas often have somatic mutations of the *NF2* gene.

Whereas humans with *NF2* germline mutations develop mostly benign tumors, *NF2+/−* knockout mice develop a range of highly malignant and metastatic tumors. In the mouse, the *p53* gene is very close to the *nf2* gene, whereas they are on separate chromosomes in humans. Mice that have the *nf2* gene knocked out only in Schwann cells show characteristics more typical of human NF2 such as schwannomas, Schwann cell hyperplasia, cataracts, and osseous metaplasia. Mice that have a mutation in the *nf2* gene, engineered to be present only in their arachnoid cap cells, develop a variety of meningiomas similar to human meningiomas. NF2 null schwannomas was shown to be highly responsive to vascular endothelial growth factor (VEGF) inhibition, which has led to encouraging studies using bevacizumab, an anti-VEGF monoclonal antibody.[22]

Tuberous Sclerosis Complex

Tuberous sclerosis complex (TSC) is an autosomal-dominant disorder in which affected individuals develop hamartomatous changes of the nervous system, skin, and other organs. Cutaneous signs of TSC include facial angiofibromas, hypopigmented ash-leaf spots, subungual fibromas, fibrous forehead plaques, and shagreen patches.[23] Brain lesions in TSC include subependymal giant cell astrocytoma (SEGA) and cortical tubers (**Fig. 42.3**).[24] A computed tomography (CT) scan is extremely characteristic because it shows multiple subependymal nodules, or candle gutterings, in the groove between the caudate nucleus and the thalamus. For unknown reasons, in the region of the foramen of Munro, some of these subependymal nodules progress to form a SEGA, whereupon they block the foramen, causing hydrocephalus. Cortical tubers can cause seizure disorders, which often lead to cognitive impairment if not well controlled. Specific criteria for a diagnosis of TSC have been published.[25] Surgery for SEGA is often curative. Some children with TSC and medically uncontrolled seizure disorders require epilepsy surgery to remove cortical tubers that are seizure foci.

Recent studies including a phase 3 randomized controlled trial have found that SEGAs have a very robust response to mTOR inhibitors, specifically RAD001 (everolimus) and as such should be strongly considered in all children with SEGAs prior to surgical intervention.[26,27] Other mTOR pathway inhibitors such as rapamycin (sirolimus) has also shown activity against SEGAs. There is also some evidence that RAD001 therapy in children with tuberous sclerosis may also reduce the frequency of seizures, although the role of mTOR inhibitors in children with TSC without SEGAs is unclear.[28]

Pearl

- Most SEGAs can be diagnosed through a combination of a history, physical examination, and appropriate imaging. Biopsy is seldom necessary, and only a very small minority of these lesions require resection.

Individuals with TSC have germline mutations in either *TSC1* (chromosome 9q34) or *TSC2* (chromosome 16p13.3).[29,30] Both genes are very large, complicating mutational analysis. Up to 60% of cases are spontaneous secondary to de novo (occurred during conception) mutation, with the rest being inherited. *TSC1* and *TSC2* likely function as true tumor suppressor genes because there is loss of heterozygosity at the TSC locus found in tumors. *TSC2* encodes the tuberin protein, which has been shown to associate with the *TSC1* gene product hamartin. Both hamartin and tuberin stabilize each other's expression. Tuberin normally switches Rap1 from its active guanosine triphosphate (GTP)-bound state to its inactive guanosine diphosphate (GDP)-bound state. Loss of function of tuberin causes increased progression through the cell cycle. Mice and rats with germline mutations of *TSC1* or *TSC2* show findings similar to human TSC with cortical tubers, brain tumors, and kidney tumors. Again, similar to NF1 and NF2, the role of genetic testing in patients with TSC is unclear, particularly in asymptomatic patients.

Von Hippel–Lindau Disease

Von Hippel–Lindau disease (VHL) is an autosomal-dominant CPS with characteristic lesions: hemangioblastoma of the CNS, retinal angiomatosis, pancreatic cysts, renal cell carcinomas, pheochromocytoma, and epididymal cysts. Hemangioblastoma is seen in about 75% of patients with VHL, often multiple, whereas up to 30% of patients with hemangioblastoma have VHL.[31,32] Consequently, most patients with a hemangioblastoma should probably have a thorough funduscopic exam and a renal ultrasound.

Patients with VHL have germline mutations in the *VHL* gene on chromosome 3q25.[33] Different types of mutations in the *VHL* gene predispose to different spectrums of disease, particularly the presence or absence of pheochromocytomas. Somatic mutations of the *VHL* gene are also seen in sporadic hemangioblastomas. Hemangioblastomas are a mixture of two

---

Pearl

- Individuals with a seemingly solitary hemangioblastoma should have a comprehensive search for the other lesions of VHL. This entails a good examination of the retina, imaging of the entire CNS, and imaging of the thorax and abdomen.

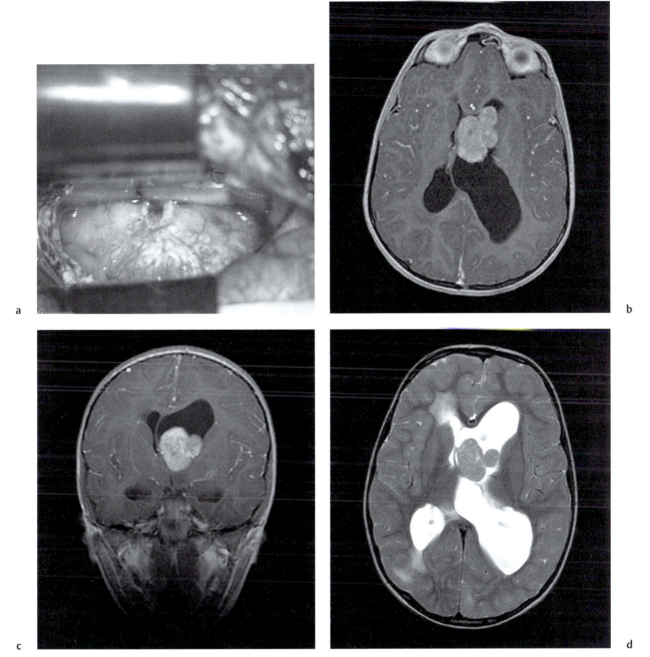

Fig. 42.3a–d Tuberous sclerosis. (**a**) Intraoperative photograph of an interhemispheric, transcallosal approach to the lateral ventricle of a child with tuberous sclerosis shows an intraventricular subependymal giant cell astrocytoma. This patient presented with hydrocephalus and papilledema that resolved with cerebrospinal fluid diversion after gross total resection. (**b**) Preoperative axial and (**c**) coronal T1 images with gadolinium enhancement show a multilobulated tumor in the region of the foramen of Munro. (**d**) T2 image of the same tumor.

cell types: stromal cells and vascular cells. The stromal cells contain the *VHL* mutation and are probably the true tumor cells, whereas the vascular cells are likely reactive. The VHL protein is involved in the cell's capability to sense hypoxia. In the face of mutant VHL, the cell constitutively senses hypoxia and thus attempts to increase its vascular supply. This explains the high vascularity seen in hemangioblastomas.

Predisposition to Rhabdoid Tumor or Atypical Teratoid/Rhabdoid Tumor

Rhabdoid tumor or atypical teratoid/rhabdoid tumor (AT/RT) is a very aggressive embryonic malignancy that can occur throughout the body but is particularly prevalent in the CNS and the kidney. Because it contains fields of small blue cells, it was often mistaken in the past for medulloblastoma. There are several reports of children or families with multiple rhabdoid tumors, often in both the kidney and the brain. Most children with multiple rhabdoid tumors, and a large subset of children with a single rhabdoid tumor, have germline mutations in the *hSNF5/INI1* gene on chromosome 22q.[34–37] In most cases the mutation is de novo and is not inherited from the parents. The hSNF5/INI1 protein is involved in controlling transcription through chromatin remodeling.

Cowden Disease and Lhermitte-Duclos Disease

Cowden disease is an autosomal-dominant CPS with affected individuals at high risk of developing breast cancer, thyroid cancer, multiple hamartomas, and Lhermitte-Duclos disease (LDD)/dysplastic gangliocytoma of the cerebellum.[38] LDD is an uncommon but characteristic mass lesion of the cerebellum that is usually readily recognized on magnetic resonance imaging (MRI) and that can be treated with observation, limited resection, or posterior fossa expansion. Individuals with Cowden disease (along with several other syndromes) have germline mutations in the important tumor suppressor gene *PTEN* on chromosome 10q23. Curiously, although the *PTEN* gene is frequently mutated in malignant gliomas, patients with Cowden disease do not develop glioblastoma. This is likely because *PTEN* mutation is a progression event, rather than an initiating event, in the pathogenesis of glioblastoma. Recognition of Cowden disease is essential due to the high risk of developing breast cancer.

Turcot's Syndrome

Turcot's syndrome (TS) is diagnosed in patients who have both colon and CNS neoplasia. TS is actually at least a couple of different CPSs whose molecular basis has been elucidated.[39] Individuals with germline mutation of the *APC* tumor suppressor gene on chromosome 5q21 develop hundreds or thousands of polyps in their colon and are diagnosed with familial polyposis coli. These patients are also at increased risk to develop brain tumors, including medulloblastoma, malignant glioma, and ependymoma. Loss of function of the APC protein results in overactivity of the Wnt signaling pathway. Interestingly, other members of the Wnt signaling pathway have been found mutated in sporadic medulloblastomas (B-catenin and Axin) that also lead to overactivity of the Wnt signaling pathway. Indeed, a specific subgroup of medulloblastoma patients has been recently identified with Wnt activation, who have an excellent prognosis relative to other subgroups.[40,41]

Individuals with hereditary nonpolyposis colon cancer (Lynch syndrome) often have germline mutations in DNA mismatch repair genes such as *hMLH1, hMSH2, hPMS1,* and *hPMS2.* Loss of function of these genes results in unstable DNA that accumulates characteristic mutations. These patients are at increased risk of developing colorectal carcinoma and malignant glial tumors. The gliomas are often diagnosed in teenagers or young adults. The prognosis for malignant glioma in the setting of a mismatch repair gene mutation appears to be much better than for other malignant gliomas.[42]

Gorlin Syndrome/Nevoid Basal Cell Carcinoma Syndrome

Nevoid basal cell carcinoma syndrome (NBCCS) is an autosomal-dominant CPS with affected patients having both developmental anomalies and a predisposition to cancer. Developmental anomalies include jaw cysts, rib abnormalities (bifid ribs), macrocephaly, characteristic facial appearance, and dural calcifications. Patients with NBCCS usually develop multiple basal cell carcinomas and are at risk of developing medulloblastoma and meningiomas.[43,44]

Most patients with NBCCS have germline mutations in the *PATCHED* gene on chromosome 9q22. A subset of sporadic medulloblastomas contains somatic truncating mutations of the *PATCHED* gene. *PATCHED* is the receptor for the mitogen Sonic hedgehog. Another Sonic hedgehog pathway inhibitor, *HSUFU,* has been demonstrated to be mutated in the germline of a subset of children with medulloblastoma.[45] Sonic hedgehog is highly mitogenic for cells of the external granular cell layer of the cerebellum, the putative cell of origin for medulloblastoma. Indeed, *ptch* +/– knockout mice develop a cerebellar tumor that is almost histologically identical to medulloblastoma. Several genes in the Sonic hedgehog pathway have been found to be somatically mutated in sporadic medulloblastoma, including *PATCHED, HSUFU,* and *SMOOTHENED.*[1] These features typify a prominent subgroup of medulloblastoma, the Shh subgroup.[40,41] Experimental therapies that block Sonic hedgehog signaling have shown some success in treating medulloblastoma in mouse models. Clinical trials are underway to study the efficacy of smoothened inhibitors in patients with both basal cell carcinoma and medulloblastoma.

Pitfall

- Radiotherapy of medulloblastoma patient with NBCCS is fraught with danger because these patients often develop hundreds, or even thousands, of basal cell carcinomas within the radiation field.

Rubinstein-Taybi Syndrome

Rubinstein-Taybi syndrome (RTS) is a complex CPS with numerous developmental manifestations, including severe developmental delay, broad thumbs and toes, and abnormal facies. Affected individuals are prone to several malignancies, including medulloblastoma, oligodendroglioma, and hematological malignancies.[46,47] RTS is secondary to germline mutations in the *CREBS binding protein (CBP)* gene on chromosome 16p. The CBP protein is thought to be a large docking protein involved in several signaling pathways, including Sonic hedgehog signaling (Gorlin's syndrome), Wnt signaling (Turcot's syndrome), and p53 signaling (LFS), so it is perhaps not surprising that children with *CBP* mutations are prone to medulloblastoma.

Trilateral Retinoblastoma

Individuals with germline mutations of the *Rb* tumor suppressor gene on chromosome 13q14 are at high risk to develop bilateral retinoblastoma. These children are also at high risk to develop several other neoplasms, including pineoblastoma and suprasellar PNET. The combination of bilateral retinoblastoma and an intracranial pineoblastoma/PNET is known as trilateral retinoblastoma.[48] Later in life individuals with germline *Rb* mutations are at risk of developing astrocytomas and sarcomas. The Rb protein plays a key role in the control of the cell cycle, and loss of function of the Rb protein leads to unrestricted cell growth.

Melanoma-Astrocytoma Syndrome

Families with a high incidence of cutaneous melanoma and astrocytoma are said to have the melanoma-astrocytoma syndrome. Melanoma has also been described as occurring in families in combination with other brain tumors, including medulloblastoma, ependymoma, meningioma, and schwannoma. Some of these families have germline mutations/deletion in the *CDKN2A* locus on chromosome 9p21.3 This important locus encodes both p16 (functions in cell cycle control with pRb) and p14ARF (functions in the p53 pathway).[49] The *CDKN2A* locus is frequently somatically deleted/mutated in several sporadic cancers, including glioblastoma multiforme.

Carney's Complex

Carney's complex is an autosomal-dominant CPS in which affected individuals are at risk for pituitary tumors, spotty skin pigmentation, cardiac myxomas, and nerve sheath tumors. The peripheral nerve lesions have a characteristic pathology because they are often melanotic. Pituitary tumors often secrete growth hormone. Some individuals with Carney's syndrome carry germline mutations in the *PRKAR1A* gene on chromosome 17 that encodes a subunit of the protein kinase A complex.[50]

Conclusion

Characterization and annotation of a range of CPSs have led to a dramatic increase in our understanding of disease pathogenesis and clinical course. The heightened susceptibility to a wide spectrum of cancers in CPS patients highlights the tremendous psychosocial and clinical challenges facing patients and caregivers. In the clinic, cancer surveillance and prevention remain important considerations when treating patients with CPS. This has paved the way for cancer genetics to become a mainstay in the clinical management and risk assessment of CPS-related tumors. Finally, new biologically targeted agents are on the horizon and some are already transforming the lives of these individuals.

Editor's Note

Familial tumor syndromes present formidable challenges for the afflicted patients and for their care teams. The CNS tumors seen in affected individuals not only occur along with other tumors, so the patient faces multiple simultaneous challenges, but also often behave more aggressively than do their sporadic counterparts. For example, hemangioblastomas in von Hippel–Lindau syndrome tend to recur more commonly or are multiple. The vestibular schwannomas occurring in neurofibromatosis type 2 are often bilateral, can grow more aggressively, be more challenging surgically, and are thought to have a higher tendency to malignant transformation after radiation, such as stereotactic radiosurgery. Quality of life of these unfortunate patients becomes important to study, as patient and caregiver understanding of these issues can improve the experience of the patients.[51] In the meantime, great hope lies in molecular biological interrogation of these tumors and syndromes, to try to illuminate new treatment strategies. (Bernstein)

References

1. Taylor MD, Mainprize TG, Rutka JT. Molecular insight into medulloblastoma and central nervous system primitive neuroectodermal tumor biology from hereditary syndromes: a review. Neurosurgery 2000; 47:888–901
2. Garber JE, Offit K. Hereditary cancer predisposition syndromes. J Clin Oncol 2005;23:276–292
3. Rechitsky S, Verlinsky O, Chistokhina A, et al. Preimplantation genetic diagnosis for cancer predisposition. Reprod Biomed Online 2002;5: 148–155
4. Simpson JL, Carson SA, Cisneros P. Preimplantation genetic diagnosis (PGD) for heritable neoplasia. J Natl Cancer Inst Monogr 2005;34: 87–90
5. Varley JM, McGown G, Thorncroft M, et al. Germ-line mutations of TP53 in Li-Fraumeni families: an extended study of 39 families. Cancer Res 1997;57:3245–3252
6. Mai PL, Malkin D, Garber JE, et al. Li-Fraumeni syndrome: report of a clinical research workshop and creation of a research consortium. Cancer Genet 2012;205:479–487

7. Malkin D. Li-Fraumeni syndrome. Genes Cancer 2011;2:475–484

8. Villani A, Tabori U, Schiffman J, et al. Biochemical and imaging surveillance in germline TP53 mutation carriers with Li-Fraumeni syndrome: a prospective observational study. Lancet Oncol 2011;12:559–567

9. Malkin D, Li FP, Strong LC, et al. Germ line p53 mutations in a familial syndrome of breast cancer, sarcomas, and other neoplasms. Science 1990;250:1233–1238

10. Iwakuma T, Lozano G, Flores ER. Li-Fraumeni syndrome: a p53 family affair. Cell Cycle 2005;4:865–867

11. Reilly KM, Loisel DA, Bronson RT, McLaughlin ME, Jacks T. Nf1;Trp53 mutant mice develop glioblastoma with evidence of strain-specific effects. Nat Genet 2000;26:109–113

12. Feldkamp MM, Gutmann DH, Guha A. Neurofibromatosis type 1: piecing the puzzle together. Can J Neurol Sci 1998;25:181–191

13. Feldkamp MM, Angelov L, Guha A. Neurofibromatosis type 1 peripheral nerve tumors: aberrant activation of the Ras pathway. Surg Neurol 1999;51:211–218

14. Ferner RE, Huson SM, Thomas N, et al. Guidelines for the diagnosis and management of individuals with neurofibromatosis 1. J Med Genet 2007;44:81–88

15. Williams VC, Lucas J, Babcock MA, Gutmann DH, Korf B, Maria BL. Neurofibromatosis type 1 revisited. Pediatrics 2009;123:124–133

16. Arun D, Gutmann DH. Recent advances in neurofibromatosis type 1. Curr Opin Neurol 2004;17:101–105

17. Ullrich NJ, Robertson R, Kinnamon DD, et al. Moyamoya following cranial irradiation for primary brain tumors in children. Neurology 2007; 68:932–938

18. Parry DM, Eldridge R, Kaiser-Kupfer MI, Bouzas EA, Pikus A, Patronas N. Neurofibromatosis 2 (NF2): clinical characteristics of 63 affected individuals and clinical evidence for heterogeneity. Am J Med Genet 1994;52:450–461

19. Baser ME, Friedman JM, Joe H, et al. Empirical development of improved diagnostic criteria for neurofibromatosis 2. Genet Med 2011; 13:576–581

20. Evans DG, Huson SM, Donnai D, et al. A genetic study of type 2 neurofibromatosis in the United Kingdom. I. Prevalence, mutation rate, fitness, and confirmation of maternal transmission effect on severity. J Med Genet 1992;29:841–846

21. Evans DG, Huson SM, Donnai D, et al. A genetic study of type 2 neurofibromatosis in the United Kingdom. II. Guidelines for genetic counselling. J Med Genet 1992;29:847–852

22. Baser ME, R Evans DG, Gutmann DH. Neurofibromatosis 2. Curr Opin Neurol 2003;16:27–33

23. Crino PB, Nathanson KL, Henske EP. The tuberous sclerosis complex. N Engl J Med 2006;355:1345–1356

24. Weiner DM, Ewalt DH, Roach ES, Hensle TW. The tuberous sclerosis complex: a comprehensive review. J Am Coll Surg 1998;187:548–561

25. Roach ES, Gomez MR, Northrup H. Tuberous sclerosis complex consensus conference: revised clinical diagnostic criteria. J Child Neurol 1998;13:624–628

26. Franz DN, Belousova E, Sparagana S, et al. Efficacy and safety of everolimus for subependymal giant cell astrocytomas associated with tuberous sclerosis complex (EXIST-1): a multicentre, randomised, placebo-controlled phase 3 trial. Lancet 2013;381:125–132

27. Krueger DA, Care MM, Holland K, et al. Everolimus for subependymal giant-cell astrocytomas in tuberous sclerosis. N Engl J Med 2010; 363:1801–1811

28. Kotulska K, Chmielewski D, Borkowska J, et al. Long-term effect of everolimus on epilepsy and growth in children under 3 years of age treated for subependymal giant cell astrocytoma associated with tuberous sclerosis complex. Eur J Paediatr Neurol 2013;17:479–485 [Epub ahead of print]

29. Kwiatkowski DJ. Tuberous sclerosis: from tubers to mTOR. Ann Hum Genet 2003;67(Pt 1):87–96

30. Jones AC, Shyamsundar MM, Thomas MW, et al. Comprehensive mutation analysis of TSC1 and TSC2-and phenotypic correlations in 150 families with tuberous sclerosis. Am J Hum Genet 1999;64:1305–1315

31. Kaelin WG Jr, Maher ER. The VHL tumour-suppressor gene paradigm. Trends Genet 1998;14:423–426

32. Maher ER, Kaelin WG Jr. von Hippel-Lindau disease. Medicine (Baltimore) 1997;76:381–391

33. Kondo K, Kaelin WG Jr. The von Hippel-Lindau tumor suppressor gene. Exp Cell Res 2001;264:117–125

34. Taylor MD, Gokgoz N, Andrulis IL, Mainprize TG, Drake JM, Rutka JT. Familial posterior fossa brain tumors of infancy secondary to germline mutation of the hSNF5 gene. Am J Hum Genet 2000;66:1403–1406

35. Biegel JA, Zhou JY, Rorke LB, Stenstrom C, Wainwright LM, Fogelgren B. Germ-line and acquired mutations of INI1 in atypical teratoid and rhabdoid tumors. Cancer Res 1999;59:74–79

36. Sévenet N, Lellouch-Tubiana A, Schofield D, et al. Spectrum of hSNF5/INI1 somatic mutations in human cancer and genotype-phenotype correlations. Hum Mol Genet 1999;8:2359–2368

37. Sévenet N, Sheridan E, Amram D, Schneider P, Handgretinger R, Delattre O. Constitutional mutations of the hSNF5/INI1 gene predispose to a variety of cancers. Am J Hum Genet 1999;65:1342–1348

38. Zhou XP, Marsh DJ, Morrison CD, et al. Germline inactivation of PTEN and dysregulation of the phosphoinositol-3-kinase/Akt pathway cause human Lhermitte-Duclos disease in adults. Am J Hum Genet 2003; 73:1191–1198

39. Hamilton SR, Liu B, Parsons RE, et al. The molecular basis of Turcot's syndrome. N Engl J Med 1995;332:839–847

40. Northcott PA, Korshunov A, Witt H, et al. Medulloblastoma comprises four distinct molecular variants. J Clin Oncol 2011;29:1408–1414

41. Taylor MD, Northcott PA, Korshunov A, et al. Molecular subgroups of medulloblastoma: the current consensus. Acta Neuropathol 2012;123: 465–472

42. Taylor MD, Perry J, Zlatescu MC, et al. The hPMS2 exon 5 mutation and malignant glioma. Case report. J Neurosurg 1999;90:946–950

43. Gorlin RJ. Nevoid basal-cell carcinoma syndrome. Medicine (Baltimore) 1987;66:98–113

44. Gorlin RJ. Nevoid basal cell carcinoma syndrome. Dermatol Clin 1995; 13:113–125

45. Taylor MD, Liu L, Raffel C, et al. Mutations in SUFU predispose to medulloblastoma. Nat Genet 2002;31:306–310

46. Miller RW, Rubinstein JH. Tumors in Rubinstein-Taybi syndrome. Am J Med Genet 1995;56:112–115

47. Taylor MD, Mainprize TG, Rutka JT, Becker L, Bayani J, Drake JM. Medulloblastoma in a child with Rubenstein-Taybi syndrome: case report and review of the literature. Pediatr Neurosurg 2001;35:235–238

48. Mouratova T. Trilateral retinoblastoma: a literature review, 1971–2004. Bull Soc Belge Ophtalmol 2005;297:25–35

49. Bahuau M, Vidaud D, Jenkins RB, et al. Germ-line deletion involving the INK4 locus in familial proneness to melanoma and nervous system tumors. Cancer Res 1998;58:2298–2303

50. Kirschner LS, Carney JA, Pack SD, et al. Mutations of the gene encoding the protein kinase A type I-alpha regulatory subunit in patients with the Carney complex. Nat Genet 2000;26:89–92

51. Hornigold RE, Golding JF, Leschziner G, et al. The NFTI-QOL: A Disease-Specific Quality of Life Questionnaire for Neurofibromatosis 2. J Neurol Surg B Skull Base 2012;73:104–111

VII   Related Issues

43 Complications of Medical Therapy

Elizabeth J. Hovey and Susan M. Chang

The treatment of patients with brain tumors remains a significant challenge. New treatment approaches have already demonstrated that combined modalities of surgery, radiotherapy, and systemic drug therapy can prolong survival without significantly adversely affecting the patients' quality of life.[1,2] However, the prognosis remains poor, and efforts to further improve patient outcome are ongoing. To optimally care for these patients, neuro-oncologists must be knowledgeable about the potential complications associated with such therapeutic modalities. Specifically, neuro-oncologists should be intimately familiar with the side effects of antitumor therapy and those associated with supportive medical treatments commonly used in this patient population. They should also appreciate the potential morbidity of the brain tumor itself on the function of the central nervous system (CNS), which can be difficult to differentiate from the neurotoxic side effects of medical intervention.

Due to the limited benefit of standard therapy on overall survival in patients with primary brain tumors, various experimental approaches are under investigation. Advances in the understanding of cell biology and cellular genetics have been translated into many complex and novel treatment strategies.[2] Some of these experimental approaches involve the direct interstitial delivery of drugs or agents into the brain parenchyma. Examples include gene therapy, immunologic therapy using monoclonal antibodies conjugated to either toxins or radiopharmaceutical analogues, and drug-impregnated biodegradable polymers. The potential side effects of these therapies include not only the operative risks and complications of interstitial delivery but also the effects of the actual agent. These are very complex approaches to therapy, and many are undergoing phase 1 evaluation of their respective toxicities. Alternative methods of improving drug intensity and drug delivery (e.g., intra-arterial administration or high-dose systemic chemotherapy with stem cell or bone marrow support) are also associated with unique risks.[3,4] It is clear that neuro-oncologists will have to remain vigilant to the potential harmful effects of a multimodality therapeutic approach to the patient.

Other unique aspects in the management of patients with brain tumors involve the use of concomitant supportive medical treatments that themselves may have direct effects on the patient. Examples include the use of anticonvulsants, corticosteroids, and anticoagulant therapies. The potential for adverse drug interactions from such supportive agents warrants special attention. The sequelae of therapy may often require drug intervention (e.g., postoperative cerebral edema requiring corticosteroid use). Similarly, some of the side effects of radiotherapy may also require medical treatment (e.g., hypothalamic and pituitary dysfunction requiring neuroendocrine replacement therapy). Patients with a malignant tumor, particularly a glioma, also have an inherently increased risk of thromboembolic disease and hence may suffer the medical complications of anticoagulant therapy.

This chapter discusses the complications of agents used in the setting of primary brain tumors rather than secondary brain tumors (metastases), emphasizing the toxicities related to the management of gliomas in adults. Some of the toxicities related to the management of other CNS tumors are briefly discussed.

■ Chemotherapy

The use of cytotoxic drugs has been shown to be beneficial for treating various histological subtypes of primary brain tumors.[5] These include anaplastic gliomas, such as grade III oligodendroglioma, grade III anaplastic astrocytoma, grade III mixed oligoastrocytoma, and grade IV glioblastoma multiforme (GBM); primitive neuroectodermal tumors (PNETs); primary germ cell tumors; and primary CNS lymphomas. Based on the international multicenter cooperative trial group data in 2005, standard treatment of newly diagnosed GBM, which accounts for 45% of primary adult brain tumors, usually consists of cytoreductive surgery followed by chemoradiation (standard radiation is 60 Gy in 30 fractions) in combination with the oral alkylating agent temozolomide, followed by adjuvant temozolomide.[6,7]

Although these results have led to general agreement on the initial treatment of GBM, in the setting of recurrent/progressive disease there is no consensus regarding the most appropriate salvage agent.[8] Regardless of this lack of accord, some patients likely benefit from additional chemotherapeutic regimens, and many patients receive agents such as

Pearl

- Anticancer drugs affect almost every organ system but especially those with rapidly dividing cells.

temozolomide given in alternate schedules (often referred to as metronomic temozolomide), lomustine (chloroethylcyclo-hexylnitrosourea [CCNU]), carboplatin, or irinotecan in the recurrent setting.[8] Another agent now approved by the Food and Drug Administration (FDA) in the recurrent GBM setting is the targeted agent bevacizumab,[9,10] a monoclonal antibody against vascular endothelial growth factor (VEGF), which, strictly speaking, is not considered to be a cytotoxic agent.

Some neurosurgeons also use chemotherapy wafers (small biodegradable polymer wafers infused with carmustine) at the time of surgery, placed in the neurosurgical cavity bed, due to evidence of improved survival in both the initial and recurrent setting.[11,12] In the initial setting of GBM, the uptake of this local chemotherapy agent is not as widespread as that of the use of systemic temozolomide. There is currently no high-level evidence to combine the use of intraoperative carmustine wafers with sequential concurrent chemoradiation with temozolomide and then adjuvant temozolomide.

Other chemosensitive CNS tumors include PNET, medulloblastoma, CNS lymphoma, and germ cell tumors. Drugs often used to treat both PNET and medulloblastoma include cisplatin, carboplatin, cyclophosphamide, vincristine, etoposide, ifosfamide, thiotepa, and methotrexate. Methotrexate and high-dose cytarabine are commonly used first-line treatments, in association with high-dose steroids, for CNS lymphoma; other drugs used in this setting are vindesine and thiotepa. Drugs commonly used in the setting of CNS germ cell tumors are ifosfamide, etoposide, carboplatin, and cisplatin.[13]

The limitations of cytotoxic drugs include the inherent and acquired resistance to these agents, the inability to deliver adequate concentrations of the drug to the tumor, and the potential complications of the agents. Most currently used anticancer drugs are selected for their ability to kill rapidly dividing tumor cells. These drugs can affect almost every organ system, but especially those with rapidly dividing cells such as bone marrow, the gastrointestinal tract, germinal epithelium, lymphoid tissue, and hair follicles.

These side effects tend to be reversible because of the capacity for stem cell renewal. Other side effects can be delayed, dose dependent, or cumulative, and may be partially reversible when therapy is stopped. It is therefore crucial to evaluate how much drug toxicity can adversely affect a patient's quality of life and to try to balance this against the therapeutic benefit to the disease process. Many of the potential side effects of anticancer therapy have been abrogated by supportive measures such as the use of antiemetic agents to control chemotherapy-related nausea and the use of colony-stimulating growth factors for cell lines of the hematopoietic system to counteract the myelosuppressive effects of anticancer agents. Another supportive measure is the use of prophylactic antibiotics to prevent infections associated with prolonged lymphopenia such as combined sulfamethoxazole and trimethoprim in the setting of newly diagnosed GBM to prevent *Pneumocystis jirovecii*.[7] As more effective supportive measures are introduced, the side-effect profile of agents can shift, and irreversible

toxicities may become more apparent. Some of the drugs introduced as supportive measures can have specific side effects associated with them, such as constipation associated with antiemetic agents and rash associated with antibiotics.

There are several important principles to be learned from the clinical toxicities of anticancer drugs. For instance, the toxicities can be schedule dependent, and patients may have variable toxic responses. Factors to consider before the administration of anticancer drugs include the age of the patient, the severity of the disease, concomitant renal and hepatic function, previous exposure to chemotherapy or radiotherapy, and concomitant medications that may affect the metabolism of other drugs.

The common side effects of chemotherapy can be conveniently divided into the categories immediate, early, delayed, and late. Immediate side effects are those that occur within the first 24 hours, such as nausea and vomiting, local tissue necrosis, phlebitis, anaphylaxis, skin rash, and renal failure. Early side effects have their onset within days to weeks and include myelosuppression, alopecia, stomatitis, and diarrhea. Delayed side effects occur within weeks to months after administration and include anemia, azoospermia (absence of sperm in the ejaculate) or teratospermia (abnormal sperm morphology), hepatocellular damage, hyperpigmentation, and pulmonary fibrosis. Late effects are less well known and are those that become evident months to years later. They include sterility, hypogonadism, premature menopause, and secondary malignancies. The chemotherapeutic agents commonly used for the treatment of malignant brain tumors and their potential risks are listed in **Table 43.1**.

In an attempt to better improve the outcome of patients with brain tumors, several phase 1 and 2 studies and a few phase 3 studies of new molecular agents are ongoing. These studies involve differentiating agents, antiangiogenic agents, anti-invasive agents, modulators of cell growth, and immune-system modulators used either alone or in combination with standard cytotoxic agents. More detailed information regarding these novel agents and how they may affect cell signaling pathways may be found elsewhere.[2,14–18] Many of their toxicity profiles are yet to be fully defined. To date, of these new molecular agents, only bevacizumab is approved for use against recurrent GBM. Nonetheless, there are some commercially available agents such as isotretinoin, tamoxifen, and erlotinib that are used in patients with brain tumors on a largely anecdotal basis. Phase 2 studies of these agents have not demonstrated significant improvement in clinical outcomes, but the agents tend to be used in refractory disease because

Table 43.1 Chemotherapeutic Agents Commonly Used for the Treatment of Malignant Brain Tumors and Their Potential Risks

Class	Agent	Side Effect
Alkylating Agents		
Imidazotetrazine derivative of dacarbazine	Temozolomide Cyclophosphamide	Fatigue and hypersomnolence, myelosuppression (particularly lymphopenia and thrombocytopenia), nausea, vomiting, constipation, acneiform rash Hemorrhagic cystitis, myelosuppression, nausea, vomiting, cardiac toxicity, secondary malignancies
Atypical alkylating agents— platinum agents	Cisplatin Carboplatin	Nausea, vomiting, peripheral neuropathy, ototoxicity, nephrotoxicity, dysgeusia, hypokalemia, hypomagnesemia, visual losses Nausea and vomiting Myelosuppression, peripheral neuropathy, hypokalemia, hypomagnesemia
Nitrosoureas	Carmustine (BCNU) Lomustine (CCNU)	Myelosuppression, nausea, vomiting, pulmonary toxicity, secondary acute leukemia Myelosuppression, nausea, vomiting, delayed renal and pulmonary toxicity
Antimetabolites		
Folic acid analogues	Methotrexate	Neutropenia, mucositis, renal toxicity, hepatotoxicity, pulmonary toxicity, pleural effusion
Pyrimidine analogues	5-Fluorouracil Cytarabine	Myelosuppression, stomatitis/mucositis, diarrhea, rash, hand–foot syndrome, cardiac toxicity (e.g., acute arterial spasm) Leukopenia, thrombocytopenia, gastrointestinal toxicity, conjunctivitis, keratitis, neurologic toxicity
Purine analogues	Thioguanine	Myelosuppression, gastrointestinal toxicity, hepatotoxicity
Natural Products		
Vinca alkaloids	Vincristine	Neurologic toxicity, constipation, hyponatremia, rash
Podophyllotoxins	Etoposide (VP-16)	Myelosuppression, allergic reaction, dermatologic effects, hepatotoxicity
Antitumor antibiotics	Bleomycin Mitomycin C	Anaphylaxis, mucositis, nausea, vomiting, pulmonary fibrosis, hyperpigmentation Myelosuppression, mucositis, alopecia, aplastic anemia, hepatotoxicity, radiation recall effects
Taxanes	Paclitaxel	Hypersensitivity reaction, myelosuppression, neurotoxicity, cardiac toxicity, alopecia, radiation recall effects
Miscellaneous		
Methylhydrazines	Procarbazine	Myelosuppression, nausea, vomiting, neurologic toxicity, allergic reaction, azoospermia, infertility, monoamine oxidase drug reaction
Novel Agents		
Protein kinase C modulators	Tamoxifen (high dose)	Hot flashes, nausea, vomiting, dizziness, thromboembolic disease, neurotoxicity, ocular toxicity
Antiangiogenic agents	Bevacizumab	Nosebleeds, hypertension, proteinuria, venous thromboembolic complications, weakness, pain, diarrhea, gastrointestinal bleeding, gastrointestinal perforation, impaired wound healing, striae, wound dehiscence (including prior craniotomy scars), intracranial bleeding (< 3% life threatening; rare and possibly not related), fatigue, skin toxicity (rare), reversible posterior leukoencephalopathy (< 2%)
Epidermal growth factor receptor tyrosine kinase inhibitors	Erlotinib	Rash on face, neck, chest, back, and arms; diarrhea; loss of appetite; inflammation of the cornea
Cell growth and migration inhibitor	Isotretinoin	Birth defects, mood disorder, muscle pain, visual changes, hyperlipidemia

of their ease of administration and relatively low side-effect profile. The mechanisms and main side effects of these agents are also listed in **Table 43.1**. Note that these molecular or target-based agents can have a variety of side effects that, due to their novel mechanism of action, may be very different from traditional cytotoxic agents. Also, one should be aware that when traditional and novel agents are combined, the side-effect profile of each agent may change in an unexpected manner.

General Neurologic Complications

An enormous range of neurologic symptoms and complications can occur in this patient population. Some may clearly be disease related, but some can also be treatment related. The nervous system is relatively protected against potentially neurotoxic effects of antitumor therapy. Most of the dose-limiting toxicities of anticancer agents are due to the effects on normally dividing cells and occur at doses that do not affect the CNS, a relatively quiescent organ in terms of dividing cells. The blood–brain barrier also protects the brain from exposure to toxic agents. However, several factors have changed the side-effect profile of these agents, resulting in an increase in clinically important neurotoxicity. These include the multimodality approach involving radiotherapy and chemotherapy, novel methods of administration such as intra-arterial or interstitial delivery, and the development of agents that are specifically targeted to the brain.

The cause of neurologic symptoms in brain tumor patients receiving chemotherapy can be difficult to elucidate and is often multifactorial. The disease process may be a direct or indirect source of these symptoms. The direct consequence of involvement of eloquent cortex can be manifest by focal neurologic deficits. General neurologic signs and symptoms include increased intracranial pressure and seizures. Vascular disorders with hemorrhage into the tumor, infarction of the tumor, or CNS infection are also possible complications related to the tumor. In patients with metastatic disease (i.e., secondary brain tumors), paraneoplastic syndromes must be considered. Adverse effects resulting from surgery or radiotherapy may also contribute to neurologic symptoms. Chemotherapeutic agents may have a direct or indirect neurotoxic effect. Direct effects can be manifest as encephalopathy, peripheral neuropathy or myopathy, cerebellar dysfunction, and, in the case of intrathecal administration of agents, myelopathy. Indirect effects include coagulopathy with hemorrhage, myelosuppression with CNS infection, and metabolic enceph-

> **Special Consideration**
>
> - Neurologic symptoms in patients receiving therapy for a brain tumor can be multifactorial.

alopathy. Certain neuropathic disorders such as diabetes mellitus or alcoholism may increase the risk of neurotoxicity from chemotherapeutic agents. Coincidental neurologic disorders and concurrent medications must be considered when evaluating neurologic signs and symptoms. Also, one cannot underestimate the psychological effects of being diagnosed and treated for a brain tumor, and the influence this may have on the manifestation of neurologic symptoms. The potential causes of neurologic symptoms in patients receiving chemotherapy are summarized in **Table 43.2**.

Neurologic Side Effects of Specific Antineoplastic Drugs

Vinca Alkaloids

The vinca alkaloids include the agents vincristine, vinblastine, and vindesine. They can all cause a progressive peripheral neuropathy with continued use. Neurotoxicity is the dose-limiting toxicity for these agents. It is manifest by an initial loss of reflexes and paresthesia in the hands and feet. Continued use of vinca alkaloids may cause muscle pains, weakness, and gait disturbance to the point of complete incapacitation. The process reverses after a period of weeks to months after stopping the drug. Vincristine and vinblastine can also affect the cranial nerves or produce an autonomic neuropathy. As

Table 43.2 Potential Neurologic Complications of Chemotherapeutic Agents Used in Patients with Malignant Brain Tumors

Agent	Type of Neurotoxicity	Clinical Manifestations
Vinca alkaloids	Peripheral	Paresthesias, hyporeflexia, motor dysfunction, gait disorder, bone pain, cranial nerve abnormalities with facial palsy and ophthalmoplegia
	Autonomic	Parasympathetic nervous system dysfunction, constipation, orthostatic hypotension
Cisplatin	Peripheral	Paresthesias, hyporeflexia, loss of vibratory sense, sensory ataxia
	Central	Seizures, encephalopathy, cortical blindness
	Autonomic	Parasympathetic nervous system dysfunction, constipation, orthostatic hypotension
Cytarabine	Central	Encephalopathy, seizures, cerebellar dysfunction
Ifosfamide	Central	Hallucinations, seizures, cerebellar dysfunction
5-Fluorouracil	Central	Confusion, cognitive deficits, cerebellar dysfunction
Methotrexate	Optic neuropathy	Visual changes
	Central	With IV administration: encephalopathy (worse with cranial irradiation)
Paclitaxel	Peripheral	Stocking glove paresthesias, loss of vibration sense, hyporeflexia, orthostatic hypotension
Procarbazine	Peripheral central	Seizures, encephalopathy
	Central	Paresthesia, hyporeflexia
		Lethargy, depression, confusion, agitation, altered mental status
Tamoxifen (high dose)	Central	Unsteady gait, dysmetria, hyperreflexia, seizures

the route of administration is through the biliary system, patients with biliary obstruction require a dose reduction because of enhanced toxicity from prolongation of high tissue levels.

Cisplatin

Cisplatin is both ototoxic and neurotoxic. The ototoxicity is dose related and is manifest as reversible tinnitus early in the course of administration. Hearing loss may be permanent. The neurotoxicity of cisplatin is manifest as a symmetrical sensory neuropathy in both upper and lower extremities and can be reversible after discontinuation of the drug.

Carboplatin

Carboplatin is a platinum agent that, like cisplatin, can be associated with as a symmetrical sensory neuropathy in both upper and lower extremities and can be reversible after discontinuation of the drug. Carboplatin is less neurotoxic than cisplatin.

Procarbazine

Procarbazine can produce several forms of neurologic toxicities ranging from a peripheral neuropathy to a central neurotoxicity manifest by altered levels of consciousness ranging from mild drowsiness to stupor. It can also potentiate the sedative effects of phenothiazines, barbiturates, and narcotics.

Paclitaxel

Paclitaxel, a microtubule toxin, can cause peripheral neuropathy manifest as a distal sensory polyneuropathy. Patients on anticonvulsant medication that can induce the hepatic metabolism of paclitaxel can tolerate higher doses of paclitaxel. In these patients, central neurotoxicity characterized by lethargy and somnolence is dose limiting and reversible.

Ifosfamide

Ifosfamide can cause acute symptoms of hallucinations, confusion, anxiety and restlessness, seizures, cerebellar and cranial nerve dysfunction, hemiparesis, coma, and death. The onset of these symptoms can occur within hours of beginning ifosfamide, and recovery occurs within a few days.

Intrathecal Drug Administration

Intrathecal administration of anticancer drugs to treat or prevent CNS metastases carries the potential for several types of adverse reactions. Methotrexate, the most commonly used intrathecal drug, can produce meningeal irritation, arachnoiditis, and, rarely, paraplegia. Cytarabine can also produce these effects. Methotrexate is also linked to chronic leuko-

---

Causes of Neurologic Symptoms in Brain Tumor Patients Receiving Chemotherapy

- Direct Neurotoxicity from the Agent
  - Encephalopathy
    - § Cisplatin, cytarabine, 5-fluorouracil, ifosfamide, procarbazine, tamoxifen, vincristine
  - Cerebellar dysfunction
    - § Cytarabine, 5-fluorouracil, procarbazine, paclitaxel
  - Peripheral neuropathy/myopathy
    - § Cisplatin, cytarabine, vinca alkaloids, paclitaxel, procarbazine, thalidomide
  - Chemical meningitis
    - § Intrathecal methotrexate, cytarabine, thiotepa
- Indirect Neurotoxicity of Chemotherapy
  - Myelosuppression with CNS infection
  - Coagulopathy with hemorrhage
  - Metabolic encephalopathy
- Tumor-Related Effects
  - Focal neurologic deficits
  - Increased intracranial pressure
  - Seizures
  - Paraneoplastic syndromes
- Complications from Other Therapies
  - Radiation
  - Surgery
  - Coincidental neurologic disorders
  - Concomitant medications
  - Psychological effects

encephalopathy, particularly when combined with cranial irradiation.

Antitumor agents have a high propensity for inducing neurotoxicity, which is evidenced by several clinical manifestations (see text box).

Radiotherapy

Although radiotherapy is the most effective treatment for malignant gliomas, doses high enough to reliably destroy the tumor would also result in brain necrosis, thereby limiting the total dose that can be safely delivered. The risk of neurologic deficits after cranial radiotherapy is associated with high dose, large fraction size, large field size, and very young or old age at time of treatment. Modern techniques with moderate total doses (50 to 54 Gy in the setting of low-grade glioma, 60 Gy in the setting of high-grade glioma), conformal radiotherapy, conventional fractionation, and advanced planning imaging and software are thought to diminish the risk of neurologic deficits. Acute side effects from radiotherapy, such as fatigue, headache, nausea, radiation skin effects such as dermatitis, myelosuppression (associated with craniospinal irradiation), and worsening of neurologic deficits related to the location of the tumor, tend to be reversible and responsive to corticosteroids. These acute side effects do not necessarily correlate with long-term side effects.

The acute radiation skin reactions can be minimized by the use of soap-free emollient cleansers and the regular application of a nonfragranced, nonirritant moisturizer. Sorbolene can relieve mild symptoms but on occasion a mild topical corticosteroid (e.g., 1% hydrocortisone) could be applied to affected skin to aid with symptoms of pruritis.[19]

Acute radiation dermatitis usually resolves over weeks to months, usually resulting in a temporary increase in skin pigmentation. High doses usually result in loss of hair follicles and sebaceous and eccrine glands. This reduces the skin's natural moisture and leads to dry, more sensitive skin that has shed and lost its hairs. Doses over 45 Gy are associated with permanent hair thinning or loss (alopecia). Recovery may take months up to a year, and in some patients the alopecia is long term. If the skin does not show signs of atrophy and thinning, hair transplant can be attempted. Over the following year the skin often becomes thinner, dryer, and semitranslucent, and the vessels are more easily seen. It is critical to protect areas treated with radiotherapy from sunlight as they are subject to accelerated photoaging and a greater risk of secondary malignancies. Many kinds of rashes, irrespective of type and etiology, can initially localize in areas of previous radiotherapy, whether this be recent (hours, days, or weeks) or months or years in the past.[19]

Determining the role of radiotherapy in long-term toxicity, especially cognitive deficits, is complex. Radiotherapy has been regarded as the principal cause of cognitive decline in brain tumor patients because children with brain tumors generally develop intellectual deterioration, presumably caused by radiotherapy. This attribution is confounded by factors such as surgery, chemotherapy, tumor characteristics, tumor progression, presence of recurrent seizures, concurrent medical illnesses, neurologic comorbidity, and medications such as anticonvulsants that can contribute to either or both neurocognitive and neurologic deficits. In fact, recent studies indicate that focal radiotherapy in patients with glioma may not be the main reason for cognitive deficits.[20,21] Instead, the tumor itself and other medical treatments may contribute in large part to cognitive deficits. As patient survival improves, more studies need to be undertaken to elucidate the degree

and cause of neurologic and cognitive deficits in patients undergoing multimodality therapy for cranial tumors. There is increasing interest in developing approaches to minimize cognitive sequelae, such as hippocampal sparing[22] to limit the effects on memory.

The most common radiation-induced endocrinopathies are hypothyroidism and growth hormone deficiency. Treatment effects on growth are multifactorial and include growth hormone deficiency, spinal shortening, precocious puberty, undetected hypothyroidism, and poor nutrition.

■ Anticonvulsant Therapy

Seizures in patients with brain tumors may occur at initial presentation and during the course of disease. The incidence of seizures at presentation of a brain tumor varies with histological subtype, ranging from 90% of patients with low-grade gliomas to 35% of patients with GBM.[23] Whether a tumor produces a seizure and what type of seizure may depend on the location and growth rate of the tumor. Seizures are more frequent when the tumor is cortical and slow growing.[24] Although the incidence of seizures in patients with brain tumors is variable, the use of antiepileptic drugs (AEDs) in this patient population is common, particularly in the peri- and postoperative settings.[25] Still, a randomized controlled study demonstrated that prophylactic AEDs are unlikely to be useful in brain tumor patients who have not had a seizure.[26] The American Academy of Neurology's practice parameters state that AEDs should be given to brain tumor patients who experience a seizure.[27] They also state that prophylactic AEDs should not be administered to patients with newly diagnosed brain tumors who have not experienced a seizure. Nonetheless, a review of practice patterns in North America indicated that most patients with brain tumors are continued on AEDs even if they have never had a seizure.[25] The following subsections discuss the adverse effects of antiepileptics, which can be divided into four categories: dose-related effects, idiosyncratic reactions, drug–drug interactions, and teratogenic effects.

Dose-Related Adverse Effects

Patients who receive too much drug exhibit subsequent dose-related side effects. This is more likely to occur when patients are taking multiple medications, especially multiple anticonvulsants. The potential additive effect of the combination of drugs and the difficulty of regulating multiple agents increase the likelihood of poor tolerance.

Idiosyncratic Reactions

Patients can exhibit idiosyncratic side effects that may occur within a few months of therapy and are not dose related. Some of these may be severe such as Stevens Johnson syndrome and require complete cessation of therapy. Other examples include skin rash and hepatotoxicity.

A rash during the first 5 days of therapy (in the first exposure) is usually due to a nondrug cause. Patients who develop a rash in the first few months of anticonvulsant therapy, particularly with phenytoin, carbamazepine, phenobarbital, and lamotrigine, need to be carefully evaluated. Rashes may only become apparent when the dexamethasone dose is decreased or stopped. The most common anticonvulsant-associated eruption is an isolated, viral-like, eruptive rash usually described as morbilliform or maculopapular in appearance; it is self-limiting. However, a clinically similar eruption may accompany rare but more serious hypersensitivity reactions. Thus, all patients who develop rash during the first few months of anticonvulsant therapy should be instructed to immediately contact their physician for consultation.[19]

Benign drug-associated eruptions typically peak within days and progressively settle over 10 to 14 days. A benign, isolated, drug-related rash is spotty, nonconfluent, and nontender. There should be only minor facial involvement and no periorbital puffiness; no facial or neck edema; and no involvement of the mucosal surfaces of the eye, lip, or mouth. The diagnosis of a benign rash is consistent with the absence of systemic symptoms such as fever, malaise, pharyngitis, anorexia, and headache. There should be no lymphadenopathy, hepatomegaly, or splenomegaly, and laboratory tests should be normal. If a benign isolated rash occurs, the anticonvulsant dose should not be increased until the rash has entirely resolved; ideally the dose should be reduced. Patients who develop a rash should be closely monitored and warned to contact medical staff should the rash worsen or new symptoms emerge. Pruritus associated with a benign rash can be treated with an antihistamine and/or topical corticosteroid. These drugs do not mask the development of a serious reaction.[19]

Serious drug rashes are usually confluent and widespread or show prominent facial, neck, and upper trunk involvement. Serious rashes may be tender or have a purple purpuric or hemorrhagic appearance that does not blanch with pressure. Serious drug rashes may involve mucosal surfaces. They are accompanied or preceded by symptoms and signs of systemic toxicity such as fever, malaise, pharyngitis, anorexia, or lymphadenopathy. Rashes with any feature suggestive of a serious reaction necessitate immediate drug cessation, and investigation and monitoring for internal organ involvement, particularly in the hepatic, renal, and hematologic systems. Involvement of different organs can occasionally occur, and the severity of internal organ toxicities may occur despite drug cessation and may necessitate hospitalization. It is important that another anticonvulsant from a different non–cross-reacting drug group be substituted as rapidly as possible, if immediate discontinuation is necessary, to reduce the risk of status epilepticus. Sodium valproate may usually be substituted safely.[19]

Drug–Drug Interactions

Other drugs may affect the metabolism of anticonvulsants, which can result in altered drug levels. An example is the induction of hepatic enzymes by phenytoin and corticosteroids, thereby affecting the phenytoin levels. In addition, some anticonvulsants may induce the hepatic cytochrome P-450 system and alter the metabolism of a treatment agent being studied. Such drug interactions may alter the type and severity of toxicity that patients experience. For example, it has been shown that patients taking paclitaxel or irinotecan while taking enzyme-inducing antiepileptic drugs (EIAEDs) may have lower than expected plasma levels and higher than expected tolerated doses. Consequently, phase 1 studies of agents known to be metabolized by this enzyme system should stratify patients into two different dose-escalation cohorts of those on and off EIAEDs. A more recent approach in early-phase neuro-oncology studies is to initiate a phase 2 study in brain tumor patients not taking EIAEDs using the established phase 2 dose from other systemic cancer patients. Only if some measure of activity is demonstrated will a phase 1 study of patients taking EIAEDs be performed.

Teratogenicity

The developing fetus can be affected by anticonvulsant medications.

Management of Symptoms

Table 43.3 outlines the dose-related, idiosyncratic, and drug–drug interactions for the common anticonvulsants phenytoin, levetiracetam, carbamazepine, phenobarbital, valproic acid, gabapentin, and lamotrigine. Insomnia has also been reported. Gastrointestinal symptoms are the most common acute effects.

The relatively newer agent levetiracetam which has a low incidence of side effects, is well tolerated and is not an EIAED. The mechanism of action is not well understood but it binds to a synaptic vesicle glycoprotein and inhibits presynaptic calcium channels. Gabapentin, which mimics the chemical structure of the neurotransmitter γ-aminobutyric acid (GABA) and likely interacts with voltage-gated calcium channels, is another agent that is well tolerated, and no serious side effects have consistently been attributed to gabapentin. Levetiracetam and gabapentin have not been associated with liver

Pearl

- Cutaneous drug eruptions with onset after 10 days of exposure to an anticonvulsant, if associated with mucosal involvement or with systemic features, may be serious and require changing the antiepileptic medication to another group or category of drugs.

Table 43.3 Dose-Related, Idiosyncratic Side Effects, and Drug–Drug Interactions for the Most Commonly Used Anticonvulsant Medications

Agent	Dose-Related Side Effects	Idiosyncratic Side Effects	Drug–Drug Interactions
Carbamazepine (CBZ)	Diplopia, ataxia, drowsiness, hyponatremia, choreoathetosis, dystonia	Myelosuppression, hepatitis, rash (and allergic skin reactions),bradycardia, endocrine side effects	*Drugs that increase plasma drug levels:* cimetidine, diltiazem, macrolide antibiotics, e.g., erythromycin and clarithromycin, metronidazole, verapamil *Drugs that decrease plasma drug levels:* cisplatin, Adriamycin, vincristine, felbamate, rifampin, phenytoin, primidone, theophylline CBZ acts as a hepatic cytochrome P-450 inducer and can enhance the metabolism of many drugs, e.g., corticosteroids, warfarin, digoxin, vitamin D, quinidine, theophylline and oral contraceptives; meaning that the dose of these drugs may need increasing Can also accelerate metabolism of various cytotoxic agents including nitrosoureas, paclitaxel, 9-amino-camptothecin, thiotepa, topotecan, and irinotecan, and newer targeted agents, e.g., imatinib, gefitinib, temsirolimus, erlotinib, and tipifarnib; this potentially reducing their effectiveness
Phenytoin (DPH)	Nystagmus, ataxia, lethargy, movement disorders	Gingival hypertrophy, megaloblastic anemia, rash (and allergic skin reactions), hepatotoxicity, endocrine side effects	*Drugs that increase plasma drug levels:* alcohol, diazepam, warfarin, estrogen, phenothiazines, isoniazid, salicylates *Drugs that decrease plasma drug levels:* carbamazepine, sucralfate, antacids, cisplatin, vincristine, and Adriamycin *Drugs whose efficacy may be impaired by DPH:* DPH acts as a hepatic cytochrome P-450 inducer and can enhance the metabolism of many drugs (see above) Can also accelerate metabolism of various cytotoxic agents including nitrosoureas, paclitaxel, 9-amino-camptothecin, thiotepa, topotecan, and irinotecan, and newer targeted agents, e.g., imatinib, gefitinib, temsirolimus, erlotinib, and tipifarnib; this potentially reducing their effectiveness Combinations of DPH with fluoropyrimidines (e.g., 5-fluorouracil increases DPH's toxic side effects)
Phenobarbital	Hypnotic properties, cognitive decline, hyperactivity, irritability, reparatory depression, nausea, vomiting	Megaloblastic anemia, allergic reaction, hepatotoxicity	Anticoagulants, corticosteroids, estrogens, doxycholine acts as a hepatic cytochrome P-450 inducer and can enhance the metabolism of many drugs (see above)
Valproic acid	Sedative effects, tremor, ataxia	Skin rash, thrombocytopenia	Acetylsalicylic acid, carbamazepine, phenytoin It inhibits the glucuronidation of SN-38, active metabolite of irinotecan *Drugs that decrease the plasma concentration:* methotrexate, Adriamycin, cisplatin Toxic effects of valproic acid can be increased when combined with cisplatin or nitrosoureas
Levetiracetam	Somnolence, asthenia, dizziness Routine therapeutic drug monitoring not currently indicated	Depression, nervousness, anxiety, emotional lability, and hostility (and rarely bizarre behavior such as suicidal ideation)	No interactions with other seizure medications or with warfarin, estrogens, or antibiotics
Lamotrigine	Mild ataxia, dizziness, headache, insomnia and sleep disturbance uncommon (6%) Routine therapeutic drug monitoring not currently indicated Skin rash	Skin rash including Stevens-Johnson syndrome Aseptic meningitis (rare) Tourette syndrome (exceedingly rare) Leukopenia	Valproate may delay elimination of lamotrigine Carbamazepine, phenytoin, and other hepatic enzyme inducing medications may shorten half-life

Table 43.3 (*continued*)

Agent	Dose-Related Side Effects	Idiosyncratic Side Effects	Drug–Drug Interactions
Gabapentin	Somnolence, dizziness, ataxia, headache, fatigue Ocular side effects Anorexia, flatulence, gingivitis	Isolated ataxia (rare) Aggression—very uncommon (e.g., in children with learning disabilities or cognitively delayed adults)	Using propoxyphene or acetaminophen together with gabapentin may increase side effects such as dizziness, drowsiness, confusion, difficulty concentrating, and other nervous system or mental effects Elderly patients in particular may experience impairment in thinking, judgment, and coordination The concurrent use of levomethadyl acetate and gabapentin may result in additive CNS and respiratory depression, hypotension, sedation, or coma Avoid gabapentin if on sodium oxybate therapy

dysfunction, serious allergic reaction, or changes in the hematopoietic system. However, levetiracetam has uncommonly been associated with depression (4%), nervousness (4%), anxiety (2%), emotional lability (2%), and hostility (2%) and rarely bizarre behavior such as suicidal ideation (0.7%).[28]

Lamotrigine, a sodium channel blocker, is another agent introduced to assist in the control of focal seizures and primary and secondary tonic-clonic seizures. It is generally well tolerated but has numerous potential side effects and drug–drug interactions (Table 43.3).

Treatment of Cerebral Edema

The development of cerebral edema as a result of direct tumor involvement or subsequent to therapeutic interventions (e.g., surgery or radiation) can be a major problem for patients with brain tumors. Injury to intracranial structures produces cerebral edema. The lack of lymphatics and the leakiness of abnormal tumor vessels predispose to the development of cerebral edema, which can be life threatening. Corticosteroids are used to reduce increased intracranial pressure and control cerebral edema associated with primary or metastatic tumors. However, corticosteroids have a significant toxicity profile and can affect many organ systems.[29,30] The goal of therapy should be to manage symptoms at the minimum steroid dose possible.

The side effects of corticosteroids include electrolyte disturbance, hypertension, hyperglycemia (which can be associated with either the development of steroid-associated diabetes, or exacerbation of underlying/preexisting diabetes), opportunis-

tic infections (especially candida), osteoporosis and fracture, aseptic bone necrosis (also termed avascular necrosis), peripheral edema, glaucoma, cataracts, gastritis and gastrointestinal hemorrhage, cushingoid state (including possible development of buffalo hump), skin fragility and increased bruising, atrophy of skin and development of striae, impaired wound healing, and acne. Corticosteroids can also cause a type of proximal myopathy, manifest as symmetrical proximal muscle weakness, which can have significant impact on the mobility of a brain tumor patient, particularly if the patient has other motor deficits due to the site of the tumor or to surgery. Central nervous system side effects of corticosteroids include mood alteration, insomnia, psychosis, and tremor. Steroids can also contribute to the development of lymphopenia in this population, which is already very common as it can be associated with radiotherapy itself and the use of temozolomide, and which can result in patients being more vulnerable to atypical or opportunistic infections such as *P. jirovecii*. Most of these side effects are reversible with reduction of the steroid dose.

Rapid steroid taper can manifest itself as a worsening of neurologic symptoms (secondary to recurrence of cerebral edema), depression, anorexia, muscle aches, and joint pains. Symptoms of adrenal insufficiency may also occur as a result of a rapid taper. Drug interactions (e.g., phenytoin) may result in decreased bioavailability of corticosteroids and alterations in drug levels.

Anticoagulants

Thromboembolic phenomena represent a major cause of morbidity and mortality in patients with brain tumors. There are increased postoperative risks, especially for patients who are immobile, as well as the general increased risk for venous thromboembolic disease among patients with cancer. Patients with malignant brain tumors can be safely anticoagulated with low molecular weight heparin such as enoxaparin or dalteparin, heparin, and warfarin, if these agents are carefully monitored.[31] Potential interactions of heparin and warfarin with other drugs must also be considered.[32]

Special Consideration

- Corticosteroids have a significant toxicity profile and can affect many organ systems. The goal of therapy should be to manage symptoms at the minimum steroid dose possible. However, rapid steroid taper should be avoided as it can be associated with worsening of neurologic and other constitutional symptoms.

The major risk associated with anticoagulants is bleeding. The most commonly affected sites are the tumor bed and the gastrointestinal or genitourinary tracts. Avoidance of nonsteroidal antiinflammatory drugs and maintaining the platelet count above 50,000 are important. Another potential reversible side effect is heparin-induced thrombocytopenia, which can also increase the risk of bleeding. Warfarin can have gastrointestinal side effects, but the alteration of the anticoagulant effect secondary to concomitant medications is a major factor for consideration in managing possible medical complications. Many agents can potentiate the anticoagulant effect, including cimetidine, acetaminophen, antibiotics, allopurinol, anabolic steroids, and aspirin. Other agents decrease the anticoagulant effect, including glucocorticoids, phenobarbital, vitamin K preparations, carbamazepine, and antacids. Some agents have an initial effect of augmenting the anticoagulant effect, but with continued use can decrease its effect. These agents include phenytoin and oral hypoglycemics. The complex interaction of multiple medications on the anticoagulant effect emphasizes the need for close monitoring of therapy.

With increasing use of bevacizumab in the setting of GBM, there was some concern that there would be increased rates of intracranial hemorrhage. Of note, despite these concerns, this has not been seen to date with the combination of bevacizumab and anticoagulants.[10]

■ Conclusion

The complications of medical therapy for patients with brain tumors include the potential side effects of antitumor agents, radiation, and supportive drug treatment. These types of treatment may cause neurologic toxicity that may be difficult to distinguish from cerebral edema or effects of the tumor. Consequently, it is important to determine whether the patients may be experiencing neurologic toxicity caused by the treatment agent or by preexisting neurologic status. If the toxicity is thought to be due to compromised neurologic status and not therapy, adverse events should be reported in the context of the patient's preexisting neurologic condition. Taking such measures will ensure that efficacious therapeutics are not inappropriately blamed for adverse events and then wrongly discontinued.

Editor's Note

Formidable foes like brain tumors call for formidable treatments. Some of these may cause complications—some expected and others less expected. Several studies in neuro-oncology over the last several decades have systematically helped to gradually decrease the complications of treatment of brain tumors. The first was the trend away from whole-brain radiotherapy to regional (e.g., parallel opposed fields), and then to conformal, thus limiting the volume of normal brain irradiated. Randomized studies of brachytherapy were negative, thus essentially removing this toxic therapy from the armamentarium of the neuro-oncologist.[33] Studies showing that prophylactic antiepileptic drugs were not beneficial for patients without seizures undergoing craniotomy for brain tumor helped decrease the use of these drugs and thus the frequency of complications, including the rare but life-threatening Stevens-Johnson syndrome.[34] Finally, the landmark randomized study of temozolomide helped replace more toxic drugs with a less toxic one as first-line chemotherapy for malignant gliomas. New drugs and treatments with new sets of complications will arise and neuro-oncologists will continue to remain vigilant about such morbidities. (Bernstein)

References

1. Van Meir EG, Bellail A, Phuphanich S. Emerging molecular therapies for brain tumors. Semin Oncol 2004;31(2, Suppl 4):38–46
2. Butowski N, Chang SM. Small molecule and monoclonal antibody therapies in neurooncology. Cancer Contr 2005;12:116–124
3. Fortin D, Desjardins A, Benko A, Niyonsega T, Boudrias M. Enhanced chemotherapy delivery by intraarterial infusion and blood-brain barrier disruption in malignant brain tumors: the Sherbrooke experience. Cancer 2005;103:2606–2615
4. Dunkel IJ, Finlay JL. High-dose chemotherapy with autologous stem cell rescue for brain tumors. Crit Rev Oncol Hematol 2002;41:197–204
5. Galanis E, Buckner JC. Chemotherapy of brain tumors. Curr Opin Neurol 2000;13:619–625
6. Stupp R, van den Bent MJ, Hegi ME. Optimal role of temozolomide in the treatment of malignant gliomas. Curr Neurol Neurosci Rep 2005; 5:198–206
7. Stupp R, Mason WP, van den Bent MJ, et al; European Organisation for Research and Treatment of Cancer Brain Tumor and Radiotherapy Groups; National Cancer Institute of Canada Clinical Trials Group. Radiotherapy plus concomitant and adjuvant temozolomide for glioblastoma. N Engl J Med 2005;352:987–996
8. Hau P, Baumgart U, Pfeifer K, et al. Salvage therapy in patients with glioblastoma: is there any benefit? Cancer 2003;98:2678–2686
9. Friedman HS, Prados MD, Wen PY, et al. Bevacizumab alone and in combination with irinotecan in recurrent glioblastoma. J Clin Oncol 2009;27:4733–4740

10. Rahmathulla G, Hovey EJ, Hashemi-Sadraei N, Ahluwalia MS. Bevacizumab in high-grade gliomas: a review of its uses, toxicity assessment, and future treatment challenges. Onco Targets Ther 2013;6:371–389

11. Valtonen S, Timonen U, Toivanen P, et al. Interstitial chemotherapy with carmustine-loaded polymers for high-grade gliomas: a randomized double-blind study. Neurosurgery 1997;41:44–48, discussion 48–49

12. Westphal M, Hilt DC, Bortey E, et al. A phase 3 trial of local chemotherapy with biodegradable carmustine (BCNU) wafers (Gliadel wafers) in patients with primary malignant glioma. Neuro-oncol 2003;5:79–88

13. Schiff D, O'Neill BP, eds. Principles of Neuro-Oncology. New York: McGraw-Hill, 2005

14. Newton HB. Molecular neuro-oncology and development of targeted therapeutic strategies for brain tumors. Part 1: Growth factor and Ras signaling pathways. Expert Rev Anticancer Ther 2003;3:595–614

15. Newton HB. Molecular neuro-oncology and development of targeted therapeutic strategies for brain tumors. Part 2: PI3K/Akt/PTEN, mTOR, SHH/PTCH and angiogenesis. Expert Rev Anticancer Ther 2004;4:105–128

16. Newton HB. Molecular neuro-oncology and the development of targeted therapeutic strategies for brain tumors. Part 3: brain tumor invasiveness. Expert Rev Anticancer Ther 2004;4:803–821

17. Newton HB. Molecular neuro-oncology and the development of targeted therapeutic strategies for brain tumors. Part 4: p53 signaling pathway. Expert Rev Anticancer Ther 2005;5:177–191

18. Newton HB. Molecular neuro-oncology and the development of targeted therapeutic strategies for brain tumors, Part 5: apoptosis and cell cycle. Expert Rev Anticancer Ther 2005;5:355–378

19. Australian Cancer Network Adult Brain Tumour Guidelines Working Party. Clinical Practice Guidelines for the Management of Adult Gliomas: Astrocytomas and Oligodendrogliomas. Cancer Council Australia, Australia Cancer Network and Clinical Oncological Society of Australia, Inc., Sydney, 2009

20. Taphoorn MJ, Klein M. Cognitive deficits in adult patients with brain tumours. Lancet Neurol 2004;3:159–168

21. Laack NN, Brown PD. Cognitive sequelae of brain radiation in adults. Semin Oncol 2004;31:702–713

22. Gondi V, Tomé WA, Mehta MP. Why avoid the hippocampus? A comprehensive review. Radiother Oncol 2010;97:370–376

23. Vecht CJ, Wagner GL, Wilms EB. Interactions between antiepileptic and chemotherapeutic drugs. Lancet Neurol 2003;2:404–409

24. Behin A, Hoang-Xuan K, Carpentier AF, Delattre JY. Primary brain tumours in adults. Lancet 2003;361:323–331

25. Chang SM, Parney IF, Huang W, et al; Glioma Outcomes Project Investigators. Patterns of care for adults with newly diagnosed malignant glioma. JAMA 2005;293:557–564

26. Forsyth PA, Weaver S, Fulton D, et al. Prophylactic anticonvulsants in patients with brain tumour. Can J Neurol Sci 2003;30:106–112

27. Glantz MJ, Cole BF, Forsyth PA, et al; Report of the Quality Standards Subcommittee of the American Academy of Neurology. Practice parameter: anticonvulsant prophylaxis in patients with newly diagnosed brain tumors. Neurology 2000;54:1886–1893

28. Mula M, Sander JW. Suicidal ideation in epilepsy and levetiracetam therapy. Epilepsy Behav 2007;11:130–132

29. Kaal EC, Vecht CJ. The management of brain edema in brain tumors. Curr Opin Oncol 2004;16:593–600

30. Nahaczewski AE, Fowler SB, Hariharan S. Dexamethasone therapy in patients with brain tumors—a focus on tapering. J Neurosci Nurs 2004; 36:340–343

31. Auguste KI, Quiñones-Hinojosa A, Berger MS. Efficacy of mechanical prophylaxis for venous thromboembolism in patients with brain tumors. Neurosurg Focus 2004;17:E3 http://www.aans.org/education/ journal/neurosurgical/oct04/ 17–4-3.pdf Accessed March 1, 2006 [serial online]

32. Knovich MA, Lesser GJ. The management of thromboembolic disease in patients with central nervous system malignancies. Curr Treat Options Oncol 2004;5:511–517

33. Laperriere NJ, Leung PMK, McKenzie S, et al. Randomized study of brachytherapy in the initial management of patients with malignant astrocytoma. Int J Radiat Oncol Biol Phys 1998;41:1005–1011

34. Glantz MJ, Cole BF, Friedberg MH, et al. A randomized, blinded, placebo-controlled trial of divalproex sodium prophylaxis in adults with newly diagnosed brain tumors. Neurology 1996;46:985–991

44 Pseudoprogression After Glioma Therapy

James Perry

Since the introduction of concomitant temozolomide chemotherapy with radiation for patients with newly diagnosed glioblastoma, there has been increased awareness of post-treatment changes detected on imaging studies, especially with magnetic resonance imaging (MRI). The appearance of increased contrast enhancement accompanied by increased cerebral edema, with or without accompanying clinical symptoms, is seen in 20 to 50% of patients who complete chemoradiation.[1,2] These changes are indistinguishable from those of true disease progression, yet some, and perhaps most, of these changes resolve over time and therefore represent a transient effect of therapy now coined pseudoprogression.[3] Most prospective case series have found that patients who experience imaging pseudoprogression have longer overall survival times, so rather than being an ominous sign of treatment resistance, the changes seen following chemoradiation are, paradoxically, sometimes a sign of improved treatment sensitivity.[2,4]

Pearl

- Pseudoprogression may be a form of treatment response. Worsening appearances on conventional imaging (computed tomography [CT], MRI) within 12 weeks of radiation therapy must be interpreted with caution as not all patients with "worse" scans will turn out to have "worse" disease.

■ Definition of Pseudoprogression

Pseudoprogression is suspected on clinical grounds when post-treatment MRI scans demonstrate features of disease progression such as increased contrast enhancement and edema that later resolve without a change in treatment (clinically suspected pseudoprogression, **Fig. 44.1**) or, in cases where surgical re-resection is performed, the tissue is found to be inflammatory without clear evidence of viable tumor cells (surgically confirmed pseudoprogression, **Fig. 44.2**). The vast majority of cases reported in the literature are clinically suspected rather than surgically confirmed; thus, there is much that remains speculative and controversial about the incidence and pathophysiology of this important posttreatment finding.

Until recently, the accepted best practice for determination of tumor response on imaging has been the comparison of measurements using the bidimensional cross-sectional area of the enhancing component of a tumor on consecutive scans.[5] These criteria rely on the presence of enhancing disease and also consider the patient's clinical condition and corticosteroid dose. These criteria have served us well in practice and as a standardized measurement across clinical trials; however, a variety of advances in neuro-oncology have called for a new definition of tumor response.[6] For example, not all tumors have contrast enhancement, such as most low-grade gliomas, and some therapies, notably the anti–vascular endothelial growth factor (VEGF) agent bevacizumab, can greatly reduce contrast enhancement, and disease progression can be due to non–contrast-enhancing tumor growth such as increases in T2 or fluid-attenuated inversion recovery (FLAIR) signal on consecutive MRI scans. For these reasons a working group developed updated criteria for response assessment in high-grade glioma termed the Response Assessment in Neuro-Oncology (RANO) criteria,[7] which specifically address the issue of pseudoprogression by calling into question the reliability of conventional MRI within 12 weeks of the completion of chemoradiation in newly diagnosed patients. Within these first 12 weeks a diagnosis of disease progression can be made only if an enlarging lesion is outside of the high-dose volume of radiation therapy (RT) or if the enlarging in-field lesion is resected and confirmed to contain viable tumor. Thus, pragmatically, pseudoprogression is an entity commonly considered within the first 3 months after chemoradiation. The cutoff of 3 months is expected to be widely incorporated into clinical trials; however, clinicians are advised to be aware that cases of both clinically suspected and surgically confirmed pseudoprogression have been observed well beyond 3 months.[3]

■ Incidence

Pseudoprogression has been widely reported from many institutions with reasonably concordant estimates of frequency. Typically, MRI scans are obtained 4 to 6 weeks following the completion of RT or chemoradiation and are compared to the postoperative MRI or MRI scan acquired at the time of RT planning. It is important for treatment centers to adopt a standardized approach to this sequence of imaging to ensure valid comparisons. For example, the imaging modality of choice is MRI with gadolinium contrast using standard anatomic imaging sequences, ideally with diffusion-weighted MRI to detect postoperative ischemia or infarction that may be confused with enhancing disease. The post-chemoradiation scan should include the same imaging parameters. Early disease progression is suspected when an increase in contrast-enhancing disease is noted. To date, there are no validated criteria to guide how best to conduct tumor measurements at the end of chemoradiation. Most series, and now most clinical trials, suggest using the RANO criteria and consider a 25% increase, or greater, in maximal biaxial diameter to be significant. No clear definition regarding changes in FLAIR imaging has emerged.

Table 44.1 lists the reported case series of patients who were found to have early imaging progression following chemoradiation for glioblastoma. Very few of these series have many patients with surgically confirmed pseudoprogression; most of them base the diagnosis of pseudoprogression on subsequent serial imaging that demonstrates stability or improvement of the lesion size over time. Thus, this collection of cases is not standardized with respect to timing of scans or definition of disease; however, recognizing these limitations, we

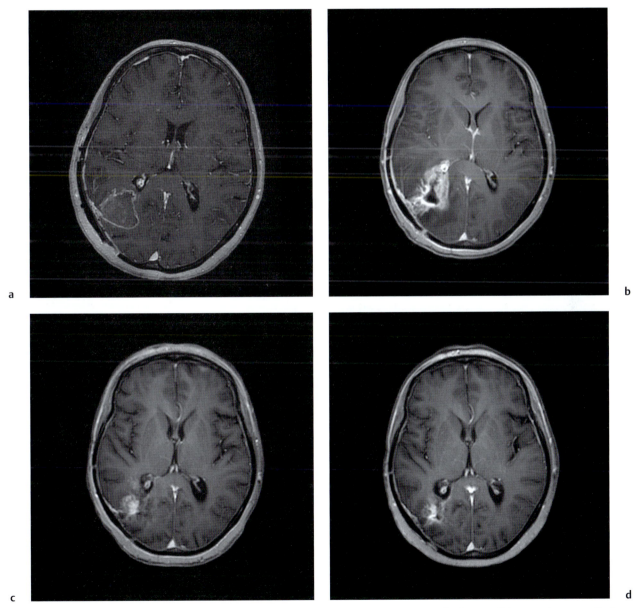

Fig. 44.1a–h Clinically suspected pseudoprogression following chemoradiation for newly diagnosed glioblastoma in a 54-year-old woman with a left parieto-occipital glioblastoma. (**a**) Axial gadolinium-enhanced images preradiotherapy. (**b**) Six weeks postradiotherapy. (**c**) Following 2 months of adjuvant temozolomide. (**d**) After completion of 6 months of adjuvant temozolomide. (*continued on next page*)

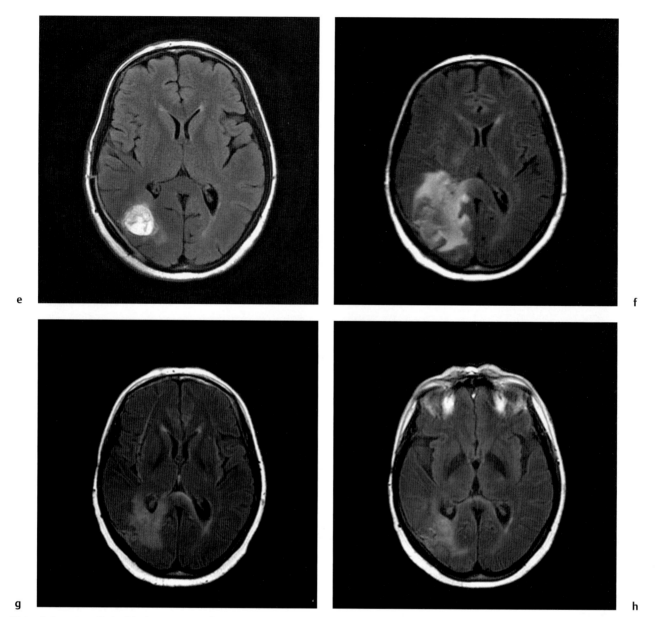

e

f

g

h

Fig. 44.1a–h (*continued*) (**e–h**) The corresponding axial fluid-attenu-ated inversion recovery (FLAIR) images. Immediately postradiother-apy there is a striking increase in enhancement and FLAIR abnormality at a time that this patient was asymptomatic and not requiring corticosteroids. The imaging changes of apparent progres-sion resolved during subsequent cycles of adjuvant chemotherapy.

attempted to pool the results across studies. Of the 2,468 pa-tients reported, 30.6% (range, 10-66%) had early progression on the first posttreatment MRI, and of the same 2,468 patients, 12.6% (range, 5.7–31%) were determined to have pseudopro-gression based on the lack of imaging progression on subse-quent scans without a change in therapy. A very instructive preliminary report from the AVAglio phase III trial of chemo-radiation with RT plus temozolomide with or without beva-cizumab versus placebo should be noted.[8] Bevacizumab is a potent monoclonal antibody against VEGF ligand and has profound effects on tumor vasculature. Some have termed this effect "vascular normalization," the net effect of which is

felt to be normalization of the "leaky" intratumoral vessels such that less contrast extravasation occurs. Some authors have termed this appearance "pseudoresponse" because MRI subsequent to bevacizumab therapy often shows significant reduction in contrast enhancement and tumor size.[9] The AVAglio trial had standardized timing and MRI sequence ac-quisition, so these data are among the most robust imaging data in the field of neuro-oncology.

Importantly, the diagnoses of pseudoprogression or true disease progression were made only in hindsight once the natural history of the patient's tumor was seen on serial im-aging. This study provides a useful working definition for

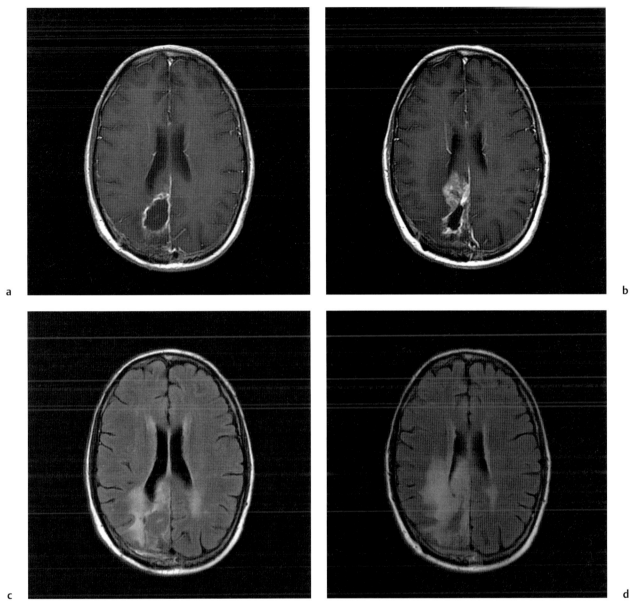

a   b   c   d

Fig. 44.2a–d Surgically confirmed pseudoprogression following chemoradiation for newly diagnosed glioblastoma in a 54-year-old woman (not the same patient as in Fig. 44.1) with partially excised right parieto-occipital glioblastoma pre- and postradiotherapy. (**a**) Axial gadolinium-enhanced MRI from the time of radiation planning. (**b**) Interval development of increased contrast enhancement 6 weeks following completion of chemoradiation. (**c,d**) Corresponding axial FLAIR images show an increase in FLAIR signal. Taken together these imaging findings are concerning for disease progression. Findings at surgical re-resection demonstrated reactive astrocytosis and inflammation with no viable tumor seen.

pseudoprogression: "a > 25% increase in index lesions and/or unequivocal progression of existing non-index lesions relative to baseline and, in the absence of clinical deterioration, was assessed as pseudoprogression, and then confirmed at the end of 2 months of continuing therapy." In this trial only 12/458 (2.6%) of patients in the bevacizumab-containing treatment arm were felt to have early progression, whereas 84/463 (18.1%) had early progression in the placebo-arm.[9] Thus, bevacizumab clearly influences the degree of contrast enhancement seen on imaging and, notably, the 18.1% incidence of early disease progression in the placebo-treated patients was lower than the simple pooled average in other series where imaging criteria were less stringent. The finding of pseudoprogression was similarly lower in the AVAglio trial than suspected from prior mixed series, and, interestingly, the patients in the bevacizumab-containing arm had a very low rate of early progression and pseudoprogression overall (less than 3%).

Table 44.1 Summary of Case Series and Clinical Trials Reporting the Incidence of Pseudoprogression

Study	No. of Patients	No. with Early Progression (%)	No. Determined as Pseudoprogression (%)
Taal et al[3]	68	31/68 (46%)	15/68 (22%)
Brandes et al[14]	103	50/103(52%)	32/103 (31%)
Chaskis et al[24]	54	25/54 (46%)	3/54 (6%)
Clarke et al[25]	85	35/85 (41%)	10/77(13%)
Fabi et al[26]	12	4/12 (33%)	2/12 (17%)
Peca et al[27]	50	15/50 (30%)	4/50 (8%)
Roldan et al[28]	43	25/43 (58%)	10/38 (26%)
Gerstner et al[29]	45	24/45 (53%)	13/45 (29%)
Sanghera et al[4]	104	27/104 (26%)	7/99 (7%)
Tsien et al[30]	27	14/27(52%)	6/27 (22%)
Yaman et al[31]	67	17/67 (25%)	4/67 (6%)
Gunjur et al[32]	68	41/68 (60%)	14/68 (21%)
Kang et al[33]	35	18/35 (51%)	8/35 (23%)
Kong et al[34]	90	59/90 (66%)	26/90 (29%)
Young et al[15]	321	93/321 (29%)	30/321(9.3%)
Park et al[35]	48	25/48 (52%)	11/48% (23%)
Pouleau et al[36]	63	33/63 (52%)	7/63 (11%)
Lee et al[16]	52	24/52 (46%)	12/52 (23%)
Topkan et al[37]	63	28/63(44%)	12/63 (19%)
Choi et al[38]	117	62/117 (53%)	28/117 (24%)
Motegi et al[39]	32	11/28 (39%)	3/32 (9.4%)
Wick et al[8]	Total, 921 Avastin arm, 458 Placebo arm, 463	96/921 (10.4%) 12/458 (2.6%) 84/463 (18.1%)	53/921 (5.7%) 10/458 (2.2%) 43/463 (9.3%)
Total, simple average, range	2,468	757/2,468 (30.6%) Range: 10–66%	310/2,468 (12.6%) Range: 5.7–31%

Source: Adapted with permission from Kruser TJ, Mehta MP, Robins IH. Pseudoprogression after glioma therapy: a comprehensive review. Exp Rev Neurother. 2013;14,4:389–403.

Pitfall

- Neuroimaging (CT or MRI) within 12 weeks of the end of radiotherapy is often unreliable. Unless changes in contrast enhancement and edema suggestive of disease progression are outside of the known radiation volume or a new distinct lesion is seen, the diagnosis of disease progression cannot be made with certainty.

■ Clinical Significance

Pseudoprogression can be seen after many types of therapeutic intervention and in brain tumor types other than glioblastoma. The landmark paper in 2005 changed the standard of care for newly diagnosed glioblastoma.[10] The addition of temozolomide chemotherapy to RT is expected to introduce a radiosensitization effect into early treatment; thus, some believe that the early adverse changes that characterize up to 30% of MRI scans after completion of chemoradiation represent an enhanced effect on tumor cell disruption, apoptosis, and inflammation. The adoption of adjuvant chemotherapy after chemoradiation created a new clinical practice of increased scrutiny of the postradiotherapy scans in order to determine if continuing with adjuvant temozolomide was appropriate. It was in this context, the putatively increased treatment effect, and the need to make an imaging-based clinical decision on adjuvant therapy, that pseudoprogression was first noticed. That said, a similar imaging phenomenon has been reported following RT alone for both low- and high-grade gliomas. In addition, a variety of other treatment interventions may increase the degree of contrast enhancement and edema seen on scans acquired posttreatment. Examples include intratumoral or intracavitary brachytherapy, convection-enhanced delivery, chemotherapy-impregnated wafers, radiosurgery, and high-intensity focused ultrasound. In addition to these effects, likely directly related to treatment, clinicians must consider other situations that might also mimic disease progression, including postoperative ischemia or infarction, postoperative

Pearl

- Pseudoprogression is best known following radiation and concomitant temozolomide chemotherapy for glioblastoma, but can be seen in both low- and high-grade gliomas following radiation alone, and following other experimental therapies such as brachytherapy, RT, and intracavitary treatment. In addition, common clinical issues such as decreasing dexamethasone dose, seizures just prior to or during MRI scans, and postoperative infarct along the surgical cavity can also mimic disease progression.

Controversy

- The MGMT methylation status is associated with pseudoprogression in some, but not all, reports. A large clinical trial with prospective determination of imaging did not find an association of MGMT methylation with pseudoprogression. In clinical practice, one should not take comfort in the assumption that a patient with a methylated MGMT promoter is more likely to have pseudoprogression as an explanation for early posttreatment imaging changes.

healing, recent seizures, and even decreases in dexamethasone dose in the days leading up to the MRI scan.[7,11,12]

Effects of Pseudoprogression on Design and Interpretation of Clinical Trials

Two areas of clinical trial design have been reconsidered since widespread recognition of pseudoprogression: the interpretation of progression-free survival (PFS), and the timing of entry into clinical trials for patients with recurrent disease.[13] Clinical trials testing novel therapy for newly diagnosed patients typically use overall survival as the most objective and meaningful end point; however, phase 1 and 2 studies designed to detect a signal of early efficacy of a compound in development might use an earlier end point such as PFS. If the study treatment itself is associated with pseudoprogression (e.g., intracavitary treatment, or a radiation sensitizer), then progression might be mistakenly determined earlier, leading to premature abandonment of the clinical trial intervention. Conversely, clinical trials testing new therapies often do so in the setting of recurrent disease; these allow entry of patients typically at the time of first progression seen on MRI scans. Obviously, if a patient is entered into such a trial but truly harbors pseudoprogression, then the effects of the new therapy would tend to be overestimated. The RANO criteria have set 12-weeks post-RT as the earliest point at which true disease progression can be assumed and the point at which a patient can be enrolled into a study testing therapy for recurrent disease.[7]

The Effect of Pseudoprogression on Prognosis and the Role of Methylguanine Methyltransferase

Although a patient who experiences true disease progression will not do as well as a patient with no disease progression, what about a patient with pseudoprogression? If part of the explanation of pseudoprogression is an enhanced antitumor effect, it stands to reason that the prognosis of patients with pseudoprogression may be better due to increased tumor sensitivity to treatment. Indeed, most reports on pseudoprogression have noticed a striking improvement in survival when comparing these patients to patients with either stable disease or true progression. Our own series of 104 patients is typical of the outcomes reported by others. We found early disease progression in 26% of patients on the first post-chemoradiation MRI and, of these, 32% were determined to have pseudoprogression.[4] Median survival, adjusted for the important prognostic variables of age and performance status, was significantly longer in the pseudoprogression group (124.9 weeks versus 36.0 weeks; $p = 0.03$)

The reason(s) for prolonged survival in patients with pseudoprogression are unknown. In 2008 it was reported that methylation of the methylguanine methyltransferase (MGMT) promoter was associated with pseudoprogression.[14] This finding was taken at the time to perhaps explain the enhanced treatment sensitivity hypothesis (methylated patients are known to respond better to temozolomide) and the prolonged survival in these patients (MGMT methylation is a strong prognostic marker for overall survival). Despite these findings, questions still loomed; the determination of pseudoprogression was made on clinical grounds, not by a tissue diagnosis, but was the apparent association of MGMT methylation with pseudoprogression the correct interpretation, or was the converse true, that nonmethylated patients were much more likely to progress earlier? Some case series have not been able to confirm the association between MGMT status and pseudoprogression, and the recent AVAglio study report found no difference in the chance of pseudoprogression based on MGMT status, leaving this finding in doubt.

Effect on Therapeutic Decisions

If the early posttreatment MRI demonstrates progression, the clinician must decide if the changes might represent true disease worsening (changes outside the high-dose margins of treatment or new nodules of disease) while recognizing that new areas of enhancement may commonly occur within the treatment field. If patients are very symptomatic, surgical resection may be indicated in selected patients to reduce mass effect and allow histological examination of the tissue.

Specialized Imaging Modalities for the Assessment of Pseudoprogression

A great deal of work is being done to develop novel imaging modalities to aid in the distinction of pseudoprogression from true disease progression. One can argue that the inflammatory posttreatment changes seen in pseudoprogression lie along a spectrum of changes ranging from mild asymptomatic reactive tissue to pseudoprogression (symptomatic or asymptomatic) to frank radiation necrosis.[2] The distinction of frank radiation necrosis from disease progression cannot be adequately made by anatomic MRI scans alone; yet, newer MRI sequences such as diffusion and perfusion mapping, and metabolic imaging such as positron emission tomography (PET), are unable to add sufficient information to obviate the need for a tissue diagnosis as the gold standard.[15-18] If pseudoprogression is simply a milder form of posttreatment radiation change, it may be similarly difficult to use advanced MRI or non-MRI techniques to assist with the diagnosis of pseudoprogression. Although a wide variety of imaging techniques have been reported and remain under investigation, none has added to the specificity of conventional MRI to the point of being useful in the clinic. Recent development of the first animal model of radiation necrosis may help to stimulate experiments correlating imaging findings with histopathology and molecular profiling of tissue.[19] This remains an important area of research, one that again is limited by the operational, rather than tissue-based, definition of pseudoprogression.

Treatment of Pseudoprogression

When pseudoprogression occurs, it can be associated with a range of imaging findings from modestly increased contrast enhancement and edema, which may or may not be clinically symptomatic, to a strikingly worse imaging appearance accompanied by clinical deterioration. In practice the clinician must use clinical judgment to determine each situation in its own right. It is important to keep in mind the mimics of progression on an MRI, such as a recent seizure, infarction around the surgical cavity, and a recent or abrupt reduction in dexamethasone dose. A patient who is asymptomatic but who has imaging changes showing modest worsening of disease on the post-chemoradiation MRI should likely continue on adjuvant temozolomide therapy and be monitored for the need for increased dexamethasone therapy based on symptom requirement. In the bigger picture, it was likely that in the past these sorts of patient situations led to overdiagnosing of disease progression early in the course of treatment. It is commonly observed that the median survival of patients with newly diagnosed glioblastoma in recent randomized trials is on the order of 18 months, whereas survival in the pivotal 2005 study (when

pseudoprogression was not widely recognized) was on the order of 14 months, perhaps in part explained by early abandonment of temozolomide therapy at a point in neuro-oncology history that few other effective therapies were available.[10]

Patients with worsening imaging findings that are most striking can be asymptomatic or symptomatic clinically. The presence of absence of symptoms does not appear to be a sensitive indicator of true progressive disease.[20] Asymptomatic patients likely can continue on adjuvant temozolomide therapy and be followed closely for clinical deterioration and with MRI. The subsequent MRI 2 months later, if the patient is clinically stable, will, according to RANO criteria, be the pivotal scan for determination of pseudoprogression versus true progression. Patients who are symptomatic clinically are more problematic to manage. Clinicians can begin by increasing the dexamethasone dose and carrying on with adjuvant treatment; however, patients already on high doses of dexamethasone or experiencing neurologic deterioration or symptoms of mass effect should be considered for early reoperation. The advantages of surgical intervention are difficult to quantify but include immediate reduction in mass effect, reduced dexamethasone requirement, and histological examination of the resected tissue. A surgical specimen revealing inflammatory changes without obvious viable tumor can be considered as evidence favoring pseudoprogression, and adjuvant chemotherapy should continue unchanged. A surgical specimen with sheets of viable tumor cells with active mitoses and high labeling indices favors a diagnosis of disease progression, and a change in postoperative therapy is indicated.

There have been preliminary reports of the use of anti-VEGF therapy, particularly bevacizumab, for the management of symptomatic pseudoprogression.[21] The mechanism of action of bevacizumab appears ideally suited to the purported mechanism of pseudoprogression and may work through vascular normalization and its profound effect on cerebral edema. To date, this is an off-label use of bevacizumab but it might be considered in individual cases, such as patients with symptomatic progression and nonresectable disease. Recently, a small randomized controlled trial of bevacizumab versus placebo was reported in the treatment of cerebral radiation necrosis following head and neck RT or RT of primary and secondary brain tumors.[22] The results strikingly favored the patients treated with bevacizumab versus placebo. Clear data such as these do not exist for pseudoprogression; however, it appears biologically intriguing as a future therapy for this condition.

Conclusion

Pseudoprogression has been increasingly recognized since the widespread adoption of concurrent radiation and temozolomide followed by adjuvant temozolomide for glioblastoma. However, pseudoprogression can occur after radiation alone, and in both high- and low-grade glioma. About 30% of patients show worsening MRI features at the time of the first post-chemoradiation scan, and in half of these patients the adverse changes will stabilize or improve over the course of continuing adjuvant therapy. It is important not to abandon adjuvant chemotherapy, such as temozolomide, too early in the case of pseudoprogression, and it is important not to enroll patients with pseudoprogression prematurely into clinical trials testing new therapies for recurrent disease. At present, novel MRI modalities such as diffusion and perfusion mapping and metabolic imaging do not add sufficient information to be useful in the clinic for the pragmatic diagnosis of pseudoprogression.[23] Treatment of pseudoprogression can range from no change in management for mild cases, to early surgical resection or perhaps anti-VEGF treatment in nonresectable cases. More work on the definition of pseudoprogression, on imaging modalities to improve case ascertainment, and on treatment is required.

Editor's Note

Pseudoprogression is the apparent worsening on imaging after treatment of a brain tumor, which later improves with no change in treatment, indicating it was not true tumor progression. This can be observed when any powerful treatment is administered that can cause swelling, lesion enlargement, or increased enhancement presumably due to alteration of vasculature. It is seen commonly after high-dose radiation as in stereotactic radiosurgery for vestibular schwannomas and for brain metastases. In the latter case the differential diagnosis of a slightly worse-looking lesion on follow-up MRI includes recurrent tumor, radiation effect, and impending radiation necrosis.

The clinical implications are significant to the neurosurgeon, radiation oncologist, and neuro-oncologist who must decide whether to wait to see what develops or to intervene. Also, there may be implications for clinical trial design, execution, and interpretation. There are some noninvasive modalities to try to sort out pseudoprogression from true progression, but they are not fail safe, and with new targeted therapies and other powerful treatments that will inevitably develop, pseudoprogression will remain a prominent challenge in the experience of neuro-oncology patients and their health care providers. (Bernstein)

References

1. Brandsma D, Stalpers L, Taal W, Sminia P, van den Bent MJ. Clinical features, mechanisms, and management of pseudoprogression in malignant gliomas. Lancet Oncol 2008;9:453–461
2. Kruser TJ, Mehta MP, Robins HI. Pseudoprogression after glioma therapy: a comprehensive review. Expert Rev Neurother 2013;13:389–403
3. Taal W, Brandsma D, de Bruin HG, et al. Incidence of early pseudo-progression in a cohort of malignant glioma patients treated with chemo-irradiation with temozolomide. Cancer 2008;113:405–410
4. Sanghera P, Perry JR, Sahgal A, et al. Pseudoprogression following chemoradiotherapy for glioblastoma multiforme. Can J Neurol Sci 2010;37:36–42
5. Macdonald DR, Cascino TL, Schold SC Jr, Cairncross JG. Response criteria for phase II studies of supratentorial malignant glioma. J Clin Oncol 1990;8:1277–1280
6. Perry JR, Cairncross JG. Glioma therapies: how to tell which work? J Clin Oncol 2003;21:3547–3549
7. Wen PY, Macdonald DR, Reardon DA, et al. Updated response assessment criteria for high-grade gliomas: response assessment in neuro-oncology working group. J Clin Oncol 2010;28:1963–1972
8. Wick W, Cloughesy TF, Nishikawa R, et al. Tumor response based on adapted Macdonald criteria and assessment of Pseudoprogression (PsPD) in the phase III AVAglio trial of bevacizumab (Bv) plus temozolomide (T) plus radiotherapy (RT) in newly diagnosed glioblastoma (GBM). Proc ASCO 2013; abstract 2002
9. Chinot OL, Macdonald DR, Abrey LE, Zahlmann G, Kerloëguen Y, Cloughesy TF. Response assessment criteria for glioblastoma: practical adaptation and implementation in clinical trials of antiangiogenic therapy. Curr Neurol Neurosci Rep 2013;13:347–358
10. Stupp R, Mason WP, van den Bent MJ, et al; European Organisation for Research and Treatment of Cancer Brain Tumor and Radiotherapy Groups; National Cancer Institute of Canada Clinical Trials Group. Radiotherapy plus concomitant and adjuvant temozolomide for glioblastoma. N Engl J Med 2005;352:987–996
11. Hyingo da Cruz LC, Rodriguez I, Domingues RC, Gasparetto EL, Sorensen AG. Pseudoprogression and pseudoresponse: imaging challenges in the assessment of posttreatment glioma. Am J Neurorad 2011;32:1978–1985
12. Rheims S, Ricard D, van den Bent M, et al. Peri-ictal pseudoprogression in patients with brain tumor. Neuro-oncol 2011;13:775–782
13. Reardon DA, Galanis E, DeGroot JF, et al. Clinical trial end points for high-grade glioma: the evolving landscape. Neuro-oncol 2011;13:353–361
14. Brandes AA, Franceschi E, Tosoni A, et al. MGMT promoter methylation status can predict the incidence and outcome of pseudoprogression after concomitant radiochemotherapy in newly diagnosed glioblastoma patients. J Clin Oncol 2008;26:2192–2197
15. Young RJ, Gupta A, Shah AD, et al. Potential utility of conventional MRI signs in diagnosing pseudoprogression in glioblastoma. Neurology 2011;76:1918–1924
16. Lee WJ, Choi SH, Park CK, et al. Diffusion-weighted MR imaging for the differentiation of true progression from pseudoprogression following concomitant radiotherapy with temozolomide in patients with newly diagnosed high-grade gliomas. Acad Radiol 2012;19:1353–1361
17. Gahramanov S, Muldoon LL, Varallyay CG, et al. Pseudoprogression of glioblastoma after enhanced perfusion MR imaging with ferumoxytol versus gadoteridol and correlation with survival. Radiology 2013;266:842–852
18. Young RJ, Gupta A, Shah AD, et al. MRI perfusion in determining pseudoprogression in patients with glioblastoma. Clin Imaging 2013;37:41–49
19. Kumar S, Arbab AS, Jain R, et al. Development of a novel animal model to differentiate radiation necrosis from tumor recurrence. J Neurooncol 2012;108:411–420

20. Singh AD, Easaw JC. Does neurologic deterioration help to differentiate between pseudoprogression and true disease progression in newly diagnosed glioblastoma multiforme? Curr Oncol 2012;19:e295–e298

21. Miyatake S, Furuse M, Kawabata S, et al. Bevacizumab treatment of symptomatic pseudoprogression after boron neutron capture therapy for recurrent malignant gliomas. Report of 2 cases. Neuro-oncol 2013; 15:650–655

22. Levin VA, Bidaut L, Hou P, et al. Randomized double-blind placebo-controlled trial of bevacizumab therapy for radiation necrosis of the CNS. Int J Radiat Oncol Biol Phys 2011;79:1487–1495

23. Shah AH, Snelling B, Bregy A, et al. Discriminating radiation necrosis from tumor progression in gliomas: a systematic review what is the best imaging modality? J Neurooncol 2013;112:141–152

24. Chaskis C, Neyns B, Michotte A, De Ridder M, Everaert H. Pseudoprogression after radiotherapy with concurrent temozolomide for high-grade glioma: clinical observations and working recommendations. Surg Neurol 2009;72:423–428

25. Clarke JL, Iwamoto FM, Sul J, et al. Randomized phase II trial of chemoradiotherapy followed by either dose-dense or metronomic temozolomide for newly diagnosed glioblastoma. J Clin Oncol 2009;27: 3861–3867

26. Fabi A, Russillo M, Metro G, Vidiri A, Di Giovanni S, Cognetti F. Pseudoprogression and MGMT status in glioblastoma patients: implications in clinical practice. Anticancer Res 2009;29:2607–2610

27. Peca C, Pacelli R, Elefante A, et al. Early clinical and neuroradiological worsening after radiotherapy and concomitant temozolomide in patients with glioblastoma: tumour progression or radionecrosis? Clin Neurol Neurosurg 2009;111:331–334

28. Roldán GB, Scott JN, McIntyre JB, et al. Population-based study of pseudoprogression after chemoradiotherapy in GBM. Can J Neurol Sci 2009;36:617–622

29. Gerstner ER, McNamara MB, Norden AD, Lafrankie D, Wen PY. Effect of adding temozolomide to radiation therapy on the incidence of pseudoprogression. J Neurooncol 2009;94:97–101

30. Tsien C, Galbán CJ, Chenevert TL, et al. Parametric response map as an imaging biomarker to distinguish progression from pseudoprogression in high-grade glioma. J Clin Oncol 2010;28:2293–2299

31. Yaman E, Buyukberber S, Benekli M, et al. Radiation induced early necrosis in patients with malignant gliomas receiving temozolomide. Clin Neurol Neurosurg 2010;112:662–667

32. Gunjur A, Lau E, Taouk Y, Ryan G. Early post-treatment pseudoprogression amongst glioblastoma multiforme patients treated with radiotherapy and temozolomide: a retrospective analysis. J Med Imaging Radiat Oncol 2011;55:603–610

33. Kang HC, Kim CY, Han JH, et al. Pseudoprogression in patients with malignant gliomas treated with concurrent temozolomide and radiotherapy: potential role of p53. J Neurooncol 2011;102:157–162

34. Kong D-S, Kim ST, Kim E-H, et al. Diagnostic dilemma of Pseudoprogression in the treatment of newly diagnosed glioblastoma: the role of assessing relative cerebral blood flow volume and oxygen-6-methylguanine-DNA methyltransferase promoter methylation status. Am J Neurorad 2011;32:382–387

35. Park C-K, Kim JW, Yim SY, et al. Usefulness of MS-MLPA for detection of MGMT promoter methylation in the evaluation of pseudoprogression in glioblastoma patients. Neuro-oncol 2011;13:195–202

36. Pouleau H-B, Sadeghi N, Balériaux D, Mélot C, De Witte O, Lefranc F. High levels of cellular proliferation predict pseudoprogression in glioblastoma patients. Int J Oncol 2012;40:923–928

37. Topkan E, Topuk S, Oymak E, Parlak C, Pehlivan B. Pseudoprogression in patients with glioblastoma multiforme after concurrent radiotherapy and temozolomide. Am J Clin Oncol 2012;35:284–289

38. Choi YJ, Kim HS, Jahng GH, Kim SJ, Suh DC. Pseudoprogression in patients with glioblastoma: added value of arterial spin labeling to dynamic susceptibility contrast perfusion MR imaging. Acta Radiol 2013; [Epub ahead of print]

39. Motegi H, Kamoshima Y, Terasaka S, et al. IDH1 mutation as a potential novel biomarker for distinguishing pseudoprogression from true progression in patients with glioblastoma treated with temozolomide and radiotherapy. Brain Tumor Pathol 2013;30:67–72

45 Quality of Life and Neurocognitive Function

Kyle Richard Noll and Jeffrey Scott Wefel

The natural history of malignant brain tumors is often a relentless neurologic deterioration to death. The tumor, the type of antineoplastic treatment the patient receives, adjuvant medications, and medical complications can all affect neurocognitive function, psychological well-being, and the ability to perform daily activities. However, a great deal can be done to improve the quality of life (QOL) of the patient and the caregiving system. Understanding the specific contribution of the effects of the tumor, of the treatment, and of other factors to the functioning of the brain and the patient's life guides the development of intervention strategies, both therapeutic and palliative.

The impact of a primary brain tumor on the individual is best conceptualized by the three-tiered system developed by the World Health Organization: *impairment* is the deficit of brain function caused by the disease and is assessed by neurologic and neuropsychological evaluations; *disability* is the impact the deficit has on the patient's ability to perform activities and is assessed by performance status and functional status measures; and *handicap* is the impact the disability has on the patient's subjective well-being and social functioning and is generally assessed by QOL questionnaires.

Similar impairments can cause greater or lesser disabilities and handicaps depending on the patient's developmental stage in life, work demands, and support systems. For instance, a young woman with a left frontal glioma was found to have a mild impairment of working memory, characterized by a reduced capacity to hold and manipulate information mentally. Because of the tumor she was more vulnerable to distraction, had difficulty performing tasks with multiple steps, and had difficulty handling more than one source of information at once (e.g., being in a room with more than one conversation going on). However, her memory, in terms of learning and retaining new information, was completely normal, as were her intellectual abilities, visuospatial and visuomotor abilities, and bilateral motor functions. Consistent with the site of her tumor, she also had mildly reduced verbal fluency and mild right visual field inattention. The impairments that this patient experienced in working memory capacity and verbal fluency were a great disability to her as a school teacher.

In addition, the disability was a great handicap because she loved her work and had difficulty adjusting to the fact that she could not maintain her previous level of performance. If she had a different career or if she did not like her job so much, the level of disability and handicap caused by the tumor might have been quite different.

Thus, interventions must be individually tailored to the patient's specific needs. This patient had the cognitive abilities necessary to successfully deal with these deficits. It is not known if she will be able to return to her former teaching occupation or if she will need to consider careers that do not place as high a demand on her areas of deficit, but it is likely that she will be able to function at a reasonable level with appropriate assistance. The assistance in this case included pharmacological treatment (stimulant therapy) and cognitive-vocational rehabilitation.

Contributions to Neurocognitive Impairment

Tumor Effects

In adult patients with primary brain cancer, presentation of neurocognitive deficits is associated with tumor location, tumor-related epilepsy, lesion type, lesion momentum (i.e., speed of tumor growth), and lesion volume. Although manifestations of the disease vary significantly across patients, glioma patients with lesions in the temporal or frontal lobes were assessed *before* initiation of any treatment, and neurocognitive dysfunction was found in 90% of patients. Executive functions were impaired in 78% and memory and attention were impaired in 60%.[1] Patients with newly diagnosed glioblastoma having tumor in heterogeneous locations who participated in a large phase 3 cooperative clinical trial demonstrated median cognitive performances that were generally 1 standard deviation (SD) below the healthy population's normative mean.[2]

Cognitive dysfunction tends to correspond with the hemispheric site of a tumor. Left hemisphere tumors are often associated with more frequent and severe deficits in verbal learning and memory, language functions, and verbally based intellectual functions. Right hemisphere tumors more frequently produce difficulties with visuospatial and visuoperceptual functions. Frontal tumors may cause marked personality changes and impairments of executive function, including problems with social judgment, frustration tolerance, ability to plan and organize activities, and working memory capacity. However, the specificity and severity of cognitive impairments related to tumor site are often less pronounced than those observed with sudden-onset neurologic conditions such as stroke.[3,4]

Effects of Chemotherapy and Radiotherapy

The adverse effects of chemotherapy are usually presumed to be acute and reversible except in the cases of intra-arterial or intraventricular administration. The neurobehavioral effects of most cancer therapy agents tend to be nonspecific and diffuse, except for those that have a mechanism of action that is expected to affect focal brain regions[5] or immunologic agents that are known to affect particular inflammatory cytokines, neurotransmitters, and neuroendocrine hormones.[6] Cognitive and emotional changes reported during and after chemotherapy include memory loss, decrease in information-processing speed, reduced attention, anxiety, depression, and fatigue. These changes are most pronounced and long lasting after high-dose treatment.[7]

Although newer agents such as temozolomide appear to enhance survival with fewer adverse symptoms,[8] emerging research has demonstrated that some patients experience worsening cognitive function while progression free and receiving temozolomide.[9,10] Specifically, a large phase 3 intergroup trial demonstrated that up to 30% of newly diagnosed glioblastoma multiforme (GBM) patients who received temozolomide evidenced decline in cognitive function across all domains assessed, despite remaining progression free on imaging.[8] Further, a small, single-institution study of standard-dose temozolomide reported cognitive decline in 3 of 13 progression-free patients after concurrent chemoradiation and three cycles of adjuvant chemotherapy.[10] It remains to be

determined if this represents the adverse effect of subclinical tumor progression or treatment-related neurotoxicity. Nonetheless, recent animal modeling suggests that such effects may be attributable, as least in part, to disruption of learning via decreased hippocampal neurogenesis and theta activity.[11] Although preliminary, these findings reflect the need for continued development of targeted chemotherapies that provide benefit with reduced toxicity.

Radiotherapy can also have deleterious effects on cognition due to a combination of vascular injury, inflammation, and damage to neuronal progenitor cells affecting neurogenesis and oligodendroglial formation.[12] Preferential disruption of frontal subcortical networks in the brain is common secondary to the effects of radiation on white matter tracts, which are particularly dense in frontal and subcortical areas. Within the first 2 weeks of treatment, patients can develop fatigue and exacerbation of preexisting neurologic deficits. Early delayed effects often develop 1 to 4 months after completion of radiation and include slowed information processing speed, executive dysfunction, diminished memory function, and motor deficits.[13] These symptoms are believed to result from transient demyelination and subsequent remyelination with variable symptom improvement.

Neuropsychological studies of patients before and after radiation treatment document neurocognitive impairments that are consistent with frontal network systems, including impaired information-processing speed, attention (e.g., working memory), mental flexibility, learning, memory, and, frequently, a decline in motor functioning bilaterally, even in patients with no evidence of disease recurrence.[14,15] Unfortunately, some patients experience late delayed encephalopathy that can involve progressive neurologic decline, dementia, leukoencephalopathy, and brain necrosis. Such late delayed problems typically emerge 6 months to 3 years following radiotherapy, though cases have reportedly occurred as early as 3 months to as late as 13 years posttreatment.[16] Several factors that contribute to the occurrence of radiation encephalopathy have been identified, including age > 60, higher total dose, dose per fraction > 2 Gy, greater brain volume irradiated, hyperfractionation schedules, shorter overall treatment time, concomitant or subsequent use of chemotherapy, and the presence of comorbid vascular risk factors.[15]

Effects of Adjuvant Medications and Medical Complications

Medical complications and adjuvant medications may cause impairments and contribute to disabilities and handicaps. For instance, glucocorticoid use is an extremely common adjuvant treatment for brain tumor patients. There are myriad neurobehavioral adverse effects of chronic steroid use in addition to the well-described gastrointestinal, dermatologic, musculoskeletal, circulatory, and immune system complications. Glucocorticoids such as dexamethasone bind to receptors in the brain that are important for controlling emotions and memory. Dexamethasone can cause memory difficulties, even in neurologically normal control subjects.[17] Reversible dementia, emotional lability, major depression, paranoia, mania, and delirium are not uncommon and are generally related to dose.

Endocrine dysfunction related to pituitary-hypothalamic injury is also very common following radiotherapy.[18] Thyroid dysfunction, loss of libido, and erectile dysfunction are present in a large proportion of patients. In fact, one study found that only 23% of brain tumor patients had normal thyroid, gonadal, and adrenal hormone levels following treatment.[19] The QOL of brain tumor patients with endocrinologic deficiency can improve greatly with replacement therapy.[20]

Seizures occur in 50 to 70% of patients at some time during their illness and have a significant impact on neurobehavioral functioning and QOL. Persistent, poorly controlled seizures cause neocortical changes, metabolic dysfunction, and hippocampal sclerosis, reducing cognitive efficiency and exacerbating underlying cognitive deficits.[21] Patients with seizures are often fearful of having them and may become socially isolated because of the possibility of having one in a public place or around people they know. In addition, many antiepileptic drugs (AEDs) have adverse constitutional and cognitive side effects. The use of phenytoin, carbamazepine, and valproic acid has been associated with impairments of attention, processing speed, and memory.[22] However, newer anticonvulsant agents including lamotrigine, oxcarbazepine, and gabapentin appear to have more favorable side-effect profiles and fewer neurocognitive side effects.[23]

Restricting brain tumor patients' driving privileges has a large impact on their feeling of independence and may place a burden on families with limited alternatives for transportation. Laws dictate how long after a grand mal seizure a person must refrain from driving, but the situation is much less clear when a person experiences focal or partial seizures without loss of consciousness, or if seizures are not an issue but cognitive impairments are. Patients with right hemisphere tumors may have visuoperceptual problems, including left visual field inattention, and are particularly at risk. If there is a question about driving safety, it is best to have the patient undergo a formal driving evaluation, which can be done by many neuropsychologists and rehabilitation psychologists. In addition, it is important for the treating physician to be aware of reporting requirements and licensing regulations.

Cancer-Related Symptoms

Fatigue and Sleep

Most brain tumor patients experience considerable cancer-related fatigue during the course of their illness. Cancer-related fatigue is a persistent, subjective sense of tiredness secondary to cancer or cancer treatment that is generally unrelieved by rest and interferes with usual functioning.[24] It is well accepted that physical, psychological, and medical factors such as anemia, cachexia, systemic illness, pain, and medications can contribute to fatigue. Across a wide variety of cancer patients, 50 to 75% reported fatigue at the time of their diagnosis, 80 to 96% reported fatigue associated with chemotherapy, and 60 to 93% reported fatigue associated with radiotherapy.[25] Several treatments can help ameliorate fatigue, including correction of anemia, treatment of depression, exercise, energy conservation, and pharmacological intervention (e.g., psychostimulants).[26]

Sleep–wake disturbance is understood as alteration in nighttime sleep followed by daytime impairment.[27] Sleep problems are estimated to occur in up to 57% of those with solid tumors, including the brain. Common problems include insomnia, sleep-related breathing disorders, parasomnias, hypersomnias, circadian rhythm disorders, and sleep-related movement disorders. Although the literature regarding sleep disturbance in primary brain tumor patients is limited, insomnias and parasomnias are the most common sleep problems in patients with solid tumors. Additionally, medications commonly used with brain tumor patients like glucocorticoids and anxiolytics may contribute to insomnia or daytime sleepiness. Management of sleep–wake disturbance often includes a combination of behavioral strategies (e.g., sleep hygiene and cognitive-behavioral therapy) as well as pharmacological treatment (i.e., hypnotics).[28]

Emotional Distress

Comprehensive studies of QOL in brain tumor patients report increased emotional reactivity, lowered frustration tolerance, depression, anxiety, and reduced family functioning in these patients.[29] Overall QOL does not appear to be closely correlated with histological diagnosis, prognosis, or age as much as the patient's social support, personality characteristics, and access to services. Approximately 93% of patients with high-grade glioma reported symptoms of depression prior to surgery and up to 6 months after resection.[30] However, physicians detected depression in only 15% of patients preoperatively and in up to 22% of patients after resection. Thus, many patients did not receive a potentially efficacious therapy to address their affective distress, and depressed patients had shorter survival times and more complications.

◼ Special Considerations for Pediatric Brain Tumor Patients

The effects of tumor and treatment in children must be considered in light of the developing brain and body. Pediatric brain tumor survivors are likely to have multiple cognitive and constitutional impairments. Children treated at a young age have significant difficulties learning and acquiring skills at a normal developmental rate.[31,32] They tend to have short stature, and, as adults, fewer marry or obtain full-time employment. The full impact of tumor and treatment on pediatric brain tumor survivors is often seen long after treatment has ended. A study of 10-year survivors of childhood medulloblastoma found that more than half of them had significant cognitive and psychosocial deficits that hampered independence as an adult, although they do not tend to report impaired QOL.[33]

Many childhood survivors develop cognitive and psychosocial deficits long after their treatments have been completed, either due to the delayed toxicities associated with radiation and chemotherapy or in association with the phenomenon of "growing into deficits." The principle of this phenomenon is that the impact of cancer and cancer therapies on certain behaviors like executive functions do not manifest themselves until the developing neural networks that subserve those functions become active (i.e., after complete myelination of the frontal lobes). At this time, the prior injury to that system is manifested as a failure to acquire a developmentally appropriate skill or ability. Pediatric brain tumor patients have been reported to demonstrate impairments in visuomotor and visuoperceptual skills, attention, memory, processing speed, language, and executive functions.[34] Impairments in core processes like attention, executive function, and processing speed have been demonstrated to be closely associated with failure to achieve expected intellectual and academic gains.[35]

■ Assessment Considerations

Assessment of Neurocognitive Impairment

The assessment of impairment includes the traditional neurologic evaluation, which usually focuses on evaluating motor and sensory function as well as the reactivity and appropriateness of response following stimulation of neural subsystems. Assessment of cognition generally involves standardized tests and questionnaires that are relatively sensitive and specific. Assessment of neurocognitive function must take into consideration the fact that tumors in different locations cause different cognitive deficits, and that there are different patterns of cognitive decline associated with radiation and chemotherapy as opposed to focal tumor progression. The particular choice of tests and the length of the assessment battery will depend on the purpose of the examination, with briefer assessments using tests that can be repeated in the clinical trial setting (e.g., tests having alternate forms or little practice effect), and more lengthy comprehensive assessments when decisions regarding issues such as the ability of the patient to go back to work are being addressed.

The Mini-Mental State Examination (MMSE), a brief screening tool for dementia, has often been used in brain tumor clinical trials. However, this tool has several drawbacks that limit

---

Pitfall

- Brief cognitive screening tests may be misleading.

---

its usefulness. Although the MMSE can detect moderate to severe global cognitive impairment, it lacks well-established sensitivity or specificity, overlaps considerably with concurrently used neurologic function scales and performance status measures, fails to measure many of the functions known to be impaired in brain tumor patients, and does not have validated alternate forms for repeated testing.[36] Further, it has been found to be insensitive to cognitive change in cancer therapy clinical trials.[5] Designed to address some of the drawbacks of the MMSE, the Montreal Cognitive Assessment (MoCA) is an alternative screening tool that more extensively measures executive functioning, delayed recall, and abstraction.[37] Despite its numerous alternate forms and superior sensitivity to the MMSE in brain tumor populations, it remains relatively insensitive to more subtle forms of cognitive dysfunction.

The results of the MMSE and similar cognitive screenings may be useful to indicate the need for a more thorough assessment of neurocognitive function. However, clinicians should be aware that, although a patient who is impaired on screening likely shows more extensive abnormalities on clinical neuropsychological evaluation, the absence of impaired performance on screening often does not correspond to an absence of cognitive dysfunction detectable with formal neuropsychological evaluation. The exclusive use of insensitive brief measures in clinical practice has the potential to lead to inappropriate expectations, to the possibility that needed interventions, resources, and support would not be appropriately offered to patients and families, as well as to misleading data for clinical trials.

Assessment of Disability

In general, disability refers to the patient's inability to perform activities of daily living (ADLs). Although used frequently to assess functional status and QOL in brain tumor patients, the Karnofsky Performance Scale (KPS) is an extremely poor assessment of QOL, as it provides a questionable assessment of patient function and does not address cognitive impairment at all. The scale has very poor interrater reliability, is more related to the age of the patient than to any other factor,

---

Special Consideration

- The Karnofsky Performance Scale is the most widely used physician-rated outcome measure in the brain tumor literature and has been used as an assessment of impairment, disability, and handicap.

and is particularly insensitive to patient function at the higher end (90 to 100).[38] There are several well-validated tools to measure patient ability to perform ADLs, including the comprehensive Functional Independence Measure and the simpler, easy to use Barthel ADL Index.[39]

Assessment of Handicap and Quality of Life

The current standard of QOL assessment is multidimensional and addresses concerns relevant for patients with a brain tumor. There are several subjective QOL instruments that have been used with patients with brain tumors, including the Functional Assessment of Cancer Therapy–Brain (FACT-Br),[40] the European Organization for Research and Treatment of Cancer Quality of Life Questionnaire–Brain Neoplasm module (EORTC QLQ-C30-BN20),[41] and the Functional Living Index–Cancer.[42] These scales differ in their development methodology. The core FACT questionnaire and EORTC QLQ-C30-BN20 address physical, family, social, emotional, and functional well-being. The items for the FACT-Br module were initially developed from interviews with patients in a neuro-oncology outpatient clinic. The QLQ-BN20 items were obtained from interviews of patients and caregivers who were participants in a brain cancer support group. Additional items for both brain tumor–specific modules were obtained from the input of health care professionals, and the methods for determining reliability, validity, and internal consistency were similar. A validated QOL tool for pediatric cancer patients (PedsQL 4.0) has been used with pediatric brain tumor patients.[43]

Some groups are defining QOL in clinical trials as a combination of survival and the amount of time patients have adverse effects of disease and treatment.[44] This approach (quality-adjusted survival analysis) provides more information on patient function beyond what is obtained from the usual tracking of KPS scores and enables better assessment of the benefit of different therapeutic strategies. However, brain tumor patients are less likely to be free of symptoms than are other cancer patients. In addition, censoring is assumed to be random and noninformative,[45] which may be misleading. Censoring of brain tumor QOL assessments may be very informative when the assessments are not done because the patient can no longer read or understand the questions. Because many cognitively impaired patients cannot complete QOL instruments, there may be substantial amounts of missing data, and information may be collected only on those patients who are cognitively more intact, biasing the interpretation of results. Thus subjective QOL questionnaires need to be supplemented by objective assessments of patient function.

Proxy assessments of patient QOL have been reported, with moderate correlations between patient and proxy.[46] However, the correlation between patient and proxy assessment is lower when patients are more cognitively impaired, which is when the proxy assessments are most likely to be done.

The QOL of the caregiver is as important as that of the patient because it will have a major impact on the person's ability to cope with the situation and provide optimal care. The

Pitfall

- Cognitive dysfunction may affect patients' ability to appraise their QOL or to cooperate with QOL assessments. Patients with brain tumors, particularly in the frontal lobe, often have diminished appreciation of their disabilities and limitations and report a level of function that is not realistic.

Caregiver Quality of Life Index–Cancer (CQOLC) is a tool designed specifically to assess the well-being of the caregivers of patients with cancer.[47]

Applications of Impairment, Disability, and Handicap Assessments

Assessing QOL, cognitive function, and the ability to perform ADLs has four broad applications: differential diagnosis, patient management, instituting and evaluating interventions, and clinical research.

Differential Diagnosis

Differential diagnosis of patient complaints and symptoms is critical for effective intervention. For instance, many patients complain of "forgetfulness." There are several underlying processes that may result in perceived forgetfulness, such as (1) restricted working memory capacity that limits the amount of information the individual is able to process, (2) impaired memory consolidation that results in rapid forgetting of information, (3) poor sustained concentration that results in distractibility, and (4) impaired language functioning that restricts the amount and complexity of information the person is able to comprehend.

There are several potential mechanisms underlying memory process malfunction, including tumor impinging on working memory or memory consolidation circuitry, the effects of radiation on white matter connections, a coexisting neurologic disease such as Alzheimer's dementia, coexisting psychiatric illness such as major depression, reactive mood and adjustment disorders, side effects of adjuvant medications, sensory impairment or general frailty, malingering (very rare), or a combination of the above (fairly common). A multidimensional assessment of neurologic, neurobehavioral, functional, and QOL issues is necessary to make these critical distinctions because interventions are quite different depending on the specific process and underlying mechanism involved.

Patient Care and Management

A description of a brain tumor patient's cognitive strengths, impairments, capabilities, and limitations is crucial for rational patient management. Decisions regarding independence in self-care activities, ability to drive, returning to work, and the suitability of the patient for rehabilitation or other interventions are based on the person's neurocognitive functioning. In addition, repeated assessments can track the patient's response to primary therapy and to targeted interventions and help design realistic goals and future plans.

Interventions

Despite the overall bleak prognosis for patients with malignant gliomas, there are several strategies that can help maximize the patient's ability to function at the highest level of independence possible for the longest duration of time.

Pharmacological Strategies

Neurobehavioral slowing is the hallmark of frontal lobe dysfunction and treatment-related adverse effects in brain tumor patients. The syndrome of neurobehavioral slowing is generally due to involvement of the monoamine pathways of the frontal brainstem reticular system. In addition, catecholamines have an important role in the modulation of attention and working memory. Stimulant treatment (e.g., methylphenidate) has been reported to be useful in the treatment of concentration difficulties, psychomotor retardation, and fatigue frequently seen in brain tumor patients, and has helped to elevate mood as well.[48] A conservative dose of 10 mg twice a day significantly improved cognitive function as assessed by objective tests, and doses in excess of 60 mg twice a day were well tolerated. Subjective improvements included improved gait, increased stamina and motivation to perform activities, and improved bladder control. There were no significant side effects, and many patients taking steroids were able to decrease their dose.

Modafinil, a novel vigilance-promoting agent, is commonly used to treat excessive daytime somnolence associated with narcolepsy and idiopathic hypersomnia. However, evidence regarding the effectiveness of modafinil for alleviating fatigue in brain tumor patients is equivocal. In a study of 37 patients with primary brain tumors, patients receiving modafinil exhibited less fatigue, better motivation, and improved working memory and processing efficiency. However, similar improvements were noted in patients receiving only placebo and no significant differences were found between groups.[49]

A recent open-label, randomized, pilot trial examined the differential efficacy of 4 weeks of methylphenidate or modafinil treatment in 24 brain tumor patients.[50] Following treatment, improvements were noted with speed of processing and executive function requiring divided attention. Those with the greatest executive dysfunction at baseline derived the greatest benefit from stimulant therapy. Additionally, there was some indication that methylphenidate differentially improves attention to a greater extent while modafinil favors processing speed. A general beneficial effect was also observed on patient-reported fatigue, mood, and quality of life. Although such findings are preliminary, further research is clearly warranted.

Although use of some AEDs is associated with reduced cognitive performances as noted above, emerging evidence suggests that postoperative treatment of brain tumor patients with newer antiepileptics may actually improve verbal memory.[51] In a study investigating the effects of AEDs in high-grade glioma, 117 postoperative patients received older, newer, or no AEDs. On a battery of cognitive tests, patients on older and newer AEDs performed as well as patients not on an AED. However, those on levetiracetam, a newer AED, performed even better on verbal memory tests than patients not on an AED. The authors speculated that levetiracetam may promote efficient storage of information by altering receptors and ion channels in glioma tissue, though additional study is needed.

Pharmacotherapies utilized in the treatment of dementia have also been examined for their possible benefit in brain tumor populations. Donepezil, an acetylcholinesterase inhibitor commonly used in the treatment of Alzheimer's disease, has been examined in a phase 2 trial. Improvement in neurocognitive functions such as attention, memory, and verbal fluency as well as in QOL were reported after 6 months of treatment with donepezil (5 to 10 mg a day) in a group of long-term survivors of partial or whole-brain radiation.[52] Memantine, an N-methyl-D-aspartate (NMDA) receptor antagonist, is another pharmacotherapy useful in the treatment of dementia. A recent phase 3 trial evaluated the potential protective effects of memantine in a large cohort of brain metastasis patients receiving whole-brain radiotherapy.[53] Those receiving memantine were administered 20 mg per day for 24 weeks and performances on neuropsychological tests were compared to a placebo control group at numerous follow-up intervals. Those treated with memantine showed longer time to cognitive decline, particularly with regard to recognition memory, executive function, and processing speed.

The effect of a megadose of α-tocopherol (vitamin E; 1,000 IU twice per day) was examined in a group of patients with nasopharyngeal carcinoma who underwent standard treatment with unilateral or bilateral temporal lobe high-dose radiation and developed temporal lobe radionecrosis.[54] Temporal lobe radionecrosis is an unfortunate but common side effect experienced by patients who receive this type of treatment. It is characterized most significantly by memory impairment and hypothesized to be related to free radical generation and tissue peroxidation in the central nervous system (CNS). Vitamin E has been demonstrated in nonhuman studies to in-

---

Pearl

- Newer generation antiepileptic drugs may actually improve neurocognitive function.

hibit lipid peroxidation, reduce cell death in hypoxic neurons, and decrease degeneration of hippocampal cells after ischemia.[55] Using an open-label, nonrandomized, treatment versus control design, improvement in memory and executive functions was demonstrated in patients with temporal lobe radionecrosis after 1 year of dietary supplementation with vitamin E.[54]

There are several strategies under development to treat radiation-induced cognitive dysfunction. Low molecular weight heparin is being investigated to prevent venous thromboembolism in brain tumor patients, which may also have a beneficial effect on cognitive function by reducing ischemia associated with brain radiation.[56] The cognitive decline seen in patients treated with brain radiation may also be due to hippocampal dysfunction resulting from decreased hippocampal neurogenesis, proliferation, and increased apoptosis, which has generated interest in developing agents that stimulate neurogenesis.[57]

Rehabilitation Strategies

Formal rehabilitation is grossly underutilized for brain tumor patients, in part because rehabilitation facilities lack experience with primary brain tumor patients. Our survey of the salient issues that caregivers of brain tumor patients cite as needing intervention include inability to perform usual activities around the home like paying bills and mowing the lawn, social isolation, and generalized slowing. Abilities not cited as particularly important included basic self-care activities, ambulation, and communication. Therefore, placement of a brain tumor patient in a program designed for stroke or severe head trauma, where the latter issues are more common, may be inappropriate.

Many patients have the ability to improve their function at home and in vocational and leisure pursuits and enjoy an improved level of independence and QOL given the right support. However, the rehabilitation strategies used must be directed toward their specific disabilities and realistic future goals. These may include physical, occupational, and speech therapy to help optimize function. For select patients, cognitive and vocational rehabilitation can be very effective, with shorter stays, lower treatment costs, and better overall outcome in terms of independence and productivity compared with traumatic brain injury patients.[58]

Although the efficacy of various cognitive rehabilitation programs has been established with stroke and trauma populations, few have been evaluated with brain tumor patients. Nonetheless, positive results have been reported for a Dutch cognitive rehabilitation program, Strategy Training and C-Car (STCC), in patients with glioma.[59] The program consists of 6 weekly sessions plus homework, integrating two approaches: (1) teaching strategies to improve attention, executive functioning, and memory; and (2) a computerized retraining module focusing on practicing attentional exercises in a game-like scenario. Utilizing a randomized control design, glioma patients who received STCC were shown to perform significantly better than a control group on tests of attention and verbal memory and also reported less mental fatigue at 6-months follow-up.

Another recent study showed promising effects for a program of advanced cognitive training in breast cancer survivors, which involved memory and speed of processing training.[60] Specifically, both treatments were associated with improvement in perceived cognitive functioning, though speed of process training also demonstrated durable gains on objective measures of processing speed and verbal memory. Accordingly, speed of process training programs may be of benefit to the cognitive functioning of patients with CNS tumors.

Patient and family education is also extremely important. Potential neurobehavioral symptoms may not be explained to the patient, sometimes because the primary physician is not aware of the impact of subtle symptoms on social and vocational functioning. Patients who experience these symptoms may wonder if they are mentally ill or may inaccurately attribute their symptoms to other causes. Patients and families may feel isolated and alone or "unusual" in experiencing neurobehavioral symptoms. The more knowledgeable patients and their families are about the disease, treatment, and expected problems, the more effective the recovery process. Even simple coping strategies, such as taking intermittent naps, writing notes, and taking special care to plan and organize activities may be of benefit.

Research has demonstrated that patients generally prefer to be fully informed by their physician about their disease and treatment. However, patient information-seeking behavior varies widely in both type and amount during medical visits. One study found that more than 90% of patients surveyed wanted to discuss the physical aspects of their disease and treatment as well as the problems in their daily lives and their feelings. In terms of physical concerns, 80 to 90% of patients were willing to initiate these discussions. However, 25% of patients were interested in discussing their feelings and problems in their daily lives but reported waiting for their doctor to initiate this discussion. Patients were, by far, much more reluctant to discuss their family and social life, with a sizable minority (20%) stating they would prefer not to do so at all.[61]

Patient characteristics that have been associated with a tendency to ask for and receive more information from their doctors include being younger, better educated, and female.[62,63] Physician communication styles that include direct questioning regarding patient physical and emotional well-being has been demonstrated to be associated with higher patient satisfaction and better health outcomes.[64] Unfortunately, although physicians uniformly felt discussions about physical health were their responsibility, only 40% felt that discussion of patients' level of functioning in daily life and patients' emotional condition was their responsibility. Moreover, very few physicians initiated discussions regarding psychosocial issues during outpatient consultations. This has been labeled a "conspiracy of silence," which leaves psychosocial issues unaddressed due to physician and patient reluctance to initiate such discussions without clear indications that each wishes and is prepared to engage in this discussion.[65] Qualitative research has shown that even patients in the terminal stages of malignant brain tumors are very willing to discuss difficult end-of-life issues if approached.[66]

Fortunately, there are effective psychosocial interventions available in most communities once these issues are identified. Support groups and counseling can be very helpful in assuring patients and families that their experiences are not unusual and can help them deal with the grief, anger, frustration, and other problems that are frequently manifested over the course of the disease. Support groups have great potential to help patients and caregivers cope and derive meaning from the illness, balance hope with realism, and maintain QOL under the most dire of circumstances.

The multidisciplinary team, in which the neuro-oncologist, radiation oncologist, and neurosurgeon consult with neuropsychologists, social workers, rehabilitation professionals, palliative care professionals, and so forth, is in the best position to make the most appropriate treatment decisions and provide individualized assistance during and after active therapy.

Research and Clinical Trials

There has been a welcome recent call for including neurocognitive and brain tumor–specific toxicity rating scales in clinical trials.[39] Neuropsychological assessments have been useful in identifying both the risks and the benefits of a variety of anticancer treatments on neurocognitive functioning and have been shown to predict survival better than clinical prognostic factors alone in patients with primary brain tumors, leptomeningeal disease, and parenchymal brain metastases.[67–69]

The potential problems and inadequacies of using brief screening measures were previously addressed. It is possible to use assessments of neurocognitive function within clinical trials in a fairly uncomplicated way as long as the assessment tools are psychometrically sound.[53] Knowing the psychometric properties of the tests is critical to determining whether real change has occurred over time. Assessments of neurocognitive function and symptoms can be done in 30 minutes and can be relatively practical in terms of training, cost, repeatability, and burden to patients in multicenter clinical trials.[39] For example, neurocognitive decline may precede magnetic resonance imaging (MRI) evidence of tumor progression, whereas the ability of the patient to perform ADLs and subjective QOL change some time after tumor progression.[69] Multifaceted end points have the potential to better define the relative risks versus benefits of different treatment regimens, particularly if they exhibit small differences in time to tumor progression (TTP) or survival. They may also provide additional helpful information in the drug approval process beyond survival and TTP. For example, a treatment that slows or stabilizes the progression of expected neurocognitive deterioration may be considered of clinical benefit to the patient even if survival or time to frank tumor progression is not improved.[67]

■ Conclusion

Primary brain cancer is often as much a progressive neurodegenerative disorder as it is a neoplastic illness. Assessments of neurocognitive function, ability to perform ADLs, and subjective QOL are indispensable to providing the best interventions for patients and the most salient information for therapeutic clinical trials. Until a clearly effective treatment is available for brain tumor patients, selection of a specific therapy needs to consider toxic side effects and effect on patient QOL. The assessment of the neurobehavioral and emotional function of brain tumor patients also helps guide the institution of appropriate adjuvant interventions. As primary therapy becomes more effective and more patients experience long-term remissions, assessment of neurobehavioral function and QOL and establishing effective treatment strategies will gain even greater importance.

Editor's Note

Quality of life is important in patients with benign tumors with long survival, because they have a long time to contend with any morbidity of their tumor or of its treatment. Quality of life is also paramount for malignant brain tumor patients whose limited time left must be of the best quality possible. Greater attention has been devoted to the study of and amelioration of QOL; it would be rare nowadays for a clinical trial to be developed, or executed without attention to study of QOL of the patients.

Randomized studies are the ideal setting to study QOL, as opposed to stand-alone studies, as comparisons in the various arms could be an important deciding factor about future treatments.[70] For example if treatment X provides modest survival benefit over treatment Y but at greater cost to QOL, it probably should not be pursued, and this type of sentiment has been articulated by patients.[66] As new and exciting treatments are innovated for patients with brain tumors, the whole neuro-oncological team of caregivers as well as clinical researchers will be bound to give due attention and resources to studying and addressing QOL issues. (Bernstein)

References

1. Tucha O, Smely C, Preier M, Lange KW. Cognitive deficits before treatment among patients with brain tumors. Neurosurgery 2000;47:324–333, discussion 333–334
2. Wefel JS, Pugh SL, Armstrong TS, et al. Neurocognitive Function (NCF) Outcomes in Patients with Glioblastoma (GBM) Enrolled in RTOG 0825. Presented at the 2013 American Society of Clinical Oncology Meeting, Chicago, May 31–June 4
3. Anderson SW, Damasio H, Tranel D. Neuropsychological impairments associated with lesions caused by tumor or stroke. Arch Neurol 1990; 47:397–405
4. Meyers CA, Berman SA, Hayman A, Evankovich K. Pathological left-handedness and preserved function associated with a slowly evolving brain tumor. Dev Med Child Neurol 1992;34:1110–1116
5. Meyers CA, Kudelka AP, Conrad CA, Gelke CK, Grove W, Pazdur R. Neurotoxicity of CI-980, a novel mitotic inhibitor. Clin Cancer Res 1997;3:419–422
6. Scheibel RS, Valentine AD, O'Brien S, Meyers CA. Cognitive dysfunction and depression during treatment with interferon-alpha and chemotherapy. J Neuropsychiatry Clin Neurosci 2004;16:185–191
7. van Dam FSAM, Schagen SB, Muller MJ, et al. Impairment of cognitive function in women receiving adjuvant treatment for high-risk breast cancer: high-dose versus standard-dose chemotherapy. J Natl Cancer Inst 1998;90:210–218
8. Macdonald DR, Kiebert G, Prados M, Yung A, Olson J. Benefit of temozolomide compared to procarbazine in treatment of glioblastoma multiforme at first relapse: effect on neurological functioning, performance status, and health related quality of life. Cancer Invest 2005;23:138–144
9. Armstrong TS, Wefel JS Wang M, et al. Net Clinical Benefit Analysis of RTOG 0525: A Phase III Trial Comparing Conventional Adjuvant Temozolomide with Dose-Intensive Temozolomide in Patients with Newly Diagnosed Glioblastoma. J Clin Oncol 2013;31(32):4076–4084
10. Hilverda K, Bosma I, Heimans JJ, et al. Cognitive functioning in glioblastoma patients during radiotherapy and temozolomide treatment: initial findings. J Neurooncol 2010;97:89–94
11. Nokia MS, Anderson ML, Shors TJ. Chemotherapy disrupts learning, neurogenesis and theta activity in the adult brain. Eur J Neurosci 2012;36:3521–3530
12. Peiffer AM, Leyrer CM, Greene-Schloesser DM, et al. Neuroanatomical target theory as a predictive model for radiation-induced cognitive decline. Neurology 2013;80:747–753
13. Armstrong CL, Gyato K, Awadalla AW, Lustig R, Tochner ZA. A critical review of the clinical effects of therapeutic irradiation damage to the brain: the roots of controversy. Neuropsychol Rev 2004;14:65–86
14. Scheibel RS, Meyers CA, Levin VA. Cognitive dysfunction following surgery for intracerebral glioma: influence of histopathology, lesion location, and treatment. J Neurooncol 1996;30:61–69
15. Lee AW, Kwong DLW, Leung SF, et al. Factors affecting risk of symptomatic temporal lobe necrosis: significance of fractional dose and treatment time. Int J Radiat Oncol Biol Phys 2002;53:75–85
16. Fink J, Born D, Chamberlain MC. Radiation necrosis: relevance with respect to treatment of primary and secondary brain tumors. Curr Neurol Neurosci Rep 2012;12:276–285
17. Wolkowitz OM, Reus VI, Weingartner H, et al. Cognitive effects of corticosteroids. Am J Psychiatry 1990;147:1297–1303
18. Darzy KH, Shalet SM. Hypopituitarism after cranial irradiation. J Endocrinol Invest 2005;28(5, Suppl):78–87
19. Arlt W, Hove U, Müller B, et al. Frequent and frequently overlooked: treatment-induced endocrine dysfunction in adult long term survivors of primary brain tumors. Neurology 1997;49:498–506
20. Mukherjee A, Tolhurst-Cleaver S, Ryder WD, Smethurst L, Shalet SM. The characteristics of quality of life impairment in adult growth hormone (GH)-deficient survivors of cancer and their response to GH replacement therapy. J Clin Endocrinol Metab 2005;90:1542–1549
21. Bronen RA. The status of status: seizures are bad for your brain's health. AJNR Am J Neuroradiol 2000;21:1782–1783
22. Taphoorn MJ, Klein M. Cognitive deficits in adult patients with brain tumours. Lancet Neurol 2004;3:159–168
23. Loring DW, Meador KJ. Cognitive side effects of antiepileptic drugs in children. Neurology 2004;62:872–877
24. Mock V. Evidence-based treatment for cancer-related fatigue. J Natl Cancer Inst Monogr 2004;32:112–118
25. Stasi R, Abriani L, Beccaglia P, Terzoli E, Amadori S. Cancer-related fatigue: evolving concepts in evaluation and treatment. Cancer 2003;98: 1786–1801
26. Cella D, Peterman A, Passik S, Jacobsen P, Breitbart W. Progress toward guidelines for the management of fatigue. Oncology (Williston Park) 1998;12:369–377
27. Armstrong TS, Gilbert MR. Practical strategies for management of fatigue and sleep disorders in people with brain tumors. Neuro-oncol 2012;14(Suppl 4):iv65–iv72
28. Schutte-Rodin S, Broch L, Buysse D, Dorsey C, Sateia M. Clinical guideline for the evaluation and management of chronic insomnia in adults. J Clin Sleep Med 2008;4:487–504
29. Weitzner MA, Meyers CA. Cognitive functioning and quality of life in malignant glioma patients: a review of the literature. Psychooncology 1997;6:169–177
30. Litofsky NS, Farace E, Anderson F Jr, Meyers CA, Huang W, Laws ER Jr; Glioma Outcomes Project Investigators. Depression in patients with high-grade glioma: results of the Glioma Outcomes Project. Neurosurgery 2004;54:358–366, discussion 366–367
31. Dennis M, Spiegler BJ, Hetherington CR, Greenberg ML. Neuropsychological sequelae of the treatment of children with medulloblastoma. J Neurooncol 1996;29:91–101

32. Packer RJ. Progress and challenges in childhood brain tumors. J Neurooncol 2005;75:239–242

33. Maddrey AM, Bergeron JA, Lombardo ER, et al. Neuropsychological performance and quality of life of 10 year survivors of childhood medulloblastoma. J Neurooncol 2005;72:245–253

34. Moore BD III. Neurocognitive outcomes in survivors of childhood cancer. J Pediatr Psychol 2005;30:51–63

35. Reddick WE, White HA, Glass JO, et al. Developmental model relating white matter volume to neurocognitive deficits in pediatric brain tumor survivors. Cancer 2003;97:2512–2519

36. Meyers CA, Wefel JS. The use of the mini-mental state examination to assess cognitive functioning in cancer trials: no ifs, ands, buts, or sensitivity. [editorial] J Clin Oncol 2003;21:3557–3558

37. Olson RA, Iverson GL, Carolan H, Parkinson M, Brooks BL, McKenzie M. Prospective comparison of two cognitive screening tests: diagnostic accuracy and correlation with community integration and quality of life. J Neurooncol 2011;105:337–344

38. Meyers CA, Brown PD. The role and relevance of neurocognitive assessment in clinical trials of patients with central nervous system tumors. J Clin Oncol 2006;24:1305–1309

39. Wade DT. Measurement in Neurological Rehabilitation. New York: Oxford University Press, 1992

40. Weitzner MA, Meyers CA, Gelke CK, et al. The Functional Assessment of Cancer Therapy (FACT) Scale: development of a brain subscale and revalidation of the FACT-G in the brain tumor population. Cancer 1995; 75:1151–1161

41. Osoba D, Aaronson NK, Muller M, et al. The development and psychometric validation of a brain cancer quality-of-life questionnaire for use in combination with general cancer-specific questionnaires. Qual Life Res 1996;5:139–150

42. Giovagnoli AR, Silvani A, Colombo E, Boiardi A. Facets and determinants of quality of life in patients with recurrent high grade glioma. J Neurol Neurosurg Psychiatry 2005;76:562–568

43. Bhat SR, Goodwin TL, Burwinkle TM, et al. Profile of daily life in children with brain tumors: an assessment of health-related quality of life. J Clin Oncol 2005;23:5493–5500

44. Murray KJ, Nelson DF, Scott C, et al. Quality-adjusted survival analysis of malignant glioma. Patients treated with twice-daily radiation (RT) and carmustine: a report of Radiation Therapy Oncology Group (RTOG) 83-02. Int J Radiat Oncol Biol Phys 1995;31:453–459

45. Scott CB. Quality-adjusted survival analysis of malignant glioma patients. Control Clin Trials 1997;18:277–285

46. Sneeuw KCA, Aaronson NK, Osoba D, et al. The use of significant others as proxy raters of the quality of life of patients with brain cancer. Med Care 1997;35:490–506

47. Weitzner MA, Jacobsen PB, Wagner H Jr, Friedland J, Cox C. The Caregiver Quality of Life Index-Cancer (CQOLC) scale: development and validation of an instrument to measure quality of life of the family caregiver of patients with cancer. Qual Life Res 1999;8:55–63

48. Meyers CA, Weitzner MA, Valentine AD, Levin VA. Methylphenidate therapy improves cognition, mood, and function of brain tumor patients. J Clin Oncol 1998;16:2522–2527

49. Boele FW, Douw L, de Groot, et al. The effect of modafinil on fatigue, cognitive functioning, and mood in primary brain tumor patients: a multicenter randomized controlled trial. NeuroOncology 2013;15:1420–1428

50. Gehring K, Patwardhan SY, Collins R, et al. A randomized trial on the efficacy of methylphenidate and modafinil for improving cognitive functioning and symptoms in patients with a primary brain tumor. J Neurooncol 2012;107:165–174

51. de Groot M, Douw L, Sizoo EM, et al. Levetiracetam improves verbal memory in high-grade glioma patients. Neuro-oncol 2013;15:216–223

52. Shaw EG, Rosdhal R, D'Agostino RB Jr, et al. Phase II study of donepezil in irradiated brain tumor patients: effect on cognitive function, mood, and quality of life. J Clin Oncol 2006;24:1415–1420

53. Brown PD, Shook S, Laack NN, et al. Memantine for the prevention of cognitive dysfunction in patients receiving whole-brain radiation therapy (WBRT): first report of RTOG 0614, a placebo-controlled, double-blind, randomized trial [abstract]. American Society for Radiation Oncology, 2012

54. Chan AS, Cheung M-C, Law SC, Chan JH. Phase II study of alpha-tocopherol in improving the cognitive function of patients with temporal lobe radionecrosis. Cancer 2004;100:398–404

55. Yoshida S, Busto R, Watson BD, Santiso M, Ginsberg MD. Postischemic cerebral lipid peroxidation in vitro: modification by dietary vitamin E. J Neurochem 1985;44:1593–1601

56. Glantz MJ, Burger PC, Friedman AH, Radtke RA, Massey EW, Schold SC Jr. Treatment of radiation-induced nervous system injury with heparin and warfarin. Neurology 1994;44:2020–2027

57. Monje ML, Mizumatsu S, Fike JR, Palmer TD. Irradiation induces neural precursor-cell dysfunction. Nat Med 2002;8:955–962

58. Sherer M, Meyers CA, Bergloff P. Efficacy of postacute brain injury rehabilitation for patients with primary malignant brain tumors. Cancer 1997;80:250–257

59. Gehring K, Sitskoorn MM, Gundy CM, et al. Cognitive rehabilitation in patients with gliomas: a randomized, controlled trial. J Clin Oncol 2009;27:3712–3722

60. Von Ah D, Carpenter JS, Saykin A, et al. Advanced cognitive training for breast cancer survivors: a randomized controlled trial. Breast Cancer Res Treat 2012;135:799–809

61. Waitzkin H. Information giving in medical care. J Health Soc Behav 1985;26:81–101

62. Greene MG, Adelman RD, Charon R, Friedmann E. Concordance between physicians and their older and younger patients in the primary care medical encounter. Gerontologist 1989;29:808–813

63. Roter DL, Hall JA. Doctors Talking with Patients/Patients Talking with Doctors: Improving Communication in Medical Settings. Westport, CT: Auburn House, 1992

64. Stewart MA. Effective physician-patient communication and health outcomes: a review. CMAJ 1995;152:1423–1433

65. Detmar SB, Aaronson NK, Wever LD, Muller M, Schornagel JH. How are you feeling? Who wants to know? Patients' and oncologists' preferences for discussing health-related quality-of-life issues. J Clin Oncol 2000;18:3295–3301

66. Lipsman N, Skanda A, Kimmelman J, Bernstein M. The attitudes of brain cancer patients and their caregivers towards death and dying: a qualitative study. BMC Palliat Care 2007;6:7

67. Meyers CA, Smith JA, Bezjak A, et al. Neurocognitive function and progression in patients with brain metastases treated with whole-brain radiation and motexafin gadolinium: results of a randomized phase III trial. J Clin Oncol 2004;22:157–165

68. Sherman AM, Jaeckle K, Meyers CA. Pretreatment cognitive performance predicts survival in patients with leptomeningeal disease. Cancer 2002;95:1311–1316

69. Meyers CA, Hess KR. Multifaceted end points in brain tumor clinical trials: cognitive deterioration precedes MRI progression. Neuro-oncol 2003;5:89–95

70. Bampoe J, Laperriere N, Pintilie M, Glen J, Micallef J, Bernstein M. Quality of life in patients with glioblastoma participating in a randomized study of boost brachytherapy. J Neurosurg 2000;93:917–926

46 End-of-Life Care and Other Ethical Issues

George M. Ibrahim and Mark Bernstein

The evolving field of neuro-oncology is replete with ethical and moral challenges that permeate virtually every aspect of patient care. In the disclosure of the diagnosis and prognosis, the initiation of standard and experimental therapies, the evaluation of patients' quality-of-life during treatment, and the initiation of end-of-life care, clinicians often face complex dilemmas that they must resolve by making difficult decisions. In contrast to law and policy, which dictate what "must" and "tends to" be done, respectively, ethics describe a set of values, principles, and beliefs that guide decisions that "should" be made (**Fig. 46.1**). Although various tools and guidelines, such as the American Medical Association (AMA) Code of Ethics,[1] are available to inform the decision-making process, the management of patients with neuro-oncological diagnoses may present unique ethical challenges (**Table 46.1**). The multifaceted ethical dilemmas encountered in the care of these patients have, in fact, considerably advanced the discipline of medical bioethics.

Individuals affected by brain tumors and other neuro-oncological diagnoses represent an especially vulnerable patient population due to the devastating disease burden, as well as the effects of the underlying pathology on patient capacity, agency, and identity. Ethical dilemmas are also introduced in clinicians' attempts to balance duties to current and future patients while conducting clinical research. Furthermore, the nascent field of cancer genetics and the emerging practice of biobanking have generated increasing questions regarding the clinician's conflicting role as both a medical provider and scientific investigator, and about privacy of patients' information. Given the prevalence of ethical conflicts in neuro-oncology, basic knowledge of ethical principles and theory is essential for the provision of care to affected individuals.

This chapter is an introduction to bioethical fundamentals that are salient in the care of patients with neuro-oncological diagnoses. The four classic principles of medical bioethics are respect for autonomy, beneficence, nonmaleficence, and justice. *Autonomy* refers to the patient's inalienable right to self-determination, whereby any intervention requires the voluntary informed consent of a capable person without undue

influence or coercion. *Beneficence* and *nonmaleficence* relate to the clinician's obligation to serve the best interest of the patient while first doing no harm. *Justice* refers to the equitable treatment of neuro-oncology patients, affording them the same opportunities as other patients.

Increasingly, clinicians and ethicists alike are also acknowledging the uniqueness of ethical challenges arising from the effects of pathological conditions on the brain, which serves as the seat of consciousness and the substrate of identity and capacity. The burgeoning field of neuroethics aims to study ethical, legal, and societal issues related to brain function and its impairment.

This chapter also explores ethical issues in the conduct of neuro-oncology research and thus can serve as a resource for clinicians throughout their interactions with patients, from diagnosis to treatment, recruitment into research studies, and during end-of-life care.

Diagnosis: Disclosure and Truth-Telling

Receiving the diagnosis of a central nervous system neoplasm is a distressing turning point in a patient's life.[2] Adjustment to the diagnosis of a brain tumor is highly individual process that may be affected by demographic and psychosocial factors.[3] Patients often view brain cancers as a unique group of neoplasms as a result of the value placed on cognitive function and mental capacity.[4]

There has been a paradigm shift in the disclosure of neuro-oncological diagnoses in Western culture. Historically, clinicians have been reluctant to disclose the full extent of brain tumor diagnoses and prognoses for various reasons, including perceived patient vulnerability or lack of understanding.[5] In 1961, 90% of physicians did not reveal a cancer diagnosis to patients,[6] but by 1979 only 2% reported that they would withhold such information.[7] With the widespread availability and

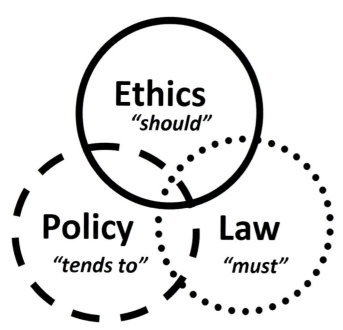

Fig. 46.1 Differentiating between ethics, policy and law. Ethics describes a set of beliefs and values regarding codes of conduct that "should" be followed, whereas policy and law describe conduct that "tends to" and "must" be followed, respectively.

accessibility of information, patients are now also increasingly empowered to play an active role in directing their medical treatment. The dissemination of medical knowledge through online venues and an increasing departure from the paternalistic model of health care has enabled patients to serve as the primary stakeholders in their own care.[8]

Disclosure of the cancer diagnosis is necessary to protect the patient's right to self-determination, that is, to enable individuals to make informed decisions regarding their care that are consistent with their own goals. Importantly, the patients themselves have consistently emphasized the necessity of honesty and candid disclosure during their care.[9] It has been previously suggested that having a sense of control over their treatment plans may provide patients with a sense of hope and optimism.[10] Furthermore, disclosure of the neuro-oncological diagnosis and expected prognosis enables patients to have realistic expectations regarding the likely outcomes and, if relevant, facilitates preparation for the process of dying. These goals cannot be overemphasized, considering that advanced cancer patients have previously been shown to overestimate their likelihood of long-term survival and often falsely

Pitfall

- Withholding information may be viewed as a form of deception, which may adversely impact the physician–patient relationship.

Special Consideration

- A "relational" view of autonomy holds that the patient's internal moderating factors must be considered during disclosure of information.

believed that the purpose of offering multiple treatment options was to maximize the chances of cure.[11,12]

To navigate their illness, patients also depend on the physician–patient relationship. Such relationships are nearly universally asymmetric with greater vulnerability on the side of patient.[5] The concept of trust is therefore central in establishing an effective therapeutic interaction. The withholding of information regarding the diagnosis or prognosis may be viewed as a form of deception.[13] Although most patients trust their physicians to make decisions in their best interest, even subtle forms of deception are viewed as unacceptable.[14] Truth telling is, therefore, a process at the center of the physician–patient relationship, which aims to empowering patients to navigate their disease course.[5]

The argument for full disclosure of the diagnosis and prognosis, however, may prioritize autonomy and the right to self-determination over other ethical principles. A traditional view of autonomy holds that capable individuals may make all necessary decisions regarding their personal care when equipped with all options, alternatives, and perceived benefits and risks. Practically speaking, there is considerably heterogeneity in the degree to which patients desire to be informed of their condition. It is also self-evident that different individuals may prioritize different treatment options, even when presented with the same information. Freedom of choice may be affected by cultural, social, and personal considerations, even when all the information is rationally presented to patients.[5] A "relational" view of autonomy has been proposed, whereby special consideration must be paid to patients' internal moderating factors that may affect their autonomy.[15,16] These may include preoperative levels of stress, willingness to participate in the decision-making process, and level of understanding of the information presented.

■ Management: Clinical Care, Research, and Therapeutic Misconception

Initiation of Nonexperimental Therapy

The patient's decision to undergo treatment, whether medical or surgical, is highly individualized and often guided by the physician's duty to maximize benefit and reduce harm. In some circumstances, there is equipoise between different therapeutic options and it remains to the patient to choose

Table 46.1 Selected Ethical Challenges in Neuro-Oncology

Category	Ethical Issue	AMA Code of Ethics Reference[1]	Specific Challenges in Neuro-Oncology
Practice Matters			
	Informed consent	8.08	Impact of disease burden on capacity
	Surrogate decision making	8.081	Definition of patient's "best interest"
	Involvement of trainees in the care of patients	8.087 and 8.088	
	Allocation of limited medical resources	2.03	Access to operative time and limited therapeutics
	Futile care	2.035 and 2.037	Continuing therapy at end-of-life
Professional Rights and Responsibilities			
	Communication with patients and their families	9.012	Disclosure and truth-telling of poor prognoses
	Evaluation of novel medical or surgical innovation	9.08 and 9.09	Definition of adequate evidence, particularly as it pertains to surgical innovations
	Racial and ethnic healthcare disparities	9.121	Inequities in access to neuro-oncological care
Research			
	Subject selection for clinical trials	2.071	Choosing the appropriate trial for neuro-oncology patients
	Ethical considerations in international research	2.077	Treatment of neuro-oncology in the developing world
	DNA databanks and genomics research	2.079	Collection, storage, and use of tumor samples
Confidentiality, Advertising, and Industry Relations			
	Conflicts in industry relations	5.09; 8.061	Industry relations with respect to novel therapeutics
Social Policy			
	Commercial use of human tissue	2.08	Ownership of brain tumor samples
	Genetic counseling	2.12	Counseling of families with different neuro-oncological disorders
	Disclosure of familial risk in genetic testing and related issues	2.131; 2.136; 2.137; 2.138; 2.139	Relevance to familial syndromes resulting in brain tumors
	Withholding life sustaining treatment, euthanasia and physician-assisted suicide	2.20; 2.21; 2.211	End-of-life care and challenges raised by a patient's wish to die
	Do not resuscitate orders and advanced directives	2.22 and 2.225	

which treatments to undertake. One example of this is the decision to undergo resection or biopsy for presumed low-grade glioma as opposed to the watch-and-wait approach. It has been shown that, in such situations, the decision to undergo surgery is moderated by the disease burden, quality of life, and fear of morbidity from the intervention as well as trust in the treating physician.[17]

In most cases, however, varying levels of evidence may support one treatment strategy over another and thus inform the options presented to patients. Most patients with brain tumors undergo surgery, and the majority of those with malignant neoplasms also receive chemotherapy and radiation therapy.[18] Informed consent for treatment requires adequate disclosure to a capable patient in the absence of any undue influence.[19] Although fully informed consent may not be feasible, given that numerous unforeseen risks may be later encountered,[20] physicians have an obligation to disclose common and material risks to patients. As defined in the landmark litigation of *Canterbury v. Spence,* a risk is said to be material "when a reasonable person in what the physician knows or should know to be the patient's position would be likely to attach significance to the risk or cluster of risks in determining whether or not to undergo the proposed therapy."[21] Therefore, informed consent is a bidirectional process that must evaluate and address the patient's position and contextualize material risks to his/her life circumstances.

One particular challenge in obtaining informed consent for treatment from patients with neuro-oncological conditions

- Informed consent is a bidirectional process that must consider the patient's unique position and life circumstances.
- Capacity is domain specific and involves understanding and appreciating the nature of the illness and the risks of intervention.

relates to how the underlying disorder may alter a patient's agency, and therefore capacity, to consent or refuse standard or experimental treatments. It has been previously shown that that the amount of information retained by patients during informed consent discussions is inversely related to the underlying disease severity.[22] One study also demonstrated that patients frequently consented to treatment with only a modest appreciation of risk, with nearly one quarter of individuals reporting no risks despite being informed of them.[23] Conversely, the presence of a cognitive deficit or the inability to perform a specific activity or task does not preclude rational decision making in all aspects of an individual's life. Capacity is domain specific, meaning that it must be evaluated independently for specific decision-making processes. Although capacity, as a socio-legal construct, varies across time and jurisdictions, there is growing consensus that two fundamental elements of capacity are the ability to "understand" and to "appreciate" risks.[24] The former describes an individual's ability to comprehend and retain information, whereas the latter refers to the decision-making process whereby personal meanings are attached to the factual information.

Clinical Trials: Recruitment and Design

Health care professionals and societies have an ethical obligation to develop novel therapies to improve survival and quality of life of future patients with brain tumors and other neuro-oncological diagnoses. The recruitment of current patients into clinical trials is widely recognized as the gold standard for the legitimization of experimental treatments. Historical failures to ethically recruit patients into clinical research have informed present practices and emphasize the importance of the ethical conduct of experimental medicine. From the Nuremburg codes to the subsequent Declaration of Helsinki and from the lessons of the Tuskegee syphilis study to the publication of the Belmont Report, high ethical standards are now enshrined in the missions of institutional review boards (IRBs) (**Table 46.2**).[25] Although seemingly simple, ethical challenges may arise during all stages of the recruitment of subjects for clinical research. The challenges that must be considered range from advertising the trials[26] to remuneration or payment of subjects involved in studies that are associated with varying degrees of risk.[27–29]

Thorough pre-enrollment discussions with prospective research subjects are necessary prior to their participation in experimental studies. Patients' assessment of experimental risk is complex and value-laden; therefore, risk perception may not be congruent with actual risk.[30] Furthermore, consent to participate in research trials differs from that for nonexperimental therapies because the risks of the latter are inherently uncertain; therefore, choices made based on perceived risk may be misguided. The challenges of ethically recruiting patients with neuro-oncological diagnoses into clinical trials are further compounded by the fact that they are

Table 46.2 Selected Seminal Guidelines on the Ethical Conduct of Research in Human Populations

Work	Year Published	Purpose
Nuremberg Code	1947	10-point statement meant to prevent future abuse of human subjects in response to inhumane experimentation on vulnerable populations during World War II
Declaration of Helsinki	Multiple revisions	Extensive work describing importance of ethical research practices, basic principles for its conduct, and the combination of research with clinical care
Vancouver Group (International Committee of Medical Editors)	Multiple revisions	Consensus guidelines regarding ethical issues in the reporting and publication of research findings, particularly pertaining to conflicts of interest, privacy and confidentiality
Belmont Report	1978	Partially published in response to the Tuskegee syphilis study, it emphasized respect for persons, with primary areas of application including informed consent, assessment of risks vs benefits, and subject selection
Common Rule	1981	Describes baseline standards of ethics to which government-funded research in the United States is held, particularly regarding institutional review boards (IRBs)
International Conference on Harmonisation of Technical Requirements for Registration of Pharmaceuticals for Human use "Guidelines for Good Clinical Practice"	1996	Defines standards for the regulation of clinical trials involving human subjects, including protection of human rights, evaluation of safety and efficacy, and responsibility of sponsors, clinicians and investigators.

often highly motivated to pursue novel treatments given the dismal prognoses with which they are often faced. These patients, therefore, may fail to recognize that the goal of experimental therapy is to benefit future patients. As such, patients often underestimate the risk and overestimate the benefit of participation in clinical research.[31,32]

Research in later stages of neuro-oncological conditions and during end-of-life stages may be further associated with unique ethical challenges. Four common objections to the conduct of research in the end-of-life setting are (1) the goals of research may conflict with care, (2) the studies may place excessive burden on patients and families, (3) there may be a lack of equipoise in this context, and (4) research in the palliative setting is inherently difficult.[33] For instance, the goals of palliation are defined by the American Academy of Hospice and Palliative Medicine (AAHPM) in the Hospice and Palliative Medicine Core Competencies as (1) pain and symptom control and addressing psychosocial, spiritual, and practical needs; (2) dissemination of information to patients and families to facilitate understanding of the condition and options; (3) provision of care in the context of a trusting physician–patient relationship; (4) communication and continuity of care; and (5) preparation of patient and families for the dying process, when it is anticipated, insofar as such preparation is desired.[34] Conversely, the goals of clinical research are often to improve the lives of future patients, and therefore the vulnerability of patients near the end of life raises concerns regarding their exploitation as research participants.[33] It has been proposed that a large proportion of patients nearing the end of life look favorably upon research studies, particularly family-focused investigations.[35] Furthermore, specific research methodologies may align the goals of the research with the patient's goals and aspirations.

Therapeutic Misconception

The enthusiasm for the development of translational therapies to provide improved care to future patients must be tempered by ethical and fiduciary duties to current patients. Physicians often play a dual role as both health care providers and clinician investigators.[36] Patients may demonstrate a "therapeutic misconception" when they fail to recognize the distinction between the competing obligations associated with these two roles.[37] Individuals affected by neuro-oncological conditions are particularly vulnerable to such misconceptions, as it has been previously shown that less optimism regarding personal

> ### Pitfall
>
> - Clinician-investigators must balance their competing obligations as both researchers and primary care providers. The inability of patients to distinguish between these roles is referred to as the therapeutic misconception.

care and hopelessness about future health states increases the probability of therapeutic misconception.[38] Investigators who practice experimental medicine involving such vulnerable patients may benefit from the use of a survey instrument that has been developed to gauge therapeutic misconception in clinical populations.[39]

■ End-of-Life Care

Transition to End-of-Life Care

The transition from active treatment to end-of-life care is often difficult for patients with neuro-oncological diagnoses and their families, and may be associated with depression, hopelessness, or anger, as patients' sentiments of hope are typically related to the pursuit of curative therapies.[40] In facing such difficulties, however, patients often report the discovery of inner strength and resilience.[4] Pursuant to their ethical duties to avoid harm, clinicians often withdraw active treatments when it is perceived that greater harm may result from treatment than benefit. Acceptance of such a transition may not be palatable to some patients, as they may view such a change as a declaration of defeat. Patient expectations may implicitly or explicitly place pressure on clinicians to continue administering therapies that may be futile. Indeed, in one study, 24% of oncologists described administering treatments that were unlikely to be efficacious in order to maintain the patients' optimism.[41] But administering therapy that may not benefit patients is ethically dubious. In fact, the AMA Code of Ethics makes it clear that physicians have no ethical obligation to administer treatments that are futile.[42]

It is important to appreciate that palliative care need not be exclusively initiated only once continued medical care is deemed futile. A greater emphasis has been placed in recent years on initiating palliative care earlier in the course of the illness. Such a strategy may place emphasis on quality of life by facilitating access to resources that may not otherwise be available to patients. To effectively transition to end-of-life care, the physician–patient relationship is of utmost importance. It has been shown that cancer patients who unrealistically overestimate their survival, in part due to breakdowns in physician–patient communication, are more likely to die under mechanical ventilation or following failed cardiopulmonary resuscitation.[43] The importance of such communication is also highlighted by one study evaluating a heterogeneous population near the end of life, which found that the strongest predictor of discharge to home hospice care was not the extent of disease and disability or the physician's perception of the patient's wishes, but rather the number of hospital beds available.[44]

One challenge that may be more commonly encountered in patients with neuro-oncological conditions is that end-of-life decisions are often made by family members because the disease course may affect a patient's capacity and agency. In circumstances where disagreements may arise regarding the ideal course of action, a common approach is to appeal to what is in the patient's best interest.[45,46] Disagreements may continue to arise regarding what constitutes "best interest." In such cases, different avenues for arbitration are available in different jurisdictions. For instance, in Ontario, physicians propose a plan of treatment to substitute decision makers for consent or refusal based on the clinical circumstances and any known prior wishes. If the substitute decision maker refuses to consent, a third, neutral party may be involved (the Consent and Capacity Board), to interpret what legally constitutes the best interest.[47] In other jurisdictions, such as the United Kingdom, the physician makes such decisions independently.

Several themes have been identified from conflicts arising from attempts to establish an incapable person's best interest.[47] First, whereas clinicians focus narrowly on the clinical condition of the patient, substitute decision makers often rely on their values and religion when interpreting what constitutes the patient's best interest. Substitute decision makers also report that patients would accept suffering as a price for living and may possess unrealistic hope for recovery. Such values may be at odds with clinicians' ethical obligations to do no harm if it is thought that additional active therapy would incur unnecessary harm to the patient with no prospect of benefit. Awareness of patients' preferences early in their disease course and counseling regarding end-of-life care, therefore, may mitigate conflicts that may arise later during their illness.

Physician-Assisted Suicide and Euthanasia

The ethical arguments and controversies related to physician-assisted suicide and euthanasia are extensive and often divisive. Although a comprehensive discussion of these controversies is beyond the scope of this chapter, it is important for clinicians working with patients with brain tumors and other neuro-oncological diagnoses to understand the concepts and regulations surrounding physician-assisted suicide and euthanasia. Whereas the latter refers to the active administration of a lethal agent to a patient to relieve intolerable and incurable suffering, the former implies that the patients themselves perform the act with necessary means or information provided by the physician. Furthermore, clinicians must recognize the distinction between a capable patient's right to forgo life-sustaining treatment and physician-assisted suicide.

Euthanasia is illegal in Canada and the United States, but there are legal provisions for physician-assisted suicide in the states of Oregon, Washington, and Montana. In a systematic review of 110 studies evaluating these topics, four themes emerged: (1) concerns about poor quality of life, (2) a desire for good quality of death, (3) concerns about abuse of assisted dying, and (4) an emphasis on the individual's stance on assisted dying.[48] Understandably, patients with neuro-oncological diagnoses may inquire about or actively seek assistance in ending their lives. One previous study capturing the attitudes of patients and their caregivers on the subject of physician-

assisted suicide and euthanasia found considerable heterogeneity in opinions regarding the means and regulation of the practice, although the general agreement was that the decision should remain in the hands of the patients and their families.[4] Although clinicians must act within their legal bounds, according to the AMA, they should also aggressively respond to the needs of patients at the end of life in order to mitigate suffering and improve quality of life.[49]

Neurologic Determination of Death

Advances in critical care and mechanical ventilation have also led to the realization that the body's physiological function can be temporarily supported in the absence of brain activity. The neurologic determination of death, the diagnosis of "brain death," is made in circumstances where an individual demonstrates no clinical evidence of brain function on physical examination. This includes absence of response to pain, lack of spontaneous respiration, no response to cranial nerve and oculocephalic reflexes, as well as negative caloric testing. Although the Uniform Determination of Death Act (UDDA) established neurologic diagnosis of death in the United States, there remains considerable heterogeneity in the criteria for determination of brain death in different jurisdictions.[50] For example, New Jersey law states the neurologic determination of death is illegal if there is "reason to believe . . . that such a declaration would violate the personal religious beliefs of the individual."[8] In many countries, the diagnosis is not possible under some or all circumstances.[50] Although the ethical issues related to diagnosing brain death as well as refusal to make the diagnosis are vast, it is sufficient to state that consensus evidence-based guidelines are necessary to standardize the diagnostic criteria and educate clinicians and the public alike regarding brain death.

Pitfall

- Palliative care need not commence only when the pursuit of curative therapy is deemed futile.

Pearl

- Addressing patients' beliefs, values, and wishes early in the course of their illness may alleviate subsequent ambiguities regarding their best interest.

◼ Emerging Ethical Challenges in Neuro-Oncology

Genomics and Biobanking

Biobanking refers to the collection of biological materials in combination with health and demographic information for the purposes of long-term storage for use in current and future research endeavors. Although biobanks initially started in the field of oncology, numerous biological specimens are now collected from other patient populations with genetic disorders. It is irrefutable that the practice of biobanking has heralded numerous scientific advances for the treatment of patients with neuro-oncological disorders. For example, an international biobanking consortium of medulloblastoma specimen recently reported genetic alterations that may have significant implications for treatment of the disease.[51] However, numerous ethical challenges are associated with biobanking, including concerns regarding control and ownership,[52] privacy and withdrawal of samples, as well as commercialization of results and management of incidental findings.[53]

Although a growing number of studies and international task forces are addressing these important topics, opinions vary considerably regarding ideal practical policies and biobanking regulations. In one study evaluating the views of patients toward specimen banking, 59.6% of patients preferred one-time consent, although a sizable minority were in favor of re-consent or a tiered consent process for future research studies using the same samples.[54] Issues of ownership and withdrawal of consent are further complicated by the fact that many patients with brain neoplasms will succumb to the disease, leaving unanswered questions regarding proxy or surrogate ownership. Although many of these issues remain open to debate, it is important to explore them with patients prior to obtaining tissue specimen for biobanking.

Patient Selection for Increasing Therapeutic and Experimental Options

Given the increasing number of treatment options and therapeutics under investigation, one patient may be eligible for several standard and experimental treatments. For example, a patient with brain metastases may be eligible for surgical resection and whole-brain radiation therapy (WBRT), WBRT with radiosurgery boost, or WBRT alone, in addition to any investigational treatments.[55] Choosing the best strategy for individual patients and presenting the treatment options available are therefore increasingly challenging. Previous authors have advocated a "participant-centered" approach to this challenge, and particularly the conduct of clinical research in this context.[56] The goals of the treatment and/or experimental therapy would be aligned with the patient's goals of care. Such a strategy may decrease attrition from clinical trials and enforce a therapeutic physician–patient relationship.

Regulation of Innovation

The regulation of novel medical and surgical therapies and procedures is also an emerging focus of ethical inquiry. The Belmont report, which outlines ethical criteria for the conduct of human research, defines an innovation as a "practice that departs significantly from the standard or accepted [practice]."[57] Innovation may also differ from other forms of research

Pitfall

- Although advances in neuro-oncology research provide hope for the provision of novel treatment options to future patients, they also introduce new and complex ethical challenges.

in that it is characterized by evolving techniques, outcome measures, and patient selection.[58] The extent to which a medical or surgical innovation requires regulation and careful oversight of its application to patient care is directly related to the extent to which it deviates from established practices.[59]

The field of neuro-oncology has benefited from several medical and surgical advances. Examples of the latter include the delineation of surgical margins using indocyanine green (ICG) staining,[60] and cortical and subcortical mapping to improve safety and resectability of tumors in eloquent cortex.[61] Conversely, innovative applications may also be identified for established procedures. For example, the use of awake craniotomy for tumors in non-eloquent cortex,[62] in the outpatient setting,[63,64] and in the developing world to conserve scarce resources has introduced different and context-specific ethical challenges.[65]

The oversight of such surgical innovations is one particular challenge. Despite the importance of sound medical and scientific evidence for supporting implementation of a particular clinical practice, the majority of surgical innovations do not undergo randomized clinical trials; it is therefore unclear what amount of evidence is sufficient to legitimize their implementations.[66,67] Furthermore, the ethical basis for sham controls in surgical trials is controversial and requires considerable foresight in trial design.[68,69] Previous authors have suggested that "one should not unnecessarily obstruct surgical innovation by always insisting on orthodox and rigid adherence to the tenets of the prospective randomized double-blind controlled trial."[70] It has been suggested that adoption of a novel surgical innovation should be preceded by observational studies, with standardization of procedures and attempts to involve multiple surgeons at different centers.[71] Although there is no consensus on how best to translate novel medical and surgical innovations to patient care, it must be performed with the utmost regard to patient safety, treatment efficacy, and ethical principles.

■ Conclusion

Patients with brain tumors and other neuro-oncological diagnoses are a vulnerable patient population due to difficulties in coping with the burden of illness as well as the effects of the disease on cognitive faculties and neurologic function. Clinicians must remain cognizant of the myriad ethical issues that may arise during the course of treatment—from diagnosis to end-of-life care. Furthermore, although medical and surgical advances have invigorated hope for the development of sorely needed treatments, they have also heralded new and complex ethical challenges that must be addressed. The ethical regulation of novel innovations, recruitment of patients into clinical trials, and storage and usage of banked biological specimen are examples of contemporary challenges that must be considered when conducting research studies. A basic ethical approach facilitates decision making during common circumstances where ethical conflicts may arise. Ultimately physicians must be able to aid their patients in confidently navigating their illness and facing uncertainties with dignity.

Editor's Note

As the art and science of neuro-oncology advances, ethical issues become even more important. Often technological and scientific advances precede our ability to know the appropriate indications and uses for them and to foresee the problems they bring. New is not always better. Some of the salient issues in neuro-oncology requiring ethical oversight include ethical conduct of clinical research, privacy of information especially with genetic profiling of tumors and maintenance of patients' tissue in tumor banks, ethical introduction of innovation especially in surgery, and end-of-life issues, among others.

The process of informed consent, the cornerstone of clinical practice, becomes more complex as more options for treatments are available, more clinical trials are begun, and patients become better informed, largely because of access to the Internet and to social media.[72] Older issues like dignified care at the end of life and new ones like assisted suicide will continue to challenge neuro-oncologists, especially as the law and public opinion shift, and we should all embrace these challenges. One way of studying ethical issues in neuro-oncology patients is to ask them their views about important issues; this is at the heart of a qualitative research methodology.[72,73] (Bernstein)

References

1. Council on Ethical and Judicial Affairs. Code of Medical Ethics of the American Medical Association. http://www.ama-assn.org/ama/pub/physician-resources/medical-ethics/code-medical-ethics.page. Accessed June 23, 2013

2. Ownsworth T, Chambers S, Hawkes A, Walker DG, Shum D. Making sense of brain tumour: a qualitative investigation of personal and social processes of adjustment. Neuropsychol Rehabil 2011;21:117–137

3. Wong J, Mendelsohn D, Nyhof-Young J, Bernstein M. A qualitative assessment of the supportive care and resource needs of patients undergoing craniotomy for benign brain tumours. Support Care Cancer 2011;19:1841–1848

4. Lipsman N, Skanda A, Kimmelman J, Bernstein M. The attitudes of brain cancer patients and their caregivers towards death and dying: a qualitative study. BMC Palliat Care 2007;6:7

5. Surbone A. Telling the truth to patients with cancer: what is the truth? Lancet Oncol 2006;7:944–950

6. Oken D. What to tell cancer patients. A study of medical attitudes. JAMA 1961;175:1120–1128

7. Novack DH, Plumer R, Smith RL, Ochitill H, Morrow GR, Bennett JM. Changes in physicians' attitudes toward telling the cancer patient. JAMA 1979;241:897–900

8. Murray E, Lo B, Pollack L, et al. The impact of health information on the internet on the physician-patient relationship: patient perceptions. Arch Intern Med 2003;163:1727–1734

9. Kutner JS, Steiner JF, Corbett KK, Jahnigen DW, Barton PL. Information needs in terminal illness. Soc Sci Med 1999;48:1341–1352

10. Slevin ML. Talking about cancer: how much is too much? Br J Hosp Med 1987;38:56, 58–59

11. Sulmasy DP, Terry PB, Weisman CS, et al. The accuracy of substituted judgments in patients with terminal diagnoses. Ann Intern Med 1998;128:621–629

12. Eidinger RN, Schapira DV. Cancer patients' insight into their treatment, prognosis, and unconventional therapies. Cancer 1984;53:2736–2740

13. Gordon EJ, Daugherty CK. "Hitting you over the head": oncologists' disclosure of prognosis to advanced cancer patients. Bioethics 2003;17:142–168

14. Yu JJ, Bernstein M. Brain tumor patients' views on deception: a qualitative study. J Neurooncol 2011;104:331–337

15. Donchin A. Understanding autonomy relationally: toward a reconfiguration of bioethical principles. J Med Philos 2001;26:365–386

16. Sherwin S. A relational approach to autonomy in health-care. In: Sherwin S, Feminist healthcare network, eds. The Politics of Women's Health: Exploring Agency and Autonomy. Philadelphia: Temple University Press, 1988:19–44

17. Hayhurst C, Mendelsohn D, Bernstein M. Low grade glioma: a qualitative study of the wait and see approach. Can J Neurol Sci 2011;38:256–261

18. Rosenblum ML. General surgical principles, alternatives, and limitations. Neurosurg Clin N Am 1990;1:19–36

19. Etchells E, Sharpe G, Walsh P, Williams JR, Singer PA. Bioethics for clinicians: 1. Consent. CMAJ 1996;155:177–180

20. Bernstein M. Fully informed consent is impossible in surgical clinical trials. Can J Surg 2005;48:271–272

21. *Canterbury v. Spence.* 464 F (2nd). 1972:772

22. Schaeffer MH, Krantz DS, Wichman A, Masur H, Reed E, Vinicky JK. The impact of disease severity on the informed consent process in clinical research. Am J Med 1996;100:261–268

23. Lidz CW, Appelbaum PS, Grisso T, Renaud M. Therapeutic misconception and the appreciation of risks in clinical trials. Soc Sci Med 2004;58:1689–1697

24. Appelbaum PS, Grisso T. Assessing patients' capacities to consent to treatment. N Engl J Med 1988;319:1635–1638

25. World Medical Association Declaration of Helsinki: ethical principles for medical research involving human subjects. JAMA 2000;284:3043–3045

26. Phillips TB. Money, advertising and seduction in human subjects research. Am J Bioeth 2007;7:88–90

27. Bernstein M. Payment of research subjects involved in clinical trials is unethical. J Neurooncol 2003;63:223–224

28. Wong JC, Bernstein M. Payment of research subjects for more than minimal risk trials is unethical. Am J Med Sci 2011;342:294–296

29. Dickert N, Emanuel E, Grady C. Paying research subjects: an analysis of current policies. Ann Intern Med 2002;136:368–373

30. Perrow C. Normal Accidents Living with High-Risk Technologies. Princeton: Princeton University Press, 1999
31. Penman DT, Holland JC, Bahna GF, et al. Informed consent for investigational chemotherapy: patients' and physicians' perceptions. J Clin Oncol 1984;2:849–855
32. Joffe S, Cook EF, Cleary PD, Clark JW, Weeks JC. Quality of informed consent in cancer clinical trials: a cross-sectional survey. Lancet 2001; 358:1772–1777
33. LeBlanc TW, Wheeler JL, Abernethy AP. Research in end-of-life settings: an ethical inquiry. J Pain Palliat Care Pharmacother 2010;24: 244–250
34. American Academy of Hospice and Palliative Medicine. Hospice and palliative medicine core competencies, version 2.3. Updated September 2009
35. Casarett D, Kassner CT, Kutner JS. Recruiting for research in hospice: feasibility of a research screening protocol. J Palliat Med 2004;7:854–860
36. Bernstein M. Conflict of interest: it is ethical for an investigator to also be the primary care-giver in a clinical trial. J Neurooncol 2003;63: 107–108
37. Appelbaum PS, Lidz CW, Grisso T. Therapeutic misconception in clinical research: frequency and risk factors. IRB 2004;26:1–8
38. Goebel S, von Harscher M, Mehdorn HM. Comorbid mental disorders and psychosocial distress in patients with brain tumours and their spouses in the early treatment phase. Support Care Cancer 2011;19: 1797–1805
39. Joffe S, Cook EF, Cleary PD, Clark JW, Weeks JC. Quality of informed consent: a new measure of understanding among research subjects. J Natl Cancer Inst 2001;93:139–147
40. Hofmann B, Håheim LL, Søreide JA. Ethics of palliative surgery in patients with cancer. Br J Surg 2005;92:802–809
41. Baile WF, Lenzi R, Parker PA, Buckman R, Cohen L. Oncologists' attitudes toward and practices in giving bad news: an exploratory study. J Clin Oncol 2002;20:2189–2196
42. Council on Ethical and Judicial Affairs. AMA Code of Medical Ethics: Opinion 2.037: Medical futility in end-of-life care. http://www.ama-assn.org/ama/pub/physician-resources/medical-ethics/code-medical-ethics/opinion2037.page? Accessed July 9, 2013
43. Weeks JC, Cook EF, O'Day SJ, et al. Relationship between cancer patients' predictions of prognosis and their treatment preferences. JAMA 1998;279:1709–1714
44. Freeborne N, Lynn J, Desbiens NA; The Study to Understand Prognoses and Preferences for Outcomes and Risks of Treatments. Insights about dying from the SUPPORT project. J Am Geriatr Soc 2000;48(5, Suppl): S199–S205
45. Baumrucker SJ, Sheldon JE, Stolick M, Morris GM, Vandekieft G, Harrington D. The ethical concept of "best interest". Am J Hosp Palliat Care 2008;25:56–62
46. The President's Commission for the Study of Ethical Problems in Medicine and Biomedical and Behavioral Research. Deciding to forgo life-sustaining treatment. Washington, DC: U.S. Government Printing Office, 1983
47. Chidwick P, Sibbald R, Hawryluck L. Best interests at end of life: an updated review of decisions made by the Consent and Capacity Board of Ontario. J Crit Care 2013;28:22–27
48. Hendry M, Pasterfield D, Lewis R, Carter B, Hodgson D, Wilkinson C. Why do we want the right to die? A systematic review of the international literature on the views of patients, carers and the public on assisted dying. Palliat Med 2013;27:13–26
49. Council on Ethical and Judicial Affairs. AMA Code of Medical Ethics: opinion 2.21: Euthanasia. http://www.ama-assn.org/ama/pub/physician-resources/medical-ethics/code-medical-ethics/opinion221.page? Accessed July 9, 2013

50. Wijdicks EF. Brain death worldwide: accepted fact but no global consensus in diagnostic criteria. Neurology 2002;58:20–25
51. Northcott PA, Shih DJ, Peacock J, et al. Subgroup-specific structural variation across 1,000 medulloblastoma genomes. Nature 2012;488: 49–56
52. Charo RA. Body of research—ownership and use of human tissue. N Engl J Med 2006;355:1517–1519
53. Wolf SM, Lawrenz FP, Nelson CA, et al. Managing incidental findings in human subjects research: analysis and recommendations. J Law Med Ethics 2008;36:219–248, 211
54. Master Z, Claudio JO, Rachul C, Wang JC, Minden MD, Caulfield T. Cancer patient perceptions on the ethical and legal issues related to biobanking. BMC Med Genomics 2013;6:8–8794
55. Ibrahim GM, Chung C, Bernstein M. Competing for patients: an ethical framework for recruiting patients with brain tumors into clinical trials. J Neurooncol 2011;104:623–627
56. Gross D, Fogg L. Clinical trials in the 21st century: the case for participant-centered research. Res Nurs Health 2001;24:530–539
57. National Commission for the Protection of Human Subjects of Biomedical and Behavioral Research. The Belmont Report: Ethical Principles and Guidelines for the Protection of Human Subjects of Research. Washington, DC: US Government Printing Office, 1978
58. McKneally MF. The ethics of innovation: Columbus and others try something new. J Thorac Cardiovasc Surg 2011;141:863–866
59. Bernstein M, Bampoe J. Surgical innovation or surgical evolution: an ethical and practical guide to handling novel neurosurgical procedures. J Neurosurg 2004;100:2–7
60. Kim EH, Cho JM, Chang JH, Kim SH, Lee KS. Application of intraoperative indocyanine green videoangiography to brain tumor surgery. Acta Neurochir (Wien) 2011;153:1487–1495, discussion 1494–1495
61. Szelényi A, Senft C, Jardan M, et al. Intra-operative subcortical electrical stimulation: a comparison of two methods. Clin Neurophysiol 2011;122:1470–1475
62. Serletis D, Bernstein M. Prospective study of awake craniotomy used routinely and nonselectively for supratentorial tumors. J Neurosurg 2007;107:1–6
63. Boulton M, Bernstein M. Outpatient brain tumor surgery: innovation in surgical neurooncology. J Neurosurg 2008;108:649–654
64. Purzner T, Purzner J, Massicotte EM, Bernstein M. Outpatient brain tumor surgery and spinal decompression: a prospective study of 1003 patients. Neurosurgery 2011;69:119–126, discussion 126–127
65. Kirsch B, Bernstein M. Ethical challenges with awake craniotomy for tumor. Can J Neurol Sci 2012;39:78–82
66. Awad IA. Innovation through minimalism: assessing emerging technology in neurosurgery. Clin Neurosurg 1996;43:303–316
67. Haines SJ. Randomized clinical trials in the evaluation of surgical innovation. J Neurosurg 1979;51:5–11
68. McDonald PJ, Kulkarni AV, Farrokhyar F, Bhandari M. Ethical issues in surgical research. Can J Surg 2010;53:133–136
69. Bernstein M. Assessing the bioethical integrity of a clinical trial in surgery. Can J Surg 2004;47:329–332
70. Gillett G. Ethics of surgical innovation. Br J Surg 2001;88:897–898
71. Gardner TJ. Are randomized trials the best way to judge the efficacy of surgical procedures? J Thorac Cardiovasc Surg 2010;140:739–742
72. Knifed E, Lipsman N, Mason W, Bernstein M. Patients' perception of the informed consent process for neurooncology clinical trials. Neurooncol 2008;10:348–354
73. Khu KJ, Doglietto F, Radovanovic I, et al. Patients' perceptions of awake and outpatient craniotomy for brain tumor: a qualitative study. J Neurosurg 2010;112:1056–1060

47 Seminal Randomized Controlled Trials in Neuro-Oncology

Ganesh M. Shankar and Fred G. Barker II

What is a seminal clinical trial? Important medical publications in any scientific field can prompt subsequent workers to build a superstructure of new knowledge on the foundations established by "seminal" studies that point out new directions for investigation. Perhaps a more characteristic function of important clinical trials is that they change clinical practice. These clinical studies move the field forward in individual and important ways. They have substantial and immediate academic impact: initial presentations in high-visibility venues such as international meetings, high citation rates by subsequent papers (**Table 47.1**), and important effects on the careers of those who designed and conducted the trials. They change clinical practice, as shown by population-based studies of changing patterns of practice and changes in treatment guidelines, and they change pharmaceutical practice by triggering regulatory approval for new agents or by finding new indications for drugs already approved for other uses. Finally, in many cases these trials include adjunct translational research that establish novel prognostic factors or biomarkers for response to the study drug.

Randomized controlled trials (RCTs) are the foundation of modern neuro-oncology. Their evidence guides important clinical questions in brain tumor surgery, radiation therapy, and chemotherapy. However, they compose a minority of the literature of neuro-oncology, which is replete with retrospective studies, nonrandomized prospective trials, and meta-analyses. Designing RCTs in neuro-oncology has historically been limited by the rarity of intracranial tumors at single institutions. In addition, as is the case for other solid tumors,[1] relatively few adult brain tumor patients in the United States enter RCTs, perhaps 5% or less of patients with eligible brain tumor histologies. In contrast, pediatric neuro-oncologists enroll the majority of patients with eligible cancer diagnoses in clinical trials.[2]

This chapter briefly reviews several landmark trials in the treatment of patients with gliomas and metastases in view of their function as studies that advanced clinical knowledge and practice.

■ Low-Grade Glioma

Treatment options for histologically proven low-grade glioma (LGG) may include surgical resection, radiation therapy, and chemotherapy. Of these, radiation therapy and chemother-

apy have been validated through an RCT to provide longer progression-free survival (PFS).

Radiation Therapy

The European Organization for Research on Treatment of Cancer (EORTC) trial 22845[3] randomized 314 patients from 24 centers to early postoperative radiation therapy (54 Gy in 1.8-Gy fractions) or to delayed radiotherapy at the time of progression. Although patients who received adjuvant radiotherapy had statistically significantly longer PFS (median PFS 5.3 years versus 3.4 years), overall survival was the same for the two groups (median 7.4 versus 7.2 years). Given the lack of an overall survival benefit, this RCT provides information that radiation therapy can be deferred until evidence of progression, especially given the potential toxicity of radiation leukoencephalopathy. EORTC trial 22844, an RCT that compared low-dose (45 Gy) and high-dose (59.4 Gy) radiation, showed no survival benefit with the higher dose, but a higher incidence of radiation necrosis in the high-dose treatment arm.[4] In addition, the high-dose arm patients had lower levels of functioning on quality-of-life testing and higher symptom burden.[5] These negative results were similar to those reported from a North American intergroup trial comparing 64.8 Gy to 50.4 Gy in 203 patients, with shorter survival and higher incidence of radiation necrosis in the high-dose group.[6]

Although EORTC trials 22844 and 22845 were disappointing from a therapeutic standpoint, showing no survival benefit for radiotherapy and higher symptom burden with higher doses, the data from these two trials were combined to establish an important system of prognostic factors for LGG. Five prognostic factors have been reported: age 40 years or older, astrocytoma histology, tumor diameter 6 cm or greater, the presence of neurologic deficits before surgery, and tumor crossing the midline. Each factor is associated with poor survival. A scoring system resulted in which two or fewer factors represent low risk and three or more represent high risk.[7] The number of patients in the two protocols was sufficient to

> **Pearl**
>
> - Randomized controlled trials show that radiation treatment at the time of diagnosis does not improve survival for adult patients with LGG and that treatment toxicity is related to radiation dose.

Table 47.1 Selected Important Randomized Controlled Trials in Neuro-Oncology

First Author (Reference)	Year	Study Type	Comparison	Neoplasm	Times Cited	Citations per Year
Stupp[26]	2005	RCT	TMZ + XRT vs XRT	HGG	3,439	430
Andrews[71]	2004	RCT	SRS + WBRT vs WBRT	Metastasis	626	70
Patchell[68]	1990	RCT	WBRT + surgery vs WBRT	Metastasis	1,202	52
Stewart[23]	2002	Meta-analysis	XRT + chemo vs XRT	HGG	570	52
Patchell[70]	1998	RCT	Surgery + WBRT vs surgery	Metastasis	553	37
Walker[42]	1980	RCT	WBRT vs chemo vs WBRT + chemo	HGG	1139	35
Fine[22]	1993	Meta-analysis	XRT + chemo vs XRT	HGG	629	31
Kondziolka[72]	1999	RCT	SRS + WBRT vs WBRT	Metastasis	407	29
van den Bent[3]	2005	RCT	Early vs late XRT	LGG	213	27
Shaw[6]	2002	RCT	Low vs high dose XRT	LGG	244	22
Vecht[69]	1993	RCT	WBRT + surgery vs WBRT	Metastasis	421	21
Karim[4]	1996	RCT	Low vs high dose XRT	LGG	273	16
Laperriere[43]	2002	Meta-analysis	XRT + surgery vs surgery	HGG	118	11
Vuorinen[14]	2003	RCT	Biopsy vs resection	HGG	97	10
Shaw[12]	2012	RCT	PCV + XRT vs XRT	LGG	8	8
Andersen[41]	1978	RCT	Surgery + XRT vs surgery	HGG	70	2

Abbreviations: RCT, randomized controlled trial; TMZ, temozolomide; chemo, chemotherapy (i.e., several agents); WBRT, whole-brain radiation therapy; XRT, radiation therapy; HGG, high-grade glioma; LGG, low-grade glioma.

Pearl

- Randomized controlled trials provide high-quality prospective outcome data not related to the investigational treatment.

---

enable the prognostic system to be developed on the 22844 patient set and then validated on the 22845 patient set, a very robust design. The North American intergroup trial, which had confirmed the negative results of the EORTC dose-response trial, was then used to validate this prognostic scoring system.[8]

Extent of Resection

Despite what many surgeons feel is a central role of initial cytoreductive surgery in the management of LGG, no RCT has yet been performed to test the value of resection on outcomes in this disease. Many prospective and retrospective nonrandomized studies, mostly single-center, have suggested a beneficial effect of extent of resection.[9] The EORTC 22844 trial,[4] an RCT that primarily assessed dose response in LGG radiotherapy, found a trend toward improved overall survival and PFS for patients undergoing gross total resection (90–100%) as compared with subtotal resection (50–89%) or biopsy (< 50%). A North American intergroup LGG radiotherapy dose-response trial also found significantly longer overall survival in patients with extensive initial resection.[6]

However, surgical resection was not the randomized treatment in these trials and it therefore cannot be concluded from their results that there is a causal relationship between resec-

tion and better outcome. This is because not all patients who entered these trials were acceptable candidates for total or even extensive surgical resection. The assignment of patients to resection versus biopsy is highly dependent on factors such as tumor size and location, including involvement of eloquent cortex, both of which have been shown to be important factors in LGG prognosis.[7,10] This bias in treatment assignment, known as confounding by indication, hinders a valid outcome between nonrandomized groups. To date, a lack of equipoise between biopsy and resection on the part of most brain tumor surgeons has prevented any RCT comparing the two modalities in LGG.

In 2008, a cohort of LGG patients entered into a nonrandomized prospective trial was exploited to circumvent this obstacle in a novel way.[11] The authors reviewed the outcome in patients from an observation-only arm of a prospective Radiation Therapy Oncology Group (RTOG) clinical trial that required neurosurgeon-defined gross total resection for entry into the study. Postsurgical scans were prospectively archived at entry into the trial. Because surgeons' assessment of extent of resection is notoriously overoptimistic, many of these patients actually had residual disease on retrospective review of the postsurgical scans. Patients with even small amounts of residual tumor (> 1 cm) as defined by enrollment magnetic

---

Pitfall

- There are no randomized studies to definitively show that gross total resection is a positive factor in outcome of adult patients with LGG.

resonance imaging (MRI) had poorer long-term PFS than patients with true gross total resections.

Chemotherapy

The recently published RTOG trial 9802[12] randomized 251 LGG patients who had undergone subtotal resection or who were more than 40 years old to receive procarbazine, chloroethylcyclohexylnitrosourea (CCNU; lomustine), and vincristine (PCV) after radiation therapy versus radiation therapy alone. Progression-free survival was significantly improved in the cohort receiving PCV. Although the initial trial report indicated no overall survival benefit, at the time of writing there is early notification of a survival benefit from PCV in a follow-up analysis of the trial (www.cancer.gov/newscenternewsfromnci/2014/RTOG9802. Accessed May 2, 2014). An earlier negative trial on CCNU in LGG was probably underpowered, including only 54 patients.[13] Although several nonrandomized studies have suggested activity and favorable toxicity profile for temozolomide (TMZ), no published RCTs to date have tested TMZ in LGG.

■ Malignant Glioma

Current treatment for high-grade (malignant) glioma (HGG) involves cytoreductive surgery followed by concurrent chemotherapy and radiation therapy. Similar to the landscape of LGG trials, RCTs in HGG have been primarily focused on assessing the role of chemotherapy and radiation therapy, but, with one exception, not the extent of surgical resection.

Extent of Resection

Determining the treatment effect of resection in HGG is hindered by the same barriers as in LGG: biased assignment of patients to the treatment based on resectability, and unwillingness of most surgeons to consider randomizing patients with resectable HGG to biopsy alone. The single RCT assessing the benefit of HGG resection was reported in 2003.[14] This study of 30 patients demonstrated a statistically significant overall survival benefit for elderly patients (> 65 years old) who underwent resection rather than biopsy (median survival after craniotomy 171 days versus 85 days after biopsy). No other RCT has been performed to address this critical question. The wealth of nonrandomized studies[9] is inherently limited by biased assignment to resection.

Several available study designs could potentially circumvent this difficulty, including randomization to resection versus observation for resectable residual disease after initial HGG resection ("second-look" surgery) or nonrandomized comparisons adjusting for a measure of resectability.[15] Indirect evidence can also be obtained from RCTs of surgical adjuncts intended to improve extent of resection. When a RCT shows a benefit for an intervention thought to act purely as a

> **Pitfall**
>
> - There does not exist good class I evidence to support the role of aggressive surgery in the treatment of patients with malignant glioma.

surgical aid, such as intraoperative MRI or fluorescence-guided surgery, this supports the value of extensive resection in improving outcome.

A RCT of 5-aminolevulinic acid (5-ALA) in improving resection by rendering residual HGG directly visible to the surgeon under blue light was reported in 2006.[16] All patients entering the trial were considered eligible for complete resection by enrolling surgeons. Fluorescence-guided surgery was superior to standard resection on the primary outcome measure of PFS; 65% of 5-ALA patients had imaging-complete resections compared with 36% of controls. A reanalysis of the study found improved survival for patients with complete resections regardless of treatment arm (16.9 months median survival after complete resection versus 11.8 months after incomplete resection), supporting more extensive resection as the reason for better survival.[17] Small trials of other surgical adjuncts, such as neuronavigation and intraoperative MRI-guided resection, have shown similar trends toward both more complete resections and longer PFS.[18] By noting the parallel between extent of resection (as "response" to surgery) and chemotherapy response, and studies linking response to chemotherapy and chemotherapy survival benefit in other solid tumors using meta-analysis,[19–21] it is possible that surgical adjunct RCTs may eventually provide stronger support for surgical resection in HGG than is currently available.

Chemotherapy

A number of RCTs have been designed to address the role of chemotherapy in anaplastic astrocytoma and glioblastoma multiforme, as reviewed by meta-analyses in 1993[22] and 2002.[23] These studies predating TMZ both found a modest, but clinically and statistically significant, improvement in overall survival when a variety of cytotoxic chemotherapeutic agents were added to the treatment of patients with HGG. The two meta-analyses included largely overlapping groups of studies (16 in one and 12 in the other), and the direction and magnitude of the overall treatment effect were similar in the two analyses. However, the earlier meta-analysis, based only on published reports of trial results, had suggested a larger and earlier survival benefit in young patients and those

> **Controversy**
>
> - Meta-analysis can identify small treatment effects not visible in single RCTs. Subgroup analyses should be treated cautiously and may only be valid in individual patient data meta-analyses.

with grade III histology, with glioblastoma patients having no survival advantage from chemotherapy until 12 months after diagnosis.[22] In contrast, the later analysis, which was based on updated individual patient data provided by the original trial investigators, showed no variation in treatment effect with either age or histology.[23]

These meta-analyses illustrate several important principles. First, the original RCTs of chemotherapy in malignant glioma were too small to demonstrate a convincing clinical benefit given the modest activity of the agents tested; six of 12 trials enrolled fewer than 200 patients. Second, meta-analysis of RCTs was useful in clarifying the presence and magnitude of the small but real benefit of chemotherapy. Third, subgroup analyses in meta-analyses should only be attempted when individual patient outcome data from the original trials are available.[24,25]

In 2005, RCT of 573 patients with newly diagnosed glioblastoma who had undergone surgical resection demonstrated a survival benefit with concurrent TMZ administration when added to focal external beam radiotherapy (median survival 14.6 months versus 12.1 months for radiation therapy alone).[26] A companion paper from the study demonstrated a larger benefit from TMZ in patients with methylation of the O^6-methylguanine-DNA methyltransferase (MGMT) promoter.[27] Both conclusions were confirmed by the final report of the study in 2009.[28] This study has been extensively cited by later papers (**Table 47.1**) and had a clear, immediate effect in changing clinical practice. Temozolomide was approved by the U.S. Food and Drug Administration (FDA) for adjuvant use in newly diagnosed glioblastoma 4 days after the study's publication date (http://www.cancer.gov/cancertopics/druginfo/fda-temozolomide; accessed July 10 2013), and a patterns-of-care study in 2006 (1 year after approval) showed that over 60% of newly diagnosed glioblastoma patients in the United States received adjuvant TMZ.[29] An Italian study showed similar rapid and widespread adoption of TMZ.[30]

Chemotherapy with PCV was found to be associated with excellent response rates in anaplastic oligodendroglioma (AO) in the 1980s. Both the RTOG and the EORTC mounted RCTs comparing PCV chemotherapy with radiotherapy to radiotherapy alone that were reported in 2006 as showing no overall survival benefit, with a modest increase in PFS with PCV, but at the cost of significant toxicity.[31,32] On longer term follow-up, both trials later found that there was a dramatic improvement in survival with PCV that was essentially limited to patients whose tumors had 1p/19q deletion.[33,34]

The reason for the discrepancy between final results and the initial reports only became clear in retrospect: the treatment was only effective in patients who already had long expected survival, even without the investigational treatment, because of positive intrinsic prognostic factors, in this case 1p/19q deletion. This finding is likely to have a profound effect on clinical practice. It may also prompt late examination of other trials with initially negative results when later study uncovers important molecular prognostic factors that might also predict a benefit of treatment. A potential parallel is the 1980s trials of radiotherapy in LGG, which showed the same pattern of PFS benefit without changing overall survival in initial results.

Some RCTs have assessed surgically delivered chemotherapy in attempts to circumvent the blood–brain barrier. Biodegradable polymer wafers loaded with bischloroethylnitrosourea (BCNU) were initially developed in the 1980s in animal models. When feasibility of manufacture and initial safety in human patients had been established, RCTs were mounted to measure efficacy. The first RCT failed when manufacturing supply was suspended and the trial was stopped early.[35] The findings suggesting a survival benefit were confirmed by a much larger multicenter trial,[36] and the drug gained FDA approval. Subsequently wafers with much higher active drug content became feasible to produce and a dose escalation trial showed adequate safety of the higher dose wafers, but these have not yet been tested in an RCT.[37] The FDA-approved wafers were implanted in a minority of patients at initial surgery in a 2006 U.S. patterns of practice study.[29]

Another surgical means of direct drug delivery developed in the early 1990s was convection-enhanced delivery (CED), in which multiple catheters are surgically implanted around a resection cavity and drug is infused over several days. As for resection itself, eligibility for this treatment would be expected to convey a survival advantage even in the absence of treatment, mandating an RCT to test efficacy. Reported CED trials to date have tested agents in the setting of recurrent glioblastoma, but post-hoc modeling based on achieved catheter placement in one RCT indicated that only a minority of the tissue volume surrounding the resections performed in the protocol was adequately perfused with the agent.[38] Clearly, future trials using CED, or locally injected treatments given immediately after resection is completed,[39,40] will need to incorporate measures of achieved drug delivery.

Radiation Therapy

The current standard of care in HGG includes postoperative external beam radiation therapy, based on the foundation of RCTs conducted in the 1970s.[41] An early report from the Brain Tumor Study Group (BTSG), a North American consortium

---

> **Pearl**
>
> • Mature trial results may uncover important benefits in good-prognosis patients.

> **Pearl**
>
> • A randomized study definitively showed a survival advantage in glioblastoma patients treated with TMZ; this study immediately changed clinical practice.

of academic centers,[42] found that patients randomized to receive 6,000 Gy with or without chemotherapy had significant improvement in median survival compared with the cohort receiving chemotherapy alone. A meta-analysis of six RCTs performed between 1978 and 1991 that compared outcome with or without radiotherapy confirmed a clinically and statistically significant improvement in survival with radiotherapy.[43] Early radiotherapy practice, before the availability of computed tomography (CT) and MRI, tended toward the use of whole-brain radiation (WBRT).

With better imaging and radiotherapy technique, focal brain irradiation to the tumor and a surrounding margin became feasible, and single-institution retrospective studies established the predominant pattern of failure as local rather than distant in the brain.[44] Two subsequent RCTs showed no benefit to whole-brain irradiation, and significant additional toxicity.[43] These trials were influential in changing practice, and WBRT for glioblastoma is unusual today.

Details of the best dose and fractionation schedule were clarified in additional RCTs conducted in the 1970s and 1980s,[43] notably a United Kingdom Medical Research Council trial[45] and an intergroup trial from the U.S. RTOG and the Eastern Cooperative Oncology Group (ECOG).[46]

When pattern-of-failure studies showed that glioblastoma recurrences after 60 Gy of fractionated external beam radiotherapy occurred mainly in the high-dose treatment volume, many efforts were made in the 1980s and 1990s to increase the delivered radiation dose in HGG. Several RCTs on hyperfractionation showed no benefit.[43] The two widely available methods of delivery of high-dose focal radiation were brachytherapy and stereotactic radiosurgery (SRS), each with promising early-phase results primarily reported from single centers, using historical controls for the comparison group.[47,48] The suggested benefit was maintained when historical controls were selected matched using the RTOG recursive partitioning analysis (RPA) classification.[48,49] Unfortunately, RCTs on both modalities showed no survival advantage, with significant toxicity.[50–52] Later studies showed that the historical control patients selected as eligible for the treatment (but who did not receive the treatment) had a survival advantage based

solely on their eligibility, which explained the overoptimistic early-phase results.[53,54] The two negative randomized studies were valuable in essentially terminating the use of high-dose brachytherapy for malignant glioma.

A similar pattern of overoptimistic comparisons using historical controls, with the therapy later shown to be ineffective in an RCT, was seen for intra-arterial BCNU chemotherapy.[55–57] The common factor appears to be the vital nature of tumor size and location for eligibility for these spatially focal therapies, an important prognostic factor that the RTOG RPA classification did not adequately adjust for.

Prognostic Factors

From the earliest cooperative group trials of the BTSG, establishment of valid prognostic factors in brain tumor patients was a stated goal,[58] and most single prognostic factors and prognosis scoring systems accepted today were first described or confirmed by secondary analyses of RCTs. Examples in both LGG and HGG include patient age, presentation with seizures, tumor location, functional status, tumor histology, molecular markers, and extent of resection.[27,59–61] The difficulty in working with multiple potentially useful prognostic factors in choosing an appropriate historical control group, or in stratifying large RCTs, led to the development of the RPA prognostic scoring system reported by the RTOG in 1993.[62] This analysis established six prognostic categories for HGG patients based on a small number of easily assessed prognostic factors. With slight modifications, this scheme is still in use today.[63]

■ Brain Metastases

Many patients with systemic cancer develop intracranial metastases during their lifetime, with reported prevalence ranging from 10 to 40%[64] and an incidence of approximately 170,000 new cases per year in the United States.[65] The management of intracranial metastasis may include surgical resection, SRS, or WBRT. Landmark RCTs have demonstrated the following points: first, that the combination of surgical resection and WBRT is superior to either alone for single brain metastases; and second, the combination of SRS and WBRT is superior to WBRT for single lesions. As for malignant glioma, RCTs in brain metastases have been used to construct RPA models that have facilitated stratification of later studies in the field.[66,67]

Surgical Resection and Whole-Brain Radiation Therapy

Two RCTs demonstrated survival benefit with surgical resection and WBRT as compared with WBRT alone for the management of a single brain metastasis.[68,69] The single RCT examining the role of postsurgical WBRT for the management of a single brain metastasis revealed decreased local recurrence and recurrence elsewhere in the brain (new metastases) in patients who received WBRT.[70] The study was not powered to assess the effect of WBRT on the secondary end point of overall survival.

Stereotactic Radiosurgery

One RCT revealed a survival benefit for patients with a single intracranial metastatic lesion who received SRS and WBRT (median survival 6.5 months in 164 patients) as opposed to WBRT alone (median survival 4.9 months in 167 patients).[71] Another small RCT reported decreased local recurrence rates after SRS and WBRT compared to WBRT alone for patients with two to four metastases (8% vs 100%).[72] The trial, which included a total of 27 patients, was not powered to address the secondary outcome of overall survival, but a nonsignificant trend toward increased survival was noted with SRS (median 11 vs 7.5 months).

▨ Conclusion

The RCTs in neuro-oncology, where available, have had substantial impact in shaping clinical practice, like TMZ for HGG, as well as the subsequent scientific literature (**Table 47.1**). Some themes that emerge in examining RCTs in neuro-oncology are the necessity for multicenter cooperative efforts (early BTSG trials), and the value of multiple similarly designed RCTs in confirming efficacy (e.g., radiotherapy for HGG, surgery for single metastases) or providing valid substrates for later meta-analysis (e.g., cytotoxic chemotherapy for HGG). Long follow-up may be necessary when a good-prognosis subgroup might benefit selectively from treatment (e.g., PCV for AO). As the best source of prospectively collected outcome data, RCTs have been important in understanding prognostic factors (e.g., BTSG HGG trials, RTOG RPAs for gliomas and metastases). Finally, RCTs have played a vital role in reducing the use of ineffective and toxic therapies (e.g., WBRT, brachytherapy, SRS, and intra-arterial chemotherapy for HGG; radiotherapy for LGG). Because clinical innovations sometimes change practice without RCT support,[73] this unique function of RCTs is a strong argument for their continued support by the neuro-oncology community.

Editor's Note

There have been many important well-designed and -executed RCTs in neuro-oncology that have changed our practice. An important positive study is the 2005 TMZ trial. An example of negative studies altering our practice include the two negative randomized trials in 1998 and 2002 showing no benefit of high-activity brachytherapy boost for de novo glioblastoma. However, much work is yet to be done.

We still have too much variability in practice for the same disease from oncologist to oncologist, surgeon to surgeon, and institution to institution, a situation that could be helped with randomized studies.[74] There are many questions yet to be answered, but arguably the most intriguing and practical question in neuro-oncology that will almost certainly never be able to be properly addressed by randomized studies is the real value of aggressive resection for both LGGs and HGGs. RCTs are expensive, time-consuming, and ethically charged for both clinicians and patients, and often further complicated by the presence of multiple competing simultaneous trials.[75] But we all must continue to strive to overcome the hurdles and do whatever it takes to obtain scientific answers to guide the best treatments for our patients. (Bernstein)

References

1. Al-Refaie WB, Vickers SM, Zhong W, Parsons H, Rothenberger D, Habermann EB. Cancer trials versus the real world in the United States. Ann Surg 2011;254:438–442, discussion 442–443
2. Bleyer WA, Tejeda H, Murphy SB, et al. National cancer clinical trials: children have equal access; adolescents do not. J Adolesc Health 1997;21:366–373
3. van den Bent MJ, Afra D, de Witte O, et al; EORTC Radiotherapy and Brain Tumor Groups and the UK Medical Research Council. Long-term efficacy of early versus delayed radiotherapy for low-grade astrocytoma and oligodendroglioma in adults: the EORTC 22845 randomised trial. Lancet 2005;366:985–990
4. Karim AB, Maat B, Hatlevoll R, et al. A randomized trial on dose-response in radiation therapy of low-grade cerebral glioma: European Organization for Research and Treatment of Cancer (EORTC) Study 22844. Int J Radiat Oncol Biol Phys 1996;36:549–556
5. Kiebert GM, Curran D, Aaronson NK, et al; EORTC Radiotherapy Cooperative Group. Quality of life after radiation therapy of cerebral low-grade gliomas of the adult: results of a randomised phase III trial on dose response (EORTC trial 22844). Eur J Cancer 1998;34:1902–1909
6. Shaw E, Arusell R, Scheithauer B, et al. Prospective randomized trial of low- versus high-dose radiation therapy in adults with supratentorial low-grade glioma: initial report of a North Central Cancer Treatment Group/Radiation Therapy Oncology Group/Eastern Cooperative Oncology Group study. J Clin Oncol 2002;20:2267–2276
7. Pignatti F, van den Bent M, Curran D, et al; European Organization for Research and Treatment of Cancer Brain Tumor Cooperative Group;

European Organization for Research and Treatment of Cancer Radiotherapy Cooperative Group. Prognostic factors for survival in adult patients with cerebral low-grade glioma. J Clin Oncol 2002;20:2076–2084

8. Daniels TB, Brown PD, Felten SJ, et al. Validation of EORTC prognostic factors for adults with low-grade glioma: a report using intergroup 86-72-51. Int J Radiat Oncol Biol Phys 2011;81:218–224

9. Sanai N, Berger MS. Glioma extent of resection and its impact on patient outcome. Neurosurgery 2008;62:753–764, discussion 264–266

10. Smith JS, Chang EF, Lamborn KR, et al. Role of extent of resection in the long-term outcome of low-grade hemispheric gliomas. J Clin Oncol 2008;26:1338–1345

11. Shaw EG, Berkey B, Coons SW, et al. Recurrence following neurosurgeon-determined gross-total resection of adult supratentorial low-grade glioma: results of a prospective clinical trial. J Neurosurg 2008;109:835–841

12. Shaw EG, Wang M, Coons SW, et al. Randomized trial of radiation therapy plus procarbazine, lomustine, and vincristine chemotherapy for supratentorial adult low-grade glioma: initial results of RTOG 9802. J Clin Oncol 2012;30:3065–3070

13. Eyre HJ, Crowley JJ, Townsend JJ, et al. A randomized trial of radiotherapy versus radiotherapy plus CCNU for incompletely resected low-grade gliomas: a Southwest Oncology Group study. J Neurosurg 1993;78:909–914

14. Vuorinen V, Hinkka S, Färkkilä M, Jääskeläinen J. Debulking or biopsy of malignant glioma in elderly people—a randomised study. Acta Neurochir (Wien) 2003;145:5–10

15. Barker FG. Brain tumor outcome studies: design and interpretation. In: Winn HR, ed. Youmans' Neurological Surgery, 6th ed, vol 2. Philadelphia: Elsevier, 2011:1243–1253

16. Stummer W, Pichlmeier U, Meinel T, Wiestler OD, Zanella F, Reulen HJ; ALA-Glioma Study Group. Fluorescence-guided surgery with 5-aminolevulinic acid for resection of malignant glioma: a randomised controlled multicentre phase III trial. Lancet Oncol 2006;7:392–401

17. Stummer W, Reulen HJ, Meinel T, et al; ALA-Glioma Study Group. Extent of resection and survival in glioblastoma multiforme: identification of and adjustment for bias. Neurosurgery 2008;62:564–576, discussion 564–576

18. Senft C, Bink A, Franz K, Vatter H, Gasser T, Seifert V. Intraoperative MRI guidance and extent of resection in glioma surgery: a randomised, controlled trial. Lancet Oncol 2011;12:997–1003

19. Buyse M, Thirion P, Carlson RW, Burzykowski T, Molenberghs G, Piedbois P; Meta-Analysis Group in Cancer. Relation between tumour response to first-line chemotherapy and survival in advanced colorectal cancer: a meta-analysis. Lancet 2000;356:373–378

20. Burzykowski T, Buyse M, Piccart-Gebhart MJ, et al. Evaluation of tumor response, disease control, progression-free survival, and time to progression as potential surrogate end points in metastatic breast cancer. J Clin Oncol 2008;26:1987–1992

21. Collette L, Burzykowski T, Carroll KJ, Newling D, Morris T, Schröder FH; European Organisation for Research and Treatment of Cancer; Limburgs Universitair Centrum; AstraZeneca Pharmaceuticals. Is prostate-specific antigen a valid surrogate end point for survival in hormonally treated patients with metastatic prostate cancer? Joint research of the European Organisation for Research and Treatment of Cancer, the Limburgs Universitair Centrum, and AstraZeneca Pharmaceuticals. J Clin Oncol 2005;23:6139–6148

22. Fine HA, Dear KB, Loeffler JS, Black PM, Canellos GP. Meta-analysis of radiation therapy with and without adjuvant chemotherapy for malignant gliomas in adults. Cancer 1993;71:2585–2597

23. Stewart LA. Chemotherapy in adult high-grade glioma: a systematic review and meta-analysis of individual patient data from 12 randomised trials. Lancet 2002;359:1011–1018

24. Clarke M, Stewart L, Pignon JP, Bijnens L. Individual patient data meta-analysis in cancer. Br J Cancer 1998;77:2036–2044

25. Koopman L, van der Heijden GJ, Hoes AW, Grobbee DE, Rovers MM. Empirical comparison of subgroup effects in conventional and individual patient data meta-analyses. Int J Technol Assess Health Care 2008;24:358–361

26. Stupp R, Mason WP, van den Bent MJ, et al; European Organisation for Research and Treatment of Cancer Brain Tumor and Radiotherapy Groups; National Cancer Institute of Canada Clinical Trials Group. Radiotherapy plus concomitant and adjuvant temozolomide for glioblastoma. N Engl J Med 2005;352:987–996

27. Hegi ME, Diserens AC, Gorlia T, et al. MGMT gene silencing and benefit from temozolomide in glioblastoma. N Engl J Med 2005;352:997–1003

28. Stupp R, Hegi ME, Mason WP, et al; European Organisation for Research and Treatment of Cancer Brain Tumour and Radiation Oncology Groups; National Cancer Institute of Canada Clinical Trials Group. Effects of radiotherapy with concomitant and adjuvant temozolomide versus radiotherapy alone on survival in glioblastoma in a randomised phase III study: 5-year analysis of the EORTC-NCIC trial. Lancet Oncol 2009;10:459–466

29. Yabroff KR, Harlan L, Zeruto C, Abrams J, Mann B. Patterns of care and survival for patients with glioblastoma multiforme diagnosed during 2006. Neuro-oncol 2012;14:351–359

30. Scoccianti S, Magrini SM, Ricardi U, et al. Patterns of care and survival in a retrospective analysis of 1059 patients with glioblastoma multiforme treated between 2002 and 2007: a multicenter study by the Central Nervous System Study Group of Airo (italian Association of Radiation Oncology). Neurosurgery 2010;67:446–458

31. van den Bent MJ, Carpentier AF, Brandes AA, et al. Adjuvant procarbazine, lomustine, and vincristine improves progression-free survival but not overall survival in newly diagnosed anaplastic oligodendrogliomas and oligoastrocytomas: a randomized European Organisation for Research and Treatment of Cancer phase III trial. J Clin Oncol 2006;24:2715–2722

32. Cairncross G, Berkey B, Shaw E, et al; Intergroup Radiation Therapy Oncology Group Trial 9402. Phase III trial of chemotherapy plus radiotherapy compared with radiotherapy alone for pure and mixed anaplastic oligodendroglioma: Intergroup Radiation Therapy Oncology Group Trial 9402. J Clin Oncol 2006;24:2707–2714

33. Cairncross G, Wang M, Shaw E, et al. Phase III trial of chemoradiotherapy for anaplastic oligodendroglioma: long-term results of RTOG 9402. J Clin Oncol 2013;31:337–343

34. van den Bent MJ, Brandes AA, Taphoorn MJ, et al. Adjuvant procarbazine, lomustine, and vincristine chemotherapy in newly diagnosed anaplastic oligodendroglioma: long-term follow-up of EORTC brain tumor group study 26951. J Clin Oncol 2013;31:344–350

35. Valtonen S, Timonen U, Toivanen P, et al. Interstitial chemotherapy with carmustine-loaded polymers for high-grade gliomas: a randomized double-blind study. Neurosurgery 1997;41:44–48, discussion 48–49

36. Westphal M, Hilt DC, Bortey E, et al. A phase 3 trial of local chemotherapy with biodegradable carmustine (BCNU) wafers (Gliadel wafers) in patients with primary malignant glioma. Neuro-oncol 2003;5:79–88

37. Olivi A, Grossman SA, Tatter S, et al; New Approaches to Brain Tumor Therapy CNS Consortium. Dose escalation of carmustine in surgically implanted polymers in patients with recurrent malignant glioma: a

New Approaches to Brain Tumor Therapy CNS Consortium trial. J Clin Oncol 2003;21:1845–1849

38. Sampson JH, Archer G, Pedain C, et al; PRECISE Trial Investigators. Poor drug distribution as a possible explanation for the results of the PRECISE trial. J Neurosurg 2010;113:301–309

39. Westphal M, Yla-Herttuala S, Martin J, et al. Adenovirus-mediated gene therapy with sitimagene ceradenovec followed by intravenous ganciclovir for patients with operable high-grade glioma (ASPECT): a randomised, open-label, phase 3 trial. Lancet Oncol 2013; (Jul):11

40. Rainov NG. A phase III clinical evaluation of herpes simplex virus type 1 thymidine kinase and ganciclovir gene therapy as an adjuvant to surgical resection and radiation in adults with previously untreated glioblastoma multiforme. Hum Gene Ther 2000;11:2389–2401

41. Andersen AP. Postoperative irradiation of glioblastomas. Results in a randomized series. Acta Radiol Oncol Radiat Phys Biol 1978;17:475–484

42. Walker MD, Green SB, Byar DP, et al. Randomized comparisons of radiotherapy and nitrosoureas for the treatment of malignant glioma after surgery. N Engl J Med 1980;303:1323–1329

43. Laperriere N, Zuraw L, Cairncross G; Cancer Care Ontario Practice Guidelines Initiative Neuro-Oncology Disease Site Group. Radiotherapy for newly diagnosed malignant glioma in adults: a systematic review. Radiother Oncol 2002;64:259–273

44. Hochberg FH, Pruitt A. Assumptions in the radiotherapy of glioblastoma. Neurology 1980;30:907–911

45. Bleehen NM, Stenning SP; Medical Research Council Brain Tumour Working Party. A Medical Research Council trial of two radiotherapy doses in the treatment of grades 3 and 4 astrocytoma. Br J Cancer 1991;64:769–774

46. Nelson DF, Diener-West M, Horton J, Chang CH, Schoenfeld D, Nelson JS. Combined modality approach to treatment of malignant gliomas—re-evaluation of RTOG 7401/ECOG 1374 with long-term follow-up: a joint study of the Radiation Therapy Oncology Group and the Eastern Cooperative Oncology Group. NCI Monogr 1988;6:279–284

47. Prados MD, Gutin PH, Phillips TL, et al. Interstitial brachytherapy for newly diagnosed patients with malignant gliomas: the UCSF experience. Int J Radiat Oncol Biol Phys 1992;24:593–597

48. Shrieve DC, Alexander E III, Black PM, et al. Treatment of patients with primary glioblastoma multiforme with standard postoperative radiotherapy and radiosurgical boost: prognostic factors and long-term outcome. J Neurosurg 1999;90:72–77

49. Videtic GM, Gaspar LE, Zamorano L, et al. Use of the RTOG recursive partitioning analysis to validate the benefit of iodine-125 implants in the primary treatment of malignant gliomas. Int J Radiat Oncol Biol Phys 1999;45:687–692

50. Laperriere NJ, Leung PM, McKenzie S, et al. Randomized study of brachytherapy in the initial management of patients with malignant astrocytoma. Int J Radiat Oncol Biol Phys 1998;41:1005–1011

51. Selker RG, Shapiro WR, Burger P, et al; Brain Tumor Cooperative Group. The Brain Tumor Cooperative Group NIH Trial 87-01: a randomized comparison of surgery, external radiotherapy, and carmustine versus surgery, interstitial radiotherapy boost, external radiation therapy, and carmustine. Neurosurgery 2002;51:343–355, discussion 355–357

52. Souhami L, Seiferheld W, Brachman D, et al. Randomized comparison of stereotactic radiosurgery followed by conventional radiotherapy with carmustine to conventional radiotherapy with carmustine for patients with glioblastoma multiforme: report of Radiation Therapy Oncology Group 93-05 protocol. Int J Radiat Oncol Biol Phys 2004; 60:853–860

53. Curran WJ Jr, Scott CB, Weinstein AS, et al. Survival comparison of radiosurgery-eligible and -ineligible malignant glioma patients treated with hyperfractionated radiation therapy and carmustine: a report of Radiation Therapy Oncology Group 83-02. J Clin Oncol 1993;11:857–862

54. Florell RC, Macdonald DR, Irish WD, et al. Selection bias, survival, and brachytherapy for glioma. J Neurosurg 1992;76:179–183

55. Greenberg HS, Ensminger WD, Chandler WF, et al. Intra-arterial BCNU chemotherapy for treatment of malignant gliomas of the central nervous system. J Neurosurg 1984;61:423–429

56. Hochberg FH, Pruitt AA, Beck DO, DeBrun G, Davis K. The rationale and methodology for intra-arterial chemotherapy with BCNU as treatment for glioblastoma. J Neurosurg 1985;63:876–880

57. Kirby S, Brothers M, Irish W, et al. Evaluating glioma therapies: modeling treatments and predicting outcomes. J Natl Cancer Inst 1995;87:1884–1888

58. Walker MD. Brain Tumor Study Group. Brain Tumor Study Group: a survey of current activities. Natl Cancer Inst Monogr 1977;46:209–212

59. Donahue B, Scott CB, Nelson JS, et al. Influence of an oligodendroglial component on the survival of patients with anaplastic astrocytomas: a report of Radiation Therapy Oncology Group 83-02. Int J Radiat Oncol Biol Phys 1997;38:911–914

60. Gehan EA, Walker MD. Prognostic factors for patients with brain tumors. Natl Cancer Inst Monogr 1977;46:189–195

61. Simpson JR, Horton J, Scott C, et al. Influence of location and extent of surgical resection on survival of patients with glioblastoma multiforme: results of three consecutive Radiation Therapy Oncology Group (RTOG) clinical trials. Int J Radiat Oncol Biol Phys 1993;26:239–244

62. Curran WJ Jr, Scott CB, Horton J, et al. Recursive partitioning analysis of prognostic factors in three Radiation Therapy Oncology Group malignant glioma trials. J Natl Cancer Inst 1993;85:704–710

63. Li J, Wang M, Won M, et al. Validation and simplification of the Radiation Therapy Oncology Group recursive partitioning analysis classification for glioblastoma. Int J Radiat Oncol Biol Phys 2011;81:623–630

64. Gavrilovic IT, Posner JB. Brain metastases: epidemiology and pathophysiology. J Neurooncol 2005;75:5–14

65. Brem S, Panattil JG. An era of rapid advancement: diagnosis and treatment of metastatic brain cancer. Neurosurgery 2005;57(5, Suppl):S5–S9, S1–S4

66. Gaspar L, Scott C, Rotman M, et al. Recursive partitioning analysis (RPA) of prognostic factors in three Radiation Therapy Oncology Group (RTOG) brain metastases trials. Int J Radiat Oncol Biol Phys 1997;37:745–751

67. Sperduto PW, Berkey B, Gaspar LE, Mehta M, Curran W. A new prognostic index and comparison to three other indices for patients with brain metastases: an analysis of 1,960 patients in the RTOG database. Int J Radiat Oncol Biol Phys 2008;70:510–514

68. Patchell RA, Tibbs PA, Walsh JW, et al. A randomized trial of surgery in the treatment of single metastases to the brain. N Engl J Med 1990; 322:494–500

69. Vecht CJ, Haaxma-Reiche H, Noordijk EM, et al. Treatment of single brain metastasis: radiotherapy alone or combined with neurosurgery? Ann Neurol 1993;33:583–590

70. Patchell RA, Tibbs PA, Regine WF, et al. Postoperative radiotherapy in the treatment of single metastases to the brain: a randomized trial. JAMA 1998;280:1485–1489

71. Andrews DW, Scott CB, Sperduto PW, et al. Whole brain radiation therapy with or without stereotactic radiosurgery boost for patients with one to three brain metastases: phase III results of the RTOG 9508 randomised trial. Lancet 2004;363:1665–1672

72. Kondziolka D, Patel A, Lunsford LD, Kassam A, Flickinger JC. Stereotactic radiosurgery plus whole brain radiotherapy versus radiotherapy alone for patients with multiple brain metastases. Int J Radiat Oncol Biol Phys 1999;45:427–434

73. Panageas KS, Iwamoto FM, Cloughesy TF, et al. Initial treatment patterns over time for anaplastic oligodendroglial tumors. Neuro-oncol 2012;14:761–767

74. Bernstein M, Khu KJ. Is there too much variability in technical neurosurgery decision-making? Virtual Tumour Board of a challenging case. Acta Neurochir (Wien) 2009;151:411–412, discussion 412–413

75. Ibrahim GM, Chung C, Bernstein M. Competing for patients: an ethical framework for recruiting patients with brain tumors into clinical trials. J Neurooncol 2011;104:623–627

48 Neuro-Oncology in the Developing World

James Ayokunle Balogun, Cara Sedney, and Mark Bernstein

A 35-year-old man with a 10-month history of headaches and blurry vision presented to the neurosurgeon at the University Teaching Hospital. He had sought help for his symptoms from a traditional medicine man. As his symptoms progressed, he had been reluctant to present at the referral center because of the distance from his village and the expected long wait to see the specialist. He has lost vision in the right eye and barely counts fingers on the left. The left fundus showed papilledema. At consultation the neurosurgeon requested a computed tomography (CT) scan, and this meant the patient had to travel back to his village to raise the funds for it. He returned after 4 weeks and had the CT scan done, which revealed a large right frontal meningioma. By this time he had become blind in both eyes. He was operated on 4 weeks later with subtotal excision of the tumor due to significant intraoperative blood loss. Due to processing delays and the fact that only one of the institution's pathologists was conversant with neuropathology, the histology of the excised tumor was reported as grade III 2 months postoperatively. The radiotherapy facility was 700 km away and there was no guarantee of its staff attending to the patient immediately due to the backlog of patients and frequent machine malfunction. This man's tumor progressed and he deteriorated clinically.

This case scenario is an example of what is often encountered in developing countries around the world. This chapter discusses the challenges in neuro-oncology in developing countries and suggests solutions.

There are various indices that have been used in the definition of a developing country. The World Bank based its classification on gross national income per capita (GNI). This stratifies countries into low-, middle- (upper and lower), and high-income countries. The term *developing* is then applied to the low- and middle-income countries. This results in a heterogeneous mix of countries, at different developmental stages with varying indices. The World Bank states, "The use of the term 'developing' is convenient; it is not intended to imply that all economies in the group are experiencing similar development or that other economies have reached a preferred or final stage of development." Classification by income does not necessarily reflect development status. Based on this category, all of Africa and the Middle East except Israel, most countries in the Caribbean and South America, and a part of Europe are classified as developing countries.[1]

Neuro-Oncology as a Subspecialty

The evolution of neurosurgery as a specialty over the last century has birthed many subspecialties including neuro-oncology, which has over the years become well established in most neurosurgical centers in the technologically advanced world. Neuro-oncology has gone further to become a distinct entity even within neurosurgical associations such as the Tumor Section of the American Association of Neurological Surgeons/Congress of Neurological Surgeons.[2] The Society of Neuro-Oncology was also formed to be a torchbearer for the subspecialty both in basic and clinical research. Neuro-oncology has not only become progressively technologically driven, but there is continued emphasis, as in most other neurosurgical subspecialties, on a multidisciplinary approach.[3] Thus, it is heavily dependent on the availability of both structural and personnel resources. The persistent pursuit of excellence in neuro-oncology practice has become part of the needed impetus for the development of new and expensive technologies directed at improving patient safety and the quality and quantity of survival.

The availability of the enormous resources at the disposal of the neuro-oncologist in the developed world is taken for granted and is viewed as a needed sine qua non for safe practice. Although patients all over the world would be appreciative of these revolutionary efforts in neuro-oncology, the state of the practice of this subspecialty in the less privileged settings is lagging behind. Central nervous system (CNS) tumors, as with every other disease, know no boundaries, and even though the precise incidence and prevalence are not as well documented in the developing world, their abundant presence in the developed world is clearly evident.[4–9]

Epidemiology of Brain Tumors in the Developing World

Although the main efforts in neurosurgery in the developing world have centered on trauma and pediatric neurosurgical care, satisfying an undeniable need for these lifesaving treatments, increasing evidence demonstrates that tumors of the CNS comprise a significant cause of morbidity and mortality in the developing world.[10] Similar epidemiology for pediatric CNS tumors in Morocco as in previously published data for developed countries has been demonstrated,[11,12] although others have reported a significantly different distribution of malignancies of childhood cancer compared with that in the developed nations.[13] The distribution of CNS tumor types among all age groups in a retrospective study of pathology specimens in Egypt demonstrated overall similar breakdown of tumor types and demographics.[14] A report of skull base operations in Nigeria seems to parallel the epidemiology of adult skull base pathology in developed nations.[15]

However, some key epidemiological differences do exist such as a preponderance of Burkitt lymphoma metastatic brain lesions reflecting the increased risk of Burkitt's lymphoma in Africa.[16] Because of delayed diagnosis, patients in developing countries often present with advanced disease, with up to 60% of patients having a Karnofsky Performance Scale score of less than 70, due to a variety of factors (**Figs. 48.1** and **48.2**).[15,17] In addition, some preliminary studies of tumor biology have suggested some geographical differences.[18]

The Surgical Neuro-Oncologist

The adequately trained surgical neuro-oncologist is the key to the surgical treatment of tumors of the CNS. The paucity of neurosurgeons in the developing world is well documented, with various efforts being implemented to increase their numbers (**Table 48.1**).[4,19–23] The ratio of neurosurgeons to the population may be as low as 1 to 10.5 million in Tanzania[23] and as high as 1 to 85,449 in the Kingdom of Saudi Arabia.[19] In Asia one neurosurgeon serves from 600,000 to 3.5 million people.[4]

Access to the few neurosurgeons is further hindered by their location within big teaching hospitals, in the urban centers.[19] The limited number of available providers and the restricted access to care with increasing patient load results in delayed presentation and resultant enormous morbidity and mortality seen in patients with CNS tumors in these countries.[4,19–23] These factors have strengthened the call for the training of more general neurosurgeons and even the training of general surgeons to manage neurosurgical conditions. It is important to note that although these calls seek to find solutions to the inadequate manpower, it has also de-emphasized subspecialty training. Neuro-oncology practice has over the years become established through the training of surgical neuro-oncologists, and the impact of this has been underscored.[20] Therefore, this may necessitate a paradigm shift in

developing countries whereby instead of focusing exclusively on basic neurosurgical needs such as trauma and hydrocephalus, one gradually entrenches surgical neuro-oncology as an established subspecialty.

Neuro-Oncology in the Preoperative Period

The effective preoperative care of the neuro-oncology patient involves timely recognition, referral, clinical evaluation, and imaging. Delay of care often occurs at each of these stages. Referral depends foremost on detection of neurologic abnormality, which is often not brought to the attention of medical personnel until at an advanced clinical stage, because of the lack of access to medical care, the lack of funds, or the initial use of traditional healing.[24] Religious, cultural, and financial factors have also been identified as all playing a role in delayed diagnosis of CNS tumors in adults in Africa.[17] The importance of educating both general practitioners and the public regarding sentinel symptoms of malignancy have included resources such as a public television campaign and translated material from international cancer organizations in their future educational projects.[25]

Imaging modalities include anatomic, physiological, and functional techniques. The availability of imaging facilities aids not just in the delineation of tumors, but also in the establishment of their spatial relationship with normal structures to help improve the accuracy of diagnosis and optimize surgical planning. Most developing countries are lacking the most basic of these facilities or have, at most, CT capability.[5,21] A report published as recently as 2001 indicates that X-ray is a common imaging modality for the diagnosis of brain tumors.[26] Available magnetic resonance imaging (MRI) machines are of low tesla strength, requiring longer imaging durations and therefore the scans are more susceptible to motion artifact.[27] In spite of this, the utility of low-field MRI in evaluating sellar lesions has been demonstrated, where pertinent anatomic relations are visible such as encasement or narrowing of the carotid in sellar meningiomas and the presence of mi-

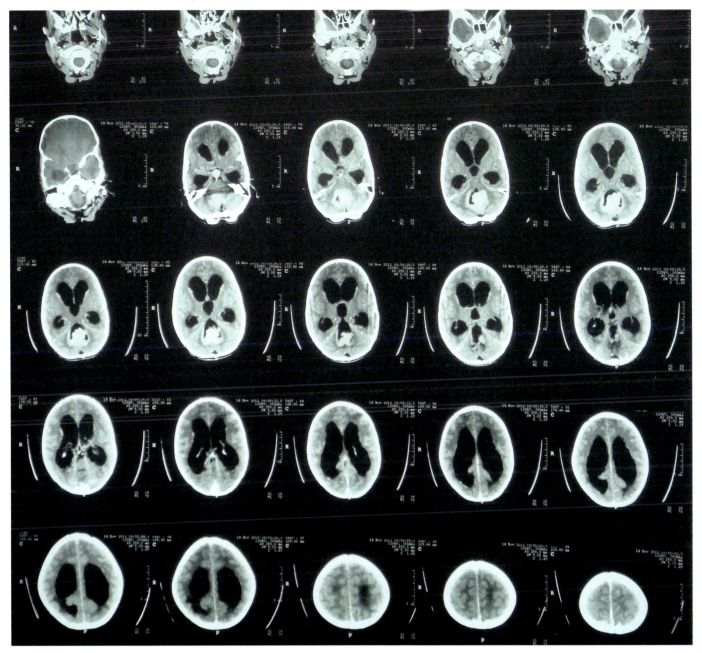

Fig. 48.1 Enhanced computed tomography (CT) scans of 10-year-old boy in a large sub-Saharan African city who presented with progressive vomiting, headache, and blindness. Delay in getting this CT was followed by a delay in getting him to surgery, and he died 2 weeks after presentation to the neurosurgery clinic unoperated. This was likely a pilocytic astrocytoma.

croadenomas.[27] Aside from access to imaging studies, the impact of unrelated disease burden may make interpretation of imaging studies more complex than in developed countries. Difficulties have been recorded in interpreting positron emission tomography (PET) scans in patients with human immunodeficiency virus (HIV) because of direct effects of both the disease and its treatment in South Africa.[28]

It is undeniable that the factors contributing to preoperative detection and workup of CNS tumors are varied and include the immense challenges of lack of funding and infra-

structure.[19,21,22,29,30] The absence of strong, coordinated, and persistent advocacy by the existing neurosurgeons in these

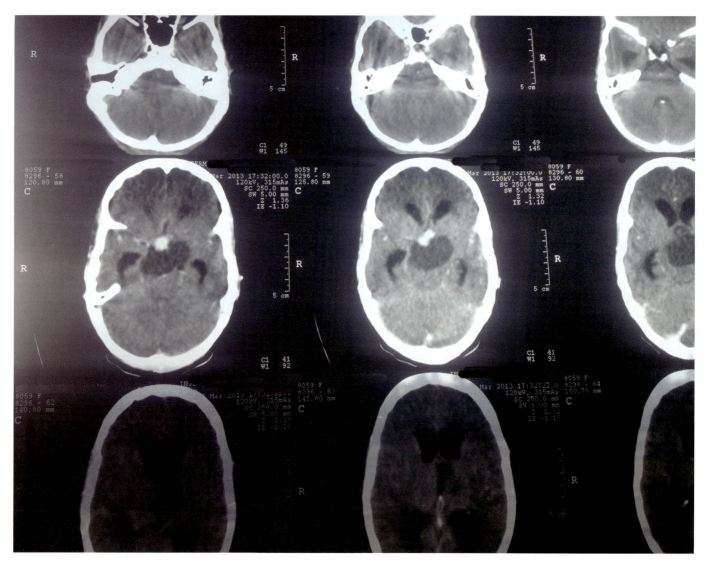

Fig. 48.2 Computed tomography scans of a 15-year-old girl in a large sub-Saharan African city who presented with visual loss progressing to complete blindness. She has hydrocephalus due to a presumed craniopharyngioma. She was treated with a ventriculoperitoneal shunt.

regions may also continue to impede development in the area of neuro-oncology.[19]

In the Operating Room

The essence of the operating room is captured in these words: "The operating room is a work of art with a choreography and emotion of its own.... The patient has trusted the neurosurgeon with his life, his person, his speech, and his memory."[31] Every precaution must be taken to reduce the risk of errors and complications, which has led to continued innovations to ensure safe surgery. Surgeons in developing countries confronted with tumors of unusual dimensions due to late presentations face this enormous challenge with the lack of

contemporary equipment. There is a persistent lack of modern equipment, necessitating the use of obsolete equipment, such as the Hudson Brace/perforator and Gigli saw instead of power drills. There are no microsurgical instruments, operating microscopes, or other adjuncts such as ultrasonic aspirators.[31] This does not encourage improved patient safety. Indeed, "the lack of an operating microscope and limited avail-

Pearl

- Traditional techniques such as split-thickness calvarial grafting or autologous grafts for dural repair are useful in a limited-resource setting.

Table 48.1 Distribution of Neurosurgeons in Africa in 1998

Groups of Countries	Total Population	No. of Neurosurgeons	Dominant Pathological Conditions	Training Needs	Equipment Needs
Group 1: Algeria, Egypt, Morocco, South Africa, Tunisia	174 million	486 neurosurgeons (1/358,000 inhabitants)	Head trauma, infections, hydrocephalus, and spinal cord pathological conditions, tumors, stroke	Workshops and seminars for neurosurgeons; short visits to European centers	Shunts and surgical instruments
Group 2: Libya, Sudan, Senegal, Nigeria, Kenya, Cameroon, Zimbabwe	188 million	52 neurosurgeons (1/3,600,000)	Same as Group 1	Course and complete training for neurosurgeons; training for general surgeons	Surgical instrument sets for craniotomies and laminectomies; CT scanners; shunts
Group 3: Ethiopia, Tanzania, Mauritius, Namibia, Botswana, Guinea, Ghana, Burkina Faso, Congo Brazzaville, Ivory Coast, Gabon, Malawi, Mozambique, Uganda, Somalia, Togo, Democratic Republic of the Congo	250 million	27 neurosurgeons (1/9 million)	Same as Group 1	Training for general surgeons; complete training for neurosurgeons	Instrument sets for craniotomies and laminectomies; CT scanners
Group 4: Niger, Mali, Equatorial Guinea, Mauritania, Guinea Bissau, Lesotho, Swaziland, Rwanda, Madagascar, Comoro Islands, Burundi	46 million	0 neurosurgeons	Same as Group 1	Training for general surgeons; complete training for neurosurgeons	Surgical instruments

Source: From El Khamlichi A. African neurosurgery: current situation, priorities, and needs. Neurosurgery 2001;48:1344–1347. Reproduced with permission.

ability of adjuvant treatments makes complex skull base procedures or resection of malignant neoplasms inappropriate."[23]

Dealing with the reality of equipment limitations in the operating room has created adaptations in surgical technique and decision making. A successful skull base surgery program has been described using surgical techniques such as extra-dural anterior clinoidectomy without the use of a drill, as well as skull base bone resections using primarily osteotomes and Leksell rongeurs.[15] Operating with loupe magnification where a microscope is unavailable is common.[15] Lack of artificial reconstructive material necessitates the use of more classic reconstructive methods such as split calvarial bone grafting as well as pericranial or fascia lata grafts for dural reconstruction.[15] Others also advocate the use of more traditional techniques as viable and useful in a limited-resource setting.[32]

Patterns of operative judgment may also differ in developing nations. Because of the lack of availability of stereotaxy in most centers, making stereotactic biopsy impossible, an initial trial of medical therapy for possible infectious etiology of mass lesions may be appropriate in some cases, as described for tuberculomas[33] and for HIV-associated mass lesions.[34] Fur-

Special Consideration

- The clinical limitations of each site and their effect on patient care must be carefully weighed. The imperative to "do no harm" must always be considered before taking on a challenging case.

thermore, a careful and realistic assessment of the capabilities of each surgeon and center should be made prior to operating on particularly advanced stage or difficult tumors to ensure patient safety and ethical medical intervention.

Arguments may be made that esoteric instruments such as a Cavitron ultrasonic aspirator (CUSA), image-guided surgery using neuronavigational devices, and intraoperative electrophysiological monitoring are not essential, yet their value cannot be denied.[31] Although there is no doubt that the high cost of purchase and maintenance of these instruments may impede their acquisition by financially challenged countries, there must also be a change from the attitude that tumor surgery can and should be done without these adjuncts. Emphasis must be not just on saving lives but also on ensuring the safety of the patients and improving their quality of life. Ideally, work with the biomedical industries will progress toward the development and manufacturing of instruments that are affordable for the neurosurgeons in these countries.

Adjuvant Care After Surgery

The postoperative care of neuro-oncology patients has impact on their outcome as much as or more so than does the surgical care. The care at this stage is multidisciplinary, with interaction among the neurosurgeon, neuropathologist, and radiation and medical oncologist. The majority of developing countries lack trained manpower in these specialties.[5,30]

There is a dearth in basic neuropathological diagnostic facilities in the developing world, in contrast to the developed world's growing standards for immunohistochemistry and genetic profiling of tumors to move toward individualized patient care.[30] A number of possibilities exist for the amelioration of this problem, although their application in developing nations remains more theoretical at the current time. A "brain smear" technique has been described for intraoperative pathological examination, which may be more viable in centers where frozen section may not be possible.[35] Additionally, telepathology is likely to be a useful adjunct to brain tumor surgery in developing nations. Comparable accuracy of a teleneuropathology program to conventional diagnosis has been demonstrated when coupled with adherence to World Health Organization (WHO) characteristics for diagnosis of astrocytoma grade.[36] Similarly, comparable accuracy of digitized tissue smears to that of frozen section at medium-power magnification has been reported.[37] Success of these techniques in a developing country setting would depend on a twinning program and a reliable method of digital information transfer.

Postoperative care is further complicated by the absence of timely and scheduled radiation therapy due to limited cobalt machines and even fewer linear accelerators.[5,29,38] Radiation has been found to play a large role in cancer care in Africa based on a previous survey[39]; however, the available facilities do not meet the projected need. The average number of teletherapy machines per million people is 1.99 for the whole world, but is 8.6 for high-income countries, contrasted with 1.6 for upper middle-income countries, 0.71 for lower-middle

Pitfall

- Radiotherapy plays a large role in neuro-oncology care, but in many limited-resource settings the demand vastly outweighs the need.

Pitfall

- Comorbidities such as HIV, malaria, tuberculosis, and chronic malnutrition may profoundly affect the efficacy of or morbidities of chemotherapy in a developing nation.

income countries, and 0.21 for low-income countries.[29] The staggering need is exemplified in Nigeria, where there are currently seven teletherapy radiotherapy machines, compared with an estimated need of 145.[29] For those centers with radiotherapy capability, some still lack simulators or treatment-planning systems.[39] There is furthermore little consensus or concordance between centers regarding radiation dosage or fractionation schedules.[39] Only two centers in one study reported the use of gamma knife radiosurgery,[39] and practically speaking this is only affordable by the very affluent within a developing society.

Also chemotherapeutic agents such as temozolomide are out of the reach of the populace in these developing nations mainly due to cost and unavailability. In a survey of radiotherapy practices in a number of African countries, the number of centers with medical oncology programs was only 29%, requiring radiation oncologists to administer chemotherapy in the majority of cases.[39] The overall cost of treatment with these adjuvant drugs, besides the cost of the drug, includes the cost for imaging and other necessary drugs, and this may well continue to take their affordability beyond the reach of the oncology patients in developing countries where health insurance coverage is lacking and patients have to pay for treatment.[40,41] For patients able to obtain these treatments, opportunistic infection may be a life-threatening complication and remains a problem in developing countries.[42]

Other challenges persist in the adjuvant care of tumors of the CNS. Comorbidities such as malaria, tuberculosis, HIV, and chronic malnutrition are significant factors affecting morbidity and mortality during adjunctive therapies.[43] The imperative need for rehabilitation and palliative care of brain tumor patients is virtually nonexistent. Furthermore, several groups have noted problems in patient compliance with the plan of care, likely related to cultural or educational factors.[17,24,25]

Ongoing Efforts and Possible Solutions

In spite of the many challenges of neuro-oncology in the developing world, interventions can make a positive impact on the lives of these patients. A significant improvement in Karnofsky Performance Scale score was reported postoperatively after skull base surgery, even with a low initial functional status.[15] Similarly, an improvement from functional blindness to useful vision was documented in over 50% of patients with large pituitary adenomas after surgery.[24] These recent studies demonstrate significantly improved patient outcomes compared with those of previous reports, wherein the mortality of brain tumor patients was as high as 83%.[26]

There are appreciable efforts that have impacted neurosurgical practice including neuro-oncology in the developing world. The contribution of the World Federation of Neurological Surgeons (WFNS) and Foundation for International Education in Neurological Surgery (FIENS) over the years, in the development of training programs, in teaching neurosurgical techniques and procedures through visiting volunteers, and in the donation of equipment, has been considerable. A number of institutions and individual surgeons in the developed world have also made concerted efforts to improve the training and practice of local surgeons in these regions through the establishment of training programs and various exchanges.

Frontiers that should continually be explored include the emphasis on training, particularly in the art and science of the management of CNS tumors. There is a more urgent need to aggressively address the shortage of neurosurgical manpower through concerted efforts that should essentially involve the local surgeons who must show a willingness and passion to see such efforts come to fruition. Surgical neuro-oncology training must no longer be seen as an unnecessary super-specialization in the developing world but as a needed tool to reduce patient suffering and improve survival in oncology patients. Opportunities for training in more established centers are ongoing but must be expanded in the form of short visits or observerships, research fellowships, and most importantly clinical fellowships.

It is important that the training be tailored to the needs of the community where the surgeon will practice, to reduce the frustrations that tend to occur following return to their home countries. This demands that there should be an understanding of the neuro-oncological needs in that community and learning directed as much as possible to these needs despite exposure to what might appear as the full neuro-oncological armamentarium available at the training site. Concerns have often been expressed regarding surgeons from developing countries using training opportunities as stepping stones to emigrate from their countries and thereby worsen the brain drain in these regions. Although there is no fool-proof solution to this problem, young surgeons with visible commitment to returning home may be identified and recruited

into these programs prior to their leaving to study. Additionally, the minimization of further brain drain may be helped through the provision of basic start-up instruments at home through the collaborative efforts of the local authorities, the training institutions, and donor agencies to the hospitals in the home of the trainees. This may alleviate trainees' frustrations on returning home, which often serves as one of the drivers for brain drain due to a lack of job satisfaction resulting from the huge disconnect between their training and practice.

It is also possible to explore the option of setting up surgical neuro-oncology training at specific designated centers to serve a particular region in the developing world. This can be facilitated by skilled and committed surgical neuro-oncologists volunteering time to teach and operate in those institutions, thereby complementing the onsite staff. This model has been utilized in pediatric neurosurgery,[44] and would validate the commitment of the visiting surgeons and dispel the idea that these visits especially by trainee surgeons are aimed at seeing the visit sites as a finishing school.[45] The "medical mission" is increasing in popularity around the world. Several ethical dilemmas have been delineated specifically regarding short-term trips to developing countries for medical work, such as the "white knight" phenomenon, sustainability concerns, complexities of informed consent, and unfair expectations, among others, and an "ethical checklist" has been proposed to deal with these issues.[46]

Through collaboration across a number of venues, the surgical evolution for CNS tumors in developing countries continues to develop. One group recently described awake craniotomy as an important tool in limited-resource settings to limit hospital stay, increase safety, and decrease anesthesia and intensive care unit requirements.[47] Through their model of surgical education, they successfully taught this technique in six neurosurgical centers in Indo-China and Africa and attempted to assess the sustainability of this teaching.[47]

There is also a need for manpower development in the other neuro-oncology specialties particularly in medical oncology and radiation oncology. A call for regional "centers of excellence" can help establish subspecialty and interdisciplinary care in developing nations.[15] However, although efforts are being directed at training and provision of services in these areas, networking between centers in the developed and developing world often referred to as twinning using tele-health facilities has proven to be very helpful.[48,49] Telepathology can serve not only as a "stop gap" to help mitigate the dearth of neuropathologists but also to provide a viable platform for teaching and collaborations.[30,50,51]

The advent of stereotactic radiosurgery has changed approaches to the management of a spectrum of brain tumors from benign to malignant. It is a versatile tool and its utility is continually being expanded; however, this modality is still uncommon in the developing world. Nevertheless, the patient with a CNS tumor should have access to radiation, and the main focus should still be on the role of conventional fractionated radiotherapy using the cobalt units, which are easier to maintain and cheaper to acquire even if as a starting point in places that lack radiotherapy facility. The efforts of the International Atomic Energy Association in achieving some equitable distribution in radiotherapy facilities require individual and institutional support.[38]

■ Conclusion

There must continually be an interchange between the developing and developed worlds, in ways that are beneficial to both and without prejudice to either side of the divide. As the African proverb states, "If you want to go far, go together. We need each other." Together, we can all be driven to pursue better quality of life and survival for all neuro-oncology patients worldwide.

Editor's Note

There are vast disparities in health care for brain tumor patients, depending on their place of birth. Arguably at least half the people on the planet do not have timely access to complete or affordable treatment of their brain tumors.

A solution to the problem, if it exists, will take many generations and dramatic changes in culture, resource distribution priorities, and political leadership in many countries. The good news is that many clinicians in underresourced countries are becoming less resigned to the problem and are trying to effect positive change, for example by obtaining fellowship training overseas. At the same time, neurosurgeons, neuro-oncologists, and organizations in more privileged and developed countries are becoming more interested in global outreach, from senior consultants to junior medical students.

There are several models to capacitate the future of this growing international educational interchange.[47,52] Some are formal partnerships between universities, site teaching visits, fellowships and observerships, equipment donations, and many other elements. Greater coordination is needed both at the resource-poor host institutions and among all the resource-rich groups visiting them, and also a more concerted effort at learning how to measure the impact of international teaching efforts. (Bernstein)

References

1. World Bank Website. How we classify countries. http://data.worldbank.org/about/country-classifications
2. Black P, Golby A, Johnson M. The emerging field of neuro-oncology. Clin Neurosurg 2007;54:36–46
3. Society of Neuro-Oncology Website. SNO history. http://www.soc-neuro-onc.org/sno-history/
4. Fairholm DJ. International education: a third alternative. Neurosurgery 1986;18:111–114
5. Baskin JL, Lezcano E, Kim BS, et al. Management of children with brain tumors in Paraguay. Neuro-oncol 2013;15:235–241
6. Qaddoumi I, Unal E, Diez B, et al. Web-based survey of resources for treatment and long-term follow-up for children with brain tumors in developing countries. Childs Nerv Syst 2011;27:1957–1961
7. Cadotte DW, Viswanathan A, Cadotte A, Bernstein M, Munie T, Freidberg SR; East African Neurosurgical Research Collaboration. The consequence of delayed neurosurgical care at Tikur Anbessa Hospital, Addis Ababa, Ethiopia. World Neurosurg 2010;73:270–275
8. Olufemi Adeleye A, Balogun JA. Bilateral deafness and blindness from a IVth ventricular medulloblastoma. Br J Neurosurg 2009;23:315–317
9. Idowu O, Akang EEU, Malomo A. Symptomatic primary intracranial neoplasms in Nigeria, West Africa. J Neurol Sci Turkish 2007;24:212–218
10. El-Gaidi MA. Descriptive epidemiology of pediatric intracranial neoplasms in Egypt. Pediatr Neurosurg 2011;47:385–395
11. Harmouch A, Taleb M, Lasseini A, Maher M, Sefiani S. Epidemiology of pediatric primary tumors of the nervous system: a retrospective study of 633 cases from a single Moroccan institution. Neurochirurgie 2012;58:14–18
12. Karkouri M, Zafad S, Khattab M, et al. Epidemiologic profile of pediatric brain tumors in Morocco. Childs Nerv Syst 2010;26:1021–1027
13. Mostert S, Njuguna F, Kemps L, et al. Epidemiology of diagnosed childhood cancer in Western Kenya. Arch Dis Child 2012;97:508–512
14. Zalata KR, El-Tantawy DA, Abdel-Aziz A, et al. Frequency of central nervous system tumors in delta region, Egypt. Indian J Pathol Microbiol 2011;54:299–306
15. Adeleye AO, Fasunla JA, Young PH. Skull base surgery in a large, resource-poor, developing country with few neurosurgeons: prospects, challenges, and needs. World Neurosurg 2012;78:35–43
16. Olasode BJ. A pathological review of intracranial tumours seen at the University College Hospital, Ibadan between 1980 and 1990. Niger Postgrad Med J 2002;9:23–28
17. Idowu OE, Apemiye RA. Delay in presentation and diagnosis of adult primary intracranial neoplasms in a tropical teaching hospital: a pilot study. Int J Surg 2009;7:396–398
18. Vasishta RK, Pasricha N, Nath A, Sehgal S. The absence of JC virus antigens in Indian children with medulloblastomas. Indian J Pathol Microbiol 2009;52:42–45
19. El-Fiki M. African neurosurgery, the 21st-century challenge. World Neurosurg 2010;73:254–258
20. Shilpakar SK. Subspecialties in neurosurgery and its challenges in a developing country. World Neurosurg 2011;75:335–337

21. El Khamlichi A. African neurosurgery: current situation, priorities, and needs. Neurosurgery 2001;48:1344–1347

22. Mukhida K, Shilpakar SK, Sharma MR, Bagan M. Neurosurgery at Tribhuvan University Teaching Hospital, Nepal. Neurosurgery 2005;57:172–180, discussion 172–180

23. Wilson DA, Garrett MP, Wait SD, et al. Expanding neurosurgical care in Northwest Tanzania: the early experience of an initiative to teach neurosurgery at Bugando Medical Centre. World Neurosurg 2012;77:32–38

24. Mezue WC, Ohaegbulam SC, Chikani MC, Achebe DN. Management of giant pituitary tumors affecting vision in Nigeria. World Neurosurg 2012;77:606–609

25. Ali AA, Elsheikh SM, Elhaj A, et al. Clinical presentation and outcome of retinoblastoma among children treated at the National Cancer Institute (NCI) in Gezira, Sudan: a single Institution experience. Ophthalmic Genet 2011;32:122–125

26. Igun GO. Diagnosis and management of brain tumours at Jos University Teaching Hospital, Nigeria. East Afr Med J 2001;78:148–151

27. Ogbole GI, Adeyinka OA, Okolo CA, Ogun AO, Atalabi OM. Low field MR imaging of sellar and parasellar lesions: experience in a developing country hospital. Eur J Radiol 2012;81:e139–e146

28. Warwick JM, Sathekge MM. PET/CT scanning with a high HIV/AIDS prevalence. Transfus Apheresis Sci 2011;44:167–172

29. Abdel-Wahab M, Bourque JM, Pynda Y, et al. Status of radiotherapy resources in Africa: an International Atomic Energy Agency analysis. Lancet Oncol 2013;14:e168–e175

30. Adesina A, Chumba D, Nelson AM, et al. Improvement of pathology in sub-Saharan Africa. Lancet Oncol 2013;14:e152–e157

31. McDermott MW, Bernstein M. Image-guided surgery. In: Neuro-Oncology, The Essentials, 2nd ed. New York: Thieme, 2008:112–125

32. Adeolu AA, Adeniji AO, Komolafe EO, et al. Review of skull base surgery in a Nigerian teaching hospital. Niger Postgrad Med J 2010;17:50–54

33. du Plessis J, Andronikou S, Wieselthaler N, Theron S, George R, Mapukata A. CT features of tuberculous intracranial abscesses in children. Pediatr Radiol 2007;37:167–172

34. Modi M, Mochan A, Modi G. Management of HIV-associated focal brain lesions in developing countries. QJM 2004;97:413–421

35. Olasode BJ, Ironside JW. The brain smear, a rapid affordable intraoperative diagnostic technique for brain tumours appropriate for Africa. Trop Doct 2004;34:223–225

36. Glotsos D, Georgiadis P, Kostopoulos S, et al. A pilot study investigating the minimum requirements necessary for grading astrocytomas remotely. Anal Quant Cytol Histol 2009;31:262–268

37. Gould PV, Saikali S. A comparison of digitized frozen section and smear preparations for intraoperative neurotelepathology. Anal Cell Pathol (Amst) 2012;35:85–91

38. Datta NR, Rajasekar D. Improvement of radiotherapy facilities in developing countries: a three-tier system with a teleradiotherapy network. Lancet Oncol 2004;5:695–698

39. Sharma V, Gaye PM, Wahab SA, et al. Patterns of practice of palliative radiotherapy in Africa, Part 1: Bone and brain metastases. Int J Radiat Oncol Biol Phys 2008;70:1195–1201

40. Wasserfallen JB, Ostermann S, Leyvraz S, Stupp R. Cost of temozolomide therapy and global care for recurrent malignant gliomas followed until death. Neuro-oncol 2005;7:189–195

41. Wasserfallen JB, Ostermann S, Pica A, et al. Can we afford to add chemotherapy to radiotherapy for glioblastoma multiforme? Cost-identification analysis of concomitant and adjuvant treatment with temozolomide until patient death. Cancer 2004;101:2098–2105

42. Saghrouni F, Ben Youssef Y, Gheith S, et al. Twenty-nine cases of invasive aspergillosis in neutropenic patients. Med Mal Infect 2011;41:657–662

43. Hadley LG, Rouma BS, Saad-Eldin Y. Challenge of pediatric oncology in Africa. Semin Pediatr Surg 2012;21:136–141

44. Albright AL, Ferson SS. Developing pediatric neurosurgery in a developing country. J Child Neurol 2012;27:1559–1564

45. Fieggen G, Mogere E. Counterpoint: Africa is not a surgical finishing school. AANS Neurosurg 2013;22

46. Howe KL, Malomo AO, Bernstein MA. Ethical challenges in international surgical education, for visitors and hosts. World Neurosurg 2013;80:751–758

47. Howe KL, Zhou G, July J, et al. Teaching awake craniotomy in resource-poor settings and implementing it sustainably. World Neurosurgery 2013;80:171–174

48. Qaddoumi I, Mansour A, Musharbash A, et al. Impact of telemedicine on pediatric neuro-oncology in a developing country: the Jordanian-Canadian experience. Pediatr Blood Cancer 2007;48:39–43

49. Augestad KM, Lindsetmo RO. Overcoming distance: video-conferencing as a clinical and educational tool among surgeons. World J Surg 2009;33:1356–1365

50. Ayad E, Sicurello F. Telepathology in emerging countries pilot project between Italy and Egypt. Diagn Pathol 2008;3(Suppl 1):S2

51. Horbinski C, Wiley CA. Comparison of telepathology systems in neuropathological intraoperative consultations. Neuropathology 2009;29:655–663

52. Haglund MM, Kiryabwire J, Parker S, et al. Surgical capacity building in Uganda through twinning, technology, and training camps. World J Surg 2011;35:1175–1182

Index

Page numbers followed by *f* or *t* indicate figures or tables, respectively.